Contemporary Nephrology Nursing

Janel Parker, Editor

Publication Management by
Anthony J. Jannetti, Inc.; East Holly Avenue/Box 56; Pitman, New Jersey 08071-0056

ISBN No. 0-9653379-0-1

In Remembrance: Ron Brady

- his clarity of thought
- his laughter
- his demand for quality
- his compassion
- his commitment
- his singing
- his intuitive sense of right and wrong
- his love of rock & roll
- his keen intellect
- his sense of humor
- his honesty
- his dancing
- his dedication
- his enjoyment of life
- his sense of fairness
- his decisiveness
- his beliefs
- his uniqueness
- his happiness.

Ron will long be remembered by those of us fortunate enough to have shared his friendship, enjoyed his larger-than-life personality, and endeavored to meet his expectations.

Janel Parker, Editor

PREFACE

CONTEMPORARY NEPHROLOGY NURSING has been written for a broad-based audience of nurses involved in the care of renal patients such as nephrology nurses, multi-organ transplant nurses, medical-surgical nurses, primary care nurses, and nursing students. The information in this book will assist the professional nurse in delivering care to renal patients and preparing for certification examinations, in particular the examination offered by the Nephrology Nursing Certification Board (NNCB). The point of view is based in the United States, but an international perspective is also reviewed since the prevention and treatment of chronic renal failure is exercised throughout the world.

The purpose of creating this textbook was to provide a current and comprehensive perspective of nephrology nursing practice as we approach a new millennium. Therefore, the content was organized into eight separate units:

Unit 1: The Nature and Scope of Nephrology Nursing.

The goal of this unit is to provide an historical perspective of nephrology nursing practice and the evolution of this practice into a nursing specialty. The American Board of Nursing Specialties (ABNS) approved nephrology nursing's application in 1992 and the components of this application, including the development of a practice base for nephrology nursing, are discussed in Chapter 1. Within this unit, the various roles occupied by nephrology nurses are also presented.

Unit 2: Conceptual Themes Basic to Nephrology Nursing.

The use of conceptual models is not new to nursing but the American Nephrology Nurses' Association (ANNA) has taken a bold step in the advancement of the nursing discipline by basing nephrology nursing practice on explicit conceptual models of nursing. The development of the Roy Adaptation Model and other nursing conceptual model-based assessment formats and intervention typologies for all categories of nephrology patients and the linkage of conceptual models of nursing with nephrology nursing practice standards, documentation, and quality monitoring is the first attempt of this kind by a nursing specialty.

Conceptual models provide a theoretical foundation for research and ethical decision making in nephrology nursing practice. The successful treatment of chronic renal failure has prompted an array of ethical dilemmas with no simple answers. Chapter 5 provides information regarding ethical foundations and strategies to assist nephrology nurses in developing plans of care for renal patients.

Chapter 6 provides an historical and current overview of research in nephrology nursing. While there is a great deal of research available, strategies to promote the application of nursing research findings into practice are needed. Throughout this textbook, nursing research utilization is highlighted to enhance the reader's understanding of this process and the development of a research-based practice.

Unit 3: The Kidney

Unit 3 is a comprehensive review of the anatomy and physiology of the renal system and the major classifications of renal diseases which provides a framework for understanding the pathogenesis and etiology of renal failure. The unit also presents the processes, manifestations, and implications of both acute and chronic renal failure. This material provides the reader with a basis for understanding the physiologic and psychosocial responses needed to effectively plan appropriate nursing interventions and evaluate patient outcomes.

Unit 4: Clinical Management of the Renal Patient

The failure of the kidney(s) to maintain their normal functions results in accumulation of metabolic waste products in body fluids and abnormalities in fluid, electrolyte homeostasis, acid-base homeostasis, and renal endocrine functions. Few diseases have such an extensive effect on the human body as chronic renal failure. The clinical management of the renal patient is multifaceted, involving every body system.

The psychosocial impact of renal disease is significant. The major stressors, coping strategies, impact on quality of life, and appropriate nursing care are reviewed in Chapter 10. Chapter 11 discusses the renal dietitian's role as a member of the renal health care team and the importance of nutrition intervention in all stages of the renal disease process and in conjunction with all treatment modalities. The kidneys are responsible for the elimination of several medications. In addition, progressive, chronic renal failure and transplant patients are treated with several medications.

Chapter 12 describes the metabolism and elimination of pharmacologic agents and pharmacokinetics, specific medications commonly utilized, and the nurse's role in the teaching and safe administration of medications. Infectious diseases were identified by nephrology nurses as the most significant area of concern while caring for transplant and ESRD patients.

The authors of Chapter 13 present an overview of the infectious diseases most commonly encountered by renal and transplant patients, including the five hepatitis viruses (A, B, C, D, E), tuberculosis, HIV/AIDS, and MRSA and VRE. These infectious diseases are explored by using an epidemiologic

PREFACE

framework. Rehabilitation was the premise on which the ESRD Program was founded and Chapter 14 presents rehabilitation as the main objective of the renal patient's plan of care and the role of the nephrology nurse as a crucial team leader.

Unit 5: Special Patient Populations

Special patient populations are defined as those patients with renal failure who differ markedly from normal adults in their physiological and psychosocial responses to renal disease, and treatment regimens differ considerably. Children are unique in that their bodies are growing and developing at a rapid rate. Elderly patients are different in that changes are occurring due to the aging process itself and the treatment of these body system failures often coexist and are interrelated with renal disease. Diabetic patients are considered as part of a special patient population for two reasons: diabetic nephropathy accounts for over one-third of the patients entering the ESRD Program, and the deleterious effects in several body organ systems caused by diabetes mellitus requires a complicated care plan to meet the special needs of diabetic ESRD patients.

Unit 6: Treatment of Renal Disease: Therapies and Approaches

The treatments for renal failure are hemodialysis, peritoneal dialysis, and transplantation. Conservative management techniques consist of therapeutic measures used to delay the progression of ongoing and irreversible destruction to the kidney structure. Recently, acute renal failure has been treated with continuous renal replacement therapy and is often the preferred treatment over hemodialysis.

Over the past two decades, the medical indications for therapeutic plasma exchange have increased beyond the scope of renal disease. Intermittent therapies have advanced to continuous flow techniques and plasma membrane separators. Nephrology nurses are recognized experts in performing extracorporeal therapies safely and effectively. Thus, their nursing care has been instrumental in the advancement of this therapy for patient care.

Unit 6 presents a thorough and contemporary description of the treatment for chronic renal failure. In addition, extracorporeal therapies are explored from the technical and patient care perspectives.

Unit 7: Public Policy and Legislative Issues

Thirty years ago, a diagnosis of chronic renal failure equated with an almost certain death. Dialysis and transplantation were experimental procedures and beyond the financial reach of most patients. The Medicare ESRD Program made life-saving treatment financially possible for several hundred thousand Americans.

As the competition for financial resources grows, nephrology nurses need to strengthen their involvement in the regulatory and legislative branches of the federal and state government. Chapter 24 provides an overview of the nephrology nurse's role in public policy development. Chapter 25 discusses the regulatory and legislative history of the ESRD Program for the purpose of establishing a foundation in which nephrology nurses can enhance participation in generating an ESRD Program for a new millennium.

Unit 8: Communication and Collaboration

As members of the renal community and nursing profession, we are aware that state-of-the-art technology is almost magical. It is anticipated that by the year 2000, almost a quarter-of-a-million people will be members of the ESRD Program. Never in the history of health care has documentation to support standards of nursing care, patient education, and the professional nurse's role as a member of the health care team been more vital.

Unit 8 presents a comprehensive discussion of the nephrology nurse's part in achieving this holistic approach to nursing care. This nursing care is offered in the context of a member of the health care team, nephrology community, and as a participant in an international specialty and global community.

Conclusion

The goal of nephrology nursing is to assist patients with renal disease to achieve their optimal state of well being. To accomplish this goal, ANNA has been instrumental in the development of a practice base for nephrology nursing and continues to endeavor toward the ultimate goal of a research-based practice.

As editor of *Contemporary Nephrology Nursing*, it is my intention that this text assists in the development of our research-based practice. State-of-the-art information has been contributed by colleagues who are at the forefront of knowledge in their areas of expertise. Nursing research that has guided the decision making of clinicians is highlighted throughout the text. Appendices have been included to exemplify information presented in several chapters.

As the specialty of nephrology nursing evolves, professional development, clinical management of renal patients, members of the health care team, and the national/international perspective of this evolution will need to be continuously evaluated. *Contemporary Nephrology Nursing* reflects a comprehensive step in evolution of this dynamic specialty as we enter a new millennium.

Janel Parker, MSN, RN, CNN
Editor

TABLE OF CONTENTS

Contemporary Nephrology Nursing
Table of Contents and Contributors

Preface III
Contributors IX
Reviewers XI
Acknowledgments XII

Unit One
Nature and Scope of Nephrology Nursing 1

Chapter 1 **Nephrology Nursing as a Specialty** 3
Janel Parker, MSN, RN, CNN

Chapter 2 **The History of Dialysis and Nephrology Nursing** 25
Anna L. Corea, MN, RN, CNAA

Chapter 3 **The Professional Roles of the Nephrology Nurse** 43
Mary Ann Gould, MSN, RN, CNN

Unit Two
Conceptual Themes Basic to Nephrology Nursing 59

Chapter 4 **Use of Conceptual Models in Nephrology Nursing Practice** 61
Jacqueline Fawcett, PhD, RN, FAAN
Marguerite F. Hartigan, MSN, RN, CNN
Marcia Keen, MS, RN
Evelyn Butera, MS, RN, CNN
Annette C. Frauman, PhD, RN, FAAN
Diane M. Breckenridge, PhD, MSN, RN
Susan Taylor Hooper, PhD, RN
Donna Mapes, DNSc, RN
Marilyn L. Neff, MBA, RN, CNN, CNAA
Linda J. Smith, MSN, RN, CNN, C

Chapter 5 **Ethical Issues in Nephrology Nursing** 83
Rosalie Starzomski, PhD, MN, RN

Chapter 6 **Research in Nephrology Nursing: Overview, Development and Future Directions** 111
Anita E. Molzahn, PhD, RN

Table of Contents

Unit Three
The Kidney 125

Chapter 7 **Renal Physiology** 127
Patricia Preisig, PhD, RN
Christine Chmielewski, MS, RN, CNN
Marcia Keen, MS, RN
Mary Jo Holechek, MS, RN, CNN
Marlys K. Ludlow, MSN, RN, CNN
Carolyn B. Yucha, PhD, RN

Chapter 8 **Diseases of the Kidney** 177
Patricia S. Jordan, MS, RN, CNA, CNN

Chapter 9 **Acute and Chronic Renal Failure** 199
Kathy P. Parker, PhD, RN, CS, ANP

Unit Four
Clinical Management of the Renal Patient 267

Chapter 10 **Psychosocial Impact of Renal Disease** 269
Anita E. Molzahn, PhD, RN

Chapter 11 **Nutritional Care of Renal Patients** 285
Sue Dickey Roberts, MS, RD, CNSD

Chapter 12 **Pharmacology in Renal Disease** 305

Chapter 12A **Pharmacologic Agents in Renal Disease** 307
Terran Warren Sims, BSN, RN, CNN
Anita E. Molzahn, PhD, RN
Robert McGory, PharmD, MS, BS

Chapter 12B **Medications in Transplant Patients** 329
Karen K. Giuliano, MSN, RN, CCRN
Anita E. Molzahn, PhD, RN
Terran Warren Sims, BSN, RN, CNN

Chapter 13 **Control of Infectious Diseases in the Renal Patient** 347
Janel Parker, MSN, RN, CNN
Linda Dickenson, BS, RN, CNN, CPHQ
Karen C. Wiseman, MSN, RN, CNN
Diane Alexander, MS, BSN, RN, CNN
Eileen Peacock, MSN, RN, CNN, CIC, CPHQ

Chapter 14 **Rehabilitation of the Renal Patient** 403
Nancy G. Kutner, PhD

Unit Five
Special Patient Populations 433

Chapter 15 **The Pediatric Patient** 435
Cyrena M. Gilman, MN, RN, CNN
Annette C. Frauman, PhD, RN, FAAN

Chapter 16 **The Diabetic Patient** 465
Marta R. Taylor, MSN, RN, NP, CNN

Chapter 17 **The Geriatric Patient** 481
Terran Mathers, MSN, BA, RN, CNN

Unit Six
Treatment of Renal Disease: Therapies and Approaches 515

Chapter 18 **Conservative Management** 517
Sally S. Russell, MN, RNC

Chapter 19 **Hemodialysis** 525
Patricia Baltz Salai, MSN, RN, CRNP, CNN

Chapter 20 **Continuous Renal Replacement Therapy** 577
Christy A. Price, RN, MSN, CNN

Chapter 21 **Therapeutic Plasma Exchange** 589
Christy A. Price, RN, MSN, CNN

Chapter 22 **Peritoneal Dialysis** 603
LaVonne Burrows, MS, RN, CNN
Barbara F. Prowant, BSN, RN, CNN

Chapter 23 **Transplantation: Introduction and Historical Perspectives** 661
Christine Mudge, MS, RN, PNPc/CNS, CNN

Chapter 23A **Immunology** 667
Christine Mudge, MS, RN, PNPc/CNS, CNN

Chapter 23B **Transplantation** 693
Christine Mudge, MS, RN, PNPc/CNS, CNN
Laurie Carlson, MSN, RN
Patricia Brennan, MSN, RN

Table of Contents

Unit Seven
Public Policy and Legislative Issues 779

Chapter 24 **The Legislative Process** 781
Kathleen Smith, BS, RN, CNN

Chapter 25 **The End Stage Renal Disease Program** 795
Janel Parker, MSN, RN, CNN

Unit Eight
Communication and Collaboration 815

Chapter 26 **Maintaining and Documenting Standards of Care: Using the Nursing Process** 817
Barbara Bednar, MHA, RN, CNN
Eileen Peacock, MSN, RN, CNN, CIC, CPHQ

Chapter 27 **Patient Education** 837
Gail S. Wick, BSN, RN, CNN
Karen C. Robbins, MS, RN, CNN

Chapter 28 **The Nephrology Community** 853
Evelyn Butera, MS, RN, CNN
Nancy Gallagher, BSN, RN, CNN

Appendices 861

Appendix A **A Chronological History of the American Nephrology Nurses' Association** 863
Appendix B **Nursing Management of the Patient with Renal Failure** 869
Appendix C **Nursing Management of the Patient with Renal Failure** 876
Appendix D **Nursing Management of the Patient with Renal Failure** 878
Appendix E **AANNT Legislative Policy Statement – November 1983** 885
Appendix F **ANNA's Health Policy Statement** 888

Glossary of Terms 893

Index 913

Contributors

Editor

Janel Parker, MSN, RN, CNN
Nephrology Nurse Consultant
Marietta, GA

Contributors

Diane Alexander, MS, BSN, RN, CNN
Quality Management Coordinator
Total Renal Care
Berwyn, PA

Barbara Bednar, MHA, RN, CNN
Vice President, Clinical Operations
Total Renal Care
Berwyn, PA

Diane M. Breckenridge, PhD, RN
Post Doctoral Fellow
University of Pennsylvania
School of Nursing
Philadelphia, PA

Patricia Brennan, MSN, RN
Transplant Outreach Director
University of California
San Francisco, CA

LaVonne Burrows, MS, RN, CNN
Staff Nurse
Kidney Disease Center of the Ozarks
Springfield, MO

Evelyn Butera, MS, RN, CNN
CQI Coordinator
Satellite Dialysis Centers, Inc.
Redwood City, CA

Laurie Carlson, MSN, RN
Clinical Nurse III
Research Study Coordinator
University of California
San Francisco, CA

Christine M. Chmielewski, MS, RN, CNN
Project Director, Orientation to the Specialty
ANNA
Pitman, NJ

Anna L. Corea, MN, RN, CNAA
Administrator
University of California at Los Angeles Dialysis
Assistant Clinical Professor
School of Nursing
University of California at Los Angeles
Los Angeles, CA

Linda Dickenson, BS, RN, CNN, CPHQ
Quality Management Coordinator
Total Renal Care
Berwyn, PA

Jacqueline Fawcett, PhD, RN, FAAN
Professor, School of Nursing
University of Pennsylvania
Philadelphia, PA

Annette C. Frauman, PhD, RN, FAAN
Chair, Family and Community Nursing
Nell Hodgson Woodruff School of Nursing
Emory University
Atlanta, GA

Nancy Gallagher, BSN, RN, CNN
Director, Nephrology Services
St. Joseph Medical Center
Tacoma, WA

Cyrena M. Gilman, MN, RN, CNN
Manager, Clinical Operations
Riley Hospital for Children
Indianapolis, IN

Karen K. Giuliano, MSN, RN, CCRN
Critical Care Clinical Nurse Specialist
Baystate Medical Center
Springfield, MA

Mary Ann Gould, MSN, RN, CNN
Nephrology Nurse Consultant
SmithKline Beecham Pharmaceuticals
Philadelphia, PA

Marguerite F. Hartigan, MSN, RN, CNN
Clinical Nurse Specialist
Outpatient Dialysis Center
University of Pennsylvania
Philadelphia, PA

Mary Jo Holechek, MS, CRNP, CNN
Transplant Nurse Practitioner
Johns Hopkins Hospital
Baltimore, MD

Susan Hooper, PhD, RN
Executive Vice President
Vintana Consulting Group
Houston, TX

Patricia S. Jordan, MS, RN, CNN, CNA
Regional Marketing Specialist
Althin Medical, Inc.
Miami Lakes, FL

Marcia Keen, MS, RN
Manager, Epogen Clinical Grants
Amgen, Inc.
Thousand Oaks, CA

Nancy G. Kutner, PhD
Professor, Rehabilitation Medicine
Emory University
Atlanta, GA

Marlys K. Ludlow, MSN, RN, CNN
Assistant Nurse Manager
Stanford University Hospital
Stanford, CA

Donna Mapes, DNSc, RN
Associate Director, Professional Services
Amgen, Inc.
Thousand Oaks, CA

Terran Mathers, MSN, BA, RN, CNN
Clinical Assistant Professor
College of Nursing
University of South Alabama
Mobile, AL

Robert McGory, PharmD, MS, BS
Transplant Pharmacist
University of Virginia Health Sciences Center
Charlottesville, VA

Anita E. Molzahn, PhD, RN
Dean, Faculty of Human & Social Development
School of Nursing
University of Victoria
Victoria, BC Canada

CONTRIBUTORS

Christine Mudge, MS, RN, PNPc/CNS, CNN
Pediatric Nurse Practitioner/Coordinator
Pediatric Transplant
University of California
San Francisco, CA

Marilyn L. Neff, MBA, RN, CNN, CNAA
Health Care Consultant
MLN Enterprises
Marietta, GA

Janel Parker, MSN, RN, CNN
Nephrology Nurse Consultant
Marietta, GA

Kathy P. Parker, PhD, RN, CS, ANP
Assistant Professor
School of Nursing
Emory University
Atlanta, GA

Eileen Peacock, MSN, RN, CNN, CIC, CPHQ
Director of Quality Assurance for Renal Service
Total Renal Care
Berwyn, PA

Patricia Preisig, PhD, RN
Associate Professor, Internal Medicine
University of Texas Southwestern Medical Center
Dallas, TX

Christy A. Price, RN, MSN, CNN
Nephrology Clinical Nurse Specialist
Total Renal Care
Salt Lake City, UT

Barbara Prowant, BSN, RN, CNN
Research Assistant
University of Missouri
School of Medicine
Dialysis Clinics, Inc.
Columbia, MO

Karen C. Robbins, MS, RN, CNN
Coordinator, CHESS Project
Hartford Hospital
Hartford, CT

Sue Dickey Roberts, MS, RD, CNSD
Renal Dietitian
TRC Union City Dialysis Center
Union City, CA

Sally S. Russell, MN, RNC
Program Coordinator
St. Elizabeth Medical Center
Lafayette, IN

Patricia Baltz Salai, MSN, RN, CRNP, CNN
Renal Clinical Specialist
VA Healthcare System
Pittsburgh, PA

Terran Warren Sims, BSN, RN, CNN
Clinician IV Transplantation
University of Virginia Hospital
Charlottesville, VA

Kathleen Smith, BS, RN, CNN
Director of Legislative Services
Nursing Economic$
Washington, DC

Linda J. Smith, MSN, RN, CNN, C
Director of Professional Development
ANNA
Pitman, NJ

Rosalie Starzomski, PhD, RN
Assistant Professor,
University of Victoria
Ethics Consultant,
Vancouver General Hospital
Vancouver, BC, Canada

Marta R. Taylor, MSN, RN, NP, CNN
Nurse Practitioner
Indiana Regional Medical Consultants
North East Indiana Kidney Center
Ft. Wayne, IN

Gail S. Wick, BSN, RN, CNN
Vice President of Clinical Quality Management Programs
Fresenius Medical Care North America
Boston, MA

Karen C. Wiseman, MSN, RN, CNN
Clinical Writer
Gambro Healthcare
Nashville, TN

Carolyn B. Yucha, PhD, RN
Assistant Professor
University of Colorado Health Sciences Center
School of Nursing
Denver, CO

ANNA National Office Staff

Gus A. Ostrum
Managing Editor

Ron Brady
Executive Director

Denise Talerico
Editorial Coordinator

Claudia Cuddy
Copy Editor

Maryanne Hatfield
Proofreader

Jack M. Bryant
Art Director

Darin Peters
Graphic Artist

Bob Taylor
Graphic Artist

Charlie Harvey
Graphic Artist

ONTEMPORARY NEPHROLOGY NURSING REVIEWERS

The Editor of *Contemporary Nephrology Nursing* wishes to thank the following professionals, who reviewed chapters in this publication for nephrology nursing content.

Debbie Ashton, BSN, RN, CNN
Gambro Healthcare
Chula Vista, CA

Marilyn Bartucci, MSN, RN
University Hospital of Cleveland
Cleveland, OH

Jeanette K. Chambers, PhD, RN, CS
Riverside Methodist Hospital
Columbus, OH

Christine Chmielewski, MS, RN, CNN
Holy Family College
Philadelphia, PA

Julie Fairman, PhD, RN
University of Pennsylvania
Philadelphia, PA

Donna Hathaway, PhD, RN, FAAN
University of Tennessee-Memphis
Memphis, TN

Nancy Hoffart, PhD, RN
University of Kansas
School of Nursing
Kansas City, KS

Bonnie Holaday, DNS, RN, FAAN
School of Nursing
Wichita State University
Wichita, KS

Mary Jo Holechek, MS, RN, CNN
Johns Hopkins Hospital
Baltimore, MD

Kathy Joyce, MSN, RN
Washington Hospital Center
Washington, DC

Eileen Peacock, MSN, RN, CNN, CIC, CPHQ
Director of Quality Assurance for Renal Service
Total Renal Care
Berwyn, PA

Karen E. Schardin, BSN, RN, CNN
RTC Sparks
Sparks, NV

Jane Scopelite, PhD, RD
New Jersey State Department of Health
Trenton, NJ

Kathleen Smith, BS, RN, CNN
Director of Legislative Services
Nursing Economic$
Washington, DC

Janette Weiner, MS, RN, CNN
University of Chicago Hospital
Chicago, IL

Rebecca L. Wingard, MSN, RN, CNN
Renal Care Group, Inc.
Nashville, TN

Acknowledgments

IN a comprehensive publication such as *Contemporary Nephrology Nursing*, there are many to whom my gratitude is expressed. My many thank you's are extended to the following people:

To **Gus Ostrum**, for his sound guidance, keen intellect, and kind perseverance; to **Anita Molzahn** for her efficiency and expertise; to the **authors** for sharing their knowledge so willingly; to the many **reviewers** for giving so freely of their time and intelligence; to **Denise Talerico** for her editorial and administrative skills; to **Robert King** for his computer expertise; to **Karen Schardin** for her tenacity; to **Evelyn Butera**, **Christy Price**, and **Nancy Gallagher** for their continued belief in my abilities; and to **Ron Brady** for pointing me in the right direction and his confidence in this project.

My affection and appreciation are also due to my children, **J.D.** and **Ellen**, who helped me see the world with a new set of eyes; my parents, **Ken** and **Peg Dager**, who long ago taught me that I could do anything I set my mind to do, and never doubted that I would; and most of all to my husband, **David**, without his encouragement and unlimited support this book would not have been completed.

Janel Parker, MSN, RN, CNN
Editor

UNIT 1

Nature and Scope of Nephrology Nursing

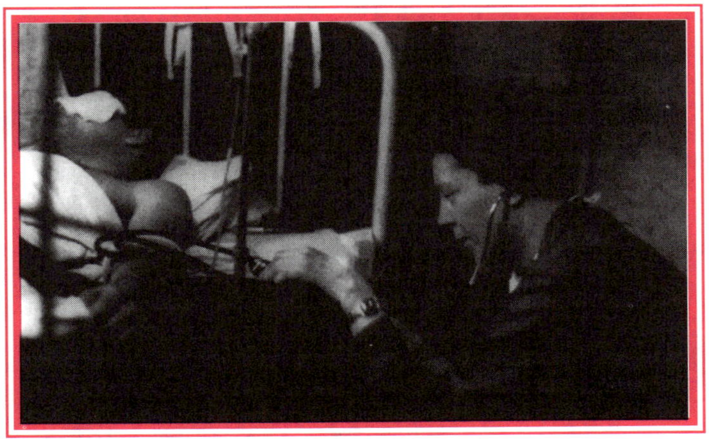

Unit Contents

Chapter 1
Nephrology Nursing as a Specialty 3
Janel Parker, MSN, RN, CNN

Chapter 2
The History of Nephrology Nursing 25
Anna L. Corea, MN, RN, CNAA

Chapter 3
The Professional Roles of the Nephrology Nurse 43
Mary Ann Gould, MSN, RN, CNN

CHAPTER 1

Nephrology Nursing as a Specialty

Janel Parker, MSN, RN, CNN

Chapter Contents

Evolution of Specialization in Nursing 5
- The Origin of Professional Nursing Practice 5
- Organized Nursing 6
- Recognition of Specialty Practice 6

The Development of Nephrology Nursing Practice 6
- The Beginning of Nephrology Nursing 6
- Influencing Factors 7

Nephrology Nursing as a Specialty: The Foundation 7
- Definition of a Specialty 7
- Foundation for Nephrology Nursing as a Specialty 8
- A Conceptual Framework 9

Nephrology Nursing as Specialty Practice: The Evolution 13
- ABNS Standards for Recognition and Approval of Nursing Specialties . . 13

Summary 21

References 22

Chapter Highlights 23

Nephrology Nursing as a Specialty

Janel Parker, MSN, RN, CNN

In spite of over 100 years of rhetoric, some of it quite elegant, nursing remains a mystery to those outside of it, including professional colleagues, administrators, public policy makers, and health care consumers. Our starched white uniforms, which once provided at least a symbol that was recognizable, have gone away. We have discarded starch for surgical scrubs and laboratory coats, skirts for pants, and caps for stethoscopes.

The reason for the existence of modern health care institutions, that is, hospitals, dialysis units, home care agencies, is to deliver nursing care. If diagnosis and management of serious medical illnesses could be done in office practices in 10 minutes, it would be. If dialysis could always be performed effectively at home, it would be. If transplant surgeries could be done safely and economically on the kitchen table, and if people could survive, they would be.

Nursing is two things: (a) caring for the sick or the potentially sick; and (b) tending to the entire environment within which care happens. What makes nursing complicated is not just the physical work of helping people – nor even the teaching, comforting, careful listening, or endless documenting – but the enormous amount of information it takes to care for people in many different diagnostic groups and different individual diagnoses (Diers, 1988).

The nursing profession has become too large and complex for any one person to master the full range of information and skills encompassed within it. Specialization enables nurses to focus in on one area of knowledge and technical skills, to provide patients with the best care possible.

One of the greatest challenges in contemporary nursing is the identification of nursing specialties. Therefore, nursing specialties originate and are recognized in a variety of ways, that is, graduate programs in nursing, state certification or secondary licensing programs, national certification programs, specialty organizations and councils, and job descriptions (Styles, 1989).

Nephrology nursing practice actually began in the 1950s when nurses worked as part of the renal research teams providing dialysis and transplant nursing care. In 1969, the American Association for Nephrology Nurses (AANN) was created. AANN has evolved to what is known today as the American Nephrology Nurses' Association (ANNA). Through ANNA, nephrology nursing has evolved into a nursing specialty. ANNA has developed the components of the practice base for nephrology nursing: the scope of practice, core curriculum, certification, standards of clinical practice, quality assurance/continuous quality improvement, and research. In 1992, the Nephrology Nursing Certification Board (NNCB) was recognized as meeting the criteria set forth by the American Board of Nursing Specialties (ABNS) to assure that national standards for specialty nursing education and practice have been met (Parker, 1994). The purpose of this chapter is to discuss the development of nephrology nursing practice as a specialty and the events that influenced its evolution.

Evolution of Specialization in Nursing

The Origin of Professional Nursing Practice

The foundation for contemporary nursing was laid by Florence Nightingale in 1860 with the opening of the Nightingale School for Nurses at St. Thomas Hospital in London. It was the first fully endowed school of nursing.

Before the 1870s, trained nurses were virtually unknown in America. Hospital nursing was a menial occupation that attracted only women who could secure no other employment. The movement for reform originated among upper-class women. As a result of their efforts, on June 13, 1861, President Lincoln signed an order creating the United States (U.S.) Sanitary Commission. Its objective was to secure healthful conditions in military camps and hospitals (Diers, 1988; Flanagan, 1976).

After the Civil War, a group of U.S. Sanitary Commission members formed the State Charities Aid Association, which in 1872 established a committee to monitor nursing care and sanitation in health care institutions. It was this committee that recommended establishment of schools of nursing to provide nursing care for sick and injured patients.

In addition to recognizing the needs of patients and nurses' roles in meeting these needs, Florence Nightingale recognized the importance of a conceptual framework in which patient care was delivered. Many of the volunteer bodies of the U.S. Sanitary Commission were counseled by Florence Nightingale, and during the Civil War a heightened interest in public sanitation, health care reform, and health education was recognized. To ensure an appropriate plan for educating nurses, the New York State Charities Aid Association sent Dr. Gill Wylie to seek the advice of Florence Nightingale. The Bellevue Training School for Nurses, founded in May 1873, was the first school in the United States to use the principles of the Nightingale School of Nursing (Flanagan, 1976; Starr, 1982).

Some physicians approved of the women's' committee to improve conditions in health care institutions and attract middle class women to schools of nursing, while other physicians were opposed. Physicians objected that educated nurses would not do as they were instructed. So the women reformers went to men of their own class who had greater authority and power. Professional nursing materialized neither from hospital administrators nor physicians, but from female consumers who recognized the need to carry out the multifarious work of caring for the sick and the injured by an educated nursing staff (Starr, 1982).

With the advent of the germ theory and antiseptic procedures during this time, the number of hospitals increased rapidly and most with an affiliated nurse training school. Each hospital developed its nurse training program to best meet its own needs. At this time, hospitals became more acceptable as institutions of care for the sick and injured instead of almshouses for the destitute and indigent.

During the late 1800s, three factors profoundly affected the development of nursing education: the campaign for women's rights, the support for public education, and the growth of schools for higher education. Nursing's stature in the health care community paralleled women's rising status in American history (Flanagan, 1976).

Organized Nursing

The first formal meeting of American nurses took place in 1893 at the Chicago World's Fair. At this meeting, 18 nursing school superintendents voted to establish the American Society of Superintendents of Training Schools for Nurses. The purpose of the organization was to promote the fellowship of its members, to establish and maintain a universal standard of training, and to further the best interests of the nursing profession (Canavan, 1996). Immediately this group recognized the lack of adequate control over its training schools and realized it would have to recruit additional members of the nursing community to establish a standardized nursing curricula and registration.

During 1886, the Superintendents Society established the Committee for the Organization of a National Association for Nurses, which was charged with preparing a constitution and bylaws for a new organization that would meet the needs of the nursing community. Later that year the Nurses' Associated Alumnae of the United States and Canada was formed and in 1911 was renamed the American Nurses Association (ANA) (Canavan, 1996; Flanagan, 1976).

Recognition of Specialty Practice

The growth of professional nursing practice was propelled by the activities of ANA. In 1966, bylaws revisions were adopted by the ANA House of Delegates to operationalize structural changes and design a more effective professional association for registered nurses...making it possible to focus on four primary areas of concern: nursing practice, nursing education, nursing services, and the economic and general welfare of nurses (Whitaker, 1968). As part of these structural changes, divisions on practice were established by the ANA Board of Directors upon evidence that a substantial number of nurses were practicing in a field with a well-defined and unique body of nursing knowledge and skills and/or upon evidence that a significant health problem existed in which nursing was involved (Flanagan, 1976). The following divisions on practice were established: community health nursing, geriatric nursing, maternal and child health nursing, medical-surgical nursing, and psychiatric and mental health nursing. The purpose of each division on practice included: establishing standards for nursing practice, conducting clinical/scientific sessions at conventions, stimulating research, disseminating relevant information in areas of practice, providing recognition for professional achievement, and establishing respective certification boards (Flanagan, 1976).

Although ANA represented all professional registered nurses and spoke collectively on their behalf, one organization was unable to satisfy the educational, technical, and regulatory requirements of the entire nursing profession. Thus, specialty organizations rapidly emerged to meet the demands of nurses requiring distinctive knowledge and skills for practice.

The Development of Nephrology Nursing Practice

The Beginning of Nephrology Nursing

Between 1915 and 1950, few articles about kidney disease appeared in nursing journals and textbooks (Hoffart, 1989 a,b). The development of the artificial kidney in the 1940s by Willem Kolff and its arrival in the United States in 1947 (McBride,

1979) spurred nurses' involvement in the treatment of patients with renal failure. The role of the nurse consisted of collecting data for medical research teams, preparing dialysis equipment, providing direct nursing care to patients, and acting as patient advocates (Hoffart, 1989 a,b).

Successful kidney transplants were not reported until 1954, when surgeons at Peter Bent Brigham performed the first of many transplants between identical twins (Merrill, Murray, Harrison, & Guild, 1956; Murray, Merrill, & Harrison, 1958). Immunosuppressive medications were administered for the first time to transplant patients in 1962 (Murray, Tilney, & Wilson, 1976). In the 1960s, hospitals began to establish transplant units and simultaneously created a specific group of nurses to care for these patients. Care of transplant patients included providing standard postoperative care, monitoring the effects of immunosuppression, treating early rejection, patient teaching, and meeting patients' psychological and emotional needs (Andrews, 1986; Shebelski, 1986; Bois, Barfield, Taylor, & Ross, 1968).

Although many nurses involved in transplantation and hemodialysis had experience with peritoneal dialysis, it was not until the late 1970s, when continuous modes were developed, that peritoneal dialysis programs were established in renal centers (Hoffart, 1989 a,b). Consequently, few nurses developed expertise in peritoneal dialysis during the formative years of nephrology nursing.

With so few nurses involved in the care of renal failure patients, there was little opportunity for sharing information and experiences. Often nephrology nurses reported directly to physicians instead of nursing administrators in the hospitals. Although this hierarchy permitted nurses to expand their knowledge and technical skills, there was little opportunity to develop peer and mentoring relationships with nurse colleagues.

The American Society for Artificial and Internal Organs (ASAIO) was established in 1955 to bring together experts who were "interested in physiological machines which stimulate the function of internal organs" (Salisbury, 1960, p. ii). During the ASAIO meetings, dialysis training nurses had opportunities to learn about new medical advances and network with nurses from other programs. Nurses who worked in transplant programs, however, recall little opportunity outside of their own hospitals to develop collegial relationships (Andrews, 1986; Cameron, 1986; Fulton, 1986; Hoffart, 1989 a,b; Shebelski, 1986).

In 1966, a formal educational program was offered for nurses at Peter Bent Brigham Hospital in Boston. The enthusiastic response to the program motivated these nurses to begin planning annual programs in conjunction with ASAIO. The involvement of nurses in this group such as Cameron and Fulton, who worked in hospitals that offered all modalities of treatment, assisted the group to focus on the educational needs of all nurses who cared for patients with kidney failure.

This core group of nurses explored the concept of a formal organization to continue educational programming and professional networking for nephrology nurses. At the 1969 conference in Atlantic City, NJ, a constitution and bylaws were adopted and an organization known as the American Association for Nephrology Nurses (AANN) was created (Hoffart, 1989 a,b). The purpose of the organization was "to promote knowledge about the care of patients with renal disease" (AANN Constitution, 1969, p. 1).

Influencing Factors

Many factors influenced the growth of nephrology nursing. The most significant of these factors was the signing of HR-1: Social Security Amendments of 1972 by President Nixon on October 30, 1972. HR-1 became Public Law 92-603 providing Medicare coverage and thereby, equal access to care for all patients with chronic renal failure. The effective date of coverage for dialysis and transplant services by Medicare's End Stage Renal Disease (ESRD) Program was July 1, 1973 (Bocchino & Burrows-Hudson, 1995).

The number of patients treated during the first year of the program was 8,000 at a cost of approximately $220 million (Bocchino & Burrows-Hudson, 1995). In 1995, 262,760 patients were treated at a cost of $13.06 billion (United States Renal Data System, 1997). The AANN was created by less than 50 people. Currently, the membership of the American Nephrology Nurses Association (ANNA) is over 11,000 registered nurses (Price, 1997).

ANNA has matured to meet the changing needs of its membership and in doing so has laid the foundation for the development of nephrology nursing as a specialty. Full membership is limited to registered nurses in an effort to appropriately represent and direct our resources to nephrology nursing practice. As the technology surrounding the care of patients with renal failure has developed so have the treatment modalities (Sims, 1994). Through expanding educational programming, chapter development, membership recruitment and retention, corporate support, professional resources, awards, scholarships, research grants, legislative involvement, and clinical and functional special interest areas, ANNA has emerged as the foundation for the development of a practice base and a strong voice for nephrology nursing specialty.

Nephrology Nursing as a Specialty Practice: The Foundation

Definition of a Specialty

The specialization of nursing practice has

Figure 1-1
Model for nephrology nursing practice base.

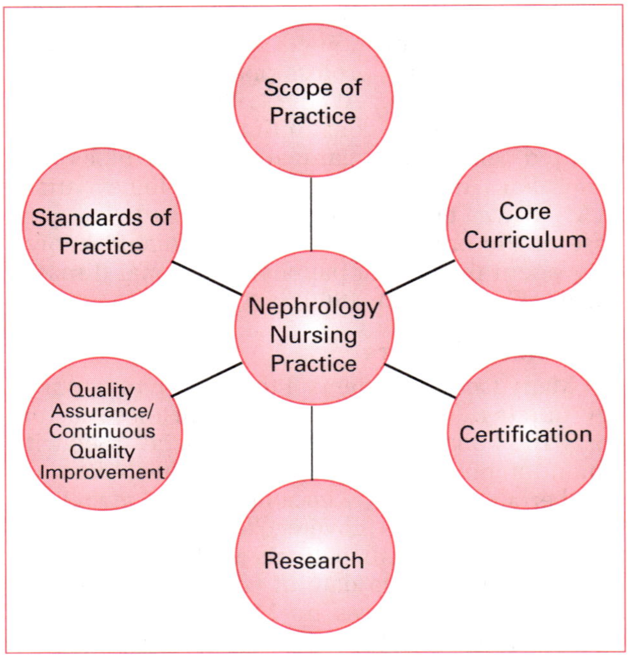

Note: Revised from Jordan, P.J. (1993). *Professional development guide* (p. 8). Pitman, NJ: American Nephrology Nurses' Association. Reprinted with permission.

occurred in response to the needs of the patients whom we care for. The rapid proliferation of medical and nursing knowledge, resulting from scientific and technological advances, and the necessary skills that must accompany this knowledge has made it impossible for any one practitioner to comprehend. Specialization provides the opportunity to focus on one area and provide the best care possible to patients.

In the U.S. and European communities, nurse scholars have studied nursing specialties. No official source for identifying nursing specialties had been recognized. Therefore, nursing specialties have originated by several methods, including educational programs, state recognition of advanced practice and/or second licensing programs, national certification programs, specialty organizations and councils, and job descriptions (Styles, 1989).

In an effort to preserve the integrity of the nursing profession and develop nursing specialties to their fullest potential, the International Council of Nurses (ICN) created and tested a set of guidelines to steer the development of nursing specialties under the direction of the profession and in accordance with the health needs of the population. The four essentials of these guidelines are:

- criteria for the development of specialties;
- establishment of an overall regulatory mechanism for specialties, preferably through the profession and not the government;
- uniform high standards of education and practice for specialties; and
- development of specialties within an overall nursing resources plan (Styles, 1991, p. 357).

Nursing in the United States is in the process of implementing some of the ICN guidelines through the establishment of the American Board of Nursing Specialties (ABNS) in 1991. The ABNS is a national peer review program that promotes the highest quality of specialty nursing practice through the recognition of approved national certification bodies and their programs. The goal of the ABNS is to serve as an advocate for consumer protection by establishing and maintaining standards of professional specialty nursing certification and to increase the consumer's awareness of the meaning and value of specialty certification (Parker, 1994; Styles, 1989). By becoming a charter member of ABNS, ANNA has participated in the identification and definition of specialty nursing practice.

Membership in ABNS is based on documentation which demonstrates that standards are met for recognition of the nursing specialty and approval of its certification program. The application is based on 12 standards and their respective criteria adopted by the charter members of ABNS. These standards were developed to encourage specialties to demonstrate the viability and effectiveness of their practice, education, research, and peer review/credentialing (Parker, 1994; Styles, 1989).

Foundation for Nephrology Nursing as a Specialty

For three decades, the nephrology nursing profession has increased in scope and numbers. Nephrology nurses were employed in hemodialysis and peritoneal dialysis units, transplant units, physician's offices, and as members of research teams and marketing programs. By the 1980s, it was no longer sufficient to be competent in delivering one modality of patient care. One patient would often experience all three modalities of care, and nephrology nurses were expected to participate in conservative management of residual renal function, preparation for hemodialysis and/or peritoneal dialysis, and planning and implementation of pretransplant and posttransplant nursing care.

Through ANNA, nephrology nurses again assessed the needs of their specialty. Realizing the importance of maintaining autonomy as professional nurses practicing in a domain requiring unique knowledge and technical skills, ANNA leaders sought to define their nursing practice. Consensus building by ANNA leaders included: ANA and National League for Nursing (NLN) forums for the purpose of identifying the components necessary to construct a practice base, surveying association membership, and developing collegial relationships with other specialty nursing organizations. ANNA designated six components to create a practice base: *Scope of Practice for Nephrology Nursing* (1986, 1995), *Core Curriculum for Nephrology Nursing* (1987, 1991, 1995), Certification Examination (1987, 1989, 1990-1996), *Quality Assurance Manual* (1988)/*Continuous Quality Improvement Manual* (1995), *Standards of Clinical Practice for Nephrology Nursing* (1988, 1993), *A Guide to Professional Development* (1993), and the establishment of a standing research committee (1990) (see Figure 1-1).

These components provide the foundation for a nephrology nursing practice base. This foundation, interrelated with the mission statement (see Table 1-1) and objectives (see Table 1-2) of ANNA, has evolved into the specialty of nephrology nursing.

A Conceptual Framework

The conceptual framework employed to analyze nephrology nursing as a specialty is the standards and criteria set forth by ABNS (see Table 1-3). These standards were developed to guide specialties in demonstrating the viability and effectiveness of their practice, education, research, and peer review/credentialing.

The standards were adapted from Styles (1989), *Criteria for Approval of Specialties*. Styles developed these criteria based on a range of sociological theories and a summary of characteristics of current nursing specialties. Nursing is seen as a social system with:

> structural elements (specialists, observing sanctions and organized by position and rank; beliefs or knowledge; systems of interactions; goals; means to achieve these goals; values to drive the system; and, conditions and norms that limit the range of choices between and among goals and available means) and functional processes (practice, research and development, education and socialization, standard setting and credentialing, organization) and internal and external boundaries. The external boundaries separate nursing from its environment; the internal boundaries define the specialties, each with its own structural elements and functional processes (Styles, 1989, pp. 11-12).

In 1985, Styles reviewed, summarized, and analyzed information from 23 nursing specialties "to determine which characteristics appeared to be related to the progress of special interest associations as a mature specialty" (Styles, 1989, p. 28). The following characteristics were acknowledged: practice, education, research and development, credentialing, organization, publications, relationship with other organizations and disciplines, and the identification of the nursing specialty through its definition of practice and the practitioner, its educational program and knowledge base, and its relationship with nursing-at-large (Styles, 1989).

The major characteristics of contemporary nursing specialties, as identified by Dr. Styles (1989) were viewed within the framework of nursing as a social system. From this analysis, it was concluded that nursing is weakened by its lack of legitimacy or recognized authority, homogeneity, and unity and internal structural-functional processes of the specialties. It was hypothesized that nursing specialties and their credentials lack the power to achieve the benefits of specialization to the public, nurses, and the profession.

Based on this problem analysis, Styles suggested four essentials for empowering nursing as a specialized social system:

- An authoritative, criterion-based professional review mechanism for specialty recognition and sanction.

Table 1-1
ANNA mission statement.

The mission of ANNA is to advance the professional development of registered nurses practicing in nephrology, transplantation and related therapies and to promote the highest standards of patient care.

Table 1-2
ANNA LRSP: Key objectives for 1996-1997.

- ☞ Implement continuing education delivery systems, formats and materials that provide appropriate teaching/learning opportunities.
- ☞ Design creative strategies that promote active participation of the learner in continuing education activities.
- ☞ Establish a research-based practice.
- ☞ Develop a high quality research program.
- ☞ Encourage policy and research initiatives that promote quality health care.
- ☞ Increase member ability to effectively participate in the legislative process.
- ☞ Promote advanced nursing practice.
- ☞ Advance collaborative practice.
- ☞ Increase the level of volunteer participation and leadership effectiveness at the local, regional, and national levels.
- ☞ Provide programs and services that reflect the cultural diversity of the membership.

Table 1-3
ABNS standards and criteria.

Definition and Scope of Nursing Specialty

Standard
The certification is based on a distinct and well-defined field of nursing practice that subscribes to the overall purpose and functions of nursing. The nursing specialty is distinct from other nursing specialties and is national in scope. There is an identified need for the specialty and nurses who devote most of their practice to the specialty.

Criteria
- Evidence of the professional and scientific status of the specialty exists.
  A body of scientific knowledge that is unique and distinct from that of basic nursing provides the theoretical underpinning for the specialty. A substantial portion of the knowledge base is not shared by other nursing specialties, although some of the components may be shared with related specialties.
  - There is evidence of a societal need for nurses in the specialty and a pool of nurses who concentrate their practice in the specialty (50% or more of their work time, functions, or professional roles are spent in the specialty).
  - A national nursing organization supports the specialty.
  - A national nursing organization has defined the specialty, explicated its core knowledge, and written a scope of specialty practice and standards for the specialty.
- The practice specialty's definition and/or standards describe how the following four essential elements of contemporary nursing practice, as detailed in the *American Nurses Association Social Policy Statement* (ANA, 1995), are operationalized.
  - attention to the full range of human experiences and responses to health and illness without restriction to a problem-focused orientation;
  - integration of objective data with knowledge gained from an understanding of the patient or group's subjective experience;
  - application of scientific knowledge to the processes of diagnosis and treatment; and
  - provision of a caring relationship that facilitates health and healing.

Research-Based Body of Knowledge

Standard
A tested body of research/data based knowledge related to the nursing specialty exists. Mechanisms are established for the support, review, and dissemination of research in the specialty. Activities within the specialty contribute to the advancement of nursing science within the specialty.

Criteria
There is a published body of literature and research on the focus of the specialty and published/stated research priorities for the specialty.

Organizational Autonomy

Standard
The certification board is an entity with organizational autonomy. However, a collaborative relationship exists between the certification body and a nursing specialty association that supports the specialty and sets standards for specialty practice.

Criteria
All policy decisions relating to certification are the sole decision of the certifying body, not subject to approval by any other entity. There is philosophical support from, and appropriate collaboration with, a specialty nursing association.

Public Representation

Standard
There is a provision for public consultation/representation on the certification board.

Criteria
The certification body has a mechanism for assuring public input into certification policies and decisions.

Eligibility Criteria for Test Candidates

Standards
The eligibility criteria for basic certification include:
- RN licensure
- Baccalaureate or higher degree in nursing
- A specified minimum educational program in the specialty

The eligibility criteria for advanced certification include:
- RN licensure
- A minimum of a graduate degree in nursing or the appropriate equivalent, including content in the specified area of specialty practice

Table 1-3
ABNS standards and criteria. (continued)

Criteria
The above listed criteria are required by the certifying body as eligibility to become certified. RN licensure must be presently required. If the educational criteria listed above are not presently required, there must be a plan in place to require them and implement them within 5 years of the initial application to ABNS. There should also be a plan to permit nurses who do not meet the educational criteria to maintain certification, if it was initially earned prior to implementation of the educational requirements.

Test Development

Standard
Certification tests are constructed and evaluated using methods that are psychometrically sound and fair to all candidates.

Criteria
The certifying body demonstrates that fair and psychometrically sound methods are used to construct and evaluate all tests.

Validity

Standard
The certifying body has conducted validation studies to assure that inferences made on the basis of test scores are appropriate and justified.

Criteria
With regard to the concept of validity, the certifying body has defined competence to practice at each level it certifies in the specialty, and assures content validity of the examination.

Reliability

Standard
The certifying body assures that test scores, including subscores, are sufficiently reliable for their intended uses.

Criteria
The certifying body has obtained measures of reliability, standard error of measurement, and classification consistency for each certification test administered. The certifying body has established equating procedures with the highest practical level of precision when scores on different test forms (editions) are intended to be comparable. When more than one testing methodology is implemented for a given examination (e.g. paper and pencil and computer based testing), the certifying body has data regarding the parallelism of the different methods.

Elimination of Bias/Sensitive Items

Standard
The certifying body does not discriminate among applicants as to age, gender, race, religion, ethnic origin, disability, marital status, or sexual orientation.

Criteria
The certifying body takes steps to detect and eliminate bias from the test to accommodate candidates with disabilities.

Test Administration

Standard
Certification tests are administered in a manner that minimizes construct-irrelevant variance.

Criteria
The certifying body has policies and procedures that assure that certification tests are administered in a fair, nondiscriminating, and standardized manner.

Test Security

Standard
Procedures are in place to maximize the security of all certification test materials.

Criteria
The certifying body has policies and procedures for the protection of the security of all test materials during every aspect of test development and administration.

Passing Scores

Standard
Passing scores for the certification examination are set in a manner that is fair to all candidates, using methods that are psychometrically sound.

Table 1-3
ABNS standards and criteria. (continued)

Criteria
The certifying body demonstrates that fair and psychometrically sound methods are used to establish passing scores.

Continued Competency

Standard
The certifying body has a mechanism in place to periodically evaluate certificate holders for continued knowledge necessary to maintain competence in the specialty.

Criteria
The certifying body has a recertification program in place that encourages certified nurses to continue those activities that support the maintenance of competence in the specialty.

Communications

Standard
The certifying body provides information that clearly describes the certification process to candidates and other stakeholders.

Criteria
The certifying body fully informs candidates and other stakeholders about the application and testing process, promptly reports test results, informs candidates of their due process rights, discloses information on certification and other activities, maintains confidentiality of nonpublic data, and provides responsive customer service.

Confidentiality

Standard
The certifying body assures that confidential information about candidates and certificate holders is protected.

Criteria
The certifying body clearly identifies categories of information available to the public and those that are held confidential. The certifying body has taken measures to protect confidential information regarding all candidates and certificate holders.

Appeals

Standard
The certifying body has an appeal process in place for nurses who have been denied access to an examination or renewal of certification, or who have had certification revoked.

Criteria
The certifying body provides evidence that an equitable and expeditious process exists for nurses seeking an amendment of a decision to deny access to initial certification, deny recertification, or to revoke active certification.

Disciplinary Action

Standard
The certifying body has a mechanism in place to respond to instances of noncompliance with eligibility criteria or certification board rules.

Criteria
When notified that individuals may not meet eligibility criteria or may not be in compliance with certification board rules, the certifying body conducts an investigation and takes disciplinary action.

Note: From American Board of Nursing Specialties. (1997). *Application for approval: Standards, rationale, criteria, required documentation*. Washington, DC: Author. Reprinted with permission.

- Criteria for accomplishing an adequate degree of homogeneity and ensuring specialty services of high quality.
- A schema within which unity of purpose and fit among the specialties can be determined.
- A plan for promoting specialists credentials (Styles, 1989, pp. 53-54).

The ABNS is recognized by the nursing profession as the professional peer review mechanism for reviewing and approving specialties. The ABNS is a voluntary system that "acknowledges the national voluntary certification of specialists as the critical mechanism for bringing quality control to specialty practice and unity, homogeneity, and authority to the development of specialties" (Styles, 1989, p. 55). Criteria for approval of specialties was proposed by Styles (1989) and adopted by ABNS in 1991 (Parker, 1994). In March 1997, criteria for approval was revised to strengthen the original standards. Some of the original standards were combined while other standards were divided and expanded. Seventeen standards were adopted by the ABNS Assembly. By complying with these criteria, nursing specialties demonstrate the effectiveness of their practice, education and socialization, research, credentialing, and organization. These criteria provide an avenue for consistency within a specialty and the nursing profession.

Nephrology Nursing as a Specialty Practice: The Evolution

ABNS Standards for Recognition and Approval of Nursing Specialties

Standard 1: The certification program is based on a distinct and well-defined field of nursing practice that subscribes to the overall purposes and functions of nursing. The nursing specialty is distinct from other nursing specialties and is national in scope. There is an identified need for the specialty and nurses who devote most of their practice to the specialty.

ANNA is the national nursing organization which has defined nephrology nursing practice. The *Scope of Practice for Nephrology Nursing* was published by ANNA in 1986 and revised in 1995. The practice of nephrology nursing was defined as nursing directed toward assessing the health needs of adult and pediatric patients and their families who are experiencing the real or threatened impact of acute and chronic renal failure, as well as to diagnose and treat their responses to these problems (ANNA, 1995). This definition is congruent with ANA's definition of nursing practice in *Nursing - A Social Policy Statement:* Nursing is the diagnosis and treatment of human responses to actual or potential health problems (ANA, 1980, p. 9).

The *ANNA Scope of Practice* defines nephrology nursing, the uniqueness of the specialty, and the essential knowledge and skills required to practice in the specialty. The working definition of nephrology nursing, as purported by the scope of practice, is: "nephrology nursing is a specialized area of nursing focused on the health needs of individuals and their families who are experiencing the real or threatened impact of renal disease" (ANNA, 1995). The scope of practice further describes the key nursing phenomena and patient population for the specialty of nephrology nursing:

Nephrology nursing focuses on the health needs of individuals and their families who are experiencing the real or threatened impact of renal disease. Because most individuals are already experiencing degrees of progressively declining renal function or have lost function completely, nephrology nursing focuses on the provision of replacement therapy, teaching self-care, assisting individuals to make informed choices regarding the type and location of therapy, and the prevention of intercurrent illnesses or complications associated with various modalities of therapy. One unique aspect of nephrology nursing is that nephrology nurses have access to and care for people over long periods of time. For nephrology nurses caring for patients with acute or chronic renal failure, this may be an interval of 2 to 6 hours three times a week for as long as patients remain on hemodialysis (usually years), or daily contact for weeks at a time during which patients may be experiencing the initiation of renal replacement therapy.

The nephrology nurse may also be responsible for intensive weekly training sessions when home and self-care is being taught, weekly home visits to supervise care, or clinic visits at which time the focus may be on preserving residual renal function or on establishing candidacy for renal transplantation. After renal transplantation occurs, the nurse evaluates the response of the patient to the transplant and related therapy on a 24-hour basis until discharge is possible. Thereafter, the nephrology nurse is also responsible for the long-term follow-up and teaching needed to maintain the health of the patient with a new kidney (ANNA, 1995).

The *Scope of Practice for Nephrology Nursing* depicts technologies unique to the specialty of nephrology nursing: "renal replacement therapy includes a variety of treatment modalities available to the patient with acute or chronic renal disease that serve to maintain life. Examples of the available modalities include conservative treatment, hemodialysis, peritoneal dialysis, hemofiltration, and renal transplantation. The degree to which renal functions are replaced by any one of these treatments varies with the patient's response to treatment" (ANNA, 1995).

The *Scope of Practice for Nephrology Nursing* identifies an essential knowledge and skill base relevant to all aspects of care for adult and pediatric renal patients and their families. This knowledge base includes:

- anatomy, physiology, and pathophysiology relevant to the care of renal patients,
- the nursing process as applied to nephrology nursing,
- knowledge of the diagnosis and treatment for patients requiring any method of renal replacement therapy,
- pharmacology,
- nutritional aspects of renal impairment,
- growth and development,
- teaching/learning theory,
- counseling/interviewing skills,
- interdisciplinary team skills,
- research processing,
- rehabilitation principles, and
- concepts related to death and dying.

In 1977, the *Standards of Clinical Practice for the Nephrology Patient* were published by our professional organization, then known as the American Association of Nephrology Nurses and Technicians (AANNT). These standards focused on the care of the nephrology patient by licensed and nonlicensed personnel. Soon after these standards were published, AANNT recognized the necessity to revise the standards using a nursing process format and in 1982, published *Nephrology Nursing Standards of Clinical Practice,* which addressed nursing care of adult and pediatric renal patients receiving treatment by conservative management, hemodialysis, peritoneal dialysis, hemoperfusion, and transplantation.

The decade of the 1980s witnessed rapid changes in methodologies for evaluation, documentation, and reimbursement of health care. In response to these changes, the 1986 ANNA Board of Directors instructed the Clinical Practice Committee to revise the existing standards to identify patient outcomes and reflect current nephrology nursing practice. The 1988 edition of the *ANNA Standards of Clinical Practice for Nephrology Nursing* includes patient outcomes based on appropriate nursing management. The quality of that management is reflected in the patient outcomes which can be evaluated by members of the nursing profession, consumer groups, accrediting and insurance agencies, and third party payers. This edition of the standards includes two major sections. First is the Structure Standards, which define the environment within which care is provided and includes organizational and management characteristics, qualifications of the nurse, staffing, the physical plant, and equipment. The second major section includes modality specific nursing process standards, conservative management, hemodialysis, peritoneal dialysis, and renal transplantation. Process standards define the actual delivery of care. The format for describing the nursing process includes a title, a description of nursing management, and patient outcomes. The title identifies a clinical problem that requires a nursing intervention. Nursing management includes assessment, nursing interventions, and patient teaching. Patient outcome(s) state the expected change in the patient or the patient's environment after nursing care has been delivered. The format of the standards provides further description of the key nursing phenomena, the patient population, and the domain of nurses practicing in the nephrology nursing specialty (Burrows-Hudson, 1993).

The 1993 revision of the *Standards of Clinical Practice for Nephrology Nursing* is based on ANA's format for Standards of Practice and Standards of Care, changes in the ESRD program, health care, and advances in technology and pharmacology. The 1993 edition also includes continuous renal replacement therapy and therapeutic plasma exchange. The 1988 Structure Standards were reorganized into Standards of Professional Performance and Standards of Care. These standards are defined as "authoritative statements that describe a level of care or performance common to the profession of nursing by which the quality of nursing practice can be judged" (Burrows-Hudson, 1993, p. 8). Standards of Professional Performance describe the competency level of professional behavior, including: quality of care, performance appraisal, education, collegiality, ethics, collaboration, research, and resource utilization. Standards of Care describe nursing care competency within the framework of the nursing process. The *Standards of Clinical Practice for Nephrology Nursing* serves as a foundation for practice guidelines, quality assessment processes, database systems, certification activities, role descriptions and performance appraisal processes, policies and procedures, educational offerings, and research agendas (Burrows-Hudson, 1993).

Evidence of the professional and distinct status of nephrology nursing exists in the literature. *The Core Curriculum for Nephrology Nursing* (1987, 1991, 1995) distinguishes the body of knowledge unique to the specialty of nephrology nursing. *The Core Curriculum* focuses on concepts and principles unique to nephrology nursing practice and includes sections on nursing diagnosis, care planning, patient education, the research process, and the history of nephrology nursing. *The Standards of Clinical Practice for Nephrology Nursing,* as previously described, provides additional documentation of the professional status of nephrology nursing.

The body of scientific knowledge that supports nephrology nursing practice exists primarily in published research performed by nurses within the specialty (Molzahn, 1992). In addition, ANNA, as the professional association for nephrology nurses, has promoted the development of a research-based practice in several ways:

- establishment of an organizational Research Committee in 1989;
- annual recognition of a nephrology nurse researcher who contributes to the advancement of nephrology nursing;
- development of a research agenda; and
- the editing, solicitation, distribution, and selection of research-related grants and awards.

The specialty of nephrology nursing has evolved in response to increasingly complex knowledge, technology, and clinical expertise required for the care of patients with actual or potential impaired renal function. The growth of the specialty has paralleled that of an expanding and recognized patient population. This trend is directly attributable to clinical and technological advances, as well as initially escalated levels of state and federal financial support. Funding for the ESRD program was first available in 1973 with 10,000 patients enrolled in the first year. Currently, the ESRD program provides funding for 627,000 patients (USRDS, 1997). The evolution of this specialty is indicative of the societal need for nephrology nursing expertise. ANNA posits that:

- Nephrology nurses play a critical role in the supervision and delivery of care for adult and pediatric patients in all treatment methods for renal disease.
- The role of nephrology nursing is to assess the real or threatened impact of renal disease in individuals and families, as well as diagnose and treat their responses to these problems. Within this context, we are also committed to helping individuals with end stage renal disease to achieve an optimal level of functioning. To achieve these goals, we believe that nephrology nurses should establish high standards of patient care that are continually updated. We believe that quality patient care is enhanced by continuing education of nephrology nurses. We further believe that sound educational programs are necessary to develop, maintain, and augment competence in practice. Because research is essential for sustaining growth and maturation, new ideas must be encouraged and tested in the field of nephrology nursing.
- The multidisciplinary approach to patient care is critical and interdisciplinary communication and cooperation are essential to achieve the highest quality of patient care. As members of the nephrology team, we believe it is our obligation to respond to issues affecting our practice in both the private and public sectors.
- Nephrology patients have the right to make choices about treatment options available to them. These choices may include an option not to accept replacement therapy. Nephrology nurses play a vital role in providing the education patients need to make informed choices (ANNA, 1995).

The specialty of nephrology nursing is national in scope and experiences a continued demand for nurses in the specialty and Certified Nephrology Nurses (CNNs) as evidenced by:

- the membership base for ANNA, the professional organization, being national in scope (see Figure 1-2 - U.S. map of members by state);
- ANNA membership profiles indicating the number of positions and roles for nephrology nurses;
- growth pattern of ANNA membership;
- an increasing trend in the number of applicants and certificates since the inception of the NNCB certification program; and
- certified nephrology nurses now totaling over 4,100, residing and practicing throughout the United States (see Figure 1-3 – U.S. map of CNNs by state).

The following is evidence that a pool of nurses exists who concentrate 50% or more of their work time and professional roles in nephrology nursing. Eligibility requirements for initial certification specify that "within 4 years prior to application, the applicant must have had a minimum of 2 years of nephrology nursing experience as a registered nurse in a general staff, administrative, teaching, or research capacity. In meeting this criterion, the applicant must have spent at least 50% of employment hours in nephrology nursing" (NNCB, 1997).

A review of employment advertisements for nephrology nurses suggest that employers prefer and in many instances require that nephrology nurses in their institutions/facilities be certified. In addition, institutions are incorporating certification into their clinical ladders. In 1989, ANNA published the *Nephrology Nursing Clinical Ladder Program* as a model program to promote the recruitment and retention of nurses in nephrology nursing. Certification by NNCB is included in this program as one of the criteria for promotion within the clinical ladder. These documents also support the enhancement of a pool of experienced clinical nurses within the specialty.

Standard 2: A tested body of research/data based knowledge related to the nursing specialty exists. Mechanisms are established for the support, review, and dissemination of research for the specialty. Activities within the specialty contribute to the advancement of nursing science within the specialty.

The knowledge base of nephrology nursing practice is well documented in various publications available to nurses practicing in the specialty. The *Core Curriculum for Nephrology Nursing* and the *Standards of Clinical Practice for Nephrology Nursing* are examples of publications that are produced and updated by ANNA. These publications, in conjunction with the *ANNA Journal*, provide state-of-the-art information for nephrology nurses. The *Journal* features research articles, research critiques, continuing education articles, and monographs on selected topics, including: AIDS, transplantation, management, vascular access, ethics, and research.

In 1989, the ANNA Research Committee was established to support a more organized effort toward the advancement of nursing science within the nephrology nursing specialty (Jordan, 1989). The purpose of the Research Committee is to provide mechanisms for the support, review, and dissemination of research and to contribute to the nephrology nursing knowledge base. The activities of this committee have contributed to the development of a research-based practice and the advancement of nursing science within the specialty. These activities include:

- the development of a long-range research agenda;
- the incorporation of the long-range research agenda into the ANNA Long-Range Strategic Plan. The final strategic plan included the establishment of six research objectives (see Table 1-2) used by the association to establish research priorities;

Figure 1-2
U.S. map of ANNA members by state.

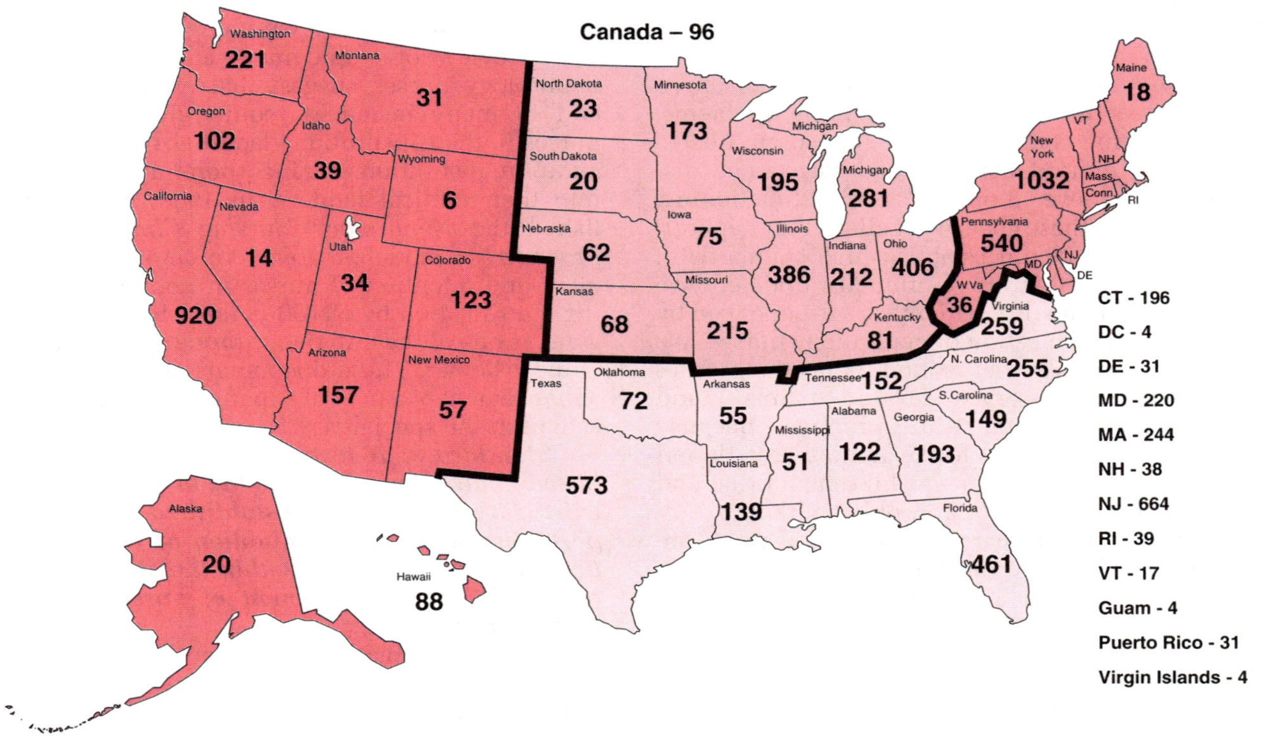

Figure 1-3
U.S. map of CNNs by state.

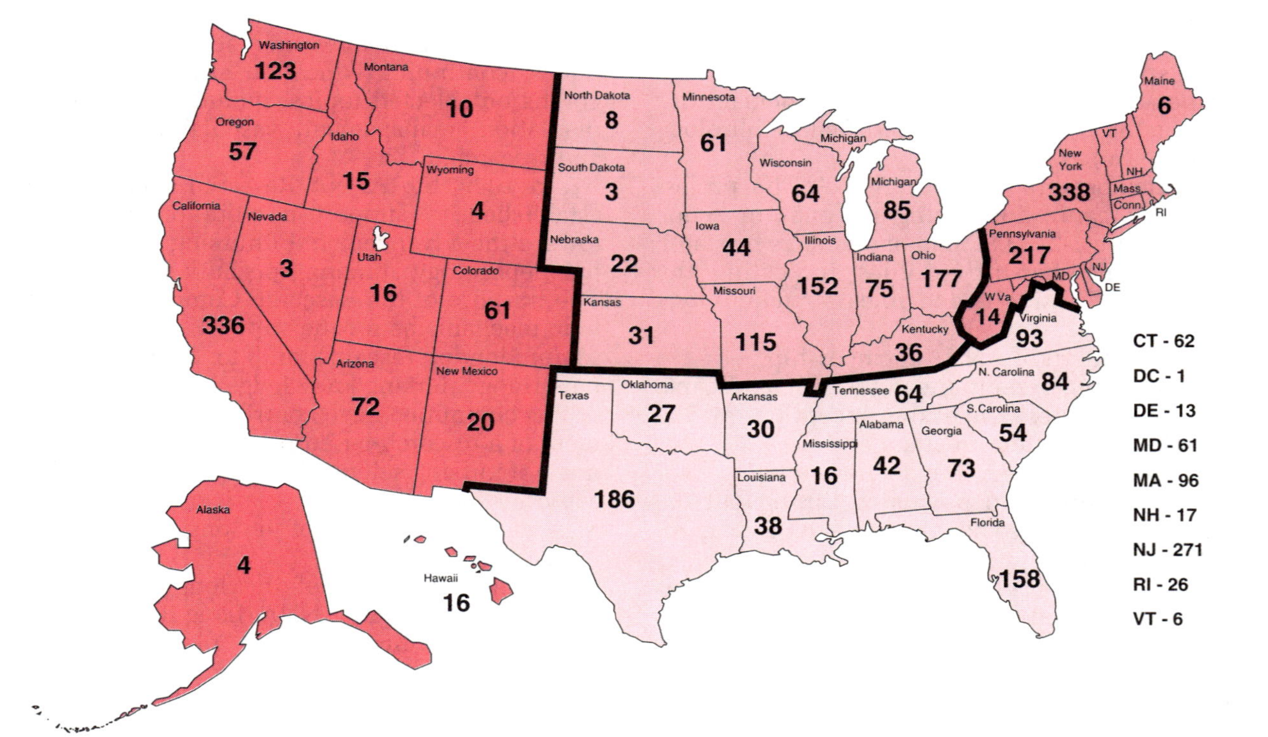

Table 1-4
NNCB eligibility criteria.

- A current license as a registered nurse in the United States or its territories.
- Within 3 years prior to application a minimum of 2 years of nephrology experience as a registered nurse.
- In meeting the above criteria, at least 50% of employment hours spent in nephrology nursing.
- Effective with the first test administration in the year 2000, candidates for certification must possess a Bachelor of Science in Nursing (BSN).
- Effective with the first test administration in the year 2000, candidates must have completed 30 hours of continuing education credit in nursing within the 3 years prior to submission of application for certification. The continuing education must be specific to nephrology nursing. These groups encompass nephrology programs awarding continuing education credits for nursing. To be acceptable, the contact hours awarded must be approved by one of the following: (1) The American Nephrology Nurses' Association (ANNA); (2) Organizations, accredited by the American Nurses' Credentialing Center-Commission on Accreditation (ANCC-COA), the credentialing body of the American Nurses Association; (3) The state boards of nursing in California, Florida, Kansas, Iowa, Nevada, Alabama, Idaho, Oklahoma, Oregon, South Dakota, and Arkansas; (4) The American Association of Critical-Care Nurses; or (5) The Council of Continuing Education. To qualify, a program must indicate that a single continuing education unit equals 10 educational contact hours, or the program must use the recognized value of CERP (continuing education recognition point) in which one educational contact hour equals one CERP. (One CEU equals 10 educational contact hours, which equal 10 CERPs. CERPs may not be converted to CEUs). A copy of the certificate awarded must be submitted as proof of attendance.
- Credit will be given according to the number of contact hours awarded. Independent study which has been approved for continuing education credit or academic credit may not constitute more than 24 contact hours of this requirement.

- financial support in the form of research grants funded by ANNA and ANNA corporate members;
- the promotion of completion, presentation, and publication of nephrology nursing research;
- the establishment of a research booth at ANNA's National Symposium, which provides the opportunity for ANNA members and meeting participants to discuss research ideas with members of the Research Committee and allow individuals to conduct surveys for their own research projects;
- a meta-analysis of existing nephrology nursing research published in 1992 (Molzahn, 1992). This project identified nephrology nursing research that was done in selected areas and a joint utilization research project with the *ANNA Journal* Editorial Board, in which short articles were published summarizing the research results in selected areas. This provided a mechanism for identifying research findings that are ready to be incorporated into practice.
- publication of the *Directory of Nephrology Nurse Researchers* in 1992 in conjunction with ANNA's Research Special Interest Group (SIG);
- SIG sessions conducted by members of ANNA's Research Committee and Research SIG during ANNA's National Symposium. Topics of special interest to novice and experienced nurse researchers are presented (Preisig, 1990, 1991, 1992).

Standard 3: The certification board is an entity with organizational autonomy. However, a collaborative relationship exists between the certification body and a nursing specialty association that supports the specialty and sets standards for specialty practice.

The NNCB was incorporated in 1987 as a corporation to develop, administer, and evaluate a program for the certification of nephrology nurses (NNCB, 1987a, p. 1). As a separate corporation for certification, NNCB maintains its own bylaws which allows it to operate autonomously in matters related to the certification program. The NNCB bylaws specify the number of directors (Article V, section 1) and the appointment method for the directors (Article V, section 2). Board members are elected to the offices of president, secretary, and treasurer in accordance with the bylaws (Article VI, section 1-3).

The NNCB accepts candidates for certification who have met the stated eligibility requirements determined by the NNCB Board of Directors (see Table 1-4). The certification examination is offered annually in conjunction with three national nephrology meetings, two ANNA regional meetings, and the ANNA chapters' test site. Certificates and wallet cards are issued to nurses who successfully pass the written examination according to policy and procedure.

The NNCB maintains a collaborative relationship with ANNA, the organization that sets standards for nephrology nursing practice. In 1986,

Table 1-5
ANNA position statements.

As a service to association members, the following ANNA Position Statements are published annually in the convention issue of the ANNA Journal. The following position statements were all recently revised or reaffirmed and are all current:

- Apolitical Educational Programs,
- BONENT Examination,
- Delegation of Nursing Care Activities,
- Folding Epoetin Reimbursement into the Composite Rate,
- HIV and HIV-Related Illnesses,
- Joint Position Statement of ANNA and NANT on Unlicensed Personnel in Dialysis,
- ANNA Legislative Policy Statement,
- Mandatory HIV Testing,
- Extending the Medicare Secondary Payor Provision for ESRD Services,
- Minimum Preparation for Entry Into Nursing Practice,
- ANNA's Resolution in Support of the Nephrology Nursing Certification Board's Certification Examination,
- Reuse of Hemodialyzer Filters and Other Dialysis Disposables,
- Solicitation of Organs and Tissues, and
- The Role of Unlicensed Assistive Personnel in Dialysis Therapy.

the ANNA Board of Directors approved a motion to pursue the development of a certification examination that would test proficiency in nephrology nursing practice. An ANNA Certification Ad Hoc Committee was appointed and the National League for Nursing (NLN) was selected to provide administrative testing services and assist in the development of the certification examination. This committee was responsible for the development of the first nephrology nursing certification examination. The *Scope of Practice for Nephrology Nursing* and the *Core Curriculum for Nephrology Nursing* were used in its development. In conjunction with NLN, a job analysis was performed and item writing workshops were conducted. A criterion-referenced examination was developed to determine an individual's status with respect to well-defined domains of behavior and to yield scores that can be directly related to articulated performance standards (Parker, 1991).

The pilot certification examination was offered in May 1987, in conjunction with the ANNA 18th National Symposium in New York City. After administration of the pilot examination, the ad hoc committee incorporated to form the NNCB. The first NNCB examination was administered at the ANNA Clinical Concerns meeting in St. Louis, Missouri in September 1987.

The original NNCB bylaws require that two ANNA Board members be members of the NNCB (Article V, section 1a) and allow the ANNA president to serve as an ex-officio member (Article V, section 1d). The NNCB bylaws also specify that any amendments to the bylaws must receive approval by the ANNA Board of Directors (Article XIII). This procedure was established so that the leadership of the professional organization would always be involved in the direction of the NNCB, but not in the daily administration.

The ANNA and NNCB collectively promote the NNCB certification program and the recognition of Certified Nephrology Nurses. For example, ANNA includes CNNs in position statements for legislative and professional nursing purposes (Table 1-5). In 1988, the ANNA Board of Directors adopted a position statement in support of NNCB examination. In 1989, the ANNA Board of Directors adopted the belief that all candidates for the ANNA Board of Directors for the 1990 elections and beyond would be required to be certified in nephrology nursing practice by the NNCB. An annual directory of CNNs is published in the *ANNA Journal* and articles, newsletter columns, and advertisements appear routinely in the journal and *ANNA Update*.

During ANNA's National Symposium and other nationally sponsored meetings, ANNA has provided opportunities for NNCB to provide information on certification to nephrology nurses attending the meetings. The following activities are examples of this collaboration:

- NNCB officers participate in the ANNA Congress of Chapters to discuss certification issues with chapter presidents;
- ANNA recognizes CNNs at their educational sessions;
- NNCB maintains an exhibit booth staffed with NNCB officers during all nationally sponsored ANNA meetings for the purpose of distributing materials and providing information regarding certification and recertification;
- invited speakers address issues related to certification and health care during ANNA scheduled programs; and
- the NNCB examination is administered in conjunction with ANNA educational programs at national, regional, and local levels.

Table 1-6
NNCB test objectives.

The objectives of the NNCB Certification Examination are to determine the nurse's ability to:
1. Recognize pathologic processes and complications that occur in renal failure and/or treatment modalities.
2. Select interventions appropriate to the pathologic processes and complications that occur in renal failure and/or treatment modalities.
3. Apply physiologic and technical principles of renal replacement therapies.
4. Select appropriate teaching/learning strategies to educate client, family, other health professionals, and the public.
5. Select appropriate actions in administering medication(s) to the patient being treated for renal failure.
6. Recognize the importance of an interdisciplinary approach to promote optimum functioning.
7. Select interventions appropriate to the psychological and sociocultural effects of renal failure.
8. Apply principles of infection control.

Test questions to measure these objectives are written within the framework of the nursing process. The questions are designed to measure proficiency in nephrology nursing across a variety of patient situations and treatment modalities. The breakdown of test items by content area is given below.

Content Area	% of Total Test
Concepts of Renal Failure	35%
Hemodialysis	30%
Peritoneal Dialysis	20%
Transplant	15%

The NNCB bylaws specify that a collaborative relationship exists between ANNA and NNCB in the statement "the NNCB shall support the American Nephrology Nurses' Association in its development and implementation of educational activities as related to certification of nephrology nurses" (Article II, Section 3).

Standard 4: There is a provision for public consultation/representation on the certification board.

The NNCB has an established policy that provides for public representation and input as required in matters related to certification policies and procedures.

Standard 5: The eligibility criteria for basic certification include:

- ***RN licensure;***
- ***Baccalaureate or higher degree in nursing; and***
- ***A specified minimum educational program in the specialty.***

The eligibility criteria for advanced certification include:

- ***RN licensure;***
- ***A minimum of a graduate degree in nursing or the appropriate equivalent, including content in the specified area of specialty practice.***

The Nephrology Nursing Certification Board (NNCB) provides a certification program for registered nurses practicing in nephrology nursing. The NNCB eligibility criteria for certification and recertification require that candidates hold a current, full, and unrestricted registered nurse license in the United States or its territories (NNCB, 1997) (see Table 1-4).

This standard is either currently in effect or a plan has been adopted for the requirement to be in effect for the new candidates no later than the year 2000.

According to the ABNS document *Levels of Certification,* NNCB provides certification at the basic level. The title Certified Nephrology Nurse (CNN) is awarded to candidates who successfully complete the certification process of meeting eligibility criteria (see Table 1-4) and pass a multiple choice written examination. In April 1991, NNCB passed two resolutions that will change the educational requirements of the eligibility criteria. With the first examination in the year 2000, all candidates for certification must possess a baccalaureate degree in nursing. Also effective in the year 2000, an educational program that prepares nurses in nephrology nursing practice must be completed and documented at the time of application for certification.

Orientation programs based on *The Core Curriculum for Nephrology Nursing* are offered in various settings. Hospitals, dialysis facilities, and local ANNA chapters sponsor programs for registered nurses entering nephrology nursing. Graduate programs that offer courses and content specific to nephrology nursing exist, but currently are few in number.

Standard 6: Certification tests are constructed and evaluated using methods that are psycho-

metrically sound and fair to all candidates.

Standard 7: The certifying body has conducted validation studies to assure that inferences made on the basis of test scores are appropriate and justified.

Standard 10: Certification tests are administered in a manner that minimizes construct-irrelevant variance.

The development of the certification examination began with a job analysis of nephrology nursing practice. This structured inventory of task and knowledge statements described job functions and knowledge specific to nephrology practice identified by nurses with expertise in the field.

The first certification examination was written in 1987, revised in 1989, and then annually. The test content areas, as well as the percentages of test questions for each area, were determined by demographic data from the job analysis survey. In 1987, content areas and percentages were as follows:

- 30% - All renal-related therapies
- 30% - Hemodialysis
- 20% - Peritoneal Dialysis
- 15% - Transplant
- 5% - Conservative Management

Test objectives for the certification examination were developed using information from the analysis of ratings of task and knowledge statements on the survey.

The current content areas and percentages are:

- 35% - Concepts of renal failure
- 30% - Hemodialysis
- 20% - Peritoneal Dialysis
- 15% - Transplant

Test objectives have been revised, in accordance with the most recent job analysis survey, to provide more accurate guidelines for examination questions that measure the nurse's current knowledge and skills (see Table 1-6).

The next step in the process of examination development was item writing. Test items were written by recognized experts in nephrology nursing practice and assisted by experts in test item construction from the NLN. The item writers followed a test blueprint. The test blueprint is a plan that ensures the test will have content validity. It is an outline of what the test will measure and serves as a guide to ensure that the course content sample included is both represented and appropriately balanced within the test. All participants in the item writing sessions were provided a copy of the test blueprint and the results of the job analysis survey. For every objective in each content area, a specific number of questions were to be written and the aspects of the nursing process that were considered important to the test were determined.

As items were written, they were coded for content area, objective, and the aspect of the nursing process that they tested. This method allowed the test forms to be assembled, conforming to the test blueprint. Each question was reviewed by the NLN Testing Service for clarity, bias, and accuracy. Two pilot test forms were assembled, each containing over 200 questions, and administered in May 1987 in conjunction with the ANNA National Symposium. Over 400 nurses participated in the pilot examinations and approximately the same number of examinees took one of the two forms. Participants in the pilot examination were required to meet the eligibility requirements for the certification examination.

The mean raw scores on the pilot examinations were similar for each form of the examination, and the mean difficulty for each item was used to determine the passing score for the certification examination. An analysis of each test item was performed following the pilot examinations to evaluate the quality and discriminatory power of each question. These evaluations allowed identification of test items that were too difficult or too simple and distractors that might have been identified too easily as wrong answers or that were not plausible to test takers. These questions were revised or eliminated as test items. Varying levels of item difficulty were included in the examination to determine the individual examinee's level of knowledge and understanding.

The two forms of the certification examination were compiled from the test questions used in the pilot examinations and were tailored specifically to reflect data obtained from the job analysis survey, the *Standards of Clinical Practice for Nephrology Nursing,* and the *Core Curriculum for Nephrology Nursing.* The final test form followed the same test blueprint as the pilot examinations and consisted of approximately 200 multiple choice items.

Standard 8: The certifying body assures that test scores, including subscores, are sufficiently reliable for their intended uses.

Standard 12: Passing scores for the certification examination are set in a manner that is fair to all candidates, using methods that are psychometrically sound.

The passing score for the examination was determined using the Angoff procedure, a criterion-based methodology, by the NNCB with the assistance of the NLN Testing Service. Each question on the final form of the examination was reviewed individually for actual examinee performance on pilot examinations and the percentage of proficient nurses who would be expected to answer the question correctly. Each individual item was given a score, and these scores were averaged to determine the overall passing summary. In order to pass, a candidate for certification is required to answer correctly 75% of the items on the examination (Parker, 1991).

Standard 9: The certifying body does not dis-

criminate among applicants as to age, gender, race, religion, ethnic origin, disability, marital status, or sexual orientation.

Standard 14: The certifying body provides information that clearly describes the certification process to candidates and other stakeholders.

The NNCB examination is designed to test proficiency in nephrology nursing practice and is administered by the Center for Nursing Education and Testing (C-NET), which specializes in test development and test administration.

The eligibility criteria set forth to determine candidates qualified to take the certification examination are published and distributed by ANNA and NNCB (see Table 1-4) and the eligibility criteria are listed in the application for certification.

The *NNCB Bylaws* and the *NNCB Policy & Procedure Manual* (NNCB, 1987 b,c) specify the credential of CNNs, which is awarded to individuals who successfully meet the eligibility criteria and pass the NNCB examination. The NNCB certificate awarded to successful candidates denotes the credential unique to the nephrology nursing specialty.

Standard 11: Procedures are in place to maximize the security of all certification test materials.

Standard 15: The certifying body assures that confidential information about candidates and certificate holders is protected.

All examination scores are forwarded to the examinee. A total score and subscores in all major test areas of concentration are provided for candidates who do not pass the examination. A total score is provided to candidates who pass the examination. A list of passing candidates and a summary of test scores are sent to NNCB, and individual scores remain confidential. Computer tapes, consisting of the complete performance record of all candidates, are retained by C-NET. Examination sheets are retained for 2 years.

Standard 13: The certifying body has a mechanism in place to periodically evaluate certificate holders for continued knowledge necessary to maintain competency in the specialty.

CNNs have two options for recertification: the examination option or continuing education option. Certification must be renewed every 3 years with candidates for recertification meeting established eligibility criteria and fulfilling the requirements of the selected option for recertification. The *NNCB Policy and Procedure Manual* (1987 c, pp. 44-45) and the handbook, *NNCB's Guide to Recertification by Continuing Education Credit,* provide detailed descriptions of the process of recertification by continuing education points of credit.

The educational programs that provide education for nurses in the specialty of nephrology nursing are primarily continuing education programs. The major provider of continuing education programs in the specialty is ANNA, which offers programs that focus on clinical nephrology, management, education, research, legislative, and professional nursing issues.

Educational programming offered by other organizations, such as the National Association of Transplant Coordinators (NATCO), National Kidney Foundation - Council of Nephrology Nurses and Technicians (NKF-CNNT), and American Society of Nephrology (ASN), also provide continuing education regarding acute, progressive, and chronic renal failure.

Standard 16: The certifying body has an appeal process in place for nurses who have been denied access to an examination or renewal of certification, or who have had certification revoked.

The *NNCB Policy & Procedure Manual* specifically describes a grievance policy (1987 c, p. 22) for applicants who question eligibility decisions and examination results. The right of appeal is printed in the Application for Certification.

Standard 17: The certifying body has a mechanism in place to respond to instances of noncompliance with eligibility or certification board rules.

The *NNCB Bylaws* maintain a formal policy and procedure for discipline of certificate holders for conduct that indicates incompetence, unethical behavior, or impairment that affects performance. This policy incorporates due process.

Summary

Specialization needs to be managed internally by the profession through a peer review process and conferring of a standardized credential that holds meaning to consumers. At the very least, the public should be able to infer from the credential, the qualifications of the provider and the relevance of the specialty practice (Joel, 1989; Styles, 1989).

Components of the practice base for nephrology nursing created a foundation for the development of a specialty nursing practice. The ANNA and NNCB have functioned collectively to demonstrate the effectiveness of their practice, education, research, and credentialing. Certification of nurse specialists is the principal means of setting standards and ensuring that these standards have been met and thus, has rendered a dominant role in the evolution of specialty nursing practice.

The ANA Social Policy Statement (ANA, 1995) suggests that the cutting edge of practice is at the point of specialization. Specialization is an inherent sign of a maturing profession and brings with it responsibility and accountability for high quality nursing care and the credibility of practitioners who offer that care.

References

American Association for Nephrology Nurses. (1969). *Constitution and bylaws.* Pitman, NJ: Author.

American Board of Nursing Specialties. (1997). *ABNS application for approval.* Washington, DC: Author.

American Nephrology Nurses' Association. (1986). *Scope of practice for nephrology nursing.* Pitman, NJ: Author.

American Nephrology Nurses' Association. (1995). *Scope of practice for nephrology nursing.* Pitman, NJ: Author.

American Nurses Association. (1980). *Nursing: A social policy statement.* Kansas City, MO: Author.

American Nurses Association. (1995). *Nursing: A social policy statement.* Washington, DC: Author.

Andrews, K. (1986, April 8). In *A history of nephrology nursing* (interview). Unpublished manuscript. Pitman, NJ: American Nephrology Nurses' Association.

Bocchino, C.A., & Burrows-Hudson, S. (1995). Other salient issues related to ESRD and its treatment. In L. Lancaster (Ed.), *Core curriculum for nephrology nursing* (3rd ed.) (pp. 423-446). Pitman, NJ: American Nephrology Nurses' Association.

Bois, M.S., Barfield, N.B., Taylor, C.E., & Ross, C.D. (1968). Nursing care of patients having kidney transplants. *American Journal of Nursing, 68,* 1238-1247.

Burrows-Hudson, S.(Ed.). (1993). *Standards of clinical practice for nephrology nursing.* Pitman, NJ: Author.

Cameron, E.M. (1986, April 11). In *A history of nephrology nursing* (interview). Unpublished manuscript. Pitman, NJ: American Nephrology Nurses' Association.

Canavan, K. (1996, June). ANA's centennial: The birth of a professional organization. *American Nurse, 28(6),* 28.

Diers, D. (1988). The mystery of nursing. In R. Coffey, D. Farley, K. Lind, & R. Wilson (Eds.), *Secretary's Commission on Nursing: Support studies & background information, 2(VIII),* 1-10.

Flanagan, L. (1976). *One strong voice: The story of the American Nurses' Association.* Kansas City, MO: American Nurses' Association.

Fulton, B.J. (1986, March 24). In *A history of nephrology nursing* (interview). Unpublished manuscript. Pitman, NJ: American Nephrology Nurses' Association.

Hoffart, N. (1989). A professional organization for nephrology nurses. *ANNA Journal, 16(3),* 197-199.

Hoffart, N. (1989). Nephrology nursing 1915-1970: A historical study of the integration of technology and care. *ANNA Journal, 16(3),* 169-178.

Joel, L. (1989, November-December). In search of a rational future for certification. *American Nurse, 21*(10).

Jordan, P. (1989). Annual report: The state of the association. *ANNA Journal, 16*(3), 143-144.

McBride, P.T. (1979). *Genesis of the artificial kidney.* Deerfield, IL: Travenol Laboratories.

Merrill, J.P., Murray, J.E., Harrison, J.H., & Guild, W.R. (1956). Successful homotransplantation of the human kidney between identical twins. *Journal of the American Medical Association, 160,* 277-281.

Molzahn, A. (1992). An evaluation of the nephrology nursing research literature: 1979-1989. *ANNA Journal, 20(4),* 395-428.

Murray, J.E., Merrill, J.P., & Harrison, J.H. (1958). Kidney transplantation between seven pairs of identical twins. *Annals of Surgery, 148,* 343-359.

Murray, J.E., Tilney, N.L., & Wilson, R.E. (1976). Renal transplantation: A twenty-five year experience. *Annals of Surgery, 184,* 565-573.

Nephrology Nursing Certification Board. (1987 a). *NNCB articles of Incorporation.* Pitman, NJ: Author.

Nephrology Nursing Certification Board. (1987 b). *NNCB bylaws.* Pitman, NJ: Author.

Nephrology Nursing Certification Board. (1987 c). *NNCB policy & procedure manual.* Pitman, NJ: Author.

Nephrology Nursing Certification Board. (1997). Don't miss your opportunity to earn the CNN credential (promotional advertisement). *ANNA Journal, 24*(3), 377.

Parker, J. (1991). The development of the nephrology nursing certification program. *ANNA Journal, 18(6),* 543-547,571.

Parker, J. (1994). The development of the American Board of Nursing Specialties. *Nursing Management 25(1),* 33-35.

Preisig, P. (1990). Annual report of the ANNA Research Committee. *ANNA Journal 17(2),* 110-111.

Preisig, P. (1991). Annual report of the ANNA Research Committee. *ANNA Journal 18(2),* 112, 137.

Preisig, P. (1992). Annual report of the ANNA Research Committee. *ANNA Journal 19(2),* 121.

Price, C.A. (1997). State of the Association. *ANNA Journal, 24*(2).

Salisbury, P.F. (1960). History: The American Society for Artificial and Internal Organs. *Transactions of the American Society for Artificial Organs, 6,* ii-vi.

Shelbelski, D. (1986, April 14). In *A history of nephrology nursing* (interview). Unpublished manuscript. Pitman, NJ: American Nephrology Nurses' Association.

Sims, T. (1994). Celebrating 25 years of nephrology nursing (editorial). In *ANNA: 1969-1994. Celebrating 25 years of service to the nephrology community* (p.1). Pitman, NJ: American Nephrology Nurses' Association.

Starr, P. (1982). *The social transformation of American medicine.* New York: Basic Books, Inc.

Styles, M. (1989). *On specialization in nursing: Toward a new empowerment.* Kansas City, MO: American Nurses' Foundation, Inc.

Styles, M. (1991). Bridging the gap between competence and excellence. *ANNA Journal, 18(4),* 353-360, 366.

United States Renal Data System (USRDS). (1997). *USRDS annual report.* Bethesda, MD: Author.

Whitaker, J. (1968). Executive director's report. *House of delegates reports, 1966- 1968.* New York: American Nurses' Association, 16.

Chapter Highlights

- The nursing profession has become too large and complex for any one person to master the full range of information and skills encompassed within them. Specialization enables nurses to focus on one area of knowledge and technical skills, and provide the patient with the best care possible.

- Through ANNA, nephrology nursing has evolved into a nursing specialty. ANNA has developed the following components of the practice base for nephrology nursing: the scope of practice, core curriculum, certification, standards of clinical practice, quality assurance/continuous quality improvement, and research.

- The first formal meeting of American nurses took place in 1893 at the Chicago World's Fair. At this meeting, 18 nursing school superintendents voted to establish the American Society of Superintendents of Training Schools for Nurses. The organization promoted the fellowship of its members, established and maintained a universal standard of training, and furthered the best interests of the nursing profession.

- During the late 1800s, three factors profoundly affected the development of nursing education: the campaign for women's rights, the support for public education, and the growth of schools for higher education.

- AANN was created by less than 50 people. Currently, the membership of the American Nephrology Nurses Association (ANNA) is over 11,000 registered nurses. ANNA has matured to meet the changing needs of its membership and in doing so has laid the foundation for the development of nephrology nursing as a specialty.

- For three decades, the profession of nephrology nursing has increased in scope and numbers. Nephrology nurses were employed in hemodialysis and peritoneal dialysis units, transplant units, physician's offices, and as members of research teams and marketing programs. By the 1980s, it was no longer sufficient to be competent in delivering one modality of patient care.

- The conceptual framework employed to analyze nephrology nursing as a specialty is the standards and criteria set forth by ABNS. These standards were developed to guide specialties in demonstrating the viability and effectiveness of their practice, education, research, and peer review/credentialing.

- The ABNS is recognized by the nursing profession as the professional peer review mechanism for reviewing and approving specialties. The ABNS is a voluntary system which acknowledges the national voluntary certification of specialists as the critical mechanism for bringing quality control to specialty practice and unity, homogeneity, and authority to the development of specialties.

- Components of the practice base for nephrology nursing created a foundation for the development of a specialty nursing practice. The American Nephrology Nurses' Association and the Nephrology Nursing Certification Board have functioned collectively to demonstrate the effectiveness of their practice, education, research, and credentialing.

CHAPTER 2

The History of Nephrology Nursing

Anna L. Corea, MN, RN, CNAA

Chapter Contents

Development of Nephrology: An Overview 27
- Prior to the 20th Century 27
- 1900 - 1959 28
- 1960 - 1972 29
- 1973 - Present 30

Industry's Contributions to Renal Care: Historical Perspectives 31
- Early to Mid-20th Century Devices 31
- 1950s and 1960s 31

Government's Role in Chronic Renal Failure Treatment 32
- VA Hospital Dialysis Program 32
- Federal Government Hemodialysis Grants 32
- The Medicare End Stage Renal Disease Program 33

Early Nephrology Nurses and Their Roles 33
- Early Nurses and Their Contributions 34
- Roles of Early Nephrology Nurses 35

A Professional Nephrology Nursing Organization: The History of ANNA 36
- Organizing of Nephrology Nurses 36
- Significant Events in ANNA History 36

Nephrology Nurses Today 38
- Career Opportunities 39
- Additional Opportunities 40

Summary 41

References 41

Chapter Highlights 42

The History of Nephrology Nursing

Anna L. Corea, MN, RN, CNAA

Nephrology nursing is a specialty practice that offers care to patients suffering from renal insufficiency. Historically, the relationship between nursing and the concept of caring has been that nursing emerged in our culture as soon as the culture was able, from an economic point of view, to afford to hire people to care (Lynaugh & Fairman, 1989). Early in our society, when people became ill, the family would nurture and provide the necessary care. The impoverished and those without families had no one to provide nursing care.

Hospitals in the 1870s were charitable institutions that served the poor, sick, and abandoned of society who were bereft of family or friends to care for them (Brodie, 1989). Dating back to the beginning of our culture, the wealthy had more access to care than the poor. Nursing in the United States began as an organized profession in 1873 when three hospitals began schools to educate women in the care of ill patients. These new students in health care, called nurses, were social activists who sought to change the deplorable conditions found in city hospitals. The women reformers of this era believed if the domestic talents of women, including housekeeping and the ability to keep their families healthy and morally fit, could be transferred to hospitals, there would be positive changes. Women of intelligence, altruism, and physical stamina were recruited into the new schools. Educating women as nurses was the change that revolutionized hospitals – for the first time since hospitals came into existence, more patients departed from them well, as compared to those who died (Brodie, 1989).

Nephrology nursing is one of several nursing specialities that has developed over the last five decades. Its beginning correlates with the growth and development of dialysis. The impetus, however, that exacerbated the growth of nephrology nursing occurred in the early 1960s when government began to provide financial support for the treatment of chronic renal failure. As the number of patients and dialysis treatments increased, the number of nephrology nurses increased as well. The purpose of this chapter is to present an overview of the development and history of the nephrology specialty and nephrology nursing, and parallel the growth of ANNA to the growth of nephrology nursing practice.

Development of Nephrology: An Overview

Historical roots of nephrology date back to the time of the early Egyptians, with numerous milestone events occurring throughout the 20th century. Not only did this chain of events play a key role in the history of dialysis care, but in the evolution of nephrology nursing as a specialty. To understand how nephrology nursing evolved into a full-fledged specialty, it is necessary to review the milestones in the treatment of renal disease prior to the 20th century, from 1900 to 1959, from 1960 to 1972, and from 1973 to the present.

Prior to the 20th Century

As far back as 3000 BC the Egyptians made note of the peritoneal cavity and other parts of the animal anatomy. Dialysis is at least as old as the ancient Romans, who discovered that steaming hot baths could remove urea from the body. The process was one that left the patient dehydrated and in a very weakened state. Although the procedure worked, the ancient Romans probably did not understand why or even what they had done. They only knew in many cases, after the weakness had passed, they felt better.

Sir William Harvey first described the circulatory system in 1600. This concept would stimulate others to look at the relationship between disease and the blood. In the next two centuries multiple physicians, physiologists, and scientists worked on methods of adding fluid into the bloodstream or removing blood from patients. The devices used and the methodology developed slowly. Of great interest, as early as the 1600s, the dangers of air embolism and clotting were identified, well recognized, and documented in the literature.

In the 17th and 18th centuries, physicians learned how to treat patients for the four liquid humors. The humors were identified as blood, phlegm, yellow bile, and black bile. Teachers taught physicians to keep the four liquid humors in balance. In the 1700s, the traditional method of treating patients with renal insufficiency was applying heat, immersing in warm baths, blood-letting, or

Figure 2-1
The first dialysis procedure in the United States.

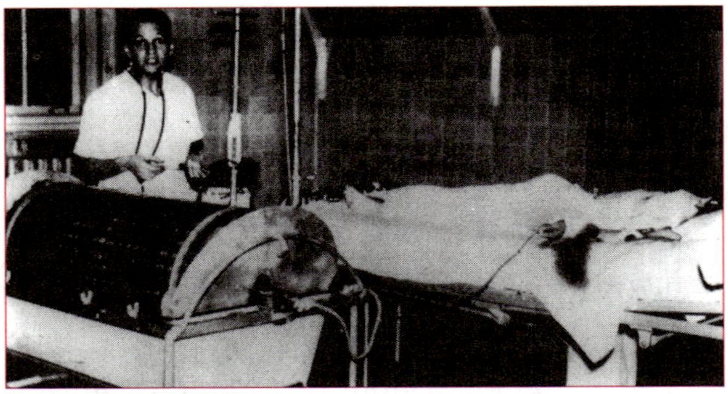

Photo courtesy of the Baxter Corporation

The first dialysis procedure in the United States was performed on a patient at Mount Sinai Medical Center in New York City in January 1948. The physician in this historic photograph is Dr. Koop, of the Brigham team in Boston. The Brigham team observed the procedure and later went on to establish its own program that cared for many of the first dialysis patients in this country.

administering diaphoretic mixtures made with nitric acid in alcohol and antimonial wine (Estes, 1981). Little is known about who administered care for these ailing patients. McBride's historical research purports that prior to 1850, there were no other treatment alternatives for patients with renal failure except those crude procedures described above.

In 1827, Richard Bright published the first volume of *Reports of Medical Cases* (Hoffart, 1989a). In these reports Bright described the association of dropsy and albuminuria with diseased kidneys. He is given credit for establishing a relationship between the symptoms and pathology of kidney failure. In 1854 Thomas Graham presented a paper on osmotic force. Graham described for the first time a process by which colloids and crystalloids could be separated. This concept, osmotic force, was of primary importance to the development of dialysis. Osmotic force was the first reference to the process of separating substances using a semipermeable membrane. Graham's definition and experimental proofs of the laws of diffusion and osmosis are classics on which the very essence of dialysis is based (McBride, 1990).

Graham is credited also for the design of the hoop form dialyzer. He suggested that animal tissue could be used as a functioning semipermeable membrane and described in specific terms that demonstrated the relationship of solute diffusion rates to molecular size, showing that the larger the molecule the slower the diffusion rate. These same principles of osmosis and diffusion are applicable today with all types of dialysis treatments. Also, in 1877, Wegmen conducted experiments using peritoneal lavage in animals; this set the foundation for other researchers to use this treatment on humans in the 20th century (Hoffart, 1995).

1900 - 1959

The first half of the 20th century brought about numerous milestones in the emerging nephrology specialty, including hemodialysis, transplantation, and peritoneal dialysis (PD). Rapid growth brought new and better treatments for renal care patients, and witnessed the introduction and development of the nephrology nursing specialty.

Hemodialysis. In 1913, Abel, Rowntree, and Turner demonstrated that a procedure called dialysis could be used to remove salicyclic acid from the blood of rabbits; this demonstration laid the groundwork for later experimentation (Hoffart, 1995, p. 470). In Holland, Willem Kolff began developing the artificial kidney. In 1938, he used in-vitro dialysis to remove urea from the blood, while in 1943 Kolff treated the first patient using the rotating drum artificial kidney (Hoffart, 1995). This was followed by another milestone, when in 1945, for the first time, a patient treated with the artificial kidney recovered from acute renal failure (Hoffart, 1995).

Kolff brought the artificial kidney to the United States in 1947, and the first dialysis procedure was performed in January 1948 on a patient at Mount Sinai Hospital in New York City (Hoffart, 1989b; McBride, 1989) (see Figure 2-1). Following this successful procedure, a few medical centers in the United States established research programs to study the use of Kolff's artificial kidney. Leading the way was John Merrill, MD, and his study team at Boston's Peter Bent Brigham Hospital, where improvements were made in the rotating artificial drum kidney. Flat plate and coil dialyzers were developed during this time period; the artificial kidney was also used successfully to treat wounded soldiers during the Korean Conflict (Hoffart, 1995).

Peritoneal dialysis (PD). Advances were made in PD throughout the first half of the 20th century. In 1923, Ganter – following the lead of Wegman's 1877 experiments – used peritoneal lavage to treat uremia in animals, and in 1927 used this procedure to treat humans (Hoffart, 1995). In 1938, Rhoads used intermittent PD to treat patients with chronic renal failure, work that was replicated by others in the 1940s (Hoffart, 1995). The first venture into intermittent home PD was undertaken by Legrain and Merrill at Peter Bent Brigham Hospital. They were able to maintain a patient on home intermittent PD for a short period (Hoffart, 1995).

PD became an acceptable treatment modality for chronic and acute renal failure by the end of the 1950s. The work of Morton and Maxwell promoted a simpler and less technological treatment. The procedure offered a treatment, without equipment, that could be used in community hospitals and required less technical training.

Renal transplantation. Several key events took place in the evolution of renal transplantation during this time period. Most surgical procedures and experiments performed were unsuccessful, but all helped researchers eventually understand the barriers they faced and how to refine their work (see Chapter 23).

In 1902, Ullmann, a Vienna researcher, performed an autotransplant of a canine kidney in demonstrating that a transplanted organ could resume normal function (Hoffart, 1995). Between 1902 and the mid-1950s, numerous attempts were made to transplant animal kidneys into humans while attempts to transplant human organs were undertaken also – all were unsuccessful. From 1950 to 1953, Hume and Murray, in Boston, performed 15 transplants between nonrelated individuals, with only 1 being successful (Hoffart, 1995). In 1954, Murray reported the first long-term success when a patient received an organ from an identical twin. This led to future successes in transplantation where twins were involved (Hoffart, 1995).

1960 – 1972

During this time period, developments in dialysis and transplantation continued and helped to improve treatments for individuals with chronic renal failure. Because of limited resources and lack of trained, qualified personnel, acceptance committees were formed at some institutions to allocate treatments. During this decade, in response to government's involvement in funding kidney treatment programs and research, the number of dialysis centers and patients rose rapidly (see Chapter 25).

Acceptance committees. In the early 1960s, hemodialysis gained immediate acceptance, but its widespread use was hampered by limited financial resources and a lack of qualified physicians and nurses who could perform the procedures. Most programs were so limited that acceptance committees were developed to allocate the scarce resources. These committees literally decided who would receive hemodialysis treatments and who would die, as was noted in a May 1962 *New York Times* article, "Panel Holds Life or Death Vote in Allotting of Artificial Kidney."

In another famous 1962 article that appeared in *Life Magazine* (see Figure 2-2), Shana Alexander's article, "They Decide Who Lives, and Who Dies," depicted the moral dilemmas faced by a small acceptance committee at the Seattle Artificial Kidney Center (Alexander, 1962). Constrained by limited funds and number of qualified personnel, the Center created The Admissions and Policies Committee to decide which patients presented by physicians would be accepted for chronic hemodialysis. Appointed by the local county medical association, the committee was composed of 7 lay persons, who included a lawyer, a minister, a banker, a housewife, a state government official, a labor leader, and a surgeon. These individuals remained anonymous and never saw the patients whom they were evaluating for dialysis treatment.

The Seattle committee had few set guidelines, but they did consider candidates' finances and standing in the community, along with marital status and number of children. All prospective patients would be prescreened by a board of physicians, who would weed out all medically or psychiatrically unsuitable candidates (Alexander, 1962, p. 103). Committee members would then hear and decide for or against the cases of all patients presented before them for limited experimental hemodialysis procedures. Alexander cited several stories within her article, including the one of John Myers, a Seattle businessman who was dialyzed two times a week, at night, with a Kiil dialyzer without a blood pump. The story also told of Myers' four other companions on dialysis. In 1962, about 100,000 patients died each year of kidney failure. "Of these 100,000 doomed patients, only 1 in 50 at present can be considered a suitable candidate for wearing Seattle new U-shaped tubes" (Alexander, 1962).

This committee set a precedent for the organization of similar groups at institutions around the country during the 1960s. Some of these committees continued until the mid-1970s. In other dialysis acceptance committees, including one that this author was a member of in 1966, patients were turned down due to limited equipment, lack of trained personnel, and in many cases a lack of financial support. When patients were not accepted, they were sent home to die. Nurses who served on these committees found themselves in difficult positions. In the conference room, they voted on who lived and who died. The next day, in the dialysis unit, the same nurses would administer dialytic care to some of these patients.

Hemodialysis. The most significant event of the decade involved the development of the arteriovenous (AV) shunt by Scribner and Quinton in Seattle in 1960. For the first time, patients with nonfunctioning kidneys could be maintained on chronic hemodialysis, a major achievement that was imperative to establish the acceptance of hemodialysis (Hoffart, 1995; McBride, 1989).

Other developments occurred as well. The first outpatient hemodialysis center in the United States was established at the Seattle Artificial Kidney Center in 1962; home hemodialysis was performed for the first time in the US in 1964 (Hoffart, 1995). The internal arterial-venous (AV) fistula, which provided a more permanent access to the blood stream, was developed by Brescia and Cimino in New York in 1966 (Hoffart, 1995).

Figure 2-2
A 1962 Life magazine article detailed an ethical dilemma of the 1960s.

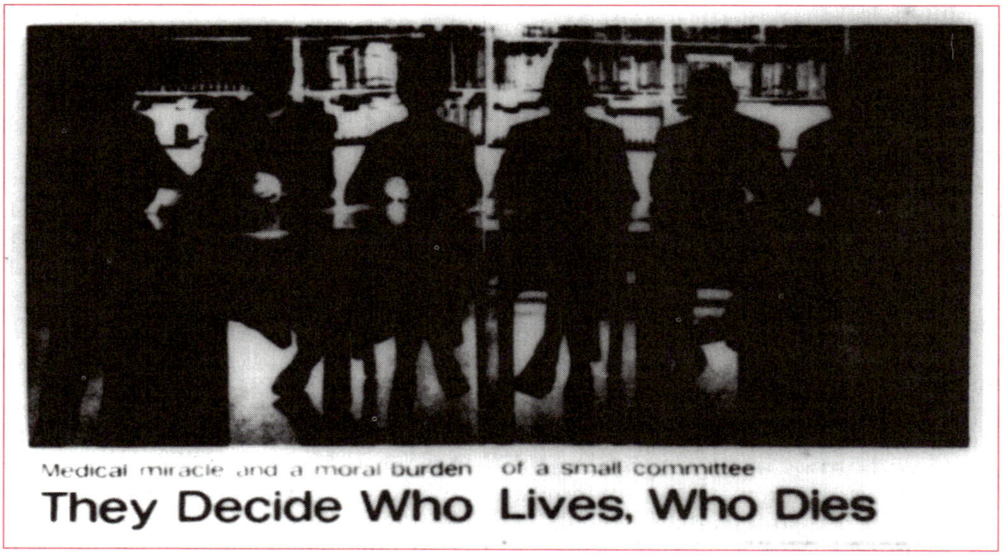
Medical miracle and a moral burden of a small committee
They Decide Who Lives, Who Dies

Peritoneal dialysis. Scribner, Boen, and Tenckhoff, all of Seattle, in conjunction with Palmer of Vancouver, British Columbia, helped to establish automated PD systems in the early 1960s (McBride, 1989). By 1968, Tenckhoff had developed a permanent catheter that allowed PD to become a chronic treatment. The Tenckhoff acute PD catheter was implanted to allow subcutaneous tissue to adhere to the catheter for permanent placement (Warren, 1989, p. 237). With the development of the Tenckhoff catheter, the number of PD patients rose rapidly, although hemodialysis continued as the most common treatment modality in the U.S. (Hoffart, 1995).

Renal transplantation. During this time period, many new drugs that successfully prevented and/or treated rejection of the grafted kidney were approved by the federal government (Hoffart, 1995). These drugs included 6-mercaptopurine (6MP), which induced immune suppression in human transplant recipients; and azathioprine, which induced immunosuppression with fewer side effects; as well as azaserine, actinomycin, and cortisone (Hoffart, 1995). In addition, in Denver, Starzl experimented with high doses of corticosteroids at the time of rejection episodes to reverse acute rejection. In 1964, Terasaki used histocompatibility testing to select the most suitable donor-recipient combinations (Hoffart, 1995).

1973 – Present

With the passage of Public Law 92-603 (H.R. 1) in 1972, which provided a universal source of funding from the federal government for the payment of renal care services, technological long-term access to maintenance care became available to all nephrology patients. Once again, this fostered new technical advances in all modalities and the number of patients grew at an astounding rate (see Chapter 25).

Hemodialysis. Many technical advances came about in this time period, including development of large surface area dialyzers, improvement in fluid delivery systems, introduction of more disposable supplies, incorporation of computer technology into delivery systems, use of kinetic modeling, and introduction of new modalities such as continuous arteriovenous hemofiltration and slow continuous ultrafiltration (Hoffart, 1995). New methods of vascular access introduced such as temporary femoral and subclavian percutaneous catheters while hemoperfusion and hemofiltration were used as alternatives or adjuncts to hemodialysis (Hoffart, 1995).

One of the most important breakthroughs came in 1987 when results of a two-phased trial were reported by Eschbach and co-investigators on the correction of anemia of chronic renal failure using recombinant human erythropoietin. This achievement was hailed as one of the most significant means of improving patients' quality of life and rehabilitation (Eschbach, Egrie, Downing, Browne, & Adamson, 1987).

Peritoneal dialysis. One key breakthrough

came in 1976 with the development of continuous ambulatory peritoneal dialysis (CAPD) by Popovich and Moncrief; a form of continuous self-care dialysis known as continuous cyclic peritoneal dialysis (CCPD) was introduced in 1981 by Diaz-Buxo. Thus, use of both CAPD and CCPD grew while use of intermittent PD declined (Hoffart, 1995).

Renal transplantation. Once again, introduction of new medications aimed at preventing and treating rejection surfaced in this time period. The most significant were cyclosporine A (1978) and OKT3® (1981). In 1978, Ting and Morris showed that HLA-DR matching improved graft survival (Hoffart, 1995). Attempts at simultaneous transplantation of multiple organs were begun while advances in immunosuppressive therapy led to an increase in kidney transplants for those patients 60 years or older (Hoffart, 1995).

Industry's Contributions to Renal Care: Historical Perspectives

Industry's contribution to the development and ongoing support of renal care has been significant throughout the 20th century. Historically, manufacturers have helped to fund the development of equipment, supplies, and treatment used in the nephrology specialty. Industry representatives have collaborated with physicians to reach many milestones during the 1900s, and in the past two decades collaboration and support have extended into nephrology nursing. Through corporate support to the American Nephrology Nurses' Association (ANNA), industry has played a key role in advancing nephrology nursing research, education, and special programs. Industry has contributed to the growth of the specialty through sponsorship of ANNA awards, scholarships, and grants along with corporate support of educational programs, journal advertisements, and special programs.

This section will examine the key historical elements in industry's contribution to the nephrology specialty. Early to mid-20th century devices and the development of equipment in contemporary dialysis will be discussed. A perspective of how industry supported the early researchers in nephrology will accompany each discussion.

Early to Mid-20th Century Devices

After their groundbreaking experiments with dialysis in 1913, Abel, Rowntree, and Turner used what was known as a vividiffusion device along with cannula and other glass components to conduct additional experiments (McBride, 1989). Their experiments may have marked the first time in nephrology when industry funded a developmental project involving well-defined dialysis principles. Abel, who hoped his experiments would eventually lead to a treatment for diabetes, had received corporate support from The Eli Lilly Company (McBride, 1989). He broke off the relationship with the Eli Lilly Company, however, because he did not want his work commercialized (McBride, 1989).

The Visking Corporation of Chicago assisted local scientist William Thalhimer, MD, of Michael Reese Hospital to develop sausage casing membrane as an ideal dialyzing membrane. This membrane was inexpensive, strong, and had excellent transport capabilities. Thalhimer's experiments of the 1930s proved beneficial to future researchers, who were convinced of the value of the membrane and the diffusion principles involved (McBride, 1989).

Dutch physician Willem Kolff, who developed the artificial kidney from 1938 to 1945, was one of the first to convince industry to support the emerging dialysis field (McBride, 1989). Near the end of World War II, Kolff received the support of The Berk Enamel Company from Holland to build the first rotating drum kidney, devices that were mechanically sound and demonstrated that a dialysis machine could overcome the problems of kidney failure. The rotating drum kidneys built by the Berk Enamel Company used the Visking membrane. Some of these machines were shipped to New York and Canada after World War II to be used in early dialysis procedures in North America (McBride, 1989).

1950s and 1960s

Industry continued to play a key role in the development of equipment used in dialysis in the early 1950s. With the help of the Brunswick Corporation and the Edward Olsen Company, Dr. Kolff teamed up with researchers at the Peter Bent Brigham Hospital to develop the Kolff-Brigham Artificial Kidney, which was the first off-the-shelf hemodialysis system that was available to the renal care community in 1956 (McBride, 1989). Other corporations that contributed to modifications and the availability of early hemodialysis systems included the Allis Chalmers Company, which built a rotating drum artificial kidney; the Westinghouse Corporation, which helped to manufacture a more compact hemodialysis machine; and Baxter Corporation, a relatively small manufacturer of specialty products for hospitals, which collaborated with 1950s researchers to improve existing hemodialysis systems (see Figure 2-3) (McBride, 1989).

The first arteriovenous Teflon shunt for continuous access to the blood stream was developed in 1960 by Belding Scribner, MD, from the University of Washington, and Wayne Quinton, who later formed Quinton Instrument Company in Seattle. Scribner and other researchers developed an automated PD system that could be used in the home as an alternative to hemodialysis; Quinton Instruments provided the permanent catheters used for PD (McBride, 1989).

The Dow Corporation supported the development of the first hollow fiber artificial kidney, constructed by Richard Stewart, MD, of the University of Michigan, and later set up a subsidiary to market these devices. In the 1960s, the Gottscho Packaging Company of New Jersey assisted Norman Lasker, MD, in the development and manufacturing of the first PD cycler. Ira Gottscho, the owner, was motivated to support development of this cycler after his daughter died of renal failure (McBride, 1989). In the 1970s and early 1980s, Baxter Corporation assisted in the development of self-care PD systems that allowed treatments to complement and not interfere with patients' lifestyles.

Industry formed an alliance with the health care community to ensure that renal care patients receive efficient and cost-effective care. The above are a few examples of how industry assisted in the movement of dialysis equipment out of the laboratory and into the renal care community. Today, trained nursing and sales personnel (see section on careers in nephrology nursing) represent industry to make treatment expertise available to clinical practitioners.

Government's Role in Chronic Renal Failure Treatment

The federal government's role in the successful treatment of renal failure patients is significant throughout most of the history of the nephrology specialty. Starting primarily in the 1960s, the government's role began in Veterans' Administration hospitals and broadened into the issuance of hemodialysis grants and the organizing of nephrology programs for nurses before the establishment of the ESRD entitlement program in 1972. This section will present an overview of government's key role in the growth of the nephrology specialty and nephrology nursing in particular.

VA Hospital Dialysis Program

In 1963, only 3 years after Scribner started treating chronic kidney failure patients with hemodialysis, the Veterans Administration (VA) announced its intention to establish approximately 30 dialysis treatment units in VA hospitals across the country (Rettig, 1986). The plan was to set up the units close to universities.

Bernice Hinckley, who helped to form what is now the American Nephrology Nurses' Association (ANNA) and who served as the organization's first president, worked in one of the first VA units opened in Washington, DC. Those first VA nurses were well respected and well educated, not to mention progressive in their practice.

Federal Government Hemodialysis Grants

In 1963, the Public Health Service (PHS) approved the first of the 14 grants to the Seattle Artificial Kidney Center from chronic disease funds. This was money needed to help pay for supplies for patients that needed dialysis. Money from private philanthropy, community fund-raising, and fund-raising for specific patients could not meet the heavy burden of the cost of hemodialysis treatment (Rettig & Marks, 1982).

After tumultuous visits to Washington by Scribner and other advocates, and extensive consultations, Congress created a second NIH research program – the Artificial Kidney-Chronic Uremia program in the National Institute of Arthritis and Metabolic Diseases. Simultaneously, it established a grant program to demonstrate the feasibility of delivering dialysis treatment, and the PHS created the Kidney Disease Control Program (KDCP) to administer the grants. Dr. Scribner was the principle investigator for the first grant that was awarded to the outpatient facility known as the Seattle Artificial Kidney Center. The second grant was awarded to Downstate Medical Center in Brooklyn in mid-1964.

As other proposals were submitted, a review process was set up and an ad hoc committee of expert reviewers was created. In 1965 and 1966, the KDCP awarded an additional 12 grants for dialysis demonstration centers, the final two being for the demonstration of home dialysis. Grants were for 3 years (Rettig & Marks, 1982). These grants established the first dialysis centers and were the first major financial contributions to CRF from the federal government. As the numbers of dialysis centers increased, the number of nurses increased proportionately. The grants were awarded to large metropolitan hospitals. Many of the PHS grants were given to university and teaching hospitals. The grant period was for 3 years based on expectation that centers would be self supporting at the end of the grant period. However, at the end of the 3 years (1967-1968) there were over 1,000 patients on hemodialysis that were supported by the government grants. Community funds were nonexistent and funds on the national level were sparse.

Scribner and associates in Seattle aggressively began to treat patients in the home in 1964. He also promoted home dialysis as a national policy (Curtis et al., 1965). Scribner argued that home treatment permitted the escape from the capacity limits of facility dialysis, was less expensive, and resulted in equally good, if not better, patient survival. Scribner, a forceful advocate, along with the growing budget constraints forced the KDCP to switch emphasis from expanding center dialysis to supporting home dialysis. Subsequently, 12 contracts were awarded to demonstrate the effectiveness of training patients for home dialysis. Each contract was for 5 years, and each grant had tapering funds.

During the next 5 years, until the 1972 Medicare amendment, centers who had been supported by state funding found that now the available monies were even less because the NIH-funded centers were losing their grants and were

Figure 2-3
The twin coil artificial kidney.

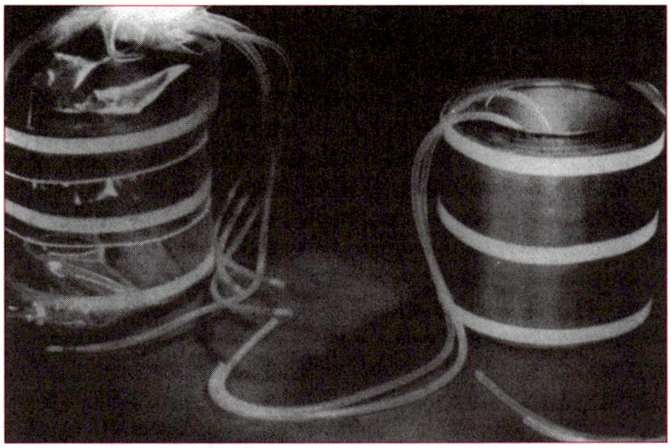

Photo courtesy of the Baxter Corporation

The Twin Coil Artificial Kidney was one of many modifications made by researchers to Kolff's original artificial kidney. Researchers and industry collaborated to help improve hemodialysis technology throughout the early days of nephrology.

Figure 2-4
The first dialysis nurse in the United States: Barbara Coleman-Wysocki.

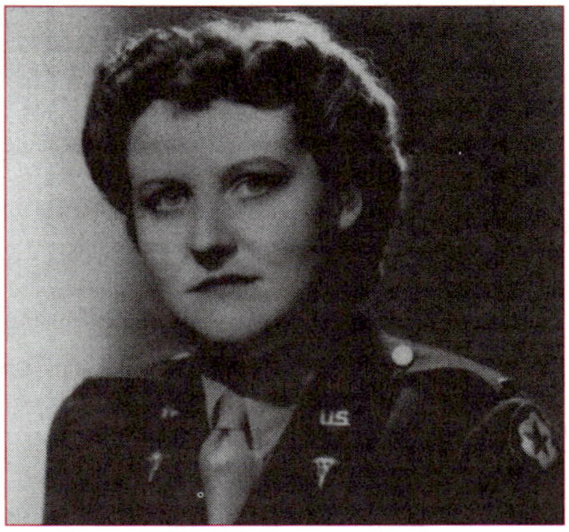

Barbara Coleman-Wysocki is recognized as the first dialysis nurse in the United States. She worked in the very first dialysis program in this country at Peter Bent Brigham Hospital in Boston from 1948 to 1954, and was the first to publish an article on the role of the dialysis nurse.

requesting state funds to support the patients already started in the KDP as they were called. The Gottschalk Committee on Chronic Kidney Disease (named after Dr. Carl Gottschalk of the University of North Carolina) convened many times during the financial crisis between 1966 and 1967. The committee published a report (U.S. Bureau of the Budget, 1967) that concluded: dialysis and transplantation were no longer experimental procedures, thus officially bringing the debate to a close. They also recommended that a national treatment program financed by Medicare be established. The Gottschalk report included a section on dialysis in the VA hospitals.

Thus, the 1960s offered many new advances in the treatment of renal disease, the emergence of home hemodialysis, NIH-sponsored dialysis centers, and the opening of VA dialysis centers. It was obvious that the number of nurses to care for these patients receiving these new modalities would need to grow, leading to the need for dialysis nurses to organize.

The Medicare ESRD Program

In 1972, Congress passed Public Law 92-603 (H.R. 1: Social Security Amendments of 1972), which amended the 1965 Medicare law to include payment for dialysis and transplantation services for patients suffering from chronic renal failure (Bocchino & Burrows-Hudson, 1995). The intent of Medicare coverage was to:

1. provide equitable access for all ESRD patients; and
2. deem patients who were certified to have chronic renal failure and require dialysis or transplantation by physicians as disabled (Bocchino & Burrows-Hudson, 1995).

With a universal source of federal funding in place, the number of facilities and nephrology nurses and technicians doubled during the mid-1970s. Experts in the mid-1970s predicted that by the mid-1980s, the total number of patients on dialysis would level out. This prediction did not hold true and today the number of patients continues to rise (see Chapter 25). In 1973, the first full year of the Medicare ESRD Program, the total number of patients was 8,000 (Bocchino & Burrows-Hudson, 1995). By 1983, the total number of dialysis patients was 71,987 in both outpatient and home settings, that number rose to 171,479 by the end of 1993 (Health Care Financing Administration [HCFA], 1993). By 1987, the total number of approved Medicare ESRD facilities was 1,701, a number that had reached 2,506 by 1993 (HCFA, 1993).

Early Nephrology Nurses and Their Roles

Hoffart's historical research explains that treatment was restricted to symptomatic relief for acute renal failure and palliative measures in cases of chronic renal disease. Rest, dietary control, diuretics, digitalis, and promotion of extrarenal elimination were the only treatments available until the 1940s (Hoffart 1989a, 1989b).

Nursing participation in nephrology in the

Figure 2-5
Nursing care for a patient on the artificial kidney.

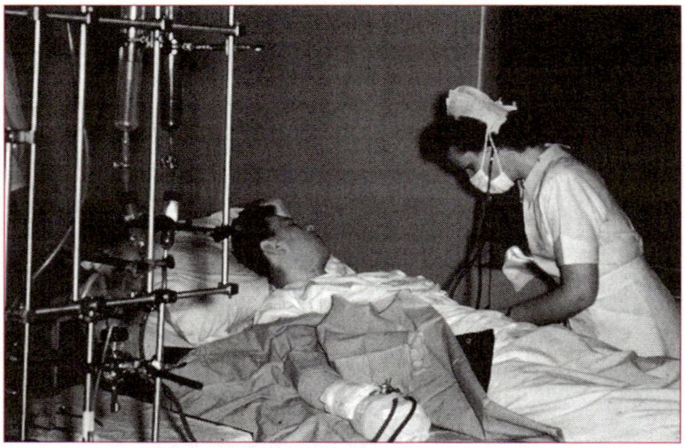

Photo courtesy of Bill Murphy, Miami, FL

Barbara Coleman-Wysocki, RN, provides nursing care for a patient on the artificial kidney at Peter Bent Brigham Hospital in Boston in 1949. The Brigham team worked on the first dialysis program in the United States.

Figure 2-6
Dialyzing a patient on the artificial kidney.

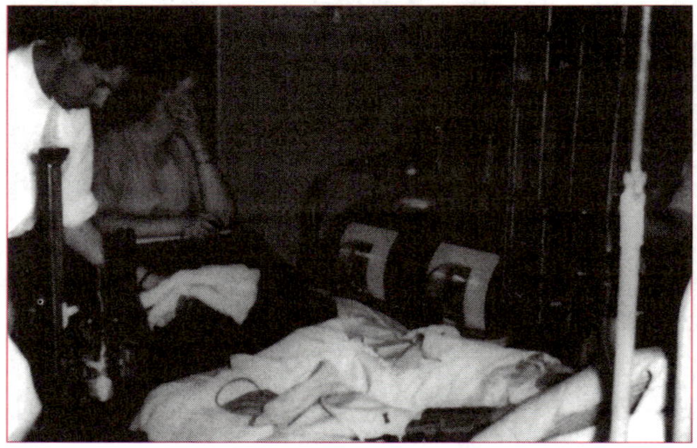

Photo by Bill Murphy, Miami, FL

At Peter Bent Brigham Hospital in Boston, around 1949, Dr. W. Goodale, Barbara Coleman-Wysocki, and Dr. John Merrill dialyze a patient with acute renal failure using a modified Kolff Rotating Drum Kidney Machine.

United States began with nursing care of hemodialysis patients in the late 1940s. The various tasks of early nephrology nurses evolved throughout the 1950s and 1960s, and included assisting physicians, making patients comfortable, keeping vigilant eyes on the dialysis procedures, and learning to institute and discontinue dialysis treatments (Hoffart, 1989a). This section will examine the nursing pioneers in the nephrology specialty and briefly describe their roles in the care of renal patients.

Early Nurses and Their Contributions

Barbara K. Coleman-Wysocki (see Figure 2-4), who worked in the first dialysis program in the U.S. at Peter Bent Brigham Hospital in Boston from 1948 to 1954, is recognized as the first dialysis nurse in the United States. Ms. Coleman-Wysocki, along with John P. Merrill, MD, were the first to publish an article that described the artificial kidney (see Figures 2-5 and 2-6). Their article, published in the March 1952 issue of the *American Journal of Nursing* (Coleman & Merrill, 1952), also described the role of the dialysis nurse. Most of the initial hemodialysis programs throughout the world had their staff educated by Ms. Coleman-Wysocki (McBride, 1989).

Many early dialysis nurses made numerous contributions to the specialty. Barbara Fulton and past ANNA President Elizabeth Cameron, both from Peter Bent Brigham Hospital, were among the first dialysis nurses involved in home training in the 1960s. These nurses worked in the Brigham dialysis unit during the day while traveling to patients' homes to dialyze them at night (Hoffart, 1989a).

Another pioneer nurse was Anna M. Smyth (see unit title page on page 1) of the Army Nurse Corps. Ms. Smyth was assigned to the Renal Insufficiency Center, 11th Evacuation Hospital, in Wonju, Korea in 1952 and 1953, to assist in providing renal care to wounded soldiers during the Korean Conflict. Only one artificial kidney machine was available, although the number of wounded soldiers who developed acute renal failure following their injuries was excessive. Ms. Smyth documented the intense pressure of trying to save the lives of soldiers using the artificial kidney under the stress of combat:

> "We were working with the prime of American youth . . . so the trauma was such an initial blow. It was very traumatizing for the nurses as our mortality rate was awful. If we saved one, we felt like we were performing a miracle. There were times we'd lose a couple in a day." (Smyth, 1986, p. 52).

With the development of many new nephrology innovations in Seattle in the late 1950s and early 1960s, many pioneer dialysis nurses also cared for patients on the West Coast. Two such nurses were Carrie Lewis and Barbara Fellows, both of the University of Washington Hospital, along with JoAnn Albers, who served as the head nurse for the Seattle Artificial Kidney Center – the nation's first

Figure 2-7
Dialysis nursing during the Korean conflict.

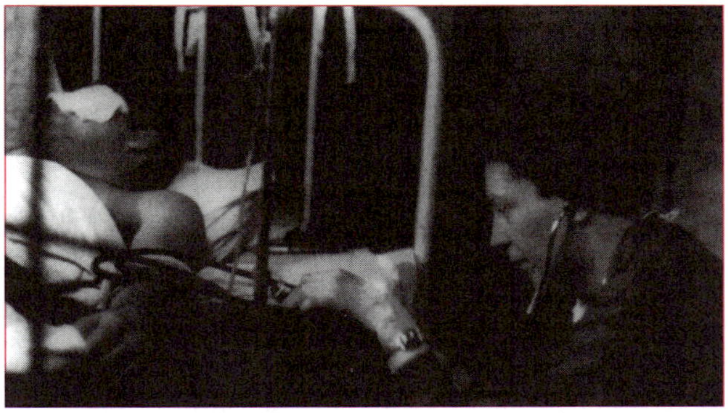

Photo courtesy of Anna M. Smyth

At the 11th Evacuation Hospital in Wonju, Korea in 1953, Anna M. Smyth, RN, monitors blood pressure during a dialysis procedure. Only one artificial kidney machine was available for numerous wounded soldiers during the Korean Conflict, making the conditions of caring for these patients difficult.

Figure 2-8
Program cover from "A Dialysis Symposium for Nurses."

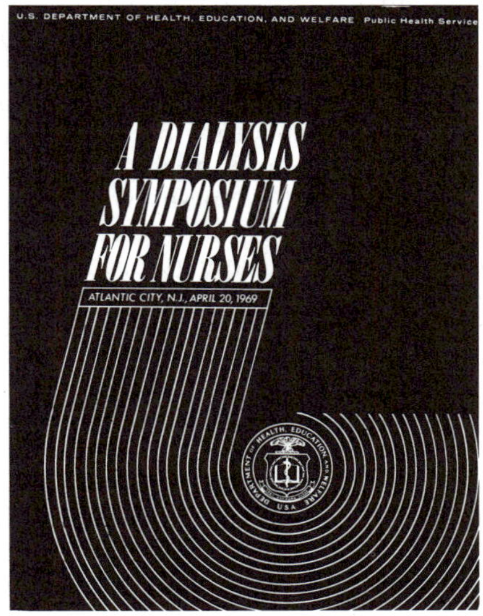

dialysis center located in a community setting (Albers, 1989). Bernice Hinckley (see Figure 2-7), who worked at one of the nation's first VA dialysis units in Washington, DC in the mid-1960s, also helped form the American Association for Nephrology Nurses (AANN), now ANNA, and served as the organization's first president in 1969.

A pioneer in transplant nursing was Dorothy Shebelski, who served as the head nurse for the transplant unit at the Denver Veterans Administration Hospital starting in 1963 (Hoffart, 1989a). At the Medical College of Virginia in Richmond, Nancye Page and Dr. David Hume worked from 1960 to 1963 to develop protocols for caring for patients who went into the sterile room after receiving total body irradiation (Hoffart, 1989a). The nurses described above were prominent transplant nurses who assisted in providing a foundation for nephrology nursing practice.

Roles of Early Nephrology Nurses

The roles of early nurses involved in the care of renal patients were varied. Barbara Coleman-Wysocki described the new, but traditional role in the early 1950s as: (a) physician assistant; (b) patient comforter; and (c) 'being vigilant,' which meant "watching what was going on all the time and protecting the patient" (Hoffart, 1989a; McCulloch, 1994). As described above, early dialysis nurses performed their duties in a number of different settings throughout the 1950s and 1960s, including the Korean Conflict, home settings, transplant units, and traditional dialysis centers.

Home dialysis. New roles for dialysis nurses that evolved in home dialysis in the 1960s were to serve as patient teachers and to provide supportive nursing care. The basic assumption of home dialysis was that patients could be taught to perform the procedure safely in their homes (Hoffart, 1989a), and nurses were responsible for providing that information to patients. Patient teaching was a new concept to nursing in the early 1960s, and textbooks on how to teach patients did not appear until 1968 (Hoffart, 1989b). Once patients were taught to perform the procedure safely, ongoing supportive nursing care was needed to address other areas such as medical, technical, socioeconomic, and psychological problems.

Transplant. Patient teaching was a key component of duties performed by early transplant nurses. Some nurses assisted physicians in developing policies and procedures for staff members to work in surgical areas, while others concentrated strictly on preparing surgical suites for transplant procedures (Hoffart, 1989a). Transplant nurses were able to administer immunosuppressive drugs to patients for the first time in 1962. Early transplant nurses were involved heavily in caring for patients postoperatively, and met great challenges in dealing with patients' emotional and psychological needs (Hoffart, 1989a). Nurses' roles evolved into serving as a primary support for patients and their families.

Peritoneal dialysis. This mode of care did not receive much attention in the early days of nephrology when compared to hemodialysis and transplantation. Nurses involved in early PD care of patients primarily served in technical, supportive, and educational roles.

After assisting the physician with the insertion of the peritoneal catheter, the nurse was responsible for maintaining and monitoring the procedure (Hoffart, 1989a, p. 175). Nurses were involved in recording intake and output, observing for patient symptoms, alleviating drainage problems, keeping the patient safe, and maintaining aseptic technique. Supportive care involved keeping patients comfortable due to lengthy procedures (Secor, 1966), while teaching helped to alleviate the fears and anxieties experienced by families and to encourage the rehabilitation process (Hoffart, 1989a).

Many early PD nurses did not develop expertise in this mode of care because so few PD programs existed in the United States, especially in the 1950s. PD care became more prominent in the 1960s following the development of the automated cycling PD machine by Scribner, Boen and colleagues at the University of Washington, and later with the development of continuous modes of PD in the late 1970s (Hoffart, 1989a).

A Professional Nephrology Nursing Organization: The History of ANNA

Nephrology nurses are represented in this country by the American Nephrology Nurses' Association (ANNA), a nonprofit, professional organization of approximately 11,000 members concerned with promoting high quality care for people with acute and chronic renal failure. Members are primarily involved in conservative management, PD, hemodialysis, transplantation, and related therapies. The purposes of ANNA are to protect the future of quality care; educate nephrology nurses; stimulate research; disseminate new ideas throughout the field; promote interdisciplinary communication and cooperation; and respond to social, governmental, and professional issues affecting the practice of nephrology nursing and its technology.

Organizing of Nephrology Nurses

Due to the initial government funding, dialysis centers expanded, home hemodialysis emerged, and the number of patients increased, thus the need for nurses to care for these patients began to parallel this growth. Thus, during the historic 1960s, dialysis nurses began to organize in the United States, eventually forming a professional organization for nephrology nurses in 1969. The first informal meeting of nephrology nurses took place in 1966 at Peter Bent Brigham Hospital in Boston, where 100 nurses gathered for an educational offering (Brennan & Jordan, 1994; Hoffart, 1989b). In 1968, a 1-day "Dialysis Symposium for Nurses," sponsored by the Public Health Service's Kidney Disease Control Program, was held at the American Society of Artificial Internal Organs (ASAIO) Meeting in Philadelphia with about 200 nurses in attendance. At this meeting, a core group of nurses pursued the idea of forming a specialty nursing organization dedicated to nephrology nursing practice (Brennan & Jordan, 1994; Hoffart, 1989b).

The next formal gathering of nephrology nurses took place in 1969 during the ASAIO Meeting in Atlantic City, NJ (see Figure 2-8). It was during this meeting that the American Association for Nephrology Nurses (AANN) was formed and officers elected. Bernice Hinckley was elected as the new association's first president, serving her term in 1969-1970 (Brennan & Jordan, 1994). In 1970, the organization changed its name to the American Association of Nephrology Nurses and Technicians (AANNT) (Sims, 1994, p. 3). In 1983, the association leaders made the decision to limit full membership to registered nurses, focusing efforts and resources toward professional nursing. As a result, the association again changed its name from AANNT to ANNA (Sims, 1994, p. 3), and has since developed into a strong, respected voice for the specialty of nephrology nursing.

Since its formation in 1969, membership has grown steadily (see Figure 2-9). As a professional organization, the majority of members are registered nurses, rising from 200 nurses in 1969 to 1,600 in 1975 (Brennan & Jordan, 1994), and to more than 11,000 members in 1997. Associate members include licensed practical nurses, dialysis technicians, registered dietitians and social workers, as well as physicians. All members are a vital part of the nephrology health care team. ANNA serves its members through a national structure, 4 regions, and over 100 local chapters. Decision-making and planning are done by the Board of Directors, local chapters, and national, regional, and local committees.

Significant Events in ANNA History

Several events in nephrology nursing and ANNA history have assisted the association's significant growth in membership, and established it as the voice for nephrology nursing (see Appendix A). These include the development of a professional journal and newsletter, along with the publication of numerous professional manuals and books; ANNA's development of a government relations program; a steady increase in educational offerings and corporate sponsorship; and development and ongoing administration of a certification examination for nephrology nurses.

Development of publications. The development of an organization newsletter and a professional journal established strong communication links to the

Figure 2-9
Growth of ANNA membership: 1987 to 1997.

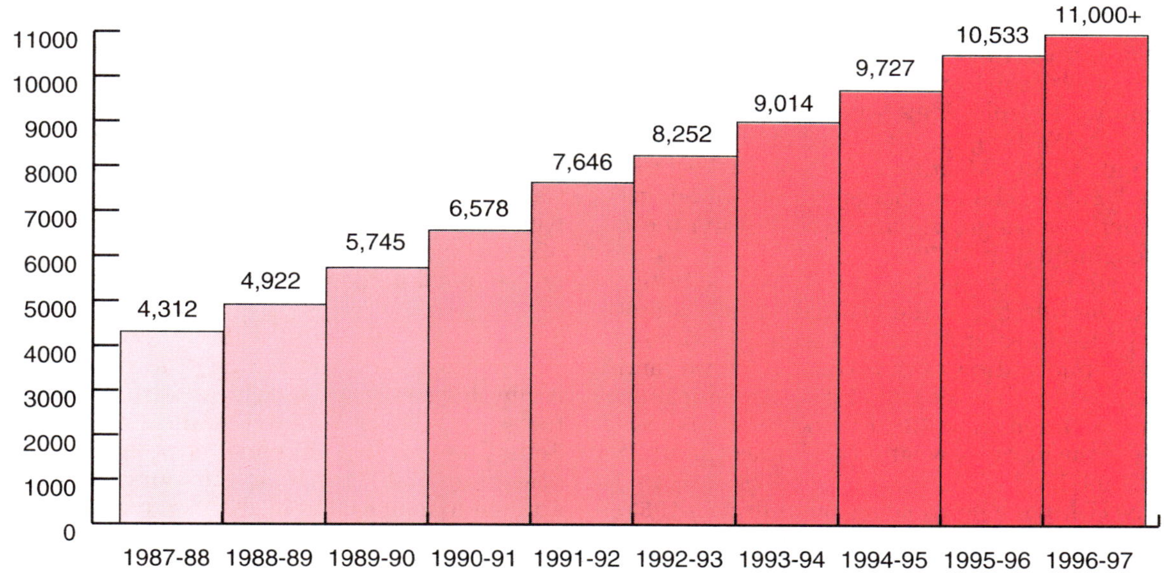

Note: From Price, C.A. (1997). ANNA annual reports: State of the Association. *ANNA Journal, 24*(2), 131-135.

membership and to nephrology nurses. This in turn helped foster growth of AANNT/ANNA members.

The association began publication of a quarterly newsletter, the *AANNT Update*, in 1972 following approval of a new organization logo (Brennan & Jordan, 1994). Now known as the *ANNA Update*, the newsletter is published six times per year and covers national, regional, and chapter news of interest to association members.

The organization's professional journal, the *AANNT Journal*, was first published in the fall of 1974. Margery Fearing served as the first editor for this new journal (McCulloch, 1994). Others who have served as the journal's editor include Marcia Keen, Jean MacMullen, and Sally D. McCulloch. Today, the *ANNA Journal* is a well-respected clinical and academic resource that provides current information on a wide variety of subjects to facilitate the practice of professional nephrology nursing.

Additional resources published through the years have also enabled ANNA to establish itself as the spokesperson for the nephrology nursing specialty. These include publication of three editions of the *Core Curriculum for Nephrology Nursing*, three editions of the *Standards of Clinical Practice for Nephrology Nursing*, along with *Continuous Quality Improvement: From Concept to Reality*, the *Nephrology Nursing Certification Review Guide*, and *A Guide to Professional Development*.

Development of government relations program. As membership grew and the complexity of specialty practice issues began to emerge, the association saw the need to become involved in the legislative and regulatory arenas. This involvement began under the leadership and direction of Past AANNT President Nancy Sharp in 1981-1982 (Smith, 1994).

The association's first Legislative Policy Statement was published in November 1983. This bold and visionary statement addressed such topics as open staffing, the use of advanced practice nurses with reimbursement for their services under Medicare, elimination of certificate of need, and support for cost-containment efforts in the ESRD Program (Smith, 1984, p. 20). Many of these and other issues addressed in this document are still appropriate in today's health care environment (Smith, 1994).

Through the years, the association has undertaken numerous activities in the legislative arena. These include the development of a State Legislative program in 1988-1989, publication of a Legislative Handbook in 1989, organization of a Legislative Committee in 1991, the first offering of the Legislative Workshop in Washington, DC in 1993, and the establishment of a legislative office in Washington, DC in 1989 (Brennan & Jordan, 1994; Smith, 1994). In addition, ANNA members have participated regularly in the Nurse in Washington

Internship in Washington since establishment of the program in 1985 (Smith, 1994).

Growth of educational offerings. The association was formed in 1969 to enable nurses to share information on nephrology nursing practice and to network with colleagues (Brennan & Jordan, 1994). In the spring of 1970, the youthful organization attracted 450 registrants to its First National Symposium for Nephrology Nurses; the convention was held in Washington, DC in conjunction with the annual ASAIO Meeting ("ANNA: 20 Years of Progress," 1989). The number and scope of educational offerings has grown significantly from these simple beginnings in 1970.

Throughout the 1970s, educational activities included the offering of the National Symposium, Regional Meetings, and Basic Learning Institutes, along with publication of the *AANNT Journal* and monographs (Smith & Binkley, 1994). An education director was hired in 1978 to work with this fast-growing segment of association activities (Smith & Binkley, 1994).

AANNT hired a new management firm in 1981, Anthony J. Jannetti, Inc., and this relationship helped to continue the growth of educational offerings. In 1981 and 1982 , the association held its first two national meetings, still in conjunction with ASAIO, under its new management firm before holding its first independent national meeting in 1983. In 1983, the association held its first independent National Symposium, with 1,000 registrants attending the meeting in Philadelphia. In 1986, the position of education director was reinstated while the first Clinical Concerns in Nephrology Meetings were held that fall. These successful meetings continued through the fall of 1994. In addition, the offering of the Nephrology Nursing Certification Board's (NNCB's) Certification Examination began in 1987; to nurses interested in recertification, more widespread CE opportunities were initiated (Smith & Binkley, 1994, p. 15).

Certification in nephrology nursing. A certification hemodialysis examination was administered beginning in 1977 by The Board of Nephrology Examiners for Nephrology Nurses and Technicians (BONENT) (Butera, 1994; Ulrich, 1985). BONENT Board members included representatives from AANNT and the American Society of Extracorporeal Technologists. Serious conceptual differences were raised with increasing concern by AANNT members and the Executive Board that the BONENT Examination did not meet current practice standards. The relationship between BONENT and AANNT also was complicated by a number of financial and organizational problems. In 1982, ANNA rescinded its endorsement of this examination (Butera, 1994; Ulrich, 1985).

Certification in nephrology nursing is now available to nurses who meet the eligibility criteria established by the NNCB. Founded in 1986, NNCB was formed by nephrology nurses to develop and administer a nephrology nursing certification examination. The purpose of NNCB is to promote the highest standards of nephrology nursing practice through the development, implementation, and coordination of all aspects of the certification process for nephrology nurses in the U.S. and its territories (Butera, 1994). Janel Parker served as NNCB's first president. Currently, there are over 4,000 certified nephrology nurses (CNNs). Certification promotes professional development as well as a commitment to the specialty. Employers often recognize certification through advancement on a clinical ladder or financial incentives.

Nephrology Nurses Today

Professional nephrology nurses and the nephrology nursing specialty have matured since the early days of dialysis and transplantation. Today, nephrology nursing is a holistic, caring-based practice in which the nursing process is applied to manage the health care needs of individuals experiencing the real or threatened impact of renal disease (ANNA, 1996).

Nephrology nursing in its broadest sense is concerned with both the prevention of disease and the care and assessment of the health needs of patients and families across the life cycle. These patients need well-educated, highly skilled, and motivated registered nurses. Nephrology nursing is a special career that offers unique professional opportunities and diverse areas of clinical practice. Nephrology is an ever-changing field as technological and educational advances are made.

Nephrology nurses have provided care for more than 40 years. In 1973, hemodialysis, peritoneal dialysis, and transplantation were funded by the federal government and these treatments became more common. Nephrology nurses worked with other health care professionals as the specialty emerged. Since then, the role of the nephrology nurse has expanded and its practice boundaries broadened. In its more limited meaning, nephrology nursing focuses on the care of people experiencing acute renal failure and the various phases of chronic renal failure. When renal failure progresses to end stage, the patient moves from conservative management to one or more of the alternative replacement therapies available. Nephrology nurses also work with patients requiring continuous renal replacement therapy (CRRT) in the acute setting, and patients requiring therapeutic plasma exchange (TPE) and multi-organ transplants. Nephrology nurses provide their experience and expertise as new extracorporeal therapies are developed. Career opportunities exist in all these treatment modalities, with the highest number of opportunities in hemodialysis and PD (ANNA, 1996).

Career Opportunities

Conservative management. Nephrology nursing does not solely consist of working with patients on dialysis or with kidney transplants. There are other areas in which the care of these patients can be extremely challenging and rewarding.

Not all nephrology patients require dialysis. Many diseases that affect the kidney are potentially treatable and curable. It is often the nurse's responsibility to educate and evaluate the patient's understanding of their disease and its prognosis, medications, and dietary interventions. Nursing care of this type of patient requires a collaborative effort among physician, nurse, and patient.

If a patient's disease does progress to chronic renal failure, it is likely that many office visits and hospitalizations have occurred in the past. In these situations, the nurse working with the nephrologist or in the hospital unit has a prime opportunity to share information with the patient and family. These patients often have multiple medical, nursing, and psychosocial problems. They learn to cope with these problems over time, with the assistance of an interested, knowledgeable and compassionate health care team. Many patients have jobs, schoolwork, home responsibilities, or other daily demands to manage beyond health issues (ANNA, 1996).

Collaboration with dialysis personnel to establish a relationship with the patient before the necessity for dialysis facilitates the transition to chronic outpatient therapy. Chapter 18 provides in-depth information on conservative management of renal patients for nephrology nurses.

Hemodialysis. Hemodialysis nurses use a general knowledge base of medical-surgical, pediatric, geriatric, and psychiatric nursing to assess patients' needs and define standards of practice. Nurses care for the health needs of chronic renal failure patients on a long-term basis. Working with a multidisciplinary team, nurses facilitate patients' adaptation to acute or chronic illness. Early hospital discharges allow hemodialysis nurses (through case management and critical pathways) to be involved with the patient's continuum of care regardless of the setting (skilled nursing facility, home health, or rehabilitation). Nurses function as educators, direct caregivers, and coordinators. Technical knowledge of dialysis equipment and good communication skills are also required.

Hospitalized renal failure patients are dialyzed either in an area specifically maintained for hemodialysis, in their hospital rooms, or in an intensive care setting. Chronic renal failure patients are treated in outpatient dialysis units. These units are either free-standing or hospital based. Greater than two-thirds of the 143,500 patients receiving hemodialysis are dialyzed at a free-standing facility (ANNA, 1996). See Chapter 19 for a complete overview of hemodialysis.

Peritoneal dialysis. PD provides several treatment options for renal failure patients. It accomplishes the same goals as hemodialysis through an internal process using the unique properties of the peritoneum as the dialysis membrane. This modality is employed in the management of both acute and chronic renal failure.

There are two forms of PD commonly used for patients with chronic renal failure. They are continuous ambulatory peritoneal dialysis (CAPD) and automated peritoneal dialysis (APD). Since the early 1980s, CAPD has gained widespread popularity for home patients. Nurses' roles in PD require flexibility and autonomy. Assessment skills are used in evaluating the patient's physical and psychosocial needs and in evaluating the effects of dialysis on the patient by interpreting monthly laboratory tests. Teaching skills are needed to provide information to the patients and their family as they learn about treatment options and about PD procedures (ANNA, 1996). See Chapter 22 for a complete overview of PD and nursing's role in this modality.

Renal transplantation. Chronic renal failure patients may choose renal transplantation as the treatment choice most appropriate for their life goals. As noted earlier in this chapter, kidney transplantation was first done in 1954 in Boston and today is an opportunity for many dialysis patients to regain a better quality of life than experienced on chronic dialysis. Successes with related donors are promising with 1-year patient survival at 97% and cadaveric graft success at 88%. Following transplants, patients generally obtain normal renal function and can resume a more normal lifestyle.

The role of nurses in the care of patients choosing renal transplantation is varied and extensive. Some centers have separate inpatient units devoted to the care of renal and/or transplant patients. Potential transplant recipients are admitted to these areas for evaluation immediately before a transplant and for postoperative care. Other institutions admit patients to general surgical units. Through continuous education and clinical training, staff nurses become very skilled in assessment, implementation of care, and evaluation of patients' progress (ANNA, 1996). Chapter 23 provides a comprehensive review of renal transplantation.

Pediatric nephrology. In the recent past, treatment for children with renal failure was not standard practice. Today, pediatric nephrology is a growing subspecialty and some form of dialysis and kidney transplantation can be offered to almost every child in renal failure. This form of nursing offers the challenge of working with children with chronic renal disease over time. Skilled pediatric nephrology nurses recognize how chronic disease affects children's growth and development and enables them to collaborate with nephrologists to establish appropriate treatment plans. These nurses not only work with children in this setting, but also with the parents, siblings, and grandparents. Family dynamics become an important factor in the care of young patients. Establishment of a relationship between social workers and nurses is imperative for providing the best possible care to pediatric patients.

PD is the most widely used form of dialysis for children with chronic renal failure, however, hemodialysis may be the treatment of choice for some patients. Basic educational information is not different in pediatric settings, however, it needs to be age appropriate for patients and all-inclusive for the parents (ANNA, 1996).

Additional Opportunities

Education. A multitude of options are available for nurses interested in nephrology education. Many facilities have a nurse educator who may be involved in patient and/or staff education. Often, the educator may serve as a resource for more than one facility. Responsibilities may include coordination of an ongoing patient education program, staff orientation to the specialty, and staff continuing education.

Nephrology nurse educators are resources in their specialty. They may be mentors for new staff or for staff in other disciplines as they care for the patient with CRF. Opportunities as nurse educators are also available on a wide variety of levels for nephrology nurses in basic nursing programs, and masters and doctoral programs (ANNA, 1996).

Management. Management positions became increasingly available to nephrology nurses in the 1980s, a trend that continued throughout the 1990s. The skills required for management positions include strong leadership, communication, and management skills, as well as superior patient care skills. As with other nephrology nursing areas, this challenging role requires previous nephrology nursing experience. Many settings also require a BSN or advanced degree. Certification in nephrology nursing may also be required.

A majority of nurses in this area have worked as staff nurses, team leaders, charge nurses, head nurses, or clinical coordinators. Nurses who stay in proprietary settings may ultimately coordinate the management of multiple dialysis units located in different cities. In large medical centers, the nurse may direct the nursing services of all the treatment alternatives, including conservative care and transplantation (ANNA, 1996).

Research. The changing health care climate in the United States is increasing the necessity for research-based practice in the nursing profession. Research opportunities in the specialized area of nephrology nursing are proliferative in all modalities: hemodialysis, PD, transplantation, and related therapies. Nephrology nursing research offers improvement of and advances in clinical practice for the benefit of patients and their families when the safety and efficacy of the practice has been established through an adequate research base and systematic investigation.

Traditionally, nephrology nursing research has been the domain of the academic setting; however, clinical nephrology nursing research is increasing as evidenced by the number of quality abstracts submitted each year and research articles published by nephrology nurses. Research funds are also available to both novice investigators and established investigators. There are currently ANNA and Corporate Research Grants available for funding nephrology nursing research. Areas qualifying for grant monies include hemodialysis, PD, transplantation, continuous quality improvement, patient outcomes, patient rehabilitation, and dialyzer reprocessing (ANNA, 1996).

Advanced practice nursing. Advance practice nurses (APNs) in nephrology nursing include clinical nurse specialists (CNSs) and nurse practitioners (NPs). Nephrology nursing APNs may provide care for individuals along the continuum of compromised renal function, as well as for populations that are modality specific. Generally, CNSs practice in acute care settings and the NPs practice in primary care. APNs hold a master's degree in nursing and, by virtue of their clinical background and academic preparation, have the expert knowledge and skills required to manage the care of individuals in both acute and chronic health care settings. Their clinical practice has a strong focus on promoting health and preventing illness and its complications. ANA certification in the specialized area of advanced practice recognizes the APN's expert knowledge and skills and is often required for many positions. The roles of APN include clinician, consultant, educator, and researcher (ANNA, 1996).

Case management. Nephrology nurse case managers are nurses who manage the quality, outcomes, and costs of patient care. The position requires clinical experience and knowledge of the specialty area as well as expert critical thinking skills. Patient advocacy and continuity of care are two important components of case management. Case managers collect patient-related data; negotiate with insurance companies; evaluate the progress of hospitalized patients; prevent problems, complications, and further hospitalizations; and educate patients, nurses, nephrology team members, and insurance companies. Specific responsibilities for patients with compromised renal function include developing a plan of care; coordinating efforts to develop and implement the critical pathway; following patients throughout the episode of illness; and managing the care of patients in both the outpatient and inpatient settings (ANNA, 1996).

Corporate/government. Career opportunities in the corporate/government arena have expanded over the years. Examples of corporate employers are national and international manufacturers and distributors of dialysis and related equipment, devices, and pharmaceuticals. Government jobs can exist at the local, state, or federal levels in offices or government-owned hospitals and facilities. Nephrology nurses have also expanded into the self-employed consulting business offering educational and management development services.

The types of positions available in the corporate/government areas are diverse and span many functional areas of nephrology nursing, including research, management, administration, and the clinical and educational arenas. Additional functional areas such as marketing, sales, regulatory, and quality management are also available. These jobs also extend across the various specialty renal areas such as acute and chronic hemodialysis, PD, transplantation, continuous renal replacement therapy, pediatrics, and conservative management (ANNA, 1996).

Summary

The history of nephrology and nephrology nursing are so intertwined that it is sometimes difficult to separate the two. Industry has supported education and technology. History, nursing, medicine, government, industry, and patients collaborate in not only the care of renal patients, but also in the fight against disease that requires renal replacement therapy.

The formation and growth of ANNA has been significant in the continued growth of the specialty and in the definition of roles and careers that nephrology nurses enjoy today.

References/Readings

Albers, J. (1989). Reflections on the first dialysis nurse training program. *ANNA Journal, 16*(3), 230-231.

Alexander, S. (1962). They decide who lives, who dies. *Life, 53,* 102-107.

American Nephrology Nurses' Association. (1986). *Scope of practice for nephrology nursing.* Pitman, NJ: Author.

American Nephrology Nurses' Association (ANNA). (1996). *Careers in nephrology nursing.* Pitman, NJ: Author.

American Nurses Association. (1980). *Nursing: A social policy statement.* Kansas City, MO: Author.

American Nurses Association (1995). *Nursing: A social policy statement.* Washington, DC: Author.

ANNA: 20 years of progress. (1989). *ANNA Journal, 16*(3), 205-209.

Bocchino, C.A., & Burrows-Hudson, S. (1995). Other salient issues related to ESRD and its treatment. In L.E. Lancaster (Ed.), *Core curriculum for nephrology nursing* (3rd edition) (pp. 423-446). Pitman, NJ: American Nephrology Nurses' Association.

Brennan, D.T., & Jordan, P.J. (1994). The history of ANNA: A chronology of events. In *ANNA: 1969-1994. Celebrating 25 years of service to the nephrology community* (p. 4). Pitman, NJ: American Nephrology Nurses' Association.

Brodie, B. (1989). A commitment to care: The development of clinical specialization in nursing. *ANNA Journal, 16*(3), 181-186.

Butera, E. (1994). Certification: A mechanism to validate nephrology nursing practice. In *ANNA: 1969-1994. Celebrating 25 years of service to the nephrology community* (pp. 21-23). Pitman, NJ: American Nephrology Nurses' Association.

Burrows-Hudson, S. (Ed.). (1993) *Standards of clinical practice for nephrology nursing.* Pitman, NJ: Author.

Coleman, B.K., & Merrill, J.P. (1952). The artificial kidney. *American Journal of Nursing, 52*(3), 327-329.

Cunningham, M. (1994). Corporate and marketing support plays a key role in ANNA growth. In *ANNA: Celebrating 25 years of service to the nephrology community.* Pitman, NJ: American Nephrology Nurses' Association.

Curtis, F.K., Cole, J.J., & Fellows, B.J. (1965). Hemodialysis in the home. *ASAIO Journal, 11,* 7-10.

Eschbach, J.W., Egrie, J.C., Downing, M.R., Browne, J.K., & Adamson, J.W. (1987). Correction of anemia of end-stage renal disease with recombinant human erythropoietin: Results of a combined phase I and II clinical trial. *New England Journal of Medicine, 316,* 73-78.

Jordan, P. (Ed.). (1993). *Nephrology nursing: A guide to professional development.* Pitman, NJ: Author.

Health Care Financing Administration (HCFA). (1993). *ESRD facility survey tables.* Washington, DC: Author.

Hoffart, N. (1989a). A professional organizational for nephrology nurses. *ANNA Journal, 16*(3), 169-178.

Hoffart, N. (1989b). Nephrology nursing 1915-1970: A historical study of the integration of technology and care. *ANNA Journal, 16*(3), 197-199.

Hoffart, N. (1995). The history of nephrology nursing. In L. Lancaster (Ed.), *Core curriculum for nephrology nursing* (pp. 467-478). Pitman, NJ: American Nephrology Nurses' Association.

Lynaugh, J.E., & Fairman, J. (1989). Caring for the chronically ill: Historical perspectives. *ANNA Journal, 16*(3), 192-196.

McBride, P. (1986). The dawn of the dialysis team and hemodialysis nursing. *Dialysis & Transplantation, 15*(1), 20-31.

McBride, P. (1989). Industry's contribution to the development of renal care. *ANNA Journal, 16*(3), 217-226.

McBride, P. (1990). The development of hemodialysis and peritoneal dialysis. In A.R. Nissenson, R.N. Fine, & D E. Gentile (Eds.), *Clinical dialysis* (2nd edition). Norwalk, CT: Appleton & Lange.

McCulloch, S.D. (1994). Celebrating ANNA's silver anniversary: 25 years of learning, sharing, caring, and growing (editorial). *ANNA Journal, 21*(3), 197-203.

Panel holds life or death vote in allotting of artificial kidney. (1962, May 6). *New York Times,* p. A1.

Price, C.A. (1997). ANNA annual reports: State of the association. *ANNA Journal, 24*(2), 131- 135.

Rettig, R. (1986). The treatment of end-stage renal disease: Some policy lessons. *Dialysis & Transplantation, 15*(1), 12-18.

Rettig, R. & Marks, E. (1982). The federal government and social planning for end-stage renal disease: past, present and future. *Seminars in Nephrology, 2*(127).

Secor, J. (1966). Peritoneal dialysis: A nursing challenge. *RN, 28*(8), 67-72, 102.

Sims, T.W. (1994). ANNA: Celebrating 25 years of promoting the interests of nephrology nurses and patients. In *ANNA: 1969-1994. Celebrating 25 years of service to the nephrology community* (p. 3). Pitman, NJ: American Nephrology Nurses' Association.

Smith, K.S. (1994). ANNA's involvement in legislative arena targets all levels of government. In *ANNA: 1969-1994. Celebrating 25 years of service to the nephrology community* (p. 20). Pitman, NJ: American Nephrology Nurses' Association.

Smith, L.J., & Binkley, L. (1994). ANNA's expanding educational activities: A brief history. In *ANNA: 1969-1994. Celebrating 25 years of service to the nephrology community* (p. 20). Pitman, NJ: American Nephrology Nurses' Association.

Smyth, A.M. (1986, April 10). In *A history of nephrology nursing* (interview). Unpublished manuscript. Pitman, NJ: American Nephrology Nurses' Association.

Ulrich, B. (1985). BONENT Revised (President's Message). *ANNA Update, 15,* p. 3.

Warren, H. (1989). Changes in peritoneal dialysis nursing. *ANNA Journal, 16*(3), 237-241.

Chapter Highlights

- Rest, dietary control, diuretics, digitalis, and promotion of extra-renal elimination were the only treatments available until the 1940s.
- In 1945, for the first time, a patient treated with the artificial kidney recovered from acute renal failure.
- Kolff brought the artificial kidney to the United States in 1947, and the first dialysis procedure was performed in January 1948 on a patient at Mount Sinai Hospital in New York City.
- PD became an acceptable treatment modality for chronic and acute renal failure by the end of the 1950s.
- In 1954, Murray then reported the first long-term success when a patient received an organ from an identical twin. This led to future successes in transplantation where twins were involved.
- The most significant event of the 1960s involved the development of the arteriovenous (AV) shunt by Scribner and Quinton in Seattle in 1960.
- The first outpatient hemodialysis center in the United States was established at the Seattle Artificial Kidney Center in 1962.
- Home hemodialysis was performed for the first time in 1964 in the U.S.
- Barbara K. Coleman-Wysocki, who worked in the very first dialysis program at Peter Bent Brigham Hospital in Boston from 1948 to 1954, is recognized as the first dialysis nurse in the United States.
- Bernice Hinckley, who worked at one of the nation's first VA dialysis units in Washington, DC in the mid-1960s, also helped form the American Association for Nephrology Nurses (AANN), now ANNA, and served as the organization's first president in 1969.
- Nephrology nurses are represented in this country by the American Nephrology Nurses' Association (ANNA), a nonprofit, professional organization of approximately 10,000 members concerned with promoting high quality care for people with acute and chronic renal failure.
- The first formal gathering of nephrology nurses took place in 1969 during the ASAIO Meeting in Atlantic City, NJ. It was during this meeting that the American Association for Nephrology Nurses (AANN) was formed and officers elected.
- The internal arteriovenous (AV) fistula, which provided a more permanent access to the blood stream, was developed in 1966 by Brescia and Cimino in New York.
- Scribner, Boen, and Tenckhoff developed a permanent catheter that allowed PD to become a chronic treatment modality.
- In 1963, the Public Health Service (PHS) approved the first of the 14 grants to the Seattle Artificial Kidney Center from chronic disease funds. This was money needed to help pay for supplies for patients that needed dialysis. Money from private philanthropy, community fund-raising, and fund-raising for specific patients could not meet the heavy burden of the cost of hemodialysis treatment (Rettig & Marks, 1982).
- Because of the passage of Public Law 92-603 (HR 1) in 1972), which provided a universal source of funding from the federal government for the payment of renal care services, long-term access to maintenance care has been available to all nephrology patients.
- One of the most important breakthroughs came in 1987 when results of a two-phase trial study were reported by Eschbach and co-investigators on the correction of anemia of chronic renal failure using recombinant human erythropoietin.
- One key breakthrough came in 1976 with the development of continuous ambulatory peritoneal dialysis (CAPD) by Popovich and Moncrief. A form of continuous self-care dialysis known as continuous cyclic peritoneal dialysis (CCPD) was introduced in 1981 by Diaz-Buxo.
- The most significant new drugs aimed at preventing and treating rejection were cyclosporine A (1978) and OKT3® (1981).
- Nephrology nursing is a special career that offers unique professional opportunities and diverse areas of clinical practice.
- APNs hold a master's degree in nursing and, by virtue of their clinical background and academic preparation, have the expert knowledge and skills required to manage the care of individuals in both acute and chronic health care settings. The roles of APN include clinician, consultant, educator, and researcher.
- Nephrology nurse case managers are nurses who manage the quality, outcomes, and costs of patient care. The position requires clinical experience and knowledge of the specialty area, as well as expert critical thinking skills.

CHAPTER 3

The Professional Roles of the Nephrology Nurse

Mary Ann Gould, MSN, RN, CNN

Chapter Contents

Theoretical Foundations of Roles 45
Types of Roles 46
  Personal Domain 46
  Interpersonal Domain 46
  System Domain 46
Patterns of Behavior 47
  Patterns of Professional Behaviors 47
  Nursing Behaviors 48
Role Relationships 49
Professional Roles in Nephrology Nursing 51
  Clinical Practice Roles 51
  Administrative Roles 53
  Educator 53
  Volunteer Role 53
  The Role of the Board of Directors 55
  The Role of Paid Staff Members 55
Role Descriptions 55
Role Evaluation 55
Summary 55
References 55
Chapter Highlights 57

The Professional Roles of the Nephrology Nurse

Mary Ann Gould, MSN, RN, CNN

The roles of the nephrology nurse are a dynamic constellation of behaviors. As a constellation, it is made up of a multitude of roles that we experience in our personal, interpersonal, and organizational interactions. Each role occupies a different priority in our life and prioritization fluctuates in relation to changing environmental influences. Roles are taken on and discarded as individuals move through life. Roles undergo metamorphosis through time. Roles defy containment within a static or narrow description.

It is important to understand the foundations of role behavior in order to understand ourselves, others, and the organizations in which we deliver nephrology nursing service. Strategies have been identified that mediate negative aspects of role performance, which reduce staff turnover, increase skill base, and motivate nurses at reduced cost. The purpose of this chapter is to promote an understanding of the roles of nephrology nurses and the complex systems in which they work. Secondarily, interventions that promote personal achievement, job satisfaction, and quality care in a cost-contained arena are explored.

The roles of the nephrology nurse are imbedded in historical and current behavior patterns. We struggle with defining these roles so that we can effectively manage our role today and be prepared to respond to the needs of society in the future.

Theoretical Foundations of Roles

The patterns of behavior or roles that we learn are dependent upon internal and external variables in relation to environmental influences. How we learn, develop, and are motivated are a primary concern of individuals and organizations as they seek to harvest every measure of productivity out of their workers. As workers, nephrology nurses' knowledge of the principles of adult learning, professional development, and motivation, empowers them to take control over the roles that they balance.

The theory of adult learning, andragogy, was described by Malcolm Knowles (1990). The andragogical model is based on several assumptions: adults learn what they need to know; adults consider themselves in control; life experiences influence the learning process; adults learn when they are ready to learn; adults learn things that are life-centered; and adults must be motivated to learn. While adults are responsive to some external motivators (better jobs, promotions, higher salaries, and the like), the most potent motivators are internal pressures (the desire for increased job satisfaction, self-esteem, quality of life and the like) (Knowles, 1990, p. 63).

Table 3-1
Maslow hierarchy of needs.

5. Self-actualization
4. Self-esteem
3. Social
2. Safety
1. Physiological

How people are motivated in their personal, interpersonal, and organizational facets of life has been hotly debated. Many people have sought to explain the process of motivation. One of the best known motivational theories is Maslow's Hierarchy of Needs. Abraham Maslow's theory is based on two assumptions. The first assumption is that different needs are active at different times. The second assumption is that these needs are in a fixed order of importance or hierarchy (see Table 3-1) in which Maslow identified five categories of needs. His theory focuses on the internal needs of the individual, but does not account for environmental influences that impact on needs.

Frederick Herzberg developed a two-factor theory that separately explained job satisfaction and dissatisfaction. Factors whose presence prevent dissatisfaction are called hygiene factors or maintenance factors. Hygiene or maintenance factors refer to aspects of work that are peripheral to the task itself and more related to the external environment (job context) (Ivancevich, Lorenzi, Skinner, & Crosby, 1994, p. 366). Hygiene factors include (a) company policy and administrative practices; (b) technical supervision by the manager; (c) interpersonal relations with the supervisor; (d) worker salary, job status, and job security; (e) the worker's personal life; and (f) physical conditions of the work setting (Ivancevich, et al., 1994, p. 366).

Factors whose presence lead to satisfaction are called satisfiers or simply, motivational factors. These factors can produce high levels of motivation when they are present. Motivational factors relate directly to the job content and the specific aspects of a job. They include: achievement, recognition, advancement, the task or work itself, the worker's potential for personal learning or growth, and the worker's responsibility for results (cited in Ivancevich et al., 1994).

Types of Roles

A role is learned through a process of socialization. Socialization of employees occurs simultaneously along with the development of skills and the performance of expected roles (Benner, 1984; Smith & Gould, 1993). To adapt to the culture, individuals need to acquire the knowledge, skills, and values of the social culture within the organization. This helps new employees to set individual expectations and their roles within the organization. In addition, nurses new to nephrology nursing, must learn the language and unspoken rules of the organizational culture (Smith & Gould, 1993).

The patterns of behaviors found in a role are shaped by the context in which the role is found. The setting where the role is found tends to form or frame the content of that role. The role of nephrology nurses delivering care is influenced by the clinical and functional setting in which nurses practice. Nephrology nurses function differently as a transplant clinical specialist than a corporate clinical specialist. Therefore, the work environment influences and is influenced by the personal, interpersonal, and system domains where they practice nephrology nursing.

Personal Domain

Individuals occupy many positions within life. Positions are classifications of people and of status. For each position, there is an expected set of behaviors. The set or pattern of expected behaviors for a given position is called a role. At any given moment in time, nephrology nurses exhibit patterns of behaviors that arise from the personal, social, or occupational roles they fulfill. All individuals occupy multiple roles and therefore have multiple sets of ways they act. Individuals at one time act as wife, daughter, friend, volunteer, and nephrology nurse. When individuals hold several roles with a similar focus, they are referred to as subroles (Creasia, 1991). For every role there are subroles. An example is the nurse, as clinical nurse specialist, fulfills the subroles of manager, consultant, clinical expert, and educator.

As the number and types of roles and subroles held by individuals increases, the risk of conflicting behavioral expectations increases. These multiple individual roles sometimes have discrete boundaries that do not overlap. On other occasions, the role behaviors overlap and can exert an effect that is neutral, in conflict, or compatible with other occupied roles. Recent studies have shown that multiple involvements do not necessarily result in role conflict and can, in fact, lead to increased privileges, resources, and rewards (Campaniello, 1988). How individuals resolve conflict between competing roles can influence nurses' abilities to manage their role in particular nephrology settings. Identification of the strategies available to resolve conflict and strategies that work in different situations is of practical value. Controlling the negative impact of competing roles on individuals can promote job satisfaction and reduce job tension, overload, and turnover.

Interpersonal Domain

Individuals occupy many different roles. These roles also interact with the roles of other individuals. In most societies, the social structure consists of positions that are reciprocal, meaning they are dependent on one or more people for appropriate enactment of the role (Creasia, 1991). Nephrology nurses interact with physicians, technicians, administrators, social workers, dietitians, and other workers to fulfill their role. Without equipment and supplies they cannot dialyze, and without transportation the patients are not available for their care. As members of the nephrology team, nephrology nurses act in partnership with other interdisciplinary team members to provide quality patient care within a cost-contained arena. Strong networks of family, friends, and colleagues are a source of advice, mentoring, information, and support. Fulfillment of single or multiple roles in the interpersonal domain both impact and are impacted by the roles of others.

System Domain

Nurses occupy roles within the systems that they practice. The system can be occupational (paid) or voluntary (unpaid) in nature. Nursing, as an occupational role, is part of the health care system. Socialization to the occupational role is imbedded in first learning and then incorporating professional behaviors. These behaviors are learned through tacit information, skill, and experience (Benner, 1984). The overall development requires recognition of a professional status together with a clear and well-defined role. Olsson and Gullberg (1991) found a significant change in the distribution of role-conceptions that occurred after the nurses had experienced their first year as registered nurses, which did not occur during the educational process. Regardless of how well new nephrology nurses are oriented to their positions, their role-conception will still continue to develop through time and experience. This confirms the necessity and importance of role modeling, role repetition, and interactions with a professional group as part of the educational process (Olsson & Gullberg, 1991, p. 30).

Patterns of Behavior

Patterns of Professional Behaviors

One must act as a professional in order to be treated as a professional. So the question is, what behaviors are accepted by society as professional behavior? Professional characteristics (see Table 3-2) in any discipline include the following factors: a social mandate for the discipline; a professional society that maintains control over the standards of practice; a defined scope of practice and a body of specialized knowledge; the ability to control entry into the discipline; and group members' acceptance of a common ideology or societal mission (Baszanger, 1985). Along with the right to perform the work as it wishes, a profession normally claims rights to exclude other workers as deemed necessary, and to dominate public definitions of the tasks on competing professions (Abbott, 1988).

All professions claim their exclusive right to diagnose, treat, and draw inference within a defined area. Diagnosis and treatment are mediating acts: Diagnosis takes information into the professional knowledge system and treatment brings instructions back out from it. Inference, by contrast, is a purely professional act. It takes the information of diagnosis and indicates a range of treatments with their predicted outcomes (Abbott, 1988). A profession's formal knowledge system is ordered by abstractions alone. Like any knowledge, it is organized into a classification system and an inferential system (Abbott, 1988).

Professional nephrology nurses are accountable for their practice. Accountability is not a vague feeling or an obscure concept. It is a clear obligation that must be manifested as a structural component of nursing practice, based on responsibility, authority, and autonomy (Kelly, 1991).

Exemplar: A clinical nurse specialist (CNS) is contracted by a hospital department of nursing to evaluate the competency of its acute hemodialysis staff. The CNS interviews each of the full-time personnel, reviews documentation, and observes care in the clinical area. Three of the four nurses have more then 8 years of hemodialysis experience. Patient volume dictates the sharing of the nurse manager with the ICU. The new nurse manager has only 3 months of limited hemodialysis experience and encourages the hemodialysis nurses to manage the hemodialysis unit themselves. The CNS observed consistent lack of predialysis equipment and patient assessment, no evidence of a treatment plan, and lack of monitoring during initiation of treatment and troubleshooting. The orientation package for new employees contained information at least 8 years old. Policies and procedures were at least 5 years outdated. Self-scheduling was employed and attempts to accomplish office work during low census days was not evidenced. When asked what part of the hemodialysis program they liked the best each nurse replied "the autonomy."

Table 3-2
Professional characteristics.

- Societal Mandate for Discipline
- Professional Society
- Defined Scope of Practice
- Controls Entry into Practice
- Common Societal Mission

To these nurses, practice in an unmonitored environment is synonymous with autonomy. They fail to make the connection between accountability for practice and the ability of individual nurses to practice autonomously.

Autonomous practice is a benefit of respected individual behavior. Self-directed practice is grounded in the trust that individuals have conscientiously practiced within a defined and current scope of practice. In a study of 320 nurses, McCloskey (1990) found that the perception of autonomy was positively linked to motivation, commitment to the organization, and satisfaction (McCloskey, 1990).

For the nurses in the exemplar, it is important to help them identify the components of nephrology nursing practice and participate in professional behavior. The behavior patterns are manifested in the performance of duties and tasks and the assumption of certain responsibilities (Creasia, 1991). Nurses can only be accountable for those duties that are clearly designated and accepted as their responsibilities. In addition, nurses must have authority to act and be expected to use judgment based on knowledge in order to fulfill their responsibilities as professionals (Kelly, 1991). In the case cited, the nurses demonstrated few of the hallmarks of professional behavior. Their practice would be enhanced through participation in a professional organization, promotion of nephrology nursing-related inservice programs, and participation in nephrology nursing-related outservice activities.

The role of nurses responsible for nursing practice in the nephrology setting is to ensure that clinical personnel know their responsibilities. Responsibilities are delineated in nursing through practice acts of individual states, standards of care developed by recognized professional nursing groups, and position descriptions of organizations

(Kelly, 1991). Promotion of an environment of professional development sets the stage for nurses to behave professionally. It is through accountability, responsibility, and autonomy that nurses practice as professionals.

Nursing Behaviors

The nursing profession remains 97% female. It inevitably reflects members' prior socialization as women. For some, the integration of professional roles produces conflict with traditional socialization. Women are not expected to display masculine characteristics of ambition, achievement, competitiveness, or autonomy (Rosenow, 1988). Stereotypically women are caught between two worlds. On one hand they are expected to fulfill their traditional roles at home as wife, mother, and daughter. On the other hand, they are supposed to achieve success in their careers outside the home. As women balance the responsibilities of these often conflicting role expectations, they learn to work smarter not harder.

Females are described in relation to the characteristics of caring and sensitivity. Benner and Wrubel (1989) asserted that motivation is based on concern and caring about specific people, projects, things, and events. Because caring sets up what matters to a person, it also sets up what counts as stressful, and what options are available for coping (Benner & Wrubel, 1989). The women's liberation movement has charted the female's course away from caregiving work and toward traditional male values of competition, power, and wealth. Intelligent, achieving young women have often had a hard time selecting nursing as a career (Fagin, 1988). Aside from those important transformative feminists who value and act upon the caring imperative, women's caregiving work has become a negative standard against which we measure our progress (Gordon, 1991).

Feminine stereotypes have prevented males from entering nursing. Men report that although friends are generally supportive, they get negative reactions from other classmates and strangers, who sometimes show a tendency to view them as homosexuals. These attitudes have created some role strain for men, as they did for women in authority (Kelly, 1991).

The nursing profession continues to struggle with the problems of image and status. Research and public opinion polls regarding societal views of nurses indicate that the public views nurses as nurturant (feminine), concerned for others, and moderately well educated. Physicians, by contrast, are characterized by both high achievement (masculine) and high educational attainment (Kaler, Levy, & Schall, 1989). The caring stereotype of nurses apparently overshadows nurses' images as intelligent and autonomous professionals (Campbell-Heider & Hart, 1993). In addition, resistance to a uniform entry to practice at the bachelor's level by some nurses, only serves to fortify those who say that nursing is not a true profession.

Society's understanding of what nurses do is still poorly understood. The societal image of nursing is still one of handmaiden and vixen. Actually, few nurses objected to being sex objects (go ahead America, eat your heart out). They did not mind if people wanted to think nurses are beautiful and desirable and even sexy. But they did resent it when nurses were portrayed as bimbos on the boob tube: that hurt – and it undermined the credibility of the profession (Curtain, 1994, p. 10). The social architecture must promote nurse status, increase identification with their professional group, and abolish media images of nurses as powerless, dependent sex objects that assist physicians (Campbell-Heider, 1993).

Professional nursing practice has its own logic and content. The nursing process is used to express the logic of nursing. Essentially, the logic of a profession refers to the way its members learn to think and make decisions, to use professional knowledge in practice. The content of nursing refers to the knowledge base for practice; the facts and principles that have been tested through research and experience and found to be useful in practice (Beyers, 1991). Professional nursing practice requires that nurses make decisions using principles, concepts, and nursing theories. The way a nurse processes this information for outcomes is the logic of nursing (Beyers, 1991, p. 62).

Each profession is bound to a set of tasks by ties of jurisdiction, the strengths and weaknesses of these ties being established in the processes of actual professional work (Abbott, 1988). The tasks are often driven by the technology, which dictates the techniques used by the profession. There are few areas of nursing that are as closely linked to technology as nephrology nursing. The advent of plastic bags heralded the choice of continuous ambulatory peritoneal dialysis (CAPD) as a treatment option. The growth of home peritoneal dialysis resulted in increased numbers of nurses practicing in this modality. No one needs to mention the impact of the membrane technology or extracorporeal equipment on the specialty of nephrology nursing. The role of the professional nurse in a technical health care system is to have an appreciation of the full range of relationships that exist between technique and technology. To promote health, nurses must understand the nature of the techniques inherent in a given technology, as well as the variety and range of techniques that clients have developed in response to the technology with which they interact (Zwolski, 1989, p. 239).

Exemplar: A nurse has been practicing in a hemodialysis unit for five years. She has an excellent attendance record and can be counted on to do overtime as needed. She is very organized and can initiate dialysis on her own four patient assignment with technical accuracy. She is excellent at cannulation and is one of the best "stickers" in the unit. Her frustration is that she does not see any difference between herself and the technical staff in the unit. She has been overheard vocalizing her frustration of having so many years of education to do the same thing as a technician. She does not attend outside continuing education programs because her employer does not pay for her time off nor pay for the registration costs to attend.

This nurse has embraced the technological advances of health care, but fails to practice within her nursing profession. As a professional nurse in a technological arena, she is responsible for sharing her knowledge of technical skills with technical and nursing colleagues. She is responsible for continuing her professional education through participation in continuing education and networking activities. The role of the professional nurse in the technological environment is not only to perform on an expert level, but to professional growth, this nurse is a candidate for "burnout."

Zwolski (1989) goes on to support nursing behaviors that have implications for nursing practice, education, and cost-effectiveness: (a) ongoing and thorough assessment of the patients' response to techniques and technology they encounter in the health care system, including the ability to appraise critically and evaluate the effect of these techniques on clients; (b) decisions about when to use alternate health-promoting techniques and the power to implement these decisions; (c) patient advocacy; (d) involvement in health policy decisions; and (e) the conduct of research relevant to these concerns (Zwolski, 1989, p. 241).

Role Relationships

From the moment individuals decide to become a nephrology nurse, they begin to learn specific patterns of behavior that are unique to the specialty. Nephrology nursing assessment skills are focused on areas related to alterations in output, knowledge deficits in the areas of bone and blood metabolism, and alterations in body defense mechanisms, just to name a few. The specialty role also exists in relationship to other roles. Members of the specialty continually renegotiate their role with the roles of other individuals and organizations. In addition, multiple roles are held by one individual, and it is easy to understand why there is such an array of individual interpretations of those we meet in the nursing role.

The relationship between two roles or patterns of behavior at any given time can be seen as satisfying, conflicting, or neutral in relation to each other. Because roles are always changing, the relationship between any two roles is never static. As one continues to add new roles, adjustments in ongoing roles must be made to make the role constellation manageable (e.g., delegating household chores to spouse or children (Cresia, 1991). A study by Campaniello in 1988 showed that nurses with more roles experience greater well-being than nurses with fewer roles. Multiple role involvements do not necessarily result in role conflict and can lead to increased privileges, resources, and rewards (Campaniello, 1988). This fact is often seen in the clinical area as nurses who occupy multiple roles can balance the negative effects of one role by emerging themselves in a role that provides more satisfaction at that time.

In order to manage nursing practice, it is important to identify positive relationships among patterns of behavior, and reduce behaviors that create conflict and stress. There is ample literature demonstrating that multiple roles are associated with competing demands, which can lead to role overload and the resulting strain (McBride, 1988, p. 43).

Exemplar: An experienced nephrology nurse was dedicated to home, work, and volunteer activities. After adopting two children, she became a full-time mother while maintaining her volunteer work. She limited herself to three volunteer associations, but participated in them with full-time enthusiasm. After several years, she found that one volunteer activity was unrewarding and participation in the board of directors meetings caused great emotional distress. Although she continued her association with the volunteer organization, she focused her attention on her home and other volunteer activities to give her the positive emotional reinforcement she needed.

Participation in more than one role allows an individual opportunity to gain satisfaction while other areas of personal and/or professional life are stressful. Multiple roles and volunteer roles allow individuals to explore and express parts of themselves while engaging in the roles that are mandatory or less satisfying.

Numerous studies have found that job satisfaction, level of training, satisfaction with pay, and opportunities for promotion all have significant effects on intent to stay on the job for registered nurses (Dailey, 1990). It is important to identify the key components of job satisfaction. Employed women who report more positive experiences at work report fewer symptoms of psychological distress (Barnett & Marshall, 1992). McCloskey, in a 1989 study, found that autonomy and social integration are job concepts that are important for job contentment of newly employed staff nurses. When nurses have both, they are more satisfied, and are more committed to the organization, have more work motivation, and are more intent to remain on the job (McCloskey, 1990). Houston, Cates, and Kelly (1992) reported that for women employed full-time, more social support received from supervisors was associated with less job-related tension, less daily stress, and less tension in general.

Table 3-3
Strategies that alleviate role stress.

1. Modify contextual conditions.
2. Redefine role.
3. Delegate some functions.
4. Set priorities.
5. Eliminate some roles.

Note: Adapted from Creasia, J.L. (1991). Professional nursing roles. In J.L. Creasia & B. Parker (Eds.), *Conceptual foundations of professional nursing practice* (p. 79). St. Louis: Mosby Year Book.

Predicting the success of perspective employees entering nephrology nursing influences the quality of patient care delivered and the cost of that care by increasing length of employment and decreasing orientation costs of new employees. Studies show that having a higher percentage of RNs on staff improves patient outcomes and lowers mortality rates (Prescott, 1993, p. 192). Promotion of positive role behaviors and providing an environment conducive to professional growth are important components in maintaining stable nursing personnel patterns.

Contradictory job expectations result in role conflict. An example is the nephrology nursing supervisor trying to provide quality patient care with an inexperienced staff. Role conflict is defined as the incongruity of expectations associated with a role, while role ambiguity, is seen as the experience of having to deal with single or multiple roles that have not been clearly articulated in terms of expected behavior or performance levels (Lambert & Lambert, 1988). Clinical decision making is one example of uncertainty in which action is taken, possibly based on incomplete information, without assured knowledge of the outcome (Creasia, 1991). In the study for women employed full-time outside the home, role conflict, as well as underutilization of skills and quantitative overload, were positively associated with job-related tension and daily stress. Thus, role conflict, quantitative overload, and underutilization skills were related not only to distress experienced in regard to the job but also to distress that pervades the day (Houston et al., 1992).

Exemplar: As the result of corporate downsizing, a nephrology nurse assume a supervisory position of a new department as a consultant. The consultant was a clinical and management expert with a successful record of performance. Although given assurances of support, she found that as a consultant, she was unable to assist her personnel with computer problems, sign time cards, order department supplies, or participate in corporate planning sessions. She persisted in the role with success, but began experiencing headaches and weight gain.

This nurse exhibits the classic examples of role ambiguity. Although she was given the title and responsibility to establish her department, she lacked the power to effectively manage its operations.

In looking at the relationship between the job role and roles outside the occupation such as mother, Barnett and Marshall (1992) found that the quality of the maternal role, and not the occupancy of the role, predicts distress among employed mothers. For women employed full-time outside the home, supervisor social support was a variable with widespread associations being negatively related not only to job tension, daily stress, and tension in general, but also tending to be positively related to marital happiness and marital adjustment (Houston et al., 1992). Therefore, the importance of a good relationship between supervisors and workers is crucial to decreasing stress found in the work environment.

Assessing, identifying, and resolving role conflicts can prevent staff turnover. Accumulating research evidence shows that conflicting and ambiguous expectations from supervisors, co-workers, and administrative hierarchies lowers job satisfaction, raises job tension, and contributes to employee turnover (Dailey, 1990). Therefore, clear unimpeded communication is encouraged. Frequent staff meetings, communication boards, books, and up-to-date policies and procedures are crucial aspects to role management.

Role stress generated by social structure is said to exist when role obligations are vague, irritating, conflicting, or unrealistic (see Table 3-3 for strategies to relieve role stress). These conditions are external to individuals, but they may result in role strain, an internal response. Role strain is described as an emotional reaction to role stress that may be experienced as feelings of frustration, anxiety, irritability, or distress (Creasia, 1991). Role strain has been measured in such terms as somatization, depression, anxiety, obsessive compulsiveness, discomfort, anger/hostility, and dissatisfaction (McBride, 1988).

If nurses' value systems embrace the belief that nursing care should be provided by nurses rather than by nonprofessionals, then there is potential for role strain because of role incongruity (Creasia, 1991). Role strain is often experienced between nurses and technicians who perform hemodialysis. When there is too much professional work, nonprofessionals do it. Boundaries between professional jurisdictions therefore tend to disappear in worksites, particularly in overworked worksites (Abbott, 1988). A study by Blegen, Gardner, and McCloskey (1992) of 1,455 staff nurses revealed that nurses on units with the highest RN vacancies and highest workloads were most likely to turn over to assistants, and that, when RN vacancy rates and workloads are high, job satisfaction is low.

Finally, when too much work is expected in the allotted time or the role becomes too complex, role overload is experienced. This is a common problem for nurses that may be attributed to structural, contextual, or role-related factors (Creasia, 1991). Too much role strain and role conflict can lead to distress or burnout (Lewis et al., 1992; Lambert & Lambert, 1988). Lewis et al. (1992) found that work load was the major contributing factor to work-related stress for dialysis nurses. The primary aspects of work load that were stressful were excessive nonnursing tasks, inadequate time to complete nursing tasks, unpredictable staffing and scheduling, and inadequate staff to cover the dialysis unit (Lewis et al., 1992). This study also found a significant positive correlation between the size of the dialysis unit (patient population > 50) and reported stress.

Those charged with managing the clinical setting must be responsive in assuring the appropriate number and type of care providers, careful and timely attention to staff and patient scheduling, and appropriate disciplinary action for those staff who are unreliable.

Professional Roles in Nephrology Nursing

Nephrology nurses at any one time reflect a dynamic mixture of roles and subroles. They assume new roles and get rid of old ones. Nurses exhibit patterns of behavior that reflect personal, interpersonal, and organizational expectations and interpretation. Personal interpretation is seen when new nurses assume a new position. Nurses who are educational coordinators for dialysis units may assure CPR training, belong to a professional organization, provide didactic and clinical teaching, and assure outservice and inservice education. Other education coordinators may be chapter leaders, send long-term staff members out to become CPR trainers for the unit and physician office staff, develop and manage a program for professional and technical growth, and host educational and business activities at units. Both nurses have filled the essence of their role behavior, but the personal interpretation determines the scope of the exhibited role behavior. Factors that influence personal interpretation are nurses' intelligence, education, maturity, socioeconomic status, and cultural experiences.

Roles in nephrology nursing are dynamic. Performance of multiple clinical (see Table 3-4) and functional roles (see Table 3-5) is usually found. Nurses perform in diverse and often unrelated clinical settings. Gone are the days of narrow specialization. Nephrology nurses manage pharmacy, laboratory, and radiology units in addition to the renal service area. Conversely, operating room managers supervise employees providing care to the renal population.

Table 3-4
Clinical roles.

- Conservative management
- Hemodialysis
- Peritoneal dialysis
- Transplantation
- Apheresis
- Continuous renal replacement therapy
- Hemoperfusion
- Medical-surgical care
- Rehabilitative and custodial care

Table 3-5
Functional roles.

- Corporate
- Government
- Research
- Education
- Administration
- Consultation
- Clinical practice

Clinical Practice Roles

Delivery of quality patient care is grounded in the provision of that nursing care. These nurses care for any individuals with real or potential deficits in renal function. They practice within the scope of the nephrology nursing arena. Nursing within the nephrology nursing clinical practice role includes nurses who care for: chronic renal failure patients admitted for access declotting in the short procedure unit; patients requiring peritoneal dialysis in the medical-surgical unit; patients requiring continuous renal replacement therapy in the critical care unit; pediatric nephrology patients requiring rehabilitation; chronic renal failure patients in an outpatient facility; acutely ill patients in the hospital setting requiring dialysis; or posttransplant recipients. They demonstrate the full range of skills from novice to expert and reflect the variety of entry levels in nursing practice. These include diploma, associate, baccalaureate, master, and doctoral degrees. Nursing in certain areas requires a high degree of crossover knowledge with nephrology nursing including: medical-surgical, pediatrics, critical care, and quality control areas. Clinical practice roles also include hospital and outpatient staff nurse, advanced practice, and case management.

Table 3-6
The volunteer process.

1. Assessing the targeted organization.
2. Identifying other volunteers(s) within the organization to act as a mentor(s).
3. Expressing your needs, expectations, and goals.
4. Participating in planning volunteer development.
5. Participating in selected activities.
6. Evaluating the fit of volunteers and the organization.

Table 3-7
Mission statements.

- Must be operational.
- Focus in on what the association really tries to do.
- Enable participants to identify their contribution.
- The mission is forever.
- Reflect the state of the art.
- Are reviewed annually.

Note: Adapted from Drucker, P. (1990). *Managing the non-profit organization.* New York: Harper and Collins.

The American Nurses Association recently defined advanced practice nurses (APN). Nurses in advanced clinical nursing practice have a graduate degree in nursing. They conduct comprehensive health assessments, and demonstrate a high level of autonomy and expert skill in diagnosis and treatment of complex responses of individuals, families, and communities to actual and potential health problems. They formulate clinical decisions to manage acute and chronic illness and promote wellness. Nurses in advanced practice perform their clinical role, and function in collegial relationships with nursing peers, physicians, professionals, and others who influence the health environment (Mirr, 1993).

Currently, advanced practice nurses are functioning in four principle roles: nurse practitioner (NP), clinical nurse specialist (CNS), certified nurse midwife, and certified registered nurse anesthetist. Each of these roles requires the performance of specialized activities requiring advanced knowledge and skills (Moore, 1993). Numerous studies show that advanced practice nurses provide a high quality of care. The Office of Technology Assessment report concluded that physicians are more effective when treatment involves the use of technical solutions, but that the APNs are superior in situations dealing with chronic illness and those requiring communication skills (Moore, 1993).

Advanced practice nurses provide cost-effective service through lower fees, less-invasive procedures, less pharmacology expenses, and increased patient compliance. Delivery of health care services by a variety of providers is planned for the future of the health care system. The increased use of APNs will help to provide individuals with direct access to a full range of qualified providers (Moore, 1993, p. 604).

Current issues related to nursing practice include (a) lack of standardization concerning educational preparation and credentialing of nursing specialists in the profession; (b) nonspecificity of labels associated with nursing specialists; (c) blurring of roles among specialist groups (Moore, 1993, p. 607); and (d) prescriptive authority. The challenges lie primarily in issues concerning titling, education, practice, and regulatory restrictions (Mirr, 1993, p. 599). Nurses prepared at the masters level were planned to provide the critical link between research and clinical practice. It is now known that many of the skills required to integrate these two roles are developed on the doctoral level. Clinical nurse specialists practice in hospital or outpatient facility-based management, education, consultation, and research. The nurse practitioner is a community-based direct care provider with a community-based practice. Traditionally, CNS's have practiced in the acute care setting, and NP's have practiced in the primary care setting (Mirr, 1993, p. 599).

Today we see a merging of these roles irrespective of setting. Currently nurse practitioners practice in emergency rooms and critical care environments. Clinical nurse specialists make rounds on their own population of dialysis or transplant patients.

Case management is an approach to balancing the needs of patients and their families with those of the health industry and society (Conti, 1989, p. 58, cited in Creasia, 1991). Case managers assess, plan, integrate, coordinate, and advocate for patients and their families requiring services (Moore, 1993). As case managers, nurses use professional expertise to ensure coordinated and cost-effective care alternatives throughout the course of treatment (Creasia, 1991). Insurance and managed health care organizations rely heavily on nurses as case managers.

Advanced practitioners are responsible for possessing clinical decision-making skills, critical and scholarly thinking, an adequate research base to promote and provide research-based nursing care, knowledge of nursing models on which to base practice, leadership skills, and adequate practicum experience to perfect advanced practice skills.

Administrative Roles

Administration of nursing services should enable professional nursing practice (Creasia, 1991). Nurse administrators must activate staff to develop new communication patterns that disrupt sex role stereotypes, enhance nurses' self-esteem, build organizational trust, and model how professional nurses are to act (Campbell-Heider & Hart, 1993, p. 138). They accomplish this work through the management process of hiring, monitoring, evaluating, and holding onto employees. Administration subroles include administrator, manager, team leader, quality assurance, coordinator, director of nursing, and nursing supervisor.

Administrators must be sensitive to ways to (a) formalize a mechanism to allow nurses to participate in unit decision making to strengthen the clarity of their job description; (b) clarify work rules that apply to nurses; and (c) develop meaningful goals for nursing units where the goals originate from a comprehensive strategic plan for the hospital and nursing division (Dailey, 1990).

Educator

Nurse educators possess clinical skills and some form of teaching experience, including academe, preceptor, or mentor. They function in many arenas, including large audiences, units, small classes, and individuals. Expectations of this role include the responsibility of assessing needs, planning, organizing, implementing, and evaluating (American Nurses Association, 1992). Fifteen key functions were grouped under the following headings: Evaluator, Group Facilitator, Individual Development Counselor, Instructional Writer, Instructor, Manager of Training and Development, Marketer, Media Specialist, Needs Analyst, Program Administrator, Program Designer, Strategist, Task Analyst, Theoretician, and Transfer Agent (Abruzzese, 1992). Education subroles include: staff educator, patient educator, and organizational educator.

The major roles of the staff development educator were reiterated in the 1978 Guideline for Staff Development as those of facilitator, teacher, and resource person (American Nurses Association, 1978, cited in Abruzzese, 1992, p. 107). Educators' effectiveness is enhanced with the utilization of adult teaching/learning strategies and expert skills in structuring cost-effective, outcome-oriented educational opportunities (Abruzzese, 1992).

Current functions and responsibilities can be derived from the ANA's 1990 Standards for Nursing Staff Development, which provides criteria for 11 standards. The standards concern organization and administration, human resources and facilities, records and reports, evaluation, consultation, climate setting, and systematic inquiry. (Abruzzese, 1992). Some of the factors that influence the responsibilities of the staff development department are the following: overall future needs of the institution; incremental needs of each department; current resources for the nursing department; turnover trends; allocation of current and future resources, and institutional strategic plans (Abruzzese, 1992). Primary evaluation of staff development educators should be through a review of their self-designed plans to increase their areas of competency (Abruzzese, 1992).

Table 3-8
Responsibilities and duties of Board of Directors.

- Determine the association's mission and set policies for its operation.
- Set the association's overall program from year to year and engage in long-range planning.
- Establish fiscal policy and boundaries.
- Provide adequate resources for the association's activities.
- Select, evaluate, and if necessary, terminate the appointment of the chief executive.
- Develop and maintain a communication link to the community.

Note: Adapted from Wolf, T. (1990). *Managing a non-profit organization* (p. 29). New York: Simon & Schuster.

Table 3-9
Purpose of role descriptions.

- Groups similar jobs into classes with pay rates by class.
- Training.
- Source of evaluation criteria.
- Provide data to personnel managers.

Volunteer Role

Nurses spend a large percentage of their time engaged in volunteer activities (see Table 3-6). The volunteer role is indigenous to the United States. Achievement is the reward for work contributed without a paycheck. Volunteers derive many benefits from commitment to charitable activities. These benefits, which vary among individuals, might include a desire to: (a) make a difference, (b) get ahead in their careers, (c) develop professional and networking skills, (d) experience a sense of community, (e) work for an achievable goal, and (f) engage in self- renewal (Gould, 1994). Volunteer activities are part of the professional volunteer experience.

Table 3-10
Elements of a role description.

- Title
- General description
- Financial impact to the company
- Functions
- Relationships (lines of communication)
- Responsibilities
- Authority
- Standards of performance
- Accountability
- Qualifications

Table 3-11
The evaluation process.

1. Gather subjective and objective information about the individual.
   - Personal.
   - Peers.
   - Subordinates.
   - Supervisor.
2. Review individual objectives developed throughout the year.
3. Put all information into behavioral terms.
4. Match responsibilities of role description with actions of the individual.
5. Review the behavior, not the character of the individual.
6. Discuss the evaluation with employee.
   - Well prepared: thought-out, no whiteouts.
   - Prearranged time: scheduled so both have a time to mentally prepare.
   - Quiet and unhurried.
   - No interruptions.
   - Open minded - leave room to negotiate individual issues when possible.
7. Evaluate the fit of the role description to the individual role evaluation.
8. Supervisor and individual update and establish new goals/objectives.
9. Adjust role description as necessary.

Volunteers are recruited to roles established through the mission of an organization. Recruitment necessarily requires an understanding of the association's mission and the roles that forward that mission (see Table 3-7). Volunteer organizations survive when they convey a mission that is worthwhile personally and professionally. There are no guarantees that any nonprofit organization will continue to grow and develop. Therefore, careful assessment is important in selecting a volunteer organization.

Six major elements of successful national volunteer-based organizations were identified at a consensus meeting of major volunteer organizations. They include: (a) values consensus, (b) clarity of volunteer and paid-staff roles, (c) constructive relationships between a national headquarters and its local affiliates, (d) inclusiveness and diversity, (e) empowerment, and (f) collaboration and partnership building (Coolsen, 1992). Commitment to long-range strategic planning provides a framework for volunteer success. Assurances that associations will continue to represent the values or beliefs of their constituents are grounded in the fact that organizations are incorporated as nonprofit organizations. As such, volunteer organizations are bound by law to fulfill specific obligations.

A nonprofit organization exists for the sake of its mission, a public service mission. It reflects the fact that the nonprofit organization exists to bring about change in individuals and society (Drucker, 1990). Drucker goes on to state that a successful mission needs three things: opportunities, competence, and commitment (Drucker, 1990). These three components are reflected in the mission statement and evidenced by the roles available within the organization.

Nonprofits are organized as not-for-profit or charitable corporations. Charitable corporations are bound by law to give away a portion of their services. Nonprofits' governance structure precludes self-interest and private financial gain. To this end, officers and appointees sign a conflict of interest statement that specifically addresses these two issues. Nonprofit organizations possess special legal status that stipulate gifts made to them are tax deductible. Nonprofits are exempt from paying federal tax as long as they in good faith attempt to fulfill their mission.

Members of volunteer organizations serve in a variety of roles: appointed volunteers, elected volunteers, paid consultants, and paid staff. Volunteer roles include: policymakers, advisors, advocates, spokespersons, direct service providers, and managers (Coolsen, 1992). Each role requires a set of behaviors that volunteers are prepared by skill and experience to exhibit. It is through the activities of volunteers that key objectives of the organization are realized and the mission supported.

The Role of the Board of Directors

The Board of Directors are elected by association members. Their major roles (see Table 3-8) include: trustee, governor, sponsor, ambassador, and consultant (Drucker, 1990). As trustees, board members are: accountable to the state government that granted the association its charter, accountable to the federal government that granted tax-exempt status, and accountable to the public (Wolf, 1990).

The Role of Paid Staff Members

The role of paid staff members in a volunteer-based organization is to provide support for volunteers and maximize volunteer involvement and productivity (Coolsen, 1992). Indeed the role of the volunteer do-gooder of the 1950s has been replaced by the unpaid professional volunteer of the 1990s. The only difference in the motivation between the paid and unpaid professional of today is a paycheck.

To be successful, the relationship between paid staff members and unpaid staff members must be nonadversarial. The paid staff member's role is to make volunteers successfully feel good about their contributions. The best relationships foster a desire for volunteers to assure that paid-staff members are also recognized for their contributions. Positive relationships between the paid staff and unpaid staff are created through: a shared vision, a positive attitude about people, mutual respect between paid staff and volunteers, clear expectations, delegation, and accountability (Coolsen, 1992).

Role Descriptions

A role description is a statement about the responsibilities of the job. Role descriptions should be clear, simple, have concise words, use outline format, and use action verbs. A good role description is 2 to 3 pages in length. Writing the position description entails defining terms, competencies, functions, tasks, skills, and knowledge required for a specific role (see Table 3-9). Clarity is essential. Competency, as defined by Benner (1984), means a defined area of skilled performance, identified and described by its intent, function, and meanings. Functions refer to the normal characteristic activities of a person; skill is defined as a present observable competence; and knowledge refers to a body of learned information.

Role descriptions detail the organizational function of individuals (see Table 3-10). These functions arise from the philosophy, goal, objectives, and mission statement of organizations. Role descriptions are general when roles are dynamic and changing. Roles that are unchanging are written in specific terms. The position description usually outlines the levels of authority, the immediate supervisor, other reporting relationships, supervisory responsibilities, working conditions, and required knowledge, skills and abilities (Abruzzese, 1992, p. 110)

Role Evaluation

Evaluation is a process (see Table 3-11). It is an ongoing interaction between the employee in a role and the superior evaluating the individual's performance of that role. Role description and role evaluation are closely linked. Without the responsibility for an action there can be no accountability. Objectives found in role evaluation are taken from the role description.

There should be no surprises in an evaluation. Both praise and reprimand are close to the action. Therefore, evaluation is ongoing and dynamic. The performance evaluation examines the professional behavior, not the individual's character.

It remains to be seen what the long-term ramifications will be of the loss of the formal evaluation process through the increased use of consultants. Lost is the mandate to perform and document the evaluation process. Poor performance by a consultant is corrected by replacement with a new consultant. In order to make individuals more secure in their role, managers relay continuous praise. Evaluation can take place in the form of self-designed plans to increase their areas of competency (Abruzzese, 1992).

The strengths and weaknesses of employees should be discussed in terms of the performance standards, productivity standards, and values of the department and institution. The goal of all evaluation should be to increase the professional growth and proficiency of staff.

Summary

What will be nurses' roles in the future? Roles are certain to be influenced by political, social, technological, and environmental forces. It can almost be assured that health promotion through education and counseling, geriatric care, ambulatory care, and rehabilitation will be key elements. The nursing role will include managing and coordinating care, consulting with self-help groups, advocating, teaching, directing, and providing direct care and referral (Fagin, 1988). Research based practice will continue to grow. With their advancing knowledge base, nurses are becoming more assertive in their communication and involvement with other health care team members in an attempt to provide improved care (England, 1986).

References

Abbott, A.D. (1988). *The system of professions.* Chicago: The University of Chicago Press.

Abruzzese, R.S. (Ed.). (1992). *Nursing staff development: Strategies for success.* St Louis: Mosby Year Book.

American Nurses Association. (1992). *Guideline for staff development.* Washington, DC: Author.

Barnett, R.C. & Marshall, N.L. (1992). Worker and mother roles, spillover effects, and psychological distress. *Women & Health. 18*(2), 9-38.

Baszanger, I. (1985). Professional socialization and social control: From medical students to general practitioners. *Social Science and Medicine,* 20, 133-143.

Benner, P. (1984). *From novice to expert excellence and power in clinical practice.* Menlo Park, CA: Addison-Wesley Publishing Company.

Benner, P., & Wrubel, J. (1989). *The primacy of caring, stress and coping in health and illness.* Menlo Park, CA: Addison-Wesley Publishing Company.

Beyers, M. (1991). Enabling professional practice. In J.L. Creasia, & B. Parker (Eds.), *Conceptual foundations of professional nursing practice* (pp. 61-72). St. Louis: Mosby Year Book.

Blegen, M.A., Gardner, D.L., & McCloskey, J.C. (1992, January). Who helps you with your work? *American Journal of Nursing,* pp. 26-31.

Campbell-Heider, N., & Hart, C.A. (1993). Updating the nurse's bedside manner. IMAGE: *Journal of Nursing Scholarship, 25*(2), 133-138.

Campaniello, J.A. (1988). When professional nurses return to school: a study of role conflict and well-being in multiple-role women. *Journal of Professional Nursing, 4*(2), 136-140.

Coolsen, P. (1992). Six keys to strong volunteer networks. *Non-profit World, 10*(6), 22-25.

Creasia, J.L. (1991). Professional nursing roles. In J.L. Creasia & B. Parker (Eds.), *Conceptual foundations of professional nursing practice* (pp. 73-86). St. Louis: Mosby Year Book.

Curtain, L. (1994, June). 25 years: A slightly irreverent retrospective. *Nursing Management,* pp. 9- 32.

Dailey, R.C. (1990). Role perceptions and job tension as predictors of nursing turnover. *Nursing Connections* 3(2), 33-42.

Drucker, P. (1990). *Managing the non-profit organization.* New York: Harper and Collins.

England, D.A. (1986). *Collaboration in nursing.* Rockville, MD: Aspen Systems Corporation.

Fagin, C.M. (1988). The visible problems of an invisible profession: the crisis and challenge for nursing. *ANNA Journal, 15*(2), 104-109.

Gordon, S. (1991, February). Fear of caring: The feminist paradox. *American Journal of Nursing,* pp. 45-48.

Gould, M.A. (1994). Volunteerism: A method of self-renewal. *ANNA Journal, 21*(5), 297-298.

Houston, B.K., Cates, D.S. & Kelly, K.E. (1992). Job stress, psychosocial strain, and physical health problems in women employed full-time outside the home and homemakers. *Women & Health, 19*(1), 1-26.

Ivancevich, J.M., Lorenzi, P., Skinner, S.J., & Crosby, P.B. (1994). *Management: Quality and competitiveness.* Boston: IRWIN Publishers.

Kaler, S.R., Levy, D.A., & Schall, M. (1989). Stereotypes of professional roles. *Image, 21,* 85-89.

Kelly, L.Y. (1991). Professional ethics and accountability. In *Dimensions of professional nursing* (pp. 200-225, sixth edition). New York: Pergamon Press.

Knowles, M.(1990). *The adult learner* (4th edition). Houston, TX: Gulf Publishing.

Lambert, C.E., & Lambert, V.A. (1988). A review and synthesis of the research on role conflict and its impact on nurses involved in faculty practice programs. *Journal of Nursing Education, 27*(2), 54-60.

Lewis, S.L., Campbell, M.A., Becktell, P.J., Cooper, C.L., Bonner, P.N., & Hunt, W.C. (1992). Work stress, burnout, and sense of coherence among dialysis nurses. *ANNA Journal, 19*(6), 545-553.

McBride, A.B. (1988). Mental health effects of women's multiple roles. *IMAGE: Journal of Nursing Scholarship,* 20(1), 41-47.

McCloskey, J.C. (1990). Two requirements for job contentment: Autonomy and social integration. *IMAGE: Journal of Nursing Scholarship, 22*(3), 140-143.

Mirr, M.P. (1993). Advanced clinical practice: A reconceptualized role. *AACN Clinical Issues, 4*(4), 599-602.

Moore, S.M. (1993). Promoting advanced practice nursing. *AACN Clinical Issues, 4*(4), 603-608.

Olsson, H.M., & Gullberg, M.T. (1991). Nursing education and definition of the professional nurse role. Expectations and knowledge of the nurse role. *Nurse Education Today, 11,* 30-36.

Prescott, P.A. (1993). Nursing: An important component of hospital survival under a reformed health care system. *Nursing Economic$, 11*(4), 192.

Rosenow, A.M. (1988). *What is achievement . Socialization, sexism, and stereotyping.* Prospect Heights, IL: Waveland Press.

Smith, L.J., & Gould, M.A. (1993). Orientation to the specialty. In P. Jordan (Ed.), *Nephrology nursing: A guide to professional development.* Pitman, NJ: American Nephrology Nurses' Association.

Wolf, T. (1990). *Managing a nonprofit organization.* New York: Simon & Schuster.

Zwolski, K. (1989). Professional nursing in a technical system. *IMAGE: Journal of Nursing Scholarship, 21*(4), 248-242.

Suggested Readings

Chimner, N.E., & Easterling, A. (1993). Collaborative practice through nursing case management. *Rehabilitation Nursing, 18*(4), 226-230.

Chitty, K.K. (1993). *Professional nursing concepts and challenges.* Philadelphia: W.B. Saunders Company.

Dixon, J.P., Dixon, J.K., & Spinner, J.C. (1991). Tensions between career and interpersonal commitments as a risk factor for cardiovascular disease among women. *Women & Health, 17*(3), 33- 57.

Gales, K.L. (1987). The recruitment process. In E.M. Lewis, & J.G. Spicer (Eds.), *Human resource management handbook.* Rockville, MD: Aspen Systems Publications.

Lewis, S.L., Bonner, P.N., Campbell, M.A., Cooper, C.L. & Willard, A. (1994). Personality, stress, coping and sense of coherence among nephrology nurses in dialysis settings. *ANNA Journal, 21*(6), 325-335.

Moloney, M.M. (1992). *Professionalization of nursing current issues and trends* (2nd edition). Philadelphia: J.B. Lippincott Company.

Rich, V.L., & Rich, A.R. (1987). Personality hardiness and burnout in female staff nurses. *IMAGE: Journal of Nursing Scholarship, 19*(2), 63-66.

Thibodeau, J.A., & Hawkins, J.W. (1994). Moving toward a nursing model in advanced practice. *Western Journal of Nursing Research, 16*(2), 205-218.

Chapter Highlights

- The roles of the nephrology nurse are a dynamic constellation of behaviors.
- The patterns of behavior or role that we learn are dependent upon internal and external variables in relation to environmental influences.
- A role is learned through a process of socialization. To adapt to the culture, individuals need to acquire the knowledge, skills, and values of the social culture within the organization.
- As the number and types of roles and subroles held by individuals increases, the risk of conflicting behavioral expectations increases.
- As members of the nephrology team, nephrology nurses act in partnership with other interdisciplinary team members to provide quality patient care within a cost-contained arena.
- Professional characteristics in any discipline include the following factors: a social mandate for the discipline; a professional society that maintains control over the standards of practice; a defined scope of practice and a body of specialized knowledge; the ability to control entry into the discipline; and group members' acceptance of a common ideology or societal mission (Baszanger, 1985).
- Autonomous practice is a benefit of respected individual behavior. Self-directed practice is grounded in the trust that individuals have conscientiously practiced within a defined and current scope of practice.
- Responsibilities are delineated in nursing through practice acts of individual states, standards of care developed by recognized professional nursing groups, and position descriptions of organizations (Kelly, 1991) . ... It is through accountability, responsibility, and autonomy that nurses practice as professionals.
- Research and public opinion polls regarding societal views of nurses indicate that the public views nurses as nurturant (feminine), concerned for others, and moderately well educated.
- Resistance to a uniform entry to practice at the bachelor's level by some nurses, only serves to fortify those who say that nursing is not a true profession.
- The content of nursing refers to the knowledge base for practice: the facts and principles that have been tested through research and experience and found to be useful in practice (Beyers, 1991).
- The relationship between two roles or patterns of behavior at any given time can be seen as satisfying, conflicting, or neutral in relation to each other.
- Multiple role involvements do not necessarily result in role conflict and can lead to increased privileges, resources, and rewards (Campaniello, 1988).
- Numerous studies have found that job satisfaction, level of training, satisfaction with pay, and opportunities for promotion all have significant effects on intent to stay on the job for registered nurses (Dailey, 1990).
- Members of volunteer organizations serve in a variety of roles: appointed volunteers, elected volunteers, paid consultants, and paid staff. Volunteer roles include: policymakers, advisors, advocates, spokespersons, direct service providers, and managers (Coolsen, 1992).
- Role description and role evaluation are closely linked; without the responsibility for an action there can be no accountability.

UNIT 2

Conceptual Themes Basic to Nephrology Nursing

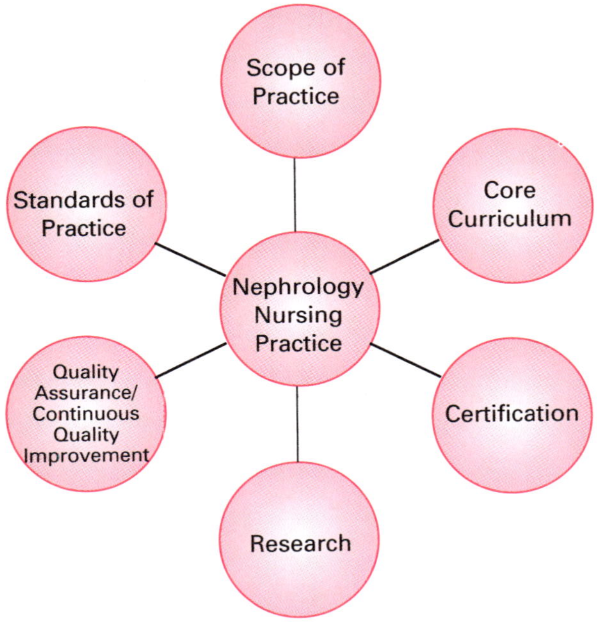

Unit Contents

Chapter 4
Use of Conceptual Models in Nephrology Nursing Practice. . . 61
Jacqueline Fawcett, PhD, RN, FAAN; Marguerite F. Hartigan, MSN, RN, CNN; Marcia Keen, MS, RN; Evelyn Butera, MS, RN, CNN; Annette C. Frauman, PhD, RN, FAAN; Diane Breckenridge, PhD, MSN, RN; Susan Taylor Hooper, PhD, RN; Donna Mapes, DNSc, RN; Marilyn L. Neff, MBA, RN, CNN, CNAA; Linda J. Smith, MSN, RN, CNN, C

Chapter 5
Ethical Issues in Nephrology Nursing 83
Rosalie Starzomski, PhD, MN, RN

Chapter 6
Research in Nephrology Nursing: Overview, Development, and Future Directions 111
Anita E. Molzahn, PhD, RN

CHAPTER 4

Use of Conceptual Models in Nephrology Nursing Practice

Jacqueline Fawcett, Consultant
Marguerite F. Hartigan
Marcia Keen, Chairperson
Evelyn Butera
Annette C. Frauman
Diane M. Breckenridge
Susan Taylor Hooper
Donna Mapes
Marilyn L. Neff
Linda J. Smith

Chapter Contents

Conceptual Models of Nursing 63
Functions of Conceptual Model 67
The Value of Conceptual Models for Nursing Practice 68
Conceptual Models of Nursing and Nephrology Nursing Practice 69
Review of the Literature 69
Accomplishments of the ANNA Conceptual Models Task Force 70
The Roy Adaptation Model of Nursing 71
Development of a Nephrology Nursing Assessment Tool 71
Development of a Typology of Nephrology Nursing Interventions 76
Linking the Assessment Tool and Intervention Typology to the ANNA Standards of Clinical Practice 76
Future Directions 76
Summary 76
References 79
Nursing Notes About Conceptual Models 81
Chapter Highlights 82

Use of Conceptual Models in Nephrology Nursing Practice

Jacqueline Fawcett, Consultant
Marguerite F. Hartigan
Marcia Keen, Chairperson
Evelyn Butera
Annette C. Frauman
Diane M. Breckenridge
Susan Taylor Hooper
Donna Mapes
Marilyn L. Neff
Linda J. Smith

The purpose of this chapter is to discuss the use of conceptual models of nursing in nephrology nursing practice. The chapter begins with a definition and description of conceptual models and a discussion of the contribution of conceptual models to clinical nursing practice. Next, a review of the literature dealing with the use of conceptual models as guides for nephrology nursing is presented. The chapter continues with a detailed discussion of the work accomplished by the American Nephrology Nurses' Association Conceptual Models Task Force. The chapter concludes with recommendations for future work with conceptual models in nephrology nursing practice.

Conceptual Models of Nursing

Conceptual models have existed since people began to think about themselves and their surroundings. They now exist in all areas of life and in all disciplines. Indeed, everything that a person sees, hears, reads, and experiences is filtered through the cognitive lens of some conceptual frame of reference (Lachman, 1993).

The term conceptual model is synonymous with the terms conceptual framework, conceptual system, paradigm, and disciplinary matrix. A conceptual model is defined as a set of abstract and general concepts and propositions that present a particular perspective about the phenomena of interest to a discipline. Conceptual models of nursing present diverse perspectives of the nursing recipient, who can be an individual, a family, or a community; the environment of the recipient, as well as the environment in which nursing occurs; the health state of the recipient; and the definition and goals of nursing, as well as nursing actions or interventions.

Concepts are words that describe mental images of phenomena. The abstract and general concepts of a conceptual model are not limited to any particular individual, group, situation, or event. Rather, they can refer to many different people in a broad range of situations. For example, the concept of an adaptive system can refer to several types of systems, including individuals, families, groups, communities, and entire societies that are experiencing a wide variety of events (Roy & Andrews, 1991).

Propositions are statements that describe or link concepts. Some conceptual model propositions are general descriptions or definitions of the conceptual model concepts. Because conceptual model concepts are abstract and general, definitions typically are broad. More specifically, definitional propositions for conceptual model concepts do not state how the concepts are empirically observed or measured, and they should not be expected to do so. Adaptation level, for example, is broadly defined as "a changing point that represents the person's ability to respond positively in a situation" (Roy & Andrews, 1991, p. 4).

Other propositions state the relationships between conceptual model concepts in a general manner. They are exemplified by the following statement: Changes in environmental stimuli are associated with changes in adaptation level (Roy & Andrews, 1991).

Conceptual models are not really new to nursing, as they have existed since Nightingale (1859) first advanced her ideas about nursing. Most early conceptualizations of nursing, however, were not presented in the formal manner of models. The works of several nurse scholars currently are recognized as conceptual models. Among the best known are Johnson's Behavioral System Model, King's General Systems Framework, Levine's Conservation Model, Neuman's Systems Model, Orem's Self-Care Framework, Rogers's Science of Unitary Human Beings, and Roy's Adaptation Model (Johnson, 1990; King, 1990; Levine, 1991; Neuman, 1995; Orem, 1995; Rogers, 1990; Roy & Andrews, 1991). An overview of the perspective of the recipient, the environment, health, and nursing presented by each of those nursing models is given in Table 4-1.

Table 4-1
Overview of seven conceptual models of nursing.

Conceptual Model	Nursing Recipient	Environment	Health	Nursing
Johnson's Behavioral System Model	A behavioral system with seven subsystems: Attachment Dependency Ingestion Elimination Sexual Aggression Achievement	Internal External	Behavioral system balance and stability. Efficient and effective behavioral functioning. Purposeful, orderly, and predictable behavior.	*Definition*: A service that is complementary to that of medicine and other health professions, but which makes its own distinctive contribution to the health and well-being of people. *Goal*: Restore, maintain, or attain behavioral system balance and stability. *Actions*: Impose external regulatory or control mechanisms. Alter set or add choices for behavior. Provide protection, nurturance, or stimulation.
King's General Systems Framework	Personal system: Focus on perception, self, growth and development, body image, time, space, learning. Interpersonal system: Focus on interaction, communication, transaction, role, stress, coping. Social system: Focus on organization, authority, power, status, decision-making, control.	Internal External	Dynamic life experiences of a human being. Ability to function in social roles.	*Definition*: Perceiving, thinking, relating, judging, and acting vís-a-vís the behavior of individuals who come to a nursing situation. *Goal*: Help individuals maintain their health so they can function in their roles. *Actions*: A process of action, reaction, interaction, and transaction directed toward establishment of goals and goal attainment.

Table 4-1 (continued)
Overview of seven conceptual models of nursing.

Conceptual Model	Nursing Recipient	Environment	Health	Nursing
Levine's Conservation Model	A holistic being, a system of systems. Organismic responses are fight or flight, stress, basic orienting system, visual system, auditory system, haptic system, taste-smell system.	Operational Perceptual Conceptual	Health and disease are patterns of adaptive change	*Definition*: A human interaction. *Goal*: Promotion of wholeness for people, sick or well. *Actions*: Conservation of energy, structural integrity, social integrity, personal integrity.
Neuman's Systems Model	A client system composed of five variables: Physiological Psychological Sociocultural Developmental Spiritual Central core surrounded by flexible and normal lines of defense and lines of resistance	Internal External Created	Client system stability	*Definition*: A unique profession that is concerned with all the variables affecting an individual's response to stressors. *Goal*: To facilitate optimal wellness through retention, attainment, or maintenance of client system stability. *Actions*: Primary prevention Secondary prevention Tertiary prevention

Table 4-1 (continued)
Overview of seven conceptual models of nursing.

Conceptual Model	Nursing Recipient	Environment	Health	Nursing
Orem's Self-Care Framework	Self-care agent Therapeutic self-care demand made up of: Universal self-care requisites Developmental self-care requisites Health deviation self-care requisites	The person's external surroundings	Soundness or wholeness of developed human structures and of bodily and mental functioning	*Definition*: A helping service, a creative effort to help people. *Goal*: Help people to meet their own therapeutic self-care demands. *Actions*: Wholly compensatory, partly compensatory, and supportive-educative nursing systems. Assist by: acting for or doing, guiding, physical and/or psychological support, providing a developmental environment, teaching.
Rogers's Science of Unitary Human Beings	A unitary human being, a patterned, open, pandimensional energy field.	A patterned, open, pandimensional energy field	An expression of the life process	*Definition*: A learned profession that is both a science and an art. *Goal*: Help people achieve maximum well-being. *Actions*: Deliberative mutual patterning that involves environmental patterning to promote helicy, integrality, and resonancy.

Table 4-1 (continued)
Overview of seven conceptual models of nursing.

Conceptual Model	Nursing Recipient	Environment	Health	Nursing
Roy's Adaptation Model	An adaptive system with four response modes: Physiological Self-Concept Role Function Interdependence Regulator and cognator coping mechanisms	Focal stimuli Contextual stimuli Residual stimuli	Being and becoming an integrated and whole person	*Definition:* A theoretical system of knowledge which prescribes a process of analysis and action related to care of the ill or potentially ill person. *Goal:* Promotion of adaptation *Actions:* Management of environmental stimuli, including increasing, decreasing, maintaining, removing, altering or changing.

Note: Adapted from Fawcett, J. (1992a). Documentation using a conceptual model of nursing. *Nephrology Nursing Today, 2*(5), 3, ©Adverceutics, Inc., 1992, with permission.

As can be seen in Table 4-1, the content of each conceptual model is stated in a distinctive vocabulary. Moreover, the meaning of each term is connected to the unique focus of the conceptual model. Thus, the same or similar terms may have different meanings in different conceptual models. For example, adaptation is defined as a response to stimuli in Roy's Adaptation Model, and as a way in which the person and the environment become congruent over time in Levine's Conservation Model.

The vocabulary of each conceptual model should not be considered jargon. Rather, the terminology used by the author of each conceptual model is the result of considerable thought about how to convey the meaning of that particular perspective to others (Biley, 1990). Furthermore, as Akinsanya (1989) pointed out, "Every science has its own peculiar terms, concepts, and principles that are essential for the development of its knowledge base. In nursing, as in other sciences, an understanding of these is a prerequisite to a critical examination of their contribution to the development of knowledge and its application to practice" (p. ii).

Functions of Conceptual Models

A conceptual model provides a distinctive frame of reference and "a coherent, internally unified way of thinking about . . . events and processes" (Frank, 1968, p. 45) that tells clinicians how to observe and interpret the phenomena of interest to their discipline. Each conceptual model, then, presents a unique focus that has a profound influence on the clinician's perceptions of people, events, and situations. The unique focus of each model is an approximation or simplification of reality that includes only those concepts that the model author considers relevant and as aids to understanding. Thus, certain aspects of the phenomena of interest to a discipline are regarded as particularly relevant, and other aspects are ignored. For example, Neuman's Systems Model focuses on preventing the deleterious impact of stressors, whereas Orem's Self-Care Framework emphasizes enhancing the person's self-care capabilities and actions. Note that Neuman's model does not deal with self-care, and Orem's does not focus on the impact of stressors.

Each conceptual model also provides a systematic structure and a rationale for practical activities. More specifically, each conceptual model gives direction to the search for relevant questions about phenomena and suggests solutions to practical problems. Each one also provides general criteria for knowing when a problem has been solved. Those features of a conceptual model are illustrated in the following example. The Roy Adaptation Model focuses on adaptation of the person to environmental stimuli, and proposes that nursing management of the most relevant stimuli leads to adaptation (Roy

& Andrews, 1991). For example, a salient clinical question is: What are the most relevant stimuli in a given situation? Clinicians who are interested in solutions to problems in adaptation would focus on the various ways of managing stimuli, and they would look for manifestations of adaptation when evaluating whether management of relevant stimuli solved the problem in adaptation.

Furthermore, conceptual models of nursing "provide [explicit] philosophical and pragmatic orientations to the service nurses provide patients—a service which only nurses can provide—a service which provides a dimension to total care different from that provided by any other health professional" (Johnson, 1987, p. 195). Conceptual models of nursing provide explicit orientations not only for nurses but also for the general public. They identify the purpose and scope of nursing and provide frameworks for objective records of the effects of nursing. Johnson (1987) explained, "Conceptual models specify for nurses and society the mission and boundaries of the profession. They clarify the realm of nursing responsibility and accountability, and they allow the practitioner and/or the profession to document services and outcomes" (pp. 196–197).

The development of conceptual models of nursing and labeling them as such is an important advancement for the discipline. Reilly's (1975) comments help to underscore this point:

> We all have a private image (concept) of nursing practice. In turn, this private image influences our interpretation of data, our decisions, and our actions. But can a discipline continue to develop when its members hold so many differing private images? The proponents of conceptual models of practice are seeking to make us aware of these private images, so that we can begin to identify commonalities in our perceptions of the nature of practice and move toward the evolution of a well-ordered concept (p. 567).

Johnson (1987) also pointed out that nurses always use some frame of reference for their activities and explained the drawbacks of implicit frameworks. She stated:

> It is important to note that some kind of implicit framework is used by every practicing nurse, for we cannot observe, see, or describe, nor can we prescribe anything for which we do not already have some kind of mental image or concept. Unfortunately, the mental images used by nurses in their practice, images developed through education and experience and continuously governed by the multitude of factors in the practice setting, have tended to be disconnected, diffused, incomplete and frequently, heavily weighted by concepts drawn from the conceptual schema used by medicine to achieve its own social mission (p. 195).

Each conceptual model of nursing, then, is the public presentation of its author's private image of nursing. Use of an explicit conceptual model facilitates communication among nurses and provides a systematic approach to nursing practice, as well as to nursing research, education, and administration.

The most tangible function of a conceptual model is its delineation of goals for nursing practice (see Table 4-1) and a nursing process format that encompasses parameters for assessment, labels for patient/client problems, a strategy for planning nursing care, a set of nursing interventions, and criteria for evaluation of the outcomes of nursing care (Fawcett, 1995). A conceptual model, therefore, provides a distinctive context and coherent format for the generic nursing process of assessment, labeling or diagnosis, planning, intervention, and evaluation. In short, a conceptual model of nursing provides a structure for documentation of all aspects of the nursing process, from patient assessment to evaluation of outcomes. Furthermore, a conceptual model also helps to identify standards of nursing practice and criteria for quality assurance reviews.

The Value of Conceptual Models for Nursing Practice

The number of nurses throughout the world who recognize the value of conceptual model-based nursing practice is rapidly increasing. As Chalmers (cited in Chalmers, Kershaw, Melia, & Kendrich, 1990) pointed out, "Nursing models have provided what many would argue is a much-needed alternative knowledge base from which nurses can practice in an informed way. An alternative, that is, to the medical model which for so many years has dominated many aspects of health care" (p. 34). Nursing models also provide an alternative to the institutional model of practice, in which "the most salient values [are] efficiency, standardized care, rules, and regulations" (Rogers, 1989, p. 113). The institutional model, moreover, typically upholds, reinforces, and supports the medical model (Grossman & Hooton, 1993).

In fact, conceptual models of nursing provide explicit frames of reference for *professional* nursing practice by delineating the scope of nursing practice and by identifying who the recipient of nursing is, what the relevant environment is, what aspects of health are to be considered, and what the steps and substance of the nursing process are. As such, conceptual models of nursing move the practice of nursing away from that driven by a medical or institutional model and, therefore, foster autonomy from medicine and a coherent purpose of practice (Bélanger, 1991; Bridges, 1991; Ingram, 1991). Furthermore, conceptual models specify innovative goals for nursing practice and introduce ideas that are designed to improve practice (Lindsay, 1990) by facilitating the identification of relevant information, reducing the fragmentation of care, and improving the coordination of care (Chalmers, cited in Chalmers et al., 1990). In particular, conceptual models provide a nursing knowledge base that has a positive effect on practice "by enabling well-coordinated care to take place, by providing a basis for the justification of care actions, and by enabling nurses to *talk nursing*" (Chalmers, cited in Chalmers et al., 1990, p. 34) and to *think nursing* (Perry, 1985).

Hayne (1992), moreover, pointed out that although some clinicians hold the "unfortunate view [that conceptual models] are the inventions and predictions only of scholars and academics [that have] little significance for their own practice environments," many other clinicians recognize the beneficial effects of conceptual models on practice (p. 105). Indeed, conceptual model-based nursing practice "help[s] nurses better communicate what they do" (Neff, 1991, p. 534) and why they do it.

The importance of communicating what nursing is and what nurses do is especially important during the current era of health care reform that is taking place in the United States and other countries. Nurses *must* be clear about their mission in relation to that of other groups of health care providers. Indeed, it is crucial that nurses explicate *what they know and why they do what they do.* In other words, it is crucial that nurses communicate *nursing* knowledge and explain how that knowledge governs the actions that they perform on behalf of or in conjunction with people who require health care.

Conceptual Models of Nursing and Nephrology Nursing Practice

Review of the Literature

A review of the literature revealed that conceptual models of nursing have been used as guides for nephrology nursing practice for more than a decade, albeit in a limited manner. Johnson's Behavioral Systems Model was the basis for a tool to measure outcome criteria for fluid and electrolyte balance in patients with chronic renal failure developed by Bruce and colleagues (1980). The tool includes items that reflect the ingestive, eliminative, and achievement subsystems, and it can be used in quality assurance programs for patients with chronic renal failure.

King's General Systems Framework was the basis for the goal-oriented nursing record (GONR). The GONR, which contains space for demographic and health data, problem list, goal list, nursing care plan, and progress notes, can be used to document the nursing care of chronic renal failure clients (King, 1984).

The Neuman Systems Model also has served as the basis for the development of tools used to document nephrology nursing practice. Breckenridge (1982) described the use of an assessment/intervention tool for both renal failure and transplant clients. Breckenridge, Cupit, and Raimondo (1982) expanded the assessment portion of the assessment/intervention tool and described its use with clients receiving continuous ambulatory peritoneal dialysis (CAPD). They later noted that the tool represents an effective measure of the quality of the CAPD client's life (Breckenridge, Cupit, & Raimondo, 1983). In a subsequent paper, Breckenridge (1989) identified potential stressors encountered by patients with renal disease and a typology of primary prevention interventions derived from the Neuman Systems Model. She also identified the major nursing diagnoses and level of prevention intervention (primary, secondary, or tertiary) required for clients with renal failure, clients receiving hemodialysis or CAPD, and postrenal transplant clients. In addition, Breckenridge (1995) explained how the Neuman Systems Model can be used to guide both qualitative and quantitative research to determine the most effective ways to prevent further deterioration in function and enhance life satisfaction of clients with chronic renal failure.

Moreover, the Neuman Systems Model has been used to guide nephrology nursing research. Herald (1994) explored the effects of aminoglycoside antibiotics (gentamicin, tobramycin, amikacin) on the physiological variables of hydration status and renal function. She found that patients who were taking the antibiotics and who were in the surgical intensive care unit were less likely to have impaired renal function than those in the medical intensive care unit.

Orem's Self-Care Framework has been used to guide the nursing care of patients with chronic renal failure. Perras and Zappacosta (1982) described the successful use of the Self-Care Framework in promoting the self-care abilities of patients who require peritoneal dialysis. Zinn (1986) and Turner (1989) explained how the Self-Care Framework can be used to guide patient teaching about chronic renal failure and peritoneal dialysis, respectively. Norris (1991) explained how the Self-Care Framework can be used to organize and direct the nursing care of adolescent renal transplant recipients in outpatient settings. Summerton (1995) described nurse-led, self-care treatment programs for patients with chronic renal failure.

Hathaway and Strong (1988) described the influence of the Self-Care Framework on nursing practice on the renal transplant unit at the University of Tennessee, Memphis, William F. Bowld Hospital. They noted that the use of the Self-Care Framework and related research to guide nursing practice is an evolutionary and subtle process that can succeed when nurses are willing to ask questions, seek answers, and be receptive to innovative approaches to practice.

In addition, Orem's Self-Care Framework has been used to guide practice-related nephrology nursing research. Miller (1986) measured predialysis and dialysis patients' perceptions of their self-care agency. The study findings revealed no differences in perceptions of self-care agency between the two groups of patients. Miller's findings also revealed that the presence of a support person enhanced the patient's perception of self-care agency. Hayward and her colleagues (1989) reported the development of a questionnaire to measure stressors experienced by new renal transplant patients. They linked the tool to the Self-Care Framework through their conceptualization of stress as a self-care deficit, reasoning that stress "may limit a person's agency (ability) to meet some or all therapeutic self-care demands" (p. 81). Beecroft (1990) investigated the effect of an 8-week program of cognitive restructuring and assertive skills training on the self-care agency of three adolescent males who were receiving hemodialysis. The study findings indicated that the young men demonstrated consistent improvement in social skills behavior. Lapp (1992) examined the effect of patient and staff education on dialysis patients' willingness to adhere to the treatment regimen. Her results revealed an increase in patients' knowledge and a decrease in morbidity. Korniewicz and O'Brien (1994) evaluated the effects of a Self-Care Framework-based program of nursing support and one-to-one teaching sessions on hemodialysis patients' physical and psychosocial responses to chronic renal failure. Their study findings indicated that the program enhanced active learning by the patients. Pressly (1994) investigated the relationship of psychosocial characteristics and the incidence of complications in patients receiving continuous ambulatory peritoneal dialysis (CAPD). She found that the psychosocial characteristic of autonomy was related to the total number of infectious complications and the length of time to the first episode of peritonitis.

Rogers' Science of Unitary Human Beings has been used to guide a study of adults waiting for a kidney transplant (Stoeckle, 1993). The investigator found that, on average, the 23 study subjects reported high health-related hardiness and low to moderate uncertainty. In addition, the subjects reported that communication with and support from physicians, nurses, family, and friends, as well as faith, were helpful environmental factors. Difficult environmental factors included the uncertainty related to the time required to wait for a transplant and the difficulty in finding a match.

The Roy Adaptation Model has been used to guide and document nephrology nursing practice. Frank (1988) explained how the Roy Adaptation Model can facilitate the integration of psychosocial assessment and intervention with the physical care of hemodialysis patients. Fawcett (1992a) presented a Roy Adaptation Model-based form for documentation of nephrology nursing practice. The form provides space to record the assessment of relevant environmental stimuli, along with the nursing diagnoses, nursing goals, and nursing interventions, for each response mode (physiological, self-concept, role function, interdependence).

Accomplishments of the ANNA Conceptual Models Task Force

Recognizing the growing importance of an explicit nursing frame of reference for nephrology nursing practice, the ANNA Board of Directors appointed a Conceptual Models Task Force in April of 1991. The Task Force convened for the first time in August of 1991 (Taylor, 1991). Discussion focused on the functions of and need for explicit conceptual models of nursing for the advancement of nephrology nursing practice. In addition, the Task Force members began to identify their own private images of nephrology nursing practice and compared the similarities and differences in those private images. The outcome of that meeting was the formulation of two recommendations, which were forwarded to and subsequently approved by the ANNA Board of Directors. The recommendations were that:

- ANNA develop a statement that nephrology nursing should be guided by a conceptual model of nursing, and
- ANNA move toward the selection of one or more conceptual models to guide nephrology nursing practice.

In addition, the Task Force members recognized the need to determine the existing private images of nephrology nursing practice held by a larger number of ANNA members prior to selection of one or more explicit conceptual models to guide nephrology nursing practice. The decision was made, therefore, to conduct a survey of ANNA members' views of the typical nephrology patient, typical nephrology nurse-patient interactions, and common nursing activities (Taylor et al., 1992). The survey respondents were 374 attendees of meetings sponsored by ANNA during the fall of 1991 and early winter of 1992. Content analysis of responses to the survey questionnaire revealed that the typical nephrology patient is elderly, has a chronic illness and negative affect, is not compliant, and is dependent on others. The typical nephrology nurse-patient interaction emphasizes teaching and support. The most common nursing activities are assessment, teaching, dialysis treatment, and psychological support.

The second Task Force meeting was held in January 1992 (Taylor, 1992). The Task Force members reviewed the results of the survey and systematically reviewed the content of several conceptual models of nursing (see Table 4-1). A comparison of the survey results with the focus and content of the various nursing models led to the selection of the Roy Adaptation Model for a demonstration project focusing on documentation of nursing care (Fawcett, 1992b).

The Roy Adaptation Model of Nursing

The Roy Adaptation Model depicts the individual as an adaptive system who interacts with constantly changing environmental focal, contextual, and residual stimuli. The focal stimulus is the one most immediately confronting the person. The focal stimulus, then, is the person's most pressing or immediate problem. The contextual stimuli are all other stimuli that might contribute to the level of adaptation, and the residual stimuli are environmental factors whose effects on adaptation cannot be directly determined. Frequently occurring contextual stimuli include cultural factors such as socioeconomic status, ethnicity, and one's belief system; family structure and tasks; developmental factors, such as age, gender, tasks, heredity, and genetic influences; changes in the environment; and use of addictive substances.

Individuals respond to stimuli through regulator and cognator coping mechanisms. The regulator mechanism encompasses basic neural, chemical, and endocrine channels that process stimuli in an automatic, unconscious manner. The cognator mechanism encompasses four cognitive-emotive channels for stimulus processing: perceptual/information processing, learning, judgment, and emotion. Regulator and cognator processes are manifested in four response modes.

The *physiological mode* emphasizes maintenance of the physical and physiological integrity of the adaptive system and encompasses oxygenation, nutrition, elimination, activity and rest, immune processes and the integument, the senses, fluids and electrolytes, neurological function, and endocrine function. The *self-concept mode* focuses on psychic integrity and deals with perception of the physical self in terms of body image and body sensation, as well as perception of the personal self, including self-consistency, self-ideal, and the moral-ethical-spiritual self. The *role function mode* deals with social integrity by focusing on performance of activities associated with the various roles one enacts throughout life. The primary role is based on age, gender, and developmental state, such as a 60-year-old male. The secondary roles are those assumed to fulfill tasks associated with each developmental stage, such as father, husband, and teacher. Tertiary roles are freely chosen, although they frequently are extensions of the secondary roles, such as Boy Scout leader or officer in a professional organization. The *interdependence mode* also deals with social integrity and emphasizes behaviors underlying the development and maintenance of satisfying affectional relationships with significant others, as well as the provision and receipt of social support.

Responses within the four modes are classified as adaptive or ineffective. Adaptive responses are those that meet the individual's goals for survival, growth, and mastery. Ineffective responses are those that do not meet those goals, and therefore, signal a need for nursing intervention.

Nursing intervention involves management of focal and contextual stimuli to achieve nursing care goals. Management encompasses altering, increasing, decreasing, removing, or maintaining relevant focal and/or contextual stimuli. The focal stimulus is selected for management whenever possible because it is the primary influence on responses. If it is not possible to manage the focal stimulus, contextual stimuli are then managed. The overarching goal of nursing intervention is to maintain adaptive responses and to convert ineffective responses to adaptive ones.

Development of a Nephrology Nursing Assessment Tool

The third meeting of the Task Force was held in September 1992. At that time, the members began to develop an assessment tool for the adult hemodialysis patient based on the Roy Adaptation Model. Tool development began by listing the components of each response mode and identifying areas of assessment within each component that are relevant for adult hemodialysis patients. A working draft of the assessment tool was completed at the fourth meeting of the Task Force in May 1993 (Breckenridge, 1993; Fawcett, 1993).

The content and format of the assessment tool were refined during the fifth, sixth, and seventh Task Force meetings, which were held in September 1993, September 1994, and July 1995, respectively. The tool is divided into four main sections, each of which contains items dealing with one of the Roy Model response modes. Information needed to complete the items can be obtained from patient interviews, physical assessment of the patient, chart reviews, and laboratory reports. Examples of items addressing each response mode are given in Table 4-2.

During the fifth meeting, the Task Force members also formulated a plan to field-test the assessment tool. The initial field test of the assessment tool was conducted during the fall of 1993 and the winter of 1994. The results were reviewed by the Task Force members and then presented to the ANNA membership at the 25th National Symposium in June 1994 (Fawcett, 1994). Five clinicians used the tool to assess a total of nine adult hemodialysis patients. The field test confirmed the Task Force members' impression that the first version of the tool was comprehensive and, as such, required a long period of time to complete. In fact, the median time for completion was 2 hours and 10 minutes. As expected, the extensive assessment of physiological mode responses required more than 1 hour, whereas assessment of self-concept, role function, and interdependence mode responses required just 15 to 20 minutes per mode.

Table 4-2
Examples from the Roy Adaptation Model assessment tool for the adult hemodialysis patient.

Physiological Mode

OXYGENATION
1. Respirations:
   a. Rate ___/minute
   b. Depth: (Check one)
      1. deep ☐ 2. moderate ☐ 3. shallow ☐
   c. Rhythm: (Check one)
      1. regular ☐ 2. irregular ☐
   d. Effort: Retraction
      1. Obvious effort ☐ 2. normal ☐

NUTRITION
1. How is your appetite?
   a. good ☐ b. moderate ☐ c. poor ☐
   1.1 How often are you genuinely hungry before or when you eat?
      a. frequently ☐ b. sometimes ☐ c. rarely ☐ d. never ☐
   1.2 Has this changed since the onset of kidney disease?
      a. yes ☐ b. no ☐
      If yes, how?
      ____
      ____
   1.3 Has this changed recently?
      a. yes ☐ b. no ☐
      If yes, how?
      ____
      ____

FLUID AND ELECTROLYTES
1. How much would you like to drink something now?
   a. extremely desirable ☐ b. very much ☐ c. would like ☐
   d. somewhat ☐ e. very little ☐ f. not at all ☐
2. How much do you want to drink at other times?
   a. extremely desirable ☐ b. very much ☐ c. would like ☐
   d. somewhat ☐ e. very little ☐ f. not at all ☐

ELIMINATION
1. How often do you normally move your bowels?
   ____
   1.1 Has this changed since onset of kidney disease?
      a. yes ☐ How?
      ____
      b. no ☐
   1.2 Has this changed recently?
      a. yes ☐ How?
      ____
      b. no ☐

2. On an average nondialysis day, how much of this cup would you fill with urine?
   a. none ☐ b. < 1/2 cup ☐ c. 1/2 cup ☐ d. 3/4 cup ☐ e. full ☐ f. > 1 cup ☐

ACTIVITY AND REST
1. What is the most physical activity in which you engage each day? ____________________
2. Do you have difficulty getting up in the morning because you feel tired?
   a. frequently ☐ b. sometimes ☐ c. rarely ☐ d. never ☐
3. How many hours of sleep do you get most nights?
   a. < 4 hours ☐ b. 4-6 hours ☐ c. 6-8 hours ☐ d. > 8 hours ☐

PROTECTION
1. What is the temperature of the skin?
   a. hot ☐ b. warm ☐ c. cool ☐ d. cold ☐
7. If cannulation sites present, the clinician should comment on the following:
   7.1 Rotation of sites: what % of access has been cannulated?
      a. < 50% ☐ b. 50-60% ☐ c. 60-70% ☐ d. > 70% ☐
   7.2 Last measured recirculation value _____%
      Date of study ____/____/_____
   7.3 Healing of cannulation sites/incisions:
      a. redness ☐ b. swelling ☐ c. drainage ☐

THE SENSES
1. Does the patient wear glasses?
   a. yes ☐ b. no ☐
2. Can the patient read the numbers on the weighing scale?
   a. yes ☐ b. no ☐
3. Does the patient answer questions appropriately if you speak in a normal voice level?
   a. yes ☐ b. no ☐
4. Is there any speech difficulty?
   a. yes ☐ b. no ☐

NEUROLOGICAL FUNCTION
1. Has there been a recent change in how alert you feel most of the time?
   a. yes ☐ b. no ☐
2. Is the person oriented to (check all that apply)
   a. person ☐ b. place ☐ c. time ☐ d. date ☐
3. Is the person able to remember events or diet of the preceding day?
   a. yes ☐ b. no ☐

3.1 If no, does this represent a recent change?
   a. yes ☐ b. no ☐

ENDOCRINE FUNCTION
1. Does the patient have diabetes?
   a. yes ☐ b. no ☐
4. Menstrual Cycle (Females)
   a. Age at the onset of menses? ____________________
   b. Age for the onset of menopause (if applicable)? ____________________
5. Laboratory bioassays: (if available)
   a. PTH level ____________________
   b. Erythropoietin level ____________________

Self-Concept Mode

PHYSICAL SELF
Body Sensation (How "tuned in" to his/her body is the patient?)
1. Pain
   a. always ☐ b. frequently ☐ c. sometimes ☐ d. rarely ☐ e. never ☐
4. Itching
   a. always ☐ b. frequently ☐ c. sometimes ☐ d. rarely ☐ e. never ☐

Body Image

1. Which of the following has been a problem for you or affected the way that you look since you developed kidney disease?
   a. vascular access ☐ b. color of skin ☐ c. changes in weight ☐
   d. height (secondary to bone disease) ☐ e. elimination ☐ f. changes in enamel of teeth ☐
   g. changes in hair texture ☐ h. changes in texture of skin (dryness/dandruff) ☐

PERSONAL SELF

Self-Consistency

1. Which of the following statements best reflects your personality?
   a. when something bothers me, I address the situation head on ☐
   b. when something bothers me, I usually discuss it with the parties involved ☐
   c. when something bothers me, I rarely discuss it with the parties involved ☐
   d. when something bothers me, I never discuss it with the parties involved ☐

Self Ideal (Hopes, expectations, desires and/or aspirations within the context of the patient's life)

1. Since you found out that you have kidney disease, how much have you had to change your goals?
   a. a lot ☐ b. somewhat ☐ c. not at all ☐

6. If some of your life goals no longer seem attainable, have you developed new ones?
   a. yes ☐ b. no ☐

Moral-Ethical-Spiritual Self (Personal beliefs, values, standards)

1. Is there anything in your personal, cultural, or spiritual beliefs that interfere with your ability to cooperate with your current treatment regimen?
   a. yes ☐ b. no ☐ c. don't know ☐

If yes, please specify:

____

____

____

Role Function Mode

PRIMARY ROLE

1. What is your date of birth? ___/___/___
   (Please check the appropriate age category below)
   ☐ trust vs. mistrust (birth to 1 yr)
   ☐ autonomy vs. shame and doubt (1 to 3 yrs)
   ☐ initiative vs. guilt (3 to 6 yrs)
   ☐ industry vs. inferiority (6 to 12 yrs)
   ☐ identity vs. role confusion (12 to 18 yrs)
   ☐ intimacy vs. isolation (18 to 35 yrs)
   ☐ generativity vs. stagnation (35 to 60 yrs)
   ☐ ego integrity vs. despair (60 yrs to death)
2. Gender:
   a. female ☐ b. male ☐

SECONDARY ROLES

6. Do you have enough time and energy to carry out your family activities?
   a. yes ☐ b. no ☐

6.1 If no, please specify which ones:

____

8. Do you work outside the home?
   a. yes ☐ b. no ☐

8.1 If yes, please describe your job.

____

8.2 If no, have you ever worked outside the home?
   a. yes ☐ b. no ☐

8.2.1 If yes, could you please describe your job.

____

8.2.2 If yes, is dialysis the reason you no longer work outside the home?
a. yes ☐ b. no ☐

TERTIARY ROLES
1. Do you participate in community activities?
a. yes ☐ b. no ☐
1.1 If yes, please list: ____________________________

SICK ROLE
Please comment on the patient's participation in treatment:
1. Does the patient express feelings about the sick role and its demands on him/her?
a. frequently ☐ b. sometimes ☐ c. rarely ☐ d. never ☐

Interdependence Mode

Please comment on the patient's interactions with the staff and fellow patients:
1. Does the patient initiate interactions with their family members, friends, co-workers, other patients, or staff?
a. frequently ☐ b. sometimes ☐ c. rarely ☐ d. never ☐
2. Is the patient receptive to the initiation of interactions by others?
a. frequently ☐ b. sometimes ☐ c. rarely ☐ d. never ☐
3. Does the patient respond to questions from the staff, other patients, or family concerning his/her health, well being, feelings of frustration?
a. frequently ☐ b. sometimes ☐ c. rarely ☐ d. never ☐
4. Does the patient express affection, pleasure, displeasure?
a. frequently ☐ b. sometimes ☐ c. rarely ☐ d. never ☐
5. Is the patient sexually active?
a. frequently ☐ b. sometimes ☐ c. rarely ☐ d. never ☐

The clinicians who participated in the initial field test provided several suggestions that have been taken into account in a revision of the assessment tool items and the directions for its use in clinical practice. The revised assessment tool has incorporated their suggestions to delete similar items in different sections and to simplify the format of the tool.

The revised assessment tool was field-tested during the winter and spring of 1995. Analysis of completed assessments conducted by six clinicians with a total of nine adult hemodialysis patients revealed no difficulties with the revised tool.

The clinicians who participated in the initial field test suggested that the actual use of the assessment tool might involve both nurses and social workers in collection of information. The clinicians also suggested that patients could be actively involved in completion of the assessment tool. More specifically, although some sections of the tool require physical assessment of the patient by the nurse or patient interviews conducted by the nurse or social worker, other sections could be given to the patient to complete during the dialysis treatment. Still other suggestions were to develop a logic tree to guide nurses to use different sections of the assessment tool in different client situations, and to distribute the assessment tool on floppy disk to facilitate computerization of information.

Furthermore, the clinicians suggested that the assessment tool should be completed over time, rather than during one sitting with the patient. As the clinicians pointed out, some items on the tool are more comfortably assessed only after an ongoing nurse-patient relationship is established. Consequently, the items for the final version of the assessment tool were prioritized for initial and ongoing assessment. A list of questions to ask for ongoing assessment was developed during the seventh Task Force meeting (see Table 4-3).

The reading and comprehension levels of the final version of the assessment tool need to be determined. In addition, inasmuch as comprehensive assessment may be the responsibility of an Advanced Practice Nurse or Clinical Specialist, and assessment of physiological mode responses may require advanced physical assessment skills, the educational preparation and the physical assessment skills required to use the final version of the assessment tool need to be determined.

Table 4-3
Questions for ongoing assessment.

Roy Adaptation Model Response Mode	Questions
Physiological	What physical problems do you have right now?
Self-Concept	How are you feeling today? How does life seem these days?
Role Function	How is your job going (if employed)? Are you able to accomplish what you would like to do each day? How are you doing with your medications?
Interdependence	How are things with your family and friends?

Development of a Typology of Nephrology Nursing Interventions

During the fourth meeting of the Conceptual Models Task Force, work was begun on the development of a typology of Roy Adaptation Model-based nursing interventions for the adult hemodialysis patient. The Task Force members first identified the primary focal stimulus that confronts the adult hemodialysis patient in each Roy Model response mode. Then, the major adaptation problems that the adult hemodialysis patient is likely to encounter were listed and prototype interventions were delineated. Further development of the typology took place at the fifth, sixth, and seventh Task Force meetings. Examples from the typology are displayed in Table 4-4.

The intervention typology obviously requires further development. In particular, specific adaptation problems and interventions for each response mode need to be refined and outcomes need to be identified.

Linking the Assessment Tool and Intervention Typology to the ANNA Standards of Clinical Practice

The Task Force also compared the completed Roy Adaptation Model-based assessment tool and intervention typology with the *ANNA Standards of Clinical Practice for Nephrology Nursing* (Burrows-Hudson, 1993). That work, which was undertaken following the seventh meeting of the Task Force, focused on comparison of the components of the Roy Adaptation Model with the standards of professional performance, standards of care, universal nephrology nursing standards of care, universal hemodialysis standards of care, and chronic patient: incenter standards.

The comparison revealed that the ANNA Standards are relatively comprehensive in relation to the Roy Adaptation Model. Although the physiological response mode of the Roy Model is clearly reflected in many standards, no standards address the senses or endocrine function aspects of the physiological mode. Furthermore, no standards address the regulator coping mechanism activity or the body sensation, self-consistency, and self-ideal aspects of the self-concept response mode. Moreover, limited attention is given in the standards to the interdependence response mode.

Future Directions

A long-range plan developed by the Conceptual Models Task Force calls for: (a) the development of Roy Adaptation Model-based assessment formats and intervention typologies for other categories of nephrology patients; (b) the development of assessment formats and intervention typologies based on other conceptual models of nursing for all categories of nephrology patients; and (c) the linkage of conceptual models of nursing with nephrology nursing practice standards, documentation, and quality monitoring. An outstanding example of linkages using the Roy Adaptation Model has already been done for perinatal nursing at the Mary Birch Hospital for Women at Sharp Memorial Hospital in San Diego, California (Weiss & Teplick, 1993). ANNA's task will be to develop the linkages using various conceptual models, for all categories of nephrology patients, and in all settings in which nephrology nursing takes place.

Summary

Johnson (1990) noted that although individual clinicians and nursing departments take risks when the decision is made to implement conceptual model-based nursing practice, the rewards far outweigh the risks. She stated:

> To openly use a nursing model is risk-taking behavior for the individual nurse. For a nursing department to adopt one of these models for unit or institution use is risk-taking behavior of an even higher order. The reward for such risk-taking for the individual practitioner lies in the great satisfaction gained from being able to specify explicit concrete *nursing* goals in the care of patients and from documenting the actual achievement of the desired outcomes. The reward

Table 4-4
Examples from a Roy Adaptation Model-based typology of nursing interventions for the adult hemodialysis patient.

Physiological Mode	
FOCAL STIMULUS:	**DISEASE—LACK OF PHYSICAL COMFORT**
PROBLEMS	**INTERVENTIONS**
OXYGENATION Inadequate oxygenation	Supplemental oxygen as necessary.
NUTRITION Inadequate nutrition	Consult with or refer patient to dietitian.
ELIMINATION Diarrhea and/or Constipation	Pharmacologic treatment as necessary.
ACTIVITY AND REST Fatigue	Discuss appropriate patterns of exercise. Promote environmental/mental techniques to facilitate rest and sleep.
PROTECTION Infections	Educate patient about good hygiene and infection control procedures.
THE SENSES Perceptual impairment	Referral to maintain optimal vision and hearing.
FLUID AND ELECTROLYTES Dehydration and/or edema.	Educate patient about the impact of environmental climate on fluid status.
NEUROLOGICAL FUNCTION Neuropathy	Educate patient about problems associated with neuropathies.
ENDOCRINE FUNCTION Ineffective hormone regulation	Educate patient about hormonal changes associated with aging and body changes.
Self-Concept Mode	
FOCAL STIMULUS:	**IDENTITY AS A PERSON REQUIRING DIALYSIS**
PROBLEMS	**INTERVENTIONS**
PHYSICAL SELF Altered body image — Altered grooming — Altered posture — Altered muscle tension/ spasm	Discuss reason for altered body image with patient. Discuss mutual goals that can be established for patient to improve his/her body image.
PERSONAL SELF Powerlessness	Discuss options to increase patient's sense of control. Give patient choices.

SELF-CONSISTENCY Altered coping with stress	Discuss feelings about life as a dialysis patient and strategies for coping with restrictions from dialysis.
SELF-IDEAL Unattainable goals due to kidney disease and dialysis	Discuss patient's goals regarding present and future aspirations and how to adapt by making changes.
MORAL-ETHICAL-SPIRITUAL SELF Problem in cooperation	Discuss with patient personal, cultural, and spiritual beliefs that interfere with his/her ability to cooperate with the current treatment regimen. Establish mutual goals that make cooperation realistic.
	Role Function Mode
FOCAL STIMULUS:	**TIME—CONFLICT BETWEEN TIME REQUIRED FOR DIALYSIS AND TIME FOR PERFORMANCE OF USUAL ROLE ACTIVITIES**
PROBLEMS	**INTERVENTIONS**
Altered secondary and tertiary roles -Job loss -Decreased time for hobbies or enjoyment	Help patient to prioritize and set realistic expectations; for example, refer patient to social worker or occupational therapist for possible retraining for an appropriate work role, refer patient to vocational rehabilitation center.
Performance of sick role	Discuss actual or potential conflicts between various role activities, the extent to which sick role activities interfere with or supersede performance of other roles, and the satisfaction gained from successful performance of sick role activities.
	Interdependence Mode
FOCAL STIMULUS:	**ACCEPTANCE AS A PERSON REQUIRING DIALYSIS**
PROBLEMS	**INTERVENTIONS**
Hemodialysis regimen requires increased dependence on significant others	Determine patient's immediate need for help. Share your perception of the patient's contribution to his/her interdependent relationships.

> for the nursing department is having a rational, cohesive, and comprehensive basis for the development of standards of nursing practice, for the evaluation of practitioners, and for the documentation of the contribution of nursing to patient welfare. (p. 32)

Anecdotal and empirical evidence is accumulating that additional rewards of conceptual model-based nursing practice include reduced staff nurse turnover (Fernandez, Brennan, Alvarez, & Duffy, 1990; Scherer, 1988), more rapid movement from novice to expert nurse (Field, 1989), and increased patient satisfaction (Scherer, 1988).

Furthermore, as the use of conceptual models moves nursing practice from a base of implicit knowledge to explicit nursing knowledge, both nurses and the recipients of nursing care are empowered. Indeed, "[nursing] knowledge is power" (Orr, 1991, p. 218), which can, as Lister (1991) and Malin and Teasdale (1991) pointed out, be used to empower health care recipients to participate fully in decisions about that care.

ANNA's decision to base nephrology nursing on explicit conceptual models of nursing represents a risk of a high order. The organizational-level reward, however, is even greater — the recognition that comes with taking the lead among nursing specialty organizations in the advancement of the nursing discipline. In fact, no other nursing specialty organization has ever undertaken such an endeavor. Once again, ANNA members have moved to the forefront in professional development and patient care.

References

Akinsanya, J.A. (1989). Introduction. *Recent Advances in Nursing, 24*, i-ii.

Beecroft, P.C. (1990). The effect of cognitive restructuring and assertion skills training on the self-efficacy and self-care agency of adolescents undergoing hemodialysis. *Dissertation Abstracts International, 51*, 5243B.

Bélanger, P. (1991). Nursing models—A major step towards professional autonomy. *AARN Newsletter, 48*(8), 13.

Biley, F. (1990). Wordly wise. *Nursing (London), 4*(24), 37.

Breckenridge, D.M. (1982). Adaptation of the Neuman Systems Model for the renal client. In B. Neuman (Ed.), *The Neuman Systems Model. Application to nursing education and practice* (pp. 267- 275). Norwalk, CT: Appleton-Century-Crofts.

Breckenridge, D.M. (1989). Primary prevention as an intervention modality for the renal client. In B. Neuman (Ed.), *The Neuman Systems Model* (2nd ed.) (pp. 397-405). Norwalk, CT: Appleton & Lange.

Breckenridge, D.M. (1993). Conceptual models task force completes development of assessment tool. *ANNA Update, 23*(3), 11.

Breckenridge, D.M. (1995). Nephrology practice and directions for research. In B. Neuman (Ed.), *The Neuman Systems Model* (3rd ed.) (pp. 499-5071). Norwalk, CT: Appleton & Lange.

Breckenridge, D.M., Cupit, M.C., & Raimondo, J.M. (1982, January/February). Systematic nursing assessment tool for the CAPD client. *Nephrology Nurse*, 24, 26-27, 30-31.

Breckenridge, D.M., Cupit, M.C., & Raimondo, J.M. (1983). *Utilization of a systematic nursing assessment tool for the CAPD client to assess quality of life.* Paper presented at the 14th National Symposium of the American Association of Nephrology Nurses and Technicians.

Bridges, J. (1991). Working with doctors: Distinct from medicine. *Nursing Times, 87*(27), 42-43.

Bruce, G.L., Hinds, P., Hudak, J., Mucha, A., Taylor, M.C., & Thompson, C.R. (1980). Implementation of ANA's quality assurance program for clients with end-stage renal disease. *Advances in Nursing Science, 2*(2), 79-95.

Burrows-Hudson, S. (Ed.). (1993). *Standards of clinical practice for nephrology nursing.* Pitman, NJ: American Nephrology Nurses' Association.

Chalmers, H., Kershaw, B., Melia, K., & Kendrich, M. (1990). Nursing models: Enhancing or inhibiting practice? *Nursing Standard, 5*(11), 34-40.

Fawcett, J. (1992a). Documentation using a conceptual model of nursing. *Nephrology Nursing Today, 2*(5), 1-8.

Fawcett, J. (1992b, May). *Enhancing practice through the use of a conceptual model for nephrology nursing.* Paper presented at the 23rd National Symposium of the American Nephrology Nurses' Association, Chicago, IL.

Fawcett, J. (1993, June). *Conceptual models and nephrology nursing practice: Report of a pilot project.* Paper presented at the 24th National Symposium of the American Nephrology Nurses' Association, Orlando, FL.

Fawcett, J. (1994, June). *Assessment of the adult hemodialysis patient: An adaptation nursing perspective.* Paper presented at the 25th National Symposium of the American Nephrology Nurses' Association, Dallas, TX.

Fawcett, J. (1995). *Analysis and evaluation of conceptual models of nursing* (3rd ed.). Philadelphia: F.A. Davis.

Fernandez, R., Brennan, M.L., Alvarez, A., & Duffy, M.R. (1990). Theory-based practice: A model for nurse retention. *Nursing Administration Quarterly, 12*(4), 47-53.

Field, P.A. (1989). Brenda, Beth, and Susan: Three approaches to health promotion. *The Canadian Nurse, 85*(5), 20-24.

Frank, D.I. (1988). Psychosocial assessment of renal dialysis patients. *ANNA Journal, 15*, 207-232.

Frank, L.K. (1968). Science as a communication process. *Main Currents in Modern Thought, 25*, 45-50.

Grossman, M., & Hooton, M. (1993). The significance of the relationship between a discipline and its practice. *Journal of Advanced Nursing, 18*, 866-872.

Hayne, Y. (1992). The current status and future significance of nursing as a discipline. *Journal of Advanced Nursing, 17*, 104-107.

Hathaway, D., & Strong, M. (1988). Theory, practice, and research in transplant nursing. *ANNA Journal, 15*, 9-12.

Hayward, M.B., Kish, J.P., Jr., Frey, G.M., Kirchner, J.M., Carr, L.S., & Wolfe, C.M. (1989). An instrument to identify stressors in renal transplant recipients. *ANNA Journal, 16*, 81-84.

Herald, P.A. (1994). Relationship between hydration status and renal function in patients receiving aminoglycoside antibiotics. *Dissertation Abstracts International, 55*, 365B.

Ingram, R. (1991). Why does nursing need theory? *Journal of Advanced Nursing, 16*, 350-353.

Johnson, D.E. (1987). Guest Editorial: Evaluating conceptual models for use in critical care nursing practice. *Dimensions of Critical Care Nursing, 6*, 195-197.

Johnson, D.E. (1990). The behavioral system model for nursing. In M.E. Parker (Ed.), *Nursing theories in practice* (pp. 23-32). New York: National League for Nursing.

King, I.M. (1984). Effectiveness of nursing care: Use of a goal oriented nursing record in end stage renal disease. *American Association of Nephrology Nurses and Technicians Journal, 11*(2), 11-17, 60.

King, I.M. (1990). King's conceptual framework and theory of goal attainment. In M.E. Parker (Ed.), *Nursing theories in practice* (pp. 73-84). New York: National League for Nursing.

Korniewicz, D.M., & O'Brien, M.E. (1994). Evaluation of a hemodialysis patient education and support program. *ANNA Journal, 21*, 33-39.

Lachman, V.D. (1993, June). *Communication skills for effective interpersonal relations.* Concurrent session presented at the 24th National Symposium of the American Nephrology Nurses' Association, Orlando, FL.

Lapp, C.L. (1992). The effect of patient and staff education on the compliance and morbidity of the dialysis patient. *Master's Abstracts International, 31*, 276.

Levine, M.E. (1991). The conservation principles: A model for health. In K.M. Schaefer & J.B. Pond (Eds.), *Levine's conservation model: A framework for nursing practice* (pp. 1-11). Philadelphia: F.A. Davis.

Lindsay, B. (1990). The gap between theory and practice. *Nursing Standard, 5*(4), 34-35.

Lister, P. (1991). Approaching models of nursing from a postmodernist perspective. *Journal of Advanced Nursing, 16*, 206-212.

Malin, N., & Teasdale, K. (1991). Caring versus empowerment: Considerations for nursing practice. *Journal of Advanced Nursing, 16*, 657-662.

Miller, M.P. (1986). Measurement of perception of self-care agency in predialysis and dialysis patients. *Master's Abstracts International, 26*, 108.

Neff, M. (1991). President's message. The future of our profession from the eyes of today. *ANNA Journal, 18*, 534.

Neuman, B. (1995). *The Neuman systems model* (3rd ed.). Norwalk, CT: Appleton & Lange.

Nightingale, F. (1859). *Notes on nursing: What it is, and what it is not.* London: Harrison. Reprinted 1946. Philadelphia: Lippincott.

Norris, M.K.G. (1991). Applying Orem's theory to the long-term care of adolescent transplant recipients. *ANNA Journal, 18*, 45-47, 53.

Orem, D.E. (1995). *Nursing: Concepts of practice* (5th ed.). St. Louis: Mosby Yearbook.

Orlando, I.J. (1961). *The dynamic nurse-patient relationship: Function, process, and principles.* New York: G.P. Putnam's Sons. [Reprinted 1990. New York: National League for Nursing.]

Orr, J. (1991). Knowledge is power. *Health Visitor, 64*, 218.

Perras, S., & Zappacosta, A. (1982). The application of Orem's theory in promoting self-care in a peritoneal dialysis facility. *ANNA Journal, 9*(3), 37-39.

Perry, J. (1985). Has the discipline of nursing developed to the stage where nurses do 'think nursing'? *Journal of Advanced Nursing, 10*, 31-37.

Pressly, K.B. (1994). Relationship of psychosocial characteristics and the occurrence of infectious complications in continuous ambulatory peritoneal dialysis patients. *Dissertation Abstracts International, 54*, 5095B.

Reilly, D.E. (1975). Why a conceptual framework? *Nursing Outlook, 23*, 566-569.

Rogers, M.E. (1989). Creating a climate for the implementation of a nursing conceptual framework. *Journal of Continuing Education in Nursing, 20*, 112-116.

Rogers, M.E. (1990). Nursing: Science of unitary, irreducible, human beings: Update 1990. In E.A.M. Barrett (Ed.), *Visions of Rogers' science-based nursing* (pp. 5-11). New York: National League for Nursing.

Roy, C., & Andrews, H.A. (1991). *The Roy adaptation model: The definitive statement.* Norwalk, CT: Appleton & Lange.

Scherer, P. (1988). Hospitals that attract (and keep) nurses. *American Journal of Nursing, 88*, 34-40.

Stoeckle, M.L. (1993). Waiting for a second chance at life: An examination of health-related hardiness, uncertainty, power, and the environment in adults on the kidney transplant waiting list. *Dissertation Abstracts International, 54*, 3000B.

Summerton, H. (1995). End-stage renal failure: The challenge to the nurse. *Nursing Times, 91*(6), 27-29.

Taylor, S. (1991). Nephrology nursing conceptual model task force. *ANNA Update, 21*(5), 21.

Taylor, S. (1992). Conceptual model task force update. *ANNA Update, 22*(6), 2.

Taylor, S., Breckenridge, D., Butera, E., Hartigan, M. F., Frauman, A. C., Keen, M., Mapes, D., Neff, M., & Fawcett, J. (1992). Images of nephrology nursing practice: Report of a survey. *ANNA Journal, 19*, 361-366.

Turner, K. (1989). Orem's model and patient teaching. *Nursing Standard, 50*(3), 32-33.

Weiss, M.E., & Teplick, F. (1993). Linking perinatal standards, documentation, and quality monitoring. *Journal of Perinatal and Neonatal Nursing, 7*(2), 18-27.

Zinn, A. (1986). A self-care program for hemodialysis patients based on Dorothea Orem's concepts. *Journal of Nephrology Nursing, 3*, 65-77.

NURSING NOTES

About Conceptual Models...

Conceptual models have existed since people began to think about themselves and their surroundings. They now exist in all areas of life and in all disciplines. Indeed, everything that a person sees, hears, reads, and experiences is filtered through the cognitive lens of some conceptual frame of reference (Lachman, 1993).

Conceptual models of nursing present diverse perspectives of the recipient of nursing, who can be an individual, a family, or a community; the environment of the recipient and the environment in which nursing occurs; the recipient's health state; and the definition and goals of nursing, as well as nursing actions or interventions.

A conceptual model provides a distinctive frame of reference and "a coherent, internally unified way of thinking about . . . events and processes" (Frank, 1968, p. 45) and tells clinicians how to observe and interpret the phenomena of interest to their discipline. Each conceptual model, then, presents a unique focus that has a profound influence on the clinician's perceptions of people, events, and situations.

Conceptual models of nursing "provide [explicit] philosophical and pragmatic orientations to the service nurses provide patients — a service which only nurses can provide — a service which provides a dimension to total care different from that provided by any other health professional" (Johnson, 1987, p. 195). Conceptual models of nursing provide explicit orientations not only for nurses but also for the general public. They identify the purpose and scope of nursing and provide frameworks for objective records of the effects of nursing.

The most tangible function of a conceptual model is its delineation of goals for nursing practice and a nursing process format that encompasses parameters for assessment, labels for patient/client problems, a strategy for planning nursing care, a set of nursing interventions, and criteria for evaluation of the outcomes of nursing care. In short, a conceptual model of nursing provides a structure for documentation of all aspects of the nursing process, from patient assessment to evaluation of outcomes. Furthermore, a conceptual model also helps to identify standards of nursing practice and criteria for quality assurance reviews.

Conceptual models of nursing move the practice of nursing away from that driven by a medical or institutional model and, therefore, foster autonomy from medicine and a coherent purpose of practice (Bélanger, 1991; Bridges, 1991; Ingram, 1991).

Conceptual models specify innovative goals for nursing practice and introduce ideas that are designed to improve practice (Lindsay, 1990) by facilitating the identification of relevant information, reducing the fragmentation of care, and improving the coordination of care (Chalmers, cited in Chalmers, et al., 1990). In particular, conceptual models provide a nursing knowledge base that has a positive effect on practice "by enabling well-coordinated care to take place, by providing a basis for the justification of care actions and by enabling nursing to *talk nursing*" (Chalmers, cited in Chalmers, Kershaw, Melia, & Kendrich, 1990, p. 34), *think nursing* (Perry, 1985), and better communicate *what they do* (Neff, 1991, p. 534) and *why they do it.*

Chapter Highlights

- A conceptual model is defined as a set of abstract and general concepts and propositions that present a particular perspective about the phenomena of interest to a discipline.
- Conceptual models of nursing present diverse perspectives of the nursing recipient; the environment of the recipient, as well as the environment in which nursing occurs; the health state of the recipient; the definition and goals of nursing, and nursing actions or interventions.
- Concepts are words that describe mental images of phenomena. The abstract and general concepts of a conceptual model are not limited to any particular individual, group, situation, or event. Rather, they can refer to many different people in a broad range of situations.
- The works of several nurse scholars currently are recognized as conceptual models. Among the best known are Johnson's Behavioral System Model, King's General Systems Framework, Levine's Conservation Model, Neuman's Systems Model, Orem's Self-Care Framework, Rogers's Science of Unitary Human Beings, and Roy's Adaptation Model.
- Each conceptual model of nursing, then, is the public presentation of its author's private image of nursing. Use of an explicit conceptual model facilitates communication among nurses and provides a systematic approach to nursing practice, as well as to nursing research, education, and administration.
- Conceptual models of nursing provide explicit frames of reference for *professional* nursing practice by delineating the scope of nursing practice and by identifying who the recipient of nursing is, what the relevant environment is, what aspects of health are to be considered, and what the steps and substance of the nursing process are.
- Johnson's Behavioral Systems Model was the basis for a tool to measure outcome criteria for fluid and electrolyte balance in patients with chronic renal failure . . . The tool includes items that reflect the ingestive, eliminative, and achievement subsystems, and it can be used in quality assurance programs for patients with chronic renal failure.
- King's General Systems Framework was the basis for the goal-oriented nursing record (GONR). The GONR, which contains space for demographic and health data, problem list, goal list, nursing care plan, and progress notes, can be used to document the nursing care of chronic renal failure clients (King, 1984).
- Orem's Self-Care Framework has been used to guide the nursing care of patients with chronic renal failure . . .
- In addition, Orem's Self-Care Framework has been used to guide practice-related nephrology nursing research.
- The Roy Adaptation Model has been used to guide and document nephrology nursing practice. Frank (1988) explained how the Roy Adaptation Model can facilitate the integration of psychosocial assessment and intervention with the physical care of hemodialysis patients. Fawcett (1992a) presented a Roy Adaptation Model-based form for documentation of nephrology nursing practice.
- A comparison of the results of a survey of ANNA members with the focus and content of the various nursing models led to the selection of the Roy Adaptation Model for a demonstration project focusing on documentation of nursing care (Fawcett, 1992b).
- The ANNA Conceptual Models Task Force has developed an assessment tool and intervention typology for adult hemodialysis patients based on the Roy Adaptation Model.

CHAPTER 5

Ethical Issues in Nephrology Nursing

Rosalie Starzomski, PhD, MN, RN

Chapter Contents

Ethical Foundations for Nephrology Nursing Practice 85
The Birth of Bioethics 85
Ethical Theories 86
The Hippocratic Period 87
The Period of Principlism 87
The Antiprinciplism Period 88
Levels of Professional Responsibility 90
Advocacy 91
Making Ethical Decisions - An Ethical Decision-Making Framework 92
Ethical Issues in Nephrology Nursing 94
Case Analysis 95
Case 1 95
Case 2 97
Case 3 99
Strategies to Enhance Ethical Decision-Making 100
Communication and Collaboration 100
Ethics at the Bedside 101
Ethics Education 101
Ethics Consultation 101
Research 102
Public and Health Care Provider Dialogue About Resource Allocation 102
Summary and Future Directions 103
References and Readings 104
Chapter Highlights 108

Ethical Issues in Nephrology Nursing

Rosalie Starzomski, PhD, MN, RN

There is no doubt that the growth of knowledge in health care, the rapid expansion of technology, and our resulting ability to treat people have generated unprecedented opportunities and challenges in the delivery of health care. At the same time, this growth and expansion have created increasingly complex ethical dilemmas for health care professionals and the general public. As a result, ethics is an area in contemporary society that is receiving growing attention, and is of interest not only to philosophers, but to everyone involved in the development and provision of health care.

The role of ethics in health care is multifaceted. Every day in our health professional or citizen roles, we are confronted with situations that require moral judgment and ability to make ethical decisions. Nowhere is this more apparent than in nephrology, where decisions about initiating, withdrawing and withholding treatment, in addition to selection of patients for treatment, are fraught with ethical dilemmas and questions about the fair and just allocation of limited resources. Although these dilemmas have been evident since the inception of dialysis and transplantation, many of these issues are becoming more problematic as we face the challenges brought on by the shrinking resources available for health care, and concomitant health care reform.

As nephrology nurses, we play an integral role in the provision of health care to people in a variety of settings, including hospitals, dialysis facilities, and in the community. The close relationship that develops between us, and the persons for whom we care, leads to many privileges and responsibilities as the people we care for allow us to enter their world and become aware of their choices, hopes, and fears. Nephrology nurses have acquired knowledge about ethics and morality due to an environment where we are constantly called upon to make decisions based on our own values and preferences. We make ethical decisions every day as we prioritize our time, determine patient assignments, interact with other health care professionals, and develop plans of care with patients and their families that are congruent with patient choices.

Knowledge about ethics and ethical decision making are essential components of nephrology nursing practice. Yet, many of us feel unprepared to resolve ethical dilemmas in patient care (Miedman, 1991). If we are to make good decisions, we must first understand the nature of the ethical problems and issues we face, and take an active role in discussing, planning, and implementing plans of care for patients. The purpose of this chapter is to provide information about ethics in nephrology nursing by highlighting the ethical foundations necessary for practice. In addition, information is provided, through the use of case studies, about many of the ethical issues facing nephrology nurses today. Strategies that will assist nurses to uphold ethical standards are presented, and future directions in ethics and nephrology nursing are explored.

Ethical Foundations for Nephrology Nursing Practice

The Birth of Bioethics

Ethics is the science or study of morals (McDonald, Stevenson, & Cragg, 1992, p. 5). The field of ethics is founded in the branch of human knowledge known as philosophy. Ethics focuses critical reflection upon actions and events from the standpoint of right and wrong, good and evil, and moral value and moral disvalue. In addition, ethics is concerned with policies, practices, duties, obligations, and rights, with fairness in the correction of wrongs (corrective justice), and with the fair distribution of benefits and burdens within society (distributive justice). Ethics is concerned with the resolution of moral disputes, controversies, and uncertainties (McDonald et al., 1992, p. 5).

Ethics reflects what ought to occur in a given situation (Omery, 1989). Ethical problems (often called dilemmas) result from areas of concern that cannot be resolved solely through an appeal to empirical data, and where there are conflicts of values, as well as uncertainty about the amount or type of information needed to make decisions (Curtin, 1982, pp. 38-39).

Previously, the focus for ethics within health care was on biomedical ethics. Currently, ethics in health care has evolved to a point where there is recognition that all health care professionals have ethical concerns and ethical responsibilities. The terms bioethics and health care ethics are being used more frequently to clarify that it is not only medical practitioners, but all health professionals, who must practice in an ethical manner (Roy, Williams, & Dickens, 1994).

Nursing organizations in North America have

Table 5-1
Ethical theory development.

Period	Time Frame
The Hippocratic Period	From the time of the Ancient Greek philosophers to the mid 1960s
The Period of Principlism	From the late 1960s to the 1980s
The Antiprinciplism Period	From the 1980s to the present
Alternative Ethical Theories Proposed	

Note: Adapted from Pellegrino, E. (1993). The metamorphosis of medical ethics. *Journal of the American Medical Association, 269*(9), 1158-1162.

developed ethical standards that provide direction for nephrology nurses and articulate clearly our role as ethical practitioners and patient advocates. The American Nurses Association (ANA) proposed a tentative code of ethics in 1926, with modifications made in subsequent years. The Canadian Nurses Association (CNA) adopted the International Council of Nurses (ICN) code as its first code of ethics in 1954 and developed its own code in 1980.

Although it is difficult to determine when bioethics emerged as an important area in health care, it is thought to have occurred after Belding Scribner used a teflon arteriovenous shunt for the continuous dialysis of Clyde Shields on March 9, 1960 (Jonsen, 1989; 1990). Following this major development, dialysis units, like the Northwest Kidney Center in Seattle, formed committees to decide which medically qualified patients would be chosen to receive dialysis in the few treatment slots available (Alexander, 1962; Fox & Swazey, 1992b). The Seattle group, called the *God Squad* by its critics, generated worldwide controversy, since, to that time, selection of patients for treatment with scarce resources was accomplished using an emergency triage system (developed in war-time and during natural disasters) where the sickest, treatable patients were given first priority for treatment (Jonsen, 1990). The Seattle committee, composed of middle and upper class members of the community, moved away from this method and in the absence of any formal principles for selection, chose patients for treatment using criteria such as the likely success of the person on dialysis, as well as criteria that rated the social worth of each potential candidate (Alexander, 1962; Fox & Swazey, 1992b; Jonsen, 1990). This selection process was described by Jonsen (1990) as using "some common sense maxims; younger rather than older patients, those with dependents rather than those without, the emotionally mature and stable, those with a record of public service and so on" (p. 46).

The story of the Seattle group illustrated one of the problems that brought bioethics into the forefront of nephrology. Because of a lack of resources, such as dialysis machines, trained personnel, and financial support, the issue of who should receive treatment, when all could not be treated, became a primary concern. The public attention given to the dialysis dilemma, coupled with discussion about concerns arising out of unethical experimentation with human subjects (Beecher, 1966), stimulated scholarly reflection on these issues, thus contributing to the evolution of the field of bioethics (Jonsen, 1990).

Ethical Theories

What provides the basis for making ethical decisions? What guides our thinking and reasoning about ethical problems? In North America, we live in a pluralistic society of many cultures, religions, and traditions, thus leading to many different moral positions. Therefore, we are unable to declare that there is one universal ethic that all persons could agree upon, rather there are a variety of diverse perspectives that guide ethical decision making.

Several components are included as we think about the right course of action when confronted with an ethical problem, issue, or dilemma. In addition to considering our values, beliefs, and attitudes, we use ethical theory to provide direction for ethical decision making. Like all theory, ethical theory has not remained stagnant, rather it is constantly progressing as challenges to existing theories are made, and new ideas are developed. The following brief review of theory development in health care ethics will provide the background context for further discussion about ethical concerns in nephrology nursing and provide direction for ethical decision making in the nephrology setting.

Pellegrino (1993) views the development of ethical theory as comprising several distinct periods (see Table 5-1). Although focusing on biomedical ethics, Pellegrino's classification is useful in understanding the development of nursing ethics, and health care ethics, as they paralleled the development of biomedical ethics and share a similar history (Yeo, 1991).

The Hippocratic Period

The first period described by Pellegrino is the interval in which the Hippocratic teachings, enhanced by contact with the Greek Stoics and religious traditions, formed the predominate ethic. During this period, ethical precepts such as obligations to do no harm, do good, and maintain confidentiality were evident in the Hippocratic Oath, an oath taken by physicians that provided direction for the practice of medicine. In addition, there were prohibitions in the Oath against abortion, euthanasia, and sexual relationships with patients. The physician was directed to follow the Oath, lead a life of virtue, and to act in conformity with the virtues of courage, temperance, and justice (Pellegrino, 1993, p.1159).

The Period of Principlism

Principle-oriented ethical theory development began the second period of theory evolution in the mid-1960s, when philosophical inquiry began to reshape the Hippocratic ethic (Pellegrino, 1993, p.1158). Philosophers brought a variety of well-established moral traditions to health care ethics, including two main ethical theories, teleological (consequentialist) and deontological theories. These theories lead to very different ways of examining ethical concerns.

Consequentialists (also called utilitarians) believe that the rightness or wrongness of an action is solely a function of the goodness or badness of the action's consequences. The whole of morality is reduced to one principle, that of utility, where actions are right if they maximize happiness. Proponents of utilitarianism believe that the end justifies the means. One major concern with this theory in contemporary practice is that it allows a person to do anything if it can be said that the act would produce the greatest net benefit for society as a whole. For example, if lying, or killing someone would produce the greatest good for society, a utilitarian would suggest that the action should be carried out (Browne, 1994; Gibson, 1993; Mappes & Zembaty, 1991).

Deontological theory, such as that formulated by the philosopher Immanuel Kant, focuses on the nature of the act to be carried out and does not look merely at consequences. In Kant's theory, there are binding obligations or duties where an act is right if, and only if, it conforms to an overriding moral duty or obligation. Kant's central idea was always to treat people with respect and never solely as a means to the end of others. A concern with this theory is that there may be circumstances where the right thing to do may not conform to following a moral duty. For instance, Kant would say that one ought not to lie or to kill, however, what if lying would protect someone from harm, or killing might protect one's child or occurred in self-defense? In these cases the theory does not provide clear direction (Browne, 1994; Mappes & Zembaty, 1991).

Table 5-2
Principles of bioethics.

Principle	Definition
Autonomy	Individual self-governance or self rule
Beneficence	Do good
Nonmaleficence	Do no harm
Justice	Treat people fairly

Table 5-3
Theories of justice.

Utilitarian Theories
Rawls' Theory of Justice
Libertarian Conception of Justice
Egalitarians

Principles of bioethics. On their own, the theories described above were not sufficient to provide guidance for ethical decision making and action. As a result, a set of duties and principles was developed by Ross (1930/1988), and later modified by Beauchamp and Childress (1983), that included four principles seen as especially appropriate for biomedical ethics. These principles — autonomy, beneficence, nonmaleficence and justice — were the cornerstone of the traditional approach to health care ethics and have become the "dominant way of doing ethics" (Pellegrino, 1993, pp. 1159-1160). The principles are viewed as codes of conduct that direct life and provide a basis for reasoning in ethics (Davis & Aroskar, 1991). (see Table 5-2).

The first principle, autonomy, is defined as self-governance or self-rule by the individual, who at the same time remains free from both controlling interferences by others and personal limitations that would prevent meaningful choices (Beauchamp & Childress, 1989, p. 68). Also known as respect for persons, autonomy directs us to see persons as worthy agents with a capacity for rational choice who are in control of their own bodies and lives (Beauchamp, 1982).

Beneficence directs us to abstain from harming others, and to help or benefit others, largely by preventing or removing possible harms (Beauchamp, 1982). Nonmaleficence is based on the Hippocratic oath and is synonymous with the Latin phrase 'primum non nocere' or 'first do no harm'. This principle directs us not to act in a manner that would harm an individual or society (Beauchamp, 1982).

Justice is defined as fairness, or providing persons with what they are entitled to or can legitimately claim. Distributive justice refers to just distribution of goods and services in society. This distribution is structured by various moral, legal, and cultural rules and principles that form the terms of cooperation for society (Beauchamp & Childress, 1989, pp. 257-258).

Justice can be viewed as a theory as well as a principle. Four major theories of justice include the utilitarian approach, Rawls' Theory of Justice as fairness (liberalism), the libertarian approach, and an egalitarian theory of justice (see Table 5-3).

Utilitarian theories reference the rightness or wrongness of actions or policies, to the good or bad consequences they generate. Right acts and policies are those that achieve the greatest net good or happiness for the greatest net number (Buchanan, 1991).

Rawls' Theory of Justice is based on the idea that inequalities in the distribution of the primary goods of a society can be condoned only if these inequalities are to everyone's benefit, especially the least advantaged. His theory is based on three central principles; (a) the principle of greatest equal liberty, (b) the principle of equality of fair opportunity, and (c) the difference principle.

With the principle of greatest equal liberty, Rawls contends that each person is to have an equal right to the most extensive system of equal basic liberties compatible with a similar system of liberty for all. In the principle of equality of opportunity, he suggests that offices and positions ought to be open to all, and that people with similar skills and abilities ought to have equal access to offices and positions. Finally, in the difference principle he proposes that social and economic institutions are to be arranged so as to benefit the maximally worst off (Rawls, 1971 as cited in Buchanan, 1991, p. 554).

In a *libertarian conception of justice,* individuals have moral rights to life, liberty, and property that any just society must recognize and respect. From a libertarian perspective, coercion may only be used to prevent harm, theft, fraud, and to enforce contracts (Buchanan, 1991, p. 556). Libertarian theorists suggest that attempts to force anyone to contribute any of his holdings for the welfare of others is a violation of property rights. However, libertarians do say that although justice does not require it, charity requires that those who seek aid are helped.

Egalitarians suggest that justice requires that social institutions work on the premise of moral equality where the life of everyone matters equally. Hence, similarities or equalities among individuals are emphasized. Distribution of health care ought to be carried out according to need, with the provision of health care of the same extent and quality to everyone in society. The underlying aim of health care should be to meet equally the health care needs of all. Different treatment is justified only where the need is different, or both needs cannot be met. Where these circumstances occur, then priority should be given to the greater need that can feasibly be met (Nielson, 1991, p. 565).

Each of the theories of justice offers a theoretical basis for answering some fundamental questions concerning justice in health care, but none of them provides unambiguous answers to all of the questions. Each depends, for its application, upon many empirical premises that are not necessarily available (Buchanan, 1991, p. 561).

The Antiprinciplism Period

The third period of ethical theory development, or anti-principle period, occurred when competing moral theories began to challenge the primacy of principles, and when nurses began to question whether biomedical ethics was the ethical foundation for their practice (Fry, 1989a; 1989b). This period led to the contemporary era of ethical theory development. Pellegrino describes the current era as... "one of crisis in which conceptual conflicts in ethics and the skepticism of moral philosophy challenge the very idea of a universal, normative ethic for medicine" (p. 1158). This same concern can be raised about health care ethics in general, where there is considerable discussion and tension among various ethical theorists.

The tension is particularly evident in the debate about the principle-oriented approach to ethics and the ethic of care. The principle-oriented approach to ethics is based on a lexical ordering and application of principles (such as autonomy, beneficence, nonmaleficence, and justice) (Veatch, 1991b). This ordering often occurs in a rational, objective, and impartial manner, where the central issue is judging whether a person's actions are right or wrong (Ackerman, 1983; Cooper, 1991; Penticuff, 1991). In this cognitive approach, an action is considered morally right if it can be justified by a valid argument appealing to a valid moral principle as instituted in the social contract (Omery, 1989; Toulmin, 1981). Principle-oriented ethics is based on a model where reliance upon rules and principles is primary in moral action and justification (Cooper, 1991). Proponents of this theory believe, generally, that principles represent the moral truth, and that there is a hierarchical ordering of principles where they are applied in a deductive, objective manner. In this ethic, there is a requirement of impartiality where the moral agent must not be influenced by personal feelings or special relationships to others. This requirement of universalizability implies that an action is right if any other person in a comparable situation ought to act in the same manner.

There has been considerable criticism, particularly in the nursing ethics literature, about the principle-based approach to ethics (Cooper, 1991; Penticuff, 1991). Principle-oriented ethics has been described as an *ethics of strangers* because of the detached way in which the theory is applied (Cooper, 1991). Critics have stated that there is a lack of consensus about the nature of fundamental ethical principles, and that a hierarchical ordering of principles applied in a prescriptive, decontextualized manner, is not practical in actual, complex ethical situations (Ackerman, 1983; Cooper, 1991). The approach has been criticized as actually representing a formula approach to ethics (Ackerman, 1983; Toulmin, 1981). Ackerman (1983) points out that principles may be more useful as heuristic devices or guidelines, rather than absolutes. As a result of the criticism, there has been a move to explore other moral theories, several of which are described below.

There is growing interest in a return to contextual ethics in moral theory development. More interest is being expressed in virtue ethics and casuistry, two theories that arose in the first period of development explicated above (Jonsen, 1990; Pellegrino, 1993; Toulmin, 1981). The first of these, virtue ethics, describes a moral theory where the character of the moral agent is considered critical to ethical decision making. According to Pellegrino, virtue ethics cannot stand alone and should be anchored in some form of prior theory of right or wrong. He suggests that virtue ethics does not provide sufficient clear action for ethical decision making. Moreover, virtue ethics is prone to individual definitions of virtue or of the virtuous person (Pellegrino, 1993, p. 1161). However, Pellegrino believes that virtue ethics ought to be part of any ethical theory that becomes predominant in modern society.

Casuistry is based on case analysis where the decision maker looks for cases that are examples of principles, then moves from these clear cases to more perplexing ones, ordering them by paradigm and analogy under a specific principle (Jonsen, 1990; Pellegrino, 1993, p. 1161). In casuistry, principles are valuable, however, they are not absolute. A criticism of casuistry stems from its development in the middle ages within Catholicism, where consensus was more easily obtained on certain principles. In a pluralistic, modern society consensus is not always possible, thus, leaving casuistry as a method of case analysis rather than a guide to moral theory or practice (Arras, 1991; Pellegrino, 1993).

Further work in contextual ethics arose when theorists postulated that a theory conceptualized around the notion of care might actually be more useful in describing a nursing ethic than the justice-based model used in principle-oriented ethics. Historically, theories about moral development and moral reasoning had been strongly influenced by the work of psychologist Kohlberg and his Piagetian-based cognitive theory of moral development (Blum, 1988). Gilligan (1982/1993) and Noddings (1984) challenged the field of moral psychology, arguing that Kohlberg's singular focus on justice in his theory of moral development obscured another dimension of the moral concerns of individuals. Gilligan suggested that issues other than rights and fairness, the concerns of justice outlined in Kohlberg's Model of Moral Development, helped to shape the way individuals frame moral conflict and choice. These included concerns about interdependence, maintaining connections and attachments among individuals, and assuring that someone not be excluded or hurt in the situation being examined (Bebeau & Brabeck, 1989; Fry, 1991). Gilligan described care as a 'different voice' and not a voice lesser than Kohlberg's justice-based voice. She found that girls and women tended to approach ethical dilemmas in a contextualized, narrative way, looking for resolution in particular details of a problem situation. She identified this orientation in her research and called it an ethic of care. In contrast, boys and men seemed inclined to try to apply general abstract principles without attention to the unique circumstances of the case (Sherwin, 1992, p. 18). Gilligan described her theory as one way of changing the voice of the world by bringing women's voices into the open, thus starting a new conversation (1993, p. xxvii).

In contrast to principle-oriented ethics, a care ethic has been described as a situational, intuitive process where the central issue is judging an action in terms of its web of relatedness (Fry, 1991). In this theory, moral concern deals with needs and responsibility as they evolve in a relationship (Cooper, 1991). Caring implies mutuality and reciprocity in relationships and is not unidirectional. An individual is considered moral when in a relationship with another, not because of a social contract as in the principled approach. The caring approach to ethics has been described as an ethic of 'intimates' versus an ethic of 'strangers' (Cooper, 1991; Fry, 1989a; 1989b; 1991; Penticuff, 1991).

There have been criticisms levied at those who suggest that caring is unique to women and to nursing, thereby excluding males and other health professionals (Gillon, 1992; Nelson, 1992). Gillon (1992) points out that Gilligan's theory describes a developmental process that involves a fundamental difference between men and women in their starting perspective on morality. He states, "... as she [Gilligan] points out in her last chapter, as men and women mature, they increasingly come to appreciate the importance of both perspectives" (p. 172). Other critics have pointed out that the ethic of care may not provide direction at the macro level of health care because of its individualistic, relativistic, and relational underpinnings (Nelson, 1992). Finally, there are concerns that an ethic of care could lead to an impoverished self if individuals

Table 5-4
Levels of professional responsibility.

Micro level - Individual level
Meso level - Institutional/Agency level
Macro level - Societal level

were required to care for all persons at all times (Fry, 1991; Nelson, 1992).

Interestingly, while principled ethics and contextual ethics are depicted in the literature as distinct theories, there are those who are proposing that there may be room for a principle-oriented ethic, woven with contextual features such as care and compassion. Recently, Bergum, Boyle, Briggs, and Dossetor (1993) have suggested that there should be a dialectic between the two processes of principled and contextual ethics. They state, "From the dialectic of close-up and distant ethics comes synthesis, and this synthesis, in the narrative of our lives and those of our patients/clients, is what ethics is all about" (p. 1). In summary, the development of ethical theory over the centuries has been progressive, with a variety of approaches being proposed to determine how we should act when confronted with an ethical problem or dilemma. Current ethical theory development in nursing is moving away from the application of principles as absolutes to consideration of the contextual features of cases and the relationships among patients, their families, and the health professionals providing their care. In this latter scenario, principles are considered guidelines rather than universal absolutes. As will be illustrated in the case studies later in this chapter, this change in focus provides nurses with ethical theory that is able to provide direction for nephrology nursing settings.

Levels of Professional Responsibility

Meeting the ethical challenges confronting us in nephrology nursing, particularly as they are confounded by issues of resource allocation, requires us to think about our professional roles as they fit into three levels of responsibility (Rodney & Starzomski, 1994, p.11) (see Table 5-4). The first of these levels is the micro level. This is the level of individual professional responsibilities for patients and families under our care. The second is the meso level, or the level of institutional responsibilities for programs of care. The third is the macro level, or the level of societal responsibilities for the health of the total population (Kluge, 1992; McDonald, 1993; Yeo & Donner, 1991) These three levels of involvement demand different types of decision making in order to arrive at ethically sound decisions. For example, at the micro level we need to look at frameworks of ethical decision making for individual patients and their family members. At the meso and macro levels of the system we need to look at health policy decision making, to assure that we develop policies that meet the needs of citizens and are, at the same time, ethical in nature (Rodney & Starzomski, 1994, p.11).

Throughout all levels of our involvement, we must keep in mind the need to foster the integrity of patient-professional relationships. Unique obligations befall health care professionals because their specialized judgment and skill is required for the good of patients. Given the trust that patients and family members place in professionals, fidelity is an important feature of professional/patient/family relationships (Beauchamp & Childress, 1989). Fidelity is based on trust, and generates rules for promise-keeping structured around respect for autonomy.

One of the most difficult challenges facing us, as we consider our roles in all three areas of professional responsibility, is our ability to act in our individual patient's best interest, while at the same time involving ourselves in discussions about how resources are to be allocated in a just manner for the aggregate. In other words, how do we uphold our bedside covenant with patients, to always act in their best interest (Pellegrino & Thomasma, 1988), and at the same time participate in decisions to allocate resources for groups of patients — decisions that may affect the care we are able to provide to individuals at the bedside?

Let us consider an illustration of these levels in nephrology nursing practice to help clarify how it is possible for nephrology nurses to be involved in micro, meso, and macro level decisions. Using the area of kidney transplantation as an illustration, at the micro level, we are concerned about how health care providers decide whether a transplant is in a particular patient's best interest. At the meso level, we are concerned about developing selection criteria for transplantation, or deciding how much of an institutional budget should be used for transplantation compared to other programs. Furthermore, at the macro level, we are concerned about how much of the health care budget is to be used for transplantation in relation to other services (Rodney & Starzomski, 1994, p.11). At the macro level, we might also be called upon to advocate on behalf of all transplant patients if a particular service was threatened. If we do not get involved in progressive planning at the meso and macro level, we shall remain caught in a fundamental tension between our obligations to benefit individual clients and our obligations to benefit society (Fry, 1985, p. 303; Kjellstrand, 1992).

Involving ourselves in meso and macro level activities does not mean that we have abandoned our patients at the micro level. On the contrary, by involvement in meso and macro level discussions, nephrology nurses may be in a better position to assure that activities at the micro level are carried out in the best interest of the patient. For example, in 1987, in Oregon, the state legislature determined there would be a budgetary shortfall in the funding of health services for Medicaid recipients (Klevit et al., 1991). The legislature decided, with little discussion and no public debate, to direct funds away from certain types of transplants in favor of prenatal and other forms of preventive and primary health care (Crawshaw, Garland, & Hines, 1989; Jennings, 1988; Welch & Larson, 1988). There was extensive public outcry when two Oregon children in the Medicaid program were denied necessary transplants. The first child denied care was an infant with neuroblastoma whose family moved to Washington state and established Medicaid eligibility there in order to receive care for their son. The second case was a 7-year old boy with leukemia, who required a bone marrow transplant, and reportedly died before his relatives could raise money needed for him to receive necessary care. Extensive lobbying and political pressure from health care providers and citizens forced the state to rethink the decision and reinstate coverage for transplantation (Boisaubin, 1988; Welch & Larson, 1988). If health care providers had not lobbied for this change they would have been unable to act in their patients interest at the micro level since some patients would have been denied transplantation. This leads to the important discussion of the role of the nephrology nurse as an advocate for people with chronic renal failure and their families.

Advocacy

Providing good nursing care at the micro, meso, or macro levels of the health care system requires that we act as advocates for people with renal disease and their families. Over the course of nursing history, we have seen the nurse's role change and evolve from being an advocate at all levels of the health care system, to focusing more attention on the micro level, leaving health policy concerns at the macro level to others. The development of the advocacy role in nursing parallels the development of nursing practice as we know it today. Winslow (1984) has described the nursing profession as moving from a military/loyalty metaphor to an advocacy metaphor over the course of modern nursing history.

Modern nursing history is often said to have begun with the work of Florence Nightingale, who is widely acknowledged as the founder of modern nursing (Peplau, 1987). Nightingale was recognized as a leader, innovator, and skilled politician in the areas of epidemiology, statistics, health policy development, and social reform areas where she believed nursing had a major role to play (Gropper, 1990; Peplau, 1987; Reed & Zurakowski, 1989). Her focus, in the late 1800s, was very similar to the areas identified as important to the practice of nursing today.

From the early 1970s to the present, the theme of the nurse as advocate has become a major part of modern nursing, thereby, impacting on how nursing ethics is conceptualized. Winslow (1984) and Starr (1982) reasoned that the move to an advocacy model in nursing was brought about, in part, by the rise of consumerism and a loss of confidence in the medical profession by consumers. Annas (1974) postulates that nurses have the potential to play key roles in becoming advocates on behalf of patients because of their unique roles with patients and their families. Other societal factors, such as rapid advances in knowledge and technology, major changes in attitudes, values, and beliefs concerning health care, as well as changes related to the role of women in society were also instrumental in moving nursing in the direction of becoming patient advocates (Cooper, 1991; Roberts, 1983).

Several nurse theorists and philosophers have attempted to describe the concept of advocacy in nursing. The models they suggest differ from the legal rights protection model proposed by Winslow (1984). Fowler (1991), in her review of advocacy models in nursing, suggests that nursing is based on an interpersonal or moral relationship with the patient. She points out that Kohnke (1980) describes a value-based model of advocacy where the nurse seeks to assist the patient in identifying or clarifying personal values. Gadow (1990) puts forward a variation of Kohnke's view of advocacy that she calls 'existential advocacy'. Gadow suggests that the philosophical foundation and ideal of nursing is advocacy. She distinguishes nursing advocacy from the type implied in the patients' rights or consumer movement and suggests that nurses assist patients to make decisions based on the patient's own value system. Gadow posits that the nurse is best suited of all professionals to claim this advocacy role because of the uniqueness of nursing's contribution to patient care, such as the amount of time nurses spend with patients and their families in their caring role (Fowler, 1991).

In the value-based models described above, the patient must be self-determining, or the patient's values should be known by others. The models exclude those persons who are unable to participate in decision making or those whose surrogate speaks for them. Fry (1987) describes a respect for persons model, in which she suggests that the nurse respects an individual's dignity and personhood, whether the person is autonomous or not. When the individual is not autonomous, and there is no surrogate to speak for him/her, then the nurse is called upon to act in the best interest of the person. If the individual is capable of self-determination, or has a surrogate, then the value-based decision model can be used. Bramlet, Gueldner, and Sowell (1990) stress the need in nursing to move from an emphasis on loyalty and obedience to institutions and physicians, to consumer-centric advocacy, where the consumer's rights in decision making are coupled with the nurse's role in supporting these rights.

Freeman (1971) proposes a practice as protest model of advocacy. According to Freeman, this form of advocacy, rooted in the concept of social justice, not only makes certain that individuals are cared for, but also calls attention to inconsistencies and inadequacies of care. Freeman suggests three ways in which nurses can enact the practice as protest model, (a) engaging in public contest and confrontation, or sharing the cause of the aggrieved; (b) acting as advocates for persons unable to fight for themselves; and (c) through the practice of nursing itself, enhancing the capabilities of patients to fend for themselves (p. 919). Freeman ends her discussion with the following comment on directions for nursing practice. It is striking to note how similar these words are to the message expressed by Florence Nightingale a century before:

> A passive or meek approach to conditions that threaten the health or integrity of individuals is no longer compatible with nursing practice. One cannot deal as a professional worker with the health and human results of public inertia and injustice while failing to take all possible action to correct the cause. Protest and social action must join ministration, education, and support as essential elements of nursing practice (p. 921).

Fowler (1991) proposes that none of the advocacy models presented above are well developed, although she suggests that the respect for persons model appears to be the most popular in nursing today. There is, however, no consensus within nursing as to which model will emerge as the definitive one for the profession and there is still debate about whether advocacy is the ideal of nursing alone, since other health professionals are obviously patient advocates as well (Abrams, 1990; Bernal, 1992; Pagana, 1990). Clearly, in many instances, advocacy is an important role for all health care professionals and certainly a central component of nursing practice.

In nephrology, where the interdisciplinary team concept is prevalent, working together with other disciplines to advocate on behalf of people with renal disease, and their families, is a common occurrence. This interdisciplinary advocacy is evident in the clinical setting, as well as at the level of organizations such as the National Kidney Foundation and the Kidney Foundation of Canada, where patients, their families, health care professionals, and the general public work together to advocate at the meso and macro levels of the system on behalf of people with kidney disease.

Making Ethical Decisions - An Ethical Decision-Making Framework

An understanding of the development of health care ethics, ethical theory, levels of professional responsibility, and the role of the nephrology nurse as a patient/family advocate provide the necessary knowledge to facilitate ethical decision making. With this foundation in place to provide direction for ethical decision making, how then does the nephrology nurse use this theory to make ethical decisions?

Ethical decision making is the application of various skills of ethical analysis and reasoning in an attempt to reach a well-grounded solution to an ethical problem or dilemma (Benjamin & Curtis, 1986, p.11). This reasoning includes the need for thoughtful, critical thinking and an understanding of personal values when making ethical decisions. Ethical decision making focuses on determining what *ought* to occur in each situation and is an important part of each health care professional's ability to make good decisions about ethical concerns. Ethical decision making in modern health care settings is not the solitary activity of one team member, but requires ongoing health care team communication and collaboration, remembering that the patient and family are integral team members, as well as nurses, physicians, technicians, social workers, dietitians, clergy, and other health professionals.

There are several frameworks that integrate various aspects of ethical theory to provide direction for decision making. Many of the models follow a process of rational deliberation similar to any decision- making process. The framework by McDonald (1994), depicted in Table 5-5, is a comprehensive ethical decision-making framework that is based on care and compassion, where ethical principles are used as guidelines to assist in developing the best solution to a particular ethical dilemma or problem. Like all frameworks, it should function as a guide, rather than a recipe, remembering that ethical decision making is a process that may vary depending on the circumstances of the case being considered. It is essential to recognize that, because real cases are complex, it will not always be possible to obtain a perfect solution to an ethical dilemma or problem. However, using a logical framework makes the process transparent to others and assures that key components have been considered.

In McDonald's framework the first step in decision making is identifying the problem and describing the case briefly with all the relevant facts and circumstances. At this stage, it is important to clarify what decisions have to be made and by whom. In addition, it is necessary to know who needs to be involved in the decision, making certain to include the appropriate individuals in the discus-

Table 5-5
An ethical decision making framework.

A decision procedure for ethical decision making. To be used as a guide, rather than a recipe, remembering that ethical decision making is a process, best done in a caring and compassionate environment.

1. Identify The Problem
   a. State the case briefly but with all the relevant facts and circumstances.
   b. What decisions have to be made?
   c. By whom? Who are the relevant decision makers?

2. Specify Feasible Alternatives
   What are the alternatives? State the options at each level of decision-making.

3. Use Your Ethics Resources To Evaluate Alternatives
   What are the critical considerations? Relevant resources?
   a. *Principles*:
      i) **Autonomy:** What does the patient want? What explicit or implicit promises have been made to the patient?
      ii) **Beneficence:** Will this benefit the patient?
      iii) **Nonmaleficence**: Will this harm the patient?
      iv) **Justice:** Consider the interests of all those - including the patient's - that have to be taken into account.
   b. *Policies:*
      Professional norms, standards and codes, legal precedents, hospital policy.
   c. *Contextual features of the case that seem important:*
      Family relationships, past history etc., spiritual and ethno-cultural considerations.
   d. *Personal judgments*:
      Yours, your colleagues, and other members of the health care team.
   e. *Organized procedures for ethical consultation:*
      Case conferences, use of an ethics committee or ethics consultant

4. Propose And Test Possible Resolutions
   a. Propose a resolution or select the best alternative, all things considered.
   b. Perform a sensitivity analysis. Consider your choice critically: Which factors would have to change to get you to alter your decision?
   c. Think about the effects of your choice upon others' choices: Are you making it easier or harder for relevant others - other health care providers, patients and their families, etc. to act ethically?
   d. Is this what a compassionate health care professional would do in a caring environment?
   e. Formulate your choice as a *general maxim for all similar cases.* Suggest cases where it does *not* apply. Consider cases where it does apply.
   f. Are you still comfortable with your decision? If you are, then go with it. If not, consider the factors that make you uncomfortable with the choice, with a view to coming up with a new general maxim that you are comfortable with. Repeat until you are convinced that you have done your best in the time you have.

Remember that you are not aiming at the perfect choice, but a good choice.

Note: Adapted from McDonald, M. (1994). *Decision making.* Unpublished manuscript, Centre for Applied Ethics, University of British Columbia, Vancouver, BC, Canada.

sion. Secondly, it is helpful to analyze the different alternatives that are practical and feasible, given the circumstances of the case. Thirdly, it is useful to consider various ethics resources to evaluate the alternatives that have been raised.

One useful ethics resource is the application of ethical principles to help sort through the problem. For instance, in regard to autonomy, we should consider what the individual wants and what explicit or implicit promises have been made to him/her. The principle of beneficence requires us to ask whether our proposal would benefit the person. One of our considerations would be whether the proposed treatment will be beneficial, useful, and reasonable for that person. The individual, in consultation with the appropriate health care professional(s), is in the best position to make this judgment.

The principle of nonmaleficence would direct us to be certain that we did no harm to the person by our actions and, therefore, not propose treatment that would be burdensome, futile, or unreasonable. Finally, the principle of justice directs us to consider that the interests of everyone — with the patient's interest being central — have been taken into account.

In addition to principles, there are other ethics resources such as policies, professional norms, standards, codes of ethics, and legal precedents that can provide valuable direction in deliberation about ethical problems. Contextual features of the case such as family relationships, past history, the illness experience, and spiritual and ethno-cultural considerations are critically important (Fry, 1989b; Jecker, Carrese, & Pearlman, 1995). All voices within the health care team must be heard, and the judgments of all team members need to be considered. There may be a need for an organized process for ethical consultation such as a case conference. Furthermore, an ethics committee or ethics consultant can provide valuable advice and assistance with the case if required.

After examining all the features of the case, a resolution to the problem can be proposed. How can we determine if we have made the best possible decision? One way is to perform a sensitivity analysis. We can consider critically the choice that was made — which factors would have to change to alter the decision? We can think about the effects the choice made upon others' choices — is it easier or harder for relevant others such as health care providers, patients, and their families to act ethically? Furthermore, we can ask ourselves if this alternative is what a compassionate health care professional would do in a caring environment.

Finally, the choice can be formulated as a general maxim (standard) for similar cases. It is useful to think about cases where it does or does not apply. The decision makers can then evaluate their level of comfort with the decision and implement the chosen alternative. If the decision makers are not comfortable with the decision then it is essential to consider the factors that make them uncomfortable with the choice, with a view to coming up with a new general standard. This process is repeated until it appears that the best decision has been made in the time available. It is important to remember that the aim is not to develop the perfect choice, but a good choice.

Ethical Issues in Nephrology Nursing

With this foundation for ethics in nephrology nursing, and some resources for decision making, let us now move to an illustration of how to use this information in the context of some of the major ethical issues facing nephrology nurses. Many of the ethical issues that nephrology practitioners encounter are representative of those that originated when dialysis and transplantation were in their infancy, and are prototypical of ethical issues raised by high technology and life-sustaining treatments in health care.

In the early years, nephrology pioneer Belding Scribner identified several ethical issues that would be problematic in the future, including patient selection, termination of treatment, suicidal patients, dying with dignity, and organ donor selection (Scribner, 1964). These concerns remain important today and have been joined by other issues, such as ensuring informed consent for treatment, deciding when to withdraw or withhold treatment, making certain that people have established advance directives, and resource allocation concerns at the micro, meso, and macro levels of the system (Long, 1994; McCormick, 1993; Moss, 1995; Moss, Rettig, & Cassel, 1993; Neu, 1994; Pfettscher, 1993; Swartz et al., 1994) .

One of the most difficult issues in nephrology nursing is the increasing number of people requiring treatment for chronic renal failure and the diminishing resources available to care for them. In the U.S., the number of patients receiving renal care has risen from a few hundred in the early 1960s to over 180,000 patients, treated in over 2,056 Medicare-approved renal facilities (U.S. Health Care Financing Administration, 1994). In Canada, in 1981, there were 5,576 patients receiving dialysis or living with a kidney transplant. Today, there are over 14,200 patients being treated (Canadian Organ Replacement Register, 1994). More liberal treatment criteria, an aging population, and an increase in patients with conditions such as Type 1 diabetes are thought to play a major role in the increasing number of people requiring treatment (Cummings, 1993). Although there are differences in how health care is funded in the U.S. and Canada, there are concerns in both systems about the ability to continue to fund renal care in a manner that allows us to provide dialysis and transplantation for all who require these treatments

(Balk, 1990; Mendez, Aswald, Dessouki, Cicciarelli, & Mendez, 1992; Moskop, 1987; Stiller, 1990).

It has been suggested that increasing kidney transplantation will resolve some of the concerns about the numbers of patients receiving expensive dialysis therapy, however, there are many unresolved ethical issues in transplantation that remain problematic. The important issues and questions arising in the transplant arena are manifested at the three levels of responsibility for health care. The community at large is faced with fundamental questions, at the macro or societal level of the health care system, about the level of resources to be allocated to life-saving technology such as organ transplantation (Benjamin, 1992; Brooks, 1993; Evans, 1992; Turcotte, 1992). Also at the macro level, a major worldwide organ shortage (Bowden & Hull, 1993; Youngner, 1992) has raised questions about changing consent for human tissue, by (a) examining strategies for presumed consent (Andrews, 1992; Childress, 1992; Cohen, 1992; Menzel, 1992b; Sadler, 1992; Veatch, 1991c; Youngner & Arnold, 1993), (b) using fetal tissue for transplantation (Martin, 1992; Nelson, 1990), (c) offering financial incentives for organ donation (Dickens, 1991; Evans, 1993), (d) engaging in buying and selling organs (Guttmann & Guttmann, 1992; Kazim et al., 1992), (e) using anencephalic infant donors (Dickens, 1988; Roy et al., 1994), and (f) considering the use of xenografts (transplanting from one species to another), as ways to solve the shortage of organs for human transplantation (Caplan, 1992; Rapaport, 1993; Reemtsma, 1992; Singer, 1992).

At the meso or institutional level of the health care system, questions are raised regarding the choice of the recipients for organ transplantation and how selection criteria should be developed (Kilner, 1988; 1990; Kluge, 1993; Seib, MacLeod, & Stiller, 1990). In addition, as transplant waiting lists grow, a question arises about the number of waiting lists on which a recipient should be listed. Another difficult question at the meso level arises when determining how decisions should be made about the proportion of an institutional budget devoted to transplantation compared to other programs (Balk, 1990).

Decisions at the micro level of the health care system are evident surrounding issues about how health care providers decide whether a transplant is in a given patient's best interest. For example, health care providers make decisions about removing kidneys from individual living donors to be transplanted into specific recipients (Hilton & Starzomski, 1994; Sells, 1992; Simmons, Marine, & Simmons, 1987). In addition, organs from unrelated donors are being considered more frequently in transplant centers around the world (Spital, 1992; 1993). Finally, there is the question of how many organs to which one individual is entitled (Evans, Manninen, Dong, & McLynne, 1993). Although this list is not exhaustive, it provides an overview of some of the most perplexing problems evident in transplantation today.

Concerns about the principles of autonomy and informed consent arise from the issues explicated above. Moreover, the critical principle of justice is embedded in many of these ethical issues about organ transplantation, exposing deep tensions about the societal sense of what is true or just (Fox & Swazey, 1992a; 1992b; Jonsen, 1985; 1989; Kjellstrand & Dossetor, 1992). These situations raise a need for a collaborative approach among health care providers and the public to define and determine legitimate and just applications of organ transplantation technology (Fox & Swazey, 1992a; 1992b; Rettig, 1989; Storch & Dossetor, 1993).

Case Analysis

The following cases, and the discussions that follow each one, highlight many of the ethical dilemmas and problems encountered by nephrology nurses, and demonstrate how an ethical decision-making framework can be used to help resolve the problems.

Case 1

Mr. B., an active 89-year-old man, has been living in a private long-term care facility for the past 5 years. He is well liked by the staff and spends most of his time reading or playing cards. His health has been good for most of his life, however, at the age of 88 he was found to have a 4 cm abdominal aortic aneurysm that was considered by his surgeon too small to repair electively. The surgeon decided, with Mr. B., to continue to monitor the size of the aneurysm and consider surgery, if necessary, in the future.

One week ago, Mr. B. was found slumped over his bed by a nurse in the long-term care facility. He was unresponsive and an ambulance was called immediately. Mr. B. was taken to the Emergency Room (E.R.) of a large, tertiary care hospital. He arrested in the ambulance enroute to the hospital and was resuscitated successfully by the ambulance attendants. In the E.R., it was confirmed that Mr. B.'s aneurysm had ruptured. He was rushed to the operating room, bumping two elective patients, and his aneurysm was repaired. In the operating room he was given 11 units of blood, and then transferred to the intensive care unit (ICU). Mr. B. did not regain consciousness, and after 3 days, it was apparent that he was in acute renal failure. The nephrologist who saw Mr. B. recommended dialysis. As Mr. B had no relatives who could be involved in the decision, his surgeon decided that dialysis would be initiated.

Mr. B. was successfully removed from the ventilator, but after 3 weeks of dialysis treatment, he remained unconscious with no improvement in his kidney function. The nurses in the dialysis unit raised concerns about whether Mr. B. should be resuscitated if he arrested, and because of his poor prognosis, wondered whether dialysis should be continued. They were told that because the decision was made to initiate treatment by repairing his aneurysm, all must now be done to treat Mr. B. The dialysis unit nurses and social worker assigned to Mr. B. were upset about this decision and did not agree with the treatment plan. They spoke to nurses at the long-term care facility who knew Mr. B. very well, and these nurses stated that they believed Mr. B. would not want to be treated if he were aware of his condition. One nurse at the facility said that, in fact, Mr. B. would not have agreed to an aneurysm repair and was going to tell his surgeon this at his next appointment.

Because of the differences in opinion about how Mr. B. should be treated, and the moral distress of the nurses caring for him, a team conference is called. Mr. B.'s family doctor and two nurses from the long-term care facility attend the conference, as well as staff from the ICU, the cardiac surgeon, the social worker, two nurses from the dialysis unit, and the nephrologist.

Discussion. One of the major ethical dilemmas to be addressed by health care professionals in this case is whether treatment should be continued. Is Mr. B.'s best interest being considered, given his prognosis and apparent wishes about surgical repair of his aneurysm (according to the nurses in the long-term care facility). Mr. B. is unable to speak for himself and has not left an advance directive or living will, nor does he have a relative or friend who could be named his surrogate decision maker. The dialysis unit nurses believe they are acting as Mr. B.'s advocates when raising the question of discontinuing dialysis, as they believe, after discussion with the nurses in the long-term care facility who have had a significant relationship with Mr. B. for many years, that he would not wish to continue the dialysis treatment.

Collecting more data about the case, and examining the four principles outlined earlier (autonomy, beneficence, nonmaleficence, and justice), provides some guidance in this case. Mr. B. is unable to exercise his autonomy in his current state. The nephrologist believes that the dialysis treatment is providing some physiological benefit to Mr. B., is not harming him, and that his condition may improve, however, he is ambivalent about what course of action should now be taken since he has heard the information from the long-term care nurses about Mr. B.'s wishes. The ICU physician believes Mr. B. may regain consciousness and be in a debilitated state, but at least he will be alive and then able to decide what treatment he wishes to have. The dialysis nurses disagree, stating that the pain and discomfort Mr. B. is currently experiencing in his weakened and debilitated state is burdensome and doing him harm. The nurses from the dialysis unit, long-term care facility, and ICU argue that the treatment is merely prolonging Mr. B.'s dying and not providing him with any real benefit. Mr. B.'s family physician, who has known him for several years, believes that Mr. B. would wish to discontinue treatment if he was unable to return to his former state and presses both the nephrologist and ICU physician for their realistic views about Mr. B.'s prognosis. When pressed, the ICU physician says he is certain that if Mr. B. does regain consciousness he would not return to his former level of health, and would very likely have significant cognitive impairment.

When considering the principle of justice, the team believed that Mr. B. was entitled to be dialyzed and that when the outcome of a critically ill individual is uncertain then a trial of dialysis is appropriate. Considering the various theories of justice they could see that all the theories would support Mr. B. receiving treatment. If, however, there was a question of limited resources, the utilitarian would say to provide care in the cases where there would be the greatest benefit. In other words, if a younger person who had a better prognosis and Mr. B. were competing for the same resource, then the person who would most benefit should receive the treatment. An individual operating from an egalitarian perspective would also *consider* examining who should receive the care if two individuals require it, however, different treatment would be justified only where the need was different, or where both needs could not be met. Where these circumstances occur, then priority would be given to the greater need that could feasibly be met. In this institution, based on the resources available, treating Mr. B. is possible.

The dialysis unit nurses suggest that they are required to send a nurse to dialyze Mr. B. in the ICU, thus taking resources away from their own unit at a time when they are extremely busy. Their first concern is with the pain and suffering that Mr. B. is enduring, and that his chances of recovery are very slim. They point out that the hospital policy, with respect to withdrawing and withholding treatment, states that there is no moral imperative to continue treatment if the treatment is futile. However, it is pointed out by another team member that futility is a very emotionally charged term and it is difficult to determine what it actually means.

The nephrologist volunteers that it is now very unlikely that Mr. B. will recover, and that he has reviewed recent data from several studies where it is suggested that in cases like this the prognosis is very poor. In the end, the team agrees to continue treatment for another 2 days, and consult with the hospital ethics committee to provide them with some guidance. In the interim, the surgeon and ICU physician agree to a 'No Code Order' as they are convinced, based on resuscitation data from similar cases, that Mr. B. is not a candidate for resuscitation.

When reviewing the case with the ethics committee, the nurses once again suggest that Mr. B. be allowed to die with dignity and that continuing treatment would only prolong his suffering. The ethics committee helps the team review the facts of the case and the different alternatives. The ICU physician and the surgeon agree that, because there has been no change in Mr. B.'s condition in the weeks he has been treated, continuing to dialyze him would only prolong his dying, and they agree that the treatment is medically futile. The team discusses whether they have made the right decision by coming to the conclusion that other caring and compassionate health professionals would make the same decision, and determining that in similar cases, circumstances being the same, they would once again choose this option. Following the case discussion, dialysis is discontinued. Mr. B. dies 2 days later without regaining consciousness.

The team members realize that the different values they held about death and dying, the absence of any relatives to speak for Mr. B., or a written advance directive, as well as their communication difficulties all made this case problematic. As a result of this case, the long-term care facility staff and the dialysis unit staff plan to develop and implement policies and programs to ensure that all patients are given the opportunity to complete an advance directive document. In addition, the team members in the agency began efforts and processes to improve their communication and decision making about ethical issues by instituting interdisciplinary ethics rounds that will be held twice a month where cases and concerns will be discussed. Moreover, they have committed to examining the outcome studies conducted about dialysis morbidity and mortality, and based on the data, determining better selection criteria for treatment. They remain committed to ensuring patient choice in treatment decisions, however, they recognize the value of providing accurate data so people are able to make their decisions based on the best outcome information available.

Case 2

Teresa is a 34-year-old former high school teacher who has had Type 1 diabetes for 22 years. She is married, with two children (a son age 10 and a daughter age 8) and a very supportive husband. Teresa has developed a variety of complications as a result of her diabetes. Currently, she is experiencing difficulty walking because of peripheral neuropathy, has frequent nausea, vomiting, and diarrhea because of gastroporesis, and has been declared legally blind as a result of retinopathy. In addition, she has developed chronic renal failure and has been receiving thrice weekly hemodialysis for the past year. Although Teresa would have preferred to do dialysis at home so she could be close to her family, she was not a candidate for continuous ambulatory peritoneal dialysis (CAPD) because of multiple abdominal surgeries and trouble placing her peritoneal catheter. When she began dialysis last year, several of her family members were tested as possible living related kidney donors and Teresa's sister was found to be compatible. Although the surgery went well, the transplanted kidney was removed 4 weeks later because of rejection. Teresa was subsequently added to the cadaveric transplant waiting list. She has been informed that a successful kidney transplant will improve her condition, and she has been anxiously waiting for a kidney to become available. She has been told that she will likely receive a kidney within about 18 months.

Because of her deteriorating condition and lack of energy, Teresa has quit her teaching job and is no longer able to golf or swim, two of her favorite activities. She feels very frustrated because she can no longer drive, do any of her housework, or socialize for any length of time with her family and friends due to her fatigue, limited mobility, and vision. She is dependent on her family and friends to drive her to and from her treatments several times a week. Teresa is hoping that she will receive a transplant soon, as she has said that she "doesn't know how much longer I can stand living like this."

Lately, Teresa has been experiencing more gastrointestinal problems that have remained resistant to any drug therapy. She has been experiencing severe chest pain, particularly during her dialysis treatments. Investigations show that she has significant coronary artery disease affecting several blood vessels. The recommended treatment is coronary artery bypass surgery. The cardiac surgeon informs Teresa that because of her unstable situation, and major diabetes complications, she is a very high-risk surgical candidate and that she may die during the operation, or be in a worsened state after the surgery. Nonetheless, he recommends she go ahead as there is a possibility things will go well. When she presses the surgeon for the success of this surgery, he quotes statistics that show a high rate of success with the surgical technique, but high complication rates with diabetic patients. Until she recovers from the surgery she will be inactive on the transplant waiting list. According to her nephrologist, there is some question about whether she will be transplantable after the surgery because of her overall deteriorating condition as a result of her diabetes.

After much thought and considerable discussion with her family and health care team members, Teresa wishes to stop dialysis and discontinue her insulin. She believes that her quality of life (QOL) has deteriorated markedly and says she is "tired of operations, pain, and discomfort." Teresa decides to stop active treatment rather than undergo a series of painful and difficult medical procedures that in the end may not make it possible for her to receive a transplant, the only hope she has had to improve her situation.

Teresa's family members are very upset about her decision and want the health care team to try and convince her to change her mind, continue treatment, and have the bypass surgery. The surgeon and nephrologist agree with the family and think Teresa is depressed and should see a psychiatrist. Teresa insists she is making a good decision, and wants the health care team to help her support her family. The nurses and social worker are impressed by her courage and are supportive of her decision. There is considerable team tension, conflict, and informal discussion about what should be done. This conflict continues even after the psychiatrist says that Teresa is mentally competent, not clinically depressed, and capable of making her own decisions.

Discussion. This case illustrates several of the concerns that emerge when individuals wish to discontinue life-saving treatment. It is often difficult for family members and health professionals to accept patients' decisions when they may conflict with their own values and wishes.

Teresa's family is having difficulty coping with the knowledge that she is dying and need emotional support to deal with this. In addition, several of the health care team members believe Teresa is refusing treatment that may improve her physical condition, albeit treatment that could potentially make her worse off than she is now. In the curative environment of dialysis and transplantation, professionals can be very uncomfortable when they are not able to provide someone with a treatment that will result in their improvement. In the pursuit of life, we may find it difficult to accept that people will die sometime, and that our job may be to help them with a good death (Starzomski, 1994).

In Teresa's situation, no one can give her the information she needs to assure her that she would have a better QOL with the proposed treatment. As a competent individual, she has the right to make choices about her own care. In considering the available information and determining the level of benefit she might receive, Teresa made her decision based on her individual circumstances and values. Teresa is able to articulate her own choices and wishes, although some team members, attempting to act in a manner that they think would not cause Teresa harm (in this case death), believe she should continue treatment. They see her as a young individual who has much to live for. On the other hand, Teresa believes the burdens of her treatment far outweigh the benefits. She believes that those who are not supporting her decision are acting in a paternalistic manner. There is a direct conflict between Teresa's individual autonomy and the autonomy of the health care professionals, who believe they are acting in accordance with the nonmaleficence, or do no harm principle.

In this case, Teresa needs the health care team to assist her and her family in preparation for her death. This is a task that some team members find particularly difficult. One way to help resolve the dilemmas that arise in this case is to encourage all team members (with Teresa and her family) to discuss the issues in an open manner, using the ethical decision-making framework to help identify the problems, determine the alternatives, and arrive at a plan that would provide the necessary support and care for all involved. The solution here is not to consider treatment for the sake of others, but to focus on what is in Teresa's best interest, and to assist the family in coping with the reality that she is dying (Starzomski, 1994). By encouraging team communication and collaboration, Teresa received the support she required, and died at home with her family 24 hours after she discontinued her dialysis and insulin treatments.

Formal discussion about withholding or withdrawing treatment in dialysis and transplant units has been infrequent. In many situations, where death is imminent, or where the potential outcome is extremely poor, there is great difficulty in shifting from a curative approach, to a palliative perspective, where palliative care principles can be applied, and support provided, thus giving people the option of dying with dignity (Starzomski, 1994). Some programs are beginning to move in the direction of using palliative perspectives, incorporating discussion of advance directives, and developing guidelines for withdrawing and withholding treatments (Colvin & Hammes, 1991; Colvin, Myhre, Welch, & Hammes, 1993; Mendelsshon & Singer, 1994). However, there is still little being done in most centers about systematically incorporating palliative care principles into programs of care. Most of the discussion about these areas occurs in an informal fashion in the coffee room, or around the nursing station, where team members discuss their frustration about treatment decisions. Many programs are left with no clear direction about how to support individuals who are turned down for transplantation, choose not to be transplanted, elect not to start dialysis, or wish to discontinue the treatment. There are concerns about where, how, and by whom care is provided to the patient and family. In most cases, dialysis success is measured by patient survival through the treatment, or as in the case of transplantation, by patient survival and success of the graft, rather than on the overall QOL for the individual (Starzomski, 1994).

How do we determine whether a treatment will in fact improve a patient's QOL? There is agreement, in most situations, that practitioners are not obligated to offer, and patients are not obligated to undergo, treatments that are futile (Roy et al., 1994, p. 394). But how do we determine futility — a heavily value-ladened term? One way of ascertaining whether a treatment is futile or beneficial is by considering whether the proposed interventions will benefit the patient as a whole, or whether the treatment will become an additional burden that the person must bear as the dying process is prolonged (Starzomski, 1994).

Schneiderman, Jacker, and Jonsen (1990) believe futility has two distinct components: physiological effect and benefit. From their point of view, some treatments can be futile because they do not produce a desired physiological effect or the anticipated goal of treatment. Although this is a useful conceptualization, it is still difficult to apply in many cases because we do not have the outcome data with which to determine the potential physiological effect. What percentage of success is considered adequate to consider a treatment beneficial? Even with outcome data, each case must be evaluated in terms of the potential benefits as seen through the patient's eyes. The patient must be the one, when presented with the information about the benefits and burdens of treatment, to make a choice based on his/her own individual interpretation of QOL. Although some clinicians might suggest that this could lead to people asking for inappropriate care, it has been this author's experience in dealing with many hundreds of patients and families that there are very few who choose a treatment that has a potentially dismal outcome when the information about what is known is presented fairly and honestly, with the risks and benefits outlined accurately. Clearly, this information disclosure must occur in a supportive and caring environment where patients, families, and clinicians are working together in a collaborative manner (Starzomski, 1994).

Case 3

Mike is a 31-year-old man who has been receiving hemodialysis in an incenter unit for 5 years. In addition to his chronic renal failure, Mike sustained a severe brain injury following an accidental cocaine overdose when he was 18. As a result of his brain injury, Mike is a paraplegic and confined to a wheelchair. He has significant cognitive impairment (according to psychological testing he has the mental capacity of a 7-year-old). He lives with his elderly parents who receive assistance caring for him from a male attendant who lives with the family. Mike cannot speak, and communicates his wishes by nodding his head yes or no when asked questions. The dialysis unit nursing staff can communicate with Mike reasonably well, and are impressed with his quiet perseverance.

Recently, Mike has had many problems with his access and is experiencing other complications on hemodialysis. Mike is an adopted, only child and his parents are concerned about his future on dialysis, and worried about how he will be cared for if anything should happen to them. They think he should have a transplant, thus requiring less medical care and potentially more care and living options if they are unable to care for him any longer. Mike seems to like the idea of not coming for dialysis and nods his head to indicate an affirmative response when asked if he wants to have a transplant.

Although the transplant team assesses Mike and believes he is physically capable of having a transplant, he has limited understanding of the implications. His parents, understanding the risks and benefits that have been outlined, and as surrogate decision makers for Mike, give consent to have him added to the waiting list.

Several members of the transplant team object to adding Mike to the list because they believe that the kidney transplant would not provide him with an improved QOL , and because of the organ shortage, people like Mike should not be transplanted. Other team members, including the clinical nurse specialist on the transplant team, and the nurses in the dialysis unit, disagree saying that Mike would benefit from a successful transplant and are concerned he is being discriminated against because of his disabilities. They state that dialysis is a scarce, expensive treatment that Mike is now receiving, therefore, they believe it follows that he should also be eligible for a transplant, if there are no medical contraindications. They think that acting in any other way would demonstrate a lack of care for Mike and would not be acting in his best interest.

Discussion. One of the ethical problems that emerges from this case is whether Mike is entitled to a kidney transplant. Using the decision-making framework presented earlier, we know that the principle of autonomy determines that individuals have the ability to make choices for themselves. In Mike's case, since his competency and ability to consent to treatment is in question, his parents are named as his surrogate decision makers. They believe Mike should have a transplant in order to improve his QOL, and they are convinced that he believes this as well. The nurses who have been caring for Mike believe he wishes to be transplanted and consider themselves his advocates to ensure his voice is heard. On the other hand, several health professionals believe that Mike is not entitled to receive a transplant, because they think it will not improve his QOL. One of the major problems is that determination of QOL is a difficult process. Research in the area of QOL is complicated by problems of definition, determination of the dimensions of QOL, whose assessments of QOL are relevant, how questions are asked, as well as assessment and measurement of the construct in the real world. Most researchers in this area agree that when determining QOL, it is the patient's assessment and perspective that is most important. Studies have shown that health care professionals, when asked to complete a questionnaire determining quality of life for patients, rate the patient's QOL differently than the patients themselves (Drummond, 1987; Evans et al., 1990; Molzahn, 1991).

Considering the various theories of justice may provide further information to assist with decision making in this case. A proponent of utilitarianism would have difficulty supporting Mike's transplant since it could be argued that because of the organ shortage, transplanting a more productive member of society might produce the greatest good for society. A proponent of Rawl's liberal theory would likely be in support of Mike's transplant as the theory focuses special attention on the least well off in society. A person operating from a libertarian perspective would not oppose the transplant as the theory supports individual rights and freedom to access needed services and resources. Finally, an egalitarian would support the transplant as the theory suggests that everyone ought to have equal access to resources if they have an equal need. Different treatment is justified only where the need is different, or both needs cannot be met. Where these circumstances occur, then priority should be given to the greater need that can feasibly be met (Nielson, 1991, p. 565). In this case, the agency has a priority list for all people having an emergent or urgent need (only two to three people are on the list at any time). Mike would be added to the regular list and would not take a kidney away from someone with a greater medical need. Determining need, other than medical need, brings us back to the difficulties of determining QOL and social worth. As all the people on the list have a similar medical need, Mike should be added to the list.

In this case, it is clear we have health care professionals who have different values and are proponents of different conceptions of justice. Of assistance would be to consider what a caring, compassionate health professional, with Mike's best interest at heart, would do. In this case, Mike was added to the transplant team after the group used the decision-making framework to help them determine what the best course of action was. They eventually agreed that at the micro level of the system, Mike's best interests had to be considered first and foremost. If a decision was to be made to exclude certain persons from receiving care, then more societal discussion was necessary.

This case illuminates some of the concerns that are raised in regard to selecting patients for treatment with life-saving technologies. As mentioned previously, when dialysis and transplantation were in their infancy, stringent selection criteria emphasizing social worth were in place to ration what was considered a scarce resource. In more recent years, selection of recipients for organ replacement therapy and dialysis has moved away from an emphasis on social worth to an assortment of criteria that vary among different programs. In addition to tissue compatibility, other selection criteria for transplantation include medical factors such as selecting those most in medical need, those who will most likely receive medical benefit from the treatment, and consideration of other factors such as length of time on the waiting list. In some centers, consideration is given to whether potential recipients have the psychological ability and the support necessary to adhere to treatment regimens, and to care for their newly transplanted organ (Kilner, 1988; 1990; Kjellstrand & Dossetor, 1992). Given these current selection criteria, there does not appear to be any reason that Mike should be denied a kidney transplant.

Strategies to Enhance Ethical Decision-Making

A variety of strategies, many of which have been mentioned briefly above, can enhance our ability to practice in an ethical manner. These strategies include team communication and collaboration, interdisciplinary education and rounds, use of resource persons for ethical decision-making assistance, research into the best methods to solve ethical problems (including the further development of outcome research), and greater public education and discussion about ethical issues.

Communication and Collaboration

Opportunities to be involved in ethical decision making at the bedside can serve to enhance the health care team's contribution to the overall care of patients and their families. Special attention must be paid to comprehensive family assessment and consideration of the families' ethno-cultural beliefs and values. Use of resource people at the bedside, such as clinical nurse specialists, ethics consultants, and/or ethics committees can enhance overall ethical decision making by encouraging interdisciplinary team communication.

As the previous cases have illustrated, a vital component of making good decisions, that are ethical in nature, is having a well-developed health care team capable of working together and respecting each other's opinions, values, and responsibilities. Often, what have been thought of as ethical problems are confounded by problems with team conflict and communication. Finding solutions to the ethical challenges faced at the micro and meso levels of the health care system will require that we expand our thinking about teamwork and look at strategies that will lead to improved team collaboration (Rodney & Starzomski, 1994). There is a growing body of research that shows that interdisciplinary collaboration requires mutual respect, and can lead to developing common goals and positive patient outcomes (Baggs, 1993; Baggs, Ryan, Phelps, Richeson, & Johnson, 1992; Mariano, 1989; Mitchell, Armstrong, Simpson, & Lentz, 1989). It is important that collaborative practice models, as opposed to vertical decision-making models, be used in health care settings to promote optimal team work leading to the best possible patient care (Rodney & Starzomski, 1993).

When nurses are caring for people who are undergoing life-prolonging treatment, they need to be free to practice in a moral manner. There is considerable research suggesting that, when nurses are constrained in their ability to practice morally, they experience moral distress. Moral distress results when persons know what ought to be done, but they are unable to translate their moral choices into moral action (Wilkinson, 1989; Jameton, 1984). Thus, moral distress can occur when nurses are not included in decision making, or when an institution or agency lacks appropriate processes or mechanisms for, or actually constrains moral action (Rodney & Starzomski, 1993; Yarling & McElmurry, 1986).

In nephrology, we have valued team work since the inception of dialysis and transplantation. Indeed, the treatments have been improved and modified by nurses, physicians, and other professionals working together to provide the best care possible to people living with kidney disease. It is imperative that we continue to foster excellent team communication and collaboration to prevent nurses from becoming morally distressed, and at the same time, promote optimal patient care. A well-functioning nephrology team can be compared to a jazz band where no one is the proclaimed leader, but at different times different instruments are heard more often, or more prominently than others. It is impossible for the saxophone player to do his job without knowing how all the other musicians are going to play. When the music is playing no one can pick out the most important instrument. All the musicians need to work together to create the magic that is their music. This is the goal we must strive for in nephrology practice. It is unacceptable for anyone on the health care team to not have a voice. Moral muteness will not lead to high quality patient care.

Ethics at the Bedside

Ethics rounds are a means of operationalizing ethical decision making on an ongoing basis, at the same time encouraging participation and communication among all team members. Using a format similar to clinical rounds, ethics rounds can be educational in nature, and/or may assist in clinical decisions. The rounds may be conducted by nursing or may be interdisciplinary. The cases reviewed may be actual cases in progress, past cases, or hypothetical cases. These rounds are an excellent way for interdisciplinary teams to work together improving communication and collaboration (Rodney & Starzomski, 1993). In many situations, it is useful to have an ethics interest group where issues can be discussed and new ideas and developments in the field of ethics explored. These can be nephrology specific or combined with other programs, depending on the needs of the individuals involved.

Ethics Education

In order to value interdisciplinary decision making and to make good ethical decisions, more work needs to be done educating health professions about ways to work together. In traditional educational settings, most professionals are socialized in the traditions and values of their own discipline. This does not always lead to a sense of understanding of what the issues are for members of other disciplines. There is not always a sense of the course of action that will lead to the most favorable outcome for the patient. Studies indicate that nurses and physicians, for example, approach patients with what are quite often divergent philosophical stances (Campbell-Heider & Pollock, 1987; Grundstein-Amado, 1992; Stein, Watts, & Howell, 1990). This suggests the need for dialogue among nurses, physicians, and other team members during professional educational preparation so that the various members of the interdisciplinary team can appreciate each others' points of view (Rodney & Starzomski, 1993).

Interdisciplinary ethics education at the undergraduate and graduate level could do much to enhance understanding of values, beliefs, and responsibilities of the various health care team members. This understanding and respect can then be transferred to the clinical settings, where the students will eventually be working together. Teaching team members about health care ethics, and business and professional ethics should lead to better team communication since health care professionals will be able to articulate their own issues and concerns more effectively, and understand the position of other team members. Finally, continuing education in the form of inservices and other educational offerings can assist team members to more effectively deal with ethical issues and situations as they arise in clinical practice (Rodney & Starzomski, 1993).

Ethics Consultation

Although ethical decision making should take place at the bedside, there are often times when consultation, advice, and guidance from resources such as ethics committees and consultants may be of value. Ethics committees are an effective resource to help team members with ethical decision making. Ethics committees are usually composed of an interdisciplinary group of physicians, nurses, administrators, clergy, ethicists, and lawyers. However, research shows that nurses are not always represented on these committees or do not access them, often because they are unaware they exist (Murphy, 1989; Storch & Griener, 1992). This situation requires change as nurses are an extremely valuable resource for ethics committees and are often in need of the assistance a committee could provide.

Most sources agree that institutional ethics committees have several roles, including education, case consultation, and policy formulation (Blake, 1992; Lo, 1987; Storch & Griener, 1992; Storch, Griener, Marshall, & Olinek, 1990). Ethics committees can play a major role in disseminating information throughout the agency and acting as an educational resource. In addition, they are able to develop policies around topics such as informed consent, resuscitation, and withdrawing and withholding treatment, that help provide guidance for ethical practice.

In many situations, ethics committees can provide consultation around individual cases and dilemmas. Sometimes this occurs with a few members of the committee or occasionally with the whole committee. In certain situations, ethics consultants are available in agencies to provide assistance with case consultation, education, and research (Singer, Pellegrino, & Sieglar, 1990). With proper institutional support, ethics committees and ethics consultants are invaluable in helping to develop healthy moral environments in hospitals and in the community.

Research

As we move into the future it is clear that activities within the health care system (including dialysis and transplantation) are undergoing considerable scrutiny, with emphasis on the need for all citizens to use resources in a responsible manner. Since an estimated 80% of medical treatments, along with surgical procedures, have never been evaluated scientifically to determine whether they are effective (Rachlis & Kushner, 1989, p. 10), there is an increasing emphasis on the development of research that focuses on the outcomes of health care and the impact of new technology on the health care system. Technology assessment and economic evaluation techniques (for example, cost effectiveness, cost benefit, and cost utility analysis) are being developed to assist with determining outcomes of health care. The resulting data are being used to help develop practice guidelines in order to assist with the diffusion of new technology and the application of various treatments in clinical settings (Boyle & Callahan, 1992; Deber, 1992; Goodman, 1992; Hadorn, 1993; Laupacis, Feeny, Detsky, & Tugwell, 1992; Moss et al., 1993; Reiser, 1992; Wennberg, 1990). It is important that this work continue, however, it should be remembered that there must be room for flexibility with guidelines when they are applied to individual cases. Practice guidelines are just that — guidelines — and should not be considered rules that must be followed in every circumstance. The value of having more accurate outcome data and information for patients to assist with their decision making cannot be emphasized enough. As Deber (1992) suggests, rarely will technology be found to be a panacea — always we are left with the question about who should receive the treatment and under what circumstances (p. 136). Economic evaluation data will always have to be considered in light of individual cases, choices and preferences.

Public and Health Care Provider Dialogue About Resource Allocation

One of the challenges for allocating resources efficiently in the health care sector is combining expert knowledge about the effectiveness of health care treatments, and the structure and financing of the system, with information about the values, preferences, and local circumstances of communities (Hurley, Birch, & Eyles, 1992). Stated another way, although health care providers possess expert knowledge about the expected effectiveness of health care in improving health status, individuals are the best judges of how these improvements affect their overall well being. Therefore, there must be a partnership between the providers of care and consumers so that all voices are heard in the debate about how resources ought to be allocated for health care. We must give great attention to include those who are most at risk, as well as those who may not have the resources and energy to be involved in the process (Starzomski, 1995).

Lay participation in health care stems from two major factors: a growing recognition that patient preferences ought to be incorporated into decision making involving individual treatment choices, and the desire to increase public accountability for health care resource allocation decisions in order to make providers more accountable to the communities they serve (Charles & DeMaio, 1992). It is believed that consumer involvement will help provide direction for health care by identifying societal needs and resolving some of the difficult ethical questions that emerge from the resource allocation debate.

One of the most extensive attempts to include consumers in resource allocation decisions occurred in Oregon, where a phenomenal amount of attention and debate was directed at Oregon's efforts to reform certain pieces of health care legislation, a debate that has come to be known as the Oregon Experiment (Nelson & Drought, 1992).
In an attempt to deal with the rationing questions that had been plaguing the state, elected officials, community leaders, consumers, and health care professionals attempted to define an adequate, minimum standard of health care for their citizens (Daniels, 1991; Eddy, 1991a; 1991c). Fox and Leichter (1991) suggested that this was a process where Oregonians sought to discover whether they shared a tradition of values about health care that

would help them define which package of health services constituted the common good. Fox and Leichter stated further, "If one was looking (searching) for a classic exercise of American democracy in the sunlight, it is Oregon's debate" (1991, p.7).

The Oregon program has become a focal point for debate on virtually every aspect of U.S. health policy: access, cost effectiveness, rationing, and basic care (Eddy, 1991b; Garland, 1992; Garland & Hasnain, 1990). The plan has sparked a major debate around the complexities and ethics related to resource allocation and involvement of citizens in developing health policy (Golenski & Thompson, 1991; Menzel, 1992a). Eddy (1991b) points out that the plan has provided "a focus for national debate, a target to shoot at, a starting point for improvement" (p. 2135). Proponents of the plan praised its boldness and suggested that it would bring discussions of appropriate care to the forefront so that the issues could be debated in the public arena (McPherson, 1991; "Oregon Reforms," 1993). Opponents suggested that the plan discriminated against poor women and children and illustrated many of the problems that arise when using QOL indicators as a means of determining how resources should be allocated (Fox & Leichter, 1991; Gore, 1990; Veatch, 1991a).

The Oregon situation illustrated that the task of prioritizing health services involves a judgment composed of facts and values. Hence, it becomes essential to incorporate citizen values about what they wish to see in a health care system, with ethical, economic, and outcome approaches to policy decision making in order to make the best possible societal decisions.

Hadorn (1993) suggests that, despite the efforts of many researchers, there are still uncertainties about how society might use outcome data to set priorities in the health care system. He says that, although the idea of determining the health outcomes associated with different treatments, determining how people feel about those outcomes, then giving priority to treatments that produce more preferred outcomes sounds simple, it is fraught with complications, not the least of which is discrimination against some individuals (Hadorn, 1991; 1992). Hadorn (1993), when speaking about the Oregon attempt to involve consumers and providers in an outcome and preference-based effort to set priorities, says:

> Unfortunately, although the Oregon project provided a wealth of experience on one possible approach to estimating and dovetailing preferences, the result of that project — a priority list containing 688 condition-treatment pairs — is of questionable utility. Because of the wide range of procedures and indications contained within each "line item" on the list, substantial additional specification will be needed before the list can be applied to actual patients (p. 2).

He goes on to say:

> An important unresolved issue in the field of resource allocation is whether people's preferences differ significantly based on demographic characteristics or, particularly, on whether they have experienced (or are experiencing) medical conditions or disabilities. Concern over such differences was the stated reason for the initial denial of the waiver needed by the State of Oregon to implement its much-discussed effort to set health care priorities in its Medicaid program (p. 5).

Although the methodology used in Oregon may have been fraught with problems, the process of opening up public discourse about resource allocation is a positive move. More public debate is needed as the health care systems of both Canada and the United States undergo reform. It is crucial that we become involved proactively in planning at the agency level as well as in the community and on the political scene. We must take initiative in discovering effective ways to maximize use of resources, while at the same time meeting the health care needs of persons with chronic renal failure and their families.

Summary and Future Directions

Ironically, the amazing success of the treatment of chronic renal failure has been the catalyst for an incredible array of ethical problems and issues. These ethical concerns will not go away. As we solve current problems, new ones will emerge. It is essential therefore, that we develop a theoretical foundation and a method for ethical decision making that can be used by nephrology nurses, regardless of the problem. Hence, a major goal of this chapter has been to provide a foundation and process for making ethical decisions that can be used by nephrology nurses wherever they practice. Ethical theory is being developed constantly and can be thought of as work in progress. In order to make good ethical decisions, we must understand the evolution and application of ethical theory, and the role theory has in helping us to make good ethical decisions.

As nephrology nurses, we have unique and pivotal roles at the micro level of the health care system as advocates for people with chronic renal failure and their families. Furthermore, we must also expand our thinking to include the patient and family in the context of the society in which they live. In other words, we must be involved in ethical decision making at the meso and macro levels of the system.

If we are to make good ethical decisions, then we need to understand and emphasize the importance of team communication and collaboration, remembering that the patient is the central member of the team. Nurses need to continue to strive for better collaborative methods of delivering care in our nephrology programs. Emphasis should be placed on the need to encourage more open, public discussion about resource allocation for health care to ensure that all societal voices are heard, values are respected, and the best decisions made about the just allocation of health care resources.

At the macro level of the system we require a collaborative approach to health care as we work together with consumers and government to improve the health status of all citizens (Klein, 1993). We need to move beyond rhetoric to a place where there is true collaboration and consultation among these three groups as we strive to open moral space for continued societal ethical discourse (Rodney & Starzomski, 1994).

In the future, allocation of resources, selection of patients for treatment, and issues around withdrawing and withholding treatment will continue to require our ability to make ethical decisions. The shortage of human organs for transplantation will continue to push us to consider alternative sources for organs. Ethical concerns about prenatal diagnosis of disease and gene therapy are not far off in nephrology as major strides are made in the identification of genes that cause specific types of kidney failure.

As we move in these new directions in nephrology, we must be vigilant, ensuring that patients and their families receive the care they require. Nurses must always remember that we have a covenant with our patients and should always act in their best interest (Pellegrino & Thomasma, 1988). This is the pivotal requirement of caring, ethical nephrology nursing practice.

There are no simple answers to the complex dilemmas confronting us in nephrology practice. As we move into the next millennium, nephrology nurses must work collaboratively using thoughtful, critical, ethical decision making, and alternatives and solutions will follow.

References and Readings

Abrams, N. (1990). A contrary view of the nurse as patient advocate. In T. Pence & J. Cantrall (Eds.), *Ethics in nursing: An anthology* (pp. 102-106). New York: National League for Nursing.

Ackerman, T. (1983). Experimentalism in bioethics research. *Journal of Medicine and Philosophy, 8*(2), 169-170.

Alexander, S. (1962, November 9). They decide who lives, who dies: Medical miracle puts a burden on a small committee. *Life*, p. 102.

Andrews, L. (1992). The body as property: Some philosophical reflections - A response to J.F. Childress. *Transplantation Proceedings, 24*(5), 2149-2151.

Annas, G. (1974). The patient rights advocate: Can nurses effectively fill the role? *Supervisor Nurse, 5*, 21-25.

Arras, J., & Rhoden, N. (1989). *Ethical issues in modern medicine.* San Francisco: Mayfield Publishing Company.

Arras, J. (1991). Getting down to cases: The revival of casuistry in bioethics. *The Journal of Medicine and Philosophy, 16*, 29-51.

Baggs, J. (1993). Collaborative interdisciplinary bioethical decision making in intensive care units. *Nursing Outlook, 41*(3), 108-112.

Baggs, J., Ryan, S., Phelps, C., Richeson, J., & Johnson, J. (1992). The association between interdisciplinary collaboration and patient outcomes in a medical intensive care unit. *Heart & Lung, 21*(1), 18-24.

Balk, R. (1990). Should transplantation be part of a health care system? *Canadian Medical Association Journal, 36*, 1129-1132.

Beauchamp, T., & Childress, J. (1983). *Principles of biomedical ethics.* New York: Oxford University Press.

Beauchamp, T., & Childress, J. (1989). *Principles of biomedical ethics* (3rd edition). New York: Oxford University Press.

Beauchamp, T. (1982). Ethical theory and bioethics. In T. Beauchamp & L. Walters (Eds.), *Contemporary issues in bioethics* (2nd edition) (pp. 1-43). Belmont, CA: Wadsworth Publishing.

Bebeau, M., & Brabeck, M. (1989). Ethical sensitivity and moral reasoning among men and women in the professions. In M. Brabeck (Ed.), *Who cares? Theory, research, and educational implications of the ethic of care.* New York: Praeger Publishers.

Beecher, H. (1966). Ethics and clinical research. *New England Journal of Medicine, 274*(24), 1354-1360.

Benjamin, M. (1992). Supply and demand for transplantable organs: The ethical perspective. *Transplantation Proceedings, 24*(5), 2139 .

Benjamin, M., & Curtis, J. (1986). *Ethics in nursing* (2nd edition). New York: Oxford University Press.

Bergum, V., Boyle, R., Briggs, M., & Dossetor, J. (1993). *Principle-based and relational ethics: Both essential features of bioethics theory and analysis.* Paper presented at The Canadian Bioethics Meeting, Montreal, Quebec.

Bernal, E. (1992). The nurse as patient advocate. *Hastings Center Report, 22*(4), 18-23.

Blake, D. (1992). The hospital ethics committee - Health care's moral conscience or white elephant? *Hastings Center Report, 22*(11), 6-11.

Blum, L. A. (1988). Gilligan and Kohlberg: Implications for moral theory. *Ethics, 98*, 472-491.

Boisaubin, E. (1988). Charity, the media, and limited medical resources. *Journal of the American Medical Association, 259*(9), 1375-1376.

Bowden, A., & Hull, A. (1993) *Controversies in organ transplantation - A summary report.* New York: National Kidney Foundation.

Boyle, P., & Callahan, D. (1992). Technology assessment: The missing human dimension. *Hastings Center Report, 22*(3), 38-39.

Bramlet, M., Gueldner, S., & Sowell, R. (1990). Consumer - Centric advocacy: Its connection to nursing frameworks. *Nursing Science Quarterly, 3*(4), 156-161.

Brooks, J. (1993). The heart of the matter: Dalton Camp and his controversial transplant. *Canadian Medical Association Journal, 149*(7), 996-1002.

Browne, A. (1994). *Ethics handout - Bridging the professions: An interdisciplinary course in health care ethics.* Vancouver: University of British Columbia.

Buchanan, A. (1989). Health care delivery and resource allocation. In R.M. Veatch (Ed.), *Medical ethics* (pp. 291-327). Boston: Jones Bartlett Publishers.

Buchanan, A. (1991). Justice: A philosophical review. In T. Mappes & J. Zembaty (Eds.), *Biomedical ethics* (pp. 552-562). Toronto: McGraw-Hill, Inc.

Campbell-Heider, N., & Pollock, D. (1987). Barriers to physician-nurse collegiality: An anthropological perspective. *Social Science & Medicine, 25*(5), 421-425.

Canadian Organ Replacement Register. (1994). *1992 Annual Report.* Don Mills, Ontario: Canadian Institute for Health Information.

Caplan, A. (1992). Is xenografting morally wrong? *Transplantation Proceedings, 24*(2), 722-727.

Charles, C., & DeMaio, S. (1992). *Lay participation in health care decision making: A conceptual framework.* Hamilton, Ontario: McMaster University (Center for Health Economics and Policy Analysis (CHEPA) Working Paper #92-16).

Childress, J. (1992). The body as property: Some philosophical reflections. *Transplantation Proceedings, 24*(5), 2143-2148.

Cohen, C. (1992). The case for presumed consent to transplant human organs after death. *Transplantation Proceedings, 24*(5), 2168-2172.

Colvin, E., & Hammes, B.(1991). If I only knew: A patient education program on advance directives. *ANNA Journal, 18*(6), 557-560.

Colvin, E., Myhre, M., Welch, J., & Hammes, B. (1993). Moving beyond the patient self-determination act: Educating patients to be autonomous. *ANNA Journal, 20*(5), 564-569.

Cooper, M. (1991). Principle-oriented ethics and the ethics of care: A creative tension. *Advances in Nursing Science, 14*(2), 22-31.

Crawshaw, R., Garland, M., & Hines, B. (1989). Organ transplants: A search for health policy at the state level. *Western Journal of Medicine, 150*(1), 361-363.

Cummings, N. (1993). Ethical considerations in end-stage renal disease. In R. Schrier & C. Gottschalk (Eds.), *Diseases of the kidney* (5th edition) (pp. 3098-3128). Boston: Little, Brown and Company.

Curtin, L. (1982). Human problems: Human beings. In L. Curtin & M.J. Flaherty (Eds.), *Nursing ethics: Theories and pragmatics* (pp. 37-42). Bowie, MD: Robert J. Brady.

Daniels, N. (1991). Is the Oregon rationing plan fair? *Journal of the American Medical Association, 265*(17), 2232-2235.

Davis, A., & Aroskar, M. (1991). *Ethical dilemmas and nursing practice.* Toronto: Appleton & Lange.

Deber, R. (1992). Translating technology assessment into policy: Conceptual choices and tough issues. *International Journal of Technology Assessment in Health Care, 8*(1), 131-137.

Dickens, B. (1988). The anencephalic organ donor and the law. *Transplantation/Implantation Today, 5*, 42-46.

Dickens, B. (1991). WHO guiding principles on human organ transplantation. *Transplantation/Implantation Today, 8*, 12-18.

Drummond, M.F. (1987). Resource allocation decisions in health care: A role for quality life assessments? *Journal of Chronic Disease, 40*(6), 605-616.

Eddy, D. (1991a). What's going on in Oregon? *Journal of the American Medical Association, 266*(3), 4117-4120.

Eddy, D. (1991b). Oregon's methods: Did cost-effectiveness analysis fail? *Journal of the American Medical Association, 266*(15), 2135-2141.

Eddy, D. (1991c). Oregon's plan: Should it be approved? *Journal of the American Medical Association, 266*(17), 2439-2445.

Evans, R.W. (1992). Need, demand, and supply in organ transplantation. *Transplantation Proceedings, 24*(5), 2152-2154.

Evans, R.W. (1993). Organ procurement and the role of financial incentives. *Journal of the American Medical Association, 269*(24), 3113-3118.

Evans, R.W., Manninen, D., Dong, F., & McLynne, D. (1993). Is retransplantation cost effective? *Transplantation Proceedings, 25*(1), 1694 1696.

Evans, R.W., Manninen, D., Dugan, M., Livak, C., McLynne, D., Raab, J., & Roder, B. (1990). *The kidney transplant health insurance study: Final report.* Seattle: Battele Research Center.

Flew, A. (Ed.). (1984). *A dictionary of philosophy* (3rd. ed.). London: Pan Books.

Fowler, M. (1991). The nurse's role: Responsibilities and rights. In T. Mappes & J.S. Zembaty (Eds.), *Biomedical ethics* (pp. 157-161). Toronto: McGraw Hill, Inc.

Fox, D., & Leichter, H. (1991). Rationing care in Oregon: The new accountability. *Health Affairs, 10*(2), 7-27.

Fox, R., & Swazey, J. (1992a). Leaving the field. *Hastings Center Report, 22*(5), 9-15.

Fox, R., & Swazey, J. (1992b). *Spare parts - Organ replacement in American society.* New York: Oxford University Press.

Freeman, R. (1971). Practice as protest. *American Journal of Nursing, 71*(5), 918-921.

Fry, S. (1985). Individual vs. aggregate good: Ethical tension in nursing practice. *International Journal of Nursing Studies, 22*(4), 303-310.

Fry, S. (1987). Autonomy, advocacy and accountability: Ethics at the bedside. In M. Fowler & J. Levine-Ariff (Eds.), *Ethics at the bedside.* Philadelphia: J.B. Lippincott Company.

Fry, S. (1989a). Toward a theory of nursing ethics. *Advances in Nursing Science, 11*(4), 9-22.

Fry, S. (1989b). The role of caring in a theory of nursing ethics. *Hypatia: A Journal of Feminist Philosophy, 4*(2), 88-103.

Fry, S. (1991). A theory of caring: Pitfalls and promises. In D. Gaut & M. Leininger (Eds.), *Caring: The compassionate healer* (pp. 161-172). New York: National League for Nursing.

Funk & Wagnalls standard dictionary. (1980). New York: Lippincott & Crowell Publishers.

Gadow, S. (1990). Existential advocacy: Philosophical foundations of nursing. In T. Pense & J. Cantrall (Eds.), *Ethics in nursing: An anthology* (pp. 41 -51). New York: National League for Nursing

Garland, M., & Hasnain, R. (1990). Health care in common: Setting priorities in Oregon. *Hastings Center Report, 20*(5), 16-18.

Garland, M. (1992). Justíce, politics and community: Expanding access and rationing health services in Oregon. *Law, Medicine & Health Care, 20*(1-2), 67-81.

Gibson, C. (1993). Underpinnings of ethical reasoning in nursing. *Journal of Advanced Nursing, 18*, 2003-2007.

Gilligan, C. (1982/1993). *In a different voice: Psychological theory and women's development.* Cambridge, MA: Harvard University Press.

Gillon, R. (1992). Caring, men and women, nurses and doctors, and health care ethics. *Journal of Medicine & Philosophy, 18*(4), 171-172.

Golenski, J., & Thompson, S. (1991). A history of Oregon's basic health services act: An insider's account. *QRB, 17*(5), 144-149.

Goodman, C. (1992). It's time to rethink health care technology assessment. *International Journal of Technology Assessment in Health Care, 8*(2), 335-358.

Gore, A. (1990). Oregon's bold mistake. *Academic Medicine, 65*, 634-635.

Gropper, E. (1990). Florence Nightingale: Nursing's first environmental theorist. *Nursing Forum, 25*(3), 30-33.

Grundstein-Amado, R. (1992). Differences in ethical decision making processes among nurses and doctors. *Journal of Advanced Nursing, 17*(2), 129-137.

Guttmann, A., & Guttmann, R. (1992). Sale of kidneys for transplantation: Attitudes of the health-care profession and the public. *Transplantation Proceedings, 24*(5), 2108-2109.

Hadorn, D. (1991). Setting health care priorities in Oregon: Cost effectiveness meets the rule of rescue. *Journal of the American Medical Association, 265*(17), 2218-2225.

Hadorn, D. (1992). The problem of discrimination in health care priority setting. *Journal of the American Medical Association, 268*(11), 1454-1459.

Hadorn, D. (1993). *Outcomes management and resource allocation: How should quality of life be measured?* Health Policy Research Unit Discussion Paper Series (HPRU 93:7D). Vancouver: University of British Columbia.

Hilton, A., & Starzomski, R. (1994). Family decision making about living related kidney donation. *ANNA Journal, 21*(6), 346-354, 381.

Hurley, J., Birch, S., & Eyles, J. (1992). *Information, efficiency, and decentralization within health care systems.* (CHEPA Working Paper # 92-21). Hamilton, Ontario: McMaster University.

Jameton, A. (1984). *Nursing practice: The ethical issues.* Englewood Cliffs, NJ: Prentice-Hall.

Jecker, N., Carrese, J.A., & Pearlman, R. (1995). Caring for patients in cross-cultural settings. *Hastings Center Report, 25*(1), 6-14.

Jennings, B. (1988). A grassroots movement in bioethics. *Hastings Center Report, 18*(3), Supplement 1-16.

Jonsen, A. (1985). Organ transplants and the principle of fairness. *Law, Medicine & Health Care, 13*(1), 37-39.

Jonsen, A. (1989). Ethical issues in organ transplantation. In R.M. Veatch (Ed.), *Medical ethics.* Boston: Jones & Bartlett Publishers.

Jonsen, A. (1990). *The new medicine and the old ethics.* Cambridge, MA: Harvard University Press.

Kazim, E., Al-Rukaimi, H., Fernandez, S., Raizada, S., Mustafa, M., & Huda, N. (1992). Buying a kidney: The easy way out? *Transplantation Proceedings, 24*(5), 2112-2113.

Ketefian, S., & Ormond, I. (1988). *Moral reasoning and ethical practice in nursing: An integrative review.* New York: National League For Nursing.

Kilner, J. (1988). Selecting patients when resources are limited: A study of U.S. medical directors of kidney dialysis and transplantation facilities. *American Journal of Public Health, 78*(2), 144-147.

Kilner, J. (1990). *Who lives? Who dies? - Ethical criteria in patient selection.* New Haven, CT: Yale University Press.

Kjellstrand, C. (1992). Disguising unjust rationing by calling it futile therapy. *The Bioethics Bulletin, 4*(2), 1-3.

Kjellstrand, C., & Dossetor, J. (1992). *Ethical problems in dialysis and transplantation.* Boston: Kluwer Academic Publishers.

Klein, R. (1993). Dimensions of rationing: Who should do what? *British Medical Journal, 307*, 309-311.

Klevit, H., Bates, A., Castanares, T., Kirk, E., Sipes-Metzler, P., & Wopat, R. (1991). Prioritization of health care services: A progress report by the Oregon health services commission. *Archives of Internal Medicine, 151*(5), 912 - 916.

Kluge, E. (1992). *Biomedical ethics in a Canadian context.* Scarborough, Ontario: Prentice-Hall Canada Inc.

Kluge, E. (1993). Age and organ transplantation. *Canadian Medical Association Journal, 149*(7), 1003.

Kohnke, M. (1980). The nurse as advocate. *American Journal of Nursing, 80*, 2030-2040.

Laupacis, A., Feeny, D., Detsky, A., & Tugwell, P. (1992). How attractive does a new technology have to be to warrant adoption and utilization? Tentative guidelines for using clinical and economic evaluations. *Canadian Medical Association Journal, 146*(4), 473-481.

Lo, B. (1987). Behind closed doors - Promises and pitfalls of ethics committees. *The New England Journal of Medicine, 317*(1), 46-50.

Long, R. (1994). Advance directives, informed consent, and the future of the ESRD program. *Contemporary Dialysis & Nephrology, 15*(5), 16-17, 21, 34.

Mappes, T., & Zembaty, J. (Eds.).(1991). *Biomedical ethics.* Toronto: McGraw-Hill, Inc.

Mariano, C. (1989). The case for interdisciplinary collaboration. *Nursing Outlook, 37*(8), 285-288.

Martin, D. (1992). Fetal tissue transplantation research: A Canadian analysis. *Health Law in Canada, 13*(1), 132-141.

McCormick, T. (1993). Ethical issues in caring for patients with renal failure. *ANNA Journal, 20*(5), 549-555.

McDonald, M. (1993, May 7). *Bio-ethical perspectives on health care cost containment.* Resource Allocation Workshop Handout, Calgary, Alberta.

McDonald, M. (1994). *A framework for ethical decision making.* Unpublished document. Centre for Applied Ethics, University of British Columbia, Vancouver, BC, Canada.

McDonald, M., Stevenson, J.T., & Cragg, W. (1992). *Finding a balance of values: An ethical assessment of Ontario Hydro's demand/supply plan.* Unpublished Report to the Aboriginal Research Coalition of Ontario.

McPherson, A. (1991). The Oregon plan: Rationing in a rational society. *Canadian Medical Association Journal, 145*(11), 1444 -1445.

Mendelsshon, D., & Singer, P. (1994). Advance directives in dialysis. *Advances in Renal Replacement Therapy, 1*(3), 240-250.

Mendez, R., Aswad, S., Dessouki, J., Cicciarelli, J., & Mendez, R. (1992). Costs and financing of kidney transplantation in the United States. *Transplantation Proceedings, 24*(5), 2127-2128.

Menzel, P. (1992a). Some ethical costs of rationing. *Law, Medicine & Health Care, 20*(1-2), 57-66.

Menzel, P. (1992b). The moral duty to contribute and its implications for organ procurement policy. *Transplantation Proceedings, 24*(5), 2175-2178.

Miedman, F. (1991). A practical approach to ethical decisions. *American Journal of Nursing, 91*(12), 20-25.

Mitchell, P., Armstrong, S., Simpson, T., & Lentz, M. (1989). American Association of Critical-Care Nurses Demonstration Project: Profile of excellence in critical care nursing. *Heart & Lung, 18*(3), 219-237.

Molzahn, A. (1991). Quality of life after organ transplantation. *Journal of Advanced Nursing, 16*, 1042-1047.

Moskop, J. (1987). The moral limits to federal funding for kidney disease. *Hastings Center Report, 17*(2), 11-15.

Moss, A. (1995). To use dialysis appropriately: The emerging consensus on patient selection guidelines. *Advances in Renal Replacement Therapy, 2*(2), 175-183.

Moss, A., Rettig, R., & Cassel, C. (1993). A proposal for patient acceptance to and withdrawal from dialysis: A follow-up to the IOM report. *ANNA Journal, 20*(5), 557-561.

Murphy, P. (1989). The role of the nurse on hospital ethics committees. *Nursing Clinics of North America, 24*(2), 551-557.

Nelson, H. (1992). Against caring. *The Journal of Clinical Ethics, 3*(1), 8-15.

Nelson, R. (1990). A policy concerning the therapeutic use of human fetal tissue in transplantation. *Western Journal of Medicine, 152*(4), 447-448.

Nelson, R., & Drought, T. (1992). Justice and the moral acceptability of rationing medical care: The Oregon experiment. *Journal of Medicine and Philosophy, 17*(1), 97-117.

Neu, S. (1994). Stopping chronic dialysis - The debate on a hot issue continues. *Contemporary Dialysis & Nephrology, 15*(5), 12-13.

Nielson, K. (1991). Autonomy, equality and a just health care system. In T. Mappes & J. Zembaty (Eds.), *Biomedical ethics* (pp. 562-567). Toronto: McGraw-Hill, Inc.

Noddings, N. (1984). An ethic of caring. In *Caring: A feminine approach to ethics and moral education* (pp. 79-103). Berkeley, CA: University of California Press.

Omery, A. (1989). Values, moral reasoning and ethics. *Nursing Clinics of North America, 24*(2), 499-506.

Oregon reforms a wake up call for Canada. (1993, March 17). *Globe & Mail*, p 1.

Pagana, K. (1990). Let's stop calling ourselves patient advocates. In T. Pence & J. Cantrall (Eds.), *Ethics in nursing: An anthology* (pp. 64-66). New York: National League for Nursing.

Pellegrino, E. (1993). The metamorphosis of medical ethics. *Journal of the American Medical Association, 269*(9), 1158-1162.

Pellegrino, E., & Thomasma, D. (1988). *For the patient's good: The restoration of beneficence in health care.* London: Oxford Press Ltd.

Penticuff, J. (1991). Conceptual issues in nursing ethics research. *Journal of Medicine & Philosophy, 16*(3), 235-258.

Peplau, H. (1987). Nursing science: A historical perspective. In R.R. Parse (Ed.), *Nursing science: Major paradigms, theories, and critiques* (pp. 13-29). Philadelphia: W.B. Saunders Company.

Pfettscher, S. (1993). Bioethics in nephrology: Definitions and practices. *ANNA Journal, 20*(5), 543-547.

Rachlis, M., & Kushner, N. (1989). *Second opinion: What's wrong with Canada's health care system and how to fix it.* Toronto: Collins Publishers.

Rapaport, F. (1993). Alternative sources of clinically transplantable vital organs. *Transplantation Proceedings, 25*(1), 42-44.

Reed, P., & Zurakowski, T. (1989). Nightingale revisited: A visionary model for nursing. In J.J. Fitzpatrick & A.L. Whall (Eds.), *Conceptual models: Analysis and application* (2nd. edition) (pp. 33-47). Norwalk, CT: Appleton & Lange.

Reemtsma, K. (1992). Xenografts. *Transplantation Proceedings, 24*(5), 2225.

Reiser, S. (1992). Consumer competence and the reform of American health care. *Journal of the American Medical Association, 267*(11), 1511-1515.

Rettig, R. (1989). The politics of organ transplantation: A parable of our time. *Journal of Health Politics, Policy and Law, 14*(1), 191-227.

Roberts, S. (1983). Oppressed group behavior: Implications for nursing. *Advances in Nursing Science, 5*(4), 21 -30.

Rodney, P., & Starzomski, R. (1993). Constraints on the moral agency of nurses. *The Canadian Nurse, 89*(9), 23-26.

Rodney, P. & Starzomski, R. (1994). Responding to ethical challenges. *Nursing BC, 26*(2), 10-13.

Ross, W. (1930/1988). *The right and the good.* Indianapolis, IN: Hackett Publishing Company.

Roy, D., Williams, J., & Dickens, B. (1994). *Bioethics in Canada.* Scarborough: Prentice Hall Canada Inc.

Sadler, B. (1992). Presumed consent to organ transplantation: A different perspective. *Transplantation Proceedings, 24*(5), 2173-2174.

Schneiderman, L., Jacker, N., & Jonsen, A. (1990). Medical futility: Its meanings and ethical implications. *Annals of Internal Medicine, 112*(12), 949-954.

Scribner, B. (1964). Ethical problems of using artificial organs to sustain human life. *ASAIO Proceedings*, 209-212.

Seib, D., MacLeod, M., & Stiller, C. (1990). A step beyond: New limits in selection criteria. *Transplantation/Implantation Today, 7*, 47-51.

Sells, R. (1992). Some ethical issues in organ retrieval, 1982 to 1992. *Transplantation Proceedings, 24*(6), 2401-2403.

Sherwin, S.(1992). Feminist and medical ethics: Two different approaches to contextual ethics. In H. Holmes & L. Purdy (Eds.), *Feminist perspectives in medical ethics* (pp. 17-31). Bloomington, IN: Indiana University Press.

Simmons, R.G., Marine, S.K., & Simmons, R.L. (1987). *Gift of life: The effect of organ transplantation on individual, family, and societal dynamics.* New Brunswick: Transaction Books.

Singer, P. (1992). Xenotransplantation and speciesism. *Transplantation Proceedings, 24*(2), 728-732.

Singer, P., Pellegrino, E., & Sieglar, M. (1990). Ethics committees and consultants. *The Journal of Clinical Ethics, 1*(14), 263-276.

Spital, A. (1992). Unrelated living donors: Should they be used? *Transplantation Proceedings, 24*(5), 2215-2217.

Spital, A. (1993). Living organ donation is still ethically acceptable. *Archives of Internal Medicine, 153*(4), 529.

Starr, P. (1982). *The social transformation of American medicine.* New York: Basic Books.

Starzomski, R. (1994). Ethical issues in palliative care: The case of dialysis and organ transplantation. *Journal of Palliative Care, 10*(3), 27-33.

Starzomski, R. (1995). What do ethics have to do with lifestyle change? *Canadian Journal of Cardiology, 11*(Suppl A), 4A-7A.

Steele, S. & Harmon, V. (1983). *Values clarification in nursing.* Norwalk, CT: Appleton-Century- Crofts.

Stein, L., Watts, D., & Howell, T. (1990). The doctor-nurse game revisited. *New England Journal of Medicine. 322*(8), 546-549.

Stiller, C. (1990). Health care funding and transplantation in Canada. *Transplantation Proceedings, 22*(3), 980-981.

Storch, J., & Dossetor, J. (1993). *Public attitudes about resource allocation in Alberta: An all Alberta study.*

Storch, J.L., & Griener, G.G. (1992). Ethics committees in Canadian hospitals: Report of the 1990 pilot study. *Healthcare Management Forum, 5*(11),19-26.

Storch, J.L., Griener, G.G. Marshall, D.A., & Olinek, B.A. (1990). Ethics committees in Canadian hospitals: Report of the 1989 survey. *Healthcare Management Forum, 3*(4),3-8.

Swartz, R., Perry, E., Schneider, C., Burdette, T., Curtis, G., & O'Neil, M. (1994). *Advances in Renal Replacement Therapy, 1*(3), 264-273.

Toulmin, S. (1981). The tyranny of principles. *Hastings Center Report, 11*, 31-39.

Turcotte, J. (1992). Supply, demand, and ethics of organ procurement: The medical perspective. *Transplantation Proceedings, 24*(5), 2140-2142.

United States Health Care Financing Administration. (1994). *National listing of Medicare providers furnishing kidney dialysis and transplant services.* Washington, DC: Bureau of Data Management.

Veatch, R. (1991a) Should basic care get priority? Doubts about rationing the Oregon way. *Kennedy Institute of Ethics Journal, 1*(3), 187-206.

Veatch, R. (1991b). *The patient-physician relation: The patient as partner - Part 2.* Indianapolis, IN: Indiana University Press.

Veatch, R. (1991c). Routine inquiry about organ donation - An alternative to presumed consent. *New England Journal of Medicine, 325*(17), 1246-1249.

Welch, G., & Larson, E. (1988). Dealing with limited resources - The Oregon decision to curtail funding for organ transplantation. *The New England Journal Of Medicine, 319*(3), 171-173.

Wennberg, J. (1990). Outcomes research, cost containment, and the fear of health care rationing. *New England Journal of Medicine, 323*, 1202-1204.

Wilkinson, J. (1989). Moral distress: A labour and delivery nurse's experience. *JOGNN, 18*(6), 513-519.

Winslow, G. (1984). From loyalty to advocacy: A new metaphor for nursing. *Hastings Center Report, 14*(3), 32-40.

Yarling, R., & McElmurry, B. (1986). The moral foundation of nursing. *Advances in Nursing Science, 8*(2), 63-73.

Yeo, M., & Donner, M. (1991). Justice. In M. Yeo (Ed.), *Concepts & cases in nursing ethics* (pp. 177-183). Peterborough, Ontario: Broadview Press.

Yeo, M. (1991). *Concepts & cases in nursing ethics.* Peterborough, Ontario: Broadview Press.

Youngner, S. (1992). Psychological impediments to procurement. *Transplantation Proceedings, 24*(5), 2159-2161.

Youngner, S., & Arnold, R. (1993). Ethical, psychosocial, and public policy implications of procuring organs from non-heart beating cadaver donors. *Journal of the American Medical Association, 269*(21), 2769-2774.

Chapter Highlights

- We are confronted daily with situations that require moral judgment and the ability to make ethical decisions. Nowhere is this more apparent than in nephrology, where decisions about initiating, withdrawing and withholding treatment, in addition to selection of patients for treatment, are fraught with ethical dilemmas and questions about the fair and just allocation of limited resources.
- Ethics focuses critical reflection upon actions and events from the standpoint of right and wrong, good and evil, moral value, and moral disvalue. In addition, ethics is concerned with policies, practices, duties, obligations, and rights, with fairness in the correction of wrongs (corrective justice), and with the fair distribution of benefits and burdens within society (distributive justice) (McDonald, Stevenson, & Cragg, 1992, p. 5).
- In North America, we live in a pluralistic society of many cultures, religions, and traditions, thus leading to many different moral positions. Therefore, we are unable to declare that there is one universal ethic that all persons could agree upon, rather there are a variety of diverse perspectives that guide ethical decision making.
- A set of duties and principles was developed by Ross (1930/1988), and later modified by Beauchamp and Childress (1983), that included four principles seen as especially appropriate for biomedical ethics. These principles — autonomy, beneficence, nonmaleficence and justice — were the cornerstone of the traditional approach to health care ethics and have become the "dominant way of doing ethics" (Pellegrino, 1993, pp. 1159-1160).
- The principle-oriented approach to ethics is based on a lexical ordering and application of principles (such as autonomy, beneficence, nonmaleficence and justice) (Veatch, 1991b). This ordering often occurs in a rational, objective, and impartial manner, where the central issue is judging whether a person's actions are right or wrong (Ackerman, 1983; Cooper, 1991; Penticuff, 1991).
- In contrast to principle-oriented ethics, a care ethic has been described as a situational, intuitive process where the central issue is judging an action in term of its web of relatedness (Fry, 1991). In this theory, moral concern deals with needs and responsibility as they evolve in a relationship (Cooper, 1991). Caring implies mutuality and reciprocity in relationships and is not unidirectional.
- Meeting the ethical challenges confronting us in nephrology nursing, particularly as they are confounded by issues of resource allocation, requires us to think about our professional roles as they fit into three levels of responsibility: the micro level, the meso level, and the macro level. . . These three levels of involvement demand different types of decision making in order to arrive at ethically sound decisions.
- From the early 1970s to the present, the theme of the nurse as advocate has become a major part of modern nursing, thereby, impacting on how nursing ethics is conceptualized. Winslow (1984) and Starr (1982) reasoned that the move to an advocacy model in nursing was brought about, in part, by the rise of consumerism and a loss of confidence in the medical profession by consumers.
- Ethical decision making is the application of various skills of ethical analysis and reasoning in an attempt to reach a well-grounded solution to an ethical problem or dilemma (Benjamin & Curtis, 1986, p.11) . . . Ethical decision making focuses on determining what *ought* to occur in each situation and is an important part of each health care professional's ability to make good decisions about ethical concerns.
- The framework by McDonald (1994) is a comprehensive ethical decision-making framework that is based on care and compassion, where ethical principles are used as guidelines to assist in developing the best solution to a particular ethical dilemma. Like all frameworks, it should function as a guide, rather than a recipe, remembering that ethical decision making is a process that may vary depending on the circumstances of the case being considered.

Chapter Highlights (continued)

- When discussing ethical situations, all voices within the health care team must be heard, and the judgments of all team members need to be considered. There may be a need for an organized process for ethical consultation such as a case conference. Furthermore, an ethics committee or ethics consultant can provide valuable advice and assistance with the case if required
- Many of the ethical issues that nephrology practitioners encounter are representative of those that originated when dialysis and transplantation were in their infancy, and are prototypical of ethical issues raised by high technology and life-sustaining treatments in health care.
- One of the most difficult issues in nephrology nursing is the increasing number of people requiring treatment for chronic renal failure and the diminishing resources available to care for them. . . There are concerns in both the U.S. and Canada about the ability to continue funding renal care in a manner that will allow us to provide dialysis and transplantation for all who require these treatments.
- It has been suggested that increasing kidney transplantation will resolve some of the concerns about the numbers of patients receiving expensive dialysis therapy, however, there are many unresolved ethical issues in transplantation that remain problematic, and it is unlikely that transplantation will be a treatment option for all patients with chronic renal failure, even if we were to solve the organ donor shortage.
- A variety of strategies can enhance our ability to practice in an ethical manner. These strategies include team communication and collaboration, interdisciplinary education and rounds, use of resource persons for ethical decision-making assistance, research into the best methods to solve ethical problems (including the further development of outcome research), and greater public education and discussion about ethical issues.

CHAPTER 6

Research in Nephrology Nursing: Overview, Development, and Future Directions

Anita E. Molzahn, PhD, RN

Chapter Contents

Historical Overview of Research in Nephrology Nursing 113
Factors Influencing the Development of Research 113
The Researchers 114
Funding Sources for Nephrology Nursing Research 114
Recent Research 114
- Volume and Form 114
- Phenomena Studied 115
- Designs of the Studies 117
- Theoretical Base 117
- Quality of the Literature 117

Research Utilization 119
ANNA's Research Agenda 120
- Establishment of a Research Grant Program 120
- Development of Review Mechanisms for Research Abstracts 120
- Directory of Nephrology Nurse Researchers/Evaluation of Research Literature 120
- Staffing Survey 120
- Patient Classification Tool 120

Future Directions for Nephrology Nursing Research 121
Summary 121
References 121
Research Brief: Definitions of Research Designs 123
Chapter Highlights 124

Research In Nephrology Nursing: Overview, Development, and Future Directions

Anita E. Molzahn, PhD, RN

Research is critical and necessary for the development of professional nephrology nursing practice. Through research and scholarly inquiry, nephrology nurses will be able to generate knowledge and theory on which to base their practice. Conversely, nephrology nursing practice provides rich data from which we can generate theory and knowledge.

The purpose of this chapter is to provide an historical overview of research in nephrology nursing, followed by a brief discussion of factors that influence nephrology nursing research, a description of the researchers, and an overview of recent research. Available funding sources for research, the need for research utilization, the American Nephrology Nurses' Association's (ANNA) research agenda, and future directions for nephrology nursing research are also addressed.

Historical Overview of Research in Nephrology Nursing

Over the past 25 years, nephrology nursing has evolved as a specialty area within nursing, and an important part of our evolution has been the movement toward research-based practice. As early as the 1950s, nurses became involved in research teams that were studying the effectiveness of dialysis and transplant therapy. In 1969, the American Association for Nephrology Nurses was formed, and in 1974, the *American Association of Nephrology Nurses and Technicians (AANNT) Journal* was first published (Brennan & Jordan, 1994). The formation of the association and the development of a professional journal provided nurses with a basis to enhance their professional practice.

There has been growth in a number of areas, not the least of which has been nephrology nursing research. The Research Special Interest Group was first established in 1982. With growth in requests from the membership regarding research-related activities, a Research Committee was formed in 1990, under the leadership of Patricia Preisig, PhD, RN. Dr. Preisig chaired the committee for 4 years during which time ANNA developed an active research agenda, which is described later.

Factors Influencing the Development of Research

Nephrology nursing research has been influenced by many of the same factors that have affected all nursing research. The numbers of qualified nurse researchers, trends in health care, and availability of funding all affect the conduct of research.

Formal educational preparation for conducting research typically is provided in graduate programs; however, it is not essential that nurses have a graduate degree to participate in research. Many nurses learn about research through informal means, and frequently, nurses are involved in research through a variety of ways other than as principal investigator, such as co-investigator, data collection, and research utilization. The number of nephrology nurses with advanced educational preparation has been rising steadily; 6.72% of ANNA's membership is prepared at the master's level and 0.3% at the doctoral level. It is this small group of people that is most likely to conduct research. As the numbers of nephrology nurses with advanced preparation increases, there is likely to be an increase in research.

Trends in health care often affect the types of research conducted. With changes in funding of health care, and a need to demonstrate cost-benefits of treatment and care, there has been a change of focus for research and evaluation. Today, greater emphasis is placed on outcomes than on process. This trend is likely to change the focus of researchers, practitioners, and funding agencies. Undoubtedly, health care reform and its impact on end stage renal disease (ESRD) programs will be a topic of considerable interest to nurse researchers in the near future.

Availability of funding is key to the conduct of research. Although some research is conducted without outside funding, the availability of research funds in a particular area will attract the interest of researchers and will increase the amount of research conducted in a particular area. Funding agencies will often establish special competitions in areas of interest or priority in anticipation that the funding will increase research in the area.

One great concern is that competition for research funding is increasing. While it is important that the number of nurse researchers increase and the amount of research conducted increases, often a lower proportion of studies are funded. For instance, in 1987, 30% of National Center for Nursing Research (NCNR, now NINR, National Institute for Nursing Research) research program grants were funded; in 1991, only 12% were funded (Kirchhoff, 1993). Similarly, ANNA has seen an increase in the number of research grant applications and there is not enough funding to support all the high-quality research that is proposed. In the future, this issue of adequacy of funding will need to be addressed by professional nursing organizations, including ANNA.

The Researchers

As noted earlier, the growth of knowledge in nephrology nursing has been limited by the small numbers of people qualified to conduct research in the field. Nancy Hoffart (1992; 1995), a former chairperson of ANNA's Research Special Interest Group, compiled a directory of nephrology nurse researchers. Responses were obtained from 96 individuals, who reported information about 137 research projects and 10 research programs. At approximately the same time, Sigma Theta Tau International reported over 3,300 active nurse researchers (McBride, 1993).

It is critical that nephrology nurses have access to the names of individuals who have research expertise. Those who have more research experience can serve as mentors, collaborators, or consultants for novice nephrology nurse researchers. The *Directory of Nephrology Nurse Researchers* (Hoffart, 1992, 1995) is a useful tool in linking potential collaborators.

Of the researchers who responded to the study, half of the nurses had a masters degree and 28 (29.2%) held doctoral degrees. Sixty nine percent of the respondents listed in the Directory were ANNA members. The employment positions of these researchers were: faculty member (26%), clinical nurse specialist or clinician (16.6%), program coordinator or head nurse (13.5%), or staff nurse (13.5%). Hoffart (1995) noted that many of the respondents had conducted only one study; it was evident from the data that many of the respondents did not hold the role of principal investigator or co-investigator, but may have been involved as research assistants or associates, project coordinators, or data collectors. Further information about research-related roles will be collected in future updates of the Directory.

Many of the nurse researchers conducted studies independently. Hoffart (1995) reported that 46.3% of the studies were conducted by solo researchers. Molzahn (1993a), in an evaluation of nephrology nursing research, found that nurses were the first (or sole) author on the reports of 68% of the studies, physicians were first author for 26.8%, and others were first author in 5.3% of the cases.

The future for nephrology nursing research is likely to be in collaborative research. For novice researchers, there are many benefits to working with experienced researchers. Through mentorship and experience, novice researchers will develop knowledge and skill about research. It is not essential that mentors be other nurses. In many settings, nurses may have more access to researchers trained in other disciplines. Also, there is a trend for large granting agencies to prefer grants from multidisciplinary research teams. Given the complexity of many research problems and the observation that multidisciplinary teams bring different and often complementary perspectives, the advantages of these approaches are difficult to dispute. Nephrology nurses will need to collaborate with other disciplines in order to secure research opportunities and funding, and to increase the likelihood that high quality research will be conducted.

Funding Sources for Nephrology Nursing Research

Hoffart (1995) noted that 43 researchers reported 154 different sources of funding for the projects that were included in the *Directory of Nephrology Nurse Researchers.* These funding sources, in decreasing order of frequency included: internal academic funds; federal agencies such as the National Institute for Nursing Research and National Institute for Health; ANNA; industry/pharmaceutical companies; other renal-related organizations (for example, the National Kidney Foundation); other nursing organizations; and internal service funds (see Table 6-1). It was interesting to note that many of the funded studies were funded by more than one agency; it was also interesting to note that 46 researchers (47.9%) assumed the costs of conducting their research themselves. In a review of the *Directory of Nurse Researchers* collated by Sigma Theta Tau International, it was also noted that a very high proportion of nurse researchers fund their studies out of pocket (McBride, 1993).

It is obvious from the proportion of researchers who fund their own research and the difficulty in securing adequate resources from a single source, that there is a need for more research grants, as well as grants of a larger magnitude. Researchers can spend many hours revising proposals to meet the specifications of different granting agencies, and much valuable time is lost in preparing multiple research grant applications so that one project can be completed.

Recent Research

Volume and Form

Both Hoffart (1992) and Molzahn (1993a) have reviewed the recent research in nephrology nursing. In Molzahn's study of nephrology nursing research studies conducted between 1979 and 1989, a total of 284 publications were identified. Of these, 258 were articles published in major journals, 25 were theses or dissertations, and one was a book.

The volume of nephrology nursing research seems to have steadily increased over the years, from 6 in 1979 (Molzahn, 1993a) to 72 in 1990 (Wilkinson, 1995). Similarly, it has been noted that the number of research manuscripts submitted to the *ANNA Journal* has increased steadily, to the point that a need has been identified by the Editorial Board to balance the research and clinical content (S.D. McCulloch, personal communication, August 1994). Clearly, there is an expanding research base for nephrology nursing.

Nephrology nursing research has been published in a variety of different publications. Molzahn reported that the highest proportion of research articles included in her study was published in the *AANNT/ANNA Journal* (33.7%), followed by *Dialysis and Transplantation* (18.6%), *American Journal of Kidney Diseases* (14.3%), and *Peritoneal Dialysis Bulletin/Peritoneal Dialysis International* (7.8%). Only 2.7% of the studies were published in *Nursing Research*. Wilkinson (1995) noted that nurses published their research in 44 different journals. While it is apparent that a considerable number of studies related to nephrology nursing are being published, Hoffart (1995) noted that 61% of researchers had not published their findings. While she did not collect data about oral or poster presentations, this observation raises some concerns. It seems that a significant proportion of the nephrology nursing research may not be disseminated. The reasons for this are not clear, but should be explored.

Phenomena Studied

Molzahn (1993a) noted that of the 284 research reports examined, 48.6% of the research related to hemodialysis, 23.9% to peritoneal dialysis, and 12.3% to renal transplantation. The remainder (15.1%) addressed end stage renal disease (ESRD) generally or addressed more than one treatment modality. Hoffart (1995) included modalities as classifiers in the *Directory of Nephrology Nurse Researchers*, but not all respondents selected a treatment modality as a classifier. For those who did, hemodialysis was the most common treatment modality studied, followed by transplant, peritoneal dialysis, and home dialysis. Only one study addressed conservative management. Wilkinson, who examined the nephrology nursing research conducted in 1990-1992, noted a higher proportion of research related to peritoneal dialysis (42.3%).

Adult ESRD patients have been the subjects for most research conducted by nephrology nurses. Only two nurse researchers reported conducting animal research (Hoffart, 1995). This is not surprising given that most nurses do not have the background to conduct animal research or are more interested in human behavior. Perhaps of greater concern is that only a few researchers have studied children with renal disease (Hoffart, 1995). Because the pediatric population of ESRD patients in each center is quite small, it is difficult to plan and conduct research that is meaningful and generalizable. Future efforts at studying this population will need to involve more than one center or unit in order to accumulate an adequate sample size. Also research with children is complicated by factors such as the lack of instruments designed for use with children, the need for different methodologies to study children, and ethical considerations, particularly in relation to informed consent.

Nephrology nursing research has covered a wide range of topic areas. Molzahn (1993a) classified research reports into 72 different categories. The most common areas of study in descending order of frequency were physiological health status; biochemical parameters; peritonitis; compliance/adherence; adaptation; urea or creatinine clearances; exit-site infections; psychological stress; quality of life; knowledge; subjective health status; morbidity/mortality; peritoneal dialysis catheter function; and transplant survival. Hoffart (1992) reported that the two major areas that respondents to the Directory addressed included psychosocial issues and quality of life. Both Molzahn (1993a) and Hoffart (1995) noted that some areas have had little if any research, including: management of symp-

Table 6–1
Sources of funding: Nephrology nursing research projects.

Source	No. of Projects
Self-funded	46
Internal academic funds	29
Federal agencies (NCNR, NIH)	21
ANNA	18
Drug companies/industry	17
Other kidney organizations (local & national, Canadian & US)	17
Other nursing organizations	15
Internal service funds	14
Other	23
No response	7

Note: From Hoffart, N. (1995). Characteristics of nephrology nurse researchers and their research. *ANNA Journal,* 22(1), 33–39. Used with permission.

toms associated with renal disease and their treatment, ethical issues, cardiovascular complications, helplessness, empowerment, sexual functioning, and courage. These are very basic and common areas of concern for patients with ESRD; yet, relatively little research has been done in these areas.

Also, there has been relatively little research that pertains to the nature of nursing care and the outcomes of nursing interventions. The nature of the nurse-patient interaction in nephrology settings has not been examined, yet it is recognized by practitioners in the field that the nature of the relationship is different in this area than in most other clinical areas of nursing. Little research in nephrology nursing has focused on the essence of nursing, that is, the caring function of nursing. Instead, much of the research focused on more easily quantifiable parameters.

It appears that there is enough research in several areas to consider a meta-analysis. Meta-analysis, which literally means analysis of analysis, refers to a statistical analysis of a number of studies (Curlette & Cannella, 1985). For the purposes of meta-analysis, individual studies are considered to be the subjects, and findings are transformed into a common statistic to examine overall effect size. This technique is particularly useful when there are a number of studies with conflicting findings, and we are unclear overall of the effect of a variable. In nephrology nursing, we could take studies completed in a particular substantive area, such as compliance, and using a meta-analysis, determine whether educational (or other) strategies are effective.

While nurse researchers have addressed questions of interest to them, one cannot help but wonder whether the research addresses the major problems encountered by practicing nephrology nurses. In order to get an accurate description of the major problems of practicing nurses, ANNA conducted a survey in 1991, of randomly selected members, to identify the major problem areas. Nurses were asked to identify five major problems that patients faced while receiving specific treatments (that is, hemodialysis, peritoneal dialysis, transplantation, and conservative management), the most difficult patient problems by age of patients (0 - 18 years, 19-40 years, 41-65 years, over 65 years), and the most difficult problems associated with specific nursing roles (clinician, educator, manager, researcher, consultant).

Several major themes recurred through all these areas, specifically: structure of the health system, social determinants of health, and complications arising from treatment. In relation to the structure of the health care system, the major concerns pertained to staffing shortages, inadequate equipment, lack of communication and support of staff from administration, lack of family support, staff training, and patient teaching. In relation to the social determinants of health, major areas of concern were noncompliance, unemployment, lack of finances and transportation, and lack of available facilities/services. In relation to complications, the major concerns related to access for hemodialysis and peritoneal dialysis, lack of available donors for transplantation, infection, and blood pressure control. Also, quite a number of psychosocial concerns were raised here, including loss of independence, time from family, friends and work, body image concerns, and treatments.

It may seem obvious that nephrology nursing research should focus on areas of greatest concern for practitioners and patients. However, researchers pursue areas that are of interest to them, and these areas may not be the ones that are of highest priority to practitioners and patients. In some areas that were identified as problems for nurses and patients, such as compliance, there has been considerable research. However, that research has not helped

Table 6-2
ANNA's research agenda.

The American Nephrology Nurses' Association (ANNA) has established a research agenda through the work of the Association's Research Committee and Board of Directors. The basic highlights of the agenda include:

Goals

- Establish research-based practice.
- Maintain and implement a research agenda for the association.
- Develop and maintain a database on nurses involved in the management and care of actual or potential patients.
- Participate in the development and maintenance of databases about actual and potential patients.
- Develop a high quality association research program.

Major Projects

- Research grant program
- Review of research abstracts
- Directory of Nephrology Nurse Researchers
- Evaluation of nephrology nursing research literature
- Staffing Survey
- Patient Classification Tool for Outpatient Hemodialysis Units

practitioners and patients reduce noncompliance. It may be, in many situations, that the wrong approach has been used to study a problem, and that there is a benefit to starting again. Using compliance as an example, it has been noted that most models or theories do not explain much more than 30% of the variance of compliance behavior (Molzahn, 1985). It seems likely that there are other variables that affect an individual's decision about whether or not they follow the directions given to them by health professionals. Future research may need to use an interview approach and qualitative methods to explore individuals' experiences with illness and the considerations involved in adhering to the medical regimen.

Also, it must be recognized that research cannot address all problems or questions; it may be that questions should be addressed in other ways. According to Carper (1978) and Belenky, Clinchy, Goldberger, and Tarule (1986), there are multiple ways of addressing issues other than the scientific/empirical ways that have traditionally been associated with research. Carper described empirics (the science of nursing), aesthetics (the art of nursing), the component of personal knowledge in nursing, and ethics or moral knowledge in nursing. Despite the value of empirical research, it is important to not discount the value of intuition, common sense, clinical judgement, peer consultation, and art in nursing practice. Hence, we should not be dismayed if answers to all our questions in nursing cannot be found in the research literature.

Some research questions may simply not be researchable. Questions about what is "right" and "wrong" are ethical questions and cannot be answered by scientific research (but philosophical inquiry may be more helpful). However, research problems that are framed within questions that start with "who," "what," "when," "where," and "why" can be addressed using one or more research methods. Determining the best method to use to answer a particular research question is often the challenge.

Designs of the Studies

In the process of knowledge development, it is common to begin with descriptive research to address the phenomenon of interest, and then move to comparative or correlational studies, and finally to experimental studies. Molzahn (1993a) noted that of the 284 publications examined, 99 (34.9%) of the studies were descriptive. Qualitative research studies were included in this category. There was also a significant proportion of analytical observational studies (129; 45.4%), which involved comparisons or correlations. Only 40 (14.1%) of the studies included in Molzahn's (1993a) (see Figure 6-1) analysis were experimental; similarly Hoffart (1995) found that 25% of the studies reported in the *Directory of Nephrology Nurse Researchers* employed experimental designs. Very few (4.9%) studies focused on methodology, instrument development, or on nursing history (2.7%). Furthermore, Hoffart (1995) noted that very few advanced statistical techniques such as factor analysis, path analysis, and structural equation modeling were used in the nephrology nursing research studies examined.

Again, the development of nephrology nursing research seems to parallel development of nursing research in general. For example, Moody et al. (1988) reported that 45% of the studies in their analysis were descriptive. Kim (1993) reported that as little as 12% of the research included in her study was prescriptive. Clearly, there is a great need to generate more knowledge about nursing and nursing interventions, but we are still in an early phase of knowledge development in nursing; as our understanding of human experience and human phenomena from a nursing perspective grows, we should be able to move to higher levels of research.

Theoretical Base

Although there is a great deal of discussion about theory-based practice and research, it seems that little nephrology nursing research has used a theoretical framework. Hoffart (1995) noted that only 34.3% of the researchers reported use of a nursing theory. Orem's Self-Care Model was the most frequently used nursing model. Another 14.6% of the researchers cited the use of nonnursing theories, such as the Health Belief Model, Lazarus' Theory of Stress and Coping, etc. Similar observations have been made in the general nursing research literature. For instance, McBride (1993), in a review of the *Directory of Nurse Researchers* published by Sigma Theta Tau, the international honor society in nursing, noted that the most popular nursing model used as a framework for research was Dorothy Orem's.

The value of use of theoretical models has been questioned by some scholars. There are many nurse researchers who believe that theory should be derived from nursing practice; that is, theory should be inductive. Other researchers advocate a deductive approach in which research questions, instruments, and analyses are guided by a theory. No single approach will answer all research questions in a discipline as complex as nursing. This author believes that the method, approach, and theoretical framework for each study should be those that are most appropriate to answer the research question that is posed. However, there are many views of the world, and the richness engendered by debates such as these should ultimately help us develop a strong knowledge base in nursing.

Quality of the Literature

In an evaluation of the nephrology nursing research literature (Molzahn, 1993a), there was an attempt to assess the quality of the research

Figure 6-1
Designs used in nephrology nursing research.

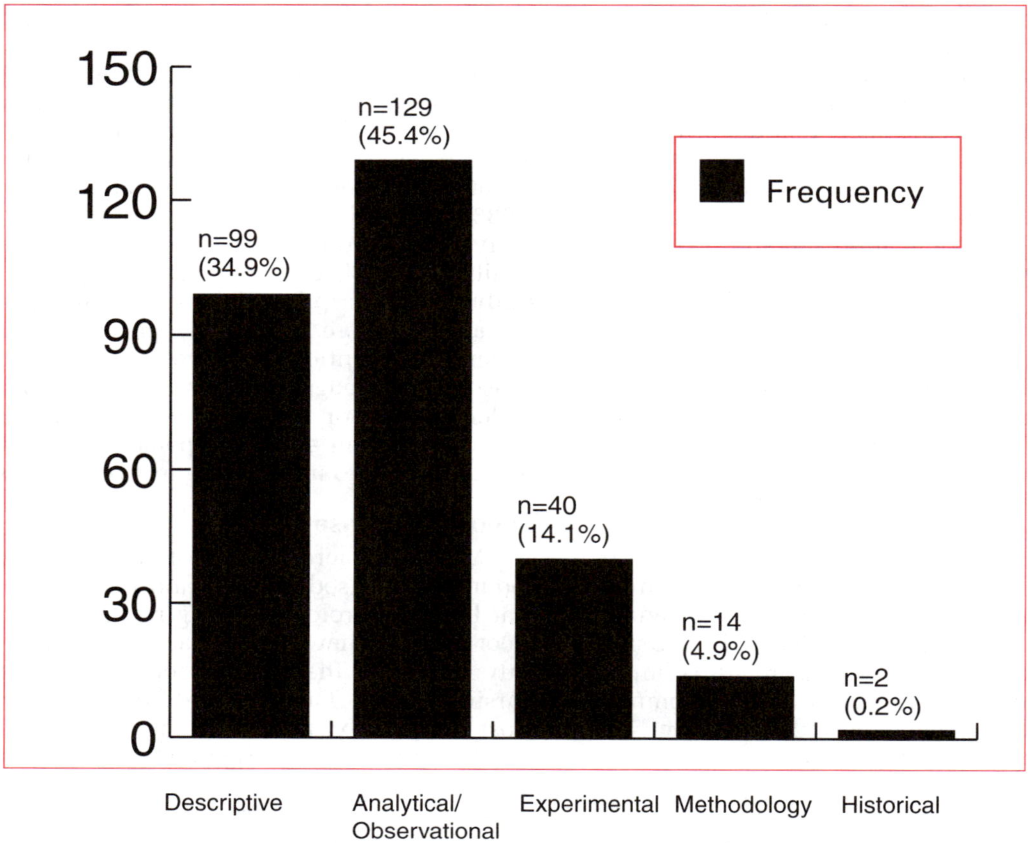

Note: From Molzahn, A.E. (1993a). An evaluation of the nephrology nursing research literature: 1979–1989. *ANNA Journal,* 20(4), 395–428. Used with permission.

involved. An instrument called the Quality Index (Georgopoulos, 1975) was used to rate the relevance, theoretical usefulness, and methodological adequacy of the papers. Of the 284 studies analyzed, 56.7% were judged to be highly relevant to nephrology nursing by reviewers. Another 32.7% were of moderate relevance, while only 10.6% were rated to be of low significance.

Theoretical usefulness was defined in the instrument as value or potential value to nephrology nursing research from a theoretical point of view (that is, treatment of concepts, theoretical emphasis, and rationale). In relation to theoretical usefulness, 36.6% of the papers were rated as high, and 35.9% were rated to be of moderate theoretical usefulness. Only 27.5% were rated as having low theoretical usefulness.

In the instrument, it was suggested that the subjective estimation of methodological adequacy was to be based on appropriateness of study design to the research problem, appropriateness of the analysis, response rates attained, measures used, and other available information about methodology. Reviewers rated 36% of the studies as having high methodological adequacy, 38.5% as having moderate or average methodological adequacy, and 22.3% as poor in terms of methodological adequacy. In only 3.6% of cases, reviewers indicated that they were unable to determine methodological adequacy from the publication.

Using the total quality score, computed by summing and averaging scores on the various items, it was found that 79% of the reports ranked in the high category, 20.6% ranked in the moderate category, and only 0.4% ranked in the low or below-average category.

In an open-ended question included on the Quality Index, reviewers were asked to comment on any particular problems in the design, method, sampling, analysis, and presentation of the study.

While many reviewers chose not to include any comments, problems were identified for 212 of the 284 studies.

There was no reference in the open-ended question to conceptual problems. Nevertheless, for 68 of the papers, 70 comments were made relating to this area. For some studies, more than one problem was identified. Of these 70 comments, 22 (31.4%) related to the lack of or inadequate theoretical framework for the study, 30 (42.9%) pertained to absent or inadequate operational definitions; 14 (20%) suggested flawed assumptions; and 4 (5.7%) related to an inadequate or outdated literature review.

Seventy-five comments, pertaining to 70 of the studies, were made relating to problems with the research design of the study. These included 39 (52%) relating to inadequate control over extraneous variables; 15 (20%) suggesting inappropriate designs; 5 (6.7%) pertaining to inappropriate timing; and 5 (6.7%) relating to lack of information regarding informed consent.

In relation to the methodology, 63 problems were identified in 59 of the studies. Most of these (42; 66.7%) related to a lack of reliability and validity. Another nine (14.3%) suggested that the tool was inappropriate, seven (11.1%) related to the timing of measurement, six (9.5%) pertained to scoring of the instrument, and six (9.5%) focused on inadequate control of extraneous variables.

With respect to sampling, the major problems identified were sample selection, sample size, and response rates. One hundred thirteen problems were identified in this area for 103 of the studies: 78 (69%) related to small sample size, 22 (28.3%) pertained to sample selection, 2 (2.2%) related to poor response rates, and 1 suggested that an inappropriate population was studied.

Only 31 comments were made regarding analyses (for 31 studies). Of these, 10 (32.3%) related to inappropriate statistical analyses, 18 (58.1%) noted no statistical analyses, and 3 (9.7%) indicated lack of statistical power.

In relation to 89 of the studies, 103 problems pertaining to presentation of the paper were identified. These problems included poor writing style (13; 12.3%); the failure to address relevance to nursing (19; 18.4%); the failure to state limitations (2; 1.9%); inconsistencies (43; 41.7%); inappropriate conclusions (28; 38.3%); lack of a purpose or hypotheses (8; 7.8%); and the failure to explain findings (6; 5.8%), analyses (10; 9.7%), and design (2; 1.9%). Wilkinson (1995) conducted similar critiques of nephrology nursing research, and although the classification scheme was different, similar findings were noted.

Assessment of quality of research is difficult. There is no well-established method to assess quality. Also, assessment of research reports may not necessarily reflect quality of research projects. Often research reports have not included important information. However, it may be that the journal did not require or wish to have this information; journal editorial policies often dictate the format of manuscripts. Reviewers of research manuscripts (and reviewers in the evaluation of nephrology nursing research) do not always rate research consistently. Some reviewers are known to be more rigorous and give more attention to detail. While the Quality Index may have indicated that most research was of reasonably good quality, it is recognized that there were numerous flaws in the studies. No research study is ever perfect, and caution needs to be used before generalizing the results of research.

While it is often assumed that research is of good quality, quality does not imply that research is ready for utilization in nursing practice. A careful review and consideration of the generalizability of each study is necessary before implementation is warranted. It is not likely that this process can be guided by the use of any particular instrument. Careful reading and critique, as well as an assessment of the practice setting are prerequisites to successful application of research to practice. Replication studies are warranted in most situations.

Research Utilization

Research is meaningless if it is not used. However, most researchers acknowledge that the findings of research are not being used extensively in clinical practice. Brett (1987) found that although most nurses knew about research-based practices and were persuaded about the benefits, they did not regularly use the innovations. This finding raises questions about what can be done to facilitate use of research findings.

Pettengill, Gillies, and Clark (1994) surveyed nurses to identify factors encouraging and discouraging research utilization. Lack of time was the factor that most discouraged research utilization. Factors that encouraged the use of nursing research included access to a library containing research journals, availability of nurse educators, and use of research newsletters. Champion and Leach (1989) and Thurstone, Tenove, and Church (1990) found similar facilitating factors, namely availability of research reports, library and consultant services, administrative support, and ongoing research in the agency. Other impeding factors included inability to understanding research reports, lack of work time to read research reports, and lack of authority to change patient care procedures (Funk, Champagne, Wiese, & Tornquist, 1991)

While studies relating to research utilization have not been conducted in nephrology nursing, it is likely that many of the same factors affect application of research findings to nephrology nursing practice. Molzahn (1993b) suggested ways to develop work environments that are conducive to research utilization. By creating environments where nurses feel safe to ask questions and where it is possible to take some risks, a positive climate for research can be created. Access to library resources, researchers, statisticians, time, money, and encouragement from colleagues will greatly assist nurses wishing to conduct research and use research findings.

There are many different models describing the research utilization process (Goode & Bulecheck, 1992; Horsley, Crane, Crabtree, & Wood, 1983; Rodgers, 1983). All of these models describe a process that includes review of research literature, critiques of the literature, and a change process to implement the research findings. A basic understanding of the research process and experience critiquing research is very helpful in applying research findings. It is beyond the scope of this chapter to describe how to conduct a research critique, but many research textbooks provide excellent guidelines and examples of critique of research. Molzahn (1993b) also outlines key questions to consider before applying research findings.

ANNA's Research Agenda

As noted earlier, the ANNA established a Research Special Interest Group in 1982, and in 1990, a Research Committee was formed. This committee worked with the Board of Directors to establish the research agenda for ANNA. The major goals of ANNA in relation to research are: to establish and maintain data bases relating to nurses practicing in the specialty and their patients; to foster development of research projects and programs in nephrology nursing research; and to promote research-based nephrology nursing practice (see Table 6-2).

ANNA has collected data about nephrology nurses through the staffing survey and through other surveys of the membership. Data relating to patients are available through other sources, such as the ESRD Networks. However, there are plans to carefully assess the data required by ANNA and the membership, and to develop or access a data base that will provide the necessary information for the future.

The goal of developing research projects and programs in nephrology nursing research has included a wide range of activities and the involvement of many people. These activities include, but are not limited to, educational programming at meetings, establishment of research grants, mentorship of novice researchers, and review of ideas or proposals for research.

Research-based practice involves the application and utilization of research in practice. As noted earlier, there is a gap between availability of research findings and application in practice. This area has been targeted for future educational programming. As well, a research utilization grant has been established to attempt to facilitate application of research findings.

Some of the major projects of the Research Committee and Special Interest Group have been (a) establishment of a research grant program, (b) development of review mechanisms for research abstracts, (c) publication of the *Directory of Nephrology Nurse Researchers* and evaluation of the nephrology nursing research literature, (d) development of a staffing survey, and (e) the development of a Patient Classification System Tool.

Establishment of a Research Grant Program

ANNA has a series of research grants available for members. In 1994-1995, there were 11 grants available, ranging in size from $500 to $5000. Some of these grants were sponsored by ANNA and others by corporate sponsors. Policies and procedures have been developed for all research-related awards, and review processes have been developed and streamlined. The number of grant applications has risen since 1989, and Research Committee members have noted improvements in the quality of the submissions.

Development of Review Mechanisms for Research Abstracts

The ANNA Research Committee reviews research abstracts for the National Symposium. The best abstracts are presented at the National Symposium, at which time the highest-rated abstract is awarded ANNA's Research Abstract Award.

Directory of Nephrology Nurse Researchers/Evaluation of Research Literature

Two of ANNA's projects, the development of the *Directory of Nephrology Nurse Researchers* and the evaluation of nephrology nursing research literature were described earlier in this chapter. Both data bases are updated regularly.

Staffing Survey

This survey of nurse managers/head nurses is conducted every 2 years to describe staffing patterns in nephrology settings. Available data include numbers and types of personnel, as well as roles and functions of the personnel. In 1992, ANNA also surveyed a random sample of 700 members regarding the major problems that faced them in their practice, as well as the major problems encountered by patients in each treatment modality. These data can be used to plan future programs.

Patient Classification Tool

The need for such an instrument was identified by the membership, and ANNA in collaboration with MECON developed and tested a tool that is now available for purchase.

Future Directions for Nephrology Nursing Research

While there has been healthy growth in the amount, and by all appearances, the quality of nephrology nursing research, there is still a need to encourage the development of more programs of research. Programs of research give investigators the opportunity to build on their findings and further develop knowledge in the field. To date, the tendency has been for most researchers to complete a single study, unrelated to past or future work.

Research in the future needs to become more closely based on and evolve from real nursing practice situations. There is a perception that research is for the academicians. Perhaps different models and methods of research and inquiry are necessary. Collaborative models could allow practitioners and researchers to work together more closely, enabling practitioners to better understand the research process and hopefully facilitate application of research findings. Furthermore, collaboration between centers could facilitate research efforts in areas where small samples are the norm (for example; pediatrics, plasma exchange). Physicians have successfully used multi-center studies for many questions; nurses could benefit from their experiences and contacts.

Participatory action research empowers practitioners and clients to control and participate in the research process. This research approach has not been used extensively in nephrology settings. However, given the emphasis on patient decision-making in nephrology, this approach has promise.

Some research questions, for example those of an ethical nature, cannot be answered by scientific means, and it may be most appropriate to use philosophical inquiry to address them. A receptiveness to different methods of inquiry could enrich our understanding of some issues.

There are many areas in our specialty that require further investigation. Unfortunately, the concerns of highest priority to nephrology nurses are not necessarily the areas that researchers examine. It would be valuable to assess and develop priorities for research, and establish research grants for projects that specifically address the priority areas. This is an area in which ANNA could demonstrate leadership in the future.

Greater efforts need to be made to disseminate nephrology nursing research. As noted earlier, much research is not published. Without availability of research findings in published form, it is unrealistic to consider progression toward research utilization.

While there are many ways that nurses can learn about research and the research process, and while ANNA is committed to offering educational opportunities related to research, there remains a need to increase the number of nurses prepared to conduct research. Supporting and assisting nephrology nurses through masters and doctoral programs will increase the number of researchers and the amount of research conducted in the future.

Summary

It is clear that there is a substantial amount of nephrology nursing research, and that our body of knowledge is growing. However, it is apparent that there are many areas that nephrology nurses need to research or continue to research. There are still many aspects of nephrology nursing research that could be improved. While it is unrealistic to expect that research will be perfect or that problems will not exist in various reports, nephrology nurses need to consider using larger sample sizes, selecting instruments that have been tested for reliability and validity, and where appropriate, using theoretical frameworks.

Nurses need opportunities to learn about the research process and application of research findings. While professional development programs and educational materials can address these areas, probably the greatest changes will occur when more nephrology nurses attain advanced degrees. Masters and doctoral programs in nursing are designed to develop nurse researchers, and as the number of nephrology nurses attaining higher degrees grows, the nephrology nursing knowledge base will undoubtedly escalate.

The research process has often been found to be frustrating and discouraging. With the help of more experienced mentors, novice researchers are more likely to survive the process and complete research of high quality. It is important that experienced researchers offer their assistance willingly and freely to promote the growth of knowledge about nephrology nursing.

The research base for nephrology nursing is strong; it is important that some of the findings are put into practice. More strategies to enhance research-based practice and promote application of research findings in practice are required. Institutions, ANNA chapters, and individuals can all facilitate research utilization through support of journal clubs and other educational programs, creating a climate conducive to innovations, and to disseminating research findings

References

Belenky, M.F., Clinchy, B.M., Goldberger, N.R., & Tarule, J.M. (1986). *Women's ways of knowing: The development of self, voice and mind.* New York: Basic Books.

Brennan, D.T., & Jordan, P.S. (1994). The history of ANNA: A chronology of events. *ANNA: Celebrating 25 years of service to the nephrology community.* Pitman, NJ: American Nephrology Nurses' Association.

Brett, J.L. (1987). The use of nursing practice research findings. *Nursing Research, 36,* 344-346.

Carper, B.A. (1978). Fundamental patterns of knowing in nursing. In L.H. Nicoll (Ed.), *Perspectives on nursing theory* (pp. 252-260). Glenview, IL: Scott Foresman.

Champion, V., & Leach, A. (1989). Variables related to research utilization in nursing: An empirical investigation. *Journal of Advanced Nursing, 14*, 705-710.

Curlette, W.L., & Cannella, K.S. (1985). Going beyond the narrative summarization of research findings: The meta-analysis approach. *Research in Nursing and Health, 8*, 293-301.

Funk, S., Champagne, M., Wiese, R., & Tornquist, E. (1991). Barriers to using research findings in practice: The clinician's perspective. *Applied Nursing Research, 4*, 90-95.

Georgopoulos, B.S. (1975). *Hospital organization research: Review and source book*. Toronto: W.B. Saunders Company.

Goode, C., & Bulecheck, G. (1992). Research utilization: An organizational process that enhances quality of care. *Journal of Nursing Care Quality*, Special Report, 27-35.

Hoffart, N. (1992). Directory of nephrology nurse researchers. *ANNA Journal, 19*, 291-320.

Hoffart, N. (1995). Characteristics of nephrology nurse researchers and their research. *ANNA Journal, 22*, 33 -39.

Horsley, J., Crane, J., Crabtree, M., & Wood, D. (1983). *Using research to improve nursing practice: A guide*. New York: Grune & Stratton.

Kim, H.S. (1993). Rethinking the typology of nursing research. In C.P. Germain & M.J. Dodd (Eds.), *Developing taxonomies for nursing research* (pp. 11-25). Washington, DC: American Nurses Association.

Kirchhoff, K. (1993). Critical care nursing research. In M.R. Kinney, D. Packa, & S. Dunbar (Eds), *AACN's Clinical reference for critical care nursing* (3rd edition). (pp. 44-53). St. Louis: Mosby Year Book.

McBride, A.B. (1993). Sigma Theta Tau International's classification system for nursing research. In C.P. Germain & M.J. Dodd (Eds.), *Developing taxonomies for nursing research* (pp. 37-44). Washington, DC: American Nurses Association.

Molzahn, A.E. (1985). *An analysis and critique of compliance theories*. Unpublished manuscript.

Molzahn, A.E. (1993a). An evaluation of the nephrology nursing research literature: 1979-1989. *ANNA Journal, 20*, 395-428.

Molzahn, A.E. (1993b). Research-based practice: Using and participating in research. In P.S. Jordan (Ed.), *Nephrology nursing: A guide to professional development* (pp. 169-206). Pitman, NJ: American Nephrology Nurses' Association.

Moody, L.E., Wilson, M.E., Smyth, K., Schwartz, R., Tittle, M., & Van Cott, M.L. (1988). Analysis of a decade of nursing practice research: 1977-1986. *Nursing Research, 37*(6), 374-379.

Pettengill, M.M., Gillies, D.A., & Clark, C.C. (1994). Factors encouraging and discouraging the use of nursing research findings. *Image: Journal of Nursing Scholarship, 26*, 143-147.

Rodgers, E. (1983). *Diffusion of innovations* (3rd edition). New York: Free Press.

Thurstone, I., Tenove, S., & Church, J. (1990). Hospital nursing research is alive and flourishing. *Nursing Management, 21*(5), 50-54.

Wilkinson, G. (1995). Analysis and evaluation of nephrology nursing research literature: 1990-1992. Unpublished master's thesis, University of Alberta.

RESEARCH BRIEF

Definitions of Research Designs

❑ Descriptive Studies

Descriptive studies are studies in which there is no comparison or control group. Some examples include: studies of the incidence, prevalence, or frequency of a disease or clinical characteristic; studies of the natural history of a disease; and studies to establish normal values of a parameter in a population. Qualitative studies also generally fall into this category.

❑ Methodological Studies

Methodological studies are studies involving the development of diagnostic procedures or techniques of measurement, including new instrumentation, comparison of various modes of measurement, development of screening techniques, studies dealing with reliability and validity of various instruments or diagnostic techniques, and studies that pertain to observer error and variation.

❑ Analytical Observational Studies

Analytical observational studies are those studies characterized by the existence of a control or comparison group and the absence of allocation of patient to control or treatment groups by the investigator. Quasi–experimental studies fit into this category. Other examples include: epidemiological studies of risk factors and disease, such as case control and cohort studies; evaluation of individual, institutional, or origram performance and outcomes; and investigations using historical controls or matched samples.

❑ Experimental Studies

Experimental studies include all studies in which the investigator manipulated the factor under investigation, in which his/her intent was to examine the direct effects of that factor. Some examples include: randomized clinical trials with concurrent controls and studies in which the investigator allocates patient to control or treatment groups.

❑ Historical Studies

Historical studies refer to "investigations to determine what happened in the past . . . in order to gain greater understanding of the present" (Trussell, Brandt, & Knapp, 1981, p. 228).

Note: From Molzahn, A.E. (1993a). An evaluation of the nephrology nursing research literature: 1979–1989. *ANNA Journal,* 20(4), 395–428. Used with permission.

Chapter Highlights

- Over the last 25 years, nephrology nursing has evolved as a specialty area within nursing, and an important part of the specialty's evolution has been a movement toward research–based practice.
- The numbers of qualified nurse researchers, trends in health care, and availability of funding all affect the conduct of nephrology nursing research.
- The future for nephrology nursing research is likely to be in collaborative research. For novice researchers, there are many benefits to working with experienced researchers.
- Multiple funding sources exist for nephrology nursing research; however, there is still a need for more research grants, as well as grants of larger magnitude.
- The volume of nephrology nursing research has steadily increased since 1979. Nephrology nursing research has been published in a variety of settings, signaling an expanding research base within the specialty.
- Of the various modalities studied, hemodialysis research has been reported on most frequently, followed by peritoneal dialysis, general ESRD issues, and renal transplantation.
- Areas having little, if any, research include management of symptoms associated with renal disease, ethical issues, cardiovascular complications, helplessness, empowerment, sexual functioning, and courage.
- The development of nephrology nursing research seems to parallel development of nursing research in general, with most studies in the literature being descriptive.
- Little nephrology research has used a theoretical framework, and the value of theoretical models, in general, has been questioned by some nursing scholars.
- While research is often assumed to be of good quality, quality does not imply that research is ready to use in practice. A careful review of the generalizability of each study is needed before implementation is warranted.
- Although research is meaningless if not used, most researchers acknowledge that research findings are not being used extensively in clinical practice.
- ANNA has established both a Research Special Interest Group and a Research Committee. The Committee has worked with ANNA's Board of Directors to develop a Research Agenda for the Association.
- Some major ANNA projects have been the establishment of a research grant program, development of review mechanisms for research abstracts, a staffing survey, and the Patient Classification System Tool.
- Research in the future needs to be based on and evolve from real nursing practice situations.
- Greater efforts need to be made to disseminate nephrology nursing research. Without availability of published research findings, progression toward use in practice will be slow.

UNIT 3

The Kidney

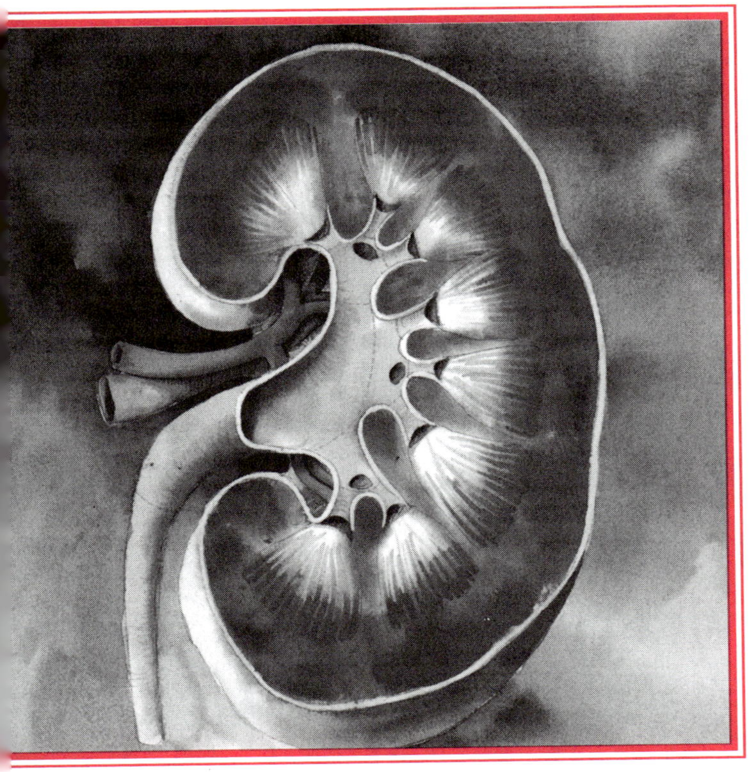

Unit Contents

Chapter 7

Renal Physiology 127

Patricia Preisig, PhD, RN; Christine Chmielewski, MS, RN, CNN; Marcia Keen, MS, RN; Mary Jo Holechek, MS, RN, CNN; Marlys K. Ludlow, MSN, RN, CNN; Carolyn B. Yucha, PhD, RN

Chapter 8

Diseases of the Kidney 177

Patricia S. Jordan, MS, RN, CNA, CNN

Chapter 9

Acute and Chronic Renal Failure 199

Kathy P. Parker, PhD, RN, CS, ANP

CHAPTER 7

Renal Physiology

Patricia Preisig, PhD, RN
Christine Chmielewski, MS, RN, CNN
Marlys K. Ludlow, MSN, RN, CNN
Marcia Keen, MS, RN
Carolyn B. Yucha, PhD, RN
Mary Jo Holechek, MS, RN, CNN

Chapter Contents

Section 1: Renal Anatomy and Overview of Nephron Function 130
- Vascular Supply 130
- Macroscopic Anatomy 130
- Microscopic Anatomy 131
- Juxtaglomerular Apparatus 133
- Renal Processes 134

Section 2: Glomerular Filtration and Renal Hemodynamics 135
- Renal Circulation 135
- Glomerular Filtration 136
- Renal Hemodynamics 138
- Intrinsic Factors 138
- Integration of Renal Hemodynamic Control Factors 141

Section 3: Urinary Concentration and Dilution 142
- Tubular Processes 142
- Other Processes 143
- Forming a Dilute and Concentrated Urine 145

Section 4: Renal Handling of Potassium 145
- Potassium Functions 145
- Sodium-Potassium ATPase Pump 146
- Extrarenal Regulation of Internal Potassium 146
- Renal Handling of Potassium 146

Section 5: Renal Control of Calcium 150
- Calcium and Its Functions 150
- Calcium Imbalances 151
- Calcium Homeostasis 151
- Renal Handling of Calcium 151

Chapter Contents

Regulation of Calcium Excretion 153
Section 6: Renal Control of Phosphorus and Magnesium 154
Phosphorus and Its Function 154
Phosphorus Homeostasis 155
Renal Handling of Phosphorus 155
Magnesium and Its Functions 157
Magnesium Homeostasis 157
Renal Handling of Magnesium 157
Section 7: Renal Acidification 158
Principles and Definitions: Acid-Base Physiology 158
Intracellular and Extracellular Buffering Systems 160
The Daily Maintenance of Acid-Base Balance 162
Renal Mechanisms Involved in the Maintenance of Acid-Base Homeostasis 162
Maintenance of Systemic Acid-Base Balance 163
Adaptations to Changes in the Magnitude of Daily Acid Load 163
Section 8: Renal Regulation of Extracellular Fluid Volume and Osmolality 164
Body Requirements for Sodium and Water 164
Homeostatic Control of Sodium and Water 165
General Renal Reabsorptive Mechanisms 168
Specific Tubular Reabsorptive Mechanisms 169
Summary 173
Readings 173
Chapter Highlights 174

Renal Physiology

Patricia Preisig, PhD, RN

Christine Chmielewski, MS, RN, CNN

Marlys K. Ludlow, MSN, RN, CNN

Marcia Keen, MS, RN

Carolyn B. Yucha, PhD, RN

Mary Jo Holechek, MS, RN, CNN

Chapter Editor's Note: This chapter is a compilation of the renal physiology series published in the ANNA Journal between February 1992 and October 1996, for which Patricia Preisig, PhD, RN, served as Editor. The individual articles have only been modified as needed to enhance the continuity of the chapter or for formatting consistency. The basic content of each article is unchanged from that published in the series and reflects the opinions and understanding of the individual authors. Textbook Editor, Janel Parker, and Dr. Preisig are indebted to the authors who wrote the individual articles, for their contributions to this book. They are: Christine Chmielewski ("Renal Anatomy and Overview of Nephron Function," February 1992 issue; Vol. 19, pp. 34-40); Mary Jo Holechek ("Glomerular Filtration and Renal Hemodynamics," June 1992 issue; Vol. 19, pp. 237-248); Patricia Preisig ("Urinary Concentration and Dilution," August 1992 issue; Vol. 19, pp. 351-355; and "Renal Acidification," August 1994 issue; Vol. 21, pp. 251-257); Marlys Ludlow ("Renal Handling of Potassium," February 1993 Issue; Vol. 20, pp. 52-58); Carolyn Yucha ("Renal Control of Calcium," August 1993 Issue; Vol. 20, pp.440-444; and "Renal Control of Phosphorus and Magnesium," August 1993 issue; Vol. 20, pp. 447-450); and Carolyn Yucha and Marcia Keen ("Renal Regulation of Body Volume and Osmolality," October 1996 issue; Vol. 23, pp. 487-495).

This chapter provides an overview of the normal anatomy and physiology of the renal system to serve as a foundation for understanding renal assessment and renal abnormalities. The chapter is divided into 8 sections, which are briefly described below.

Section 1: Renal Anatomy and Overview of Nephron Function

The kidneys are paired vascular organs that perform excretory, regulatory, and secretory functions. In order to understand how these complex organs work, the renal anatomy and renal processes involved in maintaining the body's internal milieu are reviewed in this section.

Section 2: Glomerular Filtration and Renal Hemodynamics

This section examines the unique characteristics of renal circulation, describes the physiology of glomerular filtration, reviews the extrinsic and intrinsic factors that can alter renal hemodynamics, and discusses a clinical situation in which multiple factors are interacting in an effort to maintain the renal blood flow (RBF) and glomerular filtration rate (GFR) despite systemic pressure changes.

Section 3: Urinary Concentration and Dilution

This section describes the mechanisms responsible for forming and excreting a dilute or concentrated urine. These processes specifically involve the descending and ascending limbs of the loops of Henle, the distal tubules of the juxtamedullary nephrons, the collecting tubule, and the vasa recta.

Section 4: Renal Handling of Potassium

This discussion addresses the mechanisms responsible for maintaining the K balance in the intracellular and extracellular fluid compartments of individual body cells.

Section 5: Renal Control of Calcium

The homeostasis of calcium is complex because the gastrointestinal tract, the bone, and the kidney all affect calcium balance. Accordingly, the roles and interactions of all three sites must be considered.

Section 6: Renal Control of Phosphorus and Magnesium

Phosphorus and magnesium balance is maintained by the kidney, the bone, and gastrointestinal system. Accordingly, the roles and interactions of all three sites must be considered.

Section 7: Renal Acidification

This section covers renal acidification and has been divided into two major sections. The first section reviews principles of acid-base physiology, including a description of pH and hydrogen ions, buffer systems, and intracellular and extracellular buffering mechanisms. The second section deals with the renal contribution to the maintenance of pH balance.

Section 8: Renal Regulation of Extracellular Fluid Volume and Osmolality

To function properly, cells in the body require an internal environment comprised of the correct osmolality, ionic composition, pH, and temperature. This internal environment is maintained by the cardiovascular and renal systems. Together, along with neural and endocrine input, these two systems maintain fluid and electrolyte balance within narrow limits suitable for optimal cell function. This section describes the mechanisms by which the extracellular fluid (ECF) volume and osmolality are controlled.

Section 1: Renal Anatomy and Overview of Nephron Function

The kidneys are paired vascular organs that perform excretory, regulatory, and secretory functions. To understand how these complex organs work, it is necessary to review renal anatomy and understand the renal processes involved in maintaining the body's internal milieu.

The renal system comprises the kidneys, ureters, bladder, and urethra (see Figure 7-1). Urine is formed by the kidneys and then flows through the other structures to be excreted from the body. The kidneys are located bilaterally in the retroperitoneal space at the level of T-12 to L-3. The organs are bean-shaped; measure approximately 12 cm in length, 6 cm in width, and 2.5 cm in thickness; and weigh 120 to 170 grams in the normal adult. The right kidney is slightly lower than the left because of the liver. The kidneys are protected, not only by their anatomic position within the rib cage, but also by the perinephric structures. A tough fibrous capsule covers each kidney. The renal fascia provides support, while perirenal fat acts as a cushion.

The ureters are hollow, fibromuscular tubes that begin at the renal pelvis, extend downward retroperitoneally, and join the bladder. Urine flows away from the kidneys by peristalsis. The urinary bladder, located in the pelvic region, is a spherical, muscular sac with a capacity of 300 to 500 ml in the normal adult. Urine enters via the ureteral orifices and is excreted through the urethra.

Figure 7-1
The general organizational plan of the urinary system.

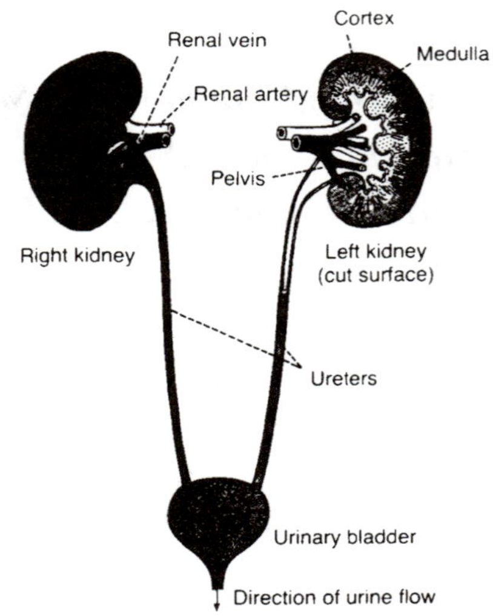

Note: From Guyton, A.C. (1991). *Textbook of medical physiology* (page 287). Philadelphia: W.B. Saunders Company. Reprinted with permission.

Vascular Supply

The kidneys are highly vascularized organs and receive approximately 20% of the resting cardiac output. Thus, renal blood flow is about 1200 ml/min. Two characteristics of the renal vasculature make it different from most other vascular beds in the body. First, there are two capillary beds in series: the glomerular capillary bed and the peritubular capillary bed. These capillary beds are separated by the efferent arteriole. This arrangement, a capillary bed surrounded by arterial vasculature, is referred to as a portal system. Second, the capillary bed is more porous. For example, it has a higher rate of fluid exudation than do the systemic capillaries. It also provides a size and charge barrier to large molecules such as albumin, unlike the systemic capillaries.

The aorta gives rise to the renal artery, which enters the kidney at the hilar region. This, in turn, branches to increasingly smaller vessels, that is, the interlobar, arcuate, and interlobular arteries. The interlobular arteries extend into the cortex and become the afferent arterioles that branch to form the glomerular capillary tufts (see Figure 7-1). The efferent arterioles receive blood from the glomerular capillaries. The presence of arteriolar structures on either end of the glomerular capillaries allows maintenance of an intracapillary pressure favoring the movement of fluid out of the capillary lumen. The efferent arterioles give rise to the second capillary bed, the peritubular network. These capillaries are a low pressure system that favors fluid movement into the capillary lumen. In the medulla, these capillaries, called the vasa recta, form long, straight loops that run parallel to the loops of Henle of the juxtamedullary nephrons and play an important role in the concentration and dilution of urine. In the cortex, the peritubular capillaries form a network surrounding nephron segments located within the cortex. This meshwork is designed to efficiently pick up water and solutes reabsorbed from the nephron structures. Blood flow in the remainder of the venous system follows the same pattern as the arterial vessels and returns to the inferior vena cava.

Macroscopic Anatomy

The renal parenchyma consists of two distinct regions, the cortex and medulla (see Figure 7-2). The cortex has a granular appearance because of the structures contained in this layer, namely, the glomeruli, proximal and distal tubules, cortical col-

Figure 7-2
Differences between a cortical and a juxtamedullary nephron.

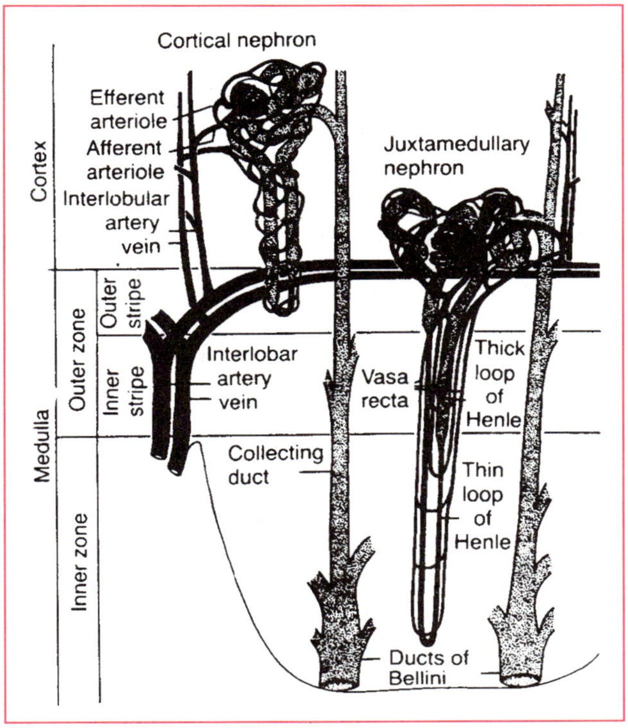

Note: From *Physiology of the kidney and body fluids* (1974) (page 287). Chicago: Year Book Medical Publishers. Reprinted with permission.

lecting tubules, and adjacent peritubular capillaries. The medulla contains triangular wedges that have a striped appearance. These wedges are the renal pyramids formed by the long loops of Henle, medullary collecting tubules, and vasa recta. The tapered end of the pyramid, the papilla, directs urine toward the minor and major calyces. Urine then enters the hollow, funnel-shaped renal pelvis, which has a volume of 5 to 10 ml, before flowing into the ureters.

Microscopic Anatomy

The nephron is the basic functional unit of the kidney. There are approximately 1 million nephrons in each kidney. There are two types of nephrons, cortical and juxtamedullary, named according to the location of their glomeruli within the renal parenchyma (see Figure 7-2). The cortical nephrons, which make up about 85% of the total nephrons, are subdivided into superficial and midcortical nephrons. The superficial cortical nephrons have their glomeruli in the outer cortex and have short loops of Henle. The midcortical nephrons, as their name suggests, have their glomeruli in the midcortex region. Their loops vary in length and may be either short (contained within the cortex) or long (extending partially into the outer medulla). The cortical nephrons perform excretory and regulatory functions. The juxtamedullary nephrons make up the remaining 15% of the nephrons. Their glomeruli are located deep in the cortex near the corticomedullary border. They have long loops of Henle that descend into the medulla, often to the tips of the pyramids. These nephrons play an important role in the concentration and dilution of urine by generating a steep interstitial fluid osmotic gradient between the cortex and deep medulla. The vasa recta are responsible for maintaining this gradient.

Glomerulus. This specialized capillary bed is a network of interconnected loops surrounded by Bowman's capsule. As described above, the glomerular capillaries have unique characteristics that contribute to its filtering capabilities. The porosity of the endothelial layer increases capillary permeability; the meshlike structure of the basement membrane provides a barrier to large molecules; and the portal structure allows maintenance of an intracapillary pressure that favors filtration.

The glomerular membrane has three layers: (a) endothelial, (b) basement membrane, and (c) epithelial. The endothelium lines the capillary lumen and contains many pores, or fenestrae, that favor the filtration of fluid and small solutes. The glomerular basement membrane (GBM) is a matrix of collagen and similar proteins that provides a size barrier to the movement of large particles out of the capillary lumen. The visceral epithelial cells of Bowman's capsule, or the podocytes, have cytoplasmic foot processes that extend over the basement membrane. Spaces between these foot processes are called slit-pores and allow the filtrate into Bowman's space. Mesangial cells are located between the capillary loops of the glomerulus and form a support network within the tuft. Some of these cells have phagocytic properties.

The glomerular membrane allows filtration of fluid and small molecules. Large molecules are prevented from entering the filtrate in two ways. First, the size of the spaces in the glomerular epithelium and basement membrane limits the passage of these larger molecules such as the white and red blood cells and albumin. Second, the podocytes and, to some extent the GBM, have a net negative charge that repels large negatively charged molecules, particularly the plasma proteins. Small anions that easily filter through the pores are not influenced by the negative electrical charge.

Bowman's capsule. Bowman's capsule is made up of two cell layers: (a) the visceral layer that forms the epithelial layer (podocytes) of the filtration barrier and (b) the parietal cell layer that forms the outer layer of the capsule. The space between the two cell layers, referred to as Bowman's space, collects the filtered fluid and solutes and directs this filtrate toward the proximal tubule.

Tubular system. The tubular system has four components: (a) proximal tubule (PT), (b) loop of Henle, (c) distal tubule (DT), and (d) collecting tubule. These components are divided further into subsegments, each with specific cellular structures and functions. The kidneys filter about 180 liters of fluid per day with an electrolyte composition similar to that of plasma. Clearly, if all of this filtrate were excreted, total body water and electrolytes would be excreted in a few hours. Thus, the nephrons have the responsibility of handling this large volume of filtrate and separating out that which must be conserved and that which needs to be excreted. The advantage of filtering such a large volume of fluid is that plasma clearance of waste products can occur rapidly. The disadvantage, however, is that the majority of the filtrate must be recycled back to the plasma, with little room for error.

To accomplish this tenuous task, the nephron is physically divided into subsegments with "assigned" specific tasks. In general, the proximal tubule can be thought of as the "bulk-phase" segment of the nephron as it transports water and solutes in bulk. It reabsorbs, and thus, returns to the plasma, almost 100% of the filtered solutes that the body does not routinely wish to discard, such as glucose, amino acids, and bicarbonate and reabsorbs a large percentage of solutes, such as sodium, potassium, chloride, calcium, and magnesium, as well as water whose amounts of excretion will vary throughout the day. This is not to say that regulation of transport of any of these solutes does not occur in the proximal tubule. In fact, transport of most of these solutes is tightly regulated, but the regulation involves a gross versus fine-tune regulation.

The distal nephron, including all subsegments between the thin descending limb of the loop of Henle and the inner-medullary collecting tubule, is the site of fine-tune regulation of all solutes and water that leave the proximal tubule. In the next sections of this chapter, the nephron segments specifically handling these solutes and water will be discussed in detail, along with discussions of the regulation of solute and water excretion. In total, these processes govern maintenance of a systemic homeostatic milieu with regard to volume regulation, acid-base balance, and electrolyte balance. The next section introduces the nephron subsegments, describing their anatomic differences and summarizing their roles in water and solute regulation.

Proximal tubule. The PT, which drains the glomerular filtrate from Bowman's space, is located in the renal cortex. The pars convoluta is the convoluted section of the PT, and the pars recta is the straight section that descends toward the medulla. The cellular structures of the PT give evidence of its high transport capacity. The flattened epithelial cells have microvilli on the luminal border, which create a brush border and increase surface area available to solute and fluid transport. The cells contain a large number of mitochondria, which are necessary for active transport.

The PT is the major site of reabsorption in the nephron. Sixty-five percent of the filtered water and sodium is reabsorbed here. Other substances reabsorbed include all of the filtered glucose and amino acids; some of the water soluble vitamins; 50% of the filtered chloride, potassium, and urea; 80%-90% of the filtered bicarbonate; 75% of the filtered phosphate; 60% of the filtered calcium; and 65% of the filtered magnesium and remaining solutes. The PT also secretes substances into the tubular fluid. Secretion occurs primarily in the pars recta and includes many endogenous and exogenous organic anions and cations. As a result of these reabsorptive and secretory processes, the osmolarity of the tubular fluid at the end of the PT is isosmotic, that is, essentially equivalent to plasma, or approximately 300 mOsm/L.

Loop of Henle. The loop of Henle is the next component of the tubular system and consists of the thin descending limb, thin ascending limb, and thick ascending limb. Of note, these segments differ between the cortical and juxtamedullary nephrons. Superficial cortical nephrons, with their short loops, do not have a thin ascending segment. This is also true of the midcortical nephrons with short loops. However, the juxtamedullary nephrons and those midcortical nephrons with loops extending into the inner medulla do have a thin ascending limb. In the juxtamedullary nephrons, the long loops of Henle together with the vasa recta are components of the countercurrent mechanism responsible for urine concentration and dilution.

In the thin descending limb and thin ascending segment, the cells are flat with few microvilli and mitochondria. Movement of solutes is by diffusion rather than by active transport. There are functional differences between the two thin segments. The thin descending limb is highly permeable to water but much less permeable to urea, sodium, and most of the other solutes. The thin ascending limb is virtually impermeable to water but transports sodium, chloride, and urea.

The epithelial cells of the thick ascending limb become thick and are similar to those in the PT but have fewer microvilli. The thick ascending limb, like the thin ascending limb, is impermeable to water. Although sodium and chloride are the major solutes reabsorbed, other ions including potassium, bicarbonate, and calcium are also reabsorbed. Because of the high solute but low water reabsorption in this segment, the tubular fluid becomes hypo-osmotic.

Distal tubule. The DT is located in the cortical region of the kidney. The initial section of the DT,

Figure 7-3
Diagram of the structural organization of the mammalian kidney demonstrating the relationships between the various segments of the nephron and the zones of the kidney, especially the medulla.

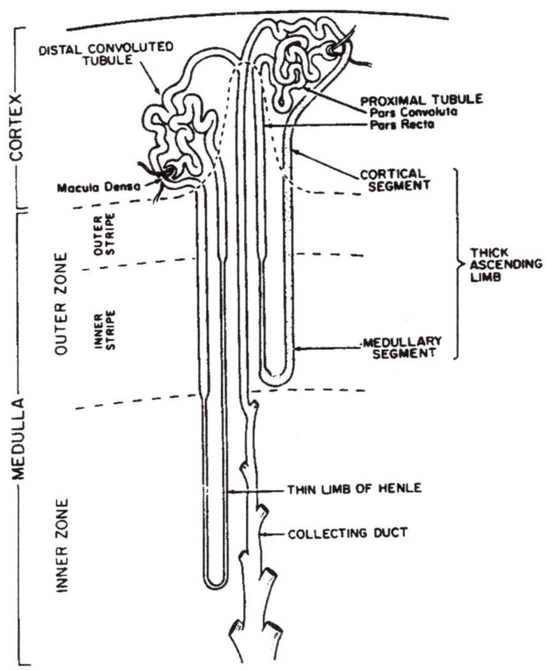

Note: From Brenner, B.M., & Rector, F.C. (1986). *The kidney* (3rd ed.). Philadelphia: W.B. Saunders Company. Reprinted with permission.

immediately after the thick ascending limb of the loop of Henle, contains specialized cells, the macula densa cells, which are a component of the juxtaglomerular apparatus. Following this specialized region, there are two sections of the DT, the distal convoluted segment or early distal tubule and the late distal segment. The tubular epithelial cells of these subsegments are thick and have both microvilli and mitochondria.

The early DT transports a number of solutes including sodium, chloride, bicarbonate, potassium, calcium, and magnesium. However, it is quite impermeable to water. With reabsorption of solutes but virtually no reabsorption of water, the tubular fluid remains hypo-osmotic.

The late DT is a site for regulation of sodium, chloride, bicarbonate, potassium, and calcium transport. These processes are regulated in a variety of manners, including hormonal, physical factors, and/or systemic acid-base or electrolyte balance.

Water permeability of the late distal tubule is influenced by antidiuretic hormone (ADH), which is produced by the hypothalamus and released in response to input by systemic baroreceptors, osmoreceptors, and angiotensin II. In the presence of ADH, water reabsorption occurs and, consequently, the tubular fluid is isosmotic as both fluid and solutes are reabsorbed. In the absence of ADH, the late DT is impermeable to water and the tubular fluid remains hypo-osmotic as solutes, not water, are reabsorbed.

Collecting tubule. A number of DTs join together to form the collecting tubules, which extend from the cortex through the medulla and empty into the papilla. The collecting tubule has three subsegments: the cortical collecting tubule, the outer medullary collecting tubule, and the inner medullary collecting tubule. For the first two subsegments, there are two predominant cell types, the principal cells and intercalated cells. The principal, or light cell, is the predominant cell in the cortical collecting tubule, making up approximately 90% of the epithelial cells. These cells are involved in the transport of sodium and potassium. The intercalated, or dark cells, are the predominant cell type in the outer medullary collecting tubules, and account for about 10% of the epithelial cells in the cortical collecting tubule. These cells are involved in the transport of hydrogen and bicarbonate and play an important role in the acidification of urine.

In the inner medullary collecting tubules, some intercalated cells are still present, but a different cell type, called the inner medullary collecting duct cell, appears. The exact role in this latter cell type is not fully known, but since sodium, chloride, potassium, and ammonia transport all occur in this segment, this cell may be involved in these processes.

All along the collecting tubule, water permeability is ADH dependent. In the absence of ADH, water absorption along the collecting tubule is minimal, and a dilute urine is excreted. In the presence of ADH, water absorption occurs. When ADH secretion is maximal, osmotic equilibration can occur between the collecting tubule fluid and the surrounding interstitium, which leads to a maximally concentrated urine of >1000 mOsm/L. Urine osmolalities between these extremes occurs with submaximal ADH secretion.

Juxtaglomerular Apparatus

This autoregulatory structure participates in maintaining systemic blood pressure and, consequently, intraglomerular pressure and glomerular filtration. It involves the interplay between vascular and tubular components in the nephron. As the ascending limb of the loop of Henle moves upward, the initial portion of the DT passes between the afferent and efferent arterioles that proceed or form from, respectively, the glomerulus of that nephron.

Specialized cells, the macula densa cells, are found in the walls of the tubule juxtapositioned to the glomerular hilus (see Figure 7-3). This region of the distal tubule "touches" the cells of the afferent arteriole, feeding the glomerular capillary associated with that nephron. At this point, the afferent arteriole basement membrane is absent so that the macula densa cells and the afferent arteriole cells "touch," forming a synsitium that allows communication between these specialized cells. These granular smooth muscle cells of the afferent arteriole are called juxtaglomerular cells, which synthesize and store renin, a proteolytic enzyme.

Figure 7-4.
Renal circulatory anatomy.
The renal artery branches into the segmental artery, interlobar artery, arcuate artery, interlobular artery, afferent artery and finally, the glomerulus.

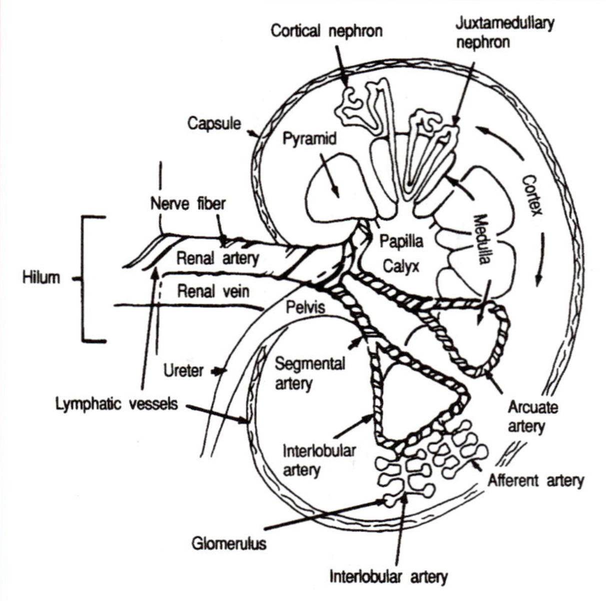

Note: Adapted from: Richard, C. (1986). *Comprehensive nephrology nursing,* (p. 12). Boston: Little, Brown & Company. Copyright 1986 by C.J. Richard. Reprinted with permission.

Renal Processes

As blood flows through the kidneys, approximately 20% of the plasma passes from the glomerulus into Bowman's space, forming the glomerular filtrate. This fluid contains no red blood cells, has approximately 0.03% small molecular weight proteins (primarily albumin), and has essentially the same concentration of electrolytes and other small molecules as the plasma. This filtrate undergoes many changes in the tubular system before it is excreted as urine.

Glomerular filtration. Glomerular filtration is the initial process in the formation of urine. The glomerular membrane is highly permeable and allows fluid and small molecular weight solute to pass into Bowman's space. The glomerular capillary tuft with its interconnected loops increases available surface area. Finally, arterioles at both ends of the glomerulus increase intraglomerular pressure.

Reabsorption. Reabsorption refers to the movement of fluid and solutes from the tubular system into the peritubular capillaries. This process allows the body to retain fluid and desired solutes. At a glomerular filtration rate of 125 ml/min, the kidneys produce 180 liters of filtrate daily. Yet the average urine output is only 1000 to 1500 ml. Through reabsorption, 99% of the glomerular filtrate is returned to the bloodstream.

The proximal tubule is the major site of reabsorption in the tubular system although reabsorption occurs throughout the nephron. Reabsorption involves both passive and active transport mechanisms. Passive transport includes osmosis and diffusion while active transport mechanisms, such as primary and secondary transport and endocytosis, require the use of energy to move substances against an electrochemical gradient. Reabsorption of fluid and solutes is regulated to meet the body's physiologic needs, through a number of hormonal and neural systems including ADH, aldosterone, angiotensin II, parathyroid hormone, prostaglandins, and alpha and beta adrenergics.

Secretion. Secretion refers to the movement of solutes from the peritubular capillaries into the tubular system. It is the process by which the body secretes unwanted or excess substances. Like reabsorption, secretion occurs by both passive and active transport mechanisms. As with reabsorption, secretion of substances is regulated by a number of factors, many of them hormonal in nature.

With regard to active transport mechanisms in both tubular reabsorption and secretion, reference is made to the maximal transport capacity (Tm). Specific carriers exist in the tubular epithelium that are responsible for the movement of substances in and out of the tubular system. However, there is a maximum rate at which substances can be transported in this way. This is known as the maximal transport capacity, or Tm, of the substance. Once the threshold or maximal solute transport rate has been reached, the presentation of larger amounts of solute results in the substance remaining in the tubular fluid (not reabsorbed) or in the plasma (not secreted). All substances actively transported have a Tm. As with all physiological processes, the Tm is subject to regulatory factors, most notably physiologic, pathologic, and pharmacologic.

Excretion. Excretion refers to the process by

Figure 7-5.
Glomerular anatomy.

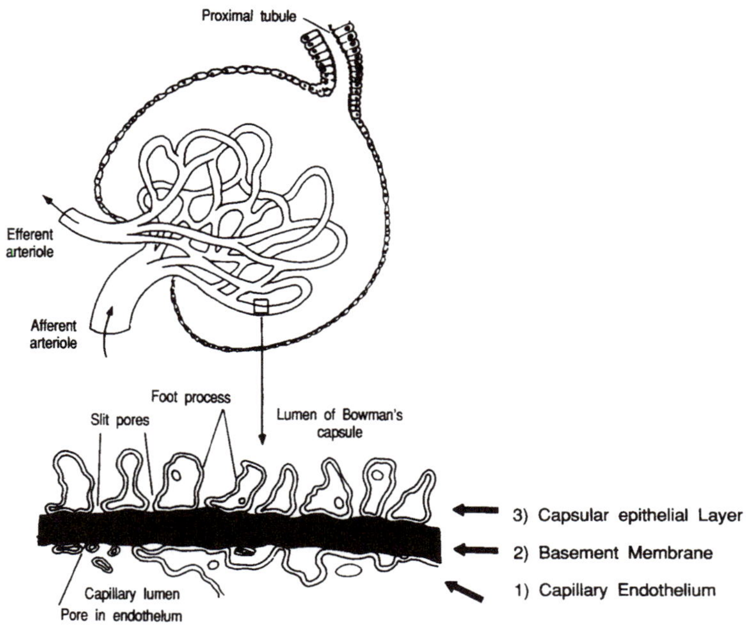

The glomerulus consists of three filtering layers: (1) the capillary endothelium; (2) the basement membrane; and (3) the capsular epithelial layer, which consists of the podocytes and foot processes.

Note: From Marsh, D.J. (1983). *Renal physiology* (page 41). New York: Raven Press. Copyright 1983 by Raven Press. Reprinted with permission.

which unwanted substances are eliminated from the body through the passage of urine. These substances include the end products of metabolism such as urea, creatinine, uric acid, drugs, and foreign chemicals and unwanted ingested substances such as sodium, potassium, and phosphate.

Summary

The kidneys are responsible for performing various roles in the maintenance of the body's internal environment. A thorough understanding of the renal system with its components and specialized functions is necessary to grasp not only its role in the healthy individual but also in the individual with renal disease.

Section 2: Glomerular Filtration and Renal Hemodynamics

Glomerular filtration is the first step in the complex process of urine formation. For adequate, efficient filtration to occur, a rapid renal blood flow at a consistent pressure is essential. There are many factors that can alter renal blood flow (RBF) and thus the rate of glomerular filtrate generation. At any given time, especially under the conditions of stress, multiple factors are acting and counteracting to maintain a normal glomerular filtration rate (GFR) despite changes in renal blood flow. This section examines the unique characteristics of the renal circulation, describes the physiology of glomerular filtration, reviews the extrinsic and intrinsic factors that can alter renal hemodynamics, and discusses a clinical situation in which multiple factors are interacting in an effort to maintain the RBF and GFR, despite systemic pressure changes.

Renal Circulation

Blood flows into the kidneys at a rate of about 1200 ml per minute, representing approximately 20% of the cardiac output. This rapid blood flow rate exceeds the metabolic and oxygen needs of the kidneys but facilitates efficient clearance of metabolic waste products.

To understand glomerular filtration, it is essential to consider the special characteristics of the renal circulation. Figure 7-4 illustrates the gross renal circulatory anatomy. The renal artery pressure is approximately 100 mmHg. This high pressure is maintained up to the afferent arteriole, the location of the first major point of vascular resistance. Across the afferent arteriole, the arterial pressure falls to about 45-60 mmHg. Although this is a significantly lower pressure than present in the systemic circulation, this pressure is higher than that in the glomerular capillary bed. Maintaining a hydrostatic pressure of about 50 mmHg is the key to glomerular filtration as it is needed to overcome other opposing pressures present in the glomerulus and Bowman's space.

The glomerulus is a capillary bundle that is

highly porous compared to systemic capillaries. The portion of the blood that is not filtered across the filtration barrier returns to the central circulation via the peritubular capillary (PTC) network.

Glomerular Filtration

Glomerular anatomy. The porous glomerular capillaries rest between the afferent and efferent arterioles (see Figure 7-5). Their function is to filter large quantities of water and solutes from the plasma. As blood flows through the glomerulus, a portion is sieved through the filtering layers of the glomerular capillaries into Bowman's space. The filtration barrier is composed of three layers that allow for the filtration of solutes and water, but prevent the loss of blood components such as red and white blood cells and plasma proteins. The three layers are the glomerular capillary endothelium, glomerular basement membrane, and visceral layer of Bowman's capsule (epithelial cell layer).

The first layer of the filtration barrier is the capillary endothelium, which has large fenestrations that allow the free filtration of substances with diameters up to 100 nm, thus excluding blood cells and large plasma proteins. The surface of the endothelial cells has a negative charge that inhibits the movement of negatively charged substances such as plasma proteins, as like-charges repel each other.

The second layer, the glomerular basement membrane, represents the major barrier to the filtration of macromolecules. The glomerular basement membrane is made of fibrous proteins such as collagen, fibrin, and laminin, which intertwine to form a meshwork. As the fibers cross each other, small openings are created through which selective filtration occurs. The crossed fibers act as a size barrier by restricting the filtration of large molecules. This layer also contains anionic sialoproteins that further inhibit filtration by repelling other negatively charged ions.

The third layer, composed of epithelial cells, is the visceral layer of Bowman's capsule. These epithelial cells, called podocytes, are attached directly to the exterior surface of the basement membrane. The podocytes branch into multiple finger-like projections called foot processes. These foot processes, which cover the outer surface of the basement membrane, are close to each other, forming narrow, elongated, slit-type openings about 25-60 nm wide. These openings, called slit pores, are covered by thin diaphragms. The foot processes have anionic sialoproteins on their borders that form the slit pores, generating a highly negatively charged region through which the filtrate must pass. These negative charges assist in preventing plasma proteins from entering the tubular fluid since plasma proteins carry negative charges. These narrow slits, combined with the negative charges of the podocytes, provide the final barrier to molecule movement through the glomerular membrane.

The glomerulus is a selective filtration membrane. The factors that determine which molecules are filtered are molecular size, electrical charge, protein binding, configuration, and rigidity. Small molecules with molecular weights (MW) less than 5,000 daltons (for example, water, MW 18, and all ions including sodium, potassium, chloride, phosphate, magnesium, and calcium) are filtered without restriction. Larger molecules, such as myoglobin with a MW of 17,000 daltons, are filtered to a lesser degree. Very large molecules, such as plasma proteins with molecular weights approaching 70,000 daltons, are restricted from passing through the normal glomerulus.

As the filtration barrier has a net negative charge, the movement of large negatively charged molecules is restricted more than positively charged or neutral molecules. As a result proteins, which are negatively charged, are not freely filtered by the glomerulus. Thus drugs, ions, or small molecules bound to protein are not filtered. Round molecules do not filter as easily as ellipsoid molecules. The more rigid a molecule, the less easily it filters. Thus, normal glomerular filtrate is essentially protein free, but contains crystalloids (for example, sodium, chloride, creatinine, urea, uric acid, and phosphate) in the same concentration as plasma.

A final anatomic aspect of the glomerulus is the mesangial cells that are located between the capillary loops. They support the capillary structures and carry out some phagocytic activities. They also demonstrate contractile properties and can alter the total filtration surface area. Mesangial cells contract when exposed to vasoconstrictive substances, such as angiotensin II, thus decreasing the effective filtration surface area and glomerular filtration rate.

Glomerular filtration rate and filtration fraction. Glomerular filtrate moves into Bowman's space and then into the tubular component of the nephron. In the average 70 kg adult, glomerular filtration rate is approximately 125 ml/minute. This means that about 180 L of glomerular filtrate is produced in a 24-hour period, which is more than 30 times the average total blood volume. All but 1 to 2 liters are reabsorbed from the nephron into the peritubular capillary and vasa recta systems. The formation of such a large amount of filtrate assures adequate filtration of plasma, but requires very efficient reabsorptive processes to prevent volume and electrolyte depletion.

GFR, which indicates the volume of filtrate moving from the glomerular capillaries into Bowman's space per unit of time, is calculated by determining the renal clearance of a marker substance. Clearance (Cl) is defined as the volume of plasma from which a substance is completely removed or cleared by the kidneys per unit of time. The ideal marker for measuring Cl is not protein bound, is freely filtered at the glomerulus, and is

Figure 7-6.
Pressures influencing normal glomerular filtration.

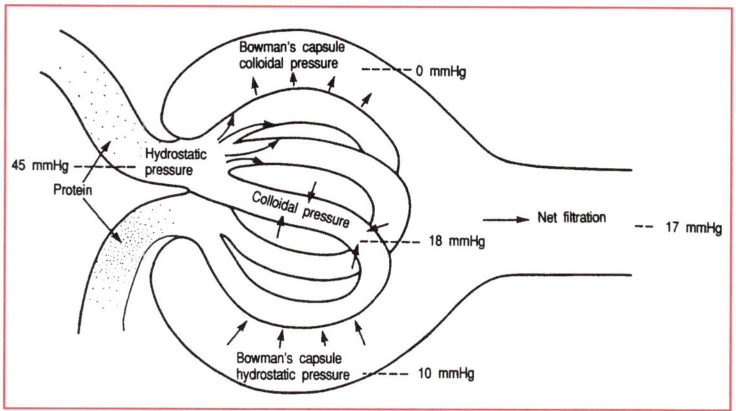

Note: Adapted from Richard, C.J. (1986). *Comprehensive nephrology nursing* (p. 23). Boston: Little, Brown & Company. Reprinted with permission.

The factor favoring filtration is capillary hydrostatic pressure (45 mmHg). The factors opposing filtration are Bowman's capsule hydrostatic pressure (10 mmHg) and capillary colloidal osmotic pressure (18 mmHg). As Bowman's capsule colloidal pressure is usually 0 mmHg, it has no effect. The net filtration pressure produced by these opposing pressures is 17 mmHg.

neither reabsorbed, secreted, synthesized, nor metabolized by the tubules. Substances that do not meet these requirements can result in falsely elevated or decreased values of GFR. As there is no naturally occurring ideal marker, endogenous creatinine (Cr) is often used to measure clearance; however, since a small amount of creatinine is secreted into the tubule, GFR measured with creatinine clearance (CrCl) will be overestimated. Since individual GFRs vary widely, a change in GFR over time is more important than the absolute value of GFR. Thus, if the CrCl method is used, it should be used for all measurements of GFR to allow for comparison of values over time.

Inulin is a marker that meets all the requirements of an ideal marker for measuring GFR, but is not often used because it is an exogenous substance that must be infused for several hours at a constant rate and thus is both impractical and costly.

To calculate the CrCl, a 24-hour urine and mid-point plasma Cr (P_{cr}) are obtained. CrCl is calculated using Equation 1 where U_{cr} is the urine creatinine concentration, mg/dl; U_v is the average urine flow rate, ml/min; and P_{cr} is the plasma creatinine concentration, mg/dl.

Equation 1

$$CrCl = \frac{U_{cr}U_v}{P_{cr}}$$

The CrCl reflects the GFR and gives a gross indication of how well the kidneys are functioning based on their ability to remove a marker substance.

Glomerular filtrate is derived from the plasma portion of whole blood. The term filtration fraction (FF) describes the percentage of the plasma that becomes glomerular filtrate. Since plasma volume is about 55% of total blood volume, normal renal plasma flow (RPF) is approximately 660 ml/min (1200 ml/min X 0.55 = 660 ml/min). The FF can then be determined using Equation 2.

Equation 2

$$FF = \frac{GFR}{RPF} = \frac{125 ml/min}{660 ml/min} = 19\%$$

Thus, almost 20% of the plasma passing through the glomerulus becomes glomerular filtrate in the average adult.

Pressures influencing normal glomerular filtration. Glomerular filtration is controlled by four pressures, the algebraic sum of which defines the net filtration pressure. These are:

1. Glomerular capillary hydrostatic pressure (P_{GC}), which is the pressure exerted against the capillary wall by fluid within the capillary lumen. This value ranges from 40 to 60 mmHg and favors the movement of fluid from the capillary lumen to Bowman's space (see Figure 7-6);
2. Glomerular capillary colloid osmotic pressure (GC), which is about 18 mmHg. This force, generated by plasma proteins within the capillaries, retards the movement of fluid out of the capillary lumen;
3. Bowman's space hydrostatic pressure (P_{BS}), which is the pressure exerted against the capillary walls by fluids within Bowman's space. This value is about 10 mmHg, and also retards the movement of fluid out of the capillary lumen; and
4. Bowman's space colloid osmotic pressure (π_{BS}), which is normally 0 mmHg because normal filtrate is void of protein.

Thus, net filtration pressure (NFP) can be calculated using Equation 3.

Equation 3

$$NFP = (P_{GC} - P_{BS}) - (\pi_{GC} - \pi_{BS})$$
$$= (45 \text{ mmHg} - 10 \text{ mmHg}) - (18 \text{ mmHg} - 0 \text{ mmHg})$$
$$= 17 \text{ mmHg}$$

These pressures are based on animal models, but are thought to be similar to those in humans. Therefore, for adequate filtration to occur, an NFP of approximately 17 mmHg is required to produce approximately 125 ml/min of glomerular filtrate.

As blood progresses through the glomerulus toward the efferent arteriole, the π_{GC} increases from 18 to approximately 35 mmHg, reflecting the removal of protein-free fluid from the glomerular capillary. P_{GC}, P_{BS}, and π_{BS} remain essentially unchanged along the capillary loop. As a result, NFP decreases along the length of the capillary and in some species is zero before or at the end of the capillary. The point at which NFP falls to zero is called filtration equilibrium and is the point at which glomerular filtration ceases.

Conditions altering glomerular filtration rate. The GFR can be altered by changes in any of the above four pressures or the ultrafiltration coefficient. Theoretically, there is a direct relationship between the renal plasma flow rate (the primary determinant of P_{GC}) and the GFR. Thus, if RPF increases due to volume expansion or other causes, GFR should also rise. However, a change in RBF rarely occurs in isolation, and is usually accompanied by changes in afferent or efferent arteriolar resistance designed to maintain P_{GC} and therefore, GFR, at normal levels. Through a process called autoregulation, the kidney is adept at maintaining normal GFRs over a wide range of vascular pressures.

Changes in the glomerular colloid osmotic pressure (π_{GC}) can also alter GFR. If π_{GC} increases, as in hypovolemic states, NFP and thus GFR will fall. If the π_{GC} decreases, as in severe liver disease, GFR can increase.

When P_{BC} increases, as in urinary tract obstruction, GFR falls. GFR decreases as glomerular filtrate outflow from the tubule is obstructed and the pressure of the increased filtrate volume in Bowman's space opposes the forces favoring filtration.

If π_{BS} rises above 0 mmHg, as it does in nephrotic conditions where protein is filtered into Bowman's space, GFR can increase. The presence of plasma proteins in Bowman's space favors increased filtration due to the increased colloid osmotic pressure within that compartment.

A final factor that can alter GFR is a change in the ultrafiltration coefficient (K_f) of the glomerular capillary membrane. The K_f is the product of the surface area and hydraulic permeability of the glomerular membrane. Vasoactive substances such as angiotensin II can cause the mesangial cells to contract, thereby decreasing the available surface area for filtration and thus decreasing GFR.

Glomerular filtration is the critical initial step in urine formation. For adequate solute and water removal to occur, glomerular filtrate must be generated at a constant rate. Changes in RPF, hydrostatic and osmotic pressures, available filtering surface area, and glomerular membrane permeability can upset the internal environment by increasing or decreasing GFR. Fortunately, a complicated system exists where factors both extrinsic and intrinsic to the kidneys act simultaneously to minimize the effects of these changes.

Renal Hemodynamics

Renal blood flow, which defines RPF, is controlled by a number of physical and humoral factors. These factors are both intrinsic and extrinsic to the kidney. Some of the intrinsic factors include an autoregulatory mechanism, intrarenal renin-angiotensin mechanism, eicosanoids, and kinins. Critical extrinsic factors include the sympathetic nervous system, angiotensin II, antidiuretic hormone, dopamine, and histamine. Three recently discovered hormones—endothelin, endothelium-derived relaxing factor (EDRF), and atrial natriuretic peptide (ANP)—also have an important role in renal hemodynamics. These multiple factors work in concert to sustain glomerular filtration despite wide variations in systemic pressures.

Intrinsic Factors

Autoregulation. The autoregulatory mechanism (ARM), an intrarenal system, maintains a consistent renal blood flow despite mean arterial pressure (MAP) fluctuations from about 80-180 mmHg, but it becomes dysfunctional when the MAP is outside this range. The ARM maintains renal perfusion at a constant level during exercise, postural changes, sleep, and emotional crises even though these conditions lead to systemic pressure changes.

There are two theories to explain this autoregulatory phenomena: the myogenic and the tubuloglomerular feedback (TGF) theories. The myogenic theory is based on the function of baroreceptors (stretch receptors) in the afferent arterioles. When the MAP increases, these receptors respond to the increased vascular wall tension or stretch and cause afferent arteriolar constriction. This constriction prevents transmission of the elevated arterial pressure to the glomerulus, thus maintaining a normal P_{GC} and GFR. Conversely, if the MAP falls, afferent arteriolar dilation occurs to allow for increased blood flow and maintenance of a normal P_{GC} and GFR.

The TGF theory relates to the function of the macula densa and juxtaglomerular cells. In conditions that increase renal blood flow and thus GFR, there is an increased delivery of sodium chloride

Figure 7-7
Renin-angiotensin mechanism: Local and systemic effects.

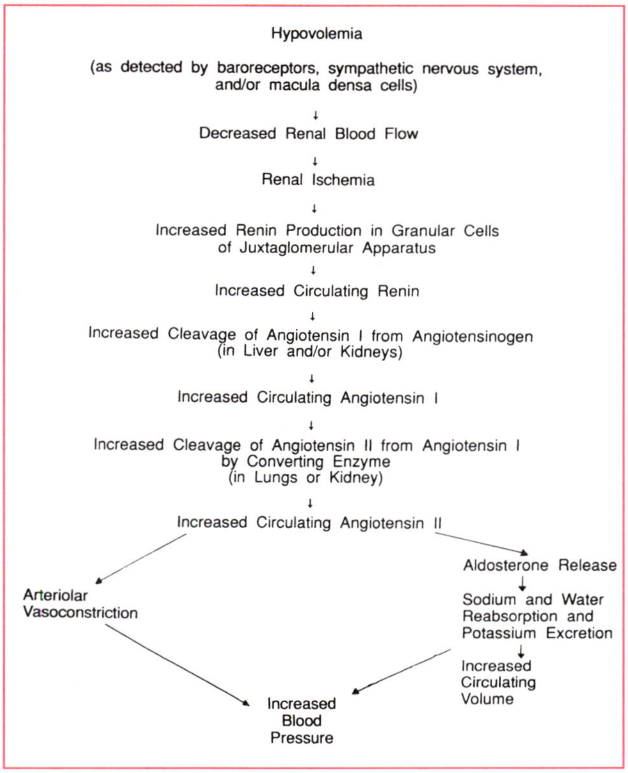

Note: From Holechek, M.J. (1992). Glomerular filtration and renal hemodynamics. *ANNA Journal, 19*(3), p. 242. Reprinted with permission.

(NaCl) to the macula densa cells in the distal nephron. When these cells detect this increased NaCl load, they mediate vasoconstriction of the afferent arteriole via an unknown messenger substance, resulting in a decrease in the glomerular blood flow, a decrease in P_{GC}, and a return of the GFR toward normal. Conversely, when there is decreased glomerular blood flow, there is decreased NaCl delivered to the macula densa cells. This leads to afferent arteriolar dilatation, increased glomerular blood flow, increased P_{GC}, and return of GFR to normal.

Neither of these theories alone fully explains the ARM, and in all likelihood several factors contribute to this phenomenon. It is important to note that the ARM cannot completely override changes in the MAP, but it can limit the degree of change transmitted to the glomerulus, and thus, the degree to which GFR changes.

Renin-angiotensin mechanism (RAM). The RAM is a critical regulator of intrarenal blood flow that is triggered by internal and external stimuli (see Figure 7-7). When renal ischemia occurs due to hypovolemia, decreased cardiac contractibility, renal artery stenosis, or other conditions, the kidney produces the proteolytic enzyme, renin, from the granular cells of the juxtaglomerular apparatus (JGA). Renin release is regulated by two intrarenal mechanisms: the afferent arteriole baroreceptors and the macula densa cells, and one extra-renal mechanism, the sympathetic nervous system (SNS). Local renal baroreceptors located in the afferent arterioles vasoconstrict in the face of decreased volume, which leads to renin release. The macula densa cells stimulate renin release when they detect a decreased NaCl load being delivered to the distal tubule because of decreased renal blood flow.

Renin facilitates the splitting of angiotensin I (Ang I) from angiotensinogen that is produced in the kidney and liver. A converting enzyme in the lungs and kidneys splits angiotensin II (Ang II), a potent vasoconstrictor, from angiotensin I. Angiotensin II is the biologically active compound and causes vasoconstriction of both the afferent and efferent arterioles, but it affects the efferent arteriole to a greater degree. Through afferent arteriole constriction, angiotensin II decreases renal blood flow. However, concurrent efferent arteriolar constriction creates a resistance to fluid leaving the glomerular capillaries, which maintains glomerular hydrostatic pressure, and thus, GFR at normal values despite the fall in RBF.

The RAM is an intrinsic system that is triggered by local and systemic stimuli. One purpose of this system is to maintain perfusion of vital organs (heart and brain) in the face of hypovolemia, an effect mediated by peripheral and intrarenal vasoconstriction. Unfortunately for the kidney, this system does not spare the kidneys, and RBF is compromised in such situations. However, the decreased RBF will to some degree be compensated for by increased efferent arteriolar resistance, preventing a proportional decrease in GFR. When the RBF returns to normal, renin production returns to normal.

Eicosanoid synthesis. Eicosanoids are vasoactive substances produced locally in the kidney by the glomerular and vascular endothelium, nephrons, and interstitial cells. Eicosanoids include prostaglandins, thromboxanes, leukotrienes, and monooxygenase products. Some prostaglandins such as PGE_1, PGE_2, and PGI_2 (prostacyclin) are vasodilators. Thromboxane, leukotrienes, and some monooxygenase products are vasoconstrictors. The physiologic role of the vasoconstrictor substances is unclear, but the vasodilatory prostaglandins play a major role in maintaining renal blood flow in individuals with impaired renal function.

Prostaglandins are produced in response to increased levels of angiotensin II and norepinephrine and attenuate the vasoconstrictive effects of these agents. The vasodilatory prostaglandins act primarily on the afferent arterioles, counteracting the vasoconstrictive effects of angiotensin II and sympathetic nervous system stimulation, and maintaining renal blood flow despite systemic arteriolar vasoconstriction. The prostaglandins also offset the angiotensin II mediated mesangial constriction, preserving adequate surface area for filtration. Thus, the vasodilatory prostaglandins perform a protective function for the kidneys in that they prevent extreme vasoconstriction in response to Ang II or norepinephrine. They have little systemic effect as they are rapidly metabolized in the pulmonary circulation. The production of vasodilatory prostaglandins is blocked by cyclooxygenase inhibitors such as aspirin, indomethacin, ibuprofen, or other nonsteroidal antiinflammatory drugs; therefore, these drugs should not be administered to individuals with renal insufficiency to prevent the loss of this crucial protective mechanism.

Kallikrein-Kinin synthesis. The kinins are inflammatory mediators produced locally in the kidney. The distal nephron cells secrete the enzyme kallikrein that initiates the process whereby bradykinin is eventually formed. Bradykinin is a vasodilator, but its physiologic role in the control of renal hemodynamics is not firmly established. It attenuates the renal ischemic effects of AII and norepinephrine. Although overall, bradykinin appears to reverse the effects of Ang II on RBF, it is ineffective in increasing GFR because of the simultaneous decrease in K_f induced by Ang II.

Extrinsic Factors. There are multiple extrarenal factors that influence renal hemodynamics. These substances or systems are based outside of the kidneys, but can directly or indirectly initiate changes in RBF and the GFR.

Sympathetic nervous system. As noted earlier, the SNS plays a role in the RAM (see Figure 7-7). The SNS detects systemic volume changes via cardiac and arterial baroreceptors and can increase or decrease renin secretion and levels of circulating catecholamines accordingly. Catecholamines act on the adrenergic receptor sites of the arterioles, causing vasoconstriction. In hypovolemic states, the SNS mediates arterial vasoconstriction, including vasoconstriction of the renal vasculature. The decreased volume detected by the stretch receptors in the afferent arteriole leads to the release of renin into the systemic circulation, resulting in the extrarenal production of Ang II.

The sympathetic nerves enter the kidney at the hilum and parallel the arterial system. The nerve endings terminate in the smooth muscle cells of the afferent and efferent arterioles. Direct stimulation of the adrenergic receptors at these locations will result in afferent and efferent arteriolar vasoconstriction. This leads to a decreased RBF, but the concurrent efferent arteriolar vasoconstriction helps maintain glomerular hydrostatic pressure so that GFR is maintained.

Angiotensin II. In addition to the afferent and efferent arteriolar vasoconstriction described earlier, Ang II mediates peripheral vasoconstriction. Ang II also stimulates the release of aldosterone that allows for sodium and water reabsorption, thus increasing circulating volume. These two effects combined allow for maintenance of systemic pressure and perfusion of critical body organs.

Antidiuretic hormone (ADH). ADH (vasopressin) in high plasma concentrations also results in renal vessel vasoconstriction, as well as mesangial cell contraction. In the presence of ADH, the RBF and GFR decrease. ADH will also trigger the production of prostaglandins, which attenuate its own vasoconstrictive effects. ADH is produced in hypovolemic states and production decreases when the serum osmolality and/or extracellular volume returns to normal.

Dopamine. Dopamine receptors within the renal vasculature respond to low-dose dopamine by increasing the renal plasma flow and the GFR. How much of a role dopamine plays in normal renal hemodynamics, however, is not clear.

Histamine. Histamine is also a vasodilator that is known to increase RBF and the GFR by dilating both the afferent and efferent arterioles. Changes in the GFR usually are minimal because decreases in arteriolar resistance and decreases in the K_f negate each other. Histamine causes the local production of Ang II, and this is what is suspected to cause the decrease in K_f.

Other factors. Three peptides that have recently gained attention for their presumed impact on the hemodynamics of the kidney are endothelin, endothelium-derived relaxing factor, and atrial natriuretic peptide. Endothelin, which is synthesized in the endothelial cells of the kidneys, lungs, cerebellum, and major arteries, is a potent vasoconstrictor produced in response to increased vessel wall tension. Endothelin works locally within the organ or vessel in which it is produced. It is thought that there are endothelin receptors in the renal vessels and that endothelin causes increased vascular resistance in both the afferent and efferent arterioles, leading to decreased RBF and GFR. Although endothelin has only recently been discovered, it is believed that it may play a role equal to that of Ang II in altering renal hemodynamics.

Endothelium-derived relaxing factor (EDRF) is a substance released from the vascular endothelium. The function of EDRF is not fully understood, but it is thought to cause the relaxation of vascular smooth muscle and possibly inhibit renin production. Specifically in the kidney, EDRF is believed to work in conjunction with other vasoactive substances to maintain basal tone in the glomerular vessels. EDRF is released in response to several vasodilators, including histamine, bradykinin, and acetylcholine. It is speculated that EDRF may be a mediator of the vasorelaxation produced by these

Figure 7-8
Integration of major renal hemodynamic factors in hemorrhage.

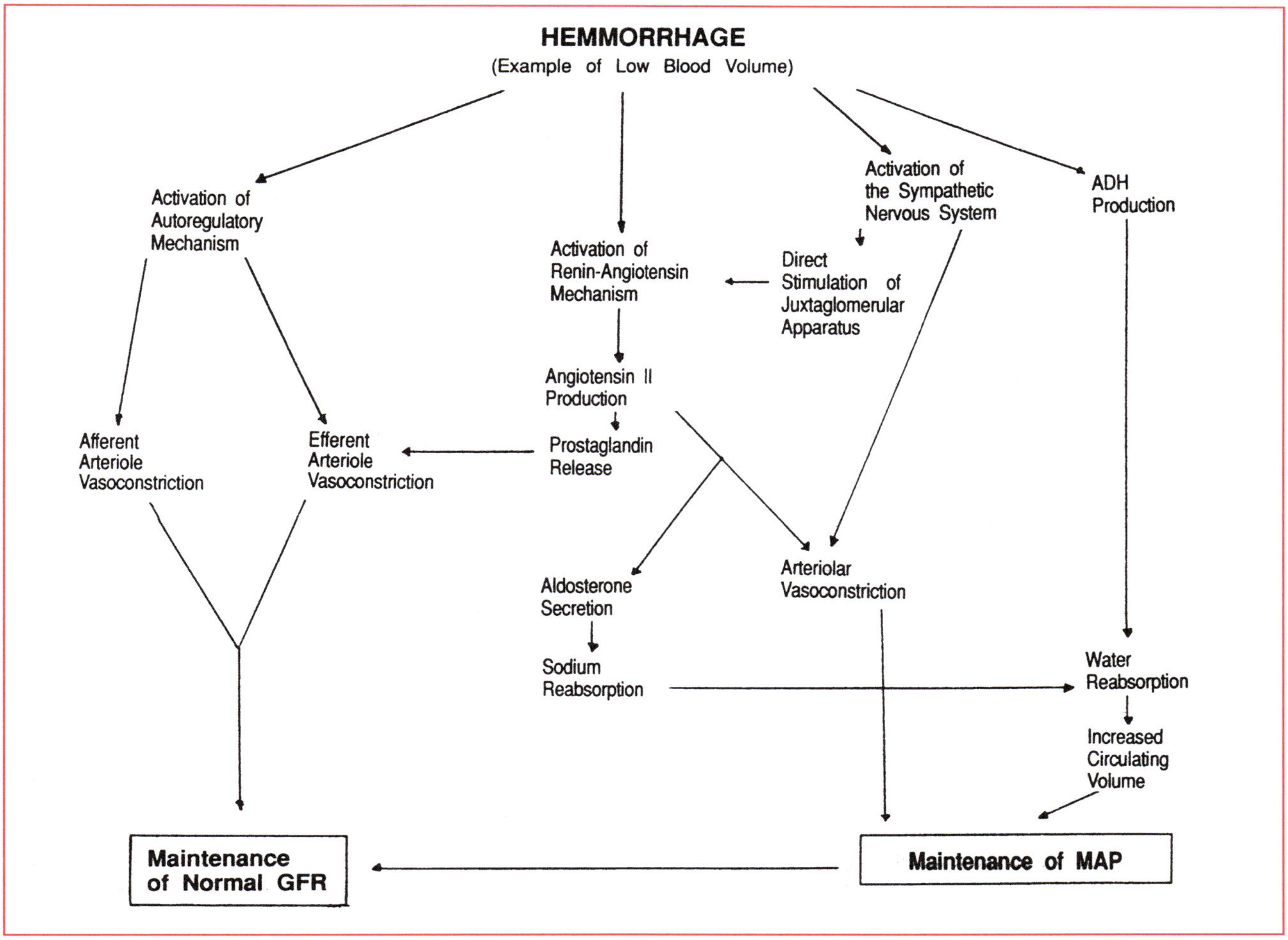

Note: From Holechek, M.J. (1992). Glomerular filtration and renal hemodynamics. *ANNA Journal, 19*(3), p. 243. Reprinted with permission.

substances. It is hoped that further research on EDRF will produce more detailed information on the delicate balance between vasodilators and vasoconstrictors in the renal vasculature and pathologic conditions that can develop as a result of imbalances.

Atrial natriuretic peptide (ANP) is secreted by specialized granular cardiocytes primarily in the right atrium in response to right atrial distention and increased right atrial pressure. ANP induces vasodilation of the afferent arteriole and vasoconstriction of the efferent arteriole, resulting in an increased GFR. Natriuresis and diuresis are enhanced because of the rise in the GFR. ANP directly blocks ADH release and interferes with aldosterone release at the adrenal gland indirectly by blocking the RAM, thus increasing sodium and water loss from the kidney. The cumulative effects are reduced peripheral and renal vasoconstriction and decreased volume. In conditions of volume overload such as congestive failure and vasoconstrictive states such as hypertension, ANP attempts to reduce the circulating volume and induce vascular relaxation.

Integration of Renal Hemodynamic Control Factors

Hemorrhage. In low volume states, such as hemorrhage, multiple alterations occur in both systemic and intrarenal hemodynamics (see Figure 7-8). Uncontrolled hemorrhage ultimately leads to hypovolemia and hypotension. At the extrarenal level, there is increased sympathetic nervous system activity and catecholamine production as a result of decreased stretch detected by the cardiac and arterial baroreceptors. These extrinsic forces result in generalized vasoconstriction, including the renal arterial system. The ARM attempts to compensate by dilating the afferent arteriole, but this becomes dysfunctional when the MAP falls below about 80 mmHg.

As a result of direct sympathetic stimulation of the juxtaglomerular cells and ischemia initiating the renin-angiotensin cascade, renin and eventually Ang II are produced. Angiotensin II causes further systemic and intrarenal vasoconstriction. All of these efforts are directed toward maintaining the MAP at the sacrifice of nonpriority organs and structures. Although the RBF falls in response to Ang II, the fall in GFR is not of equal magnitude because AII maintains pressure within the glomerular capillary by causing greater vasoconstriction of the efferent than of the afferent arteriole.

Another protective mechanism demonstrated by Ang II is that it stimulates the release of vasodilatory prostaglandins that will attenuate to a degree the intrarenal vasoconstriction induced by the RAM and SNS. Bradykinin probably also plays a minor role in attenuating the vasoconstriction. Antidiuretic hormone will also be produced, contributing to the vasoconstriction. Antidiuretic hormone also stimulates prostaglandins release in an effort to diminish its intrarenal vasoconstrictive effects.

The cumulative result of these four forces in an individual with normal renal function would be increased vascular resistance with a fall in RBF and GFR. The decrease in GFR will not be nearly as great as it would be without the protective effects of efferent arteriolar vasoconstriction, prostaglandins, and bradykinin. These mechanisms allow for the maintenance of a reasonable MAP and at the same time protection of the kidney from severe ischemia. If the hemorrhage is not controlled, eventually these protective mechanisms will be exhausted, and GFR will decline.

Summary

Glomerular filtration is a process that is impacted by numerous intrinsic and extrinsic factors that can alter renal hemodynamics and renal blood flow. These factors interact in an attempt to maintain a consistent glomerular filtration rate under a wide variety of normal and pathologic conditions. If these integrated systems fail, serious problems can develop with renal function and urine production and excretion. Understanding the physiology of glomerular filtration and the interactions of factors altering renal hemodynamics will help the nephrology nurse in predicting, identifying, and assisting in the treatment of clinical conditions that alter glomerular filtration and renal hemodynamics.

Section 3: Urinary Concentration and Dilution

The normal glomerular filtration rate is about 125 ml/min or an average of 180 liters per day. Ninety-nine percent of this tubular filtrate is reabsorbed along the nephron and returned to the systemic circulation. A smaller amount of concentrated urine is excreted in states of extracellular volume deficit. Conversely, when the fluid volume of the body is expanded above normal, the kidneys form and excrete large amounts of dilute urine, which facilitates the return of the extracellular volume to normal.

This section describes the mechanisms responsible for forming and excreting a dilute or concentrated urine. These processes specifically involve the descending and ascending limbs of the loops of Henle, distal tubules of the juxtamedullary nephrons, collecting tubule, and the vasa recta, the capillaries that surround these medullary nephron segments.

Tubular Processes

Owing to the reabsorption of proportional amounts of solutes and water in the proximal tubule, the filtrate leaving the proximal tubule and entering the descending limb of the loop of Henle has an osmolality of 290-300 mOsm, about the same as that of plasma. To understand the mechanisms responsible for altering the composition of the filtrate as it moves through the loop of Henle and collecting tubule, it is helpful to briefly review the anatomy of the kidney medulla. The loops of Henle, collecting tubules, and vasa recta all run in parallel from the cortical-medullary junction to the inner medulla. The loops of Henle and vasa recta bend in the inner medulla and return to the cortex of the kidney, while the collecting tubules continue onward into the papilla. This parallel arrangement of nephron structures and vasculature is essential to the formation of both a concentrated and dilute urine.

As will be discussed in more detail, the osmolality of the medullary interstitium surrounding the vasa recta, loops of Henle, and collecting tubules is hypertonic (>300 mOsm) relative to systemic or cortical interstitial osmolality. The degree of interstitial hypertonicity varies from just over 300 mOsm at the cortical-medullary junction to about 1200 mOsm at the medullary-papillary junction. The solutes responsible for raising the osmolality of the interstitial fluid are predominantly NaCl and urea, with minor contributions from other solutes such as potassium, ammonia, and bicarbonate.

Composition of filtrate as it passes through the loops of Henle. The fluid coming from the proximal tubule and entering the descending limb of the loop of Henle has an osmolality of about 300 mOsm, due predominantly to a NaCl concentration of about 140 mM. The descending limb of the loop of Henle is permeable to both solutes and water. Thus, in the presence of the hypertonic interstitium (interstitial osmolality >300 mOsm), as filtrate flows down the descending limb, water will be reabsorbed from the filtrate, and solutes will be secreted into the tubule lumen. Both of these processes, the addition of solute combined with the loss of water, contribute to the progressive increase in filtrate osmolality as the filtrate passes along the descending limb to the bend in the loops of Henle.

All along the descending limb, osmotic equilibration occurs, meaning that the osmolality of the tubular filtrate equals that of the surrounding interstitium, and thus, at the bend in the loops of Henle is about 1200 mOsm. When the filtrate passes the bend, it enters the ascending limb of the loops of Henle, which extends from the bend to the beginning of the distal convoluted tubule.

The ascending limb of Henle's loops can be divided into two subsegments: the thin ascending limb and the thick ascending limb. Both subsegments are impermeable to water and permeable to solutes. The mechanisms by which solutes are transported differs in the two subsegments. In the thin ascending limb solutes, predominantly NaCl and urea are passively transported, hence the name *passive diluting segment*, which is often used to refer to this nephron subsegment.

The predominant solute in the filtrate entering the thin ascending limb is NaCl (600 mM), with a lesser contribution from urea (300 mM) and even lesser contributions from other solutes such as HCO_3 and K. The very high NaCl and urea concentrations are due to the concentration of the filtrate as it passes through the descending limb, as described above. In the surrounding interstitium, the NaCl concentration is about 300 mM and the urea concentration about 600 mM. Thus, the concentration gradients are such that NaCl is reabsorbed from the tubular lumen and urea is secreted into the tubular lumen in this segment. Due to the high NaCl and low urea permeability of this segment, the net flux of NaCl out of the tubular lumen exceeds the net flux of urea into the tubular lumen, and the filtrate becomes progressively dilute as it passes from the bend up to the thick ascending limb.

In the thick ascending limb, NaCl is actively reabsorbed, hence the term *active diluting segment* is often used to refer to this subsegment. The presence of active transport processes implies that energy is being expanded to reabsorb the NaCl, and that NaCl can be transported against its concentration gradient. Thus, NaCl is transported from the tubular lumen where the NaCl concentration can be as low as 100 mM to the interstitium where the NaCl concentration is about 150 mM. As a result of this active transport process and the water impermeability of this segment, the tubular fluid achieves an osmolality of <100 mOsm by the time it reaches the distal convoluted tubule.

Filtrate composition of the distal and collecting tubules. Along the distal tubule, which is relatively water impermeable, more NaCl is reabsorbed, so that the filtrate entering the cortical collecting tubule of these juxtamedullary nephrons is about 50 mOsm. As the filtrate passes from the cortical to the papillary collecting tubule, some solute reabsorption continues. However, the major determinant of filtrate osmolality at this point is the rate of water reabsorption. Water reabsorption in the collecting tubule is antidiuretic hormone (ADH) or vasopressin dependent. In the presence of ADH, water permeability is high. Thus, water is rapidly reabsorbed due to the osmotic gradient between the tubular lumen and the surrounding interstitium (300 mOsm in the cortex to 1200 mOsm in the inner medulla).

In the presence of maximal levels of ADH, osmotic equilibration will occur between the tubular filtrate and the interstitium, resulting in a maximally concentrated urine of about 1200 mOsm by the time the filtrate enters the papilla of the kidney. And in the presence of low levels of ADH, only very small amounts of water will be reabsorbed, the osmolality will increase little along the length of the collecting tubule, and thus, a maximally dilute urine of about 50 mOsm will be excreted.

Other Processes

The ability of the above processes to result in either a dilute or a concentrated urine is dependent upon: (a) the generation and maintenance of a hypertonic medullary interstitium, and (b) the appropriate presence or absence of ADH.

The hypertonic medullary interstitium. The generation of the hypertonic medullary interstitium involves a number of nephron segments and several different transport processes, all of which result in the addition of solute to the medullary interstitium. Since only the juxtamedullary nephrons (20%-30% of nephrons with glomeruli located near the corticomedullary junction) have loops of Henle that extend into the deep medulla, only these nephrons are involved in generating and maintaining the hypertonic medullary interstitium. As mentioned above, the hypertonicity of the medullary interstitium is due to both NaCl and urea addition to the interstitial fluid, although the contribution of each solute differs along the gradient from the cortex to the inner medulla. Just below the corticomedullary junction (outer medulla), the hypertonicity of the interstitium is due predominantly to the addition of NaCl to the interstitial fluid, while in the inner medulla the hypertonicity is due to both NaCl and urea accumulation within the interstitium, with each solute contributing about half of the added osmoles.

It is well established that the thick ascending

limb of Henle's loop is responsible for the addition of the NaCl to the interstitium in the outer medulla, and that raising the NaCl concentration in this region is the first step to generating the hypertonic interstitium. In addition, it is established that the medullary collecting tubule is predominantly responsible for the urea added to the inner medullary interstitium. However, it is still controversial as to the mechanism by which NaCl is added to the inner medullary interstitium, but probably involves the passive reabsorption of NaCl from the thin ascending limb.

The actual generation process occurs in steps, dependent upon solutes being retained in the interstitium, simultaneous with the continued deliverance of additional solutes to the loop of Henle from the proximal tubule. Thus, the increase in interstitial osmolality does not occur all at once, but rather incrementally, which is why the process is often referred to as countercurrent multiplication, and the loop of Henle, the countercurrent multiplier.

Once the hypertonic gradient has been established, it is maintained throughout life unless something disrupts the maintenance process. Maintenance is dependent on the vascular bed not returning the excess solute to the systemic circulation. This is accomplished by the vasa recta being straight, as opposed to being a network as are the peritubular capillaries in the cortex, having high permeabilities to both solutes and water, and blood flow rates that are much slower than in the cortical capillaries. Thus, as blood within the vasa recta descends from the cortex into the medulla, it also becomes concentrated, as did the tubular filtrate, due to the addition of solutes and the extraction of water. Osmotic equilibration between the blood and the surrounding interstitium is achieved. Thus, the osmolality of the blood at the bend is about 1200 mOsm, as was the osmolality of the tubular filtrate at the bend in the loop of Henle.

As the blood leaves the medulla and returns to the cortex of the kidney, it returns to an osmolality close to 300 mOsm, due to the loss of solutes and the addition of water. This ability of the vasa recta to rapidly exchange both solutes and water with the surrounding interstitium, and thus, rapidly achieve osmotic equilibrium, allows reabsorbed fluid and solutes to be picked up by the vascular bed, but prevents the removal of the solute needed to maintain the hypertonic interstitium. Reflecting this rapid exchanging ability, the vasa recta are referred to as the countercurrent exchangers.

Antidiuretic hormone. The function of ADH is to regulate the water permeability of the collecting tubule and thus the rate of water reabsorption along the collecting tubule. When ADH levels are elevated, water permeability is high, water reabsorption occurs, the filtrate osmolality increases, and a concentrated urine is excreted. In the presence of low levels of ADH, the opposite occurs.

ADH is released from the posterior pituitary gland. The hormone is synthesized in the cell bodies of supraoptic and paraventricular nuclei in the hypothalamus. After synthesis, the hormone is packaged into vesicles, which are then transported down the axons of these neurons into the synaptic bulb. The synaptic bulbs, which are the tips of the neurons, are located in the posterior pituitary gland. Release of the contents of the vesicles from the bulbs results in ADH being released into the interstitium surrounding the posterior pituitary gland. The hormone then diffuses into the surrounding capillaries and is transported into the general circulation.

The release of ADH from the synaptic bulbs is under the control of other neuronal cells. These cells, called osmoreceptors, are located near the supraoptic nuclei in the hypothalamus. They are exquisitely sensitive to the surrounding interstitial fluid. When extracellular fluid osmolality increases, these osmoreceptors send signals to the supraoptic nuclei to release ADH from the synaptic bulbs. When extracellular fluid osmolality is decreased, less signals are sent to the supraoptic nuclei, and ADH secretion is reduced. Since plasma Na and its accompanying anion are the major determinants of plasma osmolality, the osmoreceptors are said to be regulated by plasma Na concentration. However, any osmol that remains in the extracellular fluid is capable and will regulate ADH secretion.

The mechanism by which ADH regulates the water permeability of the collecting tubule has been extensively studied. Receptors for ADH are located on the basolateral (interstitial) side of the collecting tubule cells. When ADH occupies those receptors, a series of enzymes are activated, which results in the movement of intracellular vesicles from the cytoplasm (center) of the cell to the apical membrane (the side of the cell that faces the tubule lumen). These vesicles, which contain preformed water channels, fuse with the apical membrane, resulting in the insertion of these water channels into the apical membrane. Water is then reabsorbed across the apical membrane through these channels, and exits the cell across the basolateral membrane (the side of the cell facing the interstitium). The water permeability of the basolateral membrane is constant and relatively high. Thus, regulation of water reabsorption occurs by regulating the water permeability of the apical membrane of the cell. Once the water exits the cell across the basolateral membrane, it enters the interstitial fluid compartment, and is picked up by the vasa recta to be returned to the systemic circulation.

In addition to affecting the water permeability of the collecting tubule, ADH also regulates NaCl reabsorption in the thick ascending limb of Henle's loop and urea reabsorption from the inner medullary collecting tubule. In the presence of

Figure 7-9
Body cell.

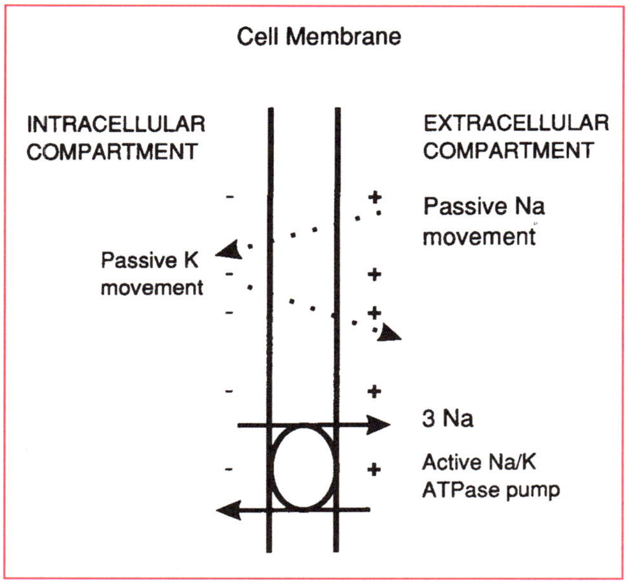

Note: From Ludlow, M. (1993). Renal handling of potassium. *ANNA Journal, 20*(1), p. 53. Reprinted with permission.

ADH, reabsorption of both solutes is increased, which contributes to the maintenance of the hypertonic interstitium.

Forming a Dilute and Concentrated Urine

Whether or not a concentrated or dilute urine will be excreted, filtrate entering the collecting tubule has an osmolality of approximately 50 mOsm. It is then the presence or absence of ADH that determines the rate of water reabsorption along the collecting tubule, and thus, the final osmolality of the fluid entering the pelvis of the kidney and passing into the bladder. Although it may seem a waste of energy to first dilute and then concentrate the tubule fluid when a concentrated urine is desired, remember that it is the reabsorption of NaCl from the ascending limb of Henle's loop that generates the hypertonic medullary interstitium necessary to extract water from the filtrate as it passes along the collecting tubule. In other words, if NaCl were not reabsorbed from the ascending limb, the medullary osmolality would be less and less water would be reabsorbed along the collecting tubule even in the presence of maximal ADH levels.

In contrast, the formation of a dilute urine is independent of the osmolality of the medullary interstitium and is totally dependent on the active diluting segment (thick ascending limb). Only within the active diluting segment, where energy is expended so that NaCl can be transported against its concentration gradient, can the osmolality of the tubule fluid become less than isosmotic (300 mOsm). As fluid enters the distal tubule and collecting tubule, the requirement for excretion of a dilute urine is that these nephron segments remain relatively water impermeable, a condition that exists when ADH levels are low.

Summary

The formation of either a concentrated or dilute urine requires coordination between the nephron and vascular structures within the medulla of the kidney. The parallel arrangement of these structures allows for the generation and maintenance of the hypertonic medullary interstitium, necessary for the formation of a concentrated urine. The solute transport processes along these nephron segments allow for the transport of NaCl out of the tubular fluid and into the interstitium, resulting in a maximally dilute filtrate by the time the fluid enters the collecting tubules. It is then the regulation of ADH secretion from the posterior pituitary that determines whether the dilute fluid entering the collecting tubule will be excreted as such or will become concentrated.

Section 4: Renal Handling of Potassium

Potassium (K) is the most abundant cation in the human body. The total body K stores in an adult are approximately 50-55 milliequivalents (mEq)/Kilogram (Kg) body weight with 98% of the K located intracellularly. Skeletal muscle has the highest K content per unit dry weight and, therefore, contains the bulk of total body K, while fat and bone have relatively low K content. The high intracellular concentration of K (150 mEq/L[L]) versus the low extracellular concentration (4-5 mEq/L) is a delicate balance critical for normal cell functions. Before reviewing how renal cells control body K content, it is important to understand how individual cells regulate K content. The following discussion addresses the mechanisms responsible for maintaining the K balance in the intracellular and extracellular fluid compartments of individual body cells.

Potassium Functions

Each body cell must regulate its internal K content and concentration in order to regulate cell growth and division, metabolic reactions, acid-base balance, and cell volume. It is also important that appropriate K concentration gradients be maintained across nerve and muscle cells so that appropriate electrical polarization of these cells is maintained for normal neuromuscular and cardiac activity. The movement of as little as 1.5%-2% of the cell K into the extracellular fluid (ECF) can result in a potentially fatal increase in the plasma K concentration.

Figure 7-10
Segmental handling of potassium.

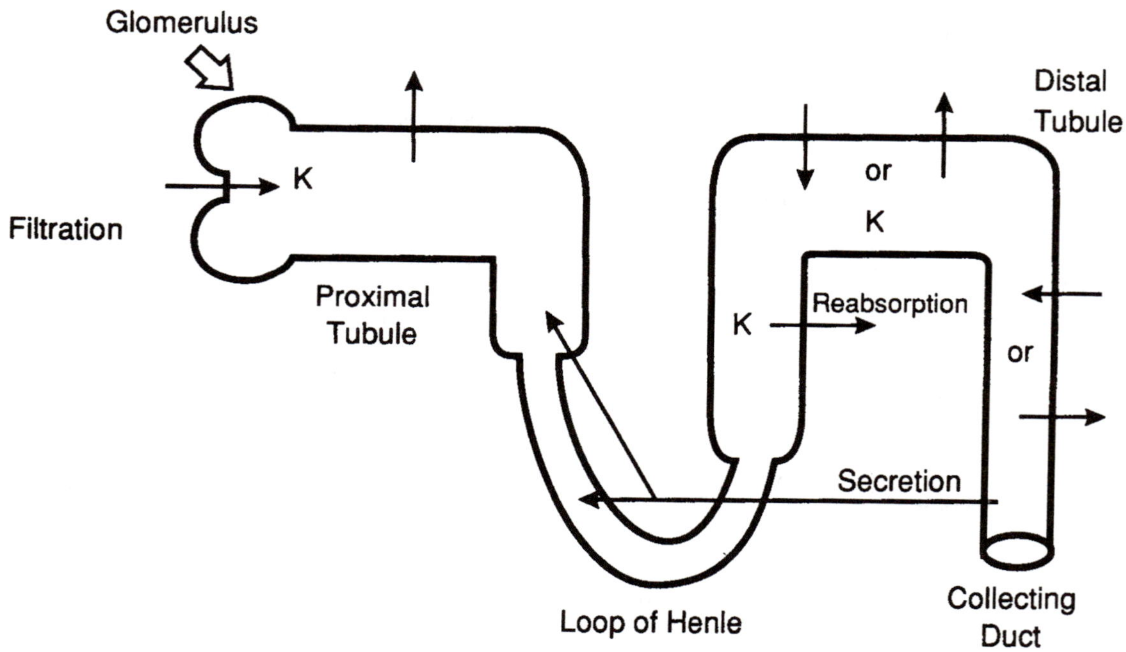

Note: From Ludlow, M. (1993). Renal handling of potassium. *ANNA Journal, 20*(1), p. 53. Reprinted with permission.

Sodium-Potassium ATPase Pump

The most important mechanism in maintaining the critical balance of K between the extracellular and intracellular compartments is the sodium-potassium Na/K ATPase pump located in the cell membrane. The Na/K ATPase pump actively transports Na out and K into the cell in a 3:2 ratio (3 Na out for every 2 K in, thus a net loss of cations). In addition to the active transport system for Na and K, the cells have tiny channels that allow for the passive movement of Na and K through the cell membrane. Because the cell membrane is 50-100 times more permeable to K than to Na, K continually diffuses down its concentration gradient from the intracellular to the extracellular compartment. Na diffuses back into the intracellular compartment but at a much slower rate than the outward movement of K, resulting in a net cation (+ charge) loss from the cell. The consequence of both the Na/K ATPase pump and the cation diffusion process both carrying net positive charges out of the cell is that the cell interior has a negative electrical potential relative to the extracellular compartment (see Figure 7-9).

Extrarenal Regulation of Internal Potassium

An average American diet includes 60-100 mEq of K per day, which requires that 60-100 mEq of K must be excreted daily to maintain a homeostatic balance. After a meal, the K absorbed from the gastrointestinal tract rapidly enters the extracellular fluid. This rise in plasma K is attenuated by the rapid uptake of K into cells to prevent life-threatening hyperkalemia. K absorption by the gastrointestinal tract stimulates insulin secretion from the pancreas, aldosterone release from the adrenal cortex, and epinephrine secretion from the adrenal medulla. These hormones promote the uptake of K into muscle, liver, bone, and red blood cells by stimulating the Na/K pumps on these cell membranes.

Renal Handling of Potassium

Although small amounts of K are lost each day in stool and sweat, the kidney plays the major role in maintenance of K balance. The kidney is able to alter the excretory rate of K in response to the quantity of K ingested. The following discussion will address the renal segmental handling of K and factors that normally regulate K transport in these segments (see Figure 7-10).

Segmental handling of potassium. The kidney

Figure 7-11
Cellular model for potassium handling by the distal nephron.

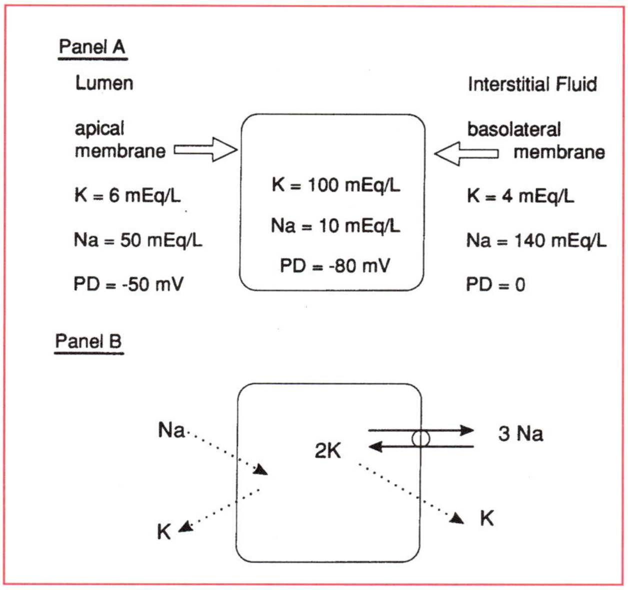

Note: From Ludlow, M. (1993). Renal handling of potassium. *ANNA Journal, 20*(1), p. 54. Reprinted with permission.

must excrete >90% of daily K intake in order for the body to remain in K balance. Because potassium is freely filtered at the glomerulus, the K concentration of the fluid entering the proximal tubule is essentially equal to that of plasma (3.5-5.0 mEq/L). Along the proximal tubule, potassium is generally reabsorbed in proportion to solute and water reabsorption. Although ~60% of filtered K is reabsorbed in the proximal tubule, the K concentration of the fluid entering the descending limb of Henle's loop, a small amount of K is secreted into the luminal fluid, and along the ascending limb, particularly the thick ascending limb of Henle's loop, K is avidly reabsorbed. Consequently, the K concentration of the fluid entering the distal convoluted tubule is lower than plasma, about 2 mEq/L.

The major site for regulating net K excretion occurs in the late distal tubule and cortical collecting tubule. The cellular mechanisms for regulating K transport are essentially the same in the two nephron segments and therefore will be discussed together using one cellular model (see Figure 7-11, Panel A, and 7-11, Panel B). Depending on the K balance of the body, these nephron segments will either reabsorb or secrete K. In conditions of K deficiency, reabsorption will occur, and when the body is in a positive K balance, secretion will occur. The latter is the normally occurring situation. To discuss regulation of K transport in these segments, it is necessary to characterize the cell responsible for K transport. The discussion will focus on K secretion, since that is the more frequent direction of net transport.

Cellular model for potassium transport. In the late distal tubule, the cell type responsible for K transport is the late distal tubule cell, and in the cortical collecting tubule, the cell type is the principal cell. The late distal tubule cell is similar in many ways to the principal cell but is so named because of its location. In these cells (see Figure 7-11B), the basolateral membrane (side of the cell facing the peritubular capillaries) contains the Na/K ATPase pump and a K channel, and the apical membrane (side of the cell facing the tubule lumen) contains both Na and K channels.

The activity of the Na/K pump transporter is exquisitely sensitive to the K concentration of blood. When extracellular K concentration increases, the pump increases its activity and more K is taken up by the cell. When plasma K concentration is decreased, the reverse is true. Due to the imbalance of charge generated by exchanging 3 Na ions for 2 K ions, there is an electrical gradient (called a potential difference or PD) across the basolateral membrane of the cell, such that the cell interior is electrically negative by about 80 mV in reference to the exterior of the cell (see Figure 7-11A).

Across the apical membrane, Na is the primary cation (positively charged ion) reabsorbed under normal conditions. Since the cell interior is negative (280 mV) and the Na concentration inside the cell (~10 mEq/L) is less than that in the tubular fluid (~50 mEq/L) (see Figure 7-11A), both the electrical and chemical driving forces for Na favor Na reabsorption from the luminal fluid into the cell. Since the anion most frequently accompanying Na is Cl, which is reabsorbed at a much slower rate than Na, the luminal compartment develops a negative PD as a consequence of Na diffusing into the cell.

As shown in Figure 7-11A, both the cell interior and the luminal compartment are negative in reference to the interstitial fluid. Because the cell is more negative than the luminal compartment, the electrical driving force between the lumen and cell interior opposes the movement of K (a positively charged ion) out of the cell, that is, K is "held" within the cell. However, because of the high intracellular K concentration (100 mEq/L) and the low luminal fluid K concentration (mean luminal ~6 mEq/L), the chemical driving force for K favors K secretion from the cell to the luminal compartment. These are opposing forces. However, the chemical driving force is larger than the electrical driving force; therefore, the net driving force favors K secretion.

In summary, the net movement of K from the extracellular fluid into the tubule lumen occurs by

Figure 7-12
Effect of luminal flow rate on potassium secretion.

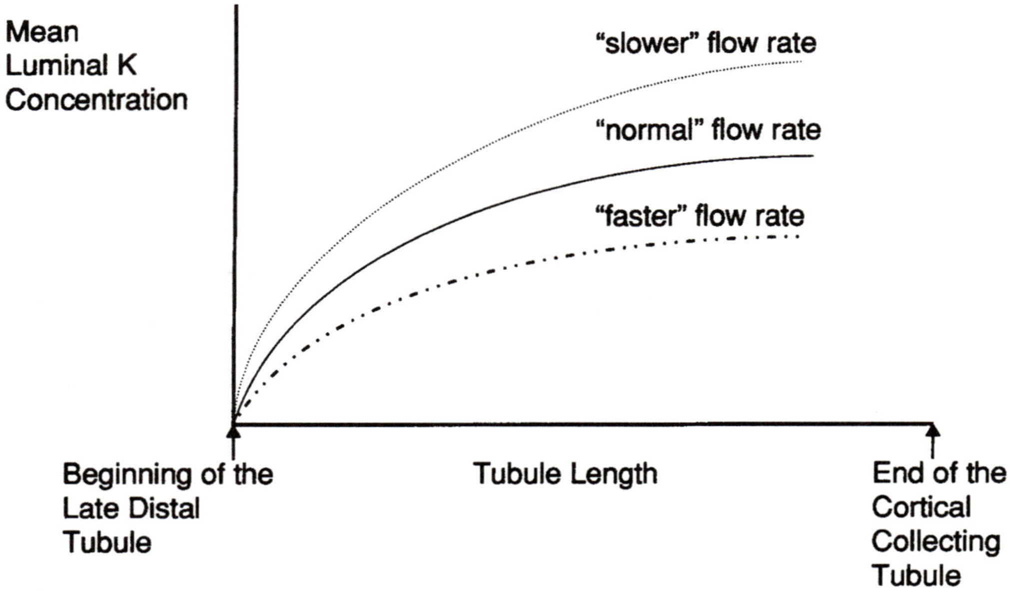

Note: From Ludlow, M. (1993). Renal handling of potassium. *ANNA Journal, 20*(1), p. 55. Reprinted with permission.

K first being actively transported from the interstitial fluid, which is in equilibrium with plasma, into the cell across the basolateral membrane on the Na/K ATPase pump, and then passively diffusing from the cell into the tubule fluid through the K channels in the apical membrane, driven by the electrochemical gradient. Changes in the rate of K secretion are secondary to changing (a) the rate of K accumulation within the cell, that is, the activity of the Na/K ATPase pump on the basolateral membrane; or (b) the magnitude and direction of the driving force for K secretion across the apical membrane. The latter involves the intracellular K concentration, luminal K concentration, and electrical gradient across the apical membrane. The influence of various factors on net K secretion will be discussed below in relationship to altering one or more of these determinants of K secretion.

Regulation of potassium secretion. Major factors that influence net K secretion include: (a) dietary K intake, (b) distal tubule flow rate, (c) distal delivery of non-reabsorbable anions, (d) aldosterone levels, and (e) acid-base balance.

Dietary potassium intake. When K intake increases, the K absorbed from the GI tract first appears in the extracellular pool (plasma and interstitial fluid). The Na/K ATPase pump on the basolateral membrane is exquisitely sensitive to the extracellular K concentration, and the uptake of K from the extracellular to the intracellular pool is a mechanism of defense against an increase in extracellular K concentration. Although this uptake of K occurs in almost all cells of the body, its occurrence in the late distal tubule and principal cells facilitate K secretion by increasing the intracellular K concentration, and therefore, the chemical gradient for K secretion into the luminal fluid (see Figure 7-11A). The increase in K secretion leads to an increase in K excretion. Increases in plasma K concentration also stimulate aldosterone secretion, which contributes to enhancing K secretion.

Distal tubule flow rate. K is secreted into the luminal fluid as the fluid flows along the distal and cortical collecting tubules. Consequently, the K concentration rises along the length of the tubule (see Figure 7-12, solid line). If luminal fluid flow rate increases, that is, transverses the distal and cortical collecting tubules in a shorter time period, the mean luminal K concentration will be less than normal due to less time available for K to be secreted into the luminal fluid (see Figure 7-12, dashed line). The reverse is true for a decrease in luminal fluid flow rate (see Figure 7-12, dotted line). When luminal flow rate is slower than normal, the mean K concentration will be higher than normal, due to the longer time available for K to enter the luminal compartment. At theoretical extremes of flow rate, luminal K concentration would remain at 2 mEq/L (infinitely fast flow rate) or become equal to intracellular K concentration (100 mEq/L) at infinitely slow flow rates.

Since the K concentration of the luminal fluid is one determinant of the net driving force governing K secretion across the apical membrane, it follows that when distal tubule fluid flow rate increases, the rate of K secretion will increase; thus excretion will increase. When distal tubule flow rate decreases, the rate of K secretion and excretion will decrease.

Although changes in extracellular fluid volume lead to changes in distal tubule flow rate, K secretion is relatively unaffected because of the offsetting effects of aldosterone. In the presence of loop diuretics, such as furosemide, or thiazide diuretics, which inhibit NaCl and secondarily water reabsorption prior to the late distal tubule, luminal flow rates increase substantially in the late distal and cortical collecting tubules. This leads to an increase in K secretion, and thus K excretion. This is the mechanism by which K depletion occurs in patients on these diuretics.

Distal delivery of non-reabsorbable anions. The anion accompanying the majority of Na delivered to the distal tubule is chloride. Although Cl is reabsorbed in these segments, the rate of reabsorption is slower than that of Na, which explains the luminal negativity of these nephron segments. If the anion accompanying Na is not Cl, then the magnitude of the luminal negativity will depend on the rate at which the anion is reabsorbed. If the anion is reabsorbed more easily than Cl, the lumen will become less negative, and if the anion is less readily reabsorbed the luminal negativity will increase. The latter situation occurs when bicarbonate or organic anions, such as penicillin, are the anions accompanying Na. These anions are less readily reabsorbed than Cl. Subsequently, luminal negativity increases and K secretion and excretion is enhanced.

Aldosterone. Aldosterone is a hormone synthesized and secreted from the adrenal cortex. Aldosterone secretion is influenced by many factors, two of which are pertinent to the regulation of K balance. These are plasma K concentration and extracellular volume. Increases in aldosterone secretion are associated with increases in plasma K concentration and decreases in extracellular volume.

Aldosterone has three major effects on the cells in the distal nephron involved in regulating K excretion. The first is to increase Na/K ATPase pump activity. This results in an increase in cellular K uptake, intracellular K content, and the magnitude of the K concentration gradient across the apical membrane. These results cause an increase in the rate of K secretion into the luminal fluid. The second effect is to increase the K permeability of the apical membrane. K transverses the apical membrane through channels. Because aldosterone increases the ease with which K can pass through the channels, more K can be secreted in a given period of time. And the third effect is to increase the rate of Na uptake across the apical membrane. The consequence is an increase in the luminal negativity, an effect that enhances K secretion by the same mechanism described above for increased delivery of non-reabsorbable anions.

Increases in dietary intake of K lead to enhanced secretion secondary to raising intracellular K concentrations. In addition, intake-induced increases in plasma K concentration stimulate aldosterone secretion, which will facilitate K secretion by the three mechanisms described above.

The effects of aldosterone associated with changes in extracellular volume are more complex. When extracellular volume is low, GFR decreases, distal delivery of solutes and water decreases, and luminal flow rate is reduced. If this were the sole effect of extracellular volume, then K secretion should be significantly impaired as previously discussed (see Figure 7-12). However, decreases in extracellular volume stimulate aldosterone secretion, which enhances K secretion. When extracellular volume is increased, the opposite occurs, that is that distal flow rate increases and aldosterone secretion is suppressed. The net effect of these two opposing factors is that changes in extracellular volume, although associated with dramatic changes in distal tubular flow rate, are not associated with dramatic effects on net K secretion. Therefore, K balance remains relatively independent of extracellular volume status.

Acid-base balance. The acid-base balance of the body is another factor that affects K secretion in the distal tubule. In acidemic states, some of the excess hydrogen (H) is buffered intracellularly. To maintain electroneutrality, K moves into the extracellular fluid, raising the plasma K concentration. The result is a decrease in the amount of K available for secretion into the luminal fluid. In addition, a decrease in cell pH (acidosis) decreases the K permeability of the apical membrane. Accordingly, at any given driving force for K secretion, less K will be secreted because of the enhanced difficulty of K passing through the K channels.

The cation shifts are reversed in alkalemia, and the plasma K+ concentration tends to fall and the intracellular K content increases. In addition, alkalosis is associated with an increase in the K permeability of the apical membrane. Therefore, during metabolic alkalosis, there is an increase in K secretion into the lumen. These changes are usually transient and of minor significance.

In general, metabolic acidosis results in a decrease in K excretion and an increase in plasma K. Conversely, metabolic alkalosis enhances K excretion and decreases plasma K. The changes in

Figure 7-13
Calcium homeostasis: Daily calcium metabolism.

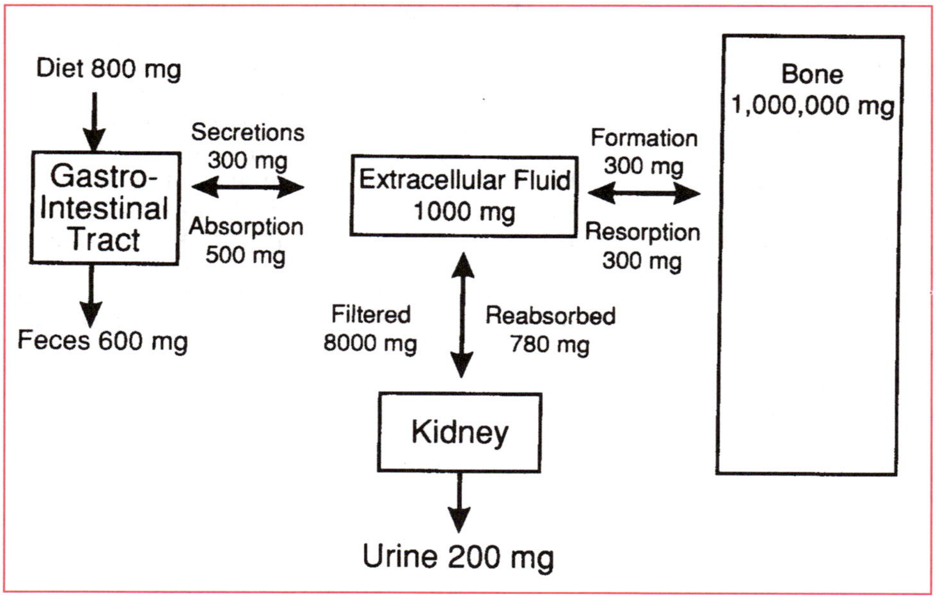

Note: From Yucha, C.B. (1993). Renal control of calcium. *ANNA Journal, 20*(4), p. 441. Reprinted with permission.

The extracellular calcium concentration is affected by the rate of formation and absorption of bone, by secretion and absorption in the GI tract, and by filtration and reabsorption by the kidneys.

plasma K concentration associated with respiratory acid-base disturbances are described as minor. The reason for this is not known.

Summary

The maintenance of a normal plasma K concentration depends upon extrarenal and renal control mechanisms. The extrarenal mechanisms (insulin, epinephrine, aldosterone) are effective in the transitory movement of K into the intracellular compartment. The renal mechanism is responsible for the chronic maintenance of a normal body K content. When these transient and chronic regulatory mechanisms are functioning in concert, large variations in K intake have relatively minor effects on plasma K concentration.

Section 5: Renal Control of Calcium

The homeostasis of calcium is complex because the gastrointestinal tract, the bone, and the kidney all affect calcium balance. Earlier sections have been concerned almost entirely with the renal handling of ions and water homeostasis. This approach is not possible when dealing with calcium because its concentration is controlled by two other major effector sites as well as the bone and the gastrointestinal system. Accordingly, the roles and interactions of all three sites are discussed in this section.

Calcium and Its Functions

Calcium is a necessary ion for many metabolic processes. It is the major cation within the structure of bone and teeth. It is involved in blood clotting, hormone secretion, cell receptor function, plasma membrane permeability, nerve impulse transmission, and muscle contraction.

The total body calcium is about 1200 g, 99% of which is located within bone as hydroxyapatite and the remainder in the plasma and body cells. The total plasma calcium (normally 4.5-5.5 mEq/L or 8.6-10.5 mg/dl) exists in three general forms:

1. **Ionized:** Approximately 45% (4.5 mg/dl) is in the free or ionized form (Ca++). This is the only biologically active form in nerve, muscle, and other target organs and is the form that is regulated.
2. **Bound:** About 40% (4.0 mg/dl) is reversibly bound to plasma proteins. When the serum protein level is reduced, more calcium is found in the ionized state; when serum proteins are elevated, more calcium may be in the bound form. Protein binding is also influenced by plasma pH. During alkalosis, hydrogen ions are released from protein, exposing more negatively charged binding sites. This increases the sites available for calcium binding and reduces the amount of free calcium in the plasma. Thus, a patient with alkalosis is susceptible to tetany. In contrast, under acidotic conditions, proteins are saturated with hydrogen. Therefore, there are fewer sites on proteins available for calcium

Figure 7-14
Calcium transport in the distal tubule.

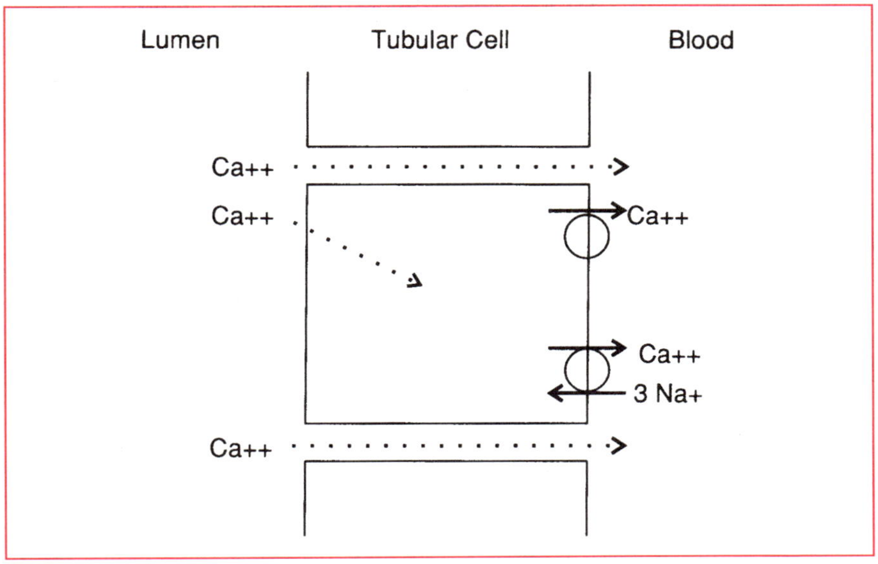

In the distal tubule, calcium diffuses across the paracellular space and the luminal membrane, driven by the chemical gradient. Transport across the basolateral membrane involves an ATP-driven calcium pump and ATP-driven Ca^{++}/Na^{+} exchange. Dashed arrows indicate passive transport; solid arrows indicate active transport.

Note: From Yucha, C.B. (1993). Renal control of calcium. *ANNA Journal, 20*(4), p. 441. Reprinted with permission.

binding, and more remains in the plasma in its ionized form. Thus, an acidotic patient may not show tetany at calcium levels low enough to produce symptoms in other people.

3. **Complexed:** Fifteen percent of the calcium in plasma (1.5 mg/dl) is complexed to anions such as chloride, citrate, and phosphate.

Calcium Imbalances

The importance of the control of calcium concentration can be illustrated by considering the consequences of abnormal concentrations of calcium. Hypercalcemia decreases the permeability of the cell membranes to sodium ions, preventing normal depolarization of nerve and muscle cells. This can lead to cardiac arrhythmias, fatigue, weakness, lethargy, anorexia, nausea, and constipation. Hypercalcemia also leads to the deposition of calcium carbonate salts in soft tissues, resulting in irritation and inflammation, or in the development of kidney stones. In contrast, hypocalcemia increases the permeability of cell membranes to sodium ions such that nerve and muscle tissues undergo spontaneous action potential generation. This may lead to confusion, muscle spasms, hyperreflexia, and intestinal cramping; it may progress to convulsions, tetany, and respiratory failure.

Calcium Homeostasis

Calcium is regulated at three different sites: the bone, the intestine, and the kidney (see Figure 7-13). Of the 800 mg ingested each day, approximately 200 mg is absorbed from the GI tract and enters the extracellular fluid. From here it may be stored in bone or excreted by the kidney, depending on the presence of parathyroid hormone, Vitamin D3, and calcitonin.

Control of calcium concentration may be divided into daily control and long-term control. The calcium ion concentration in the extracellular fluid (ECF) remains within a few percent of 2.4 mEq/L and on a day-to-day basis is controlled principally by the effect of parathyroid hormone on bone absorption. Bone is not a fixed, dead tissue; rather, it is cellular and well supplied with blood. Bone is constantly broken down (absorbed) and simultaneously reformed under the influence of the bone cells, osteoclasts and osteoblasts, respectively. Thus, bone provides a huge source or storage area for the withdrawal or deposit of calcium.

The long-term control of calcium results from the reabsorption of calcium from the kidney tubules and absorbed from the gut through the intestinal mucosa. Under normal conditions, only part of the ingested calcium is absorbed from the intestine, and the remainder is excreted in the feces. Accordingly, control of the active transport system that moves calcium from the intestinal lumen to the blood can result in large increases or decreases in net calcium absorption, thereby assisting in the regulation of total body calcium.

Renal Handling of Calcium

The kidneys control calcium by filtration and reabsorption. Only about 60% of the plasma calcium is filterable, the free calcium and that bound to anions. Protein-bound calcium is not filterable and remains in the plasma. Since calcium is both filtered at the glomerulus and reabsorbed by the tubules but is not secreted, the amount of calcium excreted can be described by the following equation:

Calcium Excreted
= Calcium Filtered – Calcium Reabsorbed

The amount of calcium filtered can be calculated by multiplying the glomerular filtration rate (GFR) by the serum concentration of filterable calcium [Ca]. To illustrate, if the GFR is 120 ml/min and the serum filterable calcium concentration is 5.0 mg/dl, the daily filtered load would be approximately 8640 mg.

Amount filtered per minute
= GFR x [Ca]
= 120 ml/min x 5.0 mg/dl
= 120 ml/min x 0.05 mg/ml
= 6 mg/min

Amount filtered per day
= 6 mg/min x 60 min/hour x 24 hours
= 8640 mg

The filtered load may be altered by changes in the GFR or the serum calcium concentration. For example, the filtered load is reduced by a decreased GFR, such as occurs in chronic renal failure or by a fall in the serum calcium concentration. Such alterations would lead to a reduction in the renal excretion of calcium if the amount reabsorbed were unchanged.

The amount of calcium excreted can also be altered by changing the amount that is reabsorbed. In many situations, both the amount filtered and the amount reabsorbed change. For example, when calcium intake rises, the plasma calcium concentration increases. This increases the amount of calcium that is filtered. In addition, the rise in plasma calcium triggers hormonal changes that cause a diminished reabsorption. The net result is an increase in calcium excretion.

Of the amount of calcium filtered, 97%-99% is reabsorbed. Approximately 50%-70% of the filtered load is reabsorbed in the proximal tubule, 25% in the thick ascending limb of Henle's loop, and 8% in the distal tubule.

Proximal tubule. Sodium is actively reabsorbed in the proximal tubule. It is followed passively by chloride and water. The ratio of the calcium concentration in tubule fluid (TF) relative to the plasma ultrafiltrate (UF) is represented by the expression $[TF/UF]_{Ca}$. This ratio remains near one along the proximal tubule, indicating that calcium reabsorption is paralleling sodium and fluid reabsorption. Changes in the rate of fluid reabsorption are accompanied by changes in calcium reabsorption. This suggests that calcium reabsorption in the proximal tubule occurs primarily through passive diffusion, probably by moving between the cells (a paracellular route), rather than through the cells (a transcellular route).

Loop of Henle. Calcium transport by thin descending and thin ascending limbs is minimal because of the low calcium permeability of these segments. In the thick ascending limb, there is evidence that calcium is reabsorbed by both passive and active mechanisms. In this segment, chloride is actively reabsorbed. Movement of a negatively charged ion out of the tubular fluid leaves behind a positive voltage in the lumen. Calcium reabsorption is driven passively as the lumen-positive voltage repels the positively charged calcium ions. When the transepithelial voltage is manipulated experimentally, the direction and rate of calcium movement is changed. That is, when the voltage is zero, there is no net calcium movement, and when the voltage is negative, calcium secretion occurs. An active transport mechanism may also exist in this nephron segment since under certain conditions

Figure 7-15
PTH regulation of calcium.
PTH increases the extracellular calcium concentration by stimulating the absorption of bone salts and by increasing the intestinal absorption and renal reabsorption of calcium.

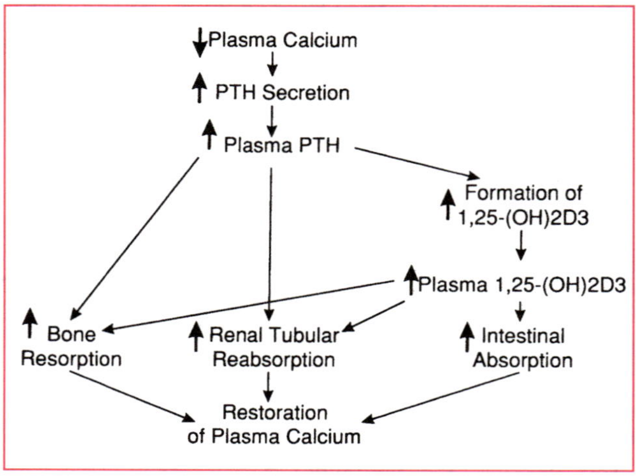

Note: From Yucha, C.B. (1993). Renal control of calcium. *ANNA Journal, 20*(4), p. 444. Reprinted with permission

calcium reabsorption occurs, even when the electrochemical driving forces are eliminated.

Distal tubule. Since more calcium than water is reabsorbed in the thick ascending limb, the calcium concentration in the fluid entering the distal tubule is less than that of plasma ultrafiltrate. The $[TF/UF]_{Ca}$ ratio is about 0.6 at the beginning of the distal tubule and falls along the length of it to 0.3 or less. This information, taken together with the lumen-negative transepithelial voltage, provides evidence for an active calcium reabsorption mechanism that proceeds against both electrical and chemical gradients.

Collecting tubule. The contribution of the cortical collecting tubule to overall calcium reabsorption is small because the calcium permeability in the cortical collecting tubule is lower than in the thick ascending limb and proximal tubule. Calcium reabsorption in this segment varies with the magnitude and direction of the transepithelial voltage.

In summary, calcium is reabsorbed passively via the paracellular pathways, driven by a chemical gradient in the proximal tubule, and by the lumen-positive transepithelial voltage in the thick ascending limb. In the distal tubule, calcium is actively reabsorbed. A simplified model illustrating the mechanisms of transfer of calcium across the membranes of the distal tubule is shown in Figure 7-14. The Ca^{++} activity within the renal cells is about four times lower than that of the extracellular fluid. Calcium moves passively from the lumen into the renal epithelial cells driven by the chemical gradient. Calcium extrusion from the cell across the basolateral membrane occurs against an electrochemical gradient. This transport involves both an ATP-driven calcium transport pump and Ca^{++}-Na^{+} exchange.

Regulation of Calcium Excretion

The renal excretion of calcium may vary considerably. In normal subjects, an average of 200 mg/day is excreted, but may reach up to 300 mg/day for men and 250 mg/day for women. In severe states of calcium depletion, it may be reduced to 50 mg/day.

Tubular calcium reabsorption may be altered by many factors. In general, those maneuvers that alter sodium transport in the proximal tubule or chloride transport in the thick ascending limb cause parallel alterations in calcium transport by interfering with the passive driving forces (concentration gradient in the proximal tubule and lumen-positive voltage in the thick ascending limb). For example, as extracellular fluid volume expansion inhibits salt and water reabsorption, calcium reabsorption in the proximal tubule is diminished. Loop diuretics, such as furosemide, decrease the lumen-positive transepithelial voltage in the thick ascending limb. The usual passive driving force for calcium reabsorption is thereby eliminated and sodium excretion is accompanied by calcium excretion.

The reabsorption that occurs in the distal tubule and collecting duct is very selective, depending upon the calcium ion concentration in the blood. In these segments of the nephron, sodium and calcium reabsorption can be dissociated from one another, suggesting that the reabsorptive mechanisms differ. This is supported by the observation that parathyroid hormone (PTH) reduces urinary excretion of calcium while enhancing urinary excretion of sodium. In addition, thiazide diuretics, acting in the early portion of the distal tubule induce a natriuresis, but cause urinary retention of calcium when administered on a chronic basis.

Calcium excretion is also affected by phosphorus levels. An increase in phosphorus may decrease urinary excretion of calcium. Presumably, this is due to deposition of calcium phosphate in the bone, thereby decreasing serum calcium levels and the filtered load. Although the mechanism has not been defined, phosphate depletion leads to an increased urinary excretion of calcium.

Parathyroid hormone. Movement of calcium into and out of the bone, gastrointestinal tract, and kidney is under the control of a hormone called parathyroid hormone (PTH). PTH is a single chain polypeptide composed of 84 amino acids, produced by the parathyroid glands. Its production is controlled directly by the calcium concentration of the fluid bathing the cells of these glands. When the extracellular calcium concentration falls too low, the parathyroid glands are directly stimulated to increase their secretion of PTH (see Figure 7-15).

PTH increases the ECF concentration of calcium by at least three distinct effects. First, it stimulates the absorption of bone salts, thereby releasing large amounts of calcium into the extracellular fluid. Second, PTH stimulates the activation of Vitamin D by the kidney, and this hormone increases bone, intestinal, and renal reabsorption of calcium. Third, it increases renal tubular calcium reabsorption in the distal nephron and thus decreases urinary calcium excretion. This enhancement of calcium reabsorption occurs primarily in the distal tubules, but also in the thick ascending limbs and collecting ducts, through activation of renal adenylate cyclase and generation of cyclic AMP within the tubular cells. PTH has little effect on calcium transport in the proximal tubules. All three effects of PTH on the bone, intestine, and kidney result in a higher ECF calcium concentration.

In contrast, when the calcium level becomes too great, PTH secretion falls and almost no bone absorption occurs. Since new bone continues to be formed by the osteoblastic system, calcium is removed from the ECF. In addition, without PTH, fecal and urinary calcium losses are increased and the ECF calcium level returns toward normal.

Vitamin D3. A second hormone that affects calcium homeostasis is 1,25 dihydroxyvitamin D3.

Figure 7-16
Phosphate transport in the proximal tubule.

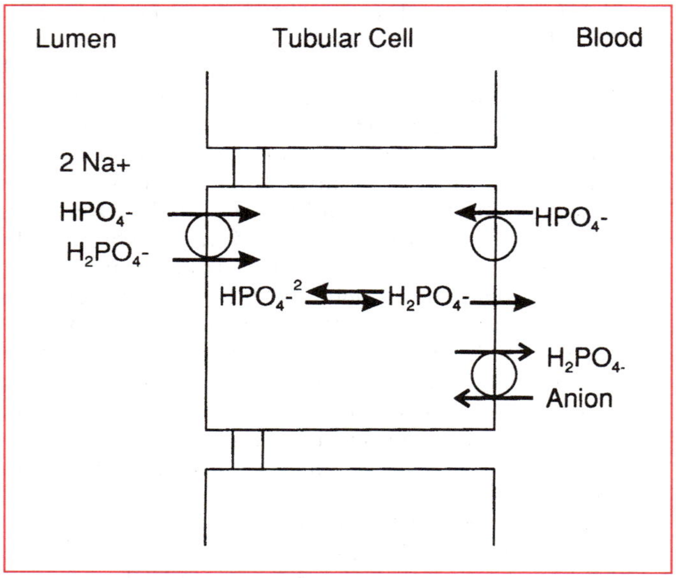

Note: From Yucha, C.B. (1993). Renal control of phosphorus and magnesium. *ANNA Journal, 20*(4), p. 449. Reprinted with permission.

In the proximal tubule, phosphate transport across the luminal membrane is dependent on the sodium gradient. Most enters the cell as divalent ($NaHPO_4^{-2}$) phosphate along with two sodium. Phosphate exits the cell by simple diffusion along its electrochemical gradient and perhaps by an anion exchange mechanism.

This hormone is metabolized from ingested Vitamin D and from Vitamin D3 (cholecalciferol) formed by the action of ultraviolet radiation on 7-dehydrocholesterol in the skin. These precursors enter the blood, and a hydroxyl group (OH-) is added in the 25 position by the liver. This chemical reaction is called hydroxylation and, in this case, involves the addition of a hydroxyl group to the 25th carbon atom of Vitamin D3. When PTH is present, 25,hydroxyvitamin D3 is further hydroxylated in the 1 position by the kidney. The end result is the formation of 1,25 dihydroxyvitamin D3, the active form of Vitamin D. This hormone stimulates active absorption of calcium (and phosphate) by the intestine, enhances bone absorption, and stimulates the renal-tubular reabsorption of calcium. The effect on Vitamin D in the kidney has been attributed to its action in the distal tubule, where a Vitamin D-dependent calcium-binding protein has been identified. All three actions on the bone, intestines, and kidney, increase the ECF calcium concentration.

Calcitonin. Calcitonin is a 24 amino acid polypeptide secreted by the parafollicular cells of the thyroid gland. It is secreted in response to hypercalcemia and tends to lower plasma calcium primarily by inhibiting bone absorption. Calcitonin also increases urinary excretion of calcium, but the mechanism for this is undefined. Its role is thought to be of minor significance in comparison to that of PTH and 1,25 dihydroxyvitamin D3.

Summary

This section has reviewed the roles, homeostasis, and renal handling of calcium. The homeostasis of calcium is complex and also involves the gastrointestinal tract and the bone as well as interaction among these three sites. The major sites of tubular reabsorption (the proximal tubule, thick ascending limb of Henle, and the distal tubule) and the presumed cellular mechanisms involved have been described.

Section 6: Renal Control of Phosphorus and Magnesium

Phosphorus and magnesium balance is maintained by the kidney, the bone, and gastrointestinal system. Accordingly, the roles and interactions of all three sites must be considered.

Phosphorus and Its Function

Phosphorus is located primarily within body cells in combination with hydrogen and oxygen, as a major intracellular anion. In this form, it is referred to as phosphate. At pH 7.4, about 28% is found in the divalent form, sodium monohydrogen phosphate ($NaHPO_4^{-2}$), and 72% is found in the monovalent form sodium dihydrogen phosphate (NaH_2PO^-). Both of these forms of phosphate play important roles as acid-base buffers because of their ability to pick up and release hydrogen. In acidosis, there is a relative increase in $NaH_2PO_4^-$ and decrease in $NaHPO_4^{-2}$. The opposite occurs when the extracellular fluid becomes alkaline.

The total quantity of phosphate includes both species and is expressed in milligrams per deciliter of blood. In the plasma, phosphate ranges from 2 to 4.5 mg/dl, but is slightly higher in children. Approximately 5%-10% of plasma phosphate is protein-bound and is therefore not filterable at the renal glomerulus. The remaining 90%-95% is filterable at the glomerulus.

Within the cells, phosphates are found combined with lipids (phospholipids) as part of the lipid bilayer of the cell membrane, combined with nucleic acids in the DNA and RNA, and as part of adenosine triphosphate (ATP), providing the energy currency of the cell. Last, the major crystalline salt found in bone, hydroxyapatite, is composed of phosphate and calcium.

The importance of phosphate homeostasis is illustrated by the effects of hypophosphatemia and hyperphosphatemia. Hypophosphatemia produces consequences secondary to a reduced capacity for oxygen transport by red blood cells and to disturbed energy metabolism. Hypoxia may occur due to reduced levels of 2,3-diphosphoglycerate and ATP. The derangement in energy metabolism may lead to nerve and muscle dysfunction, as manifested by irritability, confusion, numbness, coma, convulsions, muscle weakness, and respiratory and cardiac failure. Alternatively, hyperphosphatemia may lower calcium levels because increased amounts of phosphate and calcium are deposited in bone and soft tissues. Thus, symptoms of hyperphosphatemia are primarily those of hypocalcemia, such as confusion, muscle spasms, hyperreflexia, and intestinal cramping, and may progress to convulsions, tetany, and respiratory failure.

Phosphorus Homeostasis

Phosphates are found in meats, vegetables, and dairy products. Those ingested in foods are hydrolyzed in the gastrointestinal tract to form inorganic phosphate and are readily absorbed through the intestinal mucosa. Under normal conditions, the intestinal absorption of phosphate is unregulated in that the net absorption is directly proportional to the amount ingested.

The amount of phosphate released during bone resorption and taken up during bone formation is primarily dependent on mechanisms governing calcium homeostasis. That is, when the serum calcium level drops, bone is absorbed, releasing both phosphate and calcium into the extracellular fluids. When the serum calcium level rises, bone is formed, withdrawing both phosphate and calcium from body fluids. Thus, neither the intestines or the bone have specific means of controlling phosphorus levels that are based upon the body's needs.

Renal Handling of Phosphorus

The primary means of regulating phosphate within a normal range depends on the mechanisms that govern renal excretion of phosphate. More than 90% of the plasma phosphate is filterable at the glomerulus, and most of this is reabsorbed by the proximal tubule. Because phosphate is not thought to be secreted by the tubules, its renal excretion may be described by the following equation:

Phosphate Excreted = Phosphate Filtered – Phosphate Reabsorbed

Accordingly, phosphate excretion may be altered by changing the amount filtered and/or the amount reabsorbed. Under normal conditions, the renal tubules have a transport maximum of reabsorbing phosphate at about 0.1 mmol/min. When less than this is present in the glomerular filtrate, all of it is reabsorbed. When more phosphate is present, the excess is excreted. Because the maximal amount that can be reabsorbed is close to the normal filtered amount, even relatively small increases in plasma phosphate concentration can produce relatively large increases in phosphate excretion. Thus when plasma phosphate concentration increases due to an increase in phosphate intake, the filtered amount increases and the amount excreted increases.

Normally, 75% of this filtered phosphate is actively reabsorbed, mainly in the proximal tubule in co-transport with sodium. Nephron segments that are more distal display some capacity for additional phosphate reabsorption, but that capacity is very limited and has been demonstrated only in the acute absence of PTH (such as postparathyroidectomy) or with severe dietary phosphate restriction.

Regulation of phosphate reabsorption. The cellular mechanisms for phosphate reabsorption in the proximal tubule are shown in Figure 7-16. Phosphate transport across the luminal membrane is dependent upon the sodium gradient. Most of the phosphate enters the proximal tubule cell as divalent phosphate, along with two sodium. Via this mechanism, transport of divalent phosphate ($NaHPO_4^{-2}$) is electroneutral; whereas the smaller amount of transport of monovalent phosphate ($NaH_2PO_4^-$) is electrogenic. The presence of hydrogen in the luminal fluid alters this transport by inhibiting the sodium site and by decreasing the availability of divalent phosphate. Phosphate exits the tubular cell at the basolateral membrane by simple diffusion along its electrochemical gradient. It has also been proposed that phosphate exits the cell via an anion exchange mechanism, but this is uncertain. The rate-limiting event in phosphate reabsorption appears to be phosphate entry at the luminal membrane. In this model, phosphate entry is determined by the number or velocity of phos-

Figure 7-17
Magnesium transport in the thick ascending limb.

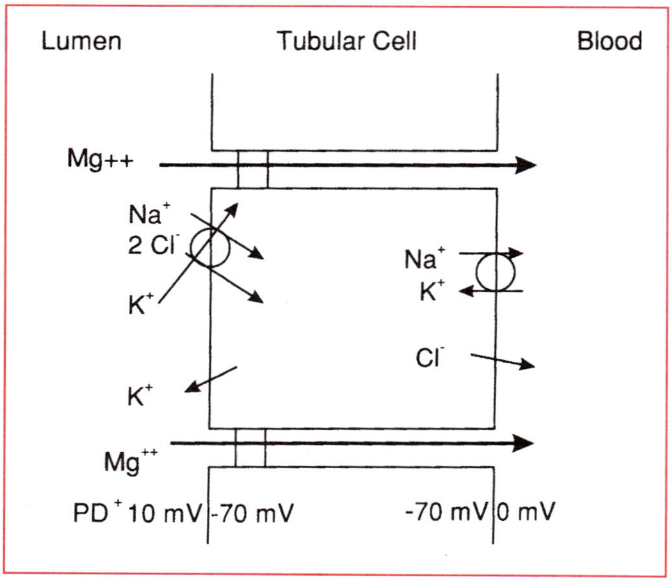

Note: From Yucha, C.B. (1993). Renal control of phosphorus and magnesium. *ANNA Journal, 20*(4), p. 449. Reprinted with permission.

In the thick ascending limb, sodium chloride transport is coupled to potassium, probably via an electroneutral $Na^+/2Cl^-/K^-$ co-transport. Selective movement of potassium back across the luminal membrane and preferential transfer of chloride across the basolateral membrane create a lumen-positive voltage. This positive voltage allows for the passive movement of magnesium through the paracellular pathway.

phate transporters located in the luminal membrane and the intensity of the inward-directed sodium gradient. Changes in the number or velocity of phosphate transporters occurs by mechanisms that modify existing transporters, insert new transporters into the luminal membrane, or delete existing transporters. This is thought to provide the physiologic basis by which phosphate excretion is regulated.

Regulation of phosphate excretion. Two major factors regulate urinary phosphate excretion, dietary adaptation, and PTH. Tubular reabsorption of phosphate changes in response to altered dietary intake. Over time, a diet low in phosphates induces an increase in the amount of phosphate reabsorbed; a diet high in phosphate reduces the amount reabsorbed. The physiologic basis for these changes in reabsorption is unknown but is not thought to be due to PTH or Vitamin D3. Since dietary adaptation changes the velocity of phosphate transport, it is likely to involve the removal of existing transporters or insertion of new transporters into the luminal membrane.

PTH also affects phosphate excretion. Whenever PTH is increased or decreased due to changes in calcium concentration, tubular phosphate reabsorption is inhibited or stimulated respectively. This phenomenon is explained if one remembers that in hypocalcemia the parathyroid gland releases PTH. PTH induces bone resorption, thereby increasing blood levels of both calcium and phosphate. Similarly, hypocalcemia stimulates activation of Vitamin D3, which enhances the intestinal absorption of both calcium and phosphate. Therefore, through its adaptive mechanisms, low calcium would produce a rise in plasma phosphate. This rise is prevented by the ability of PTH to inhibit phosphate reabsorption in the kidney, thus increasing its excretion. The major cellular action of PTH is to stimulate adenylate cyclase activity and thereby increase the production of cyclic AMP. Although cyclic AMP is known to stimulate the phosphorylation of various proteins, the mechanism by which it affects phosphate transport is unclear.

Urinary phosphate excretion is also affected by other hormonal and nonhormonal factors. Vitamin D and thyroid hormone increase phosphate reabsorption, probably by inserting new phosphate transporters into the luminal membrane. Other hormones that increase phosphate reabsorption include: somatotropin (human growth hormone), insulin, and norepinephrine. Nonhormonal factors, such as metabolic acidosis, hypercapnia, and extracellular volume expansion, decrease reabsorption, thereby increasing excretion of phosphate.

Magnesium and Its Functions

Magnesium is a major intracellular cation, being found mostly within bone (67%) and muscle (20%). Only about 2% of the magnesium in the body is found in the extracellular fluid. Plasma concentration is 1.8–2.5 mEq/L or 1.8–2.4 mg/dl, with about 20% of this bound to proteins.

Magnesium functions as a cofactor in many intracellular enzymatic reactions. While rare, hypomagnesemia increases neuromuscular excitability, producing symptoms such as behavioral changes, irritability, hyperreflexia, muscle weakness, tetany, and convulsions. Excess magnesium depresses skeletal muscle contraction and nerve function, producing nausea and vomiting, muscle weakness, hypotension, bradycardia, and respiratory depression.

Magnesium Homeostasis

Magnesium is ubiquitous in our diet and is abundant in green vegetables, seafood, grains, nuts, and meats. About 30%–40% of the dietary intake is absorbed by the gastrointestinal tract. Little is known about the mechanism of intestinal absorption, but it varies inversely with intake and does not seem to be affected by Vitamin D or PTH. Although not well understood, magnesium concentrations in the intracellular and extracellular fluid are primarily regulated by the gastrointestinal tract, the kidney, and the bone.

Renal Handling of Magnesium

With a normal dietary intake of magnesium, urinary excretion averages 100-150 mg per day. This may decrease to 10 mg per day with dietary restriction, or may increase to 600 mg per day in patients receiving magnesium-containing antacids. Thus the kidney has an excellent ability to conserve or excrete magnesium as necessary. Control of magnesium occurs primarily by filtration and tubular reabsorption, although the mechanisms involved are not yet well-defined.

Regulation of magnesium reabsorption. Seventy to 80% of the plasma magnesium is filterable. Along the length of the proximal tubule, 20%–40% of the filtered magnesium is reabsorbed. In contrast to sodium and calcium, which are reabsorbed along the proximal tubule in equivalent concentrations to plasma, tubule fluid magnesium concentration rises as a function of water abstraction. The ratio of the magnesium concentration (Mg) in tubule fluid relative to the plasma ultrafiltrate ($[TF/UF]_{Mg}$) rises along the length of the proximal tubule to a value as high as 2.0. This indicates that the proximal tubule is comparatively impermeable to magnesium.

The thick ascending limb of the loop of Henle is the principal site of magnesium reabsorption, where 50% of the filtered load is reabsorbed. In this segment, depicted in Figure 7-17, sodium chloride transport is coupled to potassium, probably via an electroneutral $Na^+/2Cl^-/K^+$ co-transport. Selective movement of potassium back across the luminal membrane and preferential transfer of chloride across the basolateral membrane accounts for the lumen-positive voltage in the thick ascending limb. This positive voltage allows for the passive movement of magnesium between the cells (through the paracellular pathway). About 70% of the magnesium reabsorption occurs through this passive mechanism. A transcellular active means of magnesium reabsorption may also exist in this segment that is able to reabsorb the remaining 20%–30%.

The distal tubule and collecting duct have a very limited role in renal magnesium conservation, reabsorbing only about 1%-2% of the filtered load. This reabsorption appears to be load dependent, but the cellular mechanisms involved are not well understood.

Regulation of magnesium excretion. No single hormone appears to regulate urinary magnesium reabsorption directly. Rather, excretion varies according to many factors such as extracellular volume and calcium and magnesium concentrations. A number of hormones, including PTH and calcitonin, also enhance magnesium reabsorption, presumably via cyclic AMP. These factors primarily affect reabsorption in the thick ascending limb.

Since transport in the thick ascending limb is dependent on sodium chloride transport and on the electrical potential, factors that alter these (for example, thiazide diuretics) also affect magnesium reabsorption. As glomerular filtration rate rises, magnesium excretion rises due to decreases in reabsorption in the proximal tubule and in the thick ascending limb.

Excretion also varies with dietary magnesium intake. With high dietary intake, reabsorption in the proximal tubule and ascending limb decrease markedly. In contrast, hypomagnesemia leads to a reduction in reabsorption in the proximal tubule corresponding to the reduction in filtered load. At the same time, the reabsorption in the thick ascending limb is enhanced, leading to excellent conservation of magnesium.

Hypercalcemia markedly increases magnesium excretion by reducing both magnesium and calcium reabsorption in the thick ascending limb. This suggests that there is some membrane interaction of calcium and magnesium in this segment. In contract, hypocalcemia decreases magnesium excretion.

Summary

In summary, the kidney is a major regulator of phosphate and magnesium levels. Phosphate reabsorption occurs primarily in the proximal tubule, driven by sodium reabsorption. Phosphate excretion is regulated by dietary adaptation and is stimulated by PTH. Magnesium reabsorption occurs predominately in the thick ascending limb, driven

Figure 7-18
Buffer pairs.

BUFFER PAIR		pKa
Proton Acceptor	Proton Donor	
$HCO_3^- + H^+ \longleftrightarrow$	$H_2CO_3 \longleftrightarrow CO_2 + H_2O$	6.1
$HPO_4^{-2} + H^+ \longleftrightarrow$	$H_2PO_4^{-1}$	6.8
$HSO_4^{-1} + H^+ \longleftrightarrow$	H_2SO_4	1.9
$NH_3 + H^+ \longleftrightarrow$	NH_4^+	9.2
Protein + $H^+ \longleftrightarrow$	Protein · H^+	varies depending on the amino acid composition of the protein

Note: From Preisig, P. (1994). Renal acidification. *ANNA Journal, 21*(5), p. 252. Reprinted with permission.

by the lumen-positive voltage. Its excretion varies with many factors. Increases in extracellular volume, dietary intake, and calcium, and use of thiazide diuretics enhance magnesium excretion.

Section 7: Renal Acidification

This section discusses renal acidification and has been divided into two major parts. The first part reviews principles of acid-base physiology, including a description of pH and hydrogen ions, buffer systems, and intracellular and extracellular buffering mechanisms. The second part deals with the renal contribution to the maintenance of pH balance, and describes (a) the reabsorption of filtered bicarbonate, (b) the regeneration of bicarbonate, (c) a description of how hydrogen ion balance is maintained over a 24-hour period, and (d) adaptations that occur in response to changes in the daily acid load.

Principles and Definitions: Acid-Base Physiology

The parameter used to define the hydrogen ion concentration of any fluid is the term pH, which is defined as the inverse log of the free hydrogen ion concentration:

$$pH = -\log [H^+]$$

Thus, hydrogen ion (H^+) concentration defines the pH of a solution. Only free hydrogen ions contribute to the measured pH. If hydrogen ions are bound to other ions (such as phosphate or bicarbonate) or proteins, and thus are not "free," they do not contribute to the measured pH. Solutes and proteins that can donate or release hydrogen ions are referred to as acids, and those that can absorb or bind hydrogen ions are referred to as bases. Another term for hydrogen ion is proton; the terms are interchangeable.

The normal plasma pH is about 7.30–7.45, meaning that the normal free hydrogen ion concen-

Figure 7-19.
The various mechanisms available to buffer an acid load, and the relative response rate of the 4 mechanisms.

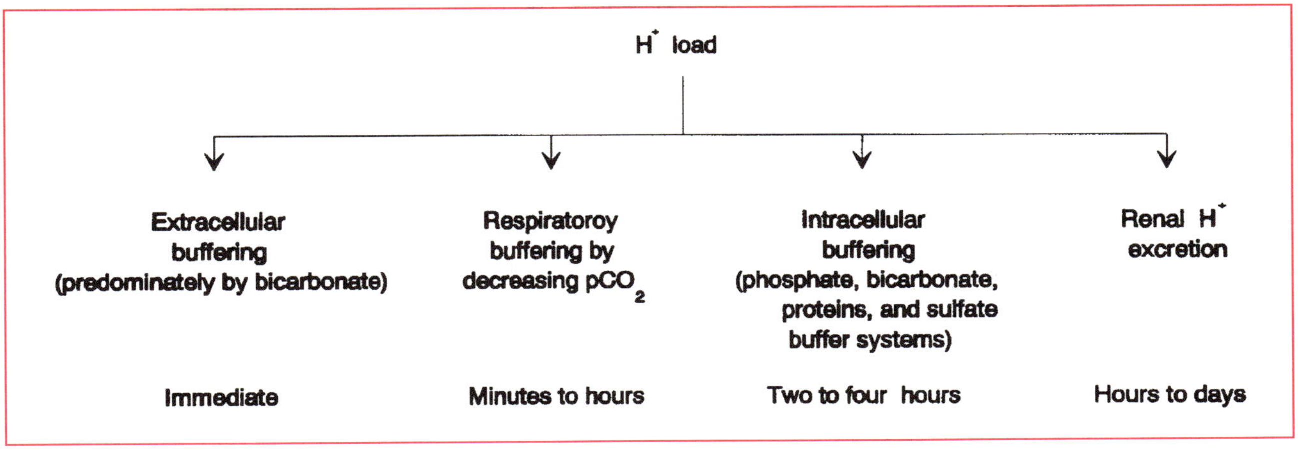

Note: From Preisig, P. (1994). Renal acidification. *ANNA Journal, 21*(5), p. 253. Reprinted with permission.

tration is 0.000045–0.000048 mEq/L. The regulatory mechanisms that will be discussed are directed toward maintaining plasma pH within this narrow range. Maintenance of a normal pH is essential because a number of physiologic processes are pH-dependent, meaning that the processes are functional and most efficient in the environment of a normal pH. Examples of pH-dependent processes are the metabolic enzymes responsible for maintaining adenosine triphosphate (ATP), or energy stores within cells, transport proteins responsible for moving substances across cell membranes, and signaling systems responsible for transmitting messages between cells or between intracellular compartments. If body pH is allowed to alter significantly in either the acid (lower pH, higher free hydrogen ion concentration), or alkaline (higher pH, lower free hydrogen ion concentration) direction, a number of physiologic processes required for life become altered and the homeostatic milieu begins to deteriorate.

The chemical systems that are responsible for maintenance of a normal pH are called buffer systems, because they "buffer" the pH and prevent it from drifting far from normal. Each buffer system is made up of two compounds, together referred to as a buffer pair. One of the members of the pair is an acid, meaning that it is capable of donating or freeing-up a proton, resulting in a lower pH. The second member of the pair is a base, meaning that it is capable of accepting or binding up a proton, resulting in a higher pH.

Figure 7-18 shows a number of buffer pairs. All the buffer systems listed, except for the ammonia system, whose primary buffering role is in the kidney and is discussed below, exist both within and outside of cells. These systems contribute to the intracellular and extracellular buffering, respectively, of the two fluid compartments. Note that each buffer system is in equilibrium, meaning that there is continual adjustment in the ratio of the acid (proton donor) to base (proton acceptor) members of the buffer pair. If the pH drops (becomes more acidic) in the environment in which the buffer exists, then the base members of the pair will accept protons, the ratio of acid:base members will increase, and the pH will increase. Conversely, if the pH increases (becomes more alkaline) in the environment in which the buffer exists, then the acid members of the pair will donate protons, the ratio of acid:base members will decrease, and the pH will decrease.

Each buffer system has an equilibrium point (pKa), defined as the pH at which 50% of the buffer members are in the acid form (capable of donating protons), and 50% are in the base form (capable of accepting protons). At this pH, the buffer system has the highest buffering potential because it has equal amounts of substrate in each form, and thus, can readily respond to either an acid or alkali load.

On the right in Figure 7-18 is the pKa for each buffer system. Note that of the systems listed, the phosphate system has a pKa closest to normal plasma pH. Thus, this is potentially the system with the greatest buffering potential for plasma. The bicarbonate system has a pKa of 6.1. Since pH is a logarithmic function of $[H^+]$, at a pH of 7.32 (normal

Figure 7-20
Bicarbonate reclamation process.

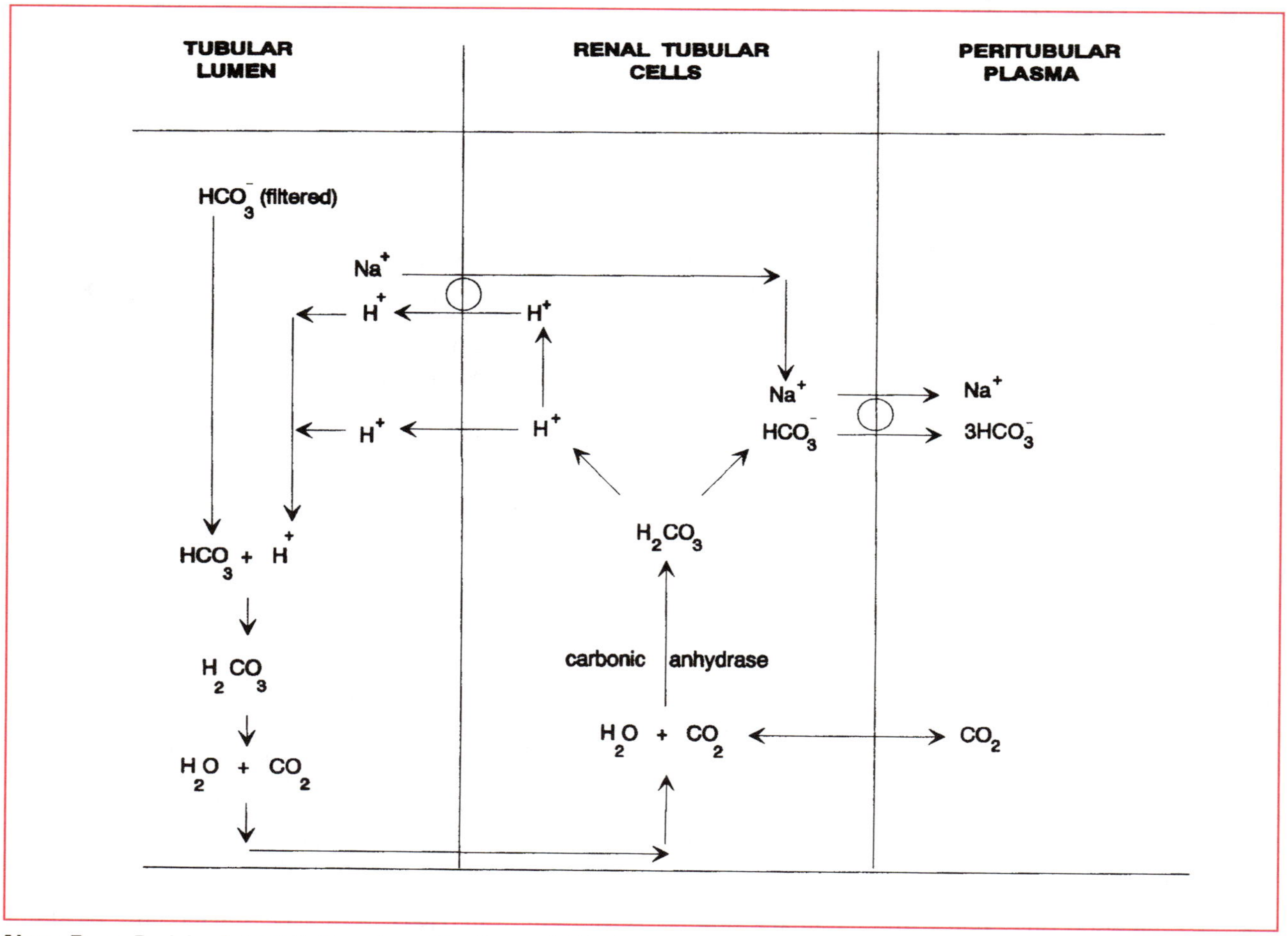

Note: From Preisig, P. (1994). Renal acidification. *ANNA Journal, 21*(5), p. 254. Reprinted with permission.

plasma pH), <10% of the members are in the acid form and >90% are in the base form. From the standpoint of balance, this is not the ideal system to defend body pH, especially in response to an alkali (hydroxyl ion) load. However, since the body is presented daily with a net acid load from metabolic processes, a buffer system with 90% of its members in the base form (capable of accepting a proton) is useful. In addition, the bicarbonate concentration is 25 mM and the phosphate concentration is around 5 mM, and thus, there is much more bicarbonate than phosphate around to contribute to the buffer pool.

Notice that the sulfate system has a pKa of 1.9, meaning that at a pH of 7.32, <0.001% of the members are in the acid form and >99.999% are in the base form. Although this system is poised to defend an acid load, it is not very versatile; it can not contribute much to the defense of an alkali load. In addition, the sulfate concentration is low, and the "supply" not well regulated. Thus, the system does not contribute much to maintaining a homeostatic environment.

The other buffer systems that play a major role in the defense of body pH are proteins. Proteins carry a large number of negative charges, some of which can readily bind hydrogen ions at physiologic pHs (7.30–7.45). Hemoglobin is one such protein. It plays an instrumental role in carrying acids (CO_2 that has been converted to a hydrogen ion and bicarbonate ion) from the peripheral tissues to the lungs, where the reaction reverses and CO_2 is expired. Other cellular and plasma proteins can also accept or donate protons and contribute significantly to the defense of body pH.

Figure 7-21.
Bicarbonate regeneration process: (A) The phosphate buffer system is entrapping the secreted proton; (B) The ammonia system is entrapping the secreted proton.

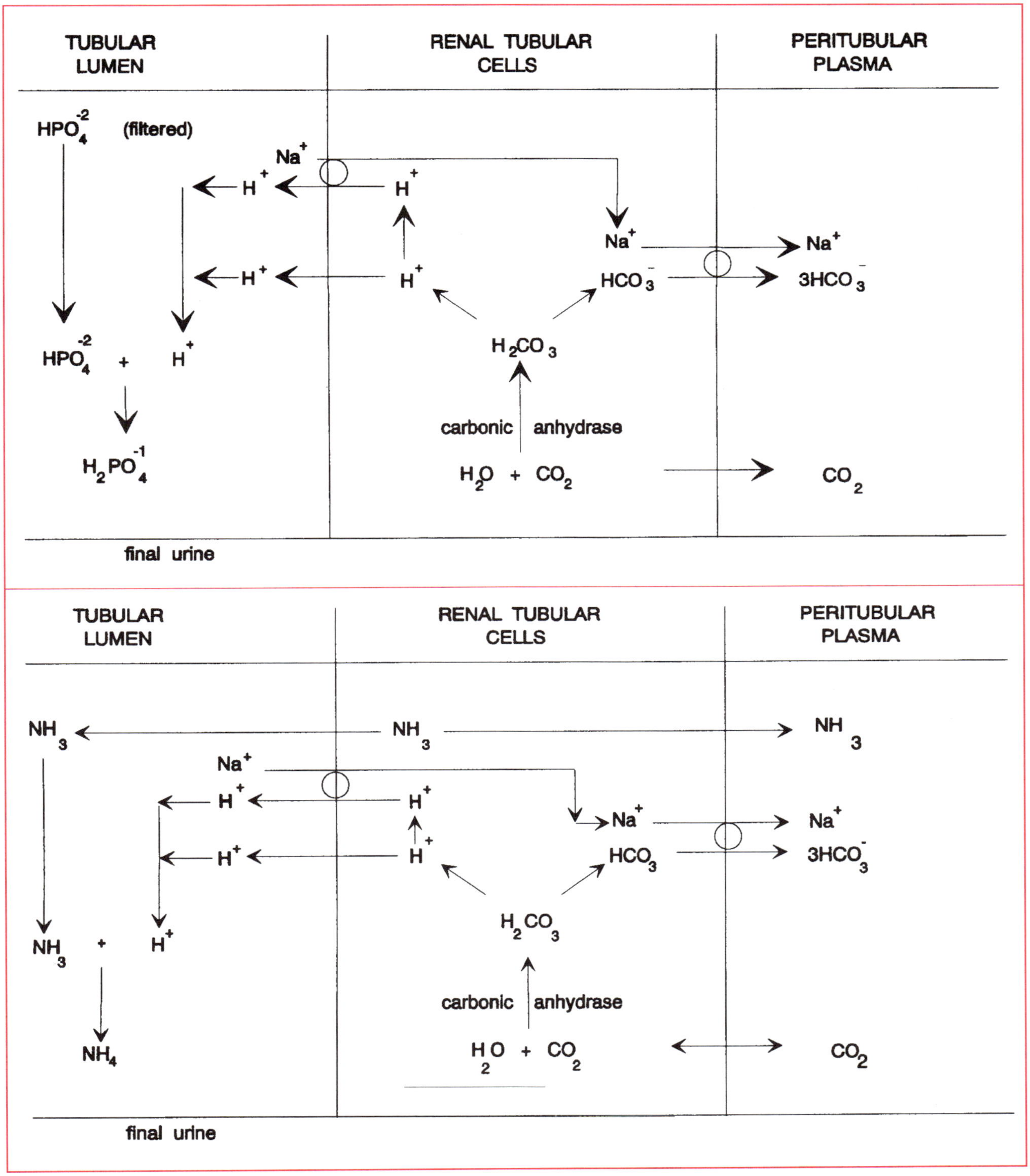

Note: From Preisig, P. (1994). Renal acidification. *ANNA Journal, 21*(5), p. 256. Reprinted with permission.

Intracellular and Extracellular Buffering Systems

Since the addition of hydrogen (acid) or hydroxyl (alkali) ions to either the intracellular or extracellular fluid will immediately change the pH if they are allowed to remain "free," there are a number of mechanisms ready to respond, ranging from ones that respond immediately to those that respond over a time span of hours-to-days. The "immediate" systems are designed to prevent minute-to-minute pH fluctuations over the course of the day in response to variations in the rate at which acidic or alkalotic compounds are added to the body fluids. The processes that take longer to respond are designed to regulate the rate of excretion of hydrogen ions from the body, and thereby replenish the buffering systems.

Thus, as seen in Figure 7-19, presented from the standpoint of an acid load, extracellular buffering (predominantly by the bicarbonate buffering system) occurs almost instantaneously when protons are added to the plasma. Second in line to respond is the respiratory system, which in response to sensing a change in plasma pH can alter respiratory rate and thereby alter plasma CO_2 in a time frame of minutes to hours. As shown in Figure 7-18, CO_2 is part of the bicarbonate buffer system. Since the members of this buffering system are all in equilibrium with each other, an increase in respiratory rate will lower plasma pCO_2 and drive the reaction to the right. This will lower free hydrogen ion concentration, and plasma pH will rise. Although the respiratory response is identified as a separate responding mechanism, this system uses the bicarbonate buffer system to provide the regulated substrate (CO_2).

Third in line of defense are the intracellular buffering systems that sometimes take a little longer to respond because of the time it takes for protons to enter the various cellular compartments. The intracellular buffering systems include the bicarbonate, phosphate, and sulfate systems, and the intracellular proteins.

The renal system regulates proton excretion on a time scale of hours-to-days. Since it takes the kidneys hours-to-days to respond to changes in acid load, body pH would fluctuate over a wide range during a 24-hour period if the buffer systems discussed above were not operating. However, although not responsible for the minute-to-minute buffering of plasma pH, the kidneys play a very important part as they are the final step in excreting protons from the body and thereby returning the net balance of protons in the body to zero.

In the steady state, for plasma pH to be maintained within a normal range over a long period of time, the rate of proton entrance into the body must equal the rate of exit from the body. The extracellular and intracellular buffering mechanisms and respiratory system that respond immediately, to within a few hours, are responsible for protecting plasma pH until the renal system is able to alter the rate of proton excretion from the body. The renal mechanisms that contribute to pH balance will be described as well as how the rate of proton excretion can be adjusted in response to changes in the rate of acid addition to the body.

The Daily Maintenance of Acid-Base Balance

The metabolism of food typical of an average diet in our culture leads to the generation of between 60 and 100 mEq of protons per day for a 70 kg person. Unless these protons are buffered, a person would become increasingly acidotic in response to normal metabolic processes. Thus, the challenge to the body each day is to buffer the acids produced from normal metabolic processes and maintain a normal pH. Similarly, if the body were faced with a daily alkali load, the base compounds would have to be buffered to prevent the individual from becoming increasingly alkalotic. The renal contribution to maintaining acid-base homeostasis from the standpoint of acid addition will be discussed, since this is the typical daily metabolic "insult" to the body.

Renal Mechanisms Involved in the Maintenance of Acid-Base Homeostasis

The kidney has two major responsibilities related to acid base balance. The first is to reabsorb any bicarbonate that is filtered at the glomerulus and return it to the plasma in order to prevent its excretion in the urine. Since bicarbonate is a small ion, it is freely filtered at the glomerulus, meaning that the bicarbonate concentration in the filtrate entering the proximal tubule is essentially equal to that in the plasma. If all of this filtered bicarbonate were excreted in the urine, the body would lose one of its first-line, predominant, extracellular and intracellular defenses against acid or alkaline loads. In fact, if all of the filtered bicarbonate were excreted, total body bicarbonate would be depleted in a matter of hours.

Bicarbonate reclamation. Bicarbonate reclamation is the process of returning filtered bicarbonate to the plasma. It occurs predominantly in the proximal tubule, with greater than 90% of filtered bicarbonate being reabsorbed before the tubular fluid enters the loop of Henle. Figure 7-20 is a schematic diagram of a renal tubule cell depicting the mechanism of bicarbonate reabsorption. On the left side of the cell is the tubular fluid; on the right side are the interstitial and peritubular capillary fluids. Bicarbonate ions are too large to be transported as such across the paracellular pathway (between the cells), and there are no transport mechanisms on the apical membrane capable of transporting bicarbonate ions as such. Therefore, the ions must be converted to some other form for transport.

As noted in the tubular fluid compartment, hydrogen (H) ions are secreted across the apical membrane (from the cell into the tubular fluid) in either a Na-independent or Na-dependent manner, where they combine with bicarbonate and are converted by the enzyme carbonic anhydrase (CA) into CO_2 and H_2O. The CO_2 readily diffuses across the apical cell membrane to the intracellular compartment. Once inside the cell, the reaction reverses and CO_2 combines with H_2O to be converted back to hydrogen (H) and bicarbonate (HCO_3) ions. The bicarbonate ion is then transported across the basolateral membrane on the Na/3HCO_3 transporter, and diffuses across the interstitium into the peritubular fluid to be returned to the systemic plasma. The generated H ion is then free to be secreted into the lumen again, and the process is repeated.

Note that this process results in the net removal of one bicarbonate ion from the tubular fluid and the addition of one bicarbonate ion to the systemic plasma, although the bicarbonate ion added to the plasma is not the "same" ion that was originally filtered at the glomerulus. While the process uses free hydrogen ions, there is no net consumption or production of hydrogen ions; the hydrogen ions merely circulate between the intracellular and tubular fluid compartments to facilitate the conversion of HCO_3 to CO_2 and H_2O, and then back to HCO_3.

Bicarbonate regeneration. The second major job the kidney has is that of bicarbonate generation. As discussed, when the bicarbonate buffer system is used, in this case to respond to an acid load, bicarbonate ions are consumed. Following addition or production of an acid, plasma bicarbonate concentration will decline as the bicarbonate molecules combine with the added protons, form carbonic acid, convert to carbon dioxide and water, and exit from the body via the respiratory system. Bicarbonate regeneration is a process that couples the excretion of protons from the body to bicarbonate generation within the kidney.

Bicarbonate generation occurs predominantly in the collecting tubule, although some occurs in earlier nephron segments. The mechanism of bicarbonate generation has many similarities to that of bicarbonate reclamation. As shown in Figure 7-21, the process again involves the secretion of protons from the intracellular to the tubular fluid compartments. This proton is generated in the cell by the combining of CO_2 and H_2O to form carbonic acid (H_2CO_3), which is then dissociated to form proton and bicarbonate ions. This process of generating intracellular protons for secretion into the luminal fluid is the same as that used in the bicarbonate reclamation process.

And as with the bicarbonate reclamation process, the bicarbonate ion formed in the cell is transported across the basolateral membrane, ultimately to be returned to the peritubular fluid and systemic circulation. The proton that is secreted into the tubular fluid combines with a base molecule, predominantly ammonia (NH_3) or dibasic phosphate (HPO_4^{-2}), forming either ammonium ($NH4^+$) or monobasic phosphate ($H_2PO_4^{-1}$), respectively. These acid forms of their respective buffer systems are then excreted in the urine. Thus, the major difference between the bicarbonate reclamation and generation processes is that the secreted proton is not excreted in the reclamation process but is excreted in the regeneration process.

It is necessary for the secreted protons to be coupled to another ion to be excreted because protons that remain "free" in the tubular fluid have the same effect on tubular fluid pH as do protons that remain "free" in the systemic plasma: the higher the free hydrogen ion concentration, the lower the pH. Due to the effects of tubular fluid pH on the ability of nephron segments to secrete protons, net proton secretion does not occur when tubular fluid pH is lower than about pH 4.0. At this point, the rate of proton secretion into the luminal fluid is balanced by the rate of proton reabsorption, so that net proton movement is zero.

The pH of the glomerular filtrate is about 7.3, essentially the same as plasma pH, and thus the free hydrogen ion concentration is 0.000050 mEq/L. At the limiting pH of 4.0, free hydrogen ion concentration will be 0.1 mEq/L. The difference between these two values is 0.09995 mEq/L. Thus, if secreted protons were not buffered within the tubular fluid, the maximum number of protons that could be excreted per day would be 0.09995 mEq, assuming a daily urine output of 1 liter. Clearly, this rate is insufficient to balance the daily addition of at least 60 mEq/day.

Maintenance of Systemic Acid-Base Balance

Systemic acid-base homeostasis will be maintained only when the net balance of protons is zero, which can be accomplished only when all protons added to the body are removed. Remember that when a proton is buffered by being picked up by one of the buffer systems, the pH is protected, but from a homeostatic standpoint, things are not the same because a buffer system has been disturbed. Thus, acid-base homeostasis is not solely defined by the pH, but also by the balance between the acid and base forms of each buffer system. The renal bicarbonate regeneration process is the primary mechanism responsible for maintaining the balance between the acid and base forms of the bicarbonate buffer system. When this system buffers a proton, a HCO_3 ion is consumed and is effectively lost from the body (since the CO_2 molecule that is generated is excreted from the body by the respiratory system). Then when the kidney regenerates a bicarbonate ion, the base molecule of the buffer system is replenished, and homeostasis is reestablished.

Adaptations to Changes in the Magnitude of Daily Acid Load

Although the typical daily acid-base insult to the body is a metabolic acid load, the magnitude of the acid load can vary widely depending on the composition of the diet. This variation in acid load will consume varying amounts of the base members

Table 7-1.
Normal routes for water and NaCl gain.

Intake	Water (ml/day)	NaCl (g/day)
Fluid	1200	
Food	1000	10.50
Metabolism	350	
Total	**2550**	**10.50**
Output		
Insensible (skin & lungs)	900	
Sweat	50	0.25
Feces	100	0.25
Urine	1500	10.00
Total	**2550**	**10.50**

of the buffer systems, and from the standpoint of the kidney, will place varying demands on the kidney for the amount of bicarbonate that must be generated daily.

As described above, bicarbonate generation is coupled and dependent on proton excretion, and predominantly uses both phosphate and ammonia as vehicles for entrapping the protons and ensuring their excretion. In an average American diet, of the 60 mEq of hydrogen that are excreted each day, 20 mEq are entrapped by phosphate and a small amount of sulfate, and 40 mEq are entrapped by ammonia. In a severe acidosis, these values can increase to about 80 mEq/day for phosphate and sulfate and 500 mEq/day for ammonia. Thus, our ability to respond to wide variations in the need to excrete acid resides predominantly in the kidneys' ability to provide varying amounts of ammonia on demand. Note in Figure 7-18 that the pKa of the ammonia system is 9.2. At a tubular fluid pH of 7.3, 99/100 synthesized and secreted ammonia (NH_3) molecules will exist as ammonium (NH_4^+). At a lower tubular fluid pH, essentially all synthesized and secreted ammonia has picked up a proton. Thus, this system is especially well poised to trap secreted protons within the tubular fluid.

Ammonia is produced by the proximal tubule cells, and its generation is regulated by enzymes whose activities are modified by the pH in the surrounding environment. Thus, when faced with a large acid load, more ammonia is produced, more secreted protons are entrapped by ammonia, and more bicarbonate is regenerated to replenish the extracellular and intracellular stores that were consumed in protecting plasma pH until the hydrogen ion was trapped in the tubular fluid. And visa versa, when faced with an alkaline load, less ammonia is produced, fewer secreted protons are entrapped by ammonia, and less bicarbonate is generated. The hour-to-hour monitoring of body pH allows renal ammonia production to be tightly regulated, and a homeostatic pH environment maintained.

Summary

The maintenance of a homeostatic pH environment is essential for normal functioning of most physiologic processes. In an attempt to achieve this goal, the body has both rapid responding and short-term approaches, along with slower responding and long-term mechanisms that each play a critical role in maintaining pH within a narrow range.

Section 8: Renal Regulation of Extracellular Fluid Volume and Osmolality

To function properly, cells in the body require an internal environment made up of the correct osmolality, ionic composition, pH, and temperature. This internal environment is maintained by the cardiovascular and renal systems. Together, along with neural and endocrine input, these two systems maintain fluid and electrolyte balance within narrow limits suitable for optimal cell function. This section describes the mechanisms by which the extracellular fluid (ECF) volume and osmolality are controlled.

The underlying goal in fluid and electrolyte homeostasis is to obtain and conserve the water and solutes necessary to maintain the constancy of the internal environment. Paramount in the control of the internal milieu is the regulation of sodium and water as they relate to extracellular fluid volume and osmolality. The osmolality is set by the ratio of solute to water so that controlling either the amount of solute or water can set the extracellular osmolality to the optimal level. The osmolality and ionic composition of extracellular fluid are controlled within very narrow limits, as illustrated by the observation that a rise in body osmolality of 1% to 2% results in a conscious desire to drink and near maximal renal water conservation.

Body Requirements for Sodium and Water

Table 7-1 shows the typical routes of water gain and loss in adults in steady state. The majority of water comes from fluid and food intake. In addition, a small amount of water is produced as a result of metabolic processes, primarily the metabolism of carbohydrates. Water loss is primarily in the form of urine. In addition, a sizable, insensible component of fluid loss occurs through evaporation from the skin and respiratory tract. This can be significantly augmented by evaporative loss from the skin in environments that induce sweating for thermal regulation. There is also a small fecal water loss. The major ways that fluid balance is con-

Table 7-2.
Major determinants of sodium and water excretion.

Net Effect	Stimulus	Modification of Signaling Pathway	Modification of Renal Response
↓Na & H_2O excretion	↓plasma volume	↓stimulation of extrarenal baroreceptors → ↑renal sympathetic nerve activity → afferent & efferent arteriole constriction	↓ RBF & GFR
		↓stimulation of intrarenal baroreceptors → ↑renin → ↑angiotensin II → ↑aldosterone	↑ Na & H_2O reabsorption
		↓stimulation of intrarenal baroreceptors → ↑renin → ↑angiotensin II → vasoconstriction	↓ GFR
		↓atrial distention → ↓release of ANH	↓ GFR ↑ Na & H_2O reabsorption
	↓ plasma volume + ↑ plasma osmolality	↑ ADH	↑ H_2O reabsorption
↑ Na & H_2O excretion	↑ plasma volume	stimulation of extrarenal baroreceptors → ↓ renal sympathetic nerve activity → afferent & efferent arteriole dilation	↑ RBF & GFR
		stimulation of intrarenal baroreceptors → ↓ renin → ↓ angiotensin II → ↓ aldosterone	↓ Na & H_2O reabsorption
		stimulation of intrarenal baroreceptors → ↓ renin → ↓ angiotensin II → vasodilation	↑ GFR
		atrial distention → ↓ release of ANH	↑ GFR ↓ Na & H_2O reabsorption
	↑ plasma volume + ↓ plasma osmolality	↓ ADH	↓ H_2O reabsorption

trolled and maintained are through fluid intake (stimulated by thirst) and urine output.

Table 7-1 also shows the normal routes for the intake and output of sodium chloride (NaCl). The majority of sodium (Na^+) and chloride (Cl^-) intake, which averages 10.5 grams per day, is through food ingestion. Sodium balance is controlled primarily by renal excretion of Na^+ and Cl^-. Since sweat is normally hypotonic, sodium chloride loss via this route is modest except in situations that produce copious sweating.

Homeostatic Control of Sodium and Water

Renal control and excretion of sodium, chloride, and water (H_2O) are the most important contributors to the control of ECF volume and osmolality. There is no minimum requirement for sodium intake to maintain extracellular fluid homeostasis unless there are significant changes in body water osmolality that result from Na^+ losses. In contrast, there is an obligatory water loss, and thus an obligatory water intake, to allow excretion of the daily waste products (e.g., urea, sulfates, and phosphates) that are produced. The typical daily production of these waste products requires a urine volume of at least 400-500 ml/day with a maximal osmolality of 1400 mOsm/L to allow for excretion.

The renal regulation of total body sodium simultaneously achieves regulation of extracellular fluid volume. This is because sodium is essentially an extracellular solute so that changes in total body sodium are accompanied by virtually identical changes in the extracellular sodium. Since sodium and its associated anions account for more than 90% of all osmotically active ECF solutes, the amount of sodium in the ECF is the major determinant of the ECF volume. Thus ECF and plasma volume normally change in the same direction as total body sodium. Plasma volume, in turn, is a major determinant of cardiovascular pressures, which control total body sodium by acting directly on the kidneys and by stimulating reflexes that alter sodi-

Figure 7-22.
The major determinants of sodium and water excretion.

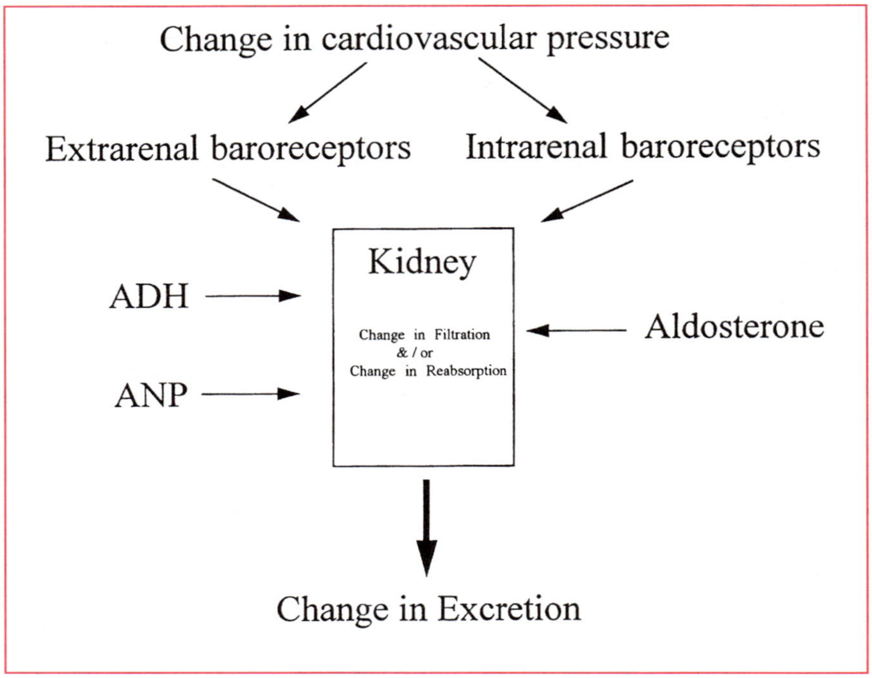

Note: From Yucha, C., & Keen, M. (1996). Renal regulation of extracellular fluid volume and osmolality. *ANNA Journal, 23*(5), p. 489. Reprinted with permission.

Neural and hormonal signals are integrated by the kidney, which alters filtration and reabsorption. This results in changes in sodium and water excretion.

um and water excretion. The regulation of sodium and water excretion is highly complex with many interactions among neurological and hormonal stimuli. The major determinants of sodium and water excretion are depicted in Figure 7-22 and outlined in Table 7-2, but are described more fully in the text.

Control of sodium filtration. The kidneys play the major role in the maintenance of body sodium and water content. Because they are small and not bound to protein, sodium, chloride, and water are all freely filtered at the glomerulus and undergo reabsorption throughout most of the nephron. Since sodium is not also secreted, the amount that is finally excreted depends on filtration and reabsorption alone:

$$\text{amount } Na^+ \text{ excreted} = \text{amount } Na^+ \text{ filtered} - \text{amount } Na^+ \text{ reabsorbed}$$

The amount of Na^+ that is filtered is equal to the glomerular filtration rate (GFR) times the plasma concentration of sodium (PNa^+). It is theoretically possible then to alter sodium excretion by altering GFR, PNa^+, and/or sodium reabsorption. Under normal conditions the plasma concentration of sodium does not change much and therefore contributes little to the regulation of sodium excretion. On the other hand, sodium reabsorption and GFR are controlled by two major types of sensors, extarenal baroreceptors and intrarenal baroreceptors, specifically the renal juxtaglomerular apparatus (JGA) and the macula densa. A rise in cardiovascular pressures (secondary to increased plasma volume, for example) stimulates extrarenal baroreceptors, which decreases the activity of renal sympathetic nerves resulting in vasodilation of afferent and efferent arterioles. Dilation of the renal arterioles allows renal blood flow (RBF) to increase, leading to a reduction in the normal rise of osmotic pressure along the glomerular capillary. The decreased osmotic pressure contributes to a higher net filtration pressure and consequently an increase in GFR.

At the same time, increased vascular pressure within the kidneys stimulates intrarenal baroreceptors, decreasing renin secretion and angiotensin II. This also contributes to the vasodilation of the afferent and efferent arterioles, supporting the rise in GFR (and rise in the amount of sodium filtered). In contrast, reduced stimulation of extrarenal and intrarenal baroreceptors leads to constriction of afferent and efferent arterioles and a reduction in renal blood flow. This results in a faster rise of osmotic pressure, which leads to the achievement of filtration pressure equilibrium prior to the efferent end of the glomerular capillary bed. The consequence of this is that glomerular filtration stops earlier in the capillary bed, resulting in a reduction in GFR (and fall in the amount of sodium filtered). These effects have been described in greater detail in an earlier section of this chapter that deals with glomerular filtration.

A last contributor to GFR is arterial oncotic pressure (the pressure due to protein concentration). As the protein concentration rises, secondary to severe sweating for example, the GFR decreases; as the protein becomes less concentrated, the GFR increases. These changes have the effect of decreasing or increasing sodium and water excretion respectively, thereby correcting the initial change in oncotic pressure.

Control of sodium reabsorption. Changes in tubular sodium reabsorption have a greater effect on sodium excretion than do changes in the amount of sodium filtered. This is because the changes in GFR are small and these changes automatically induce proportional changes in sodium reabsorption by the proximal tubule, a phenomenon known as glomerulotubular balance. That is, if GFR is decreased by 25%, the rate of sodium reabsorption also decreases by close to 25% in the proximal tubule. Glomerulotubular balance is explained in part by the fact that sodium reabsorption in the proximal tubule is by co-transport with glucose, amino acids, and other substances.

Homeostatic control of sodium excretion is achieved via changes in sodium reabsorption in the late distal and collecting tubules. This requires some explanation since more than 90% of the filtered sodium is reabsorbed before the filtrate even reaches these nephron segments. Aldosterone is the single most important controller of sodium excretion, despite the fact that only 2% of the total filtered sodium is dependent on it for reabsorption. Although this seems small, it is actually quite large because of the huge volume of sodium that is filtered. Each day, the total filtered sodium is equal to the GFR times the concentration of sodium in the plasma. This equals approximately 180 L/day times 145 mmol/L, or 26,100 mmol of sodium each day. Aldosterone controls the reabsorption of 2% of this or 522/mmol/day. This amounts to approximately 30 g NaCl per day or three times more than the average NaCl intake (see Table 7-1).

Aldosterone is secreted by the adrenal cortex in response to ACTH (adrenocorticotropic hormone released from the anterior pituitary gland), high levels of potassium, and angiotensin II. The latter stimulator of aldosterone is the most important in regard to sodium-regulating reflexes and is mediated by the renin-angiotensin system. Those factors that regulate renin secretion (intrarenal baroreceptors, the macula densa, and the renal sympathetic nerves) also regulate aldosterone secretion. In response to low plasma volume (due to low sodium intake or hemorrhage, for example), the kidney releases renin. Renin is a proteolytic enzyme that catalyzes the splitting of a decapeptide (angiotensin I) from a plasma protein known as angiotensinogen, which is produced mainly by the liver and is present in the plasma in high concentration. Next, the terminal two amino acids are split from the relatively inactive angiotensin I to yield the highly active octapeptide angiotensin II. This is catalyzed by angiotensin converting enzyme (ACE), found primarily within the pulmonary capillaries.

Although angiotensin II acts directly on the tubular cells to stimulate sodium reabsorption, it has two major additional effects: (a) it causes vasoconstriction, thereby raising blood pressure; and (b) it stimulates the release of aldosterone from the adrenal cortex. Aldosterone travels via the blood stream to the late distal tubule and collecting ducts. Being a fat-soluble steroid, aldosterone enters the cells where it combines with intracellular receptors and stimulates the synthesis of mRNA within the cell nucleus. The mRNA mediates translation of specific proteins that increase the activity and/or number of the luminal membrane sodium channels and basolateral membrane Na^+/K^+ ATPase pumps. These proteins cause more Na^+ to be reabsorbed and more K^+ to be secreted. In contrast, ingestion of a high sodium diet results in a reduction of renin secretion, plasma angiotensin II, and aldosterone secretion. Ultimately sodium and water excretion increase.

In addition to stimulating renin secretion, the renal sympathetic nerves stimulate sodium reabsorption by directly acting on proximal tubular cells. When impulses traveling through these nerves are very high, afferent and efferent arteriolar constriction occurs, resulting in a decrease in renal blood flow and GFR. Ultimately, proximal sodium reabsorption rises. The resulting decrease in fluid delivered to the macula densa is accompanied by decreased sodium and chloride concentrations in the macula densa lumen and decreased NaCl reabsorption by the macula densa cells. While the pathway by which this occurs is unclear, the decreased reabsorption by the macula densa stimulates renin secretion. The rise in renin ultimately results in vasoconstriction (due to angiotensin II) and increased sodium reabsorption (due to aldosterone). Conversely, when flow, and hence, NaCl concentration in the macula densa are high, renin secretion is inhibited.

Another hormone affecting sodium reabsorption is atrial natriuretic hormone (ANH), also known as atrial natriuretic peptide (ANP), atrial natriuretic factor (ANF), or atriopeptin. ANH is secreted from the cells in the cardiac atria in response to distention of the atria, secondary to plasma volume expansion. Its ultimate effects are opposite to those of aldosterone, inhibiting sodium reabsorption, and therefore water reabsorption.

ANH acts directly on the medullary collecting ducts and indirectly on other tubular segments (by inhibiting several steps in the renin-angiotensin-aldosterone pathway) to inhibit sodium reabsorption. It inhibits renin secretion and aldosterone secretion, and causes an increase in GFR (via its effects on the renal arterioles), all of which increase sodium and water excretion.

Other hormones also influence sodium reabsorption, but are not reflexly controlled specifically for the homeostatic regulation of sodium balance. Cortisol, estrogen, growth hormone, thyroid hormone, and insulin all increase sodium reabsorption. In contrast, glucagon, progesterone, and parathyroid hormone decrease sodium reabsorption.

Control of water excretion. Like sodium, water excretion is the difference between the amount filtered and the amount reabsorbed. Similarly, the baroreceptor-initiated reflexes controlling GFR have the same effects on water filtration as on sodium filtration described earlier, so that the major regulated determinant of water excretion is the rate of water reabsorption. Changes in ECF volume simultaneously elicit reflex changes in the excretion of both sodium and water. This works well since alterations in ECF volume are normally associated with loss or gain of sodium and water in approximately proportional amounts.

In situations whereby total body water increases without a proportional rise in total body sodium, the kidneys must be able to increase water excretion without increasing sodium excretion. This is permitted by antidiuretic hormone (ADH or vasopressin). The ADH secreting hypothalamic cells receive two inputs, from baroreceptors and from osmoreceptors. An increase in plasma volume accompanied by a decrease in osmolality inhibits ADH secretion, while a decrease in plasma volume accompanied by an increase in osmolality increases ADH secretion (see Table 7-2). In other cases, baroreceptor and osmoreceptor inputs oppose each other, if, for example, volume and osmolality are both decreased. Such situations wherein water and sodium balance are dissociated from one another occur in clinical conditions (e.g., diabetes insipidus) and will not be discussed here.

ADH is made by the hypothalamus and is stored and released by the posterior pituitary gland. It acts on principal cells within the late distal tubule and the cortical and medullary collecting ducts and markedly increases the water permeability of the luminal membrane. Receptors located in the basolateral membrane bind ADH, eliciting a second messenger that leads to the insertion of protein channels in the luminal membrane through which water can move. ADH also increases sodium reabsorption by the cortical collecting duct, appearing to synergize the effect of aldosterone in this segment. If high enough concentrations of ADH result, ADH exerts direct vasoconstrictor effects on arteriolar smooth muscle, resulting in a rise in blood pressure. Concurrent constriction of renal arterioles and mesangial cells in the glomerular membrane lowers GFR, also promoting sodium and water retention.

As shown in Table 7-1, homeostatic balance of salt and water may also be affected by altering the intake of these substances. The centers that mediate thirst are located in the hypothalamus and are stimulated by reduced plasma volume and increased body fluid osmolality (the same stimuli that increase ADH secretion). Although salt craving does occur in humans who are severely salt depleted, its contribution to sodium homeostasis is probably minimal since the typical American diet contains 20 times the amount of salt needed daily.

General Renal Reabsorptive Mechanisms

Alterations in reabsorption are the primary renal mechanism for regulation of sodium and water. The magnitude of sodium and water reabsorption can be appreciated in that approximately 180 liters of water and 630 grams of sodium are filtered per day by the kidney. In spite of this impressive filtered load, only about 0.5% to 1.0% of the filtered amounts are normally excreted in the urine.

Several pathways exist for the movement of ions and water between the tubule and the peritubular capillaries. One route is the transcellular pathway in which a solute must traverse through the epithelial cells lining the tubules, moving through both the luminal and basolateral membranes. Transcellular ionic movement generally requires the expenditure of energy. Another transport route is the paracellular pathway, between or around cells through cellular junctional complexes and lateral intercellular spaces. Ionic movement via the paracellular pathway occurs passively by diffusion along chemical and/or electrical gradients. The permeability of the junctional complexes varies among nephron segments. In those nephron sites where the permeability of the junctional complexes is high, the paracellular movement of solute may dissipate the concentration gradients between the tubular lumen and the interstitium. In contrast, in tubule segments with low permeability of the junctional complexes, large solute concentration differences may be generated between the lumen, tubular cells, and the capillaries.

In general, primary active transport of sodium provides the energy for subsequent reabsorption of chloride and water. The Na^+/K^+ ATPase pumps found on the basolateral membrane of all tubular segments are the primary active transport mechanism. Using ATP, they work diligently to exclude Na^+ from the cell while bringing K^+ into the cell. The low intracellular sodium provides the driving force for Na^+ movement across the luminal (apical) membrane. Depending on the tubular segment, the

Figure 7-23.
Sodium and chloride reabsorption in the early proximal tubule.

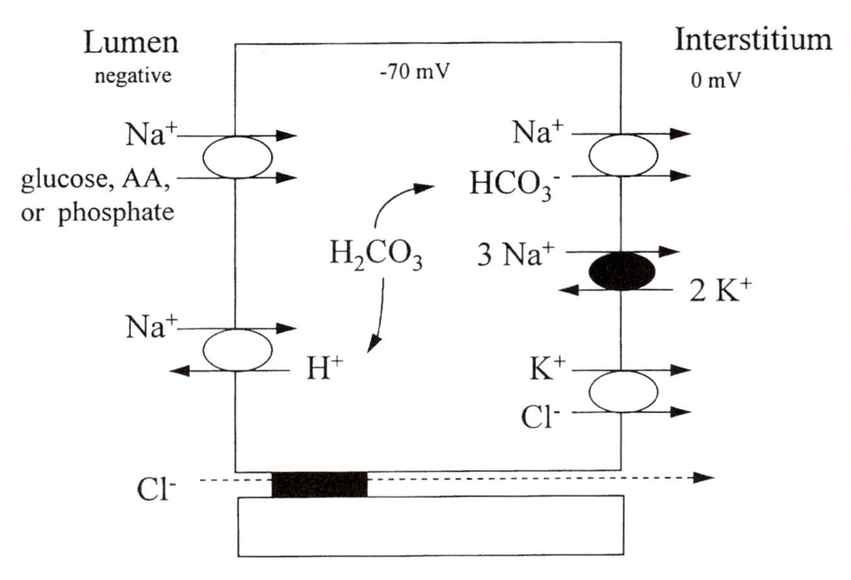

In the early proximal tubule, the lumen is negative with respect to the interstitium. Figures 7-23 through 7-26 are adapted with permission from Vander, A.J. (1995). *Renal physiology* (5th edition) (Figure 6-1, page 93). St Louis: McGraw-Hill, Inc. Filled ovals represent carriers requiring ATP (primary active transport); unfilled ovals represent carriers not requiring ATP directly, but driven by chemical or electrical gradients; dashed lines represent passive diffusion. Unless otherwise noted, all transporters transport one ion.

Note: From Yucha, C., & Keen, M. (1996). Renal regulation of extracellular fluid volume and osmolality. *ANNA Journal, 23*(5), p. 492. Reprinted with permission.

movement of Na^+ down this concentration gradient into the cell may be as a sodium ion alone, in cotransport with other organic substances such as amino acids and glucose or ions such as chloride, or in a countertransport mechanism with ions such as hydrogen. Transporters that do not require ATP directly, but are driven by the extracellular to intracellular sodium concentration gradient, are called secondary active transporters.

The mechanisms by which Na^+ reabsorption drives reabsorption of other substances are varied. The loss of Na^+ from the tubular lumen decreases the osmolality of the tubular fluid while increasing the intracellular osmolality. Depending on the water permeability, water crosses the luminal membrane to restore osmotic equilibrium between these two compartments. Movement of water out of the lumen concentrates other intraluminal substances such as urea, allowing these substances to diffuse out of the lumen along their concentration gradients. In some nephron segments, such as the collecting duct, water permeability is under hormonal control and varies according to the body's osmolality. This reabsorption of water into the peritubular capillaries is dependent upon the presence of ADH and the hypertonic medullary interstitium, as described in an earlier section of this chapter that deals with urinary concentration and dilution.

Similarly, chloride reabsorption occurs passively as a consequence of chemical and/or electrical concentration gradients between the tubular lumen, tubular cells, and the peritubular capillaries. The movement of sodium from the tubular lumen to the cell leads to the development of a lumen-negative transtubular potential difference (PD) that drives Cl^- movement. In addition, water reabsorption from the tubular lumen increases the luminal Cl^- concentration, which establishes a chemical gradient favoring Cl^- movement. In many segments, Cl^- diffuses passively via the paracellular pathway driven by both chemical and electrical gradients established secondary to the active reabsorption of sodium.

Specific Tubular Reabsorptive Mechanisms

The actual transport mechanisms differ among the various nephron segments. The segments of primary interest in sodium, chloride, and water reabsorption are the proximal tubule, the loop of Henle, the late distal tubule, and the collecting ducts.

Proximal tubule. Over the course of the convoluted and straight portions of the proximal tubules, approximately 65% of filtered Na^+, Cl, and water is reabsorbed. The large reabsorptive capacity is facilitated by the high permeability of the junctional complexes. As shown in Figure 7-23, the active movement of 3 Na^+ and 2 K^+ across the basolateral membrane by the Na^+/K^+ ATPase pump creates both a chemical gradient and an electrical gradient that

Figure 7-24.
Sodium and chloride reabsorption in the thick ascending limb of Henle.

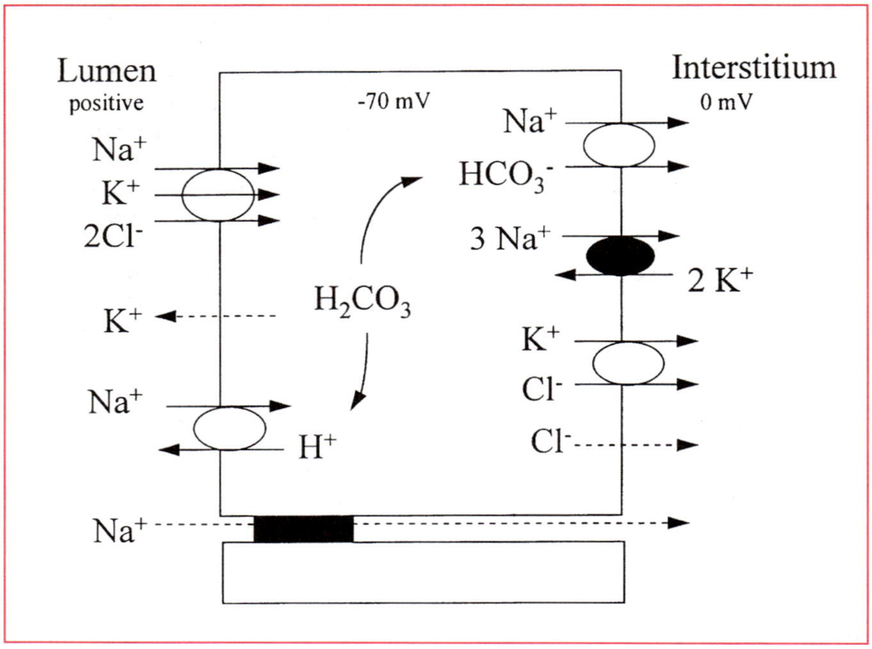

Note that the lumen is positive with respect to the interstitium. This is because potassium rapidly diffuses back into the lumen driven by the chemical gradient.

Note: From Yucha, C., & Keen, M. (1996). Renal regulation of extracellular fluid volume and osmolality. *ANNA Journal, 23*(5), p. 493. Reprinted with permission.

provide the energy needed to move Na^+ across the luminal membrane. The luminal entry of sodium requires various carriers that transport sodium coupled or in countertransport with other solutes across the luminal membrane.

In the early proximal tubule, Na^+ leaves the lumen in co-transport with phosphate or organic solutes such as amino acids and glucose. As a result, the luminal concentration of these solutes decreases, and the intracellular concentration increases. These solutes then diffuse passively across the basolateral membrane into the peritubular capillaries. In this segment, the transcellular transport rates of sodium and chloride are quite high, but because the paracellular pathway is highly permeable to water, high sodium and chloride concentration gradients between the lumen and the interstitium are not generated.

Although there is some transport of Cl^- that occurs via anion countertransport in the luminal membrane (not depicted in Figure 7-23) and co-transport with potassium across the basolateral membrane, most Cl^- is passively reabsorbed via the paracellular pathway secondary to the chemical and electrical gradients established by Na^+ movement. Luminal Cl^- concentration increases because water is reabsorbed along the proximal tubule. The loss of Na^+ from the luminal fluid leads to a lumen negative potential difference. The chemical and electrical gradients allow Cl^- to diffuse out of the lumen and into the interstitial space.

In the proximal tubule, Na^+ also crosses the luminal membrane in countertransport with hydrogen ion (H^+), thereby exchanging electropositive ions. The dissociation of H_2CO_3 within the proximal cells and subsequent movement of H^+ into the lumen, enhances the secondary active reabsorption of bicarbonate in co-transport with sodium across the basolateral membrane. Thus bicarbonate reabsorption is mostly sodium-coupled. (See the preceding section of this chapter for information on renal acidification).

As a result of the tightly coupled reabsorption of sodium, chloride, and water over the course of the proximal tubule, tubular fluid undergoes little change in Na^+ concentration or osmolality. Luminal fluid bicarbonate concentration decreases to about 20% of filtered concentration, and glucose falls to zero. In the presence of osmotic agents such as mannitol or high glucose concentration in the tubular fluid (often seen in patients with diabetes mellitus), water reabsorption may be sharply reduced, which leads to an osmotic diuresis. This situation can also lead to renal excretion of large quantities of Na^+ and Cl^- because the retardation of water reabsorption leads to a drop in luminal Na^+ concentra-

Figure 7-25.
Sodium and chloride reabsorption in the early distal tubule.

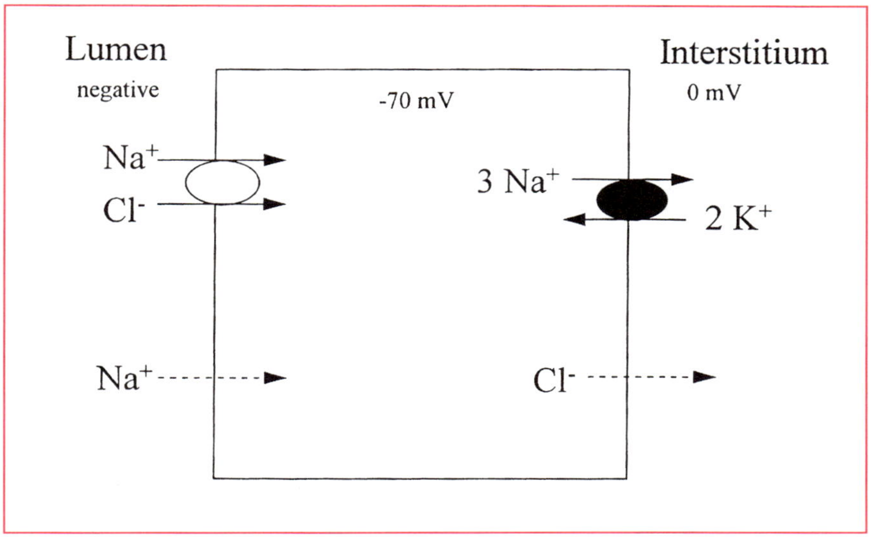

The lumen is negative with respect to the interstitium. Source and symbols as described for Figure 7-23.

Note: From Yucha, C., & Keen, M. (1996). Renal regulation of extracellular fluid volume and osmolality. *ANNA Journal, 23*(5), p. 493. Reprinted with permission.

tion, creating a concentration gradient favoring net diffusion of sodium into the tubular lumen and subsequent excretion.

Loop of Henle. The loop of Henle consists of several segments including the thin descending limb, the thin ascending limb of Henle, and the thick ascending limb. Together these segments reabsorb approximately 25% of filtered Na^+ and Cl^- and about 15% of filtered water. The individual segments have important differences in Na^+ and water reabsorption. At the beginning of the thin descending limb where the tubular fluid has an osmolality of 300 mOsm/L, the interstitial osmolality is maintained at approximately 400 mOsm/L. At the tip of the loop, the interstitial osmolality may be as high as 1200 mOsm/L. The interstitial gradient is established by Na^+ and Cl^- reabsorption in the ascending limb of the loop and the reabsorption of urea in the collecting ducts. Because the thin descending limb is highly permeable to water and relatively impermeable to Na^+ and Cl^-, water moves out of the lumen into the hypertonic medullary interstitium. As a consequence, there is an increase in tubular fluid Na^+ and Cl^- and urea concentrations as the tubular fluid travels through the descending limb.

In contrast, the thin and thick ascending limbs are highly permeable to Na^+ and Cl^- while being impermeable to water. Na^+ and Cl^- are reabsorbed, contributing to the hypertonic medullary interstitium, and the tubular fluid becomes more dilute because water is not able to follow.

As tubular fluid moves into the thick ascending limb, more Na^+ and Cl^- than water have been reabsorbed, leading to a relatively lower ion concentration and osmolality compared to plasma. As shown in Figure 7-24, Na^+ is moved across the basolateral membrane by the Na^+/K^+ ATPase pump and in co-transport with HCO_3^-. Chloride moves out of the tubular cells into the interstitium in co-transport with potassium and via diffusion. The resulting low intracellular concentrations of sodium and chloride drive a luminal membrane carrier, known as a $Na^+/K^+/2Cl^-$ co-transporter. Diffusion of potassium back across the luminal membrane (driven by the concentration gradient between the cell and the lumen) creates a lumen-positive PD. The positive voltage favors passive sodium movement through paracellular pathways. In addition, this segment contains luminal Na^+/H^+ countertransport as previously described in the proximal tubule.

By the end of the ascending limb of the loop of Henle, 90% of filtered Na^+ and Cl^- and 80% of filtered water have been reabsorbed. Under normal homeostatic conditions, Na^+ and Cl^- reabsorption continues until the final urine contains less than 1% of the filtered Na^+ and Cl^-. However, the actual Na^+ and Cl^- reabsorption is under the physiologic control of aldosterone and varies as a function of the body's salt balance.

Early distal tubule. Although the early distal convoluted tubule also serves as a diluting segment, some of the transporters differ from those in the

Figure 7-26.
Sodium and chloride reabsorption in the late distal tubule and collecting ducts.

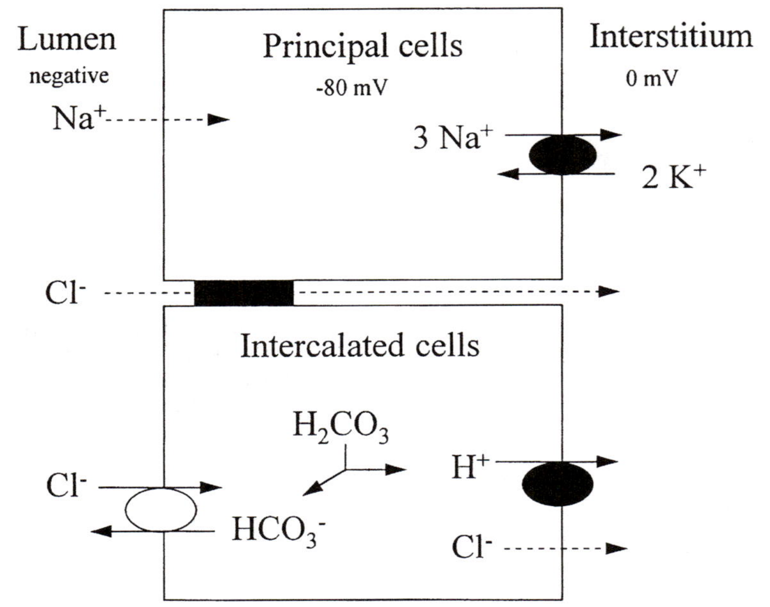

The lumen is negative with respect to the interstitium. Source and symbols as described for Figure 7-23.

Note: From Yucha, C., & Keen, M. (1996). Renal regulation of extracellular fluid volume and osmolality. *ANNA Journal, 23*(5), p. 494. Reprinted with permission.

thick ascending limb. As depicted in Figure 7-25, Na^+/K^+ ATPase pumps are again seen on the basolateral membrane, maintaining a low concentration of sodium intracellularly. Sodium crosses the luminal membrane in co-transport with Cl^- and by simple diffusion driven by the low intracellular sodium, leaving behind a negative potential. Cl^- reabsorption occurs via secondary active co-transport with Na across the luminal membrane and passive diffusion across the basolateral membrane. Since the water permeability of the distal convoluted tubule is quite low, little or no water is reabsorbed in this nephron segment, and the luminal fluid osmolality continues to decrease.

Late distal tubule and collecting duct. The late distal tubule is similar in function to the collecting duct. Two different cell types are involved in Na^+ and Cl^- reabsorption in these segments, principal cells, and intercalated cells. As shown in Figure 7-26, Na^+ enters the principal cells through sodium channels and leaves the cells via the Na^+/K^+ ATPase pump. Intercalated cells (type B) reabsorb chloride. The luminal membrane contains Cl^-/HCO_3^- countertransporters. Once inside the cell, Cl^- diffuses passively across the basolateral membrane. In addition, some Cl^- reabsorption occurs by paracellular diffusion, driven by the lumen-negative PD.

The final regulation of NaCl and water reabsorption occurs by the late distal tubule and the collecting ducts under hormonal control. In the presence of aldosterone, the principal cells synthesize proteins that increase the activity and/or number of the luminal membrane sodium channels and the basolateral Na^+/K^+ ATPase pumps, ultimately increasing sodium reabsorption. In response to plasma volume expansion, ANH inhibits sodium reabsorption in the medullary collecting duct, resulting in natriuresis. The water permeability of these segments is under control of ADH secretion. Without ADH, the late distal tubule and collecting ducts are impermeable to water, and the water that is within the tubular fluid is excreted, resulting in a dilute urine. In contrast, in the presence of ADH, the late distal tubule and collecting ducts are permeable to water and water is reabsorbed in proportion to the interstitial fluid osmolality. For a description of the mechanisms whereby the kidney is able to produce either a dilute or concentrated urine as needed, see the section of this chapter entitled "Urinary Concentration and Dilution."

Summary

In summary, regulation of sodium, chloride, and extracellular fluid volume and osmolality is complex, but very efficient. The excretion of sodium and water is altered through changes in GFR and reabsorption. As summarized in Figure 7-22, these changes are stimulated by alterations in cardiovascular pressure and are mediated by the nervous system (signals passing through extrarenal and intrarenal baroreceptors) and the endocrine system (ADH, ANH, and aldosterone). Integration of the neural and hormonal signals by the kidney results in changes in filtration and reabsorption and, therefore, changes in sodium, chloride, and water excretion.

Ninety percent of the filtered sodium, chloride, and water is reabsorbed by the proximal tubule, loop of Henle, and early distal tubule. Aldosterone, ADH, and ANH work primarily on the late distal tubule collecting duct system to fine tune sodium reabsorption in accordance with our body's needs. In normal persons, the mechanisms for regulating sodium excretion are so precise that sodium balance does not vary by more than a small percentage despite marked changes in dietary intake or losses caused by sweating, vomiting, diarrhea, hemorrhage, or burns.

Summary

In conclusion, this chapter has been designed to provide the reader with a review of our current understanding of the normal physiological functioning of the kidney. The chapter has been divided into 8 sections to 'highlight' the major functions of the kidney.

Section 1 describes the anatomical organization of the kidney, and provides and overview of the processes that mediate the functions of the kidney. Section 2 focuses on glomerular filtration and renal hemodynamics. This section provides the basis for understanding how GFR is regulated, and the renal protective mechanisms that minimize, in particular, decreases in GFR so as to preserve the homeostatic environment. Section 3 is a discussion of urinary concentrating and diluting mechanisms, and is designed to provide the reader with an understanding of how a concentrated or dilute urine is formed, and the basis for the kidney. Section 4 focuses on the current cellular model of distal nephron regulation of potassium excretion, providing the reader with an understanding of the possible mechanism(s) by which various pathological situations or drugs can lead to derangements in total body potassium balance. Sections 5 and 6 describe the handling of calcium (Section 5), magnesium (Section 6), and phosphorous (Section 6) by the kidney. In a similar style of presentation the reader is taken through a discussion of total body homeostatic state.

Section 7 is a discussion of renal acidification. This section covers basic facts about acid-base balance, then describes the mechanisms involved in both bicarbonate reclamation and regeneration, and ends with a discussion of how total body acid-base balance is maintained in the face of a daily dietary acid load. Section 8 discusses the renal regulation of sodium chloride and water excretion, focusing on the mechanisms involved in maintaining extracellular fluid volume and osmolality within normal limits. The section ends with a discussion of how derangements in extracellular volume and osmolality can occur in various pathological situations.

As mentioned, the chapter is divided into sections to 'highlight' the most important functions of the kidney, and to permit the reader to identify a section that deals with a particular renal function of interest. The level of detail in the sections varies a little, but in all cases reflects our current understanding of renal physiology. It is hoped that this chapter will provide the basis by which readers can understand the pathophysiological mechanisms involved in the development of a variety renal diseases. To that end, it is hoped that the reader will utilize the information in this chapter in conjunction with the chapters discussing the various renal pathologies.

Suggested Readings

Brenner, B.M. (Edition). (1996). *Brenner and Rector's the kidney* (5th edition). Philadelphia: W.B. Saunders Company.

Cogan, M.G. (1991). *Fluid and electrolytes: Physiology and pathophysiology*. Norwalk, CT: Appleton & Lange.

Collins, G.B., Brosnihan, K.B., Zuti, R.A., Messina, M., & Gupta, M.K. (1992). Neuroendocrine, fluid balance, and thirst responses to alcohol in alcoholics. *Alcoholism: Clinical and Experimental Research, 16*(2), 228-233.

Dolan, J.T. (Edition). (1991). *Critical care nursing: Clinical management through the nursing process*. Philadelphia: F.A. Davis Company.

Ganong, W.F. (1995). *Review of medical physiology* (17th edition). Norwalk, CT: Appleton & Lange.

Guyton, A.C. (1996). *Textbook of medical physiology* (9th edition). Philadelphia: W.B Saunders Company.

Hladsky, S.B., & Rink, T.J. (1986). *Physiological principles in medicine series: Body fluid and kidney physiology.* London: Edward Arnold Publishers Ltd.

Holechek, M.J. (1992). Glomerular filtration and renal hemodynamics. *ANNA Journal, 19*(3), 237-245.

Lancaster, L.E. (1991). Atrial natriuretic peptide: Implications for nephrology nursing. *Dialysis & Transplantation, 20*, 17-19.

Marsh, D.J. (1983). *Renal physiology*. New York: Raven Press.

Massry, S.G., & Glassock, R.J. (Eds.). (1995). *Massry and Glassock's textbook of nephrology* (3rd edition). Baltimore: Williams & Wilkins.

McCance, K.L., & Huether, S.E. (1990). *Pathophysiology: The biologic basis for disease in adults and children*. St. Louis: C.V. Mosby Company.

Miller, M. (1995). Hormonal aspects of fluid and sodium balance in the elderly. *Endocrinology and Metabolism Clinics of North America, 24*(2), 233-253.

Richard, C.J. (Ed.). (1986). *Comprehensive nephrology nursing.* Boston: Little, Brown and Company.

Rose, B.D. (1994). *Clinical physiology of acid-base and electrolyte disorders* (4th edition). New York: McGraw-Hill.

Schrier, R.W. (Ed.). (1992). *Renal and electrolyte disorders* (4th ed.). Boston: Little, Brown and Company.

Schrier, R.W., & Gottschalk, C.W. (Eds.). (1993). *Diseases of the kidney* (5th edition). Boston: Little, Brown and Company.

Seeley, R.R., Stephens, T.D., & Tate, P. (1992). *Anatomy and physiology* (2nd edition). St. Louis, MO: Mosby-Year Book, Inc.

Valtin, H., & Schafer, J.A. (1995). *Renal function: Mechanisms preserving and solute balance in health* (3rd edition). Boston: Little, Brown and Company.

Vander, A.J. (1995). *Renal physiology* (5th edition). St. Louis, MO: McGraw-Hill.

Chapter Highlights

- The kidneys are paired vascular organs that perform excretory, regulatory, and secretory functions.
- The renal system comprises the kidneys, ureters, bladder, and urethra
- At a glomerular filtration rate of 125 ml/min, the kidneys produce 180 liters of filtrate daily. Yet the average urine output is only 1000 to 1500 ml. Through reabsorption, 99% of the glomerular filtrate is returned to the bloodstream.
- The glomerulus is a selective filtration membrane. The factors that determine which molecules are filtered are molecular size, electrical charge, protein binding, configuration, and rigidity. Small molecules with molecular weights (MW) less than 5,000 daltons (for example, water, MW 18, and all ions including sodium, potassium, chloride, phosphate, magnesium, and calcium) are filtered without restriction. Larger molecules, such as myoglobin with a MW of 17,000 daltons, are filtered to a lesser degree.
- Endogenous creatinine (Cr) is often used to measure clearance; however, since a small amount of creatinine is secreted into the tubule, GFR measured with creatinine clearance (CrCl) will be overestimated.
- The CrCl reflects the GFR and gives a gross indication of how well the kidneys are functioning based on their ability to remove a marker substance.
- Glomerular filtration is the critical initial step in urine formation. For adequate solute and water removal to occur, glomerular filtrate must be generated at a constant rate.
- There are multiple extrarenal factors that influence renal hemodynamics. These substances or systems are based outside of the kidneys, but can directly or indirectly initiate changes in RBF and the GFR: sympathetic nervous system, angiotensin II, antidiuretic hormone (ADH), dopamine, and histamine.
- The function of ADH is to regulate the water permeability of the collecting tubule and thus the rate of water reabsorption along the collecting tubule. When ADH levels are elevated, water permeability is high, water reabsorption occurs, the filtrate osmolality increases, and a concentrated urine is excreted. In the presence of low levels of ADH, the opposite occurs.
- Potassium (K) is the most abundant cation in the human body. The total body K stores in an adult are approximately 50-55 milliequivalents (mEq)/Kilogram (Kg) body weight with 98% of the K located intracellularly.
- The net movement of K from the extracellular fluid into the tubule lumen occurs by K first being actively transported from the interstitial fluid, which is in equilibrium with plasma, into the cell across the basolateral membrane on the Na/K ATPase pump, and then passively diffusing from the cell into the tubule fluid through the K channels in the apical membrane, driven by the electrochemical gradient.
- The homeostasis of calcium is complex because the gastrointestinal tract, the bone, and the kidney all affect calcium balance.
- Calcium is reabsorbed passively via the paracellular pathways, driven by a chemical gradient in the proximal tubule, and by the lumen-positive transepithelial voltage in the thick ascending limb. In the distal tubule, calcium is actively reabsorbed.
- PTH increases the ECF concentration of calcium by at least three distinct effects. First, it stimulates the absorption of bone salts, thereby releasing large amounts of calcium into the extracellular fluid. Second, PTH stimulates the activation of Vitamin D by the kidney, and this hormone increases bone, intestinal, and renal reabsorption of calcium. Third, it increases renal tubular calcium reabsorption in the distal nephron and thus decreases urinary calcium excretion.
- At pH 7.4, about 28% is found in the divalent form, sodium monohydrogen phosphate ($NaHPO_4^{-2}$), and 72% is found in the monovalent form sodium dihydrogen phosphate (NaH_2PO^-). Both of these forms of phosphate play important roles as acid-base buffers because of their ability to pick up and release hydrogen. In acidosis, there is a relative increase in $NaH_2PO_4^-$ and decrease in $NaHPO_4^{-2}$. The opposite occurs when the extracellular fluid becomes alkaline.
- Magnesium is a major intracellular cation, being found mostly within bone (67%) and muscle (20%). Only about 2% of the magnesium in the body is found in the extracellular fluid.

Chapter Highlights (continued)

- The parameter used to define the hydrogen ion concentration of any fluid is the term pH, which is defined as the inverse log of the free hydrogen ion concentration: pH = -log $[H^+]$ Thus, hydrogen ion (H^+) concentration defines the pH of a solution.
- Solutes and proteins that can donate or release hydrogen ions are referred to as acids, and those that can absorb or bind hydrogen ions are referred to as bases. Another term for hydrogen ion is proton; the terms are interchangeable.
- The normal plasma pH is about 7.30–7.45, meaning that the normal free hydrogen ion concentration is 0.000045–0.000048 mEq/L.
- The chemical systems that are responsible for maintenance of a normal pH are called buffer systems, because they "buffer" the pH and prevent it from drifting far from normal.
- Extracellular buffering (predominantly by the bicarbonate buffering system) occurs almost instantaneously when protons are added to the plasma. Second in line to respond is the respiratory system, which in response to sensing a change in plasma pH can alter respiratory rate and thereby alter plasma CO_2 in a time frame of minutes to hours.
- An increase in respiratory rate will lower plasma pCO_2 and drive the reaction to the right. This will lower free hydrogen ion concentration, and plasma pH will rise.
- The major difference between the bicarbonate reclamation and generation processes is that the secreted proton is not excreted in the reclamation process but is excreted in the regeneration process.
- The renal bicarbonate regeneration process is the primary mechanism responsible for maintaining the balance between the acid and base forms of the bicarbonate buffer system. When this system "buffers" a proton, a HCO_3 ion is consumed and is effectively lost from the body (since the CO_2 molecule that is generated is excreted from the body by the respiratory system). Then when the kidney regenerates a bicarbonate ion, the base molecule of the buffer system is replenished, and homeostasis is reestablished.
- To function properly, cells in the body require an internal environment made up of the correct osmolality, ionic composition, pH, and temperature. This internal environment is maintained by the cardiovascular and renal systems. Together, along with neural and endocrine input, these two systems maintain fluid and electrolyte balance within narrow limits suitable for optimal cell function.
- The major ways that fluid balance is controlled and maintained are through fluid intake (stimulated by thirst) and urine output.
- The renal regulation of total body sodium simultaneously achieves regulation of extracellular fluid volume.
- In contrast, in the presence of ADH, the late distal tubule and collecting ducts are permeable to water and water is reabsorbed in proportion to the interstitial fluid osmolality.
- Ninety percent of the filtered sodium, chloride, and water is reabsorbed by the proximal tubule, loop of Henle, and early distal tubule. Aldosterone, ADH, and ANH work primarily on the late distal tubule collecting duct system to fine tune sodium reabsorption in accordance with our body's needs.

CHAPTER 8

Diseases of the Kidney

Patricia S. Jordan, MS, RN, CNA, CNN

Chapter Contents

Glomerular Diseases 179
Pathology of Glomerular Disease 180
Nephrotic and Nephritic Syndrome 180
 The Nephrotic Syndrome 180
 Nephritic Syndrome 181
 Postinfectious Acute Glomerulonephritis 182
 Rapidly Progressive Glomerulonephritis 183
Interstitial Diseases 183
 Acute and Chronic Interstitial Nephritis 183
Vascular Diseases 184
 Renal Artery Disorders 184
 Hypertensive Nephrosclerosis 185
Cystic and Developmental Diseases 185
 Polycystic Kidney Disease 185
 Acquired Cystic Disease 186
 Medullary Sponge Kidney 186
Obstructive Disorders 186
 Obstructive Nephropathy 186
 Diabetic Nephropathy 189
Infectious Disease of the Kidney 189
 Urinary Tract Infection 189
 Human Immunodeficiency Virus, AIDS, and Renal Disease 189
Toxic Nephropathies 190

Chapter Contents

Renal Disease in Pregnancy 192
Changes in Renal Function During Pregnancy 192
Pregnancy and Preexisting Renal Disease 192
Acute Renal Failure in Pregnancy 193
Neoplasms of the Kidney 193
Renal Cell Carcinoma 193
Summary 194
References 194
Chapter Highlights 196

Diseases of the Kidney

Patricia S. Jordan, MS, RN, CNA, CNN

Understanding the diseases of the kidney will assist nephrology nurses in the management of patients with renal disease by increasing knowledge related to the disease process, prognosis, and therapy involved in individual patient care. The purpose of this chapter is to present the major classifications of renal diseases, providing a framework for understanding of the pathogenesis and etiology of renal failure. Renal diseases have been classified as primary and secondary glomerular diseases or nonglomerular diseases, including interstitial, vascular, infectious, cystic and developmental, obstructive disorders, hypertensive nephrosclerosis, diabetic and toxic nephropathies, renal diseases in pregnancies, and neoplasms of the kidney.

Glomerular Diseases

Glomerular diseases (see Table 8-1), including those that affect both glomerular structure and function, are among the major causes of renal failure. Injury to the glomerular basement membrane (GBM) is the underlying cause of glomerular diseases. The nature and the severity of this kidney disease in individual patients is determined by the nature and severity of GBM injury. The capacity of most glomerular diseases to progress to chronic glomerular sclerosis with progressive renal failure places this category of renal disease among the most important for clinicians to understand. The plethora of glomerular diseases identified by the scientific community makes discussion of each one impossible in this chapter. Therefore, the approach will be to focus on classification for diagnosis and clinical management of glomerular disease based on clinical manifestations, and pathological and etiological factors.

The classification of glomerular diseases is constantly evolving. Some authors (Glassock, Adler, Ward, & Cohen, 1986) have classified glomerular diseases as primary or secondary disorders. Primary glomerular diseases are disorders in which glomerular tissue is the predominant or sole tissue involved. Examples of primary diseases include postinfectious glomerulonephritis, rapidly progressive glomerulonephritis, membranoproliferative glomerulonephritis, and membranous glomerulonephritis.

Table 8-1
Primary and secondary renal diseases.

Primary Glomerular Diseases
Poststreptococcal glomerulonephritis
Membranoproliferative glomerulonephritis
Rapidly progressive glomerulonephritis
IgA nephropathy (Berger's disease)
Membranous glomerulonephritis
Secondary Glomerular Diseases
Systemic lupus erythematosus
Goodpasture's syndrome
Diabetic glomerulosclerosis
Amyloidosis

Secondary disorders involve glomerular damage as the result of systemic disease or an identifiable agent such as infection, drug exposure, or neoplasm. Secondary disorders include systemic lupus erythematosus, Goodpasture's syndrome, amyloidosis, and diabetic nephropathy. More recently, the wide range of glomerulopathies are classified according to clinical manifestations and histological and pathological renal changes. Pathologically, glomerular disease is categorized as being diffuse, focal, or segmental. Diffuse disease involves all glomeruli, focal involves some glomeruli, and segmental involves portions of individual glomeruli. Rose (Rose, 1989; Rose & Appel, 1996) classifies glomerular disease according to urinary findings, narrowing the categories to three: focal nephritic, diffuse nephritic, and nephrotic. Identification and recognition of the nephrotic and nephritic syndromes are the very core of the diagnosis and clinical intervention of glomerular disease. These syndromes will be discussed in detail as they provide the framework for the understanding of this category of disease.

Table 8-2
Characteristics of nephrotic and nephritic syndromes.

Nephrotic Syndrome	Nephritic Syndrome
Proteinuria	Hematuria
Hypoalbuminemia	Modest proteinuria
Edema	Hypertension
Hyperlipidemia	Azotemia
Hypercoagulability	Edema

Pathology of Glomerular Disease

Inflammatory injury and hemodynamic injury constitute the two major pathologic categories of glomerular disease. Immunologic events inflict most glomerular inflammation, reducing the number of functioning nephrons and thus, renal function. Three categories of humoral immune-mediated glomerular diseases are immune-complex mediated, anti-GBM antibody mediated, and antineutrophil cytoplasmic auto antibody glomerulonephritis. All three mechanisms result in inflammation of the glomerulus, activating the inflammatory mediator system. This inflammation in the glomerular capillaries causes changes in the caliber of vessels, blood flow, permeability, hemostasis, leukocyte adhesion, and in severe cases, necrosis.

Hemodynamic injury to the glomeruli is the result of diminished blood flow to the glomeruli with resultant ischemic effects and loss of glomerular function. The injury to the glomeruli from immunologic and hemodynamic events results in a variety of signs and symptoms of renal disease. Proteinuria is caused by altered permeability of capillary walls; hematuria results from rupture of capillary walls; azotemia is caused by the impaired filtration of nitrogenous wastes; oliguria or anuria results from reduced urine production; edema is caused by salt and water retention; and renal regulation of blood pressure is impaired (Jennette & Falk, 1994). The signs and symptoms produced by these insults constitute the clinical presentation of patients with impaired glomerular function and are labeled as the nephrotic and nephritic syndromes.

Nephrotic and Nephritic Syndrome

An understanding of the nephrotic and nephritic syndromes will assist nephrology nurses in sorting through the plethora of glomerular renal diseases. Specific glomerular diseases characteristically produce unique findings of renal dysfunction that commonly fall under the auspices of nephrotic or nephritic syndromes. The syndromes, or collections of symptoms, may be produced by one or several glomerular diseases. The recognition of one of these syndromes along with collection of data from the history and physical examinations, assists in the diagnosis and treatment of this type of renal disease. Many diseases will manifest symptoms of both the nephrotic and nephritic syndrome, but usually one is predominate. The nephrotic syndrome has as its hallmark characteristic proteinuria, whereas the nephritic syndrome predominantly refers to hematuria. A summary of the classic characteristics of both syndromes is presented in Table 8-2. This section will define both the nephrotic and nephritic syndromes and identify characteristic glomerular diseases that behave in such a manner as to present with one of these syndromes.

The Nephrotic Syndrome

The nephrotic syndrome (NS) is defined as a clinical entity having multiple causes characterized by increased glomerular permeability resulting in proteinuria, hypoalbuminemia, edema, hyperlipidemia, and hypercoagulability (Bernard & Salant, 1991; Glassock et al., 1986; Jennette & Falk, 1994). Glomerular damage leads to increased permeability of the basement membrane, accounting for the proteinuria that distinguishes this syndrome. The leakage of large amounts of plasma proteins into the glomerular filtrate is the result of increased porosity of the glomerular basement membrane (GBM) and alteration of GBM electrical charge. Under normal conditions, 500 to 1000 mg of albumin enters the glomerular filtrate in 24 hours, but less than 150 mg of protein is excreted in the urine daily because of reabsorption and breakdown of protein in the proximal tubules. "By definition, in the nephrotic syndrome, daily urinary protein excretion is greater than 3.5 grams per 1.73 m2 of body surface area, or 50 mg per kilogram of body weight" (Bernard & Salant, 1991, pp. 258). These greater levels of proteinuria result in a loss of plasma proteins and the resultant hypoalbuminemia. Hypoalbuminemia decreases plasma oncotic pressure that facilitates the movement of fluid by osmosis into the interstitial spaces, resulting in edema. Patients with nephrotic syndrome usually seek medical intervention due to the presence of edema. Minimal change glomerulopathy, membranous glomerulopathy, amyloidosis, and diabetic glomerulosclerosis are the major glomerular diseases that commonly manifest with the nephrotic syndrome.

Minimal change disease (MCD) is almost always associated with the nephrotic syndrome at the onset of the disease. As the name indicates, MCD demonstrates little or no pathologic or histologic change in the GBM on light microscopy from that seen in normal glomeruli. However, the most common clinical manifestation is the sudden onset of the classic nephrotic syndrome. MCD frequently occurs after a nonspecific viral illness (ACP, 1994). MCD presents in both children and adults with 85%-95% of preadolescent children exhibiting nephrotic syndrome having MCD; in adults over 40 with primary nephrotic syndrome, the incidence of MCD is 20%-25%. The predominant clinical features are heavy proteinuria, low serum albumin, edema, and elevated serum cholesterol (Siegel, 1994).

The use of corticosteroids is the treatment of choice for MCD nephrotic as the nephrotic syndrome caused by MCD is particularly sensitive to steroid therapy with a high success rate in most patients, especially in children. The clinical course of MCD is usually described according to the patient's response to steroid therapy with total remission defined as complete resolution of proteinuria; partial remission is a reduction in the degree of proteinuria without complete clearing; and a relapse as the reoccurrence of proteinuria. Patients who are at the highest risk for irreversible damage are those who do not have a good response to the initial steroid therapy or who have a delayed response. Morbidity is most commonly related to complications of therapy. The majority of patients with MCD have a good response to initial steroid therapy, and although they may have relapses in their nephrotic syndrome, they have an excellent long-term prognosis (Siegel, 1994).

Membranous glomerulopathy is most commonly associated with the nephrotic syndrome in adults. It is usually idiopathic or in some cases, the consequence of infections, systemic autoimmune disease, or medication administration. The most common clinical presentation is heavy proteinuria in 80% of patients, most often associated with all other signs of the nephrotic syndrome. In contrast to MCD, membranous nephropathy's clinical course includes a more insidious, rather than abrupt onset of edema. When membranous nephropathy occurs in children, it is usually caused by an infection such as hepatitis B or by systemic lupus erythematosus (SLE). Idiopathic membranous nephropathy can occur at any age, but 80%-90% of patients are over 30 when diagnosed; in older patients, 20% of cases are associated with malignancies. Symptoms of the nephrotic syndrome may be very severe in patients with membranous disease. Anorexia, malaise, edema, and hyperlipidemia are often present. Growth retardation in children with severe nephrotic syndrome is very difficult to manage.

There are three major approaches to treatment of membranous glomerulopathy: (a) no specific treatment; (b) short-term oral prednisone; or (c) aggressive immunosuppression. Up to 30% of patients undergo spontaneous remission, especially those with less than 10 gm/day protein loss and normal renal function. In those individuals with more aggressive disease, severe proteinuria and renal insufficiency, various combinations of corticosteroids and cytotoxic therapy are employed.

Amyloidosis is a broad term for a number of diseases that have in common the extracellular deposition of insoluble fibrillar proteins (Skinner, 1991; Appel, 1994). Systemic amyloidosis is classified into four types: (a) AL, or primary, which is usually associated with myeloma; (b) AA, secondary to most commonly a chronic inflammatory or infectious disease; (c) AF, hereditary; and (d) AH, associated with long-term dialysis. The most common form of amyloidosis that causes renal insufficiency in the United States is AL, or primary amyloidosis (ACP). Approximately 25% of patients with AL amyloid present with the nephrotic syndrome, often in severe form. Although no specific therapy has been proven for treatment of AL amyloid, both chemotherapy and colchicine have demonstrated beneficial results. Some patients experience complete recovery from nephrotic syndrome, but in the majority of cases, amyloidosis is progressive and organ system involvement continues (Appel, 1994).

Nephritic Syndrome

Nephritic syndrome classically includes hematuria as its distinguishing component. Other classic symptoms include hypertension, renal insufficiency, volume overload, edema, and in some cases, mild proteinuria. Patients may present with one or all of these symptoms and may frequently have both nephrotic and nephritic symptoms. For terminology's sake, nephritic syndrome is also known as nephritis.

Hematuria may be caused by glomerular disease, but the most common cause is urinary tract disease, so diseases other than those of the glomerulus must be ruled out. The nephritic syndrome may be insidious as in patients with IgA nephropathy, or may develop into fulminant nephritis with a rapid rise in serum creatinine and consequent renal failure as in rapidly progressive glomerulonephritis. Postinfectious glomerulonephritis, acute diffuse glomerulonephritis, and crescentic glomerulonephritis are diseases that also typically exhibit the nephritic syndrome. The treatment of nephritis is aimed at correcting the cause of glomerular injury. Steroids and immunosuppression may be used, as well as management of symptoms. In most nephritic patients hypertension must be controlled with antihypertensives and a low-sodium diet. Fluid management must be employed to avert volume overload, avoiding pulmonary edema and elevated systemic arterial pressure. This is usually accomplished with sodium restriction and diuretic therapy, but in severe cases dialysis may be required. Dialysis may also be required during the resolution of acute renal failure (ARF) from a reversible disease such as poststreptococcal glomerulonephritis.

IgA nephropathy is the most common form of glomerulonephritis in the world. It occurs in benign and severe forms, including asymptomatic hematuria or proteinuria, acute nephritis, rapidly progressive nephritis, chronic nephritis, and nephrotic syndrome. Damage to the glomeruli is the result of deposition of circulating IgA-containing immune complexes in the glomerular membrane and the subsequent inflammatory response. The pathogenesis is not yet understood and there appears to be primary and in some cases secondary factors involved. The immune response is believed to arise in the respiratory or gastrointestinal tract triggered by causative antigens from infectious pathogens or ingested or inhaled material (ACP, 1994; Julian, 1994).

More than 90% of patients with IgA nephropathy have hematuria at some time and in varying degrees during the course of the disease. About 50% will have an episode of gross hematuria, especially true in children. Onset of hematuria usually occurs at the time of upper respiratory infection. More than 80% of patients will also have proteinuria, some in the nephrotic range. Presentation of other symptoms of the nephritic syndrome vary as does the degree and frequency of renal insufficiency.

IgA nephropathy is a chronic disease that accounts for approximately 10% of the CRF in the United States. Although clinical remission is possible in as many as one-third of affected patients, rarely does IgA disappear from the glomeruli. Renal function deteriorates in about 40% of patients, about half of whom reach end stage disease within 20 years. One-third of patients develop a benign course with microscopic hematuria, normal serum creatinine, and mild proteinuria. Prognostic factors that increase the chance of progression of the disease include older age, male sex, severe proteinuria, hypertension, renal insufficiency, and severe pathologic changes (Julian, 1994; ACP, 1994).

There is no proven effective therapy for IgA nephropathy. The goal of therapy is to control decline in renal function and manage related symptoms (Erickson, 1993). The approach to treatment for IgA nephropathy depends on the acute or chronic nature of the disease process. Acute renal dysfunction is treated with glucocorticoids, cytotoxic agents, anticoagulants, or plasmapheresis (Julian, 1994).

Postinfectious Acute Glomerulonephritis

The deposition of immune complexes in glomerular structures is implicated in many forms of glomerulonephritis. Infectious agents are among the most common antigens associated with immune complex-mediated glomerulonephritis (Fredrich & Jordan, 1994). Postinfectious glomerulonephritis may arise from bacterial infection, most commonly group AB-hemolytic streptococci, or from viral, parasitic, rickettsial, or fungal agents.

Poststreptococcal glomerulonephritis (PSGN) is the most common form of glomerulonephritis in children. "The relationship of acute nephritis to infection with group A streptococci was clearly established in the early 20th century" (Fredrich & Jordan, 1994, p. 88). Although rheumatic fever follows only pharyngeal infection with group A streptococci, nephritis may follow either skin or pharyngeal infection. In certain geographic areas nephritis is more common, due to streptococcal impetigo, than upper respiratory infections. Acute PSGN is an immune complex disease involving antigen derived from streptococci binding to glomerular structures. Glomerular immune complex deposition may then cause complement activation with release of chemotactic factors and acute glomerular injury.

PSGN is primarily a disease of children with an average age of onset of 6 to 7 years. The onset is usually abrupt – a latent period between the onset of pharyngeal streptococcal infection and the appearance of the first manifestation of nephritis is between 7 - 21 days, with an average of 10 days. Hematuria and edema are the most common complaints. Gross hematuria, classically described as cola-colored, is seen in about 70% of patients. Typically the edema is periorbital and is worse on first rising. The etiology of the edema is multifactoral, including reduction in glomerular filtration rate, sodium and water retention, and proteinuria. Mild or moderate hypertension is usually present in PSGN, most likely secondary to sodium and water retention. Oliguria is also common, but anuria is infrequent. Circulatory congestion secondary to expansion of extracellular fluid volume is present in the majority of patients and may result in dyspnea, orthopnea, cough, cardiomegaly, gallop rhythm, pleural effusions, and even pulmonary edema. Pallor frequently develops in patients with PSGN secondary to dilutional anemia and edema.

Acute clinical episodes of PSGN are usually self-limited and the immunologic factors return to normal within 6 weeks. Hematuria will usually disappear in 6 months; proteinuria will be present in 61% for more than 1 year and in 36% for 2 or more years. The immediate prognosis for acute PSGN is very favorable in children. The long-term prognosis is variable and appears to be closely related to the severity of the initial disease. The prognosis is excellent in patients without preexisting renal disease.

The treatment of acute PSGN is symptomatic and dependent on the clinical severity of the illness. The major goals of therapy are to control blood pressure and treat volume overload (Madaio, 1991). Treatment of established infection does not prevent the development of PSGN, but may minimize its severity. Early treatment of affected persons and immediate family members may prevent the spread of streptococcal infections. Throat cultures should be performed on all these individuals; treatment with penicillin should be undertaken as required. For patients with skin infections (impetigo), attention to personal hygiene is essential (Madaio, 1991, Fredrich & Jordan, 1994).

Nonstreptococcal postinfectious acute glomerulonephritis may be caused by a variety of bacteria, viruses, and parasites. The nephritis associated with these organisms is usually mild and often manifested only by hematuria and proteinuria, but may be difficult to distinguish between PSGN. The absence of evidence of a recent streptococcal illness and the association with viral syndromes suggests a postinfectious glomerulonephritis of nonstreptococcal origin. Other bacterial, viral, parasitic, or fungal infectious agents may produce a nonprogressive glomerulonephritis (GN), or chronic infections may cause a chronic GN. It is important to identify the causal agent/organism to determine immediate therapy and long-term prognosis.

Rapidly Progressive Glomerulonephritis

Rapidly progressive glomerulonephritis (RPGN) represents an idiopathic primary glomerular disease characterized by a rapid deterioration in renal function with distinctive glomerular crescent formation on renal biopsy (Couser, 1991; Johnson, 1994). RPGN is not a common renal disease, but holds clinical relevance as a medical emergency that warrants rapid diagnosis and intervention, dramatically impacting the outcome of the disease. This condition responds well to therapeutic intervention, but little is known of its etiology. Toxins such as hydrocarbon solvents, drugs, viral and bacterial infections, malignancies, and autoimmune mechanisms have been implicated as possible etiologic factors (Couser, 1991).

The presence of glomerular crescents on renal biopsy defines RPGN histologically and accounts for the damage to the glomerular capillary wall. These crescents represent accumulations of cells and other materials that create a disruption in the glomerular capillary wall, resulting in direct contact between plasma and cells in the circulation and elements in Bowman's capsule. Crescents vary from small capsular attachments of cells too large to circumferential aggregations that completely fill Bowman's capsule. There is some correlation among the extent of glomerular crescent formation, the severity of the disease, and the prognosis of the patient. An increase in the size and present age of crescents correlate with the progression of the disease.

Renal function declines in RPGN in a matter of days, weeks, or a few months with patients presenting with signs of progressive renal insufficiency without evidence diagnostic of any systemic disease. Clinical features of an aggressive nephritis with tea-colored urine, malaise, anorexia, low-grade fever, migratory polyarthopathy, and mild hypertension are typical (Johnson, 1994). Prodromal symptoms occur in about 50% of patients with RPGN, usually those of a viral illness with myalgias, arthralgias, back or abdominal pain, fever, and malaise. Most patients have experienced a doubling of serum creatinine in a 3-month period after the onset of symptoms or the time of diagnosis, but progression to chronic renal failure (CRF) can occur within 1 to 2 weeks (Couser, 1991).

The treatment of choice for idiopathic RPGN is steroid pulse therapy plus cytoxin; plasma exchange can be employed in resistant cases of RPGN. More than 70% of patients experience improvement in renal function with these therapies, with more positive results occurring in those treated early in the course of the disease. In those patients who progress to renal failure requiring dialysis, as many as 30% may regain enough renal function to come off dialysis with a trial of therapy. Patients with irreversible renal failure requiring dialysis should be considered candidates for transplantation since the recurrence rate in allografts is thought to be low.

Interstitial Diseases

Acute and Chronic Interstitial Nephritis

The interstitial nephropathies denote a group of diseases that cause interstitial inflammation with renal tubular damage. Usually the vascular and glomerular structures are not involved until late in the course of the disease. Acute interstitial nephritis (AIN) is usually associated with a sudden deterioration in renal function resulting from inflammation and edema in the renal interstitium. AIN accounts for approximately 10%-15% of reported cases of ARF (Meyers, 1994), with the most common cause related to drug therapy. It may also be the result of systemic or local infection, immunologic disease (such as lupus erythematosus), or of idiopathic causes. AIN occurs in all age groups, however, elderly individuals are at a higher risk for developing ARF. The severity of AIN ranges from mild changes in tubular function and glomerular filtration rate (GFR) to profound renal failure requiring dialysis.

AIN is particularly common with methicillin, affecting approximately 17% of patients who receive the drug more than 10 days. Methicillin is infrequently used currently, with the most common drugs implicated as causal agents in AIN being nonsteroidal antiinflammatory drugs (NSAIDS), penicillins, cephalosporins, rifampin, sulfonamides, cimetidine, and allopurinol (Rose, 1989). The onset of AIN after drug exposure ranges from 3 to 5 days after a second exposure to several weeks after first exposure. The latent period may be as short as 1 day with rifampin or as long as 18 months with NSAIDs.

Diagnosis of AIN is usually accomplished through clinical evaluation, but may be confirmed by renal biopsy. Treatment begins with discontinuation of the suspected drug, and in many cases renal function improves within several days.

Patients who do not regain renal function after drug discontinuation and who are poor candidates for renal biopsy undergo a trial of corticosteroids. Most patients with AIN improve with discontinuation of the offending drug within the first 6 to 8 weeks. Recovery may be incomplete, however, with a persistent rise in serum creatinine. Persistent ARF after 3 weeks increases the likelihood of irreversible injury.

Chronic interstitial disease follows a more indolent course than AIN and is characterized by tubulointerstitial fibrosis, atrophy, and in certain forms, papillary necrosis. It is most commonly associated with analgesic nephropathy, sickle cell disease, and obstructive uropathy.

Analgesic nephropathy resulting from the habitual use of combination analgesics, which usually contain acetaminophen or aspirin, accounts for 20%-30% of chronic interstitial nephritis in the United States (ACP, 1994). This is an insidious disorder, requiring a cumulative dose of 2 to 3 kg of analgesic to be ingested before the syndrome develops. It is also difficult to detect in the early stages of renal injury, with papillary necrosis as the most characteristic late finding. The cause of papillary necrosis is vascular ischemia in the papilla, which leads to generalized vasculopathy and ultimately to glomerulosclerosis, atrophy, and CRF. The characteristic symptoms of papillary necrosis are flank pain, fever, and hematuria. The papilla sloughs, obstructing the ureter, and it is difficult to distinguish papillary necrosis from nephrolithiasis.

NSAIDs, one of the most widely prescribed drugs in medicine, can produce either AIN or a long-term, less reversible lesion of interstitial fibrosis. NSAIDs mediate a number of adverse renal side effects as a result of their inhibition of renal prostaglandin synthesis. AIN has been reported with most NSAIDs currently available, but two-thirds of the cases have involved fenoprofen. AIN usually occurs after long-term exposure to NSAIDs, from 2 weeks to 18 months after a course of therapy has been initiated. Patients are usually older (60 years or over), exhibit no evidence of systemic hypersensitivity reactions, and present with hypertension, edema, and heavy proteinuria (Meyers, 1994). As with any AIN, most patients improve with the discontinuation of the NSAID and treatment with prednisone, if required. Recovery may be complete, or incomplete with a persistent elevation in serum creatinine. Diffuse interstitial infiltrates, poor response to prednisone, and persistent ARF after 3 weeks are symptoms suggesting irreversible injury.

Vascular Diseases

Renal Artery Disorders

The relationship between renal disease and systemic atherosclerosis has been increasingly recognized. Systemic atherosclerosis can adversely affect renal function by causing renal artery stenosis (RAS) and consequently, renovascular hypertension. Renovascular hypertension is defined as a "secondary elevation of blood pressure produced by various conditions that interfere with the arterial circulation to kidney tissue causing ischemia" (ACP, 1994, p. 226). This decreased perfusion of kidney tissue increases blood pressure through the renin-angiotensin-aldosterone system's release of angiotensin II, a potent vasoconstrictor. The degree of stenosis relates to the interference of renal blood flow, with 50% stenosis generally considered significant (Svetkey, 1994). Patients may have bilateral renovascular disease with or without complete occlusion of either artery.

Renal artery stenosis and renovascular hypertension are potentially curable, or reversible conditions. A history of systemic atherosclerosis, peripheral vascular disease, acute elevation of blood pressure or acceleration of previously well-controlled hypertension, refractory hypertension, accelerated retinopathy, and a systolic-diastolic abdominal bruit are among the clinical clues indicative of RAS. Diagnosis is further verified by arteriography, determining the physiologic significance of the lesion and curing of the hypertension following intervention.

Treatment of RAS and renovascular hypertension includes medical and surgical interventions, with the goal of improving tissue perfusion and controlling the effects of hypertension and improved patient survival. Antihypertensive drugs, specifically ACE inhibitors, may be used to control blood pressure in patients with bilateral RAS. Surgery to revascularize the renal tissue is generally very effective, with success rate of 85% to 90% (Rose & Appel, 1996). Percutaneous angioplasty may also be utilized, but with a lower long-term benefit.

Atheroembolic renal disease is also a possible complication of diffuse atherosclerosis. ARF may occur due to the occlusion of small arteries and arterioles of the kidney by cholesterol crystals or microemboli from atheromatous plaques that have moved downstream. This occlusion results in inflammation, ischemia, and renal dysfunction. Embolization may be spontaneous, especially in severe aortic disease, or as the result of cardiovascular surgery or angiography-induced vascular intimal trauma (ACP, 1994; Greenberg, 1994). Embolic disease can be distinguished from bilateral renal artery stenosis or nephrosclerosis by an abrupt decline in renal function, evidence of extrarenal emboli and an elevated erythrocyte sedimentation. The typical patient at risk is elderly with extensive atherosclerosis. Management focuses on supportive care during ARF, including dialysis. Some lesions improve over time, in some patients renal failure is irreversible.

Hypertensive Nephrosclerosis

A major consequence of hypertension is nephrosclerosis. Hypertensive nephropathy is the result of chronic hypertension (essential or secondary) in which the small intrarenal arteries and arterioles are affected, leading to renal insufficiency and possibly to CRF. Approximately 25% of patients requiring renal replacement therapy reach CRF due to hypertensive nephrosclerosis (ACP, 1994).

Nephrology nurses interface with a population of patients in which hypertension is extremely common. Most renal diseases produce some form of hypertension, and conversely, hypertension may cause renal insufficiency. The role of nurses in both clinical scenarios is key to the long-term survival of patients with hypertension. Assisting in the control of essential hypertension to minimize renal impairment and maintaining a level of blood pressure to prevent other organ complications such as heart disease or stroke is a major responsibility of nephrology nurses.

Hypertension is one of the most common health problems facing medical professionals today. Over 90% of patients with high blood pressure are classified as having essential or primary hypertension because the etiology is not readily definable. The etiology of essential hypertension is a complex mixture of interactions of hereditary, environmental factors, sodium homeostasis, the renin-angiotensin system, sympathetic nervous system, and other unknown factors. Approximately 5%-10% of patients may have hypertension secondary to other causes such as renal disease or endocrine disorders (Nally, 1994). Hypertension occurs in all segments of the general population with the highest incidence and prevalence being among elderly patients over age 65 and particularly in blacks. Hypertension is present in approximately 45% of whites and 60% of blacks ages 65 to 74. Blacks have the highest frequency of hypertension in the world; over age 18, 38% of blacks are hypertensive and over age 50, 66% are affected. Blacks develop high blood pressure at an earlier age than whites and it tends to be more severe than in whites. Consequently, for any given blood pressure, blacks appear to have more renal damage (ACP, 1994).

Renal damage may be sustained in individuals who have severe prolonged hypertension or episodes of accelerated hypertension and periods of poorly controlled diastolic hypertension. Renal insufficiency may also be evident in patients with moderate and mild hypertension, especially in the black population. Renal injury from hypertension occurs through the same mechanism that affects the entire vascular system of the body, that is, damage to the arteries themselves by excessive pressure. High pressure in the arteries causes sclerosis of blood vessels, causing them to become weak and to hemorrhage inside the kidneys. Large areas of the kidney can be destroyed, resulting in progressive deterioration of renal function (Guyton, 1986).

The overall goal of treatment of essential hypertension is to lower systemic blood pressure and modify other cardiovascular risks to improve morbidity and mortality. There is data to suggest that aggressive control of blood pressure can prevent or at least slow the progression of renal insufficiency due to hypertension. However, there is no clear consensus of what level of blood pressure or certain class of antihypertensives would be the most protective of renal function (ACP, 1994). The goal is to maintain blood pressure at a level that reduces the risk of end-organ damage, which is supported by several studies to be a diastolic pressure in the range of 80-90 mmHg (Brazy, 1994).

Cystic and Developmental Diseases

Renal cysts can be single or multiple, replacing vital renal tissue causing serious complications, or they can be clinically inconsequential. They occur as part of hereditary and congenital disorders or can be acquired later in life. For purposes of this section, congenital disorders are those which develop during fetal development and may or may not be hereditary (Grabow, 1994). Hereditary kidney diseases are those in which a genetic defect produces the disorder (ACP, 1994).

Polycystic Kidney Disease

Autosomal dominant polycystic kidney disease (ADPKD) is the most common hereditary renal disease. It affects approximately 500,000 adults and children in the United States and is the third most common cause of CRF in the United States. The ADPKD1 gene accounts for almost 90% of the ADPKD in the white population and is located on chromosome 6. The location of the second ADPKD gene, ADPKD2, is on chromosome 4. The genetic defect that allows cystic formation is still unknown, however, cell proliferation, epithelial secretion, and basement membrane composition have all been shown to be abnormal. The identification of the ADPKD gene's location has enabled more accurate and accessible genetic testing to be done for families with a history of ADPKD.

ADPKD, or polycystic kidney disease, is a systemic disease as well as a renal disorder. It produces diverse clinical manifestations that are both renal related and nonrenal. Renal manifestations may include hypertension, nephrolithiasis, renal cyst infection, renal concentrating defect, and renal failure (ACP, 1994; Grabow, 1994).

Hypertension is the most common renal disorder. Alteration in the intrarenal circulation, due to the existence of cysts, creates areas of renal ischemia triggering the renin-angiotensin-aldosterone system. Hypertension occurs in about 60% of adults with ADPKD prior to the onset of renal insufficiency and in about 80% of adults with CRF. Renal cyst infection is evidenced by fever, renal tenderness, positive blood cultures, and poor response to antibiotic therapy normally used with pyelonephritis. Failure to respond to antibiotic therapy is due to poor cyst penetration of the majority of antibiotics. Ciprofloxacin, chloramphenicol, and trimethoprim-sulfamethoxazole provide good cyst penetration and more effective treatment.

Chronic pain, which can be disabling in a small number of patients, can result from cyst compression. These patients can benefit from cyst decompression procedures done surgically or by percutaneous drainage. Nephrolithiasis, which also causes severe pain, occurs in approximately 20% of patients with ADPKD. Stone formation is most likely due to intrarenal urinary stasis and metabolic abnormalities, including decreased citrate excretion (Grabow, 1994).

Renal failure is the most serious renal complication of polycystic disease. About 50% of patients with ADPKD develop CRF before age 60. Factors that appear to differentiate individuals who will develop renal failure include the ADPKD1 gene, male sex, early age of onset, hypertension, black racial origin, sickle hemoglobin in black patients, episodes of gross hematuria, and larger renal size (ACP, 1994; Grabow, 1994). Patients with CRF are candidates for dialysis and transplantation and tend to tolerate both as well as nondiabetics. Nephrectomy may be warranted in cases of recurrent renal infections, gross hematuria, symptoms related to renal size, or infection at the time of renal transplantation.

Acquired Cystic Disease

Acquired cystic disease (ACD) is characterized by the development of renal cysts in the kidneys of patients with CRF originating from a noncystic renal disease. The incidence of ACD is related to the duration of renal failure or dialysis and occurs more in males and those of black racial origin. ACD occurs in 7% to 22% of patients with renal failure who are not yet on dialysis, in 40% of patients who have been dialyzed for 3 years, and in 90% who have been on dialysis for more than 10 years. The cause of ACD has not been defined, but appears to be related to epithelial hyperplasia as in polycystic disease.

The majority of patients with ACD are asymptomatic or may present with gross hematuria, flank pain, fever, cyst infection, or cyst rupture with retroperitoneal bleeding. The most serious consequence of ACD is renal cell carcinoma, which is believed to be 57 to 134 times higher in dialysis patients with ACD than in the general population. Males seem to be at higher risk, and the larger the kidney the greater the risk for development of this malignancy. The overall 5-year survival rate in patients with ACD and renal cell carcinoma is about 35%. Because both diseases are usually asymptomatic with the possibility of malignancy and metastasis, screening dialysis patients for ACD with ultrasonography has become more prevalent.

Medullary Sponge Kidney

Medullary sponge kidney (MSK) is a relatively common developmental disorder rather than an inheritable disease. Dilated intramedullary collecting ducts impart a sponge-like appearance to the kidney. MSK is often an asymptomatic, benign condition, or it may present with nephrolithiasis, hematuria, and urinary tract infection. Five percent to 21% of patients with stone formation have underlying MSK and a high incidence of hypercalcuria.

Obstructive Disorders

Obstructive Nephropathy

Obstructive nephropathy is the renal disease caused by the impairment of urine flow through the urinary tract. This nephropathy is usually caused by obstructive uropathy, or the structural or functional impediment to the normal flow of urine. Obstructive nephropathy, obstructive uropathy, and hydronephrosis are three terms often used interchangeably to describe the renal disease that results from urinary tract obstruction. However, they each reflect different clinical pathology and consequences. As described above, obstructive uropathy indicates the structural or functional impediment to normal urine flow, which results in increased pressure proximal to the point of obstruction. Obstructive uropathy may or may not result in damage to renal tissue. Hydronephrosis, or dilatation of the urinary tract, results from pressure and dilation of tissue proximal to the site of obstruction. This dilatation primarily affects the collecting duct and distal tubules. Obstructive nephropathy is the term used to describe the renal disease that results from interference of the flow of urine or tubular fluid (Brenner & Rector, 1986).

Obstructive uropathy is a common disorder that can occur at any age and is often treatable, thus preventing, minimizing, or reversing the development of nephropathy. If the obstruction is not relieved, damage to the kidney will result from increased pressure, renal ischemia, cellular atrophy and necrosis (see Figure 8-1). Causes of urinary tract obstruction are numerous and generally classified according to the location, duration, and degree of obstruction (Klahr, 1991, 1994). Table 8-3 displays the classification of obstructive uropathy.

The causes of upper urinary tract obstruction can be either intrinsic or extrinsic. Intrinsic causes are either intraluminal (usually renal calculi) or intramural, which are either anatomic or functional obstructions. Extrinsic causes may originate in the reproductive system, gastrointestinal system, the

Figure 8-1
Development of obstructive nephropathy.

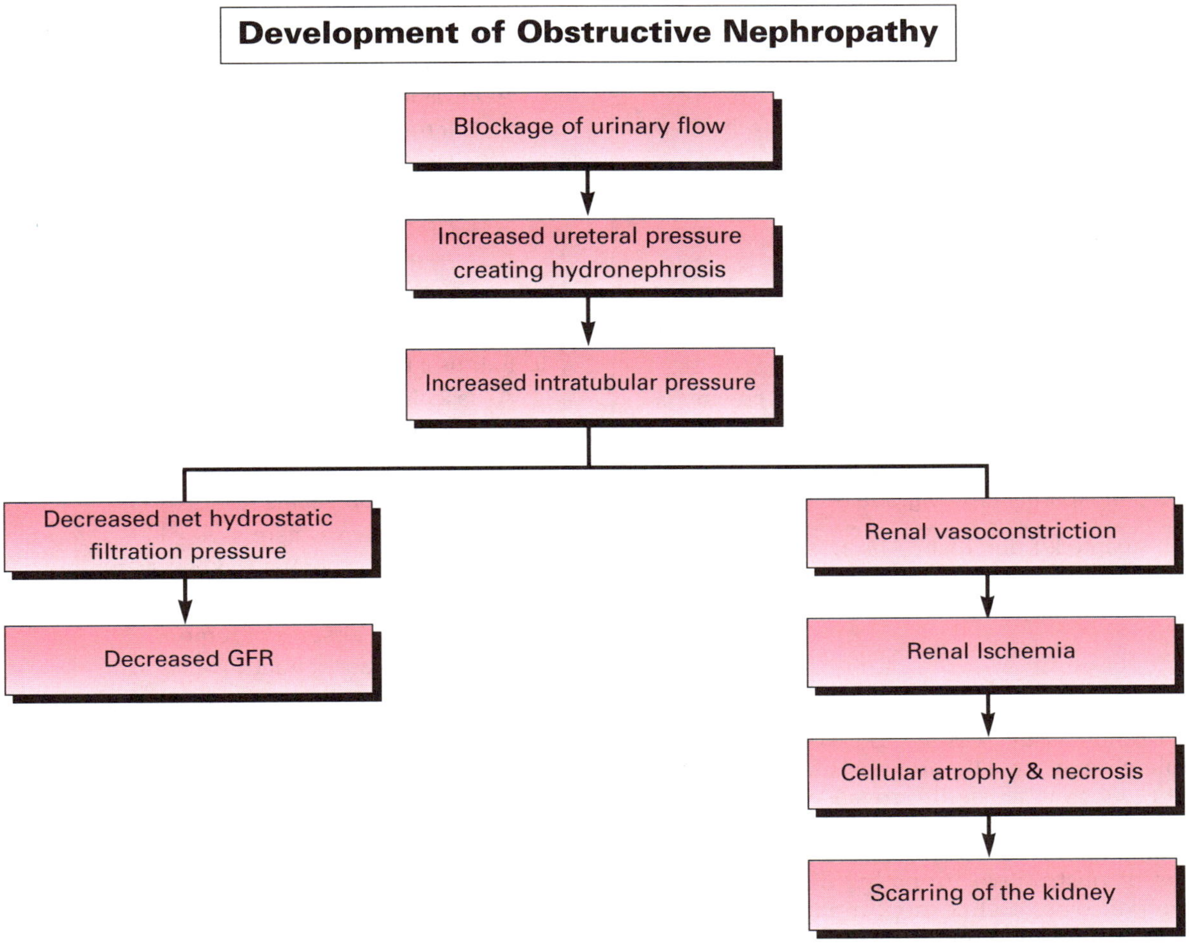

Note: Adapted from Klahr (1994); Brenner (1986).

vascular system, or the retroperitoneal space. Causes of lower urinary tract obstruction include lesions of the urethra such as urethral strictures, prostate including benign prostatic hyperplasia and prostatic cancer, and functional or anatomical abnormalities of the bladder. Table 8-4 lists the major causes of urinary tract obstruction.

Patients with obstructive uropathy present with a variety of symptoms, very often those of acute or chronic renal failure. The clinical presentation varies with the location, duration, and degree of the obstruction. In particular, the symptoms of upper and lower urinary obstruction will differ as will complete or partial obstruction. Patients with complete obstruction may present with anuria and ARF. With partial obstruction, the patient may exhibit signs of polyuria, polydipsia, or fluctuating urine output. Other symptoms that may implicate obstructive disease include recurrent urinary tract infections, abdominal flank pain, or unexplained acute or chronic renal failure (Klahr, 1994).

The approach to diagnosis and treatment of obstructive uropathy is variable and dependent upon the severity and nature of the presenting clinical syndromes. Since obstructive uropathy may result in irreversible renal damage, or obstructive nephropathy, a prompt diagnosis and appropriate intervention will improve the patient's prognosis. The site of the obstruction usually determines the therapeutic approach, which may include surgery or instrumentation to eliminate the obstruction. Relieving the obstruction often reverses renal impairment, such as in ARF due to ureteral stones. With chronic, more progressive obstruction, dam-

Table 8-3
Classification of urinary tract obstruction.

Location
Upper urinary tract (usually unilateral)
- Ureter
- Ureteropelvic junction
- Ureterovesical junction

Lower urinary tract (usually bilateral)
- Bladder and posterior urethra
- Urethra

Duration
Acute (hours - usually due to stones)
Subacute (days)
Chronic (weeks, months, years - usually congenital)

Degree
Complete (total high grade obstruction)
Incomplete (partial or low grade obstruction)

Note: Adapted from Klahr (1991, 1994); Brenner & Rector (1986).

Table 8-4
Major causes of urinary tract obstruction.

Upper urinary tract obstruction

I. Intrinsic causes
  A. Intraluminal
    1. Intratubular deposition of uric acid crystals
    2. Ureter: blood clots, stones
  B. Intramural
    1. Ureteropelvic or ureterovesical junction dysfunction
    2. Ureteral valve polyp or stricture

II. Extrinsic Causes
  A. Vascular lesions
    1. Aneurysm; abdominal aorta; iliac vessels
    2. Venous: retrocaval ureter, ovarian vein thrombophlebitis
  B. Reproductive system
    1. Pregnancy, prolapsed uterus, tumors, endometriosis
    2. Ovarian abscess or tumors
  C. Gastrointestinal tract
    1. Crohn's disease, diverticulitis, tumors
    2. Pancreatic tumors, abscess, or cysts
  D. Retroperitoneal diseases
    1. Retroperitoneal fibrosis
    2. Hematomas
    3. Tuberculosis, sarcoidosis
    4. Primary retroperitoneal tumors (lymphoma, sarcoid)
    5. Metastatic tumor (cervix, bladder, colon)

Lower urinary tract obstruction

I. Urethra: strictures, stones, diverticulum, posterior or anterior urethral valves
II. Prostate: benign prostatic hyperplasia, prostatic calculi, prostatic carcinoma
III. Bladder
  A. Neurogenic bladder
  B. Bladder neck dysfunction
  C. Bladder calculi
  D. Bladder cancer
IV. Phimosis
V. Trauma
  A. Straddle injury
  B. Pelvic fracture

Note: Adapted from Klahr (1991, 1994); Brenner (1986).

age to renal tissue may be too extensive to allow complete recovery. The prognosis for return of adequate renal function is improved with early detection of obstruction and early intervention.

Congenital renal disorders are among the major causes of obstructive uropathy, often resulting in hydronephrosis, reflux nephropathy, obstructive nephropathy, and renal failure. Urinary tract obstruction is common in utero, infancy, and childhood, and accounts for 20% of the renal failure seen in children. Hydronephrosis is frequently observed in congenital disorders, usually from obstruction, but can also be caused by nonobstructive disorders such as prune-belly syndrome. The most common site for upper tract obstruction is the ureteropelvic junction, while lower tract obstruction results from a posterior urethral valve (ACP, 1994).

Reflux nephropathy is the term used to denote the renal scarring that occurs as the result of vesicoureteral reflux (VUR). VUR is defined as "the abnormal flow of urine from the bladder into the upper urinary tract" (Velosa, 1994, p. 189) that is caused by a congenital abnormality of the vesicoureteral junction located at the insertion of the ureter into the bladder. Reflux nephropathy is the cause of CRF in 5% to 15% of adult patients under 50 years of age. The degree of reflux is graded based on the findings of voiding cystourethrographic. The severity of the reflux using this grading system ranges from grade I, being mild reflux into the ureter, to grade V, indicating severe reflux along the entire collecting system. The goal of intervention is to prevent renal tissue scarring, hypertension, and renal failure. Many lower grades resolve with urinary tract maturation, but some higher grades require surgical intervention.

Diabetic Nephropathy

Diabetic nephropathy is the leading cause of CRF in the United States, accounting for approximately 30% of all patients entering dialysis programs. The incidence of diabetic nephropathy is evenly distributed between insulin-dependent diabetic patients and noninsulin-dependent diabetics. Diabetes causes structural changes in the kidney beginning in the very early stages of the disease and continues on a progressive course to full blown diabetic glomerulopathy in approximately 25% of all diabetic patients (Goldfarb, 1994; Daniels, 1995; Manske, 1995). The specifics of this disease, its clinical course, and management are covered in detail by a separate chapter in this text.

Infectious Disease of the Kidney

Urinary Tract Infection

The majority of bacterial infections of the urinary tract occur as uncomplicated community-acquired infections, but repeated and/or complicated infections may lead to renal tissue damage and renal failure. Stamm (1991, 1994) classifies urinary tract infections (UTIs) as complicated or uncomplicated. According to Stamm, uncomplicated UTIs are community-acquired infections that occur in individuals with normal urinary tracts. Uncomplicated infections are further classified as those affecting the lower urinary tract (acute bacterial cystitis) and the upper urinary tract (acute pyelonephritis). Complicated infections are those that occur in individuals with physiologic or anatomic abnormalities of the urinary tract, including obstruction, functional disorders, calculi, instrumentation, and catheterization.

The majority of urinary tract infections (over 6-7 million annually) are diagnosed as acute cystitis, 80% of which are caused by the ascension of fecal E. coli through the urethra to the bladder. Acute cystitis responds to effective therapy in over 90% of the cases and even recurrent episodes do not appear to adversely affect renal function (Stamm, 1994).

Acute uncomplicated pyelonephritis occurs as bacteria ascend from the bladder to the kidneys via the ureter. At least 250,000 cases occur annually, most of those in females. As with acute cystitis, over 90% of the cases of acute pyelonephritis respond to antimicrobial therapy with no residual renal scarring or impairment of kidney function. However, the severity of illness associated with acute pyelonephritis may also be severe, including gram-negative septicemia, renal tissue edema with subsequent decrease in glomerular filtration rate, and necrotizing intrarenal or perinephric abscesses. Failure to improve after 72 hours of appropriate antimicrobial therapy is an indication to suspect and seek evidence of urinary obstruction or abscess. Surgical intervention may be required to relieve the urinary obstruction or drain abscesses.

Complicated urinary tract infections, like uncomplicated urinary tract infections, result from the invasion of ascending bacteria through the urinary system. The spectrum of bacteria affecting the urinary system is much broader as it may be introduced from a larger variety of mechanisms such as catheterization, instrumentation, obstruction, or functional disorders. This type of infection most commonly occurs at the extremes of life, with the vast majority occurring in older men and women and a small percentage in infants with anatomic abnormalities. Hospitalization often leads to urinary catheterization, and in men prostatic hypertrophy and urological instrumentation lead to the development of nosocomial urinary tract infection. Clinical manifestations of complicated urinary tract infections range widely from asymptomatic bacteriuria to gram-negative septicemia.

Human Immunodeficiency Virus, AIDS, and Renal Disease

Renal disease is an increasingly common complication of patients infected with the human immunodeficiency virus (HIV). Renal complications of HIV have been recognized with increasing frequency since a renal syndrome in patients with acquired immunodeficiency syndrome (AIDS) was described in 1983. The most common disorders include ARF and HIV-associated nephropathy (HIVAN) (Rao, 1995; Schoenfeld, 1994). Structural renal disease caused by infections and infiltrative diseases, including malignancies and fluid and electrolyte and acid-base disorders, are also associated with HIV infection and AIDS. Table 8-5 summarizes the most common renal disorders associated with HIV and AIDS. Renal complications can occur at any stage of HIV infection, but most often occur in patients with clinical AIDS and those who are acutely ill.

The most significant life-threatening renal problem in these patients tends to be reversible ARF, most often acute tubular necrosis (ATN) secondary to nephrotoxic agents, infection, and hypovolemic and anoxic insults to the kidney. Susceptibility to drug-induced renal failure is high in AIDS patients due to the nephrotoxic nature of many of the drugs used in the treatment of the disease. Examples of drugs causing renal failure include amphotericin B, acyclovir, aminoglycosides, foscarnet, and pentamidine. The ARF course in AIDS patients is similar to that of other patients with ARF in acute care settings. Survival and recovery are dependent on the

Table 8-5
Kidney disease associated with HIV and AIDS.

Acute Renal Failure
ATN from infection, hypovolemia, nephrotoxic agents
Crystal-induced renal failure (acyclovir and sulfadiazine)
Postinfectious immune complex glomerulonephritis
Infiltrative Diseases
Lymphoma
Kaposi's sarcoma
Amyloidosis
Calcifications
Infections of the Kidney
Cytomegalovirus lesions
Renal tuberculosis
Cryptococcosis
Abscesses from bacterial infections
Fluid, Electrolyte, Acid-Base Disorders
Hyperkalemia
Hyponatremia
Metabolic alkalosis
Abnormal secretion of antidiuretic hormone

underlying cause and other comorbidities. The majority of AIDS patients who are treated for multiple organ failure die in renal failure from the primary illness. However, some aggressively treated patients do survive the acute event(s) and may have prolonged survival (Rao, 1995).

HIVAN has been described as a renal disease unique to patients infected with the HIV virus. HIVAN occurs in 5%-10% of patients with HIV and usually progresses to CRF (Schoenfeld, 1994). The most characteristic form of HIVAN is HIV-associated focal glomerulosclerosis (FGS), which usually presents with the nephrotic syndrome. Severe damage to glomerular tissue and tubular cells are evident with this disease, but exactly how HIV infection inflicts damage is yet unclear. Patients with HIV-associated FGS typically follow a progressive course developing CRF within 1 to 4 months. The rapid decline in renal function, atypical of other FGS, is probably related to the severe damage in both glomerular and tubular cells. There is currently no effective treatment for HIV-associated FGS; in fact immunosuppressive agents can lead to an increased risk of infection. As CRF approaches, dialysis may be instituted, although survival on dialysis is short in patients with AIDS, but may exceed 1-2 years in asymptomatic carriers or in patients with AIDS-related complex (ARC) (Rose & Appel, 1996).

Toxic Nephropathies

Injury to renal tissue as the result of exposure to toxic substances is a common cause of renal insufficiency. ARF, CRF, and nephrotic syndrome may result from the toxic effects of therapeutic drugs and agents, heavy metals, and other substances primarily excreted by the kidney. The excretory function of the kidneys, the very high rate of blood flow, the regulation of blood flow upon which renal functions depend, and large epithelial surface area, inherently establishes the kidney as an organ that is susceptible for toxic injury. Excreted substances may become locally toxic as they are concentrated in the renal tubules during the normal excretory functions of the kidney. The high rate of blood flow normal to the kidneys enhances the exposure of renal epithelium to potential toxins, leading to possible tissue damage and impaired function. A drug or substance that impairs precisely regulated renal blood flow patterns may disrupt hemodynamics within the kidney, causing renal insufficiency (Coffman, 1994; Cronin, 1995).

Therapeutic agents or drugs are the most common causes of nephrotoxic renal insufficiency. Drugs inflict injury to the kidney and affect renal function through direct or indirect mechanisms. Most drugs are excreted from the body by the kidney and may damage renal tissue through direct exposure and toxicity. Others may indirectly affect renal function by causing adverse changes in renal hemodynamics. Clinical manifestation is dependent on the properties of the involved substance, the dose and duration of exposure, and the risk factors of the patient. Individual risk factors such as age, existing renal insufficiency, volume status, and coexistent conditions that may potentiate nephrotoxicity will also determine the individual patient's response to therapy with agents (Coffman, 1994; Cronin, 1995).

Nephrotoxicity presents clinically the same as ARF, CRF, and nephrotic syndrome of other causes. Coffman (1994) categorizes major nephrotoxic agents according to the type of renal syndrome they may inflict. This classification serves as a practical guide to the etiology of the major renal syndromes caused by drugs and therapeutic agents. Table 8-6 lists these major renal syndromes, the nephrotoxic agents, and the mechanism of nephrotoxicity most prevalent in each category.

ARF is the most common renal syndrome caused by nephrotoxic substances. Substances causing ARF can be classified according to the

Table 8-6
Renal failure caused by nephrotoxic agents.

Renal Syndrome/Disease	Nephrotoxic Agents	Mechanism of Nephrotoxicity
Acute Renal Failure		
Prerenal	Amphotericin B, cyclosporine, radio contrast, ACE inhibitors, NSAIDS	Renal vasoconstriction leads to reduced glomerular filtration rate (GFR).
Intrarenal		
Acute Tubular Necrosis	Aminoglycosides, cisplatin, amphotericin B	Reduced GFR due to direct toxicity of the renal tubules, renal vasoconstriction & reduced GFR may also cause insult.
Acute interstitial nephritis	Cephalosporins, penicillins, sulfonamides, NSAIDs, rifampin	Intrarenal inflammation causing reduced GFR.
Postrenal	Acyclovir, analgesic abuse, methylsergide	Intratubular, intraureteral or extrinsic drug-associated obstruction.
Chronic Renal Failure	Analgesic abuse, lithium, cisplatin, cyclosporine	Chronic tubulointerstitial process with slow increase in serum creatinine.
Nephrotic Syndrome	NSAIDs, gold, captopril	Tubular cells are damaged by direct toxicity.

mechanism by which they damage the kidney, through prerenal or hemodynamic insults, by direct toxic or intrarenal routes, and by postrenal or obstructive processes. As shown in Table 8-6, agents such as cyclosporine, radio contrast compounds, and amphotericin may cause vasoconstriction in the kidney, leading to decreased glomerular perfusion and subsequently a decease in GFR. Such renal dysfunction is usually reversible if the drug(s) are discontinued, but as in other prerenal insults, ischemic damage may occur if the insult is prolonged or severe enough. Intrarenal insults to kidney function may also result in ARF, causing ATN or AIN. ATN may be the result of the administration of drugs that are primarily excreted by the kidney such as amphotericin B, aminoglycosides, and cisplatin. Nephrotoxicity is primarily the result of direct toxic effects on the renal tubules with hemodynamic mechanisms possibly contributing to dysfunction. Agents such as cephalosporins, NSAIDs, penicillins, and sulfonimides may cause AIN through intrarenal inflammation with reduced GFR and renal blood flow. AIN is discussed in more detail in a previous section of this chapter. ATN and AIN in many cases will resolve with discontinuation of the therapeutic agent, but may result in chronic irreversible renal failure with repeated exposure or as the result of severe injury.

Clinical management to minimize the effects of nephrotoxic substances involves at the least (a) consideration of medication-induced nephrotoxicity when serum creatinine rises during drug administration; (b) inclusion of a detailed medication history when evaluating the etiology of renal failure; (c) careful planning for the effective clinical management of patients receiving known nephrotoxic agents; and (d) awareness of the impact of nephrotoxins in exacerbating renal failure in patients with existing renal impairment.

Several nontherapeutic agents/substances are also known to cause renal insufficiency of varying degrees, usually dependent on the nature and extent of exposure. Exposure to heavy metals such as lead can lead to chronic interstitial nephritis. Moonshine alcohol is a common source of lead exposure, as is workplace exposure of welders and battery workers. Cadmium toxicity is also usually the result of industrial exposure, with nephrotoxicity developing after chronic, low-level exposure. Cadmium exposure may accelerate age-related

Table 8-7
Kidney and renal function alterations during normal pregnancy.

Anatomical Changes
Renal length increases 1 to 1.5 cm
Dilatation of the ureters and renal pelvis
Increased glomerular size

Functional Changes
Effective renal plasma flow increases 75%
GFR increases 50%
BUN decreases to average of 9 mg/dl
Serum creatinine decreases to average of 0.7 mg/dl
Increased glucose excretion and glycosuria
Increased sodium reabsorption

decline in glomerular function, and damage from high level exposure may result in a chronic tubulointerstitial nephritis. Nephrolithiasis occurs in 40% of long-term cadmium workers (Thompson & Henrich, 1995).

Renal Disease in Pregnancy

Changes in Renal Function During Pregnancy

Extensive changes occur in the kidney and in renal function during the stages of normal pregnancy. The kidney size actually increases due to increased glomerular size, and dilation of the urinary tract also occurs. This physiologic dilation of the ureters may result in stasis of urine within the ureters and predisposes the pregnant woman to UTIs. UTI is the most common renal disease that occurs during pregnancy. Asymptomatic bacteriuria warrants careful screening as it has been associated with small infant size and, if left untreated, can lead to pyelonephritis (Hou, 1994).

During pregnancy increased intravascular volume elevates the cardiac output 30%-50% over nonpregnant states, which partially contributes to a 75% increase in effective renal plasma flow (ERPF). This increase in ERPF peaks at about 16 weeks and is maintained until the third trimester, when it decreases slightly. The GFR also increases early in the pregnancy so that by the end of the first trimester, it peaks at 150% of normal (Sowers et al., 1995). As GFR rises, serum levels of creatinine and urea decline to an average of 0.7 mg/dl and 9 mg/dl respectively. A blood urea nitrogen (BUN) level of 14 mg/dl or higher, or a serum creatinine level of 1 mg/dl or higher is indicative of impaired renal function (Hou, 1994). The rise in GFR is also a significant factor in the glucosuria of pregnancy. Increased GFR results in an increase in the filtered load of glucose present in the tubules and an excretion of 100 mg or more of glucose per day. This glycosuria disappears in the postpartum period as GFR returns to normal levels.

Sodium retention increases gradually, but progressively during pregnancy. Several factors appear to affect this retention, including a high level of filtered sodium load due to increased GFR, and hormonal changes, particularly estrogens and increased reabsorption at distal tubular level. Most of the increased sodium is distributed in the maternal extracellular fluid and in the amniotic fluid. Table 8-7 summarizes these changes to the kidney during a normal pregnancy.

Pregnancy and Preexisting Renal Disease

Renal function at the time of conception is the most important factor in predicting if renal function will worsen during pregnancy. Davison and Baylis (1995) contend that the "majority view is that if nonpregnant renal function is only mildly compromised and hypertension is absent or minimal, then obstetric outcome is usually successful and there is little or no adverse effect on long-term prognosis, except in a few disease entities" (p. 464). Factors contributing to renal and obstetric outcomes include several considerations for women and for health care professionals in a position to influence their care and treatment:

1. In most individuals renal impairment remains asymptomatic until a significant amount of renal function is lost and prevents counseling before pregnancy. Once the pregnancy has been established, then consideration of whether to continue the pregnancy comes into question.
2. For the individual with declining renal function, the chance for conceiving and for sustaining a successful pregnancy decreases.
3. Women with known renal impairment require counseling prior to attempts to conceive regarding the impact of pregnancy on existing renal insufficiency and risks to the pregnancy imposed by renal disease.

When considering the influence of pregnancy on different degrees of renal insufficiency, Davison and Baylis (1995) suggest looking at renal function status prior to conception. They have defined three categories of prepregnancy renal functional status according to serum creatinine levels (sCr):

1. Preserved or mildly impaired renal function: sCr œ 1.4 mg/dl
2. Moderate renal insufficiency (with or without hypertension): sCr Æ 1.4 mg/dl
3. Severe renal insufficiency (usually with hypertension) sCr Æ 2.8 mg/dl.

Pregnancy in women with mildly impaired renal function does not usually adversely affect the course of renal disease, and the pregnancy is usually a success. Diseases such as lupus nephropathy, focal glomerular sclerosis, and membranoproliferative glomerulonephritis may be more susceptible to the influence of pregnancy. In these cases, long-term renal function may be compromised by the pregnancy.

When prepregnancy renal failure is moderately impaired, risk increases for the woman and for the fetus. Major concerns are severe renal function decline, uncontrolled hypertension, and uncertain obstetric outcome. Hypertension is of special concern due to its adverse effects on the pregnant woman and the proportionately higher fetal mortality associated with it. This group is also at a higher risk for accelerated postdelivery renal deterioration.

Women in the third category of severe renal insufficiency usually do not ovulate and are amenorrheic. The possibility of conception, normal term pregnancy, and delivery is very slight. In this group, pregnancy is discouraged due to the risk of severe maternal complications, and deterioration of renal function. The goal is to preserve the renal function that remains or to introduce appropriate renal replacement therapy such as dialysis and/or transplantation. The issue of pregnancy may then be reconsidered.

Acute Renal Failure in Pregnancy

The incidence of obstetric ARF in the United States has declined significantly since the 1960s with the introduction of legalized abortion and improved prenatal care. Before the 1960s, all ARF in women was pregnancy related. Presently ARF requiring dialysis occurs in less than 1 in 10,000 to 15,000 pregnancies in the United States and other industrialized countries. The incidence remains higher in underdeveloped countries due primarily to infection and blood loss and after spontaneous and induced abortions (Hou, 1994; Chapman & Schier, 1995).

When ARF does occur, it is a life-threatening disorder that usually strikes in late pregnancy. Most commonly, ATN is seen, but cortical necrosis may also be the pathologic lesion resulting from multifactorial causes. With improved prenatal care and early detection of complications in most pregnancies, ARF during pregnancy occurs in a very complex and severe clinical situation. It usually occurs in the setting of preeclampsia with abruptio placentae, the HELLP (hemolysis, elevated liver enzymes, & low platelet) syndrome, disseminated intravascular coagulation, and antepartum hemorrhage. Other causes include amniotic fluid embolism, and retained dead fetus.

If ATN is the underlying pathologic lesion, recovery of renal function is possible and treatment in pregnancy follows the same course as in nonpregnant individuals. With cortical necrosis, permanent renal failure or incomplete recovery is more likely.

ARF may also occur after delivery as idiopathic postpartum ARF. This is a rare, but often fatal disorder that occurs between 2 and 5 weeks postpartum, usually after an uneventful pregnancy and delivery. Patients usually present with mild to moderate hypertension, microangiopathic homiletic anemia, and possibly convulsions, lethargy, and cardiomyopathy. Several causes for this ARF have been suggested, including a flu-like syndrome with respiratory and gastrointestinal symptoms, oral contraceptive use, retained placental fragments, oxytocic agents, and immunogenetic factors (Chapman & Schier, 1995). Glomerular and arteriolar lesions similar to those found in nephrosclerosis and scleroderma are most commonly seen in patients with this ARF. The severity of arterial involvement corresponds with decreased survival. Recovery of renal function is rare and slow, sometimes taking 18 months. Overall maternal mortality in this group is only 60%. The lesion has been known to recur after transplantation in cadaver kidney allografts (Hou, 1994; Chapman & Schier, 1995).

Neoplasms of the Kidney

Renal Cell Carcinoma

Tumors of the urinary organs account for over 25% of all cancers in men in the United States and significant mortality in both men and women. The most common cancer of the kidney is renal cell carcinoma, which accounts for over 90% of all solid tumors of the kidney (Smith, 1995; Bahnson, 1994). This cancer originates in the proximal convoluted tubule and has been classified as an adenocarcinoma. The sarcomatoid cell type of this carcinoma is a particularly aggressive type characterized by metastasis to the bone, aggressive clinical behavior, and a poor prognosis.

Renal carcinoma occurs most commonly in individuals over 50, but can occur at any adult age. It occurs in males three times as often as in females and is more common in smokers, but no other strong environmental or epidemiological factors have been associated with its occurrence. The classic triad of hematuria, flank pain, and palpable mass has been associated with this cancer, and occurs in 10% of patients, often indicating advanced disease. Although this triad of symptoms is rarely seen, hematuria either microscopic or gross, remains the hallmark symptom of kidney carcinoma. Most renal tumors are discovered serendipitously during computerized tomography (CT), ultrasound, and magnetic resonance imaging (MRI) (Bahnson, 1994).

When a suspicious tumor is discovered, CT scanning is used to gain information about the extent of the tumor, regional lymph node involvement, and the presence of tumor invasion of the renal vein or vena cava. Renal cell carcinoma has a propensity for vascular extension, so an important aspect of staging this type tumor is the use of MRI to determine the extent of involvement in the renal vein or vena cava. Tissue confirmation by biopsy is not usually done due to the risk of bleeding and tumor seeding along the needle tract.

The treatment for localized renal cell carcinoma is surgical excision by radical nephrectomy, including removal of the kidney's surrounding facial envelope (Gerota's fascia) and regional lymphadenectomy. Survival after surgical excision of the renal cell cancer is dependent on tumor stage. Patients who have tumors confined to the renal capsule have a 70% survival rate at 5 years; those with tumors that extend beyond the capsule, but still within Gerota's fascia, have a 50% survival rate at 5 years. Metastasis to lymph nodes decreases survival to 10% at 5 years. Metastasis to other organs (most commonly the lungs, bode, brain, and liver) brings a poor prognosis and usually rapidly progressive disease with survival rates less than 2 years. Unfortunately, chemotherapy and radiation therapy have very limited impact on this carcinoma, in fact, the cancer cells seem to be highly resistant to both. The most promising therapy has been immunotherapy with interferon and interleukin-2 (Bahnson, 1994; Smith, 1995).

Other renal neoplasms include Wilm's tumor and renal sarcoma. Wilm's tumor or nephroblastoma is one of the more common tumors of childhood comprising from 6% to 30% of malignant solid tumors in children. Most children with Wilm's tumor are asymptomatic with an abdominal mass usually found by a parent or on physical examination by a physician. Symptoms such as fatigue, malaise, and weight loss are usually late characteristics of the malignancy. Approximately 50% of patients have abdominal pain as the presenting symptom. The majority of patients are curable with a course of treatment requiring surgical excision, precise radiotherapy, and chemotherapy.

Renal sarcomas are relatively rare with an estimated incidence of only 1%-3% of all primary malignant tumors of the kidney. The most common type is fibrosarcoma, usually arising from the renal capsule. Rapid growth of the tumor is characteristic with abdominal pain as the presenting symptom. Five-year survival rates are poor and may be as low as 10%.

Summary

Renal disease continues to be a major health problem among the U.S. population. Disease states ranging from mild renal insufficiency to CRF impact the medical, psychosocial, and financial well-being of millions of patients annually. The steady increase in incidence and prevalence of ESRD is attributed to factors such as the aging of the population and the progressive loss of kidney function with age and to increased survival of patients with chronic illnesses that affect renal function. This increase will likely be sustained in the future, leading to increased social and financial costs and a diminished quality of life for millions.

Since many causes of renal insufficiency, including CRF, are preventable, it is important that a clear understanding of the etiology of renal disease be obtained by professional nurses. This knowledge is essential to the education, research, and treatment needed to decrease the incidence and prevalence of this insult to the individual's health and well-being.

References

American College of Physicians (ACP).(1994). *Medical knowledge self-assessment program in the subspecialty of nephrology and hypertension.*Philadelphia: Author.

Appel, G.B. (1994). Renal disease in the dysproteinemias. In A. Greenberg (Ed.), *Primer on kidney diseases* (pp. 117-121). San Diego, CA: Academic Press, National Kidney Foundation.

Bahnson, R.R. (1994). Renal and urinary tract neoplasia. In A. Greenberg (Ed.), *Primer on kidney diseases* (pp. 247-253). San Diego, CA: Academic Press, National Kidney Foundation.

Bernard, D.B., & Salant, D.J. (1991). Clinical approach to the patient with proteinuria and the nephrotic syndrome. In H.R. Jacobson, G.E. Striker, & S. Klahr (Eds.), *The principles and practice of nephrology* (pp. 250-261). Philadelphia: B.C. Decker, Inc.

Brazy, P.C. (1994). Therapy of hypertension. In A. Greenberg (Ed.), *Primer on kidney diseases* (pp. 355-361). San Diego, CA: Academic Press, National Kidney Foundation.

Brenner, B.M., & Rector, F.C. (1986). *The kidney.* Philadelphia: W.B. Saunders Company.

Chapman, A.B., & Schier, R.W. (1995). Acute renal failure in pregnancy. In H.R. Jacobson, G.E. Striker, & S. Klahr (Eds.), *The principles and practice of nephrology* (pp. 445-453). St. Louis: Mosby Year Book.

Coffman, T.M. (1994). Renal failure caused by therapeutic agents. In A. Greenberg (Ed.), *Primer on kidney diseases* (pp. 139-145). San Diego, CA: Academic Press, National Kidney Foundation.

Couser, W.G. (1991). Rapidly progressive glomerulonephritis. In H.R. Jacobson, G.E. Striker, & S. Klahr (Eds.), *The principles and practice of nephrology* (pp. 277-283). Philadelphia: B.C. Decker, Inc.

Cronin, R.E. (1995). Mechanisms of nephrotoxic injury. In H.R. Jacobson, G.E. Striker, & S. Klahr (Eds.), *The principles and practice of nephrology* (pp.784-787). St. Louis: Mosby Year Book.

Daniels, B.S. (1995). The natural history of renal disease in diabetes mellitus. In H.R. Jacobson, G.E. Striker, & S. Klahr (Eds.), *The principles and practice of nephrology* (pp. 336-339). St. Louis: Mosby Year Book.

Davison, J.M., & Baylis, C. (1995). Pregnancy in patients with chronic renal disease or renal transplant. In H.R. Jacobson, G.E. Striker, & S. Klahr (Eds.), *The principles and practice of nephrology* (pp. 459-473). St. Louis: Mosby Year Book.

Erickson, P. (1993). Idiopathic glomerulonephritis: Is it IgA nephropathy? *ANNA Journal, 20,* 127-132.

Fredrich, R., & Jordan, S.C. (1994). Acute poststreptococcal and postinfectious glomerulonephritis. In A. Greenberg (Ed.), *Primer on kidney diseases* (pp. 88-94). San Diego, CA: Academic Press, National Kidney Foundation.

Glassock, J., Adler, S., Ward, H., & Cohen, A. (1986). Primary glomerular diseases. In B.M. Brenner & F.C. Rector (Eds.), *The kidney* (3rd edition) (pp. 929-1013). Philadelphia: W.B. Saunders Company.

Goldfarb, S. (1994). Diabetic nephropathy. In A. Greenberg (Ed.), *Primer on kidney diseases* (pp. 112-117). San Diego, CA:

Academic Press, National Kidney Foundation.
Grabow, P.A. (1994). Polycystic and acquired cystic diseases. In A. Greenberg (Ed.), *Primer on kidney diseases* (pp. 201-206). San Diego, CA: Academic Press, National Kidney Foundation.
Greenberg, A. (1994). Cholesterol atheroembolic renal disease. In A. Greenberg (Ed), *Primer on kidney diseases* (pp. 227-229). San Diego, CA: Academic Press, National Kidney Foundation.
Guyton, A.C. (1986). *Textbook of medical physiology*. Philadelphia: W.B. Saunders Company.
Hou, S. (1994). The kidney in pregnancy. In A. Greenberg (Ed), *Primer on kidney diseases* (pp. 237-242). San Diego, CA: Academic Press, National Kidney Foundation.
Jacobson, H.R., Striker, G.E., & Klahr, S. (1991). *The principles and practice of nephrology*. Philadelphia: B.C. Decker, Inc.
Jennette, J.C., & Falk, R.J. (1994). Glomerular clinicopathologic syndromes. In A. Greenberg (Ed.), *Primer on kidney diseases* (pp. 52-59). San Diego, CA: Academic Press, National Kidney Foundation.
Johnson, J.P. (1994). Rapidly progressive glomerulonephritis. In A. Greenberg (Ed.), *Primer on kidney disease* (pp.94-99). San Diego, CA: Academic Press, National Kidney Foundation.
Julian, B.A. (1994). IgA nephropathy and related disorders. In A. Greenberg (Ed.), *Primer on kidney diseases* (pp. 83-88). San Diego, CA: Academic Press, National Kidney Foundation.
Klahr, S. (1991). Obstructive uropathy. In H.R. Jacobson, G.E. Striker, & S. Klahr (Eds.), *The principles and practice of nephrology*. (pp. 432-441). Philadelphia: B.C. Decker, Inc.
Klahr, S. (1994). Obstructive uropathy. In A. Greenberg (Ed), *Primer on kidney diseases* (pp.184-189). San Diego, CA: Academic Press, National Kidney Foundation.
Madaio, M.P. (1991). Poststreptococcal glomerulonephritis. In H.R. Jacobson, G.E. Striker, & S. Klahr (Eds.), *The principles and practice of nephrology* (pp. 262-265). Philadelphia: B.C. Decker, Inc.
Manske, C.L. (1995). End-stage renal therapy in diabetic nephropathy. In H.R. Jacobson, G.E. Striker, & S. Klahr (Eds.), *The principles and practice of nephrology* (pp. 345-351). St. Louis: Mosby Year Book.
Meyers, C.M. (1994). Acute interstitial nephritis. In A. Greenberg (Ed.), *Primer on kidney diseases* (pp.153-157). San Diego, CA: Academic Press, National Kidney Foundation.
Nally, J.V. (1994). Essential hypertension. In A. Greenberg (Ed.), *Primer on kidney diseases* (pp. 346-350). San Diego, CA: Academic Press, National Kidney Foundation.
Rao, T.K (1995). Human immunodeficiency virus disease, AIDS and the kidney. In H.R. Jacobson, G.E. Striker, & S. Klahr (Eds.), *The principles and practice of nephrology* (pp. 503-507). St. Louis: Mosby Year Book.
Rose, B., & Appel, G. (1996, May 9). Collapsing FGC and renal diseases associated with HIV infection. *UpToDate™ in Medicine*.
Rose, B.D. (1989). Clinical characteristics of glomerular disease. In E. Rubinstein & D.D. Federman (Eds.), *Scientific American Medicine,* section X (IV), 1. New York: Scientific American.
Schoenfeld, P.Y. (1994). Renal manifestations of HIV infection. In A. Greenberg (Ed.), *Primer on kidney diseases* (pp. 121-126). San Diego, CA: Academic Press, National Kidney Foundation.
Siegel, N.J. (1994). Minimal change nephropathy. In A. Greenberg (Ed.), *Primer on kidney diseases* (pp. 67-70). San Diego, CA: Academic Press, National Kidney Foundation.
Skinner, M. (1991). Amyloidosis of the kidney. In H.R. Jacobson, G.E. Striker, & S. Klahr (Eds.), *The principles and practice of nephrology* (pp. 330-335). Philadelphia: B.C. Decker, Inc.
Smith, J.A. (1995). Genitourinary tumors. In H.R. Jacobson, G.E. Striker, & S. Klahr (Eds.), *The principles and practice of nephrology* (pp. 322-335). St. Louis: Mosby Year Book.
Sowers, J.R., Mason, B.A., Dominguez, L.J., et al. (1995). Cardiovascular and renal profile in normal pregnancy. In H.R. Jacobson, G.E. Striker, & S. Klahr (Eds.), *The principles and practice of nephrology* (pp. 426-430). St. Louis: Mosby Year Book.
Stamm, W.E. (1991). Bacterial urinary tract infections. In H.R. Jacobson, G.E. Striker, & S. Klahr (Eds.), *The principles and practice of nephrology* (pp. 603-607). Philadelphia: B.C. Decker, Inc.
Stamm, W.E. (1994). Urinary tract infections. In A. Greenberg (Ed.), *Primer on kidney diseases* (pp. 243-246). San Diego, CA: Academic Press, National Kidney Foundation.
Svetkey, L.P. (1994). Renovascular hypertension. In A. Greenberg (Ed.), *Primer on kidney diseases* (pp. 351-355). San Diego, CA: Academic Press, National Kidney Foundation.
Thompson, J.R., & Henrich, W.L. (1995). Nephrotoxic agents and their effects. In H.R. Jacobson, G.E. Striker, & S. Klahr (Eds.), *The principles and practice of nephrology* (pp. 788-796). St. Louis: Mosby Year Book.
Velosa, J.A. (1994). Vesicoureteral reflux and reflux nephropathy. In A. Greenberg (Ed.), *Primer on kidney diseases* (pp. 189-192). San Diego, CA: Academic Press, National Kidney Foundation.

Chapter Highlights

- Primary glomerular diseases are disorders in which glomerular tissue is the predominant or sole tissue involved. Examples of primary diseases include postinfectious glomerulonephritis, rapidly progressive glomerulonephritis, membranoproliferative glomerulonephritis, and membranous glomerulonephritis.
- Secondary disorders involve glomerular damage as the result of systemic disease or an identifiable agent such as infection, drug exposure, or neoplasm. Secondary disorders include systemic lupus erythematosus, Goodpasture's syndrome, amyloidosis, and diabetic nephropathy.
- Identification and recognition of the nephrotic and nephritic syndromes are the very core of the diagnosis and clinical intervention of glomerular disease.
- The nephrotic syndrome has as its hallmark characteristic proteinuria, whereas the nephritic syndrome predominantly refers to hematuria.
- The nephrotic syndrome (NS) is defined as a clinical entity having multiple causes characterized by increased glomerular permeability resulting in proteinuria, hypoalbuminemia, edema, hyperlipidemia, and hypercoagulability.
- Minimal change glomerulopathy, membranous glomerulopathy, amyloidosis, and diabetic glomerulosclerosis are the major glomerular diseases that commonly manifest with the nephrotic syndrome.
- There are three major approaches to treatment of membranous glomerulopathy: no specific treatment, short-term oral prednisone, or aggressive immunosuppression.
- Nephritic syndrome classically includes hematuria as its distinguishing component. Other classic symptoms include hypertension, renal insufficiency, volume overload, edema, and in some cases, mild proteinuria.
- IgA nephropathy is the most common form of glomerulonephritis in the world. It occurs in benign and severe forms, including asymptomatic hematuria or proteinuria, acute nephritis, rapidly progressive nephritis, chronic nephritis, and nephrotic syndrome.
- IgA nephropathy is a chronic disease that accounts for approximately 10% of CRF in the United States . . . Poststreptococcal glomerulonephritis (PSGN) is the most common form of glomeronephritis in children.
- Systemic atherosclerosis can adversely affect renal function by causing renal artery stenosis (RAS) and consequently, renovascular hypertension. . . The degree of stenosis is related to the interference of renal blood flow, with 50% stenosis generally considered significant.
- A major consequence of hypertension is nephrosclerosis. Hypertensive nephropathy is the result of the chronic hypertension (essential or secondary) in which the small intrarenal arteries and arterioles are affected, leading to renal insufficiency and possibly to CRF. Approximately 25% of patients requiring renal replacement therapy reach CRF due to hypertensive nephrosclerosis.
- Hypertension is one of the most common health problems facing medical professionals today. Over 90% of patients with high blood pressure are classified as having essential or primary hypertension because the etiology is not readily definable.
- The etiology of essential hypertension is a complex mixture of interactions of hereditary, environmental factors, sodium homeostasis, the renin-angiotensin system, sympathetic nervous system, and other unknown factors.
- Autosomal dominant polycystic kidney disease (ADPKD) is the most common hereditary renal disease. It affects approximately 500,000 adults and children in the United States, and is the third most common cause of CRF in the United States.
- Obstructive nephropathy is the renal disease caused by the impairment of urine flow through the urinary tract. This nephropathy is usually caused by obstructive uropathy, or the structural or functional impediment to the normal flow of urine.

Chapter Highlights (continued)

- Obstructive nephropathy, obstructive uropathy, and hydronephrosis, are three terms that are often used interchangeably to describe the renal disease that results from urinary tract obstruction..
- Congenital renal disorders are among the major causes of obstructive uropathy, often resulting in hydronephrosis, reflux nephropathy, obstructive nephropathy, and renal failure. Urinary tract obstruction is common in utero, infancy, and childhood, and accounts for 20% of the renal failure seen in children..
- Diabetic nephropathy is the leading cause of CRF in the United States, accounting for approximately 30% of all patients entering dialysis programs. The incidence of diabetic nephropathy is evenly distributed between insulin-dependent diabetic patients and noninsulin-dependent diabetics.
- The majority of bacterial infections of the urinary tract occur as uncomplicated community-acquired infections, but repeated and/or complicated infections may lead to renal tissue damage and renal failure.
- Substances causing ARF can be classified according to the mechanism by which they damage the kidney, through prerenal or hemodynamic insults, by direct toxic or intrarenal routes, and by postrenal or obstructive processes.
- Extensive changes occur in the kidney and in renal function during the stages of normal pregnancy . . . Urinary tract infection is the most common renal disease that occurs during pregnancy.
- The most common cancer of the kidney is renal cell carcinoma, which accounts for over 90% of all solid tumors of the kidney.

CHAPTER 9

Acute and Chronic Renal Failure

Kathy P. Parker, PhD, RN, CS, ANP

Chapter Contents

Clinical Assessment: Renal Failure 201
- History 202
- Physical Examination 203
- Diagnostic Tests 207

Acute Renal Failure 214
- Prerenal Failure 214
- Postrenal Failure 218
- Intrarenal Failure 220

Chronic Renal Failure 227
- Etiology and Pathophysiology 230
- Clinical and Laboratory Features 233
- Treatment and Prevention 233

Systemic Manifestations of Acute and Chronic Renal Failure and Related Nursing Management 234
- Fluid, Electrolyte, and Acid-Base Disturbances 234
- Metabolic and Endocrine Disturbances 247
- Uremic Syndrome 249

Summary 260

References 260

Readings 264

Chapter Highlights 265

Acute and Chronic Renal Failure

Kathy P. Parker, PhD, RN, CS, ANP

The continuum of renal function (see Table 9-1) is usually defined in terms of glomerular filtration rate (GFR). Normal renal function is at one end of this continuum and is a state in which the kidneys can easily meet the metabolic demands of the body. The GFR of normal kidneys is approximately 125 ml/minute/1.73m^2 (the body surface area of an average 70 kg adult). Diminished renal reserve, defined as a GFR of 50-70 ml/minute, is a state in which the patient is asymptomatic and the small, but significant, decrease in renal function can be detected only by specific concentration and dilution tests. Loss of additional function leads to renal insufficiency (GFR 10-50 ml/min), a condition that can be identified easily with routine laboratory tests and that may produce symptoms as the kidneys become increasingly unable to meet metabolic and dietary stresses. A GFR of less than 10 ml/minute is classified as renal failure, a state in which the kidneys are unable to maintain a homeostatic internal environment (Price, 1992a; Ulrich, 1989). Because of the associated chemical and systemic effects, renal insufficiency is frequently included in the discussions of renal failure (Brezis, Rosen, & Epstein, 1991; Brezis, Rosen, & Epstein, 1993).

Renal failure is broadly classified as acute and chronic. In acute renal failure (ARF), renal function deteriorates rapidly, whereas chronic renal failure (CRF) develops slowly, sometimes over a period of years or decades. Acute renal failure may also be superimposed on preexisting chronic renal insufficiency. In all situations, the associated pathophysiology triggers multisystemic abnormalities that predispose the patient to several serious problems requiring complex medical and nursing care.

Because the needs of renal failure patients are so complex, the nurse must possess a knowledge base characterized by breadth as well as depth. The purpose of this chapter, therefore, is to provide the nurse with an overview of the processes, manifestations, and implications of both acute and chronic renal failure. The material covered will include assessment and diagnostic parameters; etiology and pathophysiologic bases of renal failure; and clinical presentation, treatment, and nursing management. Prevention strategies will also be discussed.

Clinical Assessment: Renal Failure

Patients with renal failure, both acute and chronic, may present in a variety of ways. Some have symptoms that are directly related to the kid-

Table 9-1
Continuum of renal function from normal to renal failure.

Stage	Clinical Symptoms	GFR (ml/minute/1.73m^2)/Signs
Normal		GFR: 125 ml/min
Diminished Renal Reserve	Asymptomatic	GFR: 50 to 70 ml/min Small elevations in serum creatinine Possibly proteinuria
Renal Insufficiency	Early symptoms may include nocturia. Later, signs and symptoms of uremia develop, including nausea, edema, fatigue, and hypertension	GFR: 10 to 50 ml/min Azotemia, acidosis, hyperkalemia, hypocalcemia, hyperphosphatemia, anemia
Renal Failure	Manifestations of uremic syndrome	GFR: less than 10 ml/min Azotemia, acidosis, hyperkalemia, hypocalcemia, hyperphosphatemia, anemia

Note: Adapted from Dubrow & Levin (1995); Price (1992a); Ulrich (1989).

ney, such as flank pain and gross hematuria, while others may present with associated extrarenal abnormalities such as edema, hypertension, and signs of uremia (Rose & Rennke, 1994). Patients with mild renal insufficiency, on the other hand, may be completely asymptomatic and only incidentally found to have abnormal renal function on routine screening tests. Clinical management, prevention of complications, and patient prognosis differ depending on the clinical presentation (Price, 1992b).

Once the renal abnormality is discovered, the primary goals are to establish the correct diagnosis, to assess and monitor the severity of the renal dysfunction (Rose & Rennke, 1994), to reverse or slow the progression of renal dysfunction if possible, and to address the associated nursing concerns. As part of this process, it is important to determine whether the renal failure is acute or chronic and to assess the systemic impact of the renal abnormality. This may not be simple, especially if previous data are not readily available. Thus, it is important to know how to collect and process the appropriate information.

The initial approach to the evaluation of patients with renal failure begins with the history, physical examination, and appropriate diagnostic tests. Not only is this information crucial in diagnosing the problem, but it is also important in designing an effective nursing treatment plan and in setting appropriate patient outcomes. Because the clinical presentation of renal failure may vary, nurses who work in settings ranging from walk-in clinics and emergency rooms to hospitals and critical care units are likely to be involved in the evaluation, education, follow-up, and emotional support of patients with renal function abnormalities and their families. Therefore, nurses should be knowledgeable regarding the evaluation process, including the components of the history and physical exam that are specifically related to the renal system as well as the most frequently used diagnostic tests (Baer, 1993b; Richard, 1986b).

History

The purpose of the history is to collect subjective data, or what persons say about themselves (Jarvis, 1992). A history can be divided into six components, including the chief complaint, history of present illness, past medical history, family history, social and experiential history, and a general review of body systems (Seidel, Ball, Dains, & Benedict, 1991). Although a general discussion of the health history is beyond the scope of this text, it is important to be aware that each element of the history can contain information that is relevant to the renal system (Baer, 1993b).

The chief complaint is the patient's description of the symptom or symptoms that precipitated the decision to seek medical attention (Willms, Schneiderman, & Algranati, 1994). Thus, the presentation of renal-related symptoms can provide important clues that will assist the nurse in assessing the patient. A list of these symptoms and possible associated conditions are summarized in Table 9-2. It is important to mention that many of these symptoms are seen in both acute and chronic renal failure (Baer, 1993b).

The history of present illness flows from the chief complaint and is a detailed "story" of the current problems from the patient's perspective (Willms et al., 1994). If present, each of the symptoms listed above should be evaluated regarding the onset and temporal sequence of events, the quality and quantity of the symptoms, aggravating and alleviating factors, and associated symptoms. In addition, it may also be appropriate to inquire concurrently about other ongoing medical problems (Willms et al., 1994).

The past medical history is a catalog of significant past health problems (Willms et al., 1994). Patients should describe their health history, including childhood diseases, congenital abnormalities, previous medical examinations, hospitalizations, radiation exposure, dental work, trauma, pregnancies, malignancies, and genitourinary disorders (Baer, 1993b; Richard, 1986b). Patients should also be asked about any recent illness, including history of fluid losses, recent infections, blood transfusions, and hypotensive episodes (Andreoli, Bennett, Carpenter, Plum, & Smith, 1993; Brezis et al., 1991). Because of the risk of nephrotoxicity or other adverse renal effects, information should also be collected regarding the use of medications to diagnose or treat these conditions such as dyes for vascular studies, antibiotics, antihypertensive agents, or other medications such as nonsteroidal anti-inflammatory drugs (NSAIDs) (Andreoli et al., 1993; Baer, 1993b; Brezis et al., 1991). It is especially important to obtain information related to systemic diseases, that might have a direct impact on renal function such as immunological diseases, infection, hypertension, diabetes, and disseminated intravascular coagulation. Each of these disease processes can compromise the renal system and lead to its dysfunction (Baer, 1993b).

The family history is an important component of the health history. The presence of hereditary renal diseases in the family can alert the nurse to the potential of a preexisting chronic disorder. Examples of familial renal disorders include Alport's syndrome, Fanconi's syndrome, Barter's syndrome, cystinuria, and polycystic kidney disease. This information also helps identify the need for genetic counseling (Baer, 1993b; Richard, 1986b).

The social and experiential history, often called the patient profile, is an inventory of medically relevant aspects of lifestyle. It is intended to obtain information about the patient as a member of society and family, including educational level, employment history, current living situation, family structure and support systems, hobbies, sexual activity, general health habits, and daily routine (Willms et al., 1994). There are several renal-related factors important to explore in this section of the health history, including:

1. History of exposure to environmental agents at home or work that could precipitate acute or chronic renal dysfunction;
2. Travel to particular areas of the world, which could place individuals at risk for exposure to infectious agents and subsequent renal abnormalities;
3. Illegal drug or over-the-counter medication use, as these substances are potential sources of nephrotoxicity;
4. Weight changes, which might reflect fluid gains or losses or changes in appetite;
5. Changes in activity and exercise tolerance, which could be related to the anemia associated with renal failure;
6. Allergies, as these have the potential to precipitate renal dysfunction;
7. Diet, including history of dietary (sodium, protein) or fluid restriction, which may have been prescribed for a preexisting renal condition.

General health habits should also be explored, as this information can be used to plan health promotion and disease prevention activities.

Finally, patients may present with extrarenal symptoms associated with uremia and kidney failure. Therefore, it is important to seek specific information that will reflect the degree of renal system dysfunction in relation to each body system. A summary of these symptoms appears in Table 9-3. As in the renal-related symptoms discussed above, many of these conditions can also be seen in both acute and chronic renal failure (Baer, 1993b).

Physical Examination

The physical examination consists of the process by which the clinician observes, palpates, percusses, and auscultates the patient's body and describes the findings (signs) elicited by these processes. Inspection is the informed and critical use of the examiner's eyes. Palpation is a form of touching and feeling used to assess the skin and both superficial and deep structures. Percussion is the use of sound to define structure density and content. The classical percussion method is to create vibration by tapping against the body surface and listening for differences in sound wave conduction. Auscultation is the use of the stethoscope to judge the sounds made by the movement of gases, fluid, or internal organs. Each of these modes is used to varying degrees, depending on the body region being examined (Willms et al., 1994).

The physical examination begins with a general survey or inspection of the whole person covering the general health state and any significant physical

Table 9-2
Renal-related symptoms and their correlated potential pathological conditions.

Symptoms	Potential Condition
Anuria	Obstruction Renal failure
Dysuria	Infection
Dribbling	Prostatic enlargement Strictures
Edema	Renal failure Nephrotic syndrome
Frequency	Infection Diabetes
Hematuria	Trauma Glomerular disease Neoplasia Infection
Hesitancy	Prostatic enlargement Strictures
Incontinence	Infection Neoplasia Diabetes
Nephralgia	Infection Trauma Neoplasms Ischemia Calculi Papillary necrosis
Nocturia	Infection Renal insufficiency
Oliguria	Renal insufficiency Renal failure
Polyuria	Renal insufficiency Diabetes insipidus
Frothy urine (proteinuria)	Glomerular diseases Nephrotic syndrome
Cloudy urine	Infection, crystalluria
Bloody urine	Glomerular disease
Renal colic	Calculi Papillary necrosis
Urgency	Infection Prostatic disease

Note: Adapted with permission from Baer, C. (1992). Acute renal failure. In. J.C. Hartschorn, M. Lamborn, & M.L. Noll (Eds.), *Introduction to critical care* (p. 322). Philadelphia: W.B. Saunders Company.

Table 9-3
Renal-related information to be documented in a general systems review.

Body System	Information to be Elicited	Clinical Significance
Integumentary	Dryness	Fluid volume deficit Uremia
	Pruritus	Uremia
	Ecchymosis	Uremia
	Petechiae	Uremia
	Delayed healing	Uremia
	Pallor	Uremia
	Yellowness	Uremia
Neurological	Headaches	Hypertension Fluid volume excess Uremia
	Syncope	Uremia
	Seizures	Metabolic imbalances Uremia
	Paresthesias	Hypocalcemia Uremia
	Footdrop	Uremia
	Decreased cognitive ability	Uremia Electrolyte imbalance
	Memory loss	Uremia
	Sleep disturbances	Uremia
Psychological	Apathy	Uremia
	Depression	Uremia
	Anxiety	Uremia
Visual	Blurring	Fluid volume excess Electrolytes imbalances Hypotension Malignant hypertension
Auditory	Decrease acuity	Alport's syndrome, medications
Gastrointestinal	Stomatitis	Uremia
	Ageusia	Uremia
	Dysgeusia	Uremia
	Anorexia	Uremia
	Nausea and vomiting	Uremia Electrolyte imbalances
	Constipation or diarrhea	Fluid volume changes Electrolytes imbalances Uremia
	Bloody stools	Uremia
Renal	(see Table 9-2)	
Reproductive	Impotence	Uremia
	Decreased libido	Uremia
	Amenorrhea	Uremia
Respiratory	Tenacious secretions	Fluid volume changes
	Dyspnea	Fluid volume excess
	Pneumonia	Uremia
	Hemoptysis	Good Pasture's Syndrome
Cardiovascular	Hypertension	Fluid volume excess
	Palpatations	Electrolyte imbalance
	Chest pain	Uremia
	Edema	Fluid volume excess
Musculoskeletal	Cramps	Uremia
	Muscle weakness	Uremia
	Leg movement at night	Uremia
Endocrine	Tetany	Hypocalcemia
	Thirst	Volume deficits
Hematopoietic	Fatigue	Uremia
	Malaise	Uremia
	Bleeding	Uremia

Note: Adapted with permission from Baer, C. (1993b). Renal data acquisition. In M. Kinney, D. Packa, & S. Dunbar (Eds.), *AACN's clinical reference of critical care nursing* (pp. 875-876). St. Louis: Mosby Year Book.

characteristics (Jarvis, 1992). The overall appearance of the patient can provide tremendous help in determining the health status of the individual as well as functional ability. For example, pallor, cachexia, and weariness are frequently associated with chronic illnesses. On the other hand, cyanosis and immobility related to pain are associated with acute processes. When present, many of the renal-related signs described in Table 9-4 can be observed during this part of the physical examination.

The vital signs, including blood pressure, pulse, respiratory rate, and temperature, are an important part of the physical exam and may reflect alterations in the renal system. For example, hypertension and tachycardia frequently occur in states of volume excess. Hypotension and tachycardia may accompany volume depleted states, although major changes in supine pulse and blood pressure are not seen until advanced degrees of volume contraction occur (Faber, Kupin, Krishna, & Narins, 1993). Therefore, the blood pressure and pulse, both lying and standing, should be taken approximately 2-3 minutes apart in order to check for orthostasis. If the patient is unable to stand, simply raising and lowering the head of the bed during blood pressure and pulse measurements can be helpful in checking for orthostasis. An increase in pulse of 15 beats per minutes or a drop in blood pressure of more than 15 mm/Hg indicates orthostasis (Briggs, 1995). An increase in pulse rate is frequently noted before any changes in blood pressure occur (Brezis et al., 1993).

Respiratory rate can increase with air hunger, pulmonary edema related to volume retention, pulmonary-renal syndromes, or in compensation for the metabolic acidosis that develops in renal failure (Brezis et al., 1991). Therefore, careful assessment of the rate and quality of respirations, in addition to auscultation of the lungs, is important.

For reasons poorly understood, uremic patients, particularly those with CRF, are commonly hypothermic. Several studies have reported body temperatures of less that 96° F in chronic uremic patients. In fact, body temperature may show an inverse relationship with the degree of uremia (Lewis, 1992; Schreiner & Maher, 1961; Swartz, Fitzgerald, Kalousdain, & Budd, 1983). Therefore, infection should be suspected in chronic renal failure patients who present with even small increases in temperature (98° to 99° F) (Lewis, 1992). All patients with suspected renal abnormalities should also be assessed for fever, chills, and other signs of both local and systemic infection.

The vital statistics of height and weight should also be measured, as these variables are useful in assessing fluid status and in calculating ideal body weight and nutritional requirements.

Following the collection of the preliminary data described above, a complete physical examination is performed. As the effects of renal dysfunction are multisystemic, it is important that nurses familiarize themselves with the basic approach and techniques involved. Numerous textbooks thoroughly describe the physical examination process (Jarvis, 1992; Seidel et al., 1991; Willms et al., 1994). Renal-related signs that might be identified during the examination and correlated pathological conditions appear in Table 9-4.

The kidneys, which are usually assessed during the abdominal examination, are located in the right and left upper quadrants at the midclavicular line. Because of their location, only limited information about the kidneys can be obtained by physical examination. This area should be inspected from both a standing and supine position for raised masses and unusual pulsations. During auscultation, a renal bruit may be heard slightly to the right and left of the midline in both upper quadrants using the bell of the stethoscope held lightly against the abdomen. A bruit, which can have both systolic and diastolic components, sounds like a low-pitched murmur and suggests a renal arterial stenosis (Jarvis, 1992; Richard, 1986b; Willms et al., 1994).

Renal palpation is usually attempted by elevating the flank with the nondominant hand and pressing the dominant hand deep and upward under the rib cage. The kidneys, as retroperitoneal organs, are rarely felt unless they are enlarged, as in polycystic kidney disease or ptotic kidneys. However, the right kidney lies 1-2 cm lower than the left and is occasionally palpable in the adult, even when normal in size (Willms et al., 1994). Using the technique described earlier, anterior percussion may be done to assist in assessing kidney size.

In addition, the patient should be checked for renal tenderness. This is usually done at the costovertebral angle (CVA), the area where the twelfth rib and vertebral column intersect. The palm is placed over this area and hit with the ulnar surface of the other hand that has been curled into a fist. The patient should feel a "thud." If pain occurs, renal tenderness may be present (Richard, 1986b). This physical finding is commonly seen in pyelonephritis. However, positive results may also occur in tense persons and in some musculoskeletal strains and inflammations of the midback (Willms et al., 1994).

The bladder should be examined for distention. As the bladder fills, it ascends into the abdomen. When containing more than approximately 500 cc of urine, it can be seen as an ovoid mass in the lower abdomen upon inspection. A full bladder also elicits a dull sound to percussion and can be felt as a slightly tense suprapubic mass on palpation (McConnell, 1985). A distended bladder is suggestive of obstruction while tenderness over the area (suprapubic tenderness) upon palpation is associated with infection. An assessment of postvoid resid-

Table 9-4
Systems oriented physical examination, renal-related signs, and their correlated pathological conditions.

Body System	Sign	Clinical Significance
HEENT	Dry, thin hair	Chronic renal disease
	Periorbital edema	Nephrotic syndrome
	Optic fundi - hemorrhages, exudates	Hypertension/diabetes
	Hearing loss	Drug reaction, Wegener's granulomatosis
	Epistaxis	Uremia, Wegener's granulomatosis
	Halitosis	Uremia
	Dry, cracked mucous membranes	Volume depletion
	Engorged neck veins	Volume excess
	Carotid bruits	Vascular disease
Skin	Decreased tissue turgor (forehead and sternum most reliable)	Volume depletion
	Dry, scaly skin	Uremia
	Pallor	Uremia
	Yellowness	Uremia
	Cyanosis	Cardiac failure
	Maculopapular rash	Drug reaction
	Purpura	Uremia, vasculitis
	Livedo reticularis	Vasculitis
	Pallor of nail beds	Uremia
	Butterfly rash	Lupus erythematosus
Heart	Murmurs	Valvular disease
	Pericardial friction rub	Uremia
	S_3, S_4	Congestive heart failure
Lungs	Pleural rub	Uremia
	Rales	Volume excess
	Decreased breath sounds	Uremia
	Hemoptysis	Pulmonary-renal syndromes
Abdomen	Bruits	Vascular disease
	Enlarged liver	Congestive heart failure
	Enlarged kidneys	Polycystic kidney disease, Hydronephrosis
Rectum	Enlarged prostate	Obstruction
	Tender prostate	Infection
	Occult blood	Uremia
Genitourinary Tract	Distended bladder	Obstruction
	Prostate enlargement	Prostatic hypertrophy
	Flank masses	Polycystic kidney disease
	Pelvic masses	Obstruction
Extremities	Peripheral edema	Volume excess
Musculoskeletal System	Joint pain	Immunologic disorders, uremia
	Bone pain	Uremia
	Proximal muscle weakness	Uremia
Neurologic System	Altered levels of consciousness	Uremia
	Tetany (Chvostek's/Trousseau's)	Electrolyte disturbances
	Depressed reflexes	Electrolyte disturbances, uremia

Note: Adapted from Baer (1993a); Richard (1986b).

Table 9-5
Blood and serum laboratory values and changes in renal dysfunction.

Substance	Normal Range	Renal Dysfunction
Sodium	135 - 146 mEq/L	Varies with free water load
Potassium	3.5 - 5.5 mEq/L	Increases, but may also change with acid-base balance
Chloride	98 - 110 mEq/L	Varies
CO_2 combining power	23 - 30 mEq/L	Decreases
BUN	10 - 20 mg/dl	Increases
Creatinine	0.5 - 1.5 mg/dl	Increases
Phosphorus	2.5 to 4.5 mg/dl	Increases
Calcium	8.5 - 10.5 mg/dl	Decreases
Magnesium	1.4 - 2.1 mEq/L	Increases
Hematocrit	35% - 55%	Decreases
Hemoglobin	12 - 16 g/dl	Decreases

Note: Adapted from Baer (1993b); Fischbach (1992); Yager & Harrington (1995 a,b).

ual urine to assess bladder emptying may also be done as part of the physical examination. The patient is first asked to void. Then a straight catheterization is done to determine how much urine remains in the bladder after voiding. Although an ultrasound provides more reliable information, a postvoid residual volume of more than 100 cc is suggestive of a bladder outlet obstruction or neurologic abnormality (uropathy) (Anderson, 1993). A disadvantage of this procedure is the possibility of introducing infection (Yarger, 1993).

Diagnostic Tests

Diagnostic tests are crucial in evaluating patients with renal function abnormalities. In addition to the complete history and physical, the information obtained from these tests helps to describe the degree of renal dysfunction present as well as associated systemic effects. Nurses frequently review the reports and, therefore, should know which results suggest renal abnormalities. The diagnostic tests most commonly used include analyses of the blood and urine, selected radiologic procedures, and renal biopsy.

Blood analyses. As discussed in Chapter 7, the kidneys play a major role in electrolyte balance, acid-base homeostasis, and in the regulation of the serum concentration of non-electrolyte substances such as blood urea nitrogen (BUN) and creatinine. In addition, the kidneys normally produce the hormone erythropoietin, which stimulates red blood cell production. When renal dysfunction occurs, marked changes in the amount of substances normally found in the blood and serum change. The laboratory assessments that are most commonly used in the evaluation of patients with renal failure are outlined in Table 9-5. The normal ranges of these values and changes that indicate renal function abnormalities are also listed.

Levels of BUN and serum creatinine, both by-products of metabolism, are commonly used to assess renal function. Creatinine is a waste product of muscle metabolism that originates from creatine and phosphocreatinine. It is continuously produced in amounts that depend on muscle mass. Although approximately 5% to 15% of urinary creatinine is secreted by the tubules, it is predominately filtered at the glomerular level and then excreted (Rose & Rennke, 1994; Yager & Harrington, 1995 a&b). Because of this characteristic, measurements of serum creatinine are inversely correlated with GFR. Therefore, increased serum creatinine levels occur as renal function declines. However, certain medications and muscle disorders may interfere with the measurement of serum creatinine and cause elevations without an actual decrease in GFR (see Table 9-6).

BUN is formed from the hepatic metabolism of amino acids (Rose & Rennke, 1994). When dietary protein is digested, the ammonia formed is absorbed from the intestinal tract and taken to the liver through the portal vein. The liver combines the ammonia with carbon dioxide to form urea, a much less toxic substance. Like creatinine, BUN is excreted by glomerular filtration and tends to increase as the GFR decreases (Yager & Harrington, 1995 a&b). However, the tubule reabsorbs up to

Table 9-6
Conditions causing an increase in levels of urea or creatinine in blood without a decrease in GFR.

Interference with Assays
- Cefoxitin
- Cephalothin
- Cephaloridine
- Other cephalosporins
- Ketones

Decreased Tubular Secretion of Creatinine
- Cimetidine
- Co-trimoxazole

Increased Creatinine Production
- Muscle disorders (rare)

Abnormal Renal Handling of Urea
- Familial azotemia

Increased Production of Urea
- Excessive protein intake
- Amino acid infusion
- Increased catabolism
- Tetracycline
- Corticosteroids
- Acute illness

Note: From Brezis, M., Rosen, S., & Epstein, F.H. (1991). Acute renal failure. In B.M. Brenner & F.C. Rector (Eds.), *The kidney* (4th edition) (p. 1019). Philadelphia: W.B Saunders Company. Reprinted with permission.

Table 9-7
Urinary color variations.

Color	Etiology
Orange	Pyridium Bilirubin Azulfidine
Red	Hemoglobin Red blood cells Myoglobin Porphyrin Beets
Brown to Black	Hemoglobin Mercury poisoning Lead poisoning Methyldopa Levodopa Phenylpyruvic acid
Blue, Blue Green	Methylene blue Amitriptyline Pseudomonas
White	Phosphates Chyle Lipiduria

Note: Adapted from Baer (1993b); Cooper (1993); Richard (1986b); Yager & Harrington (1995 a,b).

50% of the filtered urea. This amount can increase in physiologic states characterized by decreased tubular flow (that is, volume depletion), causing elevations in BUN. Levels of BUN also increase due to large protein loads, increased catabolic states (muscle breakdown), and renal failure. Conversely, BUN decreases due to liver dysfunction and protein restriction. Therefore, because several factors other than renal function affect BUN, it is considered a much-less reliable indicator of renal function than serum creatinine (see Table 9-6).

The normal range of BUN is 10 to 20 mg/dl while the normal value of creatinine is 0.5 to 1.5 mg/dl. The ratio of BUN:creatinine is usually 10:1 (Yager & Harrington, 1995 a&b). In most cases of renal failure, both the BUN and serum creatinine increase while maintaining this ratio. As previously discussed, however, in certain renal abnormalities characterized by low tubular flow, the BUN may increase more than the creatinine yielding an increase in BUN:creatinine ratio. Thus, it is important to note not only the absolute levels of BUN and serum creatinine, but also the ratio of BUN to creatinine (Richard, 1986b; Rose & Rennke, 1994; Yager & Harrington, 1995 a&b). A more detailed discussion of how levels of serum electrolytes and other substances change in both acute and chronic renal failure will appear later in this chapter.

Urinalysis. The urine is a very complex body fluid and contains filtrates from blood and other elements from the kidneys, ureters, and bladder. Therefore, the urinalysis is a major diagnostic tool for evaluating the patient with renal abnormalities (Rose & Rennke, 1994; Yager & Harrington, 1995 a & b). However, in order to be valid, the specimen must be appropriately collected and stored. A morning, first voided urine specimen obtained by a midstream, clean catch technique yields the most information. If urine cannot be delivered to the laboratory immediately, it should be refrigerated. After urine stands at room temperature for 1 hour, red blood cells (RBCs) hemolyze, tubercle bacilli die, and bacteria grow. In addition, bacterial action decomposes urea to ammonia and the urine becomes alkalotic, causing casts that are present to disintegrate. The analysis should ideally be conducted within 1 to 2 hours after voiding (Rose & Rennke, 1994; Yager & Harrington, 1995 a&b).

Table 9-8
Variables measured by dipstick in a urinalysis, normal and abnormal findings.

Variable	Normals	Abnormals
Specific Gravity	1.003 to 1.040	Low in ESRD and some types of ARF High in dehydration and prerenal states
pH	4.5 to 8.0	Alkaline in certain urinary tact infections such as Proteus and Klebsiella, metabolic alkalosis, potassium depletion, drugs (sodium bicarbonate), or if the specimen has sat around for a long time. Acidic in metabolic or respiratory acidosis, fever, drugs (calcium chloride).
Protein	Negative	The dipstick is sensitive to 20 to 25 mg/dl of protein (albumin) which indicates glomerular disease. Will not detect levels less than this that are clinically significant in the early detection of renal disease (particularly in diabetics).
RBCs	Negative	The dipstick will detect RBCs, hemoglobin, and myoglobin (0.3 mg/dl or 10/HPF).
WBCs	Negative	The dipstick will detect neutrophils and monocytes (10/HPF).
Bilirubin	Negative	The dipstick detects conjugated (water soluble) bilirubin. Will show up positive in obstructive liver disease.
Urobilinogen	Negative to trace	A by-product of bilirubin breakdown in the gut and can be elevated in liver disease.
Glucose	Negative	May be positive in some renal diseases that are characterized by proximal tubular defects and, of course, in diabetes when serum glucose levels exceed the renal transport maximum.
Ketones	Negative	Positive when fats are being used for energy and in insulin deficiency.
Nitrate	Negative	Nitrate is changed to nitrite by bacteria. When positive, suggests urinary tract infection. However, the urine must be in the bladder for about 4 hours for this to be positive. Will be negative in the presence of enterococcus (anaerobic streptococci in the bowel, such as Streptococcus faecalis).

Note: Adapted from Baer (1993b); Copley (1991); Farley (1989); Rose & Rennke (1994); Yager & Harrington (1995 a,b).

A urinalysis begins with inspection of the specimen for its odor, clarity, and color. Normal urine has a faint, ammonia odor. Foul-smelling urine usually indicates an infection. The sweet smell of acetone can be recognized in diabetic ketosis while some foods, such as asparagus, can produce characteristic odors. After urine stands for a long time, ammonia is formed by bacterial activity causing the decomposition of urea and producing a very pungent odor (Fischbach, 1992).

Normal urine is usually clear. However, certain types of crystals may appear or disappear in the urine and change its turbidity depending on the pH. The presence of RBCs, WBCs, bacteria, spermatozoa, prostatic fluid, and mucus can also cause cloudiness (Copley, 1991; Yager & Harrington, 1995 a&b). Foamy urine usually indicates the presence of protein.

Normal urine ranges from almost colorless to deep yellow, depending on its concentration of urochrome and urobilin pigments. The color inten-

Table 9-9
Urinary sediment and clinical significance.

Finding	Normal	Clinical Significance
CELLS		
RBCs	0-2/HPF	2 to 3 RBC's/HPF **may be** very significant. Present in urinary calculi, UTIs, urinary tract inflammation, malignancies, bleeding from trauma, glomerulopathies, renal vein thrombosis, coagulopathies, and anticoagulant drugs. Dysmorphic (malformed) cells indicate glomerular disease.
WBCs	0-4/HPF	UTI, urinary tract inflammation. Eosinophils are associated with drug-induced interstitial nephritis.
Epithelial	Occasional	Acute tubular necrosis, glomerulonephritis, pyelonephritis.
CASTS		
RBC	None	Glomerulopathies, vasculitis
WBC	None	Interstitial nephritis, pyelonephritis
Granular	Occasional	Renal parenchymal disease
Waxy	None	Advanced renal failure
Fatty	None	Heavy proteinuria
Hyaline	Occasional	Nephrotic syndrome
Epithelial cell	None	Tubular injury, glomerulonephritis, drug effects
CRYSTALS		
Uric acid	Occasional	Acid urine, acute uric acid nephropathy, hyperuricosuria
Ca phosphate	Occasional	Alkaline urine
Ca oxalate	Occasional	Acid urine, hyperoxaluria, ethylene glycol poisoning
Sulfur	None	Sulfadiazine antibiotics
Cystine	None	Cystinuria, a hereditary disorder

Note: Adapted from Baer (1993b); Copley (1991); Farley (1989); Richard (1986b); Yager & Harrington, 1995 a,b).

sity varies with the concentration of these substances. An unusually intense color might imply a normal solute load contained in a small urine volume (as in dehydration) or abnormal substances in a normal quantity (Copley, 1991). Abnormal urine colors may be a sign of disease or may indicate the presence of a pigmented drug, dye, or food (see Table 9-7).

The urine is then assessed chemically with the dipstick, a plastic strip impregnated with various reagents that detect selected substances and measures certain urine variables. These variables include specific gravity, urinary pH, protein, blood, bilirubin and urobilinogen, glucose, ketones, leukocytes, and nitrates (see Table 9-8).

Specific gravity reflects the size, weight, and number of substances in the urine in comparison to distilled water at 4% C (Richard, 1986b; Rose & Rennke, 1994). The specific gravity of water is 1.000 while normal urine specific gravity ranges from 1.003 to 1.040. The first voided specimen of the morning should be approximately 1.020 and indicates normal concentrating ability. When the kidneys lose their ability to concentrate, the first voided morning specimen is around 1.010, the specific gravity of glomerular filtrate. Specific gravity as measured by reagent strip is not affected by the presence of glycosuria or radiographic contrast media in the urine. However, these substances will raise the reading of specific gravity if it is measured by a hydrometer or urometer.

Although the measurement of specific gravity is a useful screening tool, the kidney's ability to concentrate or dilute urine is reflected in the number of particles present, not their size or weight. Thus, urine osmolality, which measures the number of dissolved solutes per unit of volume (mosm/kg), is often more clinically useful. Urine osmolality is measured by an osmometer and normally ranges from approximately 100 to 1200 mosm/kg H_2O. When the kidneys lose their ability to concentrate, as in end stage renal failure and some types of acute renal failure, both the urine specific gravity and osmolality are low and do not change appropriately with changes in volume status (Diamond, & McLaughlin, 1988; Richard, 1986b).

A microscopic examination of the urine may reveal the presence of urinary sediment, cells, casts, and crystals (see Table 9-9). Squamous, transitional, and renal tubular epithelial cells can be found in the urine. Squamous epithelial cells originate from the lower urinary tract and usually represent normal cell turnover. Transitional cells come from the renal pelvis, ureter, and bladder and, when found in the urine, indicate disorders in those areas. Renal tubular epithelial cells are found in the urine when abnormalities in the kidney occur. Oval fat bodies are a special type of renal tubular epithelial cells that have undergone fatty degeneration and indicate heavy proteinuria (Richard, 1986 a&b; Rose & Reneke, 1994).

Casts are precipitated proteins (Tamm-Horsfall mucoprotein) and cells that form within the tubular lumen and, thus, have a cylindrical shape (Yager & Harrington, 1995 a&b). When the lumen is free of cells, the casts will be composed almost entirely of this protein, are called hyaline casts, and are of little clinical significance. However, cellular casts form if there are cells in the lumen. This is a clinically important finding as it identifies the kidney as the source of the cells. Casts generally form in the collecting tubules, the site at which the urine is most concentrated and most acidic. Urinary stasis, as in poorly functioning nephrons with low flow, also promotes cast formation (Rose & Rennke, 1994; Yager & Harrington, 1995a).

Crystals are composed of salts and can be seen in the urine sediment depending on the urine composition, concentration, and pH. Uric acid and calcium crystals are found in an acid urine. Calcium phosphate and triphosphate crystals are found in alkaline urine. Urine crystals can be seen in normal subjects but may also indicate renal disease. However, an exception is the presence of cystine crystals, which are seen only in patients with cystinuria, a hereditary disorder. Sulfa crystals may be found in patients on sulfa drugs (Rose & Rennke, 1994).

Urinary electrolytes. The kidneys regulate electrolytes via several complex processes. When renal abnormalities occur, the amount of these substances found in the urine changes. To measure urinary electrolyte levels, a 24-hour sample is usually required. However, electrolytes are frequently measured using an aliquot of urine when an estimate is needed or a 24-hour collection is not practical. The results vary greatly and depend on a variety of dietary and hormonal influences. In addition, diuretics can alter test results, regardless of their site of action. The normal ranges of urinary electrolytes appear in Table 9-10.

The urine sodium is of particular clinical importance in evaluating the patient with renal function abnormalities. A urine sodium concentration less that 20 mEq/L is usually associated with volume depletion or decreased blood flow to the kidneys and suggests that renal tubular mechanisms are intact, actively conserving sodium, and able to concentrate urine. A urine sodium in excess of 40 mEq/L may indicate that the kidneys are losing their ability to concentrate as seen in some type of acute renal failure and chronic renal disease (Rose & Rennke, 1994).

Table 9-10
Normal urinary electrolytes.

Electrolyte	Normal Range
Sodium	20 - 220 mEq/L
Potassium	25 - 125 mEq/L
Chloride	100 - 250 mE/L
Calcium	110 - 250 mEq/L
Phosphorus	1g/24 hours
Magnesium	6 - 10 mEq/L

Note: Adapted from Baer (1993b); Richard (1986b); Rose & Rennke (1994); Fischbach (1992).

The fractional excretion of sodium (FENa) is an additional parameter used to assess renal tubular function. The FENa is the ratio of the amount of sodium excreted in the urine to the amount of sodium filtered by the kidney. Normally, the amount of sodium actually excreted is less that 1% because a functioning kidney reabsorbs 99% of filtered sodium. In renal failure, the FENa is greater than 1% and reflects tubular dysfunction and the inability to absorb normal amounts of sodium (Toto, 1990). To measure the FENa, a spot urine sample for sodium and creatinine is obtained simultaneously with a serum sample for sodium and creatinine (Toto, 1990). The FENa is calculated as follows:

$$\text{FENa} = \frac{U_{Na} \times P_{cr}}{U_{cr} \times P_{Na}} \times 100$$

The renal failure index (RFI) expresses the urinary sodium concentration as a function of the ratio of urine to serum creatinine concentration. The RFI is defined as (urine sodium) X (serum creatinine) divided by the urine creatinine. Renal states characterized by high tubular reabsorption will produce RFI less than 1. In states characterized by tubular dysfunction, there will be a RFI greater than 1 (Brezis et al., 1991; Diamond & McLaughlin, 1988). Although the RFI is frequently mentioned in the literature regarding acute renal failure, the FENa is generally considered to be more clinically useful.

Urine volume. The urine volume is generally of little diagnostic value. Even patients with advanced renal disease may maintain an adequate urine volume as total output is determined not by the GFR alone but by the difference between the GFR and tubular reabsorption. Thus, a patient whose GFR has fallen from the normal of 180 L/day down to near end-stage renal failure at 10 L/day will still have a urine output of 2 L if only 8 L of the filtrate are reabsorbed. In early renal failure, urine volume may actually increase as tubular function decreases and patients complain of polyuria and nocturia (Rose and Rennke, 1994).

Anuria, oliguria, and polyuria are terms used to denote the volume of urine produced. Anuria is defined as the excretion of 100 ml or less of urine a day. Oliguria is defined as the production of less than 400 ml of urine a day. Polyuria refers to normal or excess amount of urine produced despite serum chemical evidence of renal dysfunction. Nonoliguria is used to describe renal failure states accompanied by the production of significant volumes of urine (Diamond & McLaughlin, 1988; Faber et al., 1993).

Creatinine clearance. Renal clearance of a substance is that amount of blood that is cleared of that substance in a given unit of time. The clearance of any blood component that is filtered, reabsorbed, or secreted by the kidney can be calculated. However, because bodily processes affect creatinine only minimally and its excretion is regulated only by the kidney, its clearance is generally considered to be a good, reliable indicator of renal function (Moffett, Moffett, & Schauf, 1993). Creatinine clearance is usually measured by obtaining a 24-hour urine specimen for the urine volume and urine creatinine concentration and a venous blood specimen, ideally drawn at the midpoint (12 hours) of the urine collection, for the plasma creatinine concentration. The normal values for creatinine clearance in adults are 95+ 20 ml/min in women and 120 + 25 ml/min in men (Rose & Rennke, 1994). After the age of 30, there is a gradual reduction in renal mass and a subsequent decrease in creatinine clearance.

The formula for creatinine clearance (CC) is

$$CC = \frac{U_{cr} \times V}{P_{cr}}$$

U_{cr} = urine in mg/dl
V = urine volume in cc/min
P_{cr} = plasma creatinine in mg/dl

It is important to note that apparently small changes in serum creatinine can reflect marked decreases in creatinine clearance. For example, an increase in serum creatinine from 1 to 2 mg% reflects a 50% decrease in creatinine clearance.

The most common error in calculating creatinine clearance results from an incomplete urine collection leading to an underestimate of creatinine clearance. However, the relative consistent rate of creatinine production and excretion can be helpful in assessing completeness of collection. In adults, daily creatinine excretion is approximately 25 mg/kg of lean body mass for men and 20 mg/kg for women. If total creatinine excretion is less than these normal values, then an incomplete collection is likely (Rose & Black, 1988; Rose & Rennke, 1994).

Creatinine clearance can also be overestimated. In renal conditions characterized by a decrease in GFR, the creatinine secretory pump will increase secretion of creatinine and will increase clearance measurements. In this situation, creatinine clearance can markedly overestimate the true GFR and mask the severity of an abnormality (Rose & Rennke, 1994). When necessary, an inulin clearance can be performed to more accurately determine GFR. Inulin is an injectable substance that is filtered, but not secreted, by the kidney (Guyton, 1991; Moffet et al., 1993).

The Cockcroft and Gault equation can be used to estimate creatinine clearance if only the serum creatinine is known (Aronoff & Abel, 1995). The formula is as follows:

$$CC = \frac{(140\text{-}age) \times (IBW) \times (0.85 \text{ if female})}{72 \times P_{cr}}$$

IBW = ideal body weight in kg
P_{cr} = plasma creatinine in mg/dl

Radiologic studies in renal disease. Several radiologic studies are used to provide data in the evaluation of a patient with renal failure. A list of these procedures and the information they provide are outlined in Table 9-11. The following nursing interventions are important for any individual who is undergoing these procedures.

1. Explain the procedure to the individual, emphasizing the individual's responsibilities during the procedure.
2. Reinforce the explanations that have been previously provided by other health care team personnel concerning the procedure.
3. Complete any preparatory activities required for the procedure; inquire regarding any allergies to IV contrast material.
4. Provide appropriate fluids to assist the individual in maintaining an adequate hydration state before and after the procedure.
5. Assist with the procedure whenever possible or necessary.
6. Monitor the individual for any complications.
7. Document the individual's response to the procedure (Baer, 1993b, pg. 880).

Renal biopsy. A renal biopsy is performed in patients with renal parenchymal disease when other tests have been unable to identify the correct

Table 9-11
Radiologic procedures used in the evaluation of the patient with renal failure.

Test	Use
KUB	Kidney number, size, shape, and placement Diagnosis and monitoring of radiopaque stones
IVP	Kidney number, size, shape, and calyceal anatomy Detection of site and cause of obstruction (ultrasound preferable for screening)
Ultrasound & CT	Evaluation for possible urinary tract obstruction Evaluation for renal mass (cyst versus tumor) Early diagnosis of polycystic kidney disease Detection of radiolucent kidney stones
Radionuclide studies	Screening for renovascular hypertension Screening for renal thromboemboli Screening for tumors and cysts Assess symmetry of blood flow
Renal arteriography	Direct visualization of renal arterial system for renovascular hypertension, thromboemboli, or diagnosis of renal mass that seems noncystic on other studies
Voiding cystourethrogram	Detection of vesicoureteral reflux
Retrograde or antegrade pyelography	Determination of site of obstruction Relief of obstruction (catheters inserted)
Magnetic resonance imaging (MRI)	More specific than ultrasonography and CT Helpful in detection of renal masses and malformations of vessels and tubules

Note: Adapted from Borkowski (1995); Doherty (1995); Geisinger & Pohl (1995); Nally & Pohl (1995); Occhipinti & Hricak (1995); Parker, Older, Wertman, Crane, & Hidalgo (1995); Richard (1986b); Baer (1993b); Rose & Rennke (1994); Sarno (1995).

diagnosis or in order to prescribe the most appropriate therapy (Kobrin & Madaio, 1995). This is especially important in patients with glomerular disease or vasculitis when the urinalysis, serum creatinine, and serologic studies have not provided sufficient information. Indications for renal biopsy include hematuria of renal origin; proteinuria; rapidly progressing, unexplained renal failure; and acute renal failure of undetermined etiology or with a prolonged course. Contraindications to a renal biopsy include bleeding, solitary kidney, urinary tract infection, uncontrolled hypertension, and an uncooperative patient (Brezis, 1991; Faber et al., 1993; Rose & Black, 1988).

A percutaneous renal biopsy is a procedure during which a biopsy needle is inserted through the skin of the flank area under local anesthesia and directed by ultrasonography or CT. Open surgical biopsy under local or general anesthesia may be performed if a biopsy is needed and the patient has a bleeding abnormality or has some technical contraindication to the percutaneous procedure (Faber et al., 1993). Following the biopsy, the small piece of renal cortical tissue that was obtained is submitted to histological examination by light, electron microscopy, and immunofluorescence. This examination provides specific information about the glomerular basement membrane and surrounding renal tissues and greatly assists in determining the diagnosis and appropriate medical therapy.

The nurse's responsibilities in preparing the patient for a renal biopsy include:

1. Explaining the procedure, postprocedural care, and client responsibilities.
2. Demonstrating position during the test and breathing techniques, and having the patient return the demonstration.
3. Verifying that informed consent has been obtained.
4. Verifying that hematologic evaluation such as

CBC, prothrombin, bleeding and clotting time, and type and crossmatching for possible transfusion have been completed.
5. Verifying that evaluation of renal function and determination of kidney position and depth by ultrasonography or KUB has been done.
6. Providing sedation, depending on the patient (Richard, 1986b, p. 62).

Following biopsy, the major potential complications are hemorrhage and gross hematuria. These complications occur in less than 10% of patients and frequently subside after 24 hours of bed rest (Kobrin & Madaio, 1995). Perirenal hematomas radiologically develop in 50% to 80% but are rarely clinically significant. Other possible complications include laceration of the spleen, liver, gallbladder, and bowel; arteriovenous fistulae formation; and infection. The overall risk of kidney loss following biopsy is less than 0.1% (Faber et al., 1993; Madaio, 1990).

The nurse should monitor the patient frequently during the postprocedure period, checking the vital signs every 15 minutes for the first hour, every 30 minutes for the second hour, every hour for the next 4 hours, and every 4 hours for the next 24 hours (Baer, 1993b; Richard, 1986b). The nurse should also inspect all urine produced for blood. This can be done by saving specimens in clear plastic cups from one voiding to the next in order to observe the color changes closely. The biopsy site should be inspected frequently for signs of bleeding, and the patient should be assessed and treated for flank pain. In addition, fluids should be given either orally or parenterally in order to dilute the urine and prevent intrarenal clot formation (Baer, 1993b).

Acute Renal Failure

Acute renal failure may be defined as a rapid decline in GFR (greater than 50% reduction), usually causing oliguria or anuria and resulting in the accumulation of metabolic wastes in the blood (azotemia). This condition is a potentially fatal complication of critical illness, traumatic injury, and certain therapeutic regimens. Acute renal failure happens most often in acute care facilities, reaching an overall incidence of 2%-5% of hospitalized patients (Agmon & Brezis, 1993; Kellerman, 1994). The incidence increases to 10%-20% in the critically ill (Ellison & Bia, 1987; Price, 1991). Although ARF is frequently a reversible process (often self-limiting), it may also be irreversible and lead to chronic renal insufficiency or failure. As previously mentioned, ARF may occur in a patient with preexisting chronic renal insufficiency and, in this situation, is often reversible within the limits set by the preexisting disease.

The term ARF is generic and refers to a sudden impairment of kidney function without regard to a specific cause or mechanism. Renal function begins with ultrafiltration of blood, proceeds with the intrarenal processing of the filtrate, and ends with excretion of urine via the ureters, bladder, and urethra. It follows, then, that the syndrome of ARF may develop from reduced renal blood flow (RBF), prerenal ARF; from a sudden, severe renal parenchymal insult, intrarenal ARF; or from obstruction to urine flow, postrenal ARF. Although all three disturbances ultimately reduce the glomerular filtration rate, each disorder causes a different physiological response. These differences form the basis of the tests used to identify the specific disorder and subsequently to determine the appropriate treatment and nursing care (Faber, Kupin, Krishan, & Narins, 1993, p. 135).

Although renal replacement therapies have been available for over 30 years, the mortality associated with ARF continues to be approximately 50% (Wardle, 1994). Postoperative acute renal failure is reported to have an even higher mortality rate (73%-81%) (Cioffi, Ashikaga, & Gamelli, 1984). For those with ARF requiring dialysis, the mortality is as high a 90% (Henrich, 1993; Kjellstrand & Solez, 1993). Thus, the outcome of ARF is not exclusively related to the sequelae associated with failure of that organ. Rather, numerous studies have demonstrated that the outcome of ARF is dependent on age, intercurrent sepsis, hypoalbuminemia, and factors that determine failure of other organs (Groeneveld, Tran, van der Meulen, Nauta, & Thijs, 1991; Kellerman, 1994; Shusterman et al., 1987; Spiegel, Ullian, Zerbe, & Berl, 1991; Spurney, Fulkerson, & Schwab, 1991). There is considerable controversy as to whether dialysis significantly alters mortality of patients with these comorbid conditions (Alexopoulos et al., 1994; Frost, Pedersen, Bentzen, Bille, & Hansen, 1993; Spiegel et al., 1991).

Prerenal Failure

Etiology and pathophysiology. The kidneys receive approximately 20% of the cardiac output. This blood flow provides the large GFR that is necessary for efficient clearance of metabolic waste products and exceeds the metabolic needs of the kidney tissue (Holechek, 1992; Agmon & Brezis, 1993). A reduction in renal blood flow (RBF) diminishes the fundamental driving force for glomerular filtration. It also decreases the nutrients and oxygen for basic renal cellular metabolism and tubular transport systems (Agmon & Brezis, 1993; Baer & Lancaster, 1992). Thus, prerenal failure (also referred to as prerenal azotemia) results when the blood fails to reach the kidneys, causing renal hypoperfusion and a subsequent reduction in glomerular perfusion and filtration. This state is immediately reversed upon restoration of renal blood flow and is not associated with structural damage in the kidney. However, prerenal failure frequently precedes or contributes to the development of acute intrarenal failure.

Table 9-12
Causes of prerenal failure (azotemia).

Decreased Cardiac Output
Myocardial infarction
Cardiac failure
Cardiac dysrhythmias
Cardiac tamponade
Volume Depletion
Skin losses (excessive sweating or burns)
Gastrointestinal losses (vomiting and diarrhea)
Urinary losses (diuretics)
Hemorrhage
Third spacing of fluid (ascites, nephrotic syndrome, burns, acute pancreatitis)
Vasodilation
Shock
Sepsis
Anaphylaxis
Extreme acidosis
Treatment with antihypertensive agents
Renovascular Obstruction
Renal artery thrombosis (usually accompanied by renal parenchymal damage)
Renal vein thrombosis (usually accompanied by renal parenchymal damage)
Renal artery stenosis

Note: Adapted from Agmon & Brezis (1993); Faber et al. (1993); Rose & Rennke (1994); Toto (1990).

The causes of prerenal failure can be divided into four major categories, including decreased cardiac output, volume depletion, vasodilation, and obstruction of renal vessels (see Table 9-12). A decrease in effective arterial blood volume (EABV) characterizes the first three of these situations. The EABV is an unmeasurable parameter that refers to that part of the extracellular fluid in the arterial system actually available for perfusion of the tissues (Rose & Rennke, 1994). The EABV can be decreased as a result of true intravascular volume depletion from hemorrhage, diarrhea, overdiuresis, isotonic fluid losses, or from a redistribution of plasma volume to a third space. However, reductions in EABV can also occur in volume expanded states that are characterized by decreased renal perfusion, such as congestive heart failure (decreased cardiac output), advanced liver disease (pooling of blood in the portal circulation), and vasodilation from sepsis (Faber et al., 1993). Occasionally, prerenal failure can result from a vessel obstruction such as renal artery stenosis or thrombosis, or damage to small vessels and glomerular capillaries as in atherosclerosis and diabetes mellitus (Agmon & Brezis, 1993).

Under normal circumstances, the RBF and GFR are maintained in spite of changes in renal perfusion by several intrinsic and extrinsic factors that were discussed in Chapter 7. Autoregulation is an intrinsic mechanism that preserves renal perfusion and GFR through dilation of the afferent and constriction of the efferent arterioles in the face of reductions in renal perfusion pressure. This process serves as an important defense mechanism against intrarenal failure in kidneys that are underperfused. However, the autoregulation process is effective until renal perfusion pressure decreases below approximately 70 mm/Hg, at which point maximal afferent vasodilation occurs (Burnett, 1993). Below this level, renal autoregulation is severely altered by the associated intense sympathetic and renin-angiotensin activity. In response, the afferent arteriole constricts, and glomerular blood flow and GFR decrease (Baer & Lancaster, 1992).

Reduced renal perfusion also stimulates the renin-angiotensin mechanism (RAM). Renin is released and subsequently converted to angiotensin I and angiotensin II (a powerful vasoconstrictor), which also stimulates the production of aldosterone. Aldosterone increases renal absorption of sodium. The resulting increase in serum osmolality stimulates the release of antidiuretic hormone

Figure 9-1
Intrarenal responses to decreased renal perfusion.

Reduced Renal Perfusion Pressure Below Renal Autoregulation Capacity

↓

Activation of the RAM and Increased Sympathetic Activity

↓

Increased Intrarenal Vasoconstriction and Aldosterone and ADH Production

↓

Decreased GFR and Increased Sodium and Water Retention

↓

Decreased Urine Output
(characterized by a low sodium and increased SG and osmolality)

↓

PRE-RENAL FAILURE

Note: Adapted from Burnett, J.C. (1993). Acute renal failure associated with cardiac failure and hypovolemia. In J.M. Lazarus, & B.M. Brenner (Eds.) *Acute renal failure* (3rd edition) (p. 200). New York: Churchill Livingstone.

(ADH) and enhances tubular absorption of water (Holechek, 1992). The net result is renal and systemic vasoconstriction, and sodium and water retention (see Figure 9-1).

It is the ability of the kidney to successfully retain salt and water that distinguishes prerenal failure from intrarenal and the early stages of postrenal failure (Faber et al., 1993). This increased absorption causes a decrease in urine flow, a drop in urea clearance, and an increase in serum BUN. Because early prerenal failure depresses the urea clearance more than it depresses the creatinine clearance (because filtered urea is avidly absorbed by the tubules while creatinine is not), BUN increases proportionately more than serum creatinine concentration (Faber et al., 1993; Toto, 1990). Therefore, the hallmark of prerenal failure is an increase in the BUN:creatinine ratio (>15:1).

Clinical and laboratory features. Nurses should complete a thorough history and physical assessment on all patients at risk for developing prerenal failure. Risk factors include use of diuretics and antihypertensive agents, exposure to hot weather, fever, diarrhea and vomiting, wounds, burns, recent surgery, cardiac arrest, and other situations listed in Table 9-12. The presence of true volume depletion is usually evident from the history. In addition, fluid loss severe enough to decrease renal perfusion usually causes some of the physical findings associated with volume depletion such as decreased skin turgor (best assessed on the forehead and sternum) (Faber et al., 1993), dry mucous membranes, estimated jugular venous pressure less than 4 to 5 cm of water, postural tachycardia with or without hypotension, and weight loss. Those patients in hypovolemic shock may also have signs of hypoperfusion (due in part to intense peripheral vasoconstriction), such as cold, clammy extremities; cyanosis; agitation; and confusion. Those with decreased EABV from cardiac or hepatic failure may present with signs and symptoms of volume overload such as peripheral and pulmonary edema, ascites, jugular vein distention, liver congestion, and an S3 gallop (Brezis et al., 1991; Richard, 1986a). A decrease in urinary output characterizes prerenal failure, and this finding should always be reported to the physician. Anuria is rare and is more commonly seen in some types of postrenal failure.

Laboratory studies for the assessment of prerenal failure include blood and urine analyses. As previously mentioned, the hallmark of prerenal

Table 9-13
Significant laboratory findings in acute renal failure.

Laboratory Test	Pre-Renal	ATN	Post-Renal
Urine Volume	Oliguria	Oliguria, nonolguria	Anuria, oliguria, polyuria
Urine Osmolality	Concentrated	Isosmotic	Isosmotic
Urine specific gravity	High	Low, fixed	Variable
Urine Na^+	<20	>20	Variable
FeNa	<1	>1	>1
RFI	<1	>1	>1
BUN	Increased	Increased	Increased
Serum Creatinine	May be normal	Increased	Increased
BUN:Creatinine	>15:1	10:1	Normal to increased
Urine Creatinine: Plasma Creatinine	>15:1	<15:1	<15:1
Urine sediment	Normal (hyaline casts and rare granular casts)	Granular casts Epithelial casts RBC casts Cellular debris	Normal or RBCs, WBCs, and crystals

Note: Adapted from Bonaventre et al. (1995); Rose & Black (1988); Schrier (1995).

failure is an elevation in the BUN:creatinine ratio (may be as high as 40:1). Due to hemoconcentration, plasma albumin and hematocrit may increase. If volume overload is present, decreases in hematocrit and albumin may be noted. Because of the increased renal absorption of sodium and water, urinary sodium levels are characteristically less than 20 meq/L with elevated urinary specific gravity and osmolality. The renal failure index and FENa are less than 1. A summary of the serum and urinary laboratory values found in prerenal failure in comparison to other types of renal failure are summarized in Table 9-13.

Prerenal failure may also be associated with other abnormalities in electrolyte and acid-base balance. For example, elderly patients with diminished mental or physical capabilities may become hypovolemic from the inability to obtain fluid and replace insensible losses. Because of the free water deficit, hypernatremia may develop. On the other hand, the sodium level may be normal if sodium and water have been lost in proportion, as with diuretic therapy. Metabolic alkalosis may be seen with diuretic therapy or vomiting. In contrast, metabolic acidosis may be seen with diarrhea, diabetic ketoacidosis, or shock-induced lactic acidosis (Rose & Black, 1988).

A therapeutic fluid challenge is frequently given (usually 250 to 500 ml of 5% dextrose in water or normal saline over a 30-minute period) to ascertain if the renal abnormality is a result of prerenal failure from volume depletion. An attempt may also be made to increase the response of the kidney by the concurrent administration of a diuretic such as mannitol or furosemide. An increase in urinary output, 40 to 50 ml/hr after 2 to 3 hours, suggests that the cause is prerenal (Llach, 1993a). The nurse should carefully assess the patient during this procedure for side effects of the diuretics and acute changes in volume status (either volume overload or depletion, Richard, 1986a).

Treatment and prevention. Management of the patient with prerenal failure seeks to restore normal hemodynamic status and varies depending on the cause of the renal hypoperfusion (Toto, 1990). Volume-depleted patients should have their volume replaced with appropriate fluids. In patients with cardiac failure, treatment may include those interventions aimed at increasing cardiac output and normalizing fluid balance, including positive inotropic agents and/or vasodilating agents and sodium restriction. In patients with prerenal failure from vasodilation, volume replacement and use of vasoconstrictors may be successful in restoring renal perfusion. When these therapies are unsuccessful, ventricular assist devices or aortic balloon counterpulsation may be of benefit. For renal artery disease, surgery may be required to eliminate the cause (Burnett, 1993; Richard, 1986a; Toto, 1990).

Appropriate treatment frequently reverses the pathophysiologic processes of prerenal failure. However, if therapy is not instituted promptly or is not effective, prerenal failure can lead to acute intrarenal failure (Bonventre, Shah, Walker, & Humphreys, 1995). The most effective treatment for prerenal failure, therefore, is prevention, and the nurse can play a major role in implementing prevention strategies. Appropriate nursing interven-

Table 9-14
Causes of postrenal failure.

Level of Obstruction	Pathologic Process
All levels	Calculi Blood clots Papillary necrosis
Tubule	Uric acid crystals Polycystic kidneys (from cysts)
Renal pelvis	Ectopic kidney Tuberculosis Fibrous bands or strictures at the ureteropelvic junction
Ureter	Abdominal and pelvic neoplasms Lymphoma and metastatic cancer Retroperitoneal fibrosis or abscess Strictures Diverticulum Endometriosis Congenital abnormalities Inflammatory bowel disease Pregnancy
Bladder	Benign prostatic hypertrophy Foreign body Contraction of bladder neck Cancer of the prostate Cancer of the bladder Neurogenic bladder Prostatic abscesses Congenital abnormalities Anticholinergic medications Alpha-adrenergic medications
Urethra	Diverticulum Meatal stenosis Stricture Foreign body Cancer of urethra or penis Congenital abnormalities Foley catheter obstruction

Note: Adapted from Yarger (1991, 1993).

tions include the following:

1. Identify patients at risk.
2. Provide patients with adequate amounts of fluids. Unless on a volume restriction, patients should have easy access to fluids and be encouraged to drink when thirsty, as thirst is a very reliable indicator of volume depletion (Moffett et al., 1993). If a patient has mental or physical limitations, the nurse should offer fluids at regular intervals.
3. Monitor volume status. Input and output measurements provide important information. However, weight is the most reliable indicator of overall volume status and reflects insensible losses. Patients at risk for the development of prerenal failure should be weighed at least daily. If rapid weight loss occurs, the physician should be notified.
4. Monitor vital signs. Patients at risk should be checked for orthostasis at regular intervals. It is important to remember that an increase in pulse rate will frequently precede an orthostatic drop in blood pressure.
5. Monitor urine volume. Reductions in urine volume (less than 30 an hour) should be promptly reported to the physician (Anderson, 1993).
6. Monitor appropriate urine and serum analyses.
7. Assess the patient for other signs and symptoms of volume depletion and decreased EABV previously discussed in this section and outlined in Tables 9-2, 9-3, and 9-4.

Postrenal Failure

Etiology and pathophysiology. Postrenal failure results from an obstruction to urine flow that can occur anywhere within the urinary tract (Hagland, 1993; see Table 9-14). It accounts for 10% of cases of inpatient acute renal failure (Hou, Bushinsky, Wish, Cohen, & Harrington, 1983). The most common causes of postrenal failure in adults are benign prostate hypertrophy and nephrolithiasis, while obstruction secondary to congenital abnormalities occurs frequently in children (Llach, 1993b; Yarger, 1991). The obstruction may have little permanent effect on renal function, may cause progressive kidney damage over a period of months or years, or may cause rapid destruction of the kidneys (Llach, 1993b). The exact nature and site of the occlusion and its speed of onset determine the pathophysiology as well as the clinical presentation (Faber et al., 1993).

Urinary tract obstruction causes an increase in pressure proximal to the obstruction due to continued glomerular filtration. Depending on the site of the obstruction, this leads to dilation of the proximal collecting system such as the ureter (hydroureter) and the renal pelvis (hydronephrosis). (These anatomic changes are important clinically because they can be detected by ultrasonography or CT scanning.) The elevation in pressure is transmitted back to the proximal tubule. If the obstruction is complete, the increase in intratubular pressure eventually exceeds the hydrostatic pressure of the glomerulus, stopping glomerular filtration. With partial obstruction, the rise in tubular pressure may lower filtration but it will not completely stop (Yarger, 1993). Intrarenal vasoconstriction mediated by

Figure 9-2
Renal responses to bilateral urinary tract obstruction.

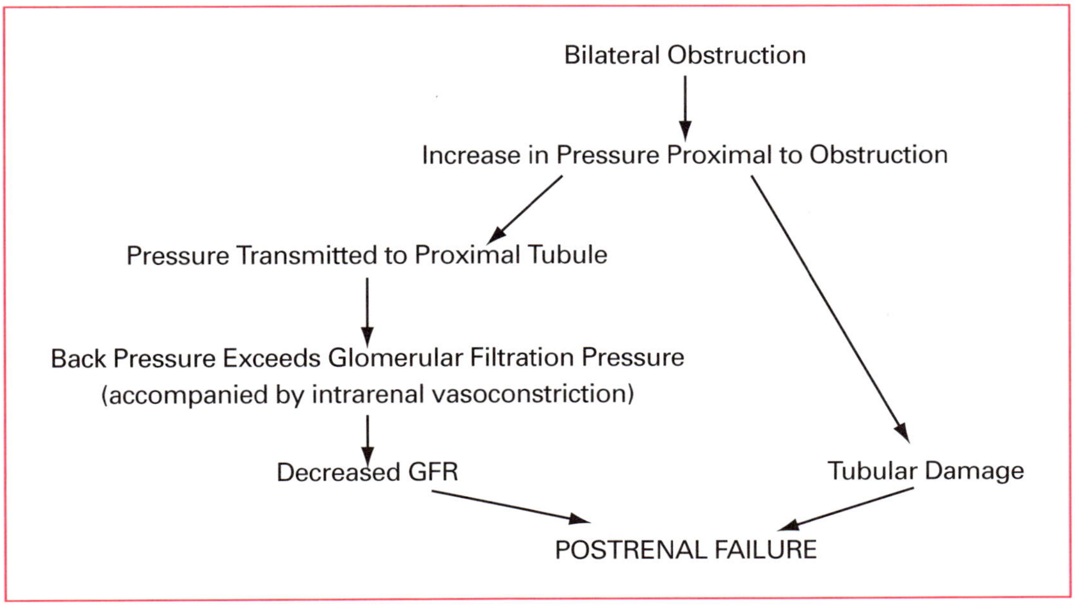

Note: Adapted from Yarger (1991, 1993); Richard (1986a).

renin, angiotensin II, and thromboxane (a vasoconstrictor eicasanoid) helps reduce GFR.

In the first 1 to 2 hours following acute obstruction, the decrease in GFR is associated with an increase in tubular absorption of sodium and water. Thus, the urine produced in this setting is decreased in volume, hypertonic, and has a low sodium concentration. The reduced GFR also results in increased urea absorption by functional tubules, leading to an elevated BUN. Following several hours of obstruction, sodium and water reabsorption decline because of tubular injury, and an isotonic urine is produced. Distal potassium and hydrogen ion secretion and water reabsorption are also diminished and frequently cause hyperkalemia, hyperchloremia, and a metabolic acidosis (see Figure 9-2). The extent of the subsequent renal damage depends on the degree, duration, and location of the obstruction as well as the presence and severity of infection (Llach, 1993a, b, c). Acute obstruction is a urological emergency. In most cases, if the obstruction is not relieved, permanent renal damage occurs.

Clinical and laboratory features. Although it may develop acutely, postrenal failure is frequently a chronic condition that has gone unnoticed or unreported by the patient (Price, 1994). However, a thorough assessment of all patients who present with renal abnormalities can frequently help identify those with postrenal abnormalities. The history may be positive for either obstructive and/or irritative symptoms of the bladder. Obstructive symptoms include hesitancy (difficulty in starting stream), decreased size and force of the urine stream, and postvoid dribbling. Irritative symptoms include dysuria, frequency, and urgency. A history positive for irritative symptoms is especially significant as urinary tract infection remains a leading cause of death in patients with ARF (Yarger, 1993). (A urine culture should always be done to rule out infection.) Pain is a common symptom if the obstruction has occurred suddenly. The pain generally begins in the flank and radiates toward the labia in women or the scrotum in men (Yarger, 1991).

The symptoms may be followed by the sudden onset of anuria or oliguria. However, some patients may present with no changes in urine flow, and it is important to note that urine volume does not necessarily reflect renal function. Depending on the type of obstruction, urine volume may vary from zero to several thousand milliliters daily. Thus, in the azotemic patient, the presence of large volumes of urine is consistent with partial, but severe, urinary tract obstruction (Yarger, 1993).

Physical examination may reveal a distended abdomen or dullness to percussion over the bladder as a result of a distention. Costovertebral (CVA) tenderness may be present if hydronephrosis or infection has developed. A large post void residual urine noted after straight catheterization indicates a lower urinary tract obstruction.

The urine and serum laboratory findings seen in

Table 9-15
Clinical settings associated with a high risk of ARF.

Patients Undergoing Surgery
Open heart surgery
Abdominal aortic surgery
Surgery in a jaundiced patient
Cadaveric Renal Transplantation
Warm and cold ischemia
Cyclosporine nephrotoxicity
Nephrotoxic agents (see Table 9-17)
Inflammatory Processes
Bacterial
Viral
Septicemia
Trauma
Penetrating
Nonpenetrating
Burns
Systemic and Vascular Disorders
Renal vein, artery, arteriolar thrombosis
Sickle cell disease
Systemic Lupus Erythematosus
Pigment Induced
Disseminated intravascular hemolysis (hemoglobin)
Transfusion reactions (hemoglobin)
Rhabdomyolysis (myoglobin)
Multiorgan Failure

Note: Adapted from Leiberthal & Levinsky (1990); Richard (1986a); Wardle (1994).

postrenal failure are summarized in Table 9-13. Microscopic hematuria and proteinuria are common. In addition, some patients may develop a salt-losing state accompanied by hyponatremia and extracellular volume contraction. Others develop hyperkalemia due to decreased levels of aldosterone and increased tubular resistance to the hormone. Patients may also have a hyperchloremic, hyperkalemic metabolic acidosis due to diminished ability of the nephron to excrete hydrogen ions (Yarger, 1993).

A plain film of the abdomen may reveal kidney enlargement and often provides clues about the cause of the obstruction. Ultrasonography and CT can be done safely to screen an azotemic patient, as contrast media is not required. An IVP can pinpoint the site and degree of obstruction. However, this study may not be useful if the GFR is markedly reduced. A anterograde or retrograde pyelogram may also help visualize the site obstruction (Faber et al., 1993; Richard, 1986b; Yarger, 1993).

Treatment and prevention. Postrenal failure is treated by relieving the obstruction, preserving renal function, and preventing and treating any complications. An acute obstruction lasting less than 24 hours is almost always accompanied by complete recovery (LaValle, 1986). In the absence of complicating infection, decompression of the urinary tract after 1 to 2 weeks of even total obstruction may still allow for complete functional recovery. However, it may take days or weeks to return to baseline renal functioning (Faber et al., 1993). The nurse plays a key role in the assessment, management, education, and support of these patients before and during relief of the obstruction.

After the obstruction has been relieved, renal concentrating abnormalities may persist such that large amount of solutes and water are excreted (generally from 8 to 20 L/day). This condition is referred to as postobstructive diuresis (Yarger, 1991, 1993). Three factors are thought to contribute to its development. First, fluid taken orally or administered intravenously before removal of the obstruction can cause volume expansion, which is later excreted. Second, solutes such as urea and electrolytes that were also retained can act as osmotic diuretics and facilitate the diuresis. Third, tubular damage may have occurred during the obstruction that inhibits the normal concentrating abilities of the kidney. The polyuria is usually associated with the excretion of large amounts of sodium, potassium, magnesium, and other electrolytes. Although the condition is self-limiting, the fluid and electrolyte losses that occur can be life-threatening (Yarger, 1991).

The nurse should carefully monitor the patient with postobstructive diuresis. Intake and output should be measured hourly and fluid replaced if needed. Daily (or more frequent) weights provide information regarding net fluid balance. Vital signs, including checks for orthostasis, should be taken every 1 to 2 hours. Electrolytes, including sodium, potassium, and magnesium, should be measured daily. Urine specific gravity and osmolality provide information regarding the ability of the kidneys to concentrate urine (LaValle, 1986; Vogel, 1979). The condition usually resolves in several days to a week (Yarger, 1991).

Activities for the prevention of postrenal failure include careful assessment of patients at risk and education of those individuals regarding symptoms, including both irritative and obstructive symptoms, which require further medical evaluation.

Intrarenal Failure

Etiology and pathophysiology. Injury to the renal tissues causes intrarenal failure and leads to the rapid decline of GFR, elevation of BUN and serum creatinine, and (frequently but not always) progressively diminishing urine output. The condition most commonly occurs in high-risk clinical settings (see Table 9-15) and in those patients with acute risk factors and preexisting renal disease (see Table 9-16). The severe insults that cause this abnormality result from damage or inflammation of the glomerulus and/or other renal vessels, the interstitial tissues, or the tubule system.

Glomerulonephritis and vasculitis result from inflammatory or immunologic disorders, such as poststreptococcal glomerulonephritis, systemic lupus erythematosus and Goodpasture's Syndrome. In these diseases, the GFR is reduced from the hemodynamic changes that result from acute immune injury as well as structural damage. Occlusion of the renal vessels from conditions such as renal thrombosis, sickle cell disease, and thrombotic thrombocytopenic purpura also cause intrarenal failure by inducing ischemia and necrosis (Bonventre et al., 1995; Brezis et al., 1993; Levine, Lieberthal, Bernard, & Salant, 1993). In contrast, interstitial nephritis, an abnormality characterized by inflammatory cell infiltrates within the renal interstitium without glomerular or tubular damage, results from certain infections, infiltrative diseases (such as lymphoma, leukemia, and sarcoidosis), and drugs (antibiotics, diuretics, analgesics (Bonventre et al., 1995; Bennett, Elzinga, & Porter, 1991; Faber et al., 1993). Approximately 5% to 20% of acute intrarenal failure is from these types of abnormalities (Anderson, 1993; Faber et al., 1993; Llach 1993a).

More commonly, intrarenal failure results from acute tubular necrosis (ATN). Although in most cases of ATN the pathology involves the renal tubules, other renal tissues may also become damaged. The major causes of ATN are ischemia and nephrotoxicity. The pathophysiology of each disorder will be discussed in the following sections. However, it is important to note that these two conditions may act in combination to produce renal damage. For example, some patients with underlying renal ischemia may develop ATN after only a brief exposure to a nephrotoxic agent (Anderson, 1993; Brezis et al., 1993).

Ischemic ATN. Renal ischemia is the most common cause of ATN. This may seem like a paradox given that the kidney is one of the best oxygenated organs of the body and receives approximately 25% of the cardiac output each minute. However, most of the renal blood flow goes to the cortex (which houses the glomeruli) for the formation of filtrate and the clearance of wastes. Only about 1/10 goes to the medulla, the minimal amount necessary for oxygen delivery while at the same time permitting urine concentration. A higher blood flow would disrupt the osmotic gradient generated in the medulla by the countercurrent system (Agmon & Brezis, 1993; Brezis et al., 1993). Therefore, when renal blood flow is reduced, the medulla (along with the tubules) is the area most severely compromised (Hays, 1992). According to Brezis et al. (1993), this susceptibility of the medulla to hypoxia and subsequent tubule damage "may be considered the price paid for an efficient urinary concentrating mechanism" (p. 214).

Table 9-16
Acute and chronic risk factors associated with the development of ARF.

Acute Risk Factors
Volume depletion
Aminoglycoside use
Radiocontrast exposure
NSAID exposure
Septic shock
Dehydration
Hypotension
Pigmenturia
Chronic Risk Factors
Preexisting renal disease
Hypertension
Congestive heart failure
Diabetes mellitus
Age
Liver cirrhosis

Note: From Brezis, M., Rosen S., & Epstein, F.H. (1993). Acute renal failure due to ischemia (acute tubular necrosis). In J.M. Lazarus & B.M. Brenner (Eds.), *Acute renal failure* (3rd edition) (pp. 210). New York: Churchill Livingstone.

The cell damage that actually occurs during periods of reduced renal perfusion depends on the extent and duration of the ischemia. When the MAP falls below 50 to 70 mm/Hg, renal blood flow and perfusion pressure decrease and ischemia begins. If this ischemia is less than 25 minutes, the damage is often mild and reversible. Ischemia of 40 to 60 minutes results in more severe damage, which may recover in 2 to 3 weeks. However, periods of ischemia of up to 60 to 90 minutes usually result in permanent kidney damage (Kjellstrand & Solez, 1993; Messmer, Kreimeier, & Hammessen, 1989; Stahl, 1986).

The initial pathophysiologic event in ischemic ATN is intrarenal vasoconstriction. As discussed previously, reduced renal blood flow causes activation of the sympathetic and renin-angiotensin systems (see Figure 9-3). In response, the afferent arteriole of the glomerulus constricts and reduces glomerular blood flow. This response may also be mediated by other vasoconstrictors such as

Figure 9-3
Ischemic and nephrotoxic ATN.

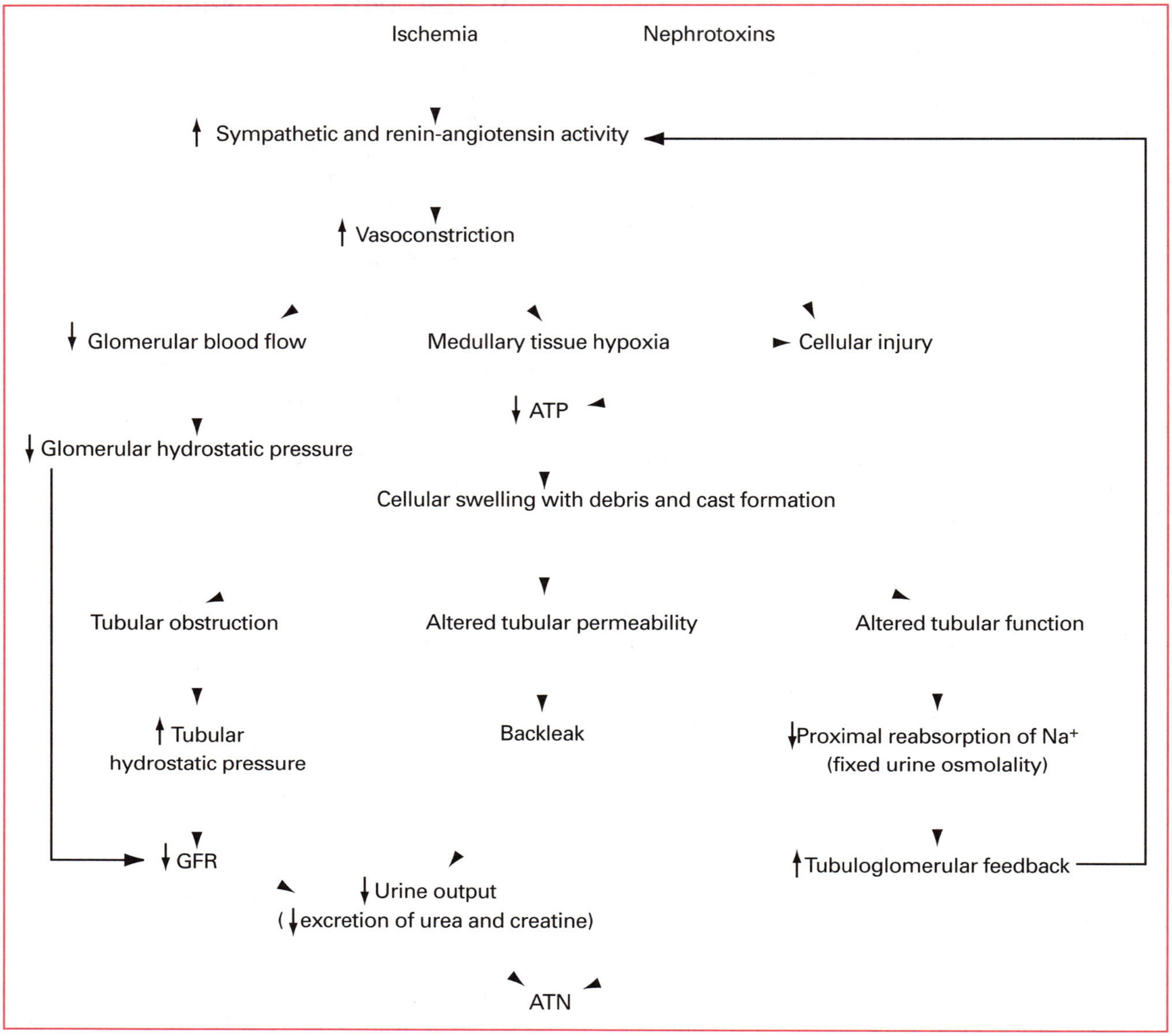

Note: Adapted from Baer & Lancaster (1992); Hays (1992); Iaina & Schwartz (1994); Stark (1994); Richard (1986a).

endothelin and thromboxane (Brezis et al., 1991; Lieberthal & Levinsky, 1990; Wardle, 1994). The reduced glomerular blood flow causes a decrease in hydrostatic pressure and a subsequent decrease in GFR. These events are in part responsible for the reduced urinary output frequently seen in ATN.

A variety of factors contribute to the development of tubular injury in ischemic ATN. These factors include cellular ATP depletion, alteration in normal polarity of the epithelial layer of the tubular walls, disruption of the basement membrane, and generation of oxygen-free radicals. The damage causes both functional impairment and cell necrosis (Rose & Rennke, 1994; Weinberg, 1995).

The presence of ATP is essential for cell homeostasis, maintenance of cellular volume and ionic concentration, and integrity of the cell membrane (Stark, 1994). Within 30 seconds of an ischemic episode, the tubular cells experience ATP depletion (Kellerman & Molitoris, 1991). This occurs because of conversion from aerobic to anaerobic metabolism, a state in which less ATP is produced (Baer,

1993a; Brezis et al., 1993; Hays, 1992). The intracellular energy depletion associated with low levels of ATP causes inactivation of the Na^+-K^+ pump, a system that helps regulate tubular cell volume. Sodium and chloride accumulate in the cell and the cells take up water and swell. The cellular swelling contributes to tubular obstruction and medullary ischemia and injury (Baer & Lancaster, 1992; Iaina & Schwartz, 1994; Stark, 1994; Weinberg, 1995). Other cellular pumps also fail, causing a decrease in intrarenal cell potassium, magnesium, and inorganic phosphates and an increase in calcium, all of which may also enhance cell injury (Stark, 1994). Sloughed necrotic cells and casts that form obstruct the tubular lumen. This obstruction to tubular flow causes an increase in Bowman's capsule hydrostatic pressure, which opposes the glomerular hydrostatic pressure. The changes cause a reduction of GFR and a decreased excretion of urea and creatinine and urinary output.

The epithelial cell membrane is composed of two different components called the apical and basolateral segments. Each segment is polarized in opposition of the other. This polarity is important in the movement of ions, water, and macromolecules between the tubular lumen and the blood compartment. ATP depletion results in a loss of the normal polarity of the epithelial layer of the tubular walls (Hays, 1992; Stark, 1994). The polarity abnormality also affects the proximal tubule, causing a decrease in proximal reabsorption of sodium. Thus, there is an increase in the delivery of sodium to the distal tubule in the area of the macula densa. In response, increased tubuloglomerular feedback produces further afferent arteriole constriction that further decreases glomerular filtration and urine output (Baer & Lancaster, 1992; Hays, 1992).

The lesion of ischemic ATN is characterized by patchy necrosis and is commonly associated with disruption of the basement membrane (Llach, 1993a). Injury to the basement membrane increases tubular permeability and allows tubular filtrate to leak back into the interstitium and peritubular capillaries. This backleak of tubular filtrate also contributes to the reduced urine output (Baer & Lancaster, 1992).

Production of oxygen-free radicals is also believed to play a major role in the development of cellular injury (Guignard, Semama, John, & Huet, 1993; Weinberg, 1995). Cells that are experiencing aerobic metabolism (with oxygen) produce oxygen-free radicals as part of the normal process. However, these substances are highly reactive and can cause disruption of cellular functioning. Usually, the cell defends itself against these normal elements by utilizing intracellular mechanisms to destroy the free radicals. However, during ischemia and anaerobic metabolism, the cell is unable to protect itself and damage occurs (Stark, 1994). Oxygen-free radicals may be particularly important in the cellular injury known to continue after reperfusion of the ischemic kidney (ischemic-reperfusion injury) (Iaina & Schwartz, 1994; Stark, 1994; Wardle, 1994).

Nephrotoxic ATN. Nephrotoxic ATN is defined as the deterioration of renal function over a matter of days to weeks following toxin exposure (see Table 9-17). This type of ATN accounts for 30% to 40% of the cases of ATN and may cause renal damage ranging from mild renal insufficiency to frank renal failure. Nephrotoxic ATN is commonly seen in hospitalized patients receiving certain antibiotics, particularly aminoglycosides. In fact, it has been estimated that an elevation in the serum creatinine concentration of 0.5 to 4.0 mg/dl occurs in 10% to 20% of patients who receive a full 7 to 10-day course of aminoglycosides (Anderson, 1993; Rose & Rennke, 1994).

The kidney is very vulnerable to toxic damage for several reasons. First, the blood circulates through the kidneys 14 times per hour. Thus, the renal tissue is repeatedly exposed to substances that are carried in the blood. Second, the kidneys play a major role in the concentration and excretion of toxic substances and are, therefore, exposed to high concentrations of these substances (Richard, 1986a; Swan & Bennett, 1993). Finally, the renal tubular cells are very susceptible to direct toxic effects of a wide variety of drugs, solvents, heavy metals, and other products (Brezis et al., 1993). Thus, the nurse should carefully monitor the renal function of any patient who has been exposed to or is receiving a potentially nephrotoxic substance.

In toxic ATN, the initial event is injury to the tubular cell from the toxic substance. Thereafter, the pathophysiology is basically the same as with ischemic ATN (see Figure 9-3). There is tubular damage, followed by necrosis and cast formation, tubular obstruction, and decreased GFR (Baer & Lancaster, 1992).

In contrast to that of ischemic ATN, the lesion of nephrotoxic ATN is uniform and may be localized to the proximal and distal tubule (Lieberthal & Levinsky, 1990; Llach, 1993a). The basement membrane of the renal tubular cells is usually not injured and remains intact. This type of lesion frequently causes a renal-concentrating defect rather than the impairment of the urinary flow seen with tubular backleak and obstruction as in ischemic ATN. As a result, dilute urine flows freely through intact, unobstructed tubules. This condition is referred to as nonoliguric ATN. The urine volume may vary from normal to as much as 2 L/h (Stark, 1992a). Nonoliguric ATN is associated with a shortened clinical course (ranging from as little as 5 to 8 days in comparison to weeks or months in the case of ischemic ATN) and a 50% to 60% reduction in mortality (Douglas, 1992; Stark, 1992a).

The severity and time course of the renal failure depends on the nature and dose of the toxin as well as a variety of host factors (Swan & Bennett, 1993).

Table 9-17
Nephrotoxic agents.

Classification	Example
Drugs	Antibacterial Antiviral Antifungal Antiprotozoal Nonsteroidal antiinflammatory Antineoplastic Angiotensin-converting enzyme inhibitors Diuretics Anti-ulcer (Cimetidine)
Anesthetics	Methoxyflurane Enflurane
Contrast Media	Diatrizoate Iothalamate Bunamiodyl
Organic Solvents	Glycols Halogenated hydrocarbons Aromatic hydrocarbons Gasoline, kerosene, turpentine
Heavy Metals	Arsenic Bismuth Barium Copper Lead Gold Mercury Lithium
Heme Pigments	Hemoglobin Myoglobin
Intrarenal Crystal Deposition	Uric acid Calcium Oxalate
Products from Multiorgan Failure	Endotoxins Tumor necrosis factor (TNF) Interleukin-1

Note: Adapted from Baer & Lancaster (1992); Brezis et al. (1991); Llach (1993a); Swan & Bennett (1993); Richard (1986a).

Thus, individual nephrotoxic insults that are tolerated by healthy persons may produce severe and prolonged injury in elderly patients or those with dehydration, vascular insufficiency, or circulatory failure (Bresiz et al., 1991). Nephrotoxic ATN is usually reversible if it is identified early and if exposure to the offending agent is removed (Brezis et al., 1991).

Clinical and laboratory features. Before the diagnosis of ATN is made, it is crucial to rule out pre- and postrenal causes of renal failure. This can be done by obtaining an indepth health history, performing a complete physical examination, and reviewing the results of appropriate urine and blood analyses. The information important to obtain was outlined in the first part of this chapter and in the sections covering pre- and postrenal failure. In addition, the laboratory analyses used to assist in distinguishing pre-, intra-, and postrenal failure are summarized in Table 9-13.

The clinical course of ATN is divided into four stages, including onset, oliguric-anuric phase, diuretic phase, and recovery. The onset begins with the precipitating event and lasts hours or days until renal cell injury occurs along with oliguria or anuria. The onset is usually a period of hours when caused by ischemia but may last 2 to 7 days when caused by a nephrotoxin (Lancaster, 1992; Rose & Rennke, 1994).

If the conditions that trigger the onset of ATN are not reversed, the oliguric-anuric phase begins. This stage is characterized by a urine output of less than 400 ml per 24 hours. Although this period usually lasts from 7 to 14 days, it can persist for weeks or months, depending on the extent of the renal injury (Stark, 1992a). The longer an individual remains in the oliguric-anuric phase, the poorer is the prognosis for recovery because of the increased risk of complications (Baer & Lancaster, 1992; Baer, 1993a; Brezis et al., 1991). Renal dysfunction persists throughout the duration of this stage, although the healing of renal tissue begins within 25 to 48 hours after the insult.

During the oliguric-anuric phase, the BUN and serum creatinine are elevated in a ratio of approximately 10:1. Daily increases in the BUN level during this stage are approximately 25 mg/dL with a daily increase in creatinine of 0.5 to 2.5 mg/dL (Douglas, 1992; Rose & Rennke, 1994). In addition, there are increases in the levels of potassium, phosphorus, and magnesium, and decreases in the levels of pH, bicarbonate, calcium, hematocrit, and hemoglobin.

As previously mentioned, the urine volume is usually less than 400 cc/24 hours. However, if the patient has nonoliguric ATN, urine volumes may be considerably greater. The urine that is produced has a low specific gravity and osmolality, a sodium level greater than 20 mEq/L, and contains granular and epithelial casts. The RFI and FENa are both greater than 1.

Because the kidney has lost most or all of its regulatory and excretory functions, the patient may develop many of the signs and symptoms of acute uremia within as few as 72 hours. The clinical problems that can occur during this phase are summarized in Table 9-18. The pathophysiology and nursing management of the uremic syndrome, in both the acute and chronic patient, are discussed in more detail in the final section of this chapter.

The diuretic phase usually lasts about 7 to 14 days and begins when the daily urinary output is greater than 400 ml per 24 hours (Baer & Lancaster, 1992; Llach, 1993a; Richard, 1986a). Although renal healing occurs during this stage, the tubule system is frequently unable to concentrate urine effectively. In addition, retained fluid and the diuretic affect of urea may facilitate the diuresis. Thus, patients may ultimately excrete large volumes of urine (in excess of 10 L/day) and lose substantial amounts of important electrolytes (Brezis et al., 1991; Llach, 1993a). Hypokalemia and metabolic alkalosis may develop. Initially the urine is comparable to plasma filtrate, but then urea excretion gradually increases and urinary sodium decreases. The BUN and serum creatinine usually slowly decrease but rapid correction may also occur.

The onset of the diuretic phase does not signify a halt to all the clinical problems associated with acute renal failure. For several days after diuresis begins, renal function remains poor, the BUN may continue to rise, infection may occur, and the uremic syndrome may become worse. In fact, 20% to 25% of the deaths occur during the diuretic phase (Brezis et al., 1991; Llach, 1993a). Thus, the nurse must carefully monitor the patient for fluid and electrolyte deficits, acid-base disorders, and the other systemic complications of uremia (Richard, 1986a).

The convalescent phase begins when the BUN is stable and lasts until the patient is able to return to normal activity. Complete recovery may require several months to a year (Lancaster, 1992; Llach, 1993a). Approximately 50% to 60% of patients with ATN fully recover their renal function. However, in the remainder of the patients, renal function never returns to baseline and some are left with significant renal impairment.

Treatment and prevention. The goals of treatment for the patient with ATN include the following: (a) prevention or correction of the primary disorder, if possible; (b) correction of fluid, electrolyte, and acid base disorders; (c) prevention of infection; (d) maintenance of an optimal nutrition state; (e) treatment of the systemic effects of uremia; (f) provision of patient and family support (Baer & Lancaster, 1992; Douglas, 1992; Kjellstrand & Barsoum, 1995; Stark, 1994).

The nurse should carefully monitor the volume status of all patients at risk for the development of ATN. Blood pressure, body weight, urinary output, central venous pressure, and pulmonary capillary wedge pressure are all valuable parameters that can help determine if a patient is volume depleted. Prompt correction of volume deficits and maintenance of cardiac output can help prevent ATN. Even when this intervention is not successful in preventing ATN, it can still contribute to the formation of a nonoliguric state by reducing renal tubular damage and thus reduce both morbidity and mortality (Stark, 1992a). The nurse should also carefully monitor patients receiving potentially nephrotoxic agents, particularly those who are elderly, diabetic, volume depleted, or receiving multiple nephrotoxic drugs. Combinations of medications, such as cephalothin and gentamicin, are particularly nephrotoxic (Douglas, 1992). Dosages of these medications should be calculated and given according to renal function and drug levels checked when appropriate.

Several pharmacologic agents are available to help prevent and treat ATN. These agents can also

Table 9-18
Acute uremia: Pathophysiology and related clinical findings.

Body System	Pathophysiology	Clinical Findings
Fluid, Electrolyte, and Acid-Base Status	Kidneys have decreased ability or are unable to regulate fluid, electrolyte, and acid-base balance.	Fluid retention, hypertension, edema, hyperkalemia, hypocalcemia, hyperphosphatemia, hypermagnesemia, and metabolic acidosis.
General Metabolic Status	Kidneys have decreased ability or are unable to excrete metabolic wastes. There is an increase in the peripheral resistance to insulin and decreased renal excretion of insulin.	Increased BUN and creatinine, and glucose intolerance.
Urinary System	Kidney damage is reflected in decreased output and presence of abnormal sediment in urine that is produced. Foley catheters are frequently in place to facilitate urine output measurement; therefore, the risk of infection is high.	Anuria or oliguria; urine sediment—red and white cells, casts, proteinuria; potential for urinary tract infection.
Gastrointestinal System	Uremic wastes are retained and exert effects on mucous membranes along GI tract. Hyper- or hypomotility can occur with electrolyte imbalances.	Anorexia, nausea and vomiting, stomatitis, constipation/diarrhea, GI bleeding, abdominal distention.
Cardiovascular System	Fluid is retained, electrolyte abnormalities (particularly hyperkalemia) are present, and uremia causes increased permeability of the pericardial membrane.	Hypertension or hypotension, congestive heart failure, pericarditis, dysrhythmias, pericardial effusion, cardiac tamponade, edema.
Respiratory System	Hyperventilation is a compensatory mechanism for metabolic acidosis. Pulmonary edema may develop with volume overload. Decreased lung expansion in patients on bed rest, along with the decreased immunologic response seen in acute renal failure, facilitates development of pneumonia.	Kussmaul respirations, pulmonary edema, pneumonia, pneumonitis. pleural effusions.
Hematologic System	Anemia is related to depressed erythropoietin secretion. Uremia decreases platelet adhesiveness and immunologic responses.	Anemia, potential for bleeding and infections.
Neurologic System	Accumulation of metabolic wastes may result in alteration of mental status.	Drowsiness, coma, convulsions, myoclonus, psychosis.
Dermatologic System	Skin changes result from accumulation of metabolic wastes, calcium and phosphate imbalances, and platelet abnormalities associated with uremia.	Dryness, pruritus, purpura, potential for infection as a result of cracking of the skin.
Skeletal System	Decreased GI absorption of calcium and decreased renal excretion of phosphate causes electrolyte imbalances.	Hypocalcemia, hyperphosphatemia, metastatic calcifications.

Note: From Parker, K.P. (1992). Disorders of the kidney. In L. Burrell, (Ed.), *Adult health nursing in hospital and community settings* (p. 1249). Norwalk, CT: Appleton Lange.

be used to create a nonoliguric ATN (Stark, 1994). Although the exact physiologic effects of many of these medications are poorly understood, potential mechanisms of action in the prevention and treatment of ARF include:

1. Improvement of renal hemodynamics by increasing blood flow, glomerular hydrostatic pressure, and GFR.
2. Decrease of tubular obstruction by reducing the formation of casts and enhancing their removal.
3. Decrease of tubular cell injury and backleak.
4. Enhancement of tubular epithelial regeneration and repair (Lieberthal & Levinsky, 1990).

A summary of these medications, their mechanism of actions, and nursing considerations appear in Table 9-19.

Infection is one of the most frequent complications of ATN and occurs in as many as 70% of patients (Kjellstrand & Barsoum, 1995; Stark, 1994). More importantly, infections have been implicated in the deaths of 29% to 72% of patients with ARF (Finn, 1993). The most common infections seen in patients with ARF include septicemia, pulmonary infections, urinary tract infections, peritonitis, and intraabdominal abscess formation (Finn, 1993). Thus, nurses should continually assess the patient for signs of infection. Interventions should include the use of aseptic technique, maintenance of skin integrity, avoidance of indwelling catheters, pulmonary toilet, and the prophylactic use of antibiotic therapy when indicated (Kjellstrand & Barsoum, 1995; Stark, 1994).

ATN frequently occurs in conjunction with other pathologic processes and is characterized by increased caloric needs and a susceptibility to catabolism. Metabolic changes caused by renal failure and the metabolic effects of the primary illness both contribute to these alterations (Finn, 1993; Takala, 1987). Therefore, patients with ARF frequently display the signs and symptoms of protein catabolism, such as negative nitrogen balance, loss of lean body mass, and enhanced production of urea with severe hyperkalemia and acidosis (Schaefer, Schaefer, & Horl, 1994). In addition, the effects of protein and calorie malnutrition are delayed wound healing and impaired immune function (Wolfson & Kopple, 1993).

Although not conclusive, the results of numerous studies suggest that a considerable amount of the morbidity and mortality associated with ARF may result from a failure to take into account these increased nutritional requirements (Kjellstrand & Barsoum, 1995; Wolfson & Kopple, 1993). Thus, adequate nutrition is essential. However, the metabolic disturbances and alterations in fluid and electrolyte excretion mandate careful planning of nutritional support. The goals of dietary management are to minimize uremic toxicity, to minimize fluid and electrolyte imbalances, and to maintain adequate nutrition (Baer & Lancaster, 1992; Kjellstrand & Barsoum, 1995).

Adequate calories should be given to meet energy needs (35 to 45 kcal/kg of IBW/day) (Druml, 1995). Protein requirements vary from 0.6 to 1.5 g/kg/day. The protein given should be of high biological value and thus contain all essential amino acids (Takala, 1987; Wolfson & Kopple, 1993.) Sodium, potassium, and phosphorous are usually restricted because the tubules are not able to secrete them. However, electrolyte replacement should be individualized based on blood levels of these substances (Wolfson & Kopple, 1993). Fluid is restricted to output plus 500 to 1000 cc for insensible losses. Water-soluble vitamin supplementation is required, but care must be taken in the administration of fat-soluble vitamins because of the risk of vitamin toxicity (Druml, 1995; Wolfson & Kopple, 1993). Whenever feasible, the GI tract should be used for nutrition. If the patient is unable to eat, administration of nutrition via enteral tubes is frequently preferred to intravenous administration (Druml, 1995). Early dialysis may be required secondary to volume overload if intravenous nutritional therapy is necessary.

The systemic effects of uremia frequently appear when the BUN level rises above 70 to 100 mg/dl (Stark, 1994; see Table 9-18). The nurse should carefully assess the patient for the development of these symptoms. Careful dietary management is helpful in preventing uremic manifestations. However, renal replacement therapy may be required. Treatment used may include hemodialysis, peritoneal dialysis, or continuous renal replacement therapies. The advantages and disadvantages of each type of therapy are listed in Table 9-20.

Patients with ARF and their families must cope with the sudden loss of health in the face of a very serious illness. The loss of renal function may require prolonged hospitalization, complex dietary and medication management, and dialysis. The nurse should continually assess the educational and emotional needs of both the patient and family, providing them with appropriate explanations of the disease process, its prognosis, and all procedures and components of treatment (Baer & Lancaster, 1992). Permitting the patient and family members to express their needs and concerns is essential. Allowing frequent family visits helps support the entire family, decreases anxiety, and provides the patient with a source of comfort (Stark, 1994).

Chronic Renal Failure

Chronic renal failure is the progressive, irreversible loss of renal function that occurs over varying periods of time ranging from a few months to decades. As previously discussed, the degree of renal functional loss is usually described in terms of GFR beginning with diminished renal reserve

Table 9-19
Pharmacologic agents potentially useful in the treatment of ARF.

Drugs	Possible Action	Nursing Considerations
Diuretics Lasix Mannitol	• Increases GFR and helps create non-oliguric ATN. • Increases tubular flow and prevents cast formation and obstruction. • Lasix produces a resting state due to blockage of Na^+-K^+ pump in ascending loop of Henle. May help preserve ATP levels. • Mannitol may help prevent cellular swelling and/or destroy oxygen-free radicals.	• Although studies disagree on whether diuretics influence the clinical course of ARF, they do increase urine flow rate. • Lasix is ototoxic. • Lasix may enhance the ototoxicity of aminoglycosides and nephrotoxicity of cephalosporins. • Mannitol may cause volume expansion. Lasix should be considered if the patient is volume overloaded. • Urine chemistries should be obtained prior to diuretic administration. • May prevent ATN if administered before or during the onset phase of ATN.
Dopamine	• Acts on the dopaminergic receptors of the renal vasculature to cause vasodilation. • Increases renal blood flow by decreasing renal vascular resistance.	• Effect decreases as the dosage requirements increase to maintain BP. • Restoration of intravascular volume is essential when using dopamine. • May be more effective if used in conjunction with Lasix. • May alter the course of ATN by increasing GFR and/or urinary output.
Atrial Natriuretic Peptide (ANP)	• Animal studies have shown that IV infusion can reverse experimental ATN. The mechanism is thought to be due to the vasodilatory action of ANP.	• A series of studies is currently being conducted at multiple sites to test its effectiveness in humans. • Causes hypotension in large doses. • ANP is rapidly degraded and quickly becomes ineffective. • May prevent ATN if administered during onset phase.
Calcium Channel Blockers	• Dilate afferent arteriole and increase GFR. • Prevent influx of calcium into the cell and thereby decrease cellular damage.	• May cause hypotension. • May prevent ATN if administered during onset phase. • May alter course of ATN by increasing GFR and urine output. • Not extensively studied in humans.
Prostaglandins	• Mechanism of action unclear but may be related to increase in renal blood flow, increased solute excretion, inhibition of platelet aggregation, and/or a direct cytoprotective effect.	• Insufficient studies in humans.
Adenine Nucleotides (ATP, ADP, or AMP complexed to $MgCl_2$)	• In animals: -decreases cell damage, -enhances GFR. • Provides ATP at cellular level and preserves cell function	• Causes of fall in systemic resistance and an increase in cardiac output. • Further research in humans needed.
Amino acids Glycine Alanine	• May be beneficial by both preventing or reducing cell injury and by enhancing regeneration and repair of tubular cells. • The mechanism of protective effect has not been established.	• Effects not well studied in humans. • Amino acids can be nephrotoxic in selected situations.
Antioxidants Allopurinol Deferoxamine	• Inhibits production of oxygen-free radicals.	• Effectiveness remains controversial.
Growth factors Insulin-like Growth Factor (IGF-1) Epidermal Growth Factor (EGF) Hepatocyte Growth Factor	In animal models: • Accelerates recovery of renal tubular cells. • May also enhance GFR and RBF	• Further study will be required in humans.

Note: Adapted from Dolleris (1992); Fischereder et al. (1994); Hammerman & Miller (1994); Hays (1992); Lieberthal & Levinsky (1990); Nouwen, Verstrepen, & DeBroe (1994); Shilliday & Allison (1994); Stark (1994); Strupp (1988).

Table 9-20
Renal replacement therapies used in the treatment of ARF.

Renal Replacement Therapy Options	Indications	Contraindications	Advantages	Disadvantages
Hemodialysis (HD) - removal of soluble substances and water from the blood into a dialysate bath across a semi-permeable membrane by diffusion, filtration, and use of a transmembrane pressure gradient.	• uremia and related symptoms • electrolyte imbalances • volume overload • symptomatic acidosis • contraindications to other forms of dialysis • availability of highly trained staff and equipment	• hemodynamic instability • lack of access to circulation • inability to anticoagulate • lack of highly trained staff and/or equipment	• rapid and efficient • intermittent treatment usually sufficient	• hemodynamic instability • rapid fluid and solute shifts • membrane incompatibility • blood loss • anticoagulation needed • access to circulation • equipment/personnel
Peritoneal Dialysis (PD) - removal of soluble substances and water from the body by transfer across the peritoneum through diffusion, filtration, and osmosis using a dialysate solution that is intermittently introduced into and removed from the peritoneal cavity.	• uremia • electrolyte imbalance • volume overload • blood access failure • hemodynamic instability • inability to anticoagulate • contradiction to hemodialysis	• need for rapid removal of fluid or solute • presence of abdominal adhesions • traumatized abdomen • consider postoperative abdomen • consider peritonitis • history of ineffective clearances	• slow, gradual dialysis • indicated for unstable or bleeding patients • requires less technical support and equipment • no anti-coagulation needed	• slow fluid and solute removal • less predictable • infection • drainage failure • respiratory compromise • hyperglycemia
Continuous Renal Replacement Therapies (CRRT) - an extracorporeal process for removing fluid, electrolytes, and small to medium-sized molecules from the blood by ultrafiltration or combinations of ultrafiltration, fluid replacement, and dialysis. (Ultrafiltration is the removal of soluble substances and water from the blood across a semipermeable membrane)	• hypervolemia • need to remove large volumes of fluid in hemodynamically unstable patients • oliguric patients requiring large quantities of volume replacement • contraindication to hemo/peritoneal dialysis • lack of hemodialysis staff	• hematocrit over 45% • inability of anticoagulate	• maintains consistent homeostasis • avoids hypotensive episodes • permits continuous control of fluid balance	• nursing time involved • technical problems

Note: Adapted from Daugirdas & Ing (1994); Mehta (1994); Price (1992b); Stark (1992b, pp. 40-44).

Table 9-21
Major causes of ESRD in order of their prevalence from 1988-1991.

Major causes of ESRD
Diabetes
Hypertension
Glomerulonephritis
Cystic Kidney Diseases
Interstitial Nephritis
Obstructive Nephropathy
Collagen Vascular Diseases
Malignancies
Metabolic Diseases
Congenital/Other Hereditary Diseases
Sickle Cell Disease
AIDS-Related

Note: From *United States Renal Data System Annual Report.* (1994). The National Institutes of Health, The National Institutes of Diabetes and Digestive and Kidney Diseases, Division of Kidney, Urologic, and Hematologic Diseases, Bethesda, MD.

and proceeding from renal insufficiency to end stage renal disease (ESRD) (see Table 9-1). Once renal insufficiency is established, renal disease is almost always progressive and, if the patient survives long enough, ultimately leads to renal failure (Hunsicker & Levey, 1995).

Chronic renal failure continues to be a significant health problem in the U.S. population. By the end of 1992, there were over 220,000 patients with chronic renal failure in the United States, and the number of patients receiving treatment for kidney failure is increasing at a rate of approximately 10% per year (United States Renal Data System, 1994). The incidence of chronic renal failure is higher in the elderly. This finding may be related to the overall aging of the general population, the progressive loss of renal function with age, and the improved survival of patients with chronic diseases with renal complications such as diabetes mellitus and hypertension. Although the reasons are unclear, the incidence of ESRD is higher in African Americans, Native Americans, and possibly Hispanic Americans. Gender may also be a risk factor, as both the prevalence and incidence rates of ESRD are consistently higher in males than in females (Agodoa, Jones, & Striker, 1995; USRDS, 1994).

Whether conservative medical management or treatment with dialysis or transplantation is indicated, chronic renal failure remains a condition that extracts a serious toll from those with the illness and from society as a whole. As renal function diminishes, patients experience a myriad of physical and psychosocial problems that literally affect every aspect of their lives. In addition, the monetary cost of chronic renal failure is substantial. Hospitalization is often required as part of treatment. Dialysis, if needed, must be provided on a regular basis. Drug regimens are expensive. The total estimated direct medical charges for ESRD alone, excluding the costs of care for patients with renal insufficiency, was over $8.6 billion during 1991 (USRDS, 1994).

Nurses are being called upon with increasing frequency to play key roles in the management of patients with chronic renal failure. In addition, effective management of these patients requires continual collaboration, coordination, and communication between all members of the health care team (Price, 1992a). It is vital for all members of the health team to work together to obtain a clear understanding of the causes of renal disease, to place emphasis on its prevention, and to investigate ways to provide cost-effective, high-quality care for patients with renal disease (Agodoa et al., 1995).

Etiology and Pathophysiology

Chronic renal failure leading to ESRD may be caused by a progressive primary renal disease such as glomerulonephritis, kidney damage due to other diseases such as diabetes or hypertension, or acute irreversible damage resulting in permanent renal failure (see Table 9-21). The specific pathophysiology of many of these abnormalities was discussed in Chapter 8. As described, each entity is associated with a particular pathophysiological process. However, there are similar histologic features that are shared by many of the chronic renal diseases. These include glomerular sclerosis, periglomerular and interstitial fibrosis, and chronic interstitial inflammation characterized by the infiltration of macrophages and lymphocytes. Research has demonstrated that these changes occur progressively. Knowledge regarding the progression process can assist nurses in helping prevent disease progression, anticipating the development of clinical signs and symptoms, educating and preparing patients with renal disease and their families, and planning appropriate and comprehensive nursing care.

An extremely important clinical observation is that patients with progressive chronic renal failure survive with only minimal symptoms until the GFR is reduced to approximately 10% of normal (Fine et al., 1993; Lakkis & Martinez-Maldonado, 1995; Meyer, Scholey, & Brenner, 1991). In spite of the disease process, the kidneys of these individuals obviously continue to excrete water, nitrogenous wastes, and mineral solutes without notable alterations in diet and other forms of treatment (Meyer et al., 1991). Robert Platt (1900-1978), who is considered to be the "Father of Renal Pathophysiology," was the first to propose an explanation for this observation. He suggested that although nephrons were progressively lost due to the disease process, the remaining functioning nephrons underwent adaptive changes and became able to maintain a relatively homeostatic environment. He based this theory on observations that, in spite of progressive renal destruction, the kidney was still able to excrete relatively constant amounts of sodium, urea, and creatinine (Fine et al., 1993).

These concepts served as the impetus for Bricker and his colleagues to investigate the functional adaptation of the kidney to disease (Bricker, 1972; Bricker & Fine, 1978). Using animal models, they studied the function of a partially removed kidney in comparison to a normal contralateral kidney. They found that the nephrons in the artificially diseased kidney underwent adaptations that enabled it to function similarly to the normal kidney and that appeared to be directed toward conservation of normal body fluid composition. The term "intact nephron" was coined to describe this phenomenon and, thus, the intact nephron hypothesis was born (Fine et al., 1993).

Subsequent studies have demonstrated that, in the face of nephron destruction, compensatory mechanisms elevate the GFR and enlarge the tubules of normal and less-damaged nephrons (Meyer et al., 1991). Key mechanisms involved in this process are glomerular hypertrophy and hyperfiltration. Therefore, in the face of progressive loss of glomerular function, individual nephrons adapt to maintain the aggregate GFR. After a critical level of nephron destruction is reached, however, the GFR declines progressively and linearly over time (see Figure 9-4).

The biological price of this nephron adaptation appears to be the deterioration of the remaining nephrons. The very hemodynamic changes that cause nephron hyperfiltration seem to injure the glomeruli. Increases in intraglomerular pressure (glomerular hypertension) frequently lead to progressive glomerulosclerosis. Glomerular hypertrophy also seems to accelerate the development of glomerular sclerosis and may be related to the increased susceptibility of hypertrophied glomeruli to the hemodynamic stresses of glomerular hypertension or from growth factors that stimulate cell proliferation (Hunsicker & Levey, 1995).

Other mechanisms implicated in progressive glomeruli destruction include systemic hypertension; hyperlipidemia with glomerular lipid deposition; proteinuria; glomerular capillary thrombosis; glomerular deposition of calcium secondary to phosphate metabolism abnormalities; and tubulointerstitial injury mediated by certain hormones, growth factors, cytokines, and biologically active lipids. Research is being directed toward interrupting these processes in an attempt to halt the progression of chronic renal failure. A summary of the specific progression risk factors, their proposed pathophysiologic mechanisms, interventions being tested, and related nursing considerations appears in Table 9-22.

It is likely that a combination of several or all of the above factors contribute to the ultimate progression of chronic renal disease leading to CRF (Fine et al., 1993; Hunsicker & Levey, 1995; Meyer et al., 1991). Data from studies that assess the impact of these risk factors on the progression of renal disease suggest that clinical predictors of progression are the patient's underlying renal disease (specifically polycystic kidney disease), higher baseline proteinuria, lower baseline transferrin levels, black race, higher baseline mean arterial blood pressure, and lower baseline level of high-density lipoprotein (HDL) cholesterol. However, other factors not yet identified may also play a role. Thus, further research in this area needs to be conducted.

The progression of chronic renal failure can be monitored clinically by plotting the reciprocal of serum creatinine (1/serum creatinine) across time. The slope of this line is an estimate of the rate of loss of renal function and tends to fall linearly with time

Figure 9-4
Renal response to loss of glomerular mass.

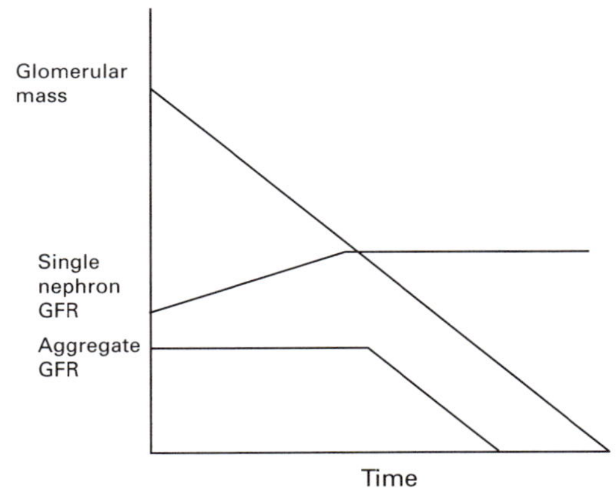

Note: From Andreoli, T.E., Bennett, J.C., Carpenter, C.C.J., Plum, F., & Smith, L.H. (1993). *Cecil's essential of medicine* (3rd edition) (p. 246). Philadelphia: W.B. Saunders Company. Reprinted with permission.

Table 9-22
Risk factors that mediate progression of chronic renal disease.

Risk Factor	Pathophysiology	Treatment and Nursing Considerations
Systemic and Glomerular Hypertension	• May damage kidney by increasing arteriolar wall thickness leading to glomerulosclerosis. • May directly damage glomerulus. • May also cause focal detachment of endothelial and epithelial cells from glomerular basement membrane.	• Reduction in mean arterial blood pressure correlates significantly with the decrease in rate of loss of renal function. • ACE inhibitors may be more effective than other agents in delaying CRF because they also decrease intraglomerular pressure. • Patients on ACE inhibitors should be observed closely for acute changes in renal function and hyperkalemia. • Calcium channel blockers have also been shown to have a beneficial effect.
Proteinuria/High Protein Intake	• Proteinuria may be injurious to the glomerulus because of macromolecular traffic through the mesangium. • Proteinuria may also lead to cast formation in the distal nephron and epithelial damage with interstitial inflammation. • High phosphate levels in protein may cause tissue damage from calcium-phosphate deposition. • Dietary protein restriction reduces renal hypertrophy and hyperplasia in remaining nephrons.	• Moderately low protein diets (0.6 to 8 gm/kg) reduce urine protein in short-term studies; long-term data are not available. • ACE inhibitors seem to be more effective than other agents in reducing proteinuria by decreasing intraglomerular pressure. • Low protein diets may be more effective in decreasing disease progression when coupled with phosphate restriction. • Phosphate binders can be used to treat hyperphosphatemia.
Hyperlipidemia	• Glomerulosclerosis, a histologic hallmark of CRF, has many similarities to atherosclerosis. • There is an increased amount of cholesterol in the end stage kidney. • Lipid droplets are present in glomerular sclerotic lesions in humans and experimental animals.	• Lipid-lowering drugs decrease degree of glomerulosclerosis in animal models. • Major lipid abnormality in patients with renal disease is hypertriglyceridemia. Medications used to lower triglycerides have serious side effects and doses must be adjusted for level of renal failure. Dietary modification and exercise may be safer in patients with renal failure. • Lipid lowering agents that have reduced renal injury in animal models include: -cholestyramine -clofibrate -lovastation -probucol
Intraglomerular Coagulation	• The presence of fibrin in kidneys of patients with rapidly progressive acute glomerulonephritis suggests that coagulation might be important in glomerular damage. • Capillary thrombosis may be precipitated by glomerular endothelial cell injury.	• Agents that prevent platelet aggregation such as aspirin and dipyridamole may slow the progressive course of CRF. • Anticoagulants, such as heparin and coumadin, have also been reported to slow disease progression.
Infiltration of Renal Parenchyma by Immune Cells	• Interstitial infiltrates are seen in most glomerular diseases that progress to CRF. • Mechanisms underlying this process are poorly understood. The process may be mediated by certain hormones, growth factors, and cytokines.	• Fatty acid deficient diets are effective in decreasing tubulointerstitial infiltrates in animal models. • No systematic studies in humans have examined methods of preventing or decreasing renal infiltration by immune cells. • Antibodies to growth factors may prove helpful in decreasing infiltration.

Note: Adapted from Fine et al. (1993); Jacobson (1991); Keane & Levey (1995); Klaher (1991); Llach (1993b); Meyer et al. (1991).

in individual patients with different types of renal disease (see Figure 9-5). This information is extremely useful in predicting when dialysis will be needed (Mitch, Walser, Buffington, & Lemann, 1976). It is also helpful in identifying the presence of certain acute conditions that may accelerate the expected rate of loss of residual renal function such as the development of hypertension, loss of fluids, congestive heart failure, presence of urinary tract infection, sepsis, pregnancy, nephrotoxins, and metabolic derangements (for example, hypercalcemia or hyperuricemia) (Klahr, 1991; Llach, 1993b).

Clinical and Laboratory Features

Renal function may deteriorate without clinical symptoms over variable periods of time. Depending on the particular pathophysiologic process, this may occur over months to many years (Llach, 1993b). In most patients with chronic renal failure, the signs and symptoms of the disease begin to develop when the GFR decreases to less than 15 to 20 ml/min (Lakkis & Martinez-Maldonado, 1995; Meyer et al., 1991) (see Figure 9-6). These symptoms are related to fluid, electrolyte, and acid-base imbalances, disordered regulatory functions, and the multisystem complications associated with the uremic syndrome. A thorough discussion of these changes, their pathophysiologic bases, associated laboratory findings, and nursing care appears in the last section of this chapter. The reader is also referred to Table 9-5 for a summary of the blood and serum laboratory values that commonly occur with renal failure.

These issues can greatly affect patients' clinical status, general well-being, and overall quality of life. A complete discussion of the psychosocial impact of renal disease and related nursing considerations and interventions is presented in Chapter 10.

Treatment and Prevention

Progressive loss of renal function ultimately leads to uremia. As mentioned previously, the signs and symptoms associated with chronic renal failure begin to develop once the GFR declines to less than 15 to 20 ml/min. Conservative management of the patient with chronic renal insufficiency not yet requiring dialysis has three goals:

1. to control the rate of progression of renal disease;
2. to prevent further damage to the kidneys; and
3. to manage complications from the uremic syndrome (Lakkis & Martinez-Maldonado, 1995).

Strategies for accomplishing these goals include control of hypertension, dietary protein and phosphate restriction, reduction of proteinuria, and management of hyperlipidemia (see Table 9-22). When the GFR reaches a level lower than 5 ml/min, renal replacement therapy becomes necessary (Lakkis & Martinez-Maldonado, 1995). A detailed discussion of the conservative management of chronic renal failure, renal replacement options, and related nursing care is presented in Chapter 18.

Figure 9-5
Rate of loss of renal function in patients with three types of renal disease.

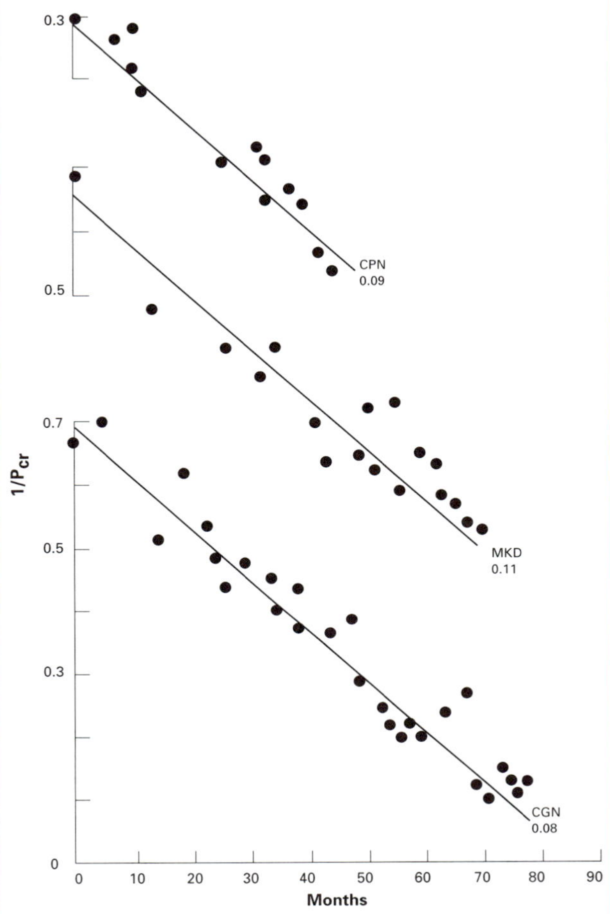

Key: Composite plot of the reciprocal of the P_{cr} vs. months of observation in 3 patients with progressive renal disease due to chronic pyelonephritis (CPN), the medullary cystic kidney disease (MKD), and chronic glomerular nephritis (CGN).

Note: From Llach, F. (1993b). Chronic renal failure. In F. Llach, (Ed.), *Papper's clinical nephrology* (3rd edition) (p. 71). Boston: Little, Brown and Company. Reprinted with permission.

The nurse should also continually monitor the patient with chronic renal insufficiency for those risk factors that might lead to the development of acute renal failure. These risk factors include hypertension, diabetes mellitus, age, and liver cirrhosis (see Table 9-16). In addition, conditions that predispose patients to reduced renal perfusion such

Figure 9-6
The relationship of clinical manifestations to renal function.

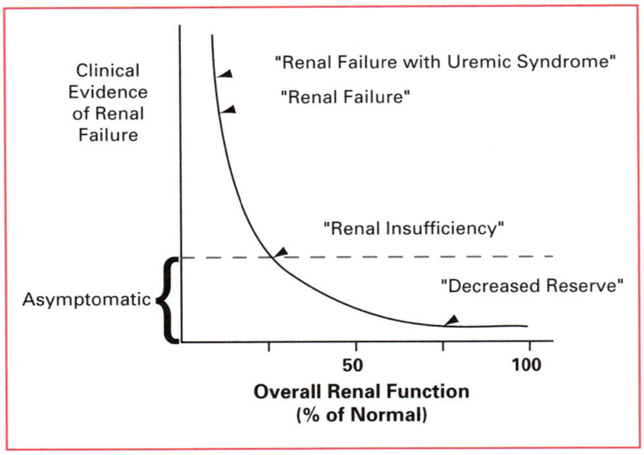

Note: From Llach, F. (1993b). Chronic renal failure. In F. Llach, (Ed.), *Papper's clinical nephrology* (3rd edition) (p. 70). Boston: Little, Brown and Company. Reprinted with permission.

Figure 9-7
Ionic composition of major body-fluid compartments.

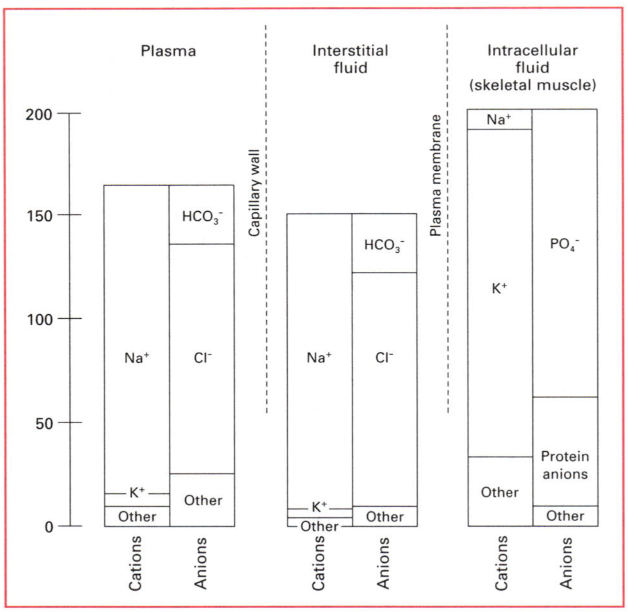

Note: From Sherwood, L. (1993). *Human physiology: From cells to systems* (p. 513). New York: West Publishing Company. Reprinted with permission.

as vigorous diuretic therapy, congestive heart failure, gastrointestinal losses from vomiting or diarrhea, blood loss, or salt and water restriction can cause an acute decrease in residual renal function. Patients on potentially nephrotoxic agents such as aminoglycosides, nonsteroidal antiinflammatory drugs, and angiotensin-converting enzyme inhibitors (ACEIs) should also be closely monitored. Nursing interventions used in the prevention of acute loss of renal function in the patient with chronic renal insufficiency include awareness of risk factors, accurate assessment of volume status, knowledge of nephrotoxic agents, and appropriate patient teaching (Zorzanello, 1989).

Systemic Manifestations of Acute and Chronic Renal Failure and Related Nursing Management

The patient in renal failure is at risk for developing a wide variety of systemic abnormalities. Although existing medical treatments, including dialysis, correct many of these problems, they cannot reverse several of the maladaptive physiologic changes induced by renal failure (Lazarus & Hakin, 1991). In addition, the psychosocial responses to the disease are profound. Thus, patients with renal failure and their families require complex nursing care.

In general, the manifestations of renal failure can be divided into four areas including:

1. manifestations specifically related to disorders of fluid and electrolyte excretion and acid-base disturbances;
2. manifestations related to disordered metabolic and regulatory functions;
3. alterations related to the effects of uremia (uremic syndrome); and
4. psychosocial responses of the patient and family to acute/chronic illness.

The nursing management of the systemic manifestations of both acute and chronic renal failure is considered in this section. Although these two groups of patients share many of the same problems, significant differences also exist. Therefore, appropriate comparisons and contrasts are covered in the discussions. The pathophysiologic basis, clinical presentation, and medical treatment for each of the first three areas listed above are covered in the text. Assessment parameters, nursing interventions, and expected outcomes are covered in tables at the end of this textbook (see Appendices B, C, and D). A thorough discussion of the psychosocial problems facing these patients appears in Chapter 10.

Fluid, Electrolyte, and Acid-Base Disturbances

Body water represents approximately 60% of the total body weight in a young, lean adult. As the water content of fat is less than that of lean body mass, the percentage of body weight that is water is

Table 9-23
Classification of body fluid.

Compartment	Volume of fluids (in liters)	Percentage of body fluid	Percentage of body weight
Total body fluid	42	100%	60%
Intracellular fluid (ICF)	28	67	40
Extracellular fluid (ECF)	14	33	20
Plasma	2.8	6.6 (20% of ECF)	4
Interstitial fluid	11.2	26.4 (80% of ECF)	16
Lymph	negligible	negligible	negligible
Transcellular fluid	negligible	negligible	negligible

Note: From Sherwood, L. (1993). *Human physiology: From cells to systems* (p. 512). New York: West Publishing Company. Reprinted with permission.

lower in obese individuals and in women (who typically have a higher body fat content) than men. In a newborn, water may account for as much as 75% of the total body weight. In contrast, total body water decreases with age and may compose as little as 50% of the body weight in the elderly.

Body water is divided into two major compartments. Fluids outside the cells are in the extracellular fluid compartment (ECF). This compartment can be further divided into interstitial fluids (fluid in between cells) and intravascular fluid (plasma water). Intracellular fluid is that volume inside the cells and accounts for 28 of the 42 liters in the body (see Table 9-23). Although the composition of the intravascular and interstitial fluids are very similar, the electrolyte concentration of the intracellular fluid compartment differs significantly (see Figure 9-7).

Fluid balance is determined by daily gains and losses. Most of the daily intake of water enters orally, two-thirds of which is in the form of pure water. The remainder is in food. A small amount is also produced in the body as a result of oxidation processes associated with metabolism. A majority of body fluid losses normally occur in the form of urine (sensible fluid loss). Hidden water losses through the skin and respiratory tract (insensible water loss) also occur and typically amount to 300 to 500 cc/day (Guyton, 1991; Sherwood, 1993).

The kidneys, in association with hormones such as aldosterone and antidiuretic hormone (ADH), are the primary organs responsible for the regulation of the volume and composition of body fluids (see Chapter 7). Until renal function falls below 25% of normal, body fluid volume and composition are generally within the normal range. The ability to regulate fluid balance is maintained by several intrarenal and humoral adaptations that augment renal tubular function (Suki & Eknoyan, 1995). In this situation, however, the kidneys have a limited capacity to deal with excess fluid, electrolytes, and metabolic loads, as well as stressors associated with volume and electrolyte loss.

Because of compromised renal function, patients with acute and chronic renal abnormalities are very prone to retain fluid. However, as the damaged kidney may be unable to conserve as well as excrete water, volume depletion from renal and/or extrarenal losses can also occur. Sodium excess and depletion may develop, depending on the free water load. Imbalances of other electrolytes, including potassium, phosphate, calcium, and magnesium, are common. Although metabolic acidosis related to retention of fixed acids is more likely, metabolic alkalosis can develop in selected situations because the kidneys are unable to excrete bicarbonate loads. Thus, the nurse should be knowledgeable regarding the physiologic bases for

Table 9-24
Major causes of hyper- and hypovolemia.

Hypervolemia—Volume Excess	Hypovolemia—Volume Deficit
Renal Insufficiency Renal Failure Congestive Heart Failure Cirrhosis Nephrotic Syndrome	Renal Losses of Salt and Water • Diuretics • Postobstructive diuresis • Renal tubular defects GI Losses • Vomiting • Diarrhea Skin Losses • Diaphoresis • Burns • Insensible losses Third-Spacing of Fluid • Ascites Blood Loss

Note: Adapted from Bicket & Gougoux (1995); Briggs (1995); Gougoux & Bicket (1995); Rose & Rennke (1994).

all potential abnormalities, their clinical presentation, and appropriate nursing interventions (Baer, 1993b; Jacobsson & McNatt, 1986; Lancaster, 1995; Price, 1994; Stark, 1994; see Appendix B).

Alterations in fluid balance. Fluid overload is a serious complication of acute renal failure and may develop insidiously or abruptly (O'Meara & Bernard, 1995). Control of volume intake may be especially difficult to manage if the patient is receiving hyperalimentation, blood products, multiple IV medications, and drips. Therefore, medications should be given in the smallest volume possible, and this may necessitate the use of double-, triple-, or quadruple-strength solutions (Price, 1992a). Although IV medications are frequently given in 5% dextrose solution (D_5W), large amounts of this fluid can precipitate hyponatremia, and, therefore, normal saline may be a more-appropriate medium. Treatment of volume overload in acute renal failure usually includes an attempt to induce diuresis through the use of high-dose furosemide and low-dose dopamine (to enhance renal blood flow). Generally, an increasing dose of furosemide 2-5-10 mg/kg is infused over 30 minutes with the simultaneous infusion of dopamine 1 to 2 micrograms/kg/min. Although patients may not respond to this treatment with increased urine output, some may show some resolution of pulmonary edema, if present, as the furosemide increases large vein capacitance and shunts blood away from the pulmonary circulation (Kjellstrand & Barsoum, 1995). Dialysis with ultrafiltration may be required if attempts to induce diuresis are not successful. When the blood pressure is low, a slow continuous renal replacement therapy may be the treatment of choice (see Chapter 20).

Fluid management in the patient with chronic renal failure on dialysis is often a challenge for both the patient and the nurse (Shapiro, Deshetler, & Stockard, 1994). The daily fluid allowance is usually 1 L plus the volume of urine produced. Sodium is also restricted to 2 g/day. Thirst can cause significant distress, particularly following dialysis, due to volume removal and increases in serum osmolality. Patients can be advised to chew gum and suck on hard candy to help relieve this symptom. Ice chips can also be used to moisten the mucous membranes of the mouth and throat. However, the volume of fluid given with ice must be included in that volume permitted per day (the water volume of ice chips is approximately one-half of the measured volume). Good oral care is also crucial.

Although volume overload is more common in patients with acute and chronic renal failure, volume depletion may also occur. In the acute setting, fluid losses can develop from acute blood loss, fluid loss secondary to burns and vomiting/diarrhea, and increased insensible losses. Fluid losses should be replaced as soon as possible with solutions similar in composition to the lost fluid (Gougoux & Bichet, 1995). Chronic renal failure patients can develop volume deficits for many of the same reasons (see Table 9-24). In addition, these patients may have increased insensible losses during elevations in ambient temperature and increased activity. In most cases, fluid losses can usually be replaced orally or during dialysis.

Although fluid intake and output are valuable guides, weight remains the most important indicator of overall fluid status. However, the information obtained from frequent measurements of weight does have its limitations. It is important to remember that acute and chronic renal failure patients easily become catabolic and develop protein wasting, and that dry body weight can be lost and replaced with fluid weight. Thus, it is important to complete a thorough assessment of the patient's fluid status, as outlined previously, on a regular basis. For the patient with acute renal failure, an assessment may need to be done every 4 hours. For the individual with chronic renal failure, this should be done at clinic visits and prior to each dialysis treatment.

Alterations in sodium balance. Sodium is a major determinant of serum osmolality. It also plays an essential role in nerve conduction, acid-base balance, and numerous chemical reactions. Because water is freely permeable across cell membranes, changes in the extracellular sodium concentration result in shifts in water distribution in ECF and ICF compartments (DeVita & Michelis, 1993). For example, a decrease in the sodium concentration of the intravascular compartment results in a shift of water into the cells, causing an increase in cell volume. On the other hand, an increase in intravascular sodium concentration produces a shift of water from the intracellular to the extracellular compartment, and cells shrink.

As nephrons are progressively lost, the ability to excrete sodium becomes limited. In the damaged kidney, however, the ability to conserve sodium is also lost and major salt wasting states can develop. Therefore, although sodium restriction is commonly necessary in the treatment of patients with acute or chronic renal failure, the dietary prescription of sodium should be individualized and based on urinary sodium losses.

Hyponatremia, defined as a serum sodium concentration less than 135 mEq/L, is a state in which there is a decrease in sodium relative to water. Depending on the etiology of the hyponatremia, this condition may be seen in association with hypervolemia, hypovolemia, and euvolemia (DeVita & Michelis, 1993; Schrier, 1995; see Table 9-25). Pseudohyponatremia may been seen in association with hyperlipidemia, hyperproteinemia, and hyperglycemia as these substances are osmotically active and pull water into the intravascular space. In this case, correction of the underlying problem also corrects the hyponatremia.

The symptoms of hyponatremia are caused by the decreased osmolality of the extracellular fluid and generally correlate with the rate of development of the abnormality. Early manifestations include gastrointestinal symptoms such as anorexia, nausea, and vomiting. Generalized weakness and muscle cramps can also occur. The later and more severe signs and symptoms relate to the central nervous system (cerebral edema) and include malaise, headache, confusion, lethargy, seizures, and coma. These symptoms usually develop when the sodium decreases rapidly to 120 to 125 mEq/L (Veis & Berl, 1995).

The medical management of hyponatremia is determined by the degree of symptoms exhibited as well as by the onset and duration of the abnormality. Treatment may include water restriction, administration of IV sodium chloride solutions, or discontinuation of diuretic therapy. In the renal failure patient, the sodium content of the dialysate bath in hemodialysis can be increased (Daugirdas & Ing, 1994). However, overly rapid correction of hyponatremia may cause shrinkage of the brain tissue, resulting in severe neurologic signs and symptoms and even death (central pontine myelinolysis) (DeVita & Michelis, 1993; Rose & Rennke, 1994).

Hypernatremia, defined as a serum sodium concentration above 146 mEq/L, is extremely dangerous. This condition rarely occurs, but when it does, it is associated with a 10% to 40% mortality rate (Lanese & Teitelbaum, 1995). Hypernatremia occurs when there is an increase in sodium or loss of free water. Like hyponatremia, hypernatremia can occur with decreased, normal, or increased total body water (see Table 9-25). This condition is most commonly seen in patients with no access to fluid, such as the elderly or critically ill, or with impaired thirst regulation. In the patient with renal failure, hypernatremia may also occur during peritoneal dialysis when high-dextrose, short-dwell exchanges are used to remove fluid quickly (Daugirdas & Ing, 1994).

The symptoms associated with hypernatremia vary with the speed of onset and result from the loss in intracellular fluid stores (Lanese & Teitelbaum, 1995). Manifestations include dry mucous membranes, intense thirst, flushed skin, fever, and oliguria. CNS symptoms include lethargy, altered mentation, and seizures related to cerebral shrinking. Physical examination may be unremarkable.

The treatment of hypernatremia depends on two very important factors: (a) the ECF volume status of the patient; and (b) the rate of development of the hypernatremia. The overall goal of treatment is to restore normal osmolality. If the imbalance is caused by water deficits, it is important to replace volume with free water, hypotonic sodium chloride, or D_5W. If it is associated with volume expansion, diuretics may be used to enhance sodium excretion if renal function permits.

Severe neurologic signs and symptoms are associated with the rapid correction of hypernatremia and may result in cerebral edema, seizures, and death. In general, the serum sodium level should be reduced no faster than 2 mEq/L/hour

Table 9-25
Major causes of hyper- and hyponatremia.

Hypernatremia - Serum Na⁺ > 146 mEq/L	Hyponatremia - Serum Na⁺ < 135 mEq/L
Hypovolemic • GI losses of water • Renal losses of water • Skin losses of water	Hypovolemic • Vomiting • Diarrhea • Diuretics • Salt-loosing nephritis
Euvolemic • Renal losses of water • Skin and respiratory water losses • Inability to gain access to fluids	Euvolemic • Drugs • Pain • Emotional distress
Hypervolemic • Hypertonic saline administration • Infants given hypertonic feedings	Hypervolemic • Congestive heart failure • ARF • CRF • Cirrhosis

Note: Adapted from DeVita & Michelis (1993); Felver (1995); Lanese & Teitelbaum (1995); Rose & Rennke (1994); Schrier (1995); Veis & Berl (1995).

during the first 48 hours (Lanese & Teitelbaum, 1995). If dialysis is being used, the safest approach is to dialyze a patient with a dialysis solution sodium level close to that of the plasma and then correct the hypernatremia by slow administration of isotonic saline (Daugirdas & Ing, 1994).

Alterations of potassium balance. Approximately 150 mEq of potassium are present in each liter of intracellular fluid while only 4.0 mEq are present in each liter of extracellular fluid. Thus, more than 98% of total body potassium is present inside of the cells (Schrier, 1995). As the major intracellular cation, potassium helps maintain intracellular osmolality; regulates skeletal, cardiac, and smooth muscle activity; influences acid-base balance; and participates in many intracellular enzyme reactions (Porth, 1994).

Changes in the serum potassium concentration can have important effects on neuronal membrane excitability. A fall in extracellular potassium concentration (hypokalemia) lowers the resting membrane potential (E_m) of the cell, leading to hyperpolarization and decreased neuronal excitability. A rise in potassium concentration (hyperkalemia) increases the resting membrane potential, bringing it closer to the threshold potential (E_t) for neuronal firing. Hyperkalemia, therefore, causes increased neuronal excitability (see Figure 9-8). The effects of alterations in potassium levels on neuromuscular transmission are clinically important because they are largely responsible for the most serious symptoms associated with disturbances in potassium balance: muscle weakness, potentially fatal cardiac arrhythmias, and disturbances in cardiac conduction (Rose & Rennke, 1995).

Hypokalemia is defined as a serum potassium level less than 3.5 mEq/L. Generally, this condition occurs in one of four major situations: decreased dietary intake, excessive GI losses, increased urinary losses, or increased entry of potassium into the cells (see Table 9-26). This electrolyte disturbance is commonly seen in the ARF patient with nonoliguric renal failure caused by diuretics, cisplatin, or amphotericin B (O'Meara & Bernard, 1995) and as a complication of TPN (Daugirdas & Ing, 1994). In the CRF patient, hypokalemia commonly occurs when food intake is poor or the patient has diarrhea (Daugirdas & Ing, 1994).

As previously mentioned, the clinical manifestations of hypokalemia result from hyperpolarization of cellular membranes of nerve and muscle cells, which decrease neuromuscular excitability. The most significant effect of hypokalemia is on the heart. Manifestations include alterations in the electrocardiogram (ECG) (see Figure 9-9), predisposition to digitalis toxicity, and atrial and ventricular arrhythmias. Hypomotility of the gastrointestinal tract leading to constipation also occurs. Patients may experience malaise, weakness, fatigue, and myalgia. Paralysis of the extremities and respiratory muscles has been described with a serum potassium < 2.0 (Latta, Hisano, & Chan, 1993; Linas & Singh, 1995).

Table 9-26
Major causes of hyper- and hypokalemia.

Hyperkalemia - Serum K^+ > 5.5 mEq/L	Hypokalemia - Serum K^+ < 3.5 mEq/L
Increased Dietary Intake • Rapid IV K^+ infusion • Transfusion of stored blood • Salt substitutes Decreased Renal Excretion • ARF • CRF • Adrenal insufficiency • Potassium sparing diuretics • Angiotensin converting enzyme inhibitors • Nonsteroidal anti-inflammatory drugs Release of Intracellular K^+ • Hemolysis • Catabolism • Burns • Rhabdomyolysis Shift of K^+ From Cells to ECF • Insulin deficiency • Acidosis • Beta blockers	Decreased Dietary Intake • Anorexia • Alcoholism Renal Losses • Diuretics • Steroids GI Losses • Vomiting • Diarrhea • Laxative abuse Shift of K^+ From ECF into Cells • Alkalosis • Insulin • Hypothermia

Note: Adapted from Copstead (1995); Latta, Hisono, & Chan (1993); Linas & Singh (1995); Rosa & Batlle (1995); Rose & Rennke (1994); Schrier (1995).

Treatment for hypokalemia usually involves replacement of the deficit with potassium salts either orally or IV. The oral route is preferable if tolerated by the patient (particularly with foods high in potassium such as orange juice). However, a common complication of oral potassium chloride supplementation is gastrointestinal bleeding (Latta et al., 1993). Phlebitis may occur with IV administration of potassium chloride, especially when the concentration exceeds 40 mEq/L. The major risk of potassium replacement in patients with renal impairment is the development of hyperkalemia. If the patient is receiving dialysis, the potassium content of the dialysate should be increased, particularly if the patient is on digitalis (Daugirdas & Ing, 1994).

Hyperkalemia, defined as a serum potassium greater than 5.5 mEq/L, is caused by factors that increase potassium intake, shift potassium from the cells into the extracellular fluid, and decrease potassium excretion (see Table 9-26). Pseudohyperkalemia may be seen when blood is hemolyzed or an excessively tight tourniquet is used during the blood collection procedures (Latta et al., 1993).

Hyperkalemia in ARF is a serious complication and may be aggravated by release of intracellular stores with hypercatabolism, extensive tissue injury, or hemolysis (O'Meara & Bernard, 1995). In the chronic renal failure patient, acute hyperkalemia occurs most often in the noncompliant individual who has failed to report for dialysis for several days or to follow the prescribed dietary regimen. In both groups, diabetes may aggravate hyperkalemia because of insulin deficiency or resistance. Medications that can impair potassium entry into cells such as alpha-adrenergic receptor agonists (nasal sprays), nonselective beta-blockers or agents that interfere with potassium secretion such as NSAIDS, angiotensin-converting enzyme inhibitors, and potassium-sparing diuretics can also increase potassium levels in the patient with compromised renal function (Suki & Eknoyan, 1995).

As hyperkalemia develops, the smooth muscle and skeletal muscle become hypopolarized and more reactive to stimuli. Early hyperkalemia is associated with mild intestinal cramping and diarrhea, nausea, and vomiting. Later, muscle weakness and flaccid paralysis are common. Ultimately, hyperkalemia decreases the duration and rate of rise of cardiac action potential and decreases conduction velocity in the heart (see Figure 9-9).

Acute hyperkalemia is potentially life-threatening because of the risk of cardiac arrest. The various treatments for acute hyperkalemia are outlined in

Figure 9-8
Effects of potassium and calcium on membrane excitability.

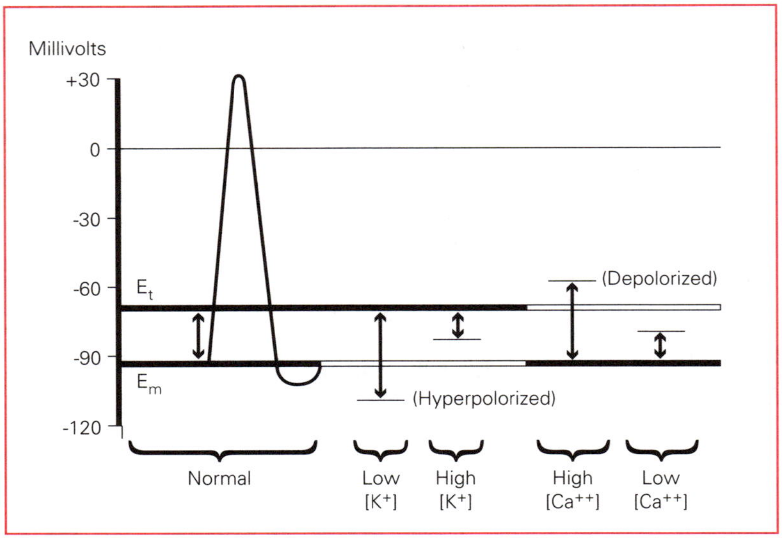

Note: From McCance, K.L., & Huether, S.E. (1994). *Pathophysiology: The biologic basis for disease in adults and children* (p. 105). St. Louis, MO: Mosby Yearbook. Reprinted with permission.

Figure 9-9
Electrocardiogram abnormalities associated with potassium changes.

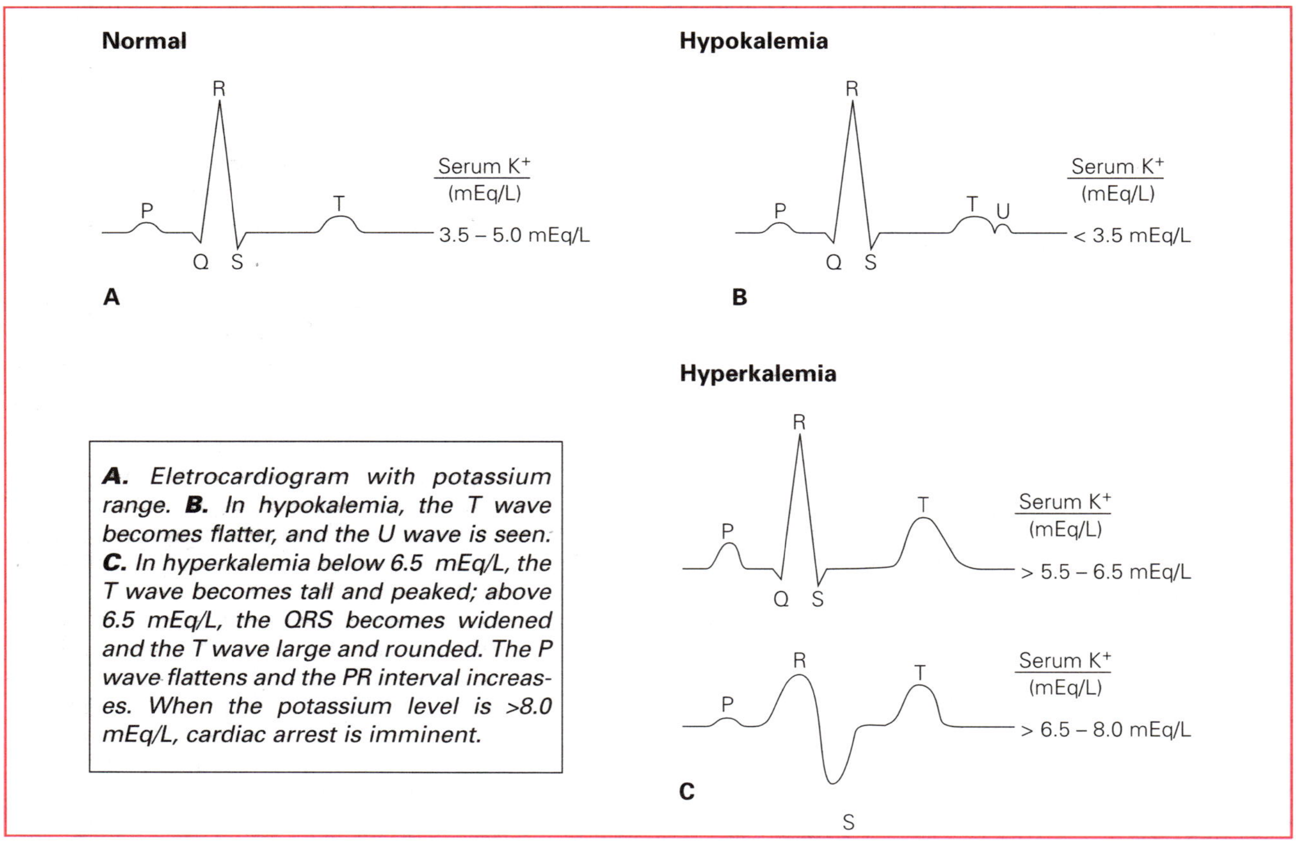

A. *Eletrocardiogram with potassium range.* ***B.*** *In hypokalemia, the T wave becomes flatter, and the U wave is seen.* ***C.*** *In hyperkalemia below 6.5 mEq/L, the T wave becomes tall and peaked; above 6.5 mEq/L, the QRS becomes widened and the T wave large and rounded. The P wave flattens and the PR interval increases. When the potassium level is >8.0 mEq/L, cardiac arrest is imminent.*

Note: From Bullock, B.L. (1996). *Pathophysiology: Adaptations and alterations in function* (p. 201). Philadelphia: J.B. Lippincott Company. Reprinted with permission.

Table 9-27
Treatment of hyperkalemia.

Mechanism	Onset of Action
Antagonism of membrane actions	
A. Calcium	Several minutes and then rapidly wanes
Increased potassium entry into cells	
A. Insulin and glucose B. β-2 adrenergic agonists C. Sodium bicarbonate	Each of these modalities works within 30-60 minutes, lowers the serum potassium concentration by 0.5-1.5 mEq/L, and lasts for several hours
Potassium removal from the body	
A. Diuretics	Several hours but many patients have advanced renal failure and show little response
B. Cation exchange resin	2-3 hours
C. Dialysis	Several hours

Note: From Rose, B.D. & Rennke, H.G. (1994). *Renal pathophysiology - The essentials* (p. 183). Baltimore: Williams & Wilkins. Reprinted with permission.

Table 9-27. When hyperkalemia is mild and chronic, therapeutic measures should address the specific cause. In the patient with chronic renal insufficiency, compliance with diet is often the problem. In some patients with renal insufficiency, treatment with diuretics may be helpful (Rose & Batlle, 1995).

Alterations in calcium and phosphorous balance. There is a close link between the regulation of calcium and phosphate in the body. A change in the concentration of one leads to a change in the concentration of the other. Thus, both calcium and phosphate are discussed together in this section.

Calcium plays a major role in many important metabolic and physiologic processes. In addition to being a major constituent of bone, calcium ions are important in intracellular and enzymatic reactions and in blood coagulation. Calcium is also critical for neuromuscular transmission (Kumar, 1995). About 99% of the calcium in the body is found in the skeleton and teeth. Of the remaining 1%, about 0.9% is found intracellularly with less than 0.1% being present in the ECF. Approximately half of the plasma calcium is bound to plasma proteins. The other half of the plasma calcium is ionized and, therefore, can freely diffuse through cell membranes. Only the free, or ionized, calcium is biologically active (Sherwood, 1993). Natural cheeses, milk, and milk products are major sources of dietary calcium.

Phosphorous is the sixth most abundant element in the human body (Hruska & Kovach, 1995). Approximately 80% of this phosphorous is also found in the bones. Only a small amount is found in the ECF, the normal levels being 2.5 mg/dl to 4.5 mg/dl. Phosphorous is the major anion in the ICF, where it functions primarily as a cofactor in many metabolic reactions (Workman, 1992). In the ECF, phosphorus plays an important roll in acid-base buffering and calcium homeostasis. Milk and its products are the richest source of phosphorus. However, it is also found in other foods, such as meat, fish, poultry, whole grains, eggs, and peanuts (Brunier, 1994; Hruska & Kovach, 1995).

Serum calcium and phosphate are maintained within their normal ranges via regulatory mechanisms involving the gastrointestinal tract, the skeleton, and the kidneys under the influence of parathyroid hormone (PTH) and vitamin D (Bourke & Delany, 1993; Brunier, 1994). PTH, a substance produced by the parathyroid glands, is sensitive to the level of serum calcium. When serum calcium levels drop, PTH is released, causing enhanced renal absorption of calcium and increased activity of bone osteoclasts (bone breakdown cells), which liberate ionized calcium. The result is an increase in serum calcium.

PTH also activates the production of the most active form of vitamin D (1,25-$(OH)_2D_3$; 1, 25- dihydroxycholecalciferol; or calcitriol) by the kidney. This substance facilitates the absorption of calcium from the GI tract, which also increases the serum calcium level. However, a series of metabolic changes must occur before calcitriol is produced. Initially, Vitamin D_3 (cholecalciferol, a fat-soluble steroid ingested in food or synthesized in the skin in the presence of ultraviolet light) is converted by the liver into 25-$(OH)D_3$ (calcifediol). This substance is subsequently converted into calcitriol [1,25-$(OH)_2D_3$] by the kidney. Thus, both normal liver and kidney function are required for these

Table 9-28
Major causes of hyper- and hypocalcemia.

Hypercalcemia - Serum Ca^{++} > 10.5 mg/dl	Hypocalcemia - Serum Ca^{++} < 8.5 mg/dl
Increased GI Absorption of Ca^{++} • Milk-alkali syndrome • Vitamin D intoxication	Decreased Intake or Poor GI Absorption of Ca^{++} • Poor diet • Malabsorption • Renal failure
Increased Release of Ca^{++} From Bone • Hyperparathyroidism • Malignancies • Immobilization	Increased Urinary Losses of Ca^{++} • Renal defects
Increased Physiologic Availability of Ca^{++} • Acidosis	Disturbances of Parathyroid System • Hypoparathyroidism • Pseudohypoparathyroidism
Medications • Thiazide diuretics • Lithium carbonate • Estrogens	Decreased Physiologic Availability of Ca^{++} • Alkalosis • Massive transfusion with citrated blood • Hypoalbuminemia

Note: Adapted from Bourke & Delaney (1993); Munday & Reasner (1995a, 1995b); Schrier (1995).

Figure 9-10
Hormonal regulation of calcium balance.

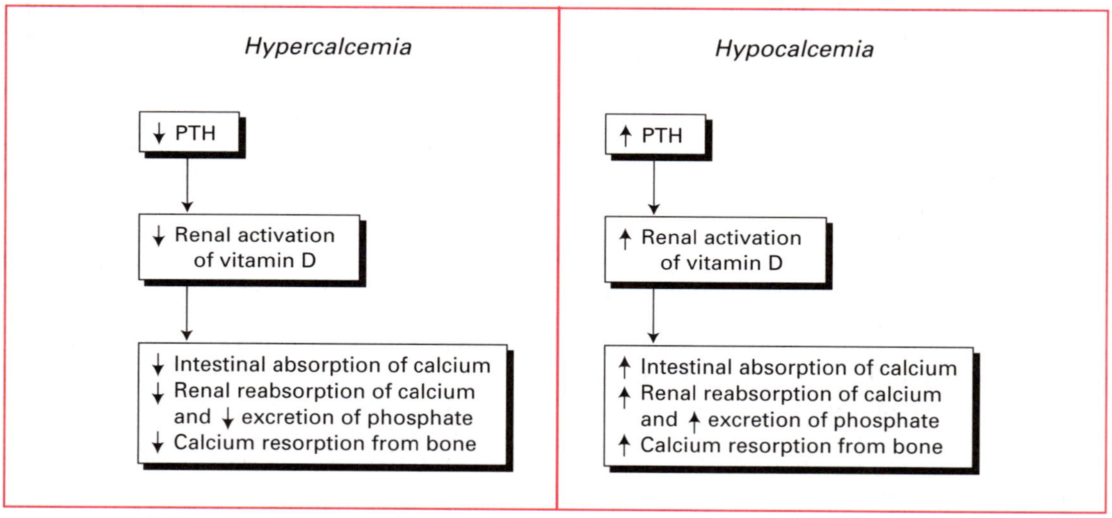

Note: From McCance, K.L. & Huether, S.E. (1994) *Pathophysiology: The biological basis for disease in adults and children* (p. 107). St. Louis: Mosby Yearbook. Reprinted with permission.

processes to occur.

Although PTH also increases the absorption of phosphorous from the GI tract, it enhances renal phosphate excretion. This action is very important in calcium-phosphate regulation. Elevated phosphate levels actually lower ionized calcium because phosphate binds with calcium, forming a complex that precipitates out of solution. These calcium-phosphate complexes can deposit anywhere in the body, a process called metastatic calcification. Thus, maintenance of normal calcium and phosphate levels is important in preventing calcium-phosphate deposition. Under normal circumstances, the calcium phosphate product (calcium in mg/dl X phosphate in mg/dl) is approximately 40. If the product exceeds 70, complex deposition may occur (Brunier, 1994).

In summary, three principal mechanisms

Figure 9-11
Position of the hand in hypocalcemic tetany (Trousseau's Sign).

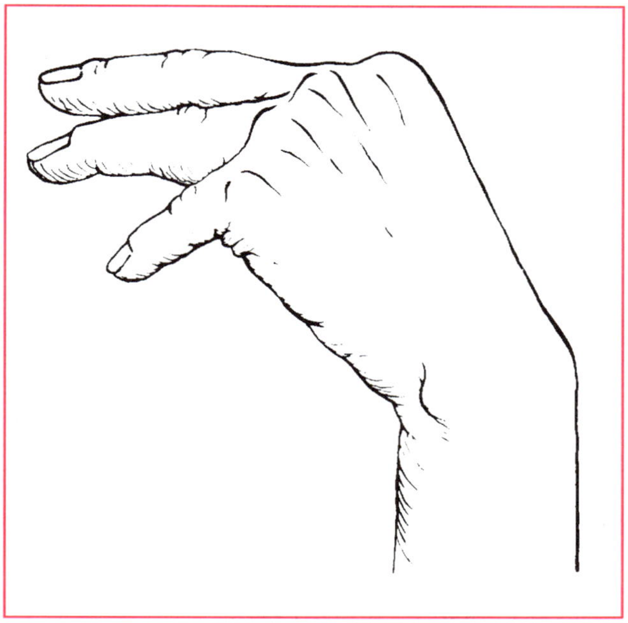

Note: From Ganong, W.F. (1993). *Review of medical physiology* (p. 357). Norwalk, CT: Appleton & Lange. Reprinted with permission.

Figure 9-12
EKG abnormalities associated with alterations in calcium levels.

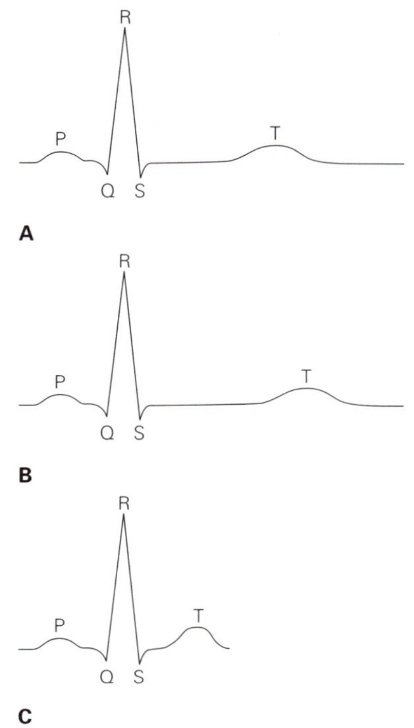

A. *Normal electrocardiogram tracing.* ***B.*** *Prolongation of the QT interval in hypocalcemia may increase risk of dysrhythmias or heart block and may be associated with poor contractility.* ***C.*** *Shortening of QT in hypercalcemia may cause severe dysrhythmias that may result from increased cardiac irritability.*

Note: From Bullock, B.L. (1996). *Pathophysiology: Adaptations and alterations in function* (p. 203). Philadelphia: J.B. Lippincott Company. Reprinted with permission.

involving the bone, the kidney, and the GI tract, all controlled by PTH, bring a low calcium level back to within its normal range (Brunier, 1994). The processes reverse in the presence of high calcium levels (Hruska & Kovach, 1995; Kumar, 1995; McCance & Huether, 1994) (see Figure 9-10). Alterations in the levels of calcium and phosphate and their product occur frequently in renal failure and are related to abnormalities in the excretion, absorption, and metabolism of the electrolytes. In patients with chronic renal failure, these alterations may lead to metastatic calcifications, secondary hyperparathyroidism, and renal bone disease. A thorough discussion of these abnormalities appears later in this chapter.

Hypocalcemia is defined as a serum calcium level below 8.5 mg/dL (Mundy & Reasner, 1995 a,b). Calcium deficits cause partial depolarization of neuronal cells, resulting in an increase in neuromuscular irritability (McCance & Huether, 1994) (see Figure 9-8). The major causes of hypocalcemia include decreased intake or GI absorption of calcium, decreased physiologically available calcium, increased urinary excretion of calcium, and parathyroid abnormalities (see Table 9-28). As mentioned previously, hypocalcemia in renal failure occurs predominantly because of abnormalities in the absorption and metabolism of calcium (Llach, 1993b).

The clinical features of hypocalcemia depend on the rapidity of onset and duration of the abnormality. Circumoral and acral (fingers and toes) paresthesias are frequently the initial manifestations of hypocalcemia-induced increased neuromuscular excitability. Latent tetany may be detected by tapping over the facial nerve to produce a facial twitch (Chvostek's sign) or by inflation of a blood pressure cuff to a level between systolic and diastolic pressure for more than 5 minutes to produce carpopedal spasm (Trousseau's sign) (see Figure 9-11). In more severe cases, laryngeal stridor and convulsions can occur (Schrier, 1995). Neuropsychiatric manifestations range from emotional lability to depression or frank psychosis. Weakness and fatigue may also be present. The characteristic electrocardiographic finding is a prolonged QT interval (see Figure 9-12). In chronic cases, papilledema, cataracts, dental caries, rickets, and osteomalacia may be present (Bourke & Delaney, 1995; Mundy & Reasner, 1995a). The skin may also become dry and scaly, the nails brittle, and the hair coarse.

Decreased calcium levels are frequently seen in association with hypoalbuminemia, a condition often seen in renal failure patients (Bourke & Delaney, 1993). This decrease occurs in the protein-bound fraction of the calcium, with a negligible change in the ionized component. Thus, one way of correcting the measured serum calcium level when the concentration of albumin is low is to add 0.8 mg/dl to the patient's calcium for every 1.0 g/dl that the serum albumin is below 4.0 g/dl (Mundy & Reasoner, 1995a). Acid-base disturbances also affect the ionized fraction of calcium. A drop in pH of 0.1 units results in a reciprocal rise in ionized calcium of approximately 0.1 mEq/L (Kumar, 1995). Therefore, renal failure patients who have acidosis may be asymptomatic from hypocalcemia because metabolic acidosis increases the level of ionized calcium and counterbalances its effect on the neuromuscular system (O'Meara & Bernard, 1995).

Therapy for acute hypocalcemia is replacement with intravenous calcium salts such as calcium chloride, calcium citrate, and calcium gluconate. Replacement should be done slowly and carefully if the patient is on digitalis or hypokalemia is present. Treatment of chronic hypocalcemia in the renal failure patient includes oral calcium, vitamin D supplementation, and control of hyperphosphatemia.

Hypercalcemia is defined as a total serum calcium greater than 10.5 mg/dl. Hypercalcemia causes the threshold potential to become more positive and depresses neuromuscular excitability (McCance & Huether, 1994) (see Figure 9-8). The major causes of hypercalcemia include increased GI absorption, increased calcium release from bone, and increased physiologically available calcium (see Table 9-28). Hypercalcemia may be seen in the ARF patient with a malignancy, such as multiple myeloma or a solid tumor, because of bone destruction and release of intracellular stores (O'Meara & Bernard, 1995). Hypercalcemia may also occur in patients with chronic renal failure and is usually attributable to secondary hyperparathyroidism or aluminum toxicity (Mundy & Reasner, 1995 a,b).

The neuropsychiatric manifestations of hypercalcemia range from subtle personality changes to acute psychosis. There may also be weakness, lethargy, confusion, and coma. Vomiting and constipation may occur. Hypercalcemia shortens the QT interval on electrocardiogram (see Figure 9-12), potentiates the action of cardiac glycosides, and may cause arrhythmias. When hyperphosphatemia is also present, calcium will bind with the phosphate, precipitate, and deposit in soft tissues.

In the acute care setting, symptomatic patients usually have a calcium greater than 13 mg/dl and require prompt treatment. If renal function permits, the administration of saline and diuretics can assist in increasing calcium excretion in the urine. To maintain normocalcemia, pamidronate may be used to inhibit osteoclastic bone resorption. Calcitonin may also be used. In addition, therapy for renal failure patients includes reducing calcium in dialysis bath and withdrawing vitamin D therapy and calcium containing binders (Daugirdas & Ing, 1994).

A serum phosphate concentration of 2.5 mg/dl or less indicates hypophosphatemia. This condition can be caused by (a) decreased intestinal absorption of phosphorous, (b) increased urinary losses, and (c) a shift of phosphorus from extracellular to intracellular compartments (such as during nutritional repletion or in alkalosis (see Table 9-29). Hypophosphatemia may be seen in some patients with acute renal failure, particularly those with burns, alcoholics, and those on hyperalimentation (Kjellstrand & Barsoum, 1995). In CRF patients, this abnormality can be seen in association with poor nutritional intake or excessive phosphorous-binder therapy (Daugirdas & Ing, 1994).

Mild or moderate hypophosphatemia frequently has no clinical manifestations (Bourke & Yanagawa, 1993). Symptoms usually do not occur until serum phosphate levels approach or fall below 1 mg/dl. The mechanisms believed to be responsible for the clinical manifestations include diminished ATP production, decreased concentrations of 2,3 diphosphoglycerate in erythrocytes (causing a decreased binding affinity for oxygen), and stimulation of other electrolyte imbalances (Kjellstrand & Barsoum, 1995).

Neurologic manifestations of hypophosphatemia include encephalopathy, paresthesias, and hyperreflexia. Skeletal muscles become weak, possibly leading to respiratory failure. Hematologic abnormalities include decreased platelet aggregation, loss of erythrocyte oxygen binding capacity, hemolysis, and immunosuppression. Acute hypophosphatemia can also result in impaired leukocyte function and increase the risk of infections (Bourke & Yanagawa, 1993; Kovach & Hruska, 1995a; Workman, 1992).

The appropriate treatment of hypophosphatemia requires identification and correction of the underlying cause. When supplementation is necessary, it can be done with milk, an excellent source of phosphorus. Neutraphos tablets can also be used. Intravenous supplementation may be necessary for severe cases. Complications of treatment include diarrhea, hyperphosphatemia, and hypocalcemia with metastatic calcifications (Kovach & Hruska, 1995a).

Hyperphosphatemia is defined as a serum phosphate concentration above 4.5 mg/dl. A

Table 9-29
Major causes of hyper- and hypophosphatemia.

Hyperphosphatemia - Serum $PO_4^=$ > 4.5 mg/dl	Hypophosphatemia - Serum $PO_4^=$ < 2.5 mg/dl
Decreased Renal Excretion • Renal failure • Hypoparathyroidism Increased $PO_4^=$ Loads or GI Absorption • IV, oral, or rectal administration of $PO_4^=$ • Vitamin D administration Release of Intracellular $PO_4^=$ Into ECF • Catabolism • Infections • Crush injuries • Cytotoxic therapy	Decreased Intake or Poor GI Absorption of $PO_4^=$ • Alcoholism • Malabsorption • Vitamin D deficiency • Starvation Increased Urinary Losses • Hyperparathyroidism • Acidosis • Renal tubular defects • Drugs - diuretics, calcitonin Shift of $PO_4^=$ From ECF Into Cells • Nutritional repletion • Alkalosis • Salicylate poisoning • Insulin

Note: Adapted from Bourke & Yanagawa (1993); Kovach & Nruska (1995a, 1995b); Schrier (1995).

decrease in the GFR accounts for more than 90% of the cases of hyperphosphatemia and is a common complication of both acute and chronic renal failure. In ARF, levels rarely rise above 7 mg/dl but very high levels may be seen with severe tissue breakdown as in rhabdomyolysis and tumor lysis syndrome (O'Meara & Bernard, 1995) (see Table 9-29). The most important short-term consequence of hyperphosphatemia is hypocalcemia. Calcium phosphate crystals form and deposit in soft tissues including the joints, myocardium, brain, lungs, skin, blood vessels, and the conjunctiva, a process known as metastatic calcification.

Treatment for hyperphosphatemia in the renal failure patient includes dietary restriction of phosphorus (600 to 1000 mg/day) (Kovach & Hruska, 1995 a,b). Intestinal absorption is frequently blocked with an aluminum antacid. However, aluminum-containing agents have been shown to be toxic to bone, brain, and the myocardium of patients and are not ideal for long-term use (constipation is also a major complication.) Calcium salts, in the form of calcium carbonate or calcium acetate, are the preferred maintenance binders. Maximal binding occurs when these binders are taken with meals. Dialysis also assists in removing phosphorous (Bourke & Yanagawa, 1993; Kovach & Hruska, 1995b).

Alterations in magnesium balance. Magnesium is the fourth most abundant cation in the body and is involved in enzymatic reactions and the maintenance of cellular permeability and neuromuscular excitability (Sutton & Sakhaee, 1995a). The normal serum level of magnesium ranges between 1.4 to 2.1 mEq/L (1.7 to 2.6 mg/dl).

Hypomagnesemia is defined as a serum magnesium less than 1.4 mEq/L (1.7 mg/dl) (see Table 9-30). The major causes of hypomagnesemia are increased GI and urinary losses. The clinical manifestations depend on the total body deficit and the rate of the development of the deficiency. Tetany is a common finding, Chvostek's sign more frequently positive than Trousseau's sign. Other neuromuscular and psychiatric manifestations include tremors, asterixis, myoclonus, and seizures. Cardiac dysrythmias, including ventricular tachycardia, fibrillation, and asystolic arrest, can occur. By causing intracellular potassium loss, a magnesium deficiency will increase the risk of digitalis toxicity (Sutton & Sakhaee, 1995b).

Hypomagnesemia may occasionally be seen in patients with renal tubular injury from nephrotoxic agents such as cisplatin, amphotericin B, and aminoglycoside antibiotics. Such hypomagnesemia is usually asymptomatic, though severe depletion may result in neuromuscular side effects (O'Meara & Bernard, 1995). Hypomagnesemia also occurs in malnourished dialysis patients, including those receiving TPN (Daugirdas & Ing, 1994). Treatment involves oral or IV supplementation with magnesium sulfate.

Hypermagnesemia is defined as a serum magnesium greater than 2.1 mEq/L (2.6 mg/dl) and can result from increased magnesium absorption (see

Table 9-30
Major causes of hyper- and hypomagnesemia.

Hypermagnesemia - Serum Mg^{++} > 2.1 mEq/L (2.6 mg/dl)	Hypomagnesemia - Serum Mg^{++} < 1.4 mEq/L (1.7 mg/dl)
Increased Intake • Oral or parenteral Mg^{++} administration Decreased Renal Excretion • Renal failure	Increased GI Loss of Mg^{++} • Steatorrhea • Diarrhea Increased Renal Excretion • Renal tubular defects • Diuretics • Aminoglycosides • Cisplatin

Note: Adapted from Sutton & Sakhaee (1995b, 1995c).

Table 9-30). Symptoms of hypermagnesemia are related to diminished neuromuscular transmission and cardiac conduction. Therefore, patients have nausea, vomiting, lethargy, confusion, respiratory depression, and absent tendon reflexes. Cardiovascular effects include hypotension, bradycardia, heart block, and cardiac arrest.

Mild degrees of asymptomatic hypermagnesemia are common in patients with renal failure, though higher levels may be seen with the injudicious use of magnesium-containing antacids, enemas, or laxatives (Daurgirdas & Ing, 1994; O'Meara & Bernard, 1995). Treatment is to stop ingestion of magnesium-containing compounds. In symptomatic patients, urgent treatment with intravenous calcium gluconate as a magnesium antagonist and insulin and glucose to promote entry of magnesium into cells is required. Dialysis quickly improves the condition (Daugirdas & Ing, 1994; Sutton & Sakhaee, 1995c).

Alterations in acid-base balance. The pH of a solution is a measurement of its hydrogen ion concentration and is expressed as the logarithm (log) to the base 10 of the reciprocal of the hydrogen ion concentration $[H^+]$:

$$pH = \log 1/[H^+]$$

Under normal circumstances, systemic acid-base balance is well regulated within a relatively narrow range (7.36 to 7.44) by buffering systems in the blood and renal and respiratory mechanisms (Hamm, 1995). The maintenance of this narrow range is very important because small changes in $[H^+]$ have dramatic effects on normal cell function. The effects of changes in pH include: (a) changes in the excitability of nerve and muscle cells, (b) alterations in the rate and direction of enzymatic reactions, and (c) changes in the K^+ levels in the ICF and ECF (Sherwood, 1993).

Acidosis is present when the blood pH falls below 7.35, while alkalosis occurs when the blood pH is above 7.45. Acidosis and alkalosis can both be caused by metabolic and respiratory abnormalities. A detailed explanation of these abnormalities is beyond the scope of this discussion but can be found in numerous textbooks. Each of the acid-base disorders can potentially occur in the renal failure patient. However, because metabolic derangements in acid-base balance are more common, a brief discussion of metabolic acidosis and alkalosis will be presented here.

Metabolic acidosis results from an excess of hydrogen ions in the body fluids. Three major defects cause this condition, including renal abnormalities in hydrogen ion excretion, an increase in acid burden, or a loss of bicarbonate (see Table 9-31). The most striking clinical manifestation of metabolic acidosis is an increase in the rate and depth of respiration. This change in the pattern of breathing is termed "Kussmaul's respirations" (Bushinsky, 1995) and assists in compensating for the acidosis by lowering the pCO_2. In severe acidosis, the respiratory rate may increase so much as to cause extreme fatigue. Hyperkalemia may develop or worsen as potassium ions move from the ICF to the ECF in exchange for hydrogen ions, also in an attempt to compensate.

In ARF, acidosis may be severe and occur in conjunction with diabetic ketoacidosis, lactic acidosis, or septic catabolism. In addition to displaying Kussmaul's respirations, the patient may develop myocardial depression and hypotension, insulin resistance, impaired carbohydrate utilization, and increased protein degradation (O'Meara & Bernard, 1995). In contrast, the patient with chronic renal failure may exhibit a slow progressive retention of acid, which can also become severe (Bushinsky, 1995).

Decreasing acid production by reducing dietary protein is frequently the first line of treatment in

Table 9-31
Major causes of metabolic acidosis and alkalosis.

Metabolic Acidosis - A Decrease in Systemic pH	Metabolic Alkalosis - An Increase in Systemic pH
Decreased Renal Excretions of H^+ • Renal failure • Renal tubular acidosis	Increased Intake of Alkali • Sodium bicarbonate administration
Increased Production of H^+ • Lactic acidosis • Ketoacidosis • Starvation	Gastric Losses of H^+ • Vomiting • Gastric suction
Bicarbonate Loss • Renal defects • Diarrhea	Renal Losses of H^+ • Diuretics • Renal tubular defects • Mineralocorticoid excess
Ingestions • Salicylate • Ethylene glycol • Methanol	Movement of H^+ From ECF Into Cells • Hypokalemia

Note: Adapted from Bushinsky (1995); Gennari (1995); Rose & Rennke (1994).

the renal failure patient. Depending on the severity of the acidosis, oral or IV sodium bicarbonate can also be administered. Dialysis is an effective treatment and may be used on an emergent basis for the patient in ARF with severe acidosis.

Metabolic alkalosis is an acid-base disorder characterized by an elevated bicarbonate concentration, an alkaline blood pH, and an increase in pCO_2 (Gennari, 1995). The major causes of metabolic alkalosis include increased loads of alkali such as bicarbonate, gastric or renal losses of hydrogen ions, and potassium depletion (see Table 9-31). In ARF, the most common cause is administered lactate or acetate, especially with TPN (Daugirdas & Ing, 1994). Dialysis usually assists in correcting this abnormality. A custom dialysate bath with a lower acetate or bicarbonate level can be used depending on the degree of the alkalosis. Metabolic alkalosis rarely occurs in the chronic renal failure patient but may occur in several of the situations listed in Table 9-31.

Metabolic and Endocrine Disturbances

In renal failure, the homeostasis of metabolic and endocrine systems depends on a variety of adaptive mechanisms, many of which are poorly understood. Unfortunately, these adaptations have numerous adverse systemic effects that result in the development of metabolic and regulatory disorders. The major abnormalities that occur include glucose intolerance, disturbances in protein and lipid metabolism, and alterations in endocrine function. In order to plan appropriate care, nurses should develop an understanding of the pathophysiologic basis and psychosocial responses associated with these changes (see Appendix C).

Glucose intolerance. Glucose intolerance develops in most patients with acute and chronic renal failure. Although baseline insulin levels are increased and the degradation of insulin is reduced when GFR falls to less than 20%, there is a decreased response or resistance to insulin at the tissue level (Suki & Eknoyan, 1995). Other factors that may also contribute to glucose intolerance include delayed insulin secretion after glucose ingestion and altered cellular metabolism secondary to acidosis (Llach, 1993b). Although insulin and glucose metabolism are improved with regular dialysis, complete normalization does not occur (Lazarus & Hakim, 1991). However, the glucose intolerance is seldom severe enough to result in extreme hyperglycemia and ketoacidosis (Llach, 1993b).

Although glucose intolerance develops in many patients, the reduced metabolic clearance and degradation of insulin may actually decrease the insulin requirements of diabetics who develop renal failure, leading to hypoglycemia. This may be complicated by the fact that diabetic dialysis patients may also have a blunted response to the effects of low blood sugar. Thus, unless this problem is recognized and the insulin dosage is reduced, symptomatic hypoglycemia can develop (Suki & Eknoyan, 1995). Appropriate nursing management of these patients includes a careful assessment of glucose levels and insulin requirements, maintenance of an adequate oral intake prior to dialysis, and use of a hemodialysate glucose level of 200 mg/dl to avoid hypoglycemia (Lazarus & Hakim, 1991) (see Appendix C).

Alterations of protein metabolism. Protein synthesis is generally normal in early renal insufficiency but gradually decreases with progressive renal failure. Malnutrition, insulin resistance, metabolic acidosis, and hyporesponsiveness to growth hormone are possible causes (Suki & Eknoyan, 1995). Clinical markers of poor protein metabolism include low serum levels of albumin, transferrin, and complements, all of which are reliable indicators of overall nutritional status.

Although protein restriction is often an important component of the treatment plan, it is important that patients with acute and chronic renal failure have adequate protein intake in order to avoid depleting their protein stores. Negative-nitrogen balance is associated with increased mortality in both groups (Kellerman, 1994; Lazarus & Hakim, 1991). Adequate energy intake in the form of calories is also important. In a restricted protein diet, as much of the protein as possible should be of high biological value (containing essential amino acids, such as meat and fish). These essential amino acids are vital for protein synthesis. On the other hand, low biological value proteins (bread and cereals) provide few essential amino acids and their breakdown increases the BUN. Adequate dialysis is also important in the maintenance of appropriate protein metabolism (Lazarus & Hakim, 1991).

Nursing care should begin with a careful assessment of eating habits, dietary preferences, and cultural influences on eating patterns (Lancaster, 1995). A dietary or nutritional support team consult is often crucial in conducting a thorough nutritional evaluation. Oral supplements or total parenteral nutrition are then prescribed after assessing the patient's unique needs (Price, 1992a). Multivitamin supplements are also frequently recommended. Nurses should continually monitor indicators of nutritional status, including weight, electrolytes, and albumin levels. Sources of protein depletion such as losses from wounds, drainage, or peritoneal dialysis should be identified and replaced. Patients and their families should also be educated regarding the importance of adequate nutritional intake (see Appendix C).

Alterations of lipid metabolism. Although serum cholesterol is usually normal or only slightly elevated, serum triglyceride levels are frequently high in the chronic renal failure patient (a condition referred to as Type IV hyperlipoproteinemia) (Suki & Eknoyan, 1995). The development of hypertriglyceridemia is believed to be related to decreased lipoprotein lipase activity and a reduced conversion of VLDL to LDL (Suki & Eknoyan, 1995). The use of high concentrations of glucose in peritoneal dialysate leads to an increase in the carbohydrate load and has been reported to aggravate hypertriglyceridemia in some patients. However, the glucose concentration of 100 to 200 mg/dl in hemodialysate does not appear to add to the carbohydrate load and has not been shown to make a significant contribution to lipid abnormalities (Lazarus & Hakim, 1991). Other factors that may aggravate lipid abnormalities in some patients include the use of beta blockers and diuretics (Lazarus & Hakim, 1991).

The treatment of hypertriglyceridiemia is important in the chronic patient because of its relationship to the development of atherosclerosis and coronary artery disease, major causes of morbidity and mortality. Lowering the dietary intake of saturated fats and carbohydrates may be helpful. However, because of other dietary restrictions used in the treatment of renal failure patients, the usefulness of these additional dietary modifications may be limited. A carefully monitored program of exercise can help reduce triglyceride levels as can avoidance of drugs known to exacerbate hyperlipidemia, such as beta adrenergic blocking agents (Daugirdas & Ing, 1994). The use of antilipemic agents, such as gemfibrozil or lovastatin, has not been reported in large numbers of patients with chronic renal failure (Lazarus & Hakim, 1991).

Endocrine disorders. Endocrine changes in ARF patients have not been well studied. However, decreases in follicle-stimulating hormone (FSH) and testosterone levels, and increases in prolactin levels have been described. Low levels of T_4 and a blunted response to thyroid releasing hormone (TSH) have also been reported. These changes appear to resolve after recovery of renal function (O'Meara & Bernard, 1995).

A wide variety of endocrine abnormalities are known to develop in patients with chronic renal failure as changes occur in the synthesis, secretion, and metabolism of various hormones, as well as alterations in their biologic activity (Daugirdas & Ing, 1994; Lazarus & Hakim, 1991) (see Table 9-32). Several of these abnormalities are covered in other appropriate sections of this chapter. For example, changes in insulin metabolism were previously discussed in the section entitled Glucose Intolerance. Because alterations in erythropoietin and parathyroid hormone production cause numerous clinical symptoms contributing to the uremic syndrome, these abnormalities are covered in that section. Two additional endocrine-related problems commonly seen in the chronic renal failure population are hypothyroidism and sexual dysfunction, both of which are discussed in this section.

Although most dialysis patients are euthyroid, hypothyroidism occurs with increased frequency in this population. Symptoms include cold intolerance, lethargy, hoarseness, dry skin, and weight gain. However, the diagnosis is difficult to make on clinical features because dialysis patients often have cold intolerance and lethargy related to the uremic syndrome. T_3 and T_4 levels are of limited usefulness in making the diagnosis of hypothyroidism as baseline levels are commonly low in the dialysis patient. A TSH level over 20 microunits/ml is usually sufficient evidence that hypothyroidism is present and indicates the need from thyroxine therapy (Daugirdas & Ing, 1994).

Of the clinical complications that result from endocrine alterations, sexual dysfunction is one of the most upsetting to chronic renal failure patients. Although not well understood, the abnormalities are caused by dysfunction of the hypothalamic-pituitary-adrenal axis and are characterized by: (a) elevated levels of luteinizing hormone (LH), follicle-stimulating hormone (FSH), prolactin, and LH-releasing hormone; and (b) decreased levels of testosterone in men and progesterone in women (Suki & Eknoyan, 1995). Symptoms of sexual dysfunction include impotence, decreased libido, testicular atrophy, and reduced sperm count in men and amenorrhea, dysmenorrhea, and decreased libido in women (Binik & Mah, 1994; Rickus, 1987; Suki & Eknoyan, 1995; Zarifian, 1992). Reproductive abnormalities also occur. Pregnancy is rare in uremic women who have a GFR less than 30 ml/min and spontaneous abortions, amenorrhea, and dysfunctional uterine bleeding are common. Men are frequently infertile from absent or decreased spermatogenesis. Elevated prolactin levels may cause galactorrhea in both sexes as well as amenorrhea in women and impotence in men (Dubrow & Levin, 1995). Agents such as bromocryptine decrease prolactin levels and may improve sexual functioning in men.

Treatment for sexual dysfunction should begin with a thorough history and physical examination. Laboratory tests that are frequently ordered include a complete blood count, a biochemical panel, a urinalysis and culture and sensitivity, and thyroid, testosterone, prolactin, FSH, and LH levels (Zarifian, 1992). Correction of anemia with erythropoietin has also been shown to improve sexual function in some patients (Lakkis & Martinez-Maldonado, 1995). Vacuum devices used to achieve erection may be effective (Zarifian, 1992). Psychological counseling of the patient and partner is often helpful. It is also very important that nurses, themselves, obtain the education necessary to ensure that they are comfortable in discussing and are knowledgeable regarding issues of sex and sexuality (Ulrich, 1987; Zarifian, 1992).

Uremic Syndrome

The term uremia was first coined by P.A. Piorry

Table 9-32
Summary of endocrine abnormalities in dialysis patients.

- Pancreas
  - Insulin
    - Postreceptor defect, insulin resistance
    - Insulin binding, normal or reduced
    - Impaired insulin secretion
    - Decreased insulin catabolism
  - Hyperglucagonemia
    - Impaired glucagon degradation
    - Augmented gluconeogenesis?
- Renin-angiotensin, aldosterone
  - Angiotensin II, aldosterone levels usually normal or reduced
- Catecholamines
  - Controversial; resting levels high or low
  - Reduced renal excretion and enzymatic degradation
  - Decreased neuronal uptake
  - Increased sympathetic nerve traffic (not found in nephrectomized patients)
- Cortisol
  - Increased total and free plasma levels
  - Decreased degradation
  - Decreased binding to cortisol-binding globulin
  - IV dexamethasone required to suppress cortisol secretion
- Thyroid
  - Increased incidence of goiter and hypothyroidism
  - Thyroxine and triiodothyronine levels tend to be low
  - Thyroid-stimulating hormone usually normal; best test for hypothyroidism
- Gonadal
  - Serum total and free testosterone reduced (decreased production)
  - Seminal fluid volume, sperm motility reduced
  - Plasma luteinizing hormone and follicle-stimulating hormone levels normal
    - Increase appropriately after clomiphene
    - Fail to increase after estrogen stimulation
    - Reduced gonadotropin pulsatility
  - Serum prolactin levels 3-6 times normal.
- Growth hormone
  - Immunoreactive growth hormone levels increased
  - Insulin-like growth factor levels normal or increased, but bioactivitiy is reduced
  - Recombinant human growth hormone therapy for children and malnourished adults
- Parathyroid hormone, 1,25-dihydroxyvitamin D3
  - Serum levels of parathyroid hormone increased
    - Early cause is hypocalcemia
    - Late cause is gland hypertrophy
  - Serum levels of calcitriol reduced
    - Reduced 1-hydroxylation by the kidney
      - Structural damage
      - Hyperphosphatemia

Note: From Daugirdas, J.T., & Ing, T.S. (1994). Handbook of dialysis (p. 492). Boston: Little, Brown and Company. Reprinted with permission.

Table 9-33
Potentially toxic compounds that accumulate in renal failure.

Urea	Pyridine Derivatives
Phenols	Guanidino Compounds
Hormones	Beta 2 Microglobulin
Polyamines	Middle Molecules
Trace Elements	Serum Proteases

Note: From May, R.C., Kelly, R.A., & Mitch, W.E. (1991). Pathophysiology of uremia. In B.M. Brenner, & F.C. Rector (Eds.), *The kidney* (4th edition) (p. 1999). Philadelphia: W.B. Saunders Company. Reprinted with permission.

to describe a condition caused by "contaminating the blood with urine" (May, Kelly, & Mitch, 1991, p. 1997). Currently, the term uremic syndrome is used to describe the constellation of signs and symptoms associated with renal failure. This condition affects multiple organ systems and thus reflects the complex role that the kidneys play in systemic regulation.

Uremia results from the retention of substances that are normally excreted by the kidneys, including the end products of protein metabolism such as BUN. However, kidney failure is also associated with the accumulation of several other potentially toxic substances. For example, much attention has been focused on the possible role of the middle molecules, compounds with a molecular weight of 500 to 2000 daltons, in the development of uremic symptoms. Although it is known that these middle molecules are retained in patients with renal disease, their exact nature and pathophysiologic role remain to be defined. Elevated PTH (parathyroid hormone) may also play an important role, especially in chronic renal failure (Dunbrow & Levin, 1995) in addition to several other potentially toxic compounds (see Table 9-33). However, to date, no single substance has been implicated as the uremic toxin (Dunbrow & Levin, 1995; May et al., 1991).

The clinical features of the uremic patient may vary depending on the cause of the renal problem, the severity of the renal injury, and the speed with which it develops (O'Meara & Bernard, 1995). The symptoms are generally more severe and develop more rapidly in ARF patients as adaptive mechanisms have not had time to occur. In CRF patients, the number and severity of symptoms may vary considerably depending on the rate of disease progression and compliance with medical therapy (Fraser & Arieff, 1993). The nurse must, therefore, carefully assess the patient's overall status and be very knowledgeable regarding the multisystemic manifestations of the uremic syndrome (see Appendix D).

Neurologic manifestations. A variety of neurologic complications affecting the central, peripheral, and autonomic nervous systems are seen in patients with both acute and chronic renal failure. These abnormalities are believed to be related to the retention of uremic toxins, decreased cerebral blood flow, and reduced cerebral oxygen utilization (Suki & Eknoyan, 1995). Neurological changes vary directly with the rate at which renal dysfunction develops and usually respond favorably to dialysis.

The earliest central nervous system (CNS) effects usually noted include reduced cerebral activity and alterations in mentation and cognition. EEG abnormalities include a diffuse slowing of electrical activity accompanied by spike activity (Moe & Sprague, 1994; O'Meara & Bernard, 1995; Suki & Eknoyan, 1995). Other CNS effects include headache, lassitude, apathy, drowsiness, and insomnia accompanied by daytime drowsiness. As uremia worsens, somnolence, confusion, asterixis, seizures, and coma can develop. Behavioral alterations include personality changes, increased irritability, emotional lability, and depression. In patients with acute renal failure, these changes can occur within 48 hours of onset of renal failure and are not usually affected by dialysis within the first 3 weeks of treatment (Fraser & Arieff, 1993).

Although CNS effects are more apparent with increasing levels of uremia, encephalopathy, including seizures, may develop in severely uremic patients who are initially dialyzed too aggressively. This condition, referred to as dialysis disequilibrium syndrome, is believed to be related to a rapid fall in the osmolality of the blood during dialysis, resulting in cerebral edema, and can usually be avoided by altering the dialysis technique (see Chapter 19) (O'Meara & Bernard, 1995). Less-severe manifestations of this syndrome also occur in chronic dialysis patients causing symptoms such as headache, nausea, blurring of vision, muscular twitching and cramps, and disorientation (Fraser & Arieff, 1993).

Dialysis dementia, a progressive, frequently fatal neurologic disease, was first described in chronic patients in the mid 1970s when contamination of the dialysis water with aluminum was determined to be the cause (Moe & Sprague, 1994). Although it is seen less frequently today, isolated incidents still occur. Early manifestations of this problem include dysarthria and apraxia of speech with slurring, stuttering, and hesitancy. Later symptoms include personality changes, dementia, and seizures. Usually, the disease progresses to death within 6 months. Although the etiology of this syndrome remains controversial, an increase in brain aluminum content remains a likely contributing factor (Fraser & Arieff, 1993; Moe & Sprague, 1994).

Chronic dialysis patients report that sleep alter-

Figure 9-13
Etiologic factors of the cardiovascular manifestations.

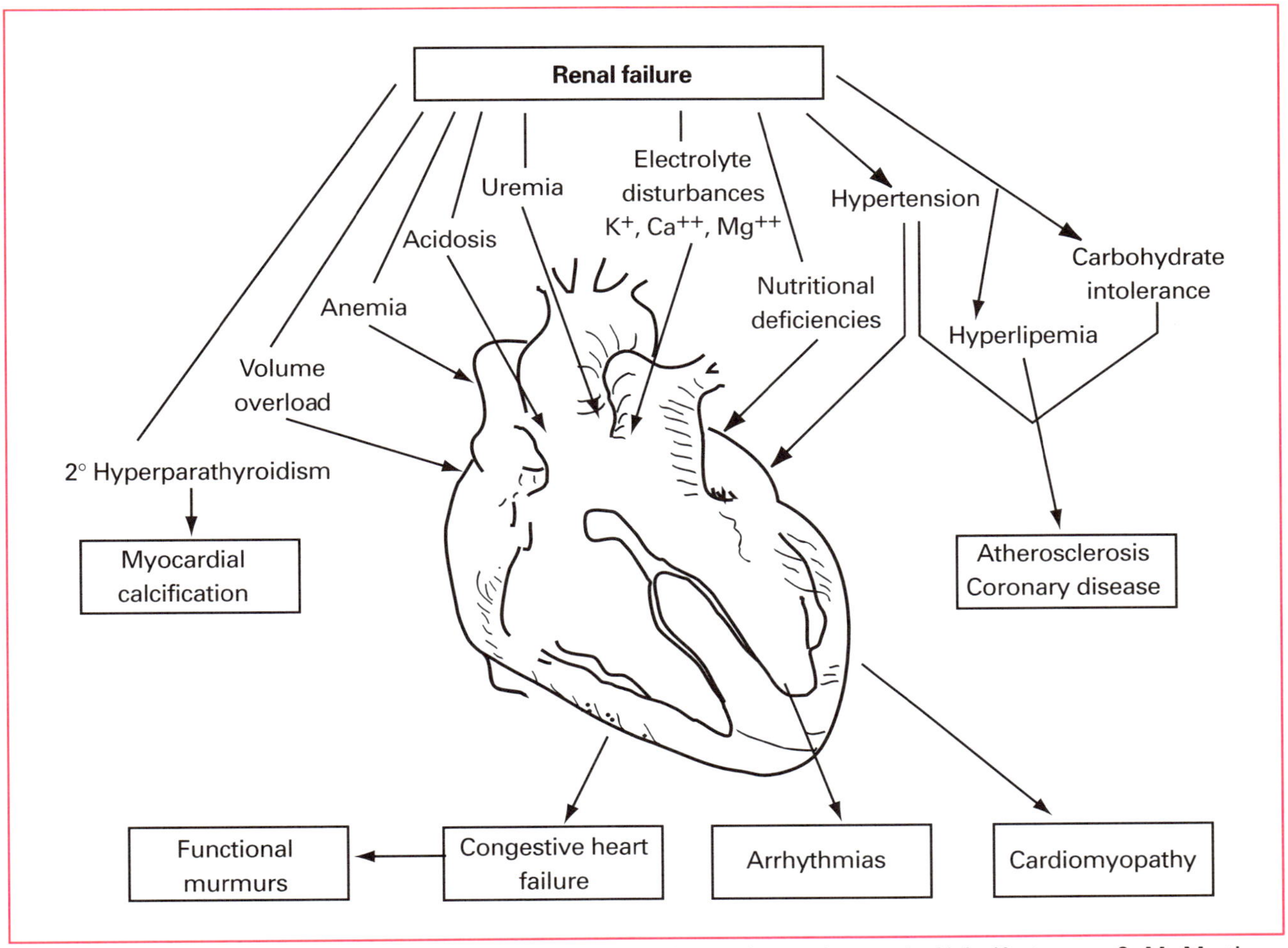

Note: From Eknoyan, G. (1977). Chronic renal failure and uremic syndrome. In N.A. Kurtzman, & M. Martinez-Maldonado (Eds.), *Pathophysiology of the kidney* (p. 856). Springfield, IL: Charles C. Thomas Publishers. Reprinted with permission.

ations are major sources of stress and problems adversely affecting the quality of their lives (Eichel, 1986; Health Care Financing Administration, 1986; Parker, 1990). Between 65% and 85% of dialysis patients report sleep alterations that are characterized by diminished sleep efficiency (time asleep/time in bed) and more fragmented sleep (Walker, Fine, & Kryger, 1995). Daytime sleepiness is a common complaint, and most patients report daily naps (Holley, Nespor, & Rault, 1992; Walker et al., 1995). Results from some polysomnographic studies reveal that sleep apnea syndrome (SAS) is prevalent in this population (Mendelson, Wadhwa, Greenberg, Gujavarty, & Bergofsky, 1990; Kimmel, Miller, & Mendelson, 1989; Wadhwa & Mendelson, 1992). Others have found that the prevalence of restless leg syndrome (RLS) and periodic leg movements (PLMs), which cause multiple arousals and disturb nocturnal rest, is also high (Winkelman & Lazarus, 1994; Pressman, Benz, & Peterson, 1995).

Peripheral nervous system effects include paresthesias in the lower extremities that are symmetrical, slowly progressive, begin distally, and spread proximally. Typically, paresthesias affect the lower before the upper extremities. Other complications include painful dysthesias (burning feet syndrome), decreases in deep tendon reflexes, gait changes, and foot drop. Muscle twitching and myoclonic jerks are painful, annoying, and interfere with sleep. These abnormalities are related to demyelinization of the neural axon and can be present in both ARF and CRF patients. Electrophysiologic studies reveal decreased nerve conduction time. Remyelinzation of peripheral nerves occurs with restoration of renal

Table 9-34
Checking for a paradoxical pulse by sphygmomanometer.

A paradox is often cited as specific for pericardial effusion. Normally, on inspiration, increased venous return to the right heart and increased pulmonary vascular capacity results in less blood in the left heart and a small decrease in cardiac output. This change in cardiac output is evidenced as the arterial blood pressure falls as much as 10 mm/Hg during inspiration. A paradoxical pulse is an exaggeration of this normal event. On inspiration, the arterial blood pressure falls more than 10 mm/Hg. The pericardial effusion limits or restricts cardiac filling and decreases cardiac output. The result is a marked fall in blood pressure on inspiration (paradoxical pulse; Lancaster, 1983, p. 44).

1. Ask the patient to breathe as easily and normally as possible.
2. Apply sphygmomanometer and inflate it until no sounds are audible.
3. Deflate the cuff gradually until sounds are audible only during expiration. Note the pressure.
4. Deflate the cuff further until sounds are also audible during inspiration. Note the pressure.

The difference in systolic pressure between expiration and inspiration should be 5 mm/Hg. If it is greater than 10 mm/Hg, the paradoxical pulse is exaggerated. Associated findings include low blood pressure and weak and rapid pulse (Seidel et al., 1991, p. 343).

function, dialysis, or renal transplantation (Suki & Eknoyan, 1995).

Autonomic nervous system abnormalities are probably related to a decreased responsiveness of the baroreceptors, including failure to develop tachycardia in response to hypotension (Suki & Eknoyan, 1995). Depression of the cough reflex and decreased sweating may also occur (Fraser & Arieff, 1993). The cranial nerves are also often affected, causing transient nystagmus, miosis, and facial asymmetry (Fraser & Arieff, 1993).

Nursing care should begin with a careful assessment of the patient's cognitive and neurologic function. It is important to identify those factors that would aggravate or cause deterioration of the neurologic status such as concomitant abnormalities in fluid, electrolyte, and acid-base disturbances. Changes in neurologic status are also associated with severe hypertension and cerebrovascular events. Deficiency of certain vitamins such as B_{12} and B_6 can precipitate neurologic abnormalities. Adverse reactions to drugs such as antibiotics, antihypertensive agents, ritalin, and cimetidine can cause a variety of central and peripheral nervous system effects.

Cardiovascular manifestations. The cardiovascular system is greatly affected by renal failure and dialysis (Lazarus & Hakim, 1991). Salt and water retention, anemia, hypertension, and numerous metabolic abnormalities are contributing factors. These complications occur in ARF patients and are a leading cause of morbidity and mortality in those with CRF (Suki & Eknoyan, 1995) (see Figure 9-13).

Hypertension occurs in approximately 10% to 30% of patients with ARF (O'Meara & Bernard, 1995) and 80% of those with CRF (Suki & Eknoyan, 1995) and is usually volume dependent (related to the retention of salt and water). However, it may be complicated by decreased renal perfusion and activation of the renin-angiotensin system, excess aldosterone secretion, increased sympathetic tone, diminished production of vasodepressor hormones, and excess release of vasoconstrictor natriuretic factors (Suki & Eknoyan, 1995). For the CRF patient, untreated hypertension represents a major risk factor in the development of coronary artery disease, congestive heart failure, and cerebrovascular disease (Suki & Eknoyan, 1995). Blood pressure medications are, therefore, an important component of treatment. However, most antihypertensive agents may increase vascular instability and can cause profound hypotension during dialysis. Therefore, the administration of these drugs should be timed to minimize their action during the procedure (Lazarus & Hakim, 1991).

Congestive heart failure is often present in varying degrees depending on volume status and may be aggravated by other problems such as hypertension, anemia, electrolyte abnormalities, and acidosis (Suki & Eknoyan, 1995). Reduction of blood pressure and correction of acidosis and hyperkalemia often have marked effects on the stabilization of cardiac function (O'Meara & Bernard, 1995).

Serious disturbances in cardiac rhythm may develop secondary to hyperkalemia, hypermagnesemia, hypocalcemia, and severe acidosis. In the ARF patient, hypomagnesemia and hypokalemia frequently occur after diuretic administration, predisposing the individual to digitalis intoxication (O'Meara & Bernard, 1995; Suki & Eknoyan, 1995). In CRF patients, metastatic calcifications can also cause intraventricular conduction defects, complete heart block, and calcification of the valvular annulus, causing murmurs (Suki & Eknoyan, 1995).

Uremic pericarditis, an inflammation of the membrane surrounding the heart, is a condition often accompanied by the collection of varying amounts of fluid and/or blood in the pericardial sac (Suki & Eknoyan, 1995). In most cases, the inflammation is aseptic, although some cases of bacterial and viral pericarditis have been reported (Becker, 1988; Suki & Eknoyan, 1995). Clinical manifestations include pain, fever, and a pericardial friction

Figure 9-14
Factors contributing to uremic pneumonitis.

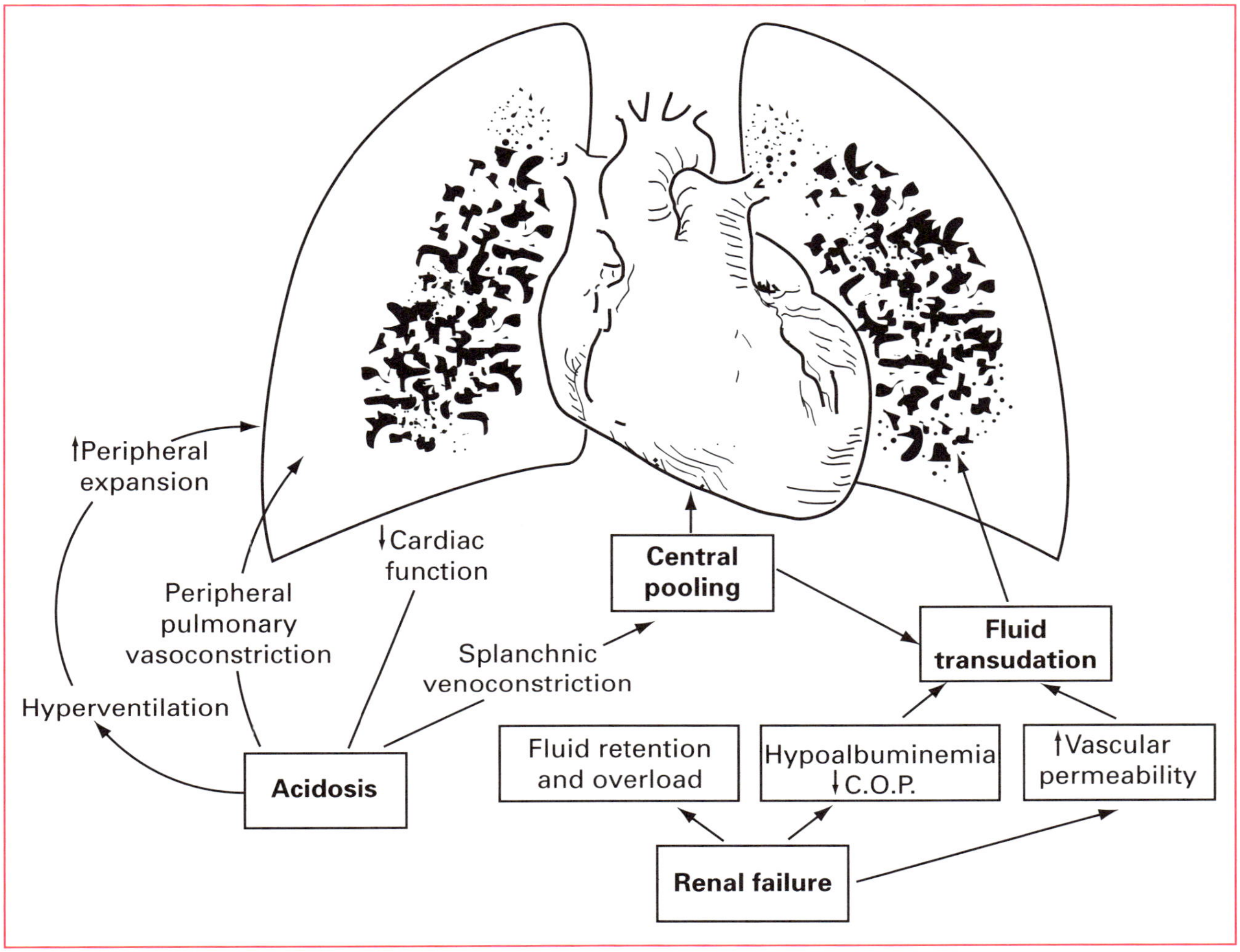

Note: From Eknoyan, G. (1977). Chronic renal failure and uremic syndrome. In N.A. Kurtzman, & M. Martinez-Maldonado (Eds.), *Pathophysiology of the kidney* (p. 859). Springfield, IL: Charles C. Thomas Publishers. Reprinted with permission.

rub (a harsh leathery sound heard over the precordium). The friction rub may precede the pain, often persists when the pain has subsided, and may disappear when fluid begins collecting. Other symptoms include tachycardia, low-grade fever, hypotension, narrowing pulse pressure, and a paradoxical pulse (see Table 9-34). About 50% of patients will have the EKG changes of pericarditis (elevated and upwardly concave ST segments). Tamponade may also occur with the development of severe right ventricular failure, requiring pericardiocentesis or tube pericardiostomy. Treatment usually includes daily dialysis. Minimal doses of heparin or regional anticoagulation should be used during dialysis to minimize the risk of pericardial bleeding and tamponade (O'Meara & Bernard, 1995). Antiinflammatory agents such as indomethacin and corticosteroids may also be effective in relieving the pericardial inflammation. In CRF patients, constrictive pericarditis may develop and necessitate complete or partial pericardiectomy (Suki & Eknoyan, 1995).

Appropriate nursing management includes a careful assessment of the cardiovascular status of the patient and careful monitoring of fluid, electrolyte, and acid-base balance. Many cardiac medications require dosage adjustments in renal failure, and patients' responses to these agents may vary with electrolyte levels. Assessing CRF patients for other cardiovascular risk factors and providing education regarding risk factor reduction is also important.

Respiratory manifestations. A variety of pulmonary complications are associated with the uremic syndrome. These complications include pulmonary edema, pleuritis with or without pleural effusion, and increased susceptibility to pulmonary infection. In addition, Kussmaul respirations secondary to metabolic acidosis are frequently encountered. Thus, a careful assessment of the pulmonary system is crucial in the management of these patients as prompt treatment is often required.

Pulmonary edema occurs frequently in patients with renal failure and is generally related to congestive heart failure and volume overload. Associated symptoms include shortness of breath, frothy sputum, and rales and rhonchi over lung fields. Although invasive monitoring is of great help in assessing volume status, pulmonary edema may occur in some patients with normal central venous or pulmonary artery pressures as acute uremia may damage capillaries, causing the leakage of fluid (Kjellstrand & Barsoum, 1995). In addition, a low serum albumin level resulting in decreased colloidal osmotic pressure (C.O.P.) of the blood may favor the formation of pulmonary edema in some patients. Central fluid collection, a phenomenon associated with metabolic acidosis, may also contribute to the problem (Suki & Eknoyan, 1995) (see Figure 9-14). X-rays often reveal a characteristic pattern in which opacities of the central perihilar areas of the chest give a bat wing appearance (uremic pneumonitis). Pulmonary edema usually resolves after treatment with diuretics and/or dialysis (Suki & Eknoyan, 1995).

Pleuritis, an inflammation of the pleura, can occur in both acute and chronic renal failure patients and may be accompanied by effusion. The etiology is believed to be similar to that of pericarditis and the two conditions frequently coexist. Symptoms include chest pain on inspiration and dyspnea. Decreased breath sounds over the area and a pleural friction rub are common physical findings (Suki & Eknoyan, 1995). Treatment with intensive dialysis is frequently helpful. Diagnostic thoracentesis may be necessary to exclude other causes of effusion, such as malignancy (Daugirdas & Ing, 1994).

Uremic patients exhibit an increased susceptibility to infection, including pneumonia and pulmonary tuberculosis. When infection is present, the sputum is often thick and tenacious. The cough reflex may also be depressed. Prompt treatment with antibiotics is required. Those patients with CRF should receive vaccinations against the influenza virus (annually) and pneumococcus (revaccination dependent on antibody response) (Daugirdas & Ing, 1994) to enhance their immunity against some of the more common pneumonias.

Hematologic manifestations. Anemia is a well-known complication of renal failure, generally worsens as renal function deteriorates, and is related to a decreased production of erythropoietin. In ARF, anemia can occur as early as 10 days after the onset. The hematocrit gradually falls, stabilizing in the 20% to 30% range (O'Meara & Bernard, 1995). In CRF, the hematocrit usually ranges between 15% and 30 % (Eschbach & Adamson, 1993). Other factors that may contribute to the anemia of renal failure include bone marrow suppression, bleeding, hemodilution, decreased red blood cell survival, gastrointestinal hemorrhage, perioperative blood loss, and intravascular hemolysis (Eschbach & Adamson, 1993; Lazarus & Hakim, 1991; O'Meara & Bernard, 1995). The anemia is usually normocytic (normal RBC size) and normochromic (normal RBC color) unless it is complicated by iron deficiency, folate deficiency, or aluminum overload secondary to the administration of aluminum-containing phosphate binders (Daugirdas & Ing, 1994; Eschbach & Adamson, 1993; Suki & Eknoyan, 1995). Associated symptoms include fatigue, reduced exercise tolerance, depression, decreased appetite, increased angina, cold intolerance, and hypotension.

Administration of recombinant human erythropoietin (r-HuEPO) has dramatically improved most patients by correcting anemia, increasing exercise tolerance, and improving subjective well-being, appetite, cognitive functioning, and overall quality of life. When administered in doses of 50 to 150 U/kg IV or SQ from one to three times a week, it causes an increase in hematocrit approaching normal limits within about 8 to 14 weeks. (Because of the length of time required for full effects, transfusions may be used instead of r-HuEPO to treat the anemia of ARF.) Adequate assessment of iron stores through measurements of ferritin, iron saturation, and transferrin are important, and iron adequate replacement (oral and IV) is essential (Daugirdas & Ing, 1994). In addition, supplementation of folic acid, iron, and amino acids is often given to patients with renal failure to replace suspected dietary deficiencies or extra losses due to dialysis (Eschbach & Adamson, 1993). Androgens can increase the red cell mass in some anemic dialysis patients. However, because of the high incidence of side effects, r-HuEPO should be the primary therapy. Other interventions that may assist include improving dialysis clearance and increasing exercise (Eschbach & Adamson, 1991).

A bleeding tendency related to platelet dysfunction also develops in uremia manifested by easy bruising, GI bleeds, epistaxis, bleeding gums, and spontaneous ecchymosis (Jacobsson & McNatt, 1986). Uremic platelets display defective aggregation and adhesiveness related to a decreased availability of platelet factor 3 and an altered platelet response to clotting factor VIII (von Willebrand's factor) (Lazarus & Hakim, 1991; Suki & Eknoyan,

Table 9-35
Protocols for pharmacologic reduction of the bleeding time in uremia.

Agent	Usual dosage	Onset of action	Peak action	Duration of effect	Comments
Cryoprecipitate (IV)	10 units over 30 min	1 h	4-12 h	24-36 h	Effective on repeat dosing; hepatitis or HIV risk equivalent to transfusion of 10 units of blood.
DDAVP	0.3 μg/kg IV or SC	1 h	2-4 h	6-8 h	May not be effective on repeated dosing.
Intranasal DDAVP[a]	3.0 μg/kg	Same?	Same?	Same?	Convenient, but only limited clinical experience.
IV estrogen[b]	0.6 mg/kg/day for 5 days (days 1-5)	6 h (day 1)	Day 5-7	21-30 days	No reported adverse effects.

[a] Desmopressin (DDAVP) is available from Armour Pharmaceutical Co., Kankakee, IL.
[b] Conjugated estrogen (Emopreparin) is available from Ayerst Pharmaceutical Co., New York, NY.

Note: From Daugirdas, J.T., & Ing, T.S. (1994). Handbook of dialysis (p. 465). Boston: Little, Brown and Company. Reprinted with permission.

1995). The platelet count is usually only slightly reduced but may be very low in patients with hemolytic uremic syndrome or disseminated intravascular coagulation (DIC) (O'Meara & Bernard, 1995). The most reliable test to evaluate this bleeding tendency and its response to therapeutic interventions is the bleeding time (Suki & Eknoyan, 1995). Interventions that can improve the bleeding time include intensive dialysis (especially in the acute setting), increasing the hematocrit, and treatment with cryoprecipitate, desmopressin, and estrogen (Daugirdas & Ing, 1994; Eschbach & Adamson, 1993) (see Table 9-35). Cryoprecipitate and desmopressin are believed to improve the bleeding time by supplying or inducing other forms of factor VIII. The action of estrogen is not known (Daugirdas & Ing, 1994).

Uremia also induces impairment of several aspects of lymphocyte and granulocyte function (Daugirdas & Ing, 1994; Eschbach & Adamson, 1993). These immunologic defects include suppression of both humoral and cellular immunity (Dubrow & Levin, 1995). Although the leukocyte count is normal and increases appropriately in response to infection, the phagocytic capacity of the cell is compromised. A moderate lymphopenia may also be present in patients with CRF. In addition, the absolute number of circulating T cells is reduced, and suppressor cell activity seems to be increased while helper cell activity is decreased (Suki & Eknoyan, 1995). These factors increase the susceptibility of the patients to infections. In those patients with ARF, sepsis and infectious complication account for much of the morbidity and mortality (O'Meara & Bernard, 1995). In CRF, patients are likewise more susceptible to infections, have increased severity of infection, and are predisposed to chronic infections such as hepatitis and tuberculosis (Daugirdas & Ing, 1994). There is also some evidence that CRF patients have an increased incidence of malignancies, particularly renal cell carcinoma, cancer of the uterus and prostate, and myeloma related to immune defects (Daugirdas & Ing, 1994; Port, Ragheb, Schwartz, & Hawthorne, 1989).

In summary, the hematologic manifestations of uremic syndrome have the potential to profoundly affect the health outcomes of patients with acute and chronic renal failure. Nursing management should begin with a careful assessment of hematologic parameters and evaluation of related signs and symptoms. Evaluation of the patient's status and response to treatment is an ongoing process.

Table 9-36
Treatment for chronic pruritus.

Treatment	Dosage	Side Effects
General measures		
Topical emollients		
Lubricating solutions (such as Keri lotion)		
Camphor and menthol-containing creams		
Switch from ethylene oxide to gamma ray-sterilized dialyzer?		
Phototherapy		
UV light	UV-B or UV-A light delivered in a conventional light box giving 2 treatments/week for 4 weeks	Sunburn
Calcium and phosphorus metabolism		
Control of hyperphosphatemia:		
Control of hyperparathyroidism:		
Correction of iron deficiency:		
Drug therapy		
Antihistamines		
Diphenhydramine	25-50 mg q8-24h	Drowsiness
Hydroxyzine	10 mg q8-12h	
Oral activated charcoal	6 g of activated charcoal daily	Black stools
Topical capsaicin	0.025% cream	
Erythropoietin		
Renal transplantation		

Note: From Daugirdas, J.T., & Ing, T.S. (1994). Handbook of dialysis (p. 586). Boston: Little, Brown and Company. Reprinted with permission.

Dermatologic manifestations. Although integumentary problems are more frequently described in CRF than in ARF, they are particularly uncomfortable for both groups of patients (Baer, 1993a). Pruritus, a tickling or crawling sensation experienced by 60% to 80% of patients with CRF, causes scratching and may lead to skin breakdown (Daugirdas & Ing, 1994). Sleep deprivation and suffering to the point of committing suicide are possible outcomes from severe itching in these patients (Balaskas & Oreopoulos, 1992). The exact etiology of pruritus in renal failure is unknown but may be related to skin dryness from decreased sebaceous gland oil production, urochrome and metabolic waste retention, deposition of calcium phosphate and magnesium phosphate crystals, increased plasma calcium ions, allergic reactions, and histamine (Shoop, 1994). Intractable pruritus, a manifestation of secondary hyperparathyroidism, may disappear after parathyroidectomy in some patients (Suki and Eknoyan, 1995).

Treatment for pruritus includes efforts to relieve dry skin with topical emollients that are best applied following a bath or shower when the skin is still wet. Exposure to ultraviolet light, both UVA and UVB bands, has been reported to provide some relief. In addition, controlling hyperphosphatemia may assist in decreasing symptoms. Medications that are useful in some patients include diphenhydramine hydroxyzine and oral charcoal (see Table 9-36). The different therapies are useful in individual patients to varying degrees. Often, the most successful treatment is renal transplantation (Daugirdas & Ing, 1994).

Uremic frost, a white, powderlike substance resulting from the precipitation of urea crystals secreted in the sweat, may be seen on the face and trunk. However, this condition is rarely seen today as dialysis is usually initiated before it develops. The skin color may be altered to a bronze or tan hue because of the collection of urochrome pigments and urea that are normally excreted in the urine. Pallor from anemia and purpura and ecchymoses secondary to increased capillary fragility are common (Suki & Eknoyan, 1995).

Nail changes are occasionally seen in chronic dialysis patients. The nails become thin and brittle and are characterized by a white proximal nail bed

Figure 9-15
Factors contributing to the development of gastrointestinal bleeding in renal failure.

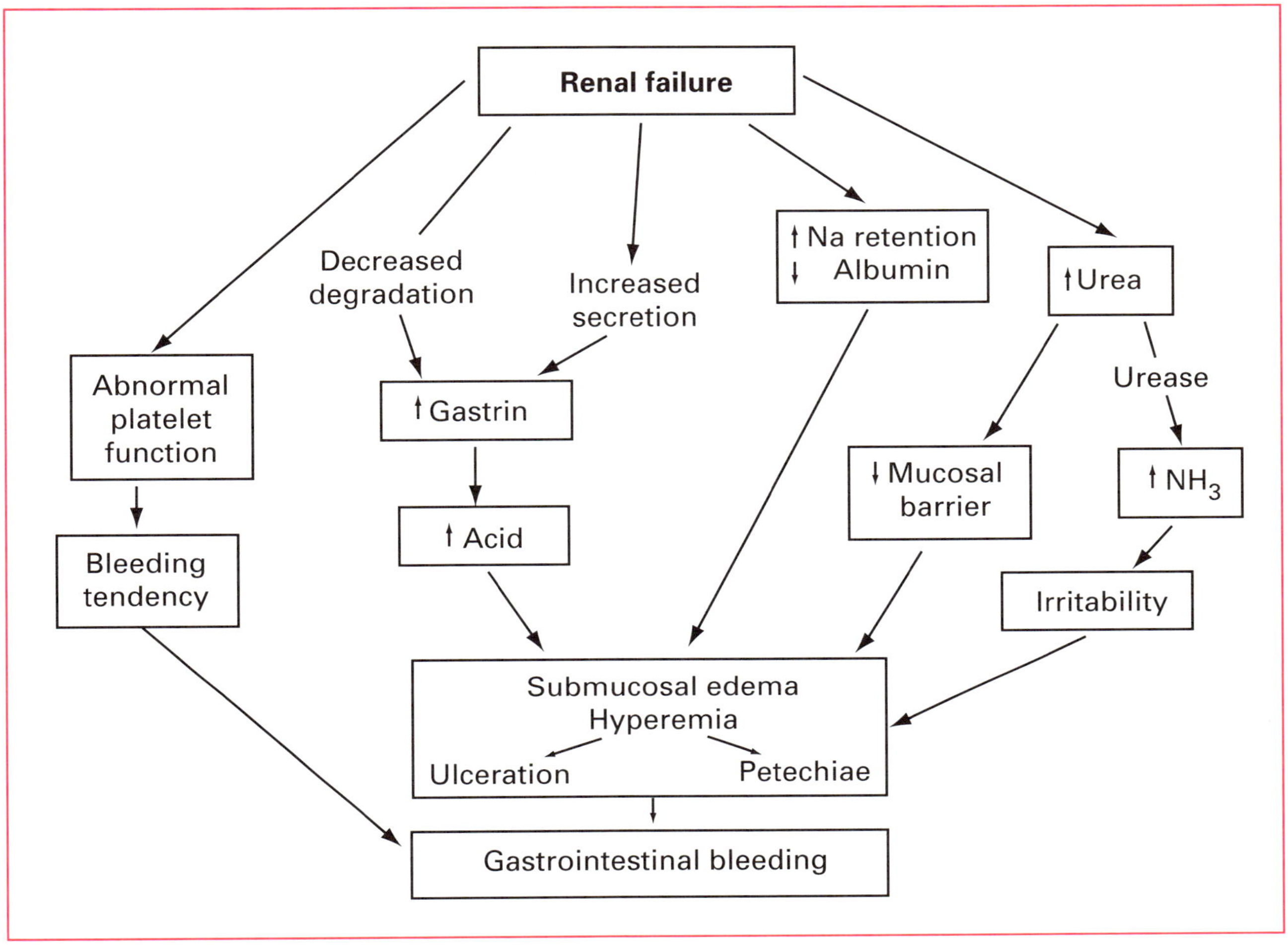

Note: Adapted with permission from Eknoyan, G. (1977). Chronic renal failure and uremic syndrome. In Kurtzman, N.A., & Martinez-Maldonado, M. (Eds.), *Pathophysiology of the Kidney* (p. 854). Springfield, IL: Charles C. Thomas.

and a red or brown discoloration of the distal nail bed (half-and-half nail). The cause of the nail changes is unknown but may be due to hypoalbuminemia or metabolic and humoral factors (Jacobsson & McNatt, 1986).

A thorough nursing assessment of the skin is critical in both acute and chronic renal failure patients. Prevention of skin breakdown from scratching is especially important as broken areas can provide a portal of entry for infection. Keeping the skin clean and moisturized and the finger nails short and well trimmed are important, basic nursing interventions.

Gastrointestinal manifestations. Patients with ARF and CRF commonly manifest a variety of gastrointestinal symptoms related to mucosal alterations from uremia such as anorexia, nausea, dyspepsia, and vomiting. Hiccups also occur but are usually a late sign occurring in patients with advanced uremia (O'Meara & Bernard, 1995). Although diarrhea may be severe (especially if secondary to diabetic autonomic neuropathy), constipation is very common and a side effect of the aluminum binders patients often take with meals to decrease serum phosphate levels (Daugirdas & Ing, 1994). Patients may also complain of a metallic or salty taste in the mouth that is probably related to the high concentration of urea in the saliva. Halitosis and stomatitis are common. Spontaneous gingival bleeding often occurs and may be related to abnormalities in clotting mechanisms and high circulating levels of gastrin (Suki & Eknoyan, 1995). High amylase levels occur in both ARF and CRF and are related to reduced renal excretion of the

Figure 9-16
Mechanisms involved in the development of hyperparathyroidism in renal failure.

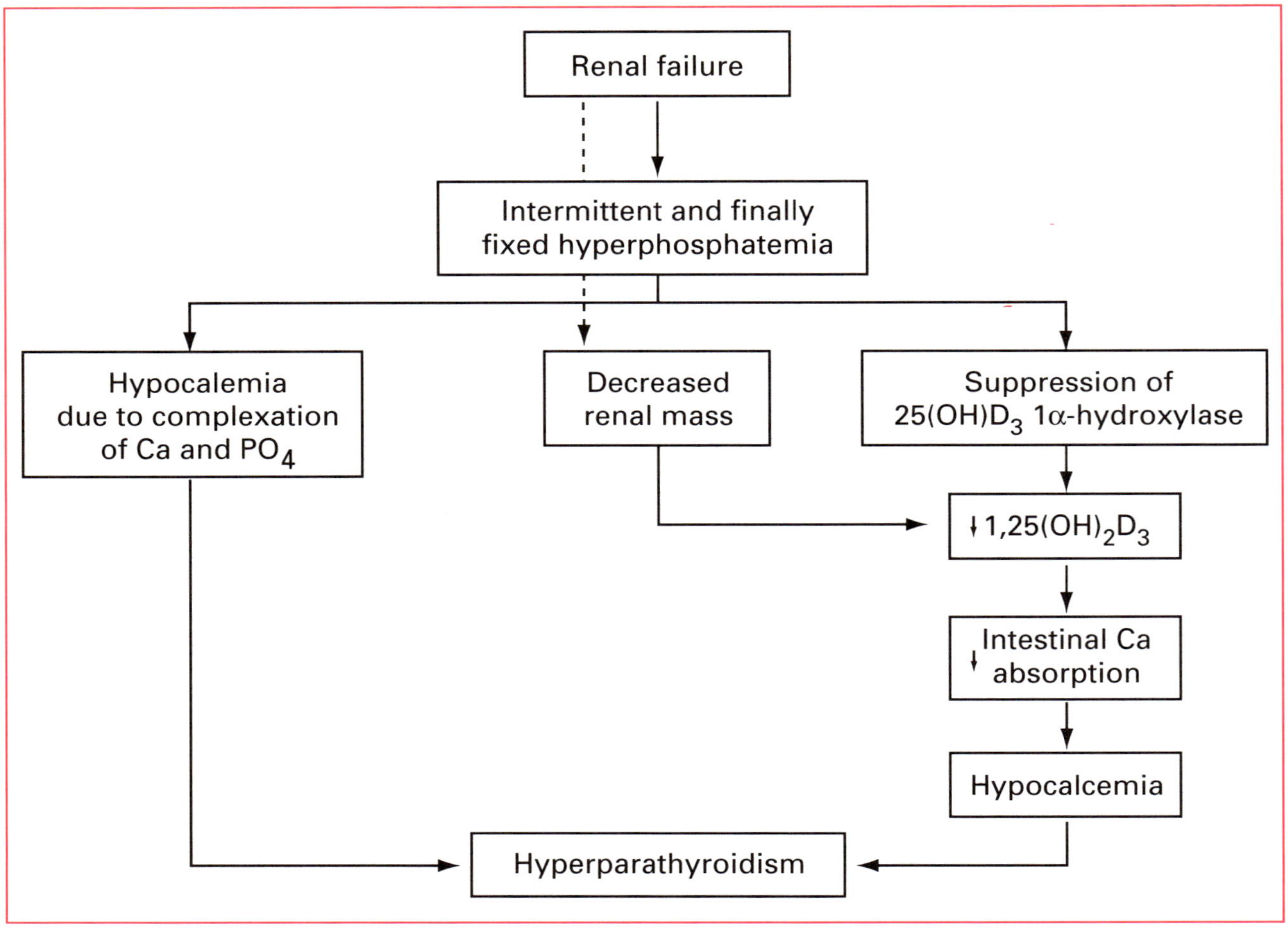

Note: From McCarthy, J.T., & Kumar, R. (1995). Renal osteodystrophy. In H.R. Jacobson, G.E. Striker, & S. Klahr (Eds). *The principles and practice of nephrology* (p. 1034). St. Louis: Mosby Yearbook. Reprinted with permission.

enzyme, but levels rarely exceed twice the upper limit of normal (O'Meara & Bernard, 1995; Suki & Eknoyan, 1995).

As renal failure progresses, patients may develop gastritis, duodenitis, ileitis, colitis, or proctatitis. Pathologic examination of the gastrointestinal system frequently reveals mucosal abnormalities such as edema, capillary hyperemia, angiodysplasia, multiple superficial shallow areas of ulceration, and necrotic lesions (Suki & Eknoyan, 1995). Although the pathophysiological basis is not fully understood, the formation of these alterations seems to be related to elevated levels of serum urea nitrogen. Urea diffuses into the bowel lumen and is converted by bacterial enzymes into ammonia and carbon dioxide (Suki & Eknoyan, 1995) (see Figure 9-15). Mucosal and submucosal edema may also contribute to decreased gastric peristalsis with prolonged emptying time, a common problem in the CRF patient (Suki & Eknoyan, 1995).

ARF is associated with gastrointestinal bleeding in up to 25% of the cases (O'Meara & Bernard, 1995). The acute erosive ulcerations may affect any part of the upper or lower GI tract. Gastrointestinal blood loss may be exacerbated by the bleeding tendency or uremia and the use of heparin during hemodialysis. Early institution of dialysis and prophylactic antacids and H_2 blockers may prevent problems.

Treatment with a medication such as metoclopramide can control nausea and enhance gastric emptying. Because of the increased tendency to bleed, medications such as steroids and NSAIDs should be avoided. Diets high in fiber and laxatives free of magnesium or phosphate can be safely used for patients with constipation (Lakkis & Martinez-

Maldonado, 1995). Diarrhea is often successfully treated with diphenoxylate hydrochloride (Lomotil). Nursing care should begin with a thorough assessment of the oral cavity, abdomen, and bowel patterns. All vomitus and stool should be checked for occult blood, the presence of which can potentially increase the BUN. Good oral hygiene not only makes the patient more comfortable, but may also help enhance the appetite.

Skeletalmuscular manifestations. A serious, potential complication of renal failure is bone disease (renal osteodystrophy). Although this problem can potentially occur in ARF, it rarely develops because of the short duration of the renal abnormality (Baer & Lancaster, 1992). However, bone disease occurs frequently in the CRF patient. The condition is both painful and debilitating but with proper medical and nursing care and compliance with medical therapy on the part of the patient, the devastating effects of renal bone disease can be prevented.

The two major classifications of renal osteodystrophy most commonly seen in the chronic renal failure patient are high turnover or hyperparathyroid bone disease and low turnover bone disease. High turnover bone disease is characterized by increased activity and number of osteoclasts (bone breakdown cells) and osteoblasts (bone deposition cells). Under normal circumstances, the activity of these cells is in equilibrium, maintaining both normal bone integrity and serum calcium levels under the control of PTH. In renal failure, however, a series of pathophysiologic events disrupt this normal process.

As functional renal mass and GFR decrease, normal calcium and phosphorus balance (discussed previously) are disturbed by several mechanisms (see Figure 9-16). The initial event is hyperphosphatemia, resulting from decreased renal phosphate excretion. In the presence of elevated phosphate levels, calcium ions bind with the phosphate forming a calcium-phosphate complex. This complex precipitates out of solution, depositing in the soft tissues (metastatic calcifications), and causing hypocalcemia. Elevated phosphate levels and loss of functional renal mass also suppress the action of 25-hydroxyvitamin D_3 1α- hydroxylase, an enzyme in the renal tubules that forms the active type of Vitamin D, $1,25(OH)_2D_3$ (calcitriol), causing impaired intestinal absorption of calcium. Thus, hypocalcemia resulting from (a) calcium/phosphate complex formation; and (b) low $1,25(OH)_2D_3$ levels stimulate PTH production, increasing release of calcium from bone (Brunier, 1994; McCarthy & Kumar, 1995).

If left unchecked, these abnormalities can lead to parathyroid gland hypertrophy, increased secretion of PTH, and the development of hyperparathyroidism secondary to renal failure (McCarthy & Kumar, 1995). High PTH levels continue to "pull" calcium out of the bone, leading to bone weakness, further calcium/phosphate complex formation with metastatic calcifications, and worsened hypocalcemia. The result of this vicious cycle is high turnover renal osteodystrophy. In its mild form, patients may be asymptomatic. However, as the condition worsens, patients experience bone pain, fractures, muscle weakness (particularly of the proximal muscles), myalgias, and arthralgias. Rupture of the Achilles tendon or quadriceps tendon can occur from metastatic calcification. Severe pruritus and cutaneous gangrene may also be seen (McCarthy & Kumar, 1995).

Laboratory changes associated with high turnover renal bone disease include marked elevations of alkaline phosphatase levels from bone destruction, elevated phosphorus levels, and increased PTH. Although hypocalcemia is typical, severe hypercalcemia can develop with progressive parathyroid disease (Andress & Sherrard, 1993; Brunier, 1994). X-rays reveal subperiosteal bone reabsorption (bone thinning) most easily noted in the hands and clavicles. A definitive diagnosis is made by bone biopsy of the iliac crest following double tetracycline labeling. The patient is given two separate oral doses of tetracycline (a fluorescent marker that is deposited at the mineralization fronts of bones and forms a band). A measurement of bone formation rate is calculated by subsequent histologic examination of the distance between the two bands (Brunier, 1994; Daugirdas & Ing, 1994).

There are two major types of low turnover bone disease. Osteomalacia, a condition characterized by decreased numbers of osteoblasts and osteoclasts, results in decreased bone turnover with increased formation of unmineralized bone tissue (Brunier, 1994; McCarthy & Sherrard, 1995). The second type is aplastic renal osteodystrophy, which is characterized by decreased bone matrix. Common symptoms of both disorders include muscle weakness, severe bone pain, and fractures most often involving the ribs, hips, pelvis, and vertebrae (McCarthy & Sherrard, 1995).

Bone aluminum accumulation is believed to be a major cause of osteomalacia and aplastic bone disease because it impairs the function of osteoblasts, suppresses PTH production, and results in impaired bone formation (Brunier, 1994). The most common source of aluminum intake in the renal failure patient is in the form of aluminum antacids used to control phosphate levels. Thus, these medications should be used only when necessary. Aluminum toxicity is treated with deferoxamine, which binds with the aluminum and moves it out of the tissues into the blood where it can be removed by dialysis (Brunier, 1994).

A major focus of treatment for both high and low turnover renal osteodystrophy should be on prevention. Dietary phosphate reduction is crucial with a restriction of 600 to 1000 mg/day (McCarthy & Kumar, 1995). Phosphate control with binders should be done to keep levels within normals limits. Aluminum antacids are very potent phosphate binders and are frequently use to obtain initial control. However, medications such as calcium carbonate or calcium acetate should be used for maintenance to limit aluminum intake and prevent toxicity. Vitamin D supplements are given to enhance absorption of calcium from the GI tract and may also help suppress the secretion of parathyroid hormone. Because Vitamin D therapy can cause hypercalcemia, patients should be followed closely. Furthermore, it is crucial that hyperphosphatemia be corrected before vitamin D supplements are initiated to avoid extraskeletal deposition of calcium/phosphate (Brunier, 1994; Lakkis & Martinez-Maldonado, 1995). Surgical removal of the parathyroid glands may be required for high turnover renal osteodystrophy if medical treatment is not effective.

Summary

Developments in the field of nephrology have presented the nursing profession with great challenges. Not only is the scientific and theoretical basis of the discipline exceedingly complicated, but the nursing management required by patients with renal failure continues to grow in complexity with further scientific developments. A thorough understanding of the physiologic basis and human responses, both systemic and psychosocial, is essential in order to effectively plan appropriate nursing interventions and evaluate patient outcomes.

References

Agmon, Y., & Brezis, M. (1993). Acute renal failure: A multifactorial syndrome: Pathogenesis and prevention strategies. In E. Bourke, N.P. Mallick, & V.E. Pollak (Eds.), *Moving Points in Nephrology. Contributions to Nephrology, 102,* 23-36.

Agodoa, L.Y.C., Jones, C.A., & Striker, G.E. (1995). Scope, prevalence, and incidence of renal disease. In H.R. Jacobson, G.E. Striker, & S. Klahr (Eds.), *The principles and practice of nephrology* (2nd edition) (pp. 2-5). St. Louis: Mosby Year Book.

Alexopoulos, E., Vakianis, P., Kokolina, E., Koukoudis, P., Sakellariou, G., Memmos, D., & Papadimitriou, M. (1994). Acute renal failure in the medical setting: Changing patterns and prognostic factors. *Renal Failure, 16*(2), 273-284.

Anderson, R. J. (1993). Prevention and management of acute renal failure. *Hospital Practice 28*(8), 61-75.

Andreoli, T.E., Bennett, J.C., Carpenter, C.C.J., Plum, F., & Smith, L.H. (1993). *Cecil's essentials of medicine* (3rd edition). Philadelphia: W.B. Saunders Company.

Andress, D.L., & Sherrard, D.J. (1993). The osteodystrophy of chronic renal failure. In R.W. Schrier & C.W. Gottschalk (Eds.), *Disease of the kidney* (pp. 2759-2788). Boston: Little, Brown, and Company.

Aronoff, G.R., & Abel, S.R. (1995). Practical guidelines for drug dosing in patients with renal impairment. In R.W. Schrier (Ed.), *Manual of nephrology* (pp. 173-185). Boston: Little, Brown and Company.

Baer, C. (1993a). Acute renal failure. In M. Kinney, D. Packa, & S. Dunbar (Eds.), *AACN's clinical reference of critical care nursing* (pp. 885-901). St. Louis: Mosby Year Book.

Baer, C. (1993b). Renal data acquisition. In M. Kinney, D. Packa, & S. Dunbar (Eds.), *AACN's clinical reference of critical care nursing* (pp. 873-883). St. Louis: Mosby Year Book.

Baer, C.L., & Lancaster, L.E. (1992). Acute renal failure. *Critical Care Nursing Quarterly, 14*(4), 1-21.

Balaskas, E.V., & Oreopoulos, D.G. (1992). Uremic pruritus. *Dialysis and Transplantation, 21*(5), 278-284.

Becker, R.C. (1988). Cardiovascular disease in patients with chronic renal failure. *Cleveland Clinic Journal of Medicine, 55*(6), 521-530.

Bennett, W.M., Elzinga, L.W., & Porter, G.A. (1991). Tubulointerstitial disease and toxic nephropathy. In B.M. Brenner & F.C Rector (Eds.), *The kidney* (4th edition) (pp. 1430-1496). Philadelphia: W.B. Sunders Company.

Bichet, D.G., & Gougoux, A. (1995). Extracellular fluid volume expansion. In H.R. Jacobson, G.E. Striker, & S. Klahr (Eds.), *The principles and practice of nephrology* (2nd edition) (pp. 880-883). St. Louis: Mosby Year Book.

Binik, Y.M., & Mah, K. (1994). Sexuality and end-stage renal disease: Research and clinical recommendations. *Advances in Renal Replacement Therapy, 1*(3), 198-209.

Bonventre, J.V., Shah, S.V., Walker, P.D., & Humphreys, M.H. (1995). Acute renal failure: Ischemic, toxic, other. In H.R. Jacobson, G.E Striker, & S. Klahr (Eds.), *The principles and practice of nephrology* (2nd edition) (pp. 564-576). St. Louis: Mosby Year Book.

Borkowski, G.P. (1995). Computed tomography of the kidney. In H.R. Jacobson, G.E. Striker, & S. Klahr (Eds.), *The principles and practice of nephrology* (2nd edition) (pp. 29-39). St. Louis: Mosby Year Book.

Bourke, E., & Delaney, V. (1993). Assessment of hypocalcemia and hypercalcemia. *Clinics in Laboratory Medicine, 13*(1), 157-177.

Bourke, E., & Yanagawa, N. (1993). Assessment of hyperphosphatemia and hypophosphatemia. *Clinics in Laboratory Medicine, 13*(1), 183-205.

Brezis, M., Rosen, S., & Epstein, F.H. (1991). Acute renal failure. In B.M. Brenner, & F.C. Rector (Eds.), *The kidney* (4th edition) (pp. 993-1061). Philadelphia: W.B. Sunders Company.

Brezis, M., Rosen, S., & Epstein, F.H. (1993). Acute renal failure due to ischemia (acute tubular necrosis). In J.M. Lazarus & B.M. Brenner (Eds.), *Acute renal failure* (3rd edition) (pp. 207-229). New York: Churchill Livingstone.

Bricker, N.S. (1972). On the pathogenesis of the uremic state: An exposition of the "trade-off hypothesis". *New England Journal of Medicine, 286*(20), 1093-1099.

Bricker, N.S., & Fine, L.G. (1978). The trade-off hypothesis. Current status. *Kidney International, 13,* 55.

Briggs, J.P. (1995). Introduction to body fluids. In H.R. Jacobson, G.E Striker, & S. Klahr (Eds.). *The principles and practice of nephrology* (2nd edition) (pp. 864-872). St. Louis: Mosby Year Book.

Brunier, G.M. (1994). Calcium/phosphate imbalances, aluminum toxicity, and renal osteodystrophy. *ANNA Journal, 21*(4), 171-177.

Bullock, B. (1996). *Pathophysiology: Adaptations and alterations in function* (4th edition). Philadelphia: J.B. Lippincott Company.

Burnett, J.C. (1993). Acute renal failure associated with cardiac failure and hypovolemia. In J.M. Lazarus, & B.M. Brenner (Eds.), *Acute renal failure* (3rd edition) (pp.193-206). New York: Churchill Livingstone.

Bushinsky, D.A. (1995). Metabolic acidosis. In H.R. Jacobson, G.E. Striker, & S. Klahr (Eds.), *The principles and practice of nephrology* (pp. 924-932). St. Louis: Mosby Year Book.

Cioffi, W.G., Ashikaga, T., & Gamelli, R.L. (1984). Probability of surviving postoperative acute renal failure. Annals of Surgery, 200(27), 205-211.

Cooper, C. (1993). What color is that urine specimen? *American Journal of Nursing, 93*(8), 37.

Copley, J.B. (1991). What can be learned from urinalysis? *Physician Assistant, 15*(3), 21-34.

Copstead, L.C. (1995). *Perspectives on pathophysiology.* Philadelphia: W.B. Saunders Company.

Daugirdas, J.T., & Ing, T.S. (1994). *Handbook of dialysis* (2nd edition) Boston: Little, Brown and Company.

DeVita, M.V., & Michelis, M.F. (1993). Perturbation in sodium balance - Hyponatremia and hypernatremia. *Clinics in Laboratory Medicine, 13*(1), 135-148.

Diamond, J.R., & McLaughlin, M.L. (1988). Urinary parameters to assess renal function. *Clinics in Laboratory Medicine, 8*(3), 493-505.

Doherty, F.J. (1995). Ultrasound of the kidney. In H.R. Jacobson, G.E. Striker, & S. Klahr (Eds.), *The principles and practice of nephrology* (2nd edition) (pp. 13-22). St. Louis: Mosby Year Book.

Dolleris, P.M. (1992). Diuretic and vasopressor usage in acute renal failure: A synopsis. *Critical Care Nursing Quarterly, 14*(4), 28-31.

Douglas, S. (1992). Acute tubular necrosis: Diagnosis, treatment, and nursing implication. *ACCN Clinical Issues, 3*(3), 688-697.

Druml, W. (1995). Nutritional management of acute renal failure. In H.R. Jacobson, G.E. Striker, & S. Klahr (Eds.), *The principles and practice of nephrology* (2nd edition) (pp. 745-753). St. Louis: Mosby Year Book.

Dubrow, A., & Levin, N. (1995). Biochemical and hormonal alterations in chronic renal failure. In H.R. Jacobson, G.E Striker, & S. Klahr (Eds.), *The principles and practice of nephrology* (2nd edition) (pp. 596-603). St. Louis: Mosby Year Book.

Eichel, C.J. (1986). Stress and coping in patients on CAPD compared to hemodialysis patients. *ANNA Journal, 13*(1), 9-13.

Ellison, D., & Bia, N. (1987). Acute renal failure in critically ill patients. *Journal of Intensive Care Medicine 2*(8), 8-24.

Eknoyan, G. (1977). Pathophysiology of chronic renal failure and the uremic syndrome. In N.A. Kurtzman, & M. Martinez-Maldonado (Eds.), *Pathophysiology of the kidney* (pp. 842-888). Springfield, IL: Charles C. Thomas Publishers.

Eschbach, J.W., & Adamson, J.W. (1991). Hematologic consequences of renal failure. In B.M. Brenner, & F.C. Rector (Eds.), *The kidney* (4th edition) (pp. 2019-2031). Philadelphia: W.B. Saunders Company.

Eschbach, J.W., & Adamson, J.W. (1993). Anemia in renal disease. In R.W. Schrier, & C.W. Gottschalk (Eds.), *Diseases of the kidney* (5th edition) (pp. 2743-2758). Boston: Little, Brown, and Company.

Faber, M.D., Kupin, W.L., Krishna, G.G., & Narins, R.G. (1993). The differential diagnosis of acute renal failure. In J.M. Lazarus, & B.M. Brenner (Eds.), *Acute renal failure* (3rd edition) (pp. 133-192). New York: Churchill Livingstone.

Farley, D. (1989, October). Looking into the void. *FDA Consumer,* pp, 17-21.

Felver, L. (1995). Fluid and electrolyte homeostasis and imbalances. In L.E.C. Copstead (Ed.), *Perspectives on pathophysiology* (pp. 524-537). Philadelphia: W.B. Saunders Company.

Fine, L.G., Kurtz. I., Woolf, A.S., Danovitch, G.M., Emmons, C., Kujubu, D.A., & Norman, J.T. (1993). Pathophysiology and nephron adaptation in chronic renal failure. In R.W. Schrier, & C.W. Gottschalk (Eds.), *Diseases of the kidney* (5th edition) (pp. 2703-2741). Boston: Little, Brown and Company.

Finn, W.F. (1993). Recovery from acute renal failure. In J.M. Lazarus, & B.M. Brenner (Eds.), *Acute renal failure* (3rd edition) (pp. 553-596). New York: Churchill Livingstone.

Fischbach, F. (1992). *A manual of laboratory & diagnostic tests* (4th edition). Philadelphia: J.B. Lippincott Company.

Fischereder, M., Trick, W., & Nath, K.A. (1994). Therapeutic strategies in the prevention of acute renal failure. *Seminars in Nephrology, 14*(1), 41-52.

Fraser, C.L., & Arieff, A.I. (1993). Nervous system manifestations of renal failure. In R.W. Schrier, & C.W. Gottschalk (Eds.), *Diseases of the kidney* (5th edition) (pp. 2789-2816). Boston: Little, Brown, and Company.

Frost, L., Pedersen, R.S., Bentzen, S., Bille, H., & Hansen, H.E. (1993). Short and long-term outcome in a consecutive series of 419 patients with acute dialysis-requiring renal failure. *Scandinavian Journal of Urology & Nephrology, 27*(4), 453-62.

Ganong, W.F. (1993). *Review of medical physiology* (16th Edition). Norwalk, CT: Appleton- Century Crofts.

Gennari, F.J. (1995). Metabolic alkalosis. In H.R. Jacobson, G.E. Striker, & S. Klahr (Eds.), *The principles and practice of nephrology* (2nd edition) (pp. 932-941). St. Louis: Mosby Year Book.

Geisinger, M.A., & Pohl, M.A. (1995). Renal angiography. In H.R. Jacobson, G.E. Striker, & S. Klahr (Eds.), *The principles and practice of nephrology* (2nd edition) (pp. 55-64). St. Louis: Mosby Year Book.

Gougoux, A., & Bichet, D.G. (1995). Extracellular fluid volume contraction. In H.R. Jacobson, G.E. Striker, & S. Klahr (Eds),*The principles and practice of nephrology* (2nd edition) (pp. 876-879). St. Louis: Mosby Year Book.

Groeneveld, A.B. Tran, D.D., van der Meulen, J., Nauta, J.J., & Thijs, L.G. (1991). Acute renal failure in the medical intensive care unit: Predisposing, complicating factors and outcome. *Nephron, 59*(4) 602-610.

Guignard, J.P., Semama, D., John, E.J., & Huet, F. (1993). Acute renal failure. *Critical Care Medicine, 21*(9), S349-351.

Guyton, A.C. (1991). *Textbook of medical physiology* (8th edition). Philadelphia: W.B. Saunders Company.

Hagland, M.R. (1993). The management of acute renal failure in the intensive therapy unit. *Intensive and Critical Care Nursing, 9*(4), 237-241.

Hamm, L.L. (1995). Regulation of acid-base balance. In H.R. Jacobson, G.E. Striker, & S. Klahr (Eds.), *The principles and practice of nephrology* (2nd edition) (pp. 917-923). St. Louis: Mosby Year Book.

Hammerman, M.R., & Miller, S.B. (1994). Therapeutic use of growth factors in renal failure. *Journal of the American Society of Nephrology, 5*(1), 1-11.

Hays, S.R. (1992). Southwestern Internal Medicine Conference: Ischemic acute renal failure. *American Journal of the Medical Sciences, 304*(2), 93-108.

Health Care Financing Administration. (1986). *Special Report: Findings from the National Kidney Dialysis and Kidney Transplantation Study.* Baltimore: Author.

Henrich, W. (1993). Arteriovenous or venovenous continuous therapies are not superior to standard hemodialysis in all patients with acute renal failure. *Seminars in Dialysis, 6,* 174- 176.

Holechek, M.J. (1992). Glomerular filtration and renal hemodynamics. *ANNA Journal, 19*(3), 237-248.

Holley, J.L., Nespor, S., & Rault, R. (1992). A comparison of reported sleep disorders in patients on chronic hemodialysis and continuous peritoneal dialysis. *American Journal of Kidney Diseases, 19*(2), 156-161.

Hou, S.H., Bushinsky, D.A., Wish, J.B., Cohen, J.J., & Harrington, J.T. (1983). Hospital-acquired renal insufficiency: A prospective study. *American Journal of Medicine, 74*(2), 243- 248.

Hruska, K.A., & Kovach, K.L. (1995). Phosphate balance and metabolism. In H.R. Jacobson, G.E. Striker, & S. Klahr (Eds.), *The principles and practice of nephrology* (pp. 986-992). St. Louis: Mosby Year Book.

Hunsicker, L.G., & Levey, A.S. (1995). Progression of chronic renal disease: Mechanisms, risk factors, and testing of intervention. In H.R. Jacobson, G.E. Striker, & S. Klahr (Eds.), *The principles and practice of nephrology* (2nd edition) (pp. 622-631). St. Louis: Mosby Year Book.

Iaina, A., & Schwartz, D. (1994). Renal tubular cellular and molecular events in acute renal failure. *Nephron, 68,* 413-418.

Jacobson, H.R. (1991). Chronic renal failure: Pathophysiology. *The Lancet, 338*(8764), 419- 423.

Jacobsson, P.K. & McNatt, G.E. (1986). Holistic nursing of the client with end-stage renal disease. In C.J. Richard (Ed), *Comprehensive nephrology nursing* (pp. 225-249). Boston: Little, Brown and Company.

Jarvis, C. (1992). *Physical examination and health assessment.* Philadelphia: W.B. Saunders Company.

Keane, W.F., & Levey, A.S. (1995). Effects of diet and lipid-lowering agents on the progression of renal disease. In H.R. Jacobson, G.E Striker, & S. Klahr (Eds.), *The principles and practice of nephrology* (2nd edition) (pp. 640-647). St. Louis: Mosby Year Book.

Kellerman, P.S. (1994). Perioperative care of the renal patient. *Archives of Internal Medicine, 154*(15), 1674-1688.

Kellerman, P.S., & Molitoris, B.A. (1991). Pathogenetic mechanisms of ischemic acute renal failure. In H.R. Jacobson, & G.E. Striker (Eds.), *The principles and practice of nephrology* (pp. 626-631). Philadelphia: Decker Publishers.

Kimmel, P.L., Miller, G., & Mendelson, W.B. (1989). Sleep apnea in chronic renal disease. *American Journal of Medicine, 86,* 308-314.

Kjellstrand, C.M., & Barsoum, R. (1995). Management of acute renal failure. In H.R. Jacobson, G.E. Striker, & S. Klahr (Eds.), *The principles and practice of nephrology* (pp. 584-594). St. Louis: Mosby Year Book.

Kjellstrand, C.M., & Solez, K. (1993). Treatment of acute renal failure. In R. Schrier, & C. Gottschalk (Eds.), *Diseases of the kidney* (5th edition) (pp. 1371-1404). Boston: Little Brown and Company.

Klahr, S. (1991). Chronic renal failure: Management. *The Lancet, 338*(8764), 423-427.

Kobrin, S., & Madaio, M.P. (1995). Renal biopsy. In H.R. Jacobson, G.E. Striker, & S. Klahr (Eds.), *The principles and practice of nephrology* (2nd edition) (pp. 65-71). St. Louis: Mosby Year Book.

Kovach, K. L., & Hruska, K. A. (1995a). Hypophosphatemia. In H.R. Jacobson, G.E. Striker, & S. Klahr (Eds.), *The principles and practice of nephrology* (pp. 993-999). St. Louis: Mosby Year Book.

Kovach, K. L., & Hruska, K.A. (1995b). Hyperphosphatemia. In H.R. Jacobson, G.E. Striker, & S. Klahr (Eds.), *The principles and practice of nephrology* (pp. 1000-1005). St. Louis: Mosby Year Book.

Kumar, R. (1995). Calcium metabolism. In H.R. Jacobson, G.E. Striker, & S. Klahr (Eds.), *The principles and practice of nephrology* (2nd edition) (pp. 964-971). St. Louis: Mosby Year Book.

Lakkis, F.G., & Martinez-Maldonado, M. (1995). Conservative management of chronic renal failure and the uremic syndrome. In H.R. Jacobson, G.E. Striker, & S. Klahr (Eds.), *The principles and practice of nephrology* (2nd edition) (pp. 614-620). St. Louis: Mosby Year Book.

Lancaster, L. (1983, March/April). Renal failure: Pathophysiology, assessment and intervention. *Nephrology Nurse*, pp. 38-51.

Lancaster, L.E. (1992). Acute renal failure. In V.B. Huddleston (Ed.), *Multisystem organ failure: Pathophysiology and clinical implications* (pp. 222-235). St. Louis: Mosby Year Book.

Lancaster, L. (1995). *ANNA's core curriculum for nephrology nursing* (3rd edition). Pitman, NJ: American Nephrology Nurses' Association.

Lanese, D.M., & Teitelbaum. (1995). Hypernatremia. In H.R. Jacobson, G.E. Striker, & S. Klahr (Eds.), *The principles and practice of nephrology* (pp. 893-898). St. Louis: Mosby Year Book.

Latta, K., Hisano, S., & Chan, J.C.M. (1993). Perturbations in potassium balance. *Clinics in Laboratory Medicine, 13*(1), 149-156.

LaValle, S. (1986). Infectious and obstructive disease of the kidney. In C. Richard (Ed.), *Comprehensive nephrology nursing* (pp. 85-98). Boston: Little, Brown and Company.

Lazarus, J.M., & Hakim, R.M. (1991). Medical aspects of hemodialysis. In B.M. Brenner, & F.C. Rector (Eds.), *The kidney* (4th edition) (pp. 2223-2298). Philadelphia: W.B. Saunders Company.

Lewis, S. (1992). Fever: Thermal regulation and alterations in end stage renal disease patients. *ANNA Journal, 19*(1), 13-18.

Levine, J.S., Lieberthal, W., Bernard, D.B., & Salant, D.J. (1993). Acute renal failure associated with renal vascular disease, vasculitis, glomerulonephritis, and nephrotic syndrome. In J.M. Lazarus, & B.M. Brenner (Eds.), *Acute renal failure* (3rd edition) (pp. 247- 355). New York: Churchill Livingstone.

Lieberthal, W., & Levinsky, N.G. (1990). Treatment of acute tubular necrosis. *Seminars in Nephrology, 10*(6), 571-583.

Linas, S.L., & Singh, H. (1995). Hypokalemia. In H.R. Jacobson, G.E. Striker, & S. Klahr (Eds), *The principles and practice of nephrology* (2nd edition) (pp. 903-910). St. Louis: Mosby Year Book.

Llach, F. (1993a). Acute renal failure. In F. Llach (Ed.), *Papper's clinical nephrology* (3rd edition) (pp. 109-134). Boston: Little, Brown and Company.

Llach, F. (1993b). Chronic renal failure. In F. Llach (Ed.), *Papper's clinical nephrology* (3rd edition) (pp. 67-107). Boston: Little, Brown and Company.

Madaio, M.P. (1990). Renal biopsy. *Kidney International, 38*(3), 529-543.

May, R.C., Kelly, R.A., & Mitch, W.E. (1991). Pathophysiology of uremia. In B.M. Brenner, & F.C. Rector (Eds.), *The kidney* (4th edition) (pp. 1997-2017). Philadelphia: W.B. Saunders Company.

McCance, K.L., & Huether, S.E. (1994). *Pathophysiology: The biological basis for disease in adults and children* (2nd edition). St. Louis: Mosby Year Book.

McCarthy, J.T., & Kumar, R. (1995). Renal osteodystrophy. In H.R. Jacobson, G.E. Striker, & S. Klahr (Eds.), *The principles and practice of nephrology* (2nd edition) (pp. 1032-1045). St. Louis: Mosby Year Book.

McConnell, E. A. (1985). Assessing the bladder. *Nursing 85, 15*(11), 44-46.

Mehta, R.L. (1994). Therapeutic alternatives to renal replacement for critically ill patients in acute renal failure. *Seminars in Nephrology, 14*(1), 64-82.

Mendleson, W.B., Wadhwa, N.K., Greenberg, H.E., Gujavarty, K., & Bergofsky, E. (1990). Effects of hemodialysis on sleep apnea syndrome in end-stage renal disease. *Clinical Nephrology, 33*(5), 247-251.

Messmer, K., Kreimeier, U., & Hammessen, F. (1989). Changes in microcirculation in sepsis and septic shock. In K. Reinhart & K. Eyrich (Eds.), *Sepsis - An interdisciplinary challenge* (pp. 148-159). Berlin: Springer-Verlag.

Meyer, T.W., Scholey, J.W., & Brenner, B.M. (1991). Nephron adaptation to renal injury. In B.M. Brenner, & F.C. Rector

(Eds.), *The kidney* (4th edition) (pp. 1871-1908). Philadelphia: W.B. Saunders Company.

Mitch, W.E., Walser, M., Buffington, G.A., & Lemann, J. (1976, December, 18). A simple method of estimating progression of chronic renal failure. *Lancet, 2*(7999), 1326-1328.

Moe, S.M., & Sprague, S.M. (1994). Uremic encephalopathy. *Clinical Nephrology, 42*(4), 251- 256.

Moffett, D.F., Moffett, S.B., & Schauf, C.L. (1993). *Human physiology: Foundations & frontiers.* St. Louis: Mosby Year Book.

Mundy, G.R., & Reasner, C.A. (1995a). Hypocalcemia. In H.R. Jacobson, G.E. Striker, & S. Klahr (Eds.), *The principles and practice of nephrology* (2nd edition) (pp. 971-977). St. Louis: Mosby Year Book.

Mundy, G.R., & Reasner, C.A. (1995b). Hypercalcemia. In H.R. Jacobson, G.E. Striker, & S. Klahr (Eds.), *The principles and practice of nephrology* (2nd edition) (pp. 977-986). St. Louis: Mosby Year Book.

Nally, J.V., & Pohl, M.A. (1995). Radionuclide renography. In H.R. Jacobson, G.E. Striker, & S. Klahr (Eds.), *The principles and practice of nephrology* (2nd edition) (pp. 23-29). St. Louis: Mosby Year Book.

Nouwen, G.J., Verstrepen, W.A., & DeBroe, M.E. (1994). Epidermal growth factor in acute renal failure. *Renal Failure, 16*(1), 44-60.

Occhipinti, K.A., & Hricak, H. (1995). Magnetic resonance imaging of the kidneys. In H.R. Jacobson, G.E. Striker, & S. Klahr (Eds.), *The principles and practice of nephrology* (2nd edition) (pp. 46- 54). St. Louis: Mosby Year Book.

O'Meara, Y. M., & Bernard, D.B. (1995). Clinical presentation, complications, and prognosis of acute renal failure. In H.R. Jacobson, G.E. Striker, & S. Klahr (Eds.), *The principles and practice of nephrology* (2nd edition) (pp. 577-584). St. Louis: Mosby Year Book.

Parker, K. (1990). Sleep and dream patterns of end-stage renal disease patients on chronic dialysis. *Journal of the American Society of Nephrology, 1*(4), 371.

Parker, M.D., Older, R.A., Wertman, D.E., Crane, L.M., & Hidalgo, H.S. (1995). Use of radiologic techniques in the patient with renal problems. In R.W. Schrier (Ed.), *Manual of nephrology* (pp. 250-275). Boston: Little, Brown and Company.

Port, F.K., Ragheb, N.E., Schwartz, A.G., & Hawthorne, V.M. (1989). Neoplasms in dialysis patients: A population based study. *American Journal of Kidney Disease, 14*(2), 119-123.

Porth, C.M. (1994). *Pathophysiology: Concepts of altered health states* (4th edition). Philadelphia: J.B. Lippincott Company.

Pressman, M.R., Benz, R.L., & Peterson, D.D. (1995). High incidence of sleep disorders in end stage renal disease. *Sleep Research, 24,* 417.

Price, C.A. (1991). Continuous renal replacement therapy: The treatment of choice of acute renal failure. *ANNA Journal, 18*(3), 239-244.

Price, C. A. (1992a). Issues related to the care of critically ill patients with end stage renal failure. *AACN Clinical Issues, 3*(3), 585-596.

Price, C.A. (1992b). An update on continuous renal replacement therapies. *AACN Clinical Issues, 3*(3), 597-604.

Price, C.A. (1994). Acute renal failure: A sequelae of sepsis. *Critical Care Nursing Clinics of North America, 6*(2), 359-372.

Richard, C.J. (1986a). Acute renal failure. In C.J. Richard (Ed.), *Comprehensive nephrology nursing* (pp. 178-221). Boston: Little, Brown and Company.

Richard, C.J. (1986b). Renal assessment with nursing implications. In C.J. Richard (Ed.), *Comprehensive nephrology nursing* (pp. 41-65). Boston: Little, Brown and Company.

Rickus, M.A. (1987). Sexual dysfunction in the female ESRD patient. *ANNA Journal, 14*(3), 184-188.

Rosa, R.M., & Battle, D. (1995). Hyperkalemia. In H.R. Jacobson, G.E. Striker, & S. Klahr (Eds.), *The principles and practice of nephrology* (2nd Edition) (pp. 911-917). St. Louis: Mosby Year Book.

Rose, B.D. & Black, R.M. (1988). *Manual of clinical problems in nephrology.* Boston: Little, Brown and Company.

Rose, B.D., & Rennke, H.G. (1994). *Renal pathophysiology - The essentials.* Baltimore: Williams & Wilkins.

Sarno, R.C. (1995). Urography. In H.R. Jacobson, G.E. Striker, & S. Klahr (Eds.), *The principles and practice of nephrology* (2nd edition) (pp. 39-46). St. Louis: Mosby Year Book.

Schaefer, R.M., Schaefer, L., & Horl, W.H. (1994). Mechanisms for protein catabolism in acute renal failure. *Nephrology Dialysis Transplantation, Suppl 3,* 44-47.

Schreiner, G.E., & Maher, J.F. (1961). Uremia and body temperature. In *Uremia: Biochemistry, pathogenesis, and treatment* (pp. 380-384). Springfield, IL: Charles C. Thomas Publishers.

Schrier, R.W. (1995). *Manual of nephrology* (4th edition). Boston: Little, Brown and Company.

Seidel, H.M., Ball, J.W., Dains, J.E., & Benedict, G.W. (1991). *Mosby's guide to physical examination.* St. Louis: Mosby Year Book.

Shapiro, R.S., Deshetler, N., & Stockard, H.E. (1994). Fluid overload again! A technique to enhance fluid compliance. *Dialysis & Transplantation, 23*(6), 303-305.

Sherwood, L. (1993). Human physiology: From cells to systems. Minneapolis/St. Paul: West Publishing Company.

Shilliday, I, & Allison, ME. (1994). Diuretics in acute renal failure. *Renal Failure, 16*(1), 3-17.

Shoop, K.L. (1994). Pruritus in end stage renal disease. *ANNA Journal, 21*(2), 147-153.

Shusterman, N., Strom, B.L., Murray, T.G., Morrison, G., West, S.L., & Maislin, G. (1987). Risk factors and outcome of hospital-acquired acute renal failure: Clinical epidemiologic study. *The American Journal of Medicine, 83*(1), 65-71.

Spiegel, D.M., Ullian, M.E., Zerbe, G.O., & Berl, T. (1991). Determinants of survival and recovery in acute renal failure patients dialyzed in intensive-care units. *American Journal of Nephrology, 11*(1), 44-47.

Spurney, R.F., Fulkerson, W.J., & Schwab, S.J. (1991). Acute renal failure in critically ill patients: Prognosis for recovery of kidney function after prolonged dialysis support. *Critical Care Medicine, 19*(1), 8-11.

Stahl, W. (1986). Kidney in shock. In J. Barrett, & L.M. Nyhus (Eds.), *Treatment of shock: Principles and practice* (2nd edition) (pp. 137-149). Philadelphia: Lea & Febiger.

Stark, J. (1992a). Acute tubular necrosis: Differences between oliguria and nonoliguria. Critical Care Nursing Quarterly, 14(4), 22-27.

Stark, J. (1992b). Dialysis options in the critically ill patient: Hemodialysis, peritoneal dialysis, and continuous renal replacement therapy. *Critical Care Nursing Quarterly, 14*(4), 40-44.

Stark, J. (1994). Acute renal failure in trauma: Current perspectives. *Critical Care Nursing Quarterly, 16*(4), 49-60.

Strupp, T.W. (1988). Postshock resuscitation of the trauma victim: Preventing and managing acute renal failure. *Critical Care Nursing Quarterly, 11*(2), 1-9.

Suki, W.N., & Eknoyan, G. (1995). Pathophysiology and clinical manifestations of chronic renal failure and the uremic syndrome. In H.R. Jacobson, G.E. Striker, & S. Klahr (Eds.), *The principles and practice of nephrology* (2nd edition) (pp. 603-614). St. Louis: Mosby Year Book.

Sutton, R.A., & Sakhaee, K. (1995a). Magnesium balance and metabolism. In H.R. Jacobson, G.E. Striker, & S. Klahr (Eds), *The principles and practice of nephrology* (2nd edition) (pp. 1005-1008). St. Louis: Mosby Year Book.

Sutton, R.A., & Sakhaee, K. (1995b). Hypomagnesemia. In H.R. Jacobson, G.E. Striker, & S. Klahr (Eds.), *The principles and practice of nephrology* (2nd edition) (pp. 1008-1012). St. Louis: Mosby Year Book.

Sutton, R.A., & Sakhaee, K. (1995c). Hypermagnesemia. In H.R. Jacobson, G.E. Striker, & S. Klahr (Eds), *The principles and practice of nephrology* (2nd edition) (pp. 1013-1014). St. Louis: Mosby Year Book.

Swan, S.K., & Bennett, W.M. (1993). Nephrotoxic acute renal failure. In J.M. Lazarus, & B.M. Brenner (Eds.), *Acute renal failure* (3rd edition) (pp. 357-392). New York: Churchill

Livingstone.

Swartz, R.D., Fitzgerald, F.T., Kalousdain, S., & Budd, M. (1983). Hypothermia in the uremic patient. *Dialysis and Transplantation, 12,* 584-590.

Takala, J. (1987). Nutrition in acute renal failure. *Critical Care Clinics, 3*(4), 155-166.

Toto, K. (1990). Prerenal azotemia. In B.C. Mims (Ed.), *Case studies in critical care nursing* (pp. 312-317). Baltimore: Williams & Wilkins.

Ulrich, B.T. (1987). Sexual knowledge of nephrology personnel. *ANNA Journal, 14*(3), 179-183.

Ulrich, B.T. (1989). *Nephrology nursing concepts and strategies.* Norwalk, CT: Appleton & Lange.

United States Renal Data System Annual Report. (1994). The National Institutes of Health, The National Institutes of Diabetes and Digestive and Kidney Diseases, Division of Kidney, Urologic, and Hematologic Diseases, Bethesda, MD.

Veis, J.H., & Berl, T. (1995). Hyponatremia. In H.R. Jacobson, G.E. Striker, & S. Klahr (Eds.), *The principles and practice of nephrology* (2nd edition) (pp. 888-893). St. Louis: Mosby Year Book.

Vogel, C.H. (1979). Keeping patients alive in spite of post-obstructive diuresis. *Nursing 79, 79*(9), 50-56.

Walker, S., Fine, A., & Kryger, M.H. (1995). Sleep complaints are common in a dialysis unit. *American Journal of Kidney Diseases, 26*(5), 751-756.

Wardle, E.N. (1994). Acute renal failure and multiorgan failure. *Nephron, 66*(4), 380-385.

Weinberg, J.M. (1995). Pathogenetic mechanisms of ischemic acute renal failure. In H.R. Jacobson, G.E. Striker, & S. Klahr (Eds.), *The principles and practice of nephrology* (2nd edition) (pp. 544-555). St. Louis: Mosby Year Book.

Willms, J.L., Schneiderman, H., & Algranati, P.S. (1994). *Physical diagnosis: Bedside evaluation of diagnosis and function.* Baltimore: Williams & Wilkins.

Winkelman, J.W., & Lazarus, J.M. (1994). Restless legs syndrome in patients on hemodialysis: Association with sleep disorders and dialysis intolerance. *Sleep Research, 23,* 402.

Wolfson, M., & Kopple, J.D. (1993). Nutritional management of acute renal failure. In J.M. Lazarus, & B.M. Brenner (Eds.), *Acute renal failure* (3rd edition) (pp. 467-485). New York: Churchill Livingstone.

Workman, M.L. (1992). Magnesium and phosphorus: The neglected electrolytes. *AACN Clinical Issues, 3*(3), 655-663.

Yager, H.M., & Harrington, J.T. (1995a). Evaluation of serum electrolytes, creatinine, and blood urea nitrogen. In H.R. Jacobson, G.E. Striker, & S. Klahr (Eds.), *The principles and practice of nephrology* (2nd edition) (pp. 85-89). St. Louis: Mosby Year Book.

Yager, H.M., & Harrington, J.T. (1995b). Urinalysis and urine electrolytes. In H.R. Jacobson, G.E. Striker, & S. Klahr (Eds.), *The principles and practice of nephrology* (2nd edition) (pp. 90-100). St. Louis: Mosby Year Book.

Yarger, W.E. (1991). Urinary tract obstruction. In B.M. Brenner, & F.C. Rector (Eds.), *The kidney* (4th edition) (pp. 1768-1808). Philadelphia: W.B. Saunders Company.

Yarger, W.E. (1993). Obstructive urinary tract disease as a cause of acute renal failure. In J.M. Lazarus, & B.M. Brenner (Eds.), *Acute renal failure* (3rd edition) (pp. 393-415). New York: Churchill Livingstone.

Zarifian, A.A. (1992). Sexual dysfunction in the male end stage renal disease patient. *ANNA Journal, 19*(6), 527-534.

Zorzanello, M.M. (1989). Preventing acute renal failure in patients with chronic renal insufficiency: Nursing implications. *ANNA Journal, 16*(6), 433-436.

Readings

Alfrey, A.C. (1995). Chronic renal disease. In R.W. Schrier (Ed.), *Manual of nephrology* (pp. 152-160). Boston: Little, Brown and Company.

Brundage, D. (1980). *Nursing management of renal problems* (2nd edition). St. Louis: C.V. Mosby Company.

Cadnapaphornchai, P., Alavalapati, R.K., & McDonald, F.D. (1995). Differential diagnosis of acute renal failure. In H.R. Jacobson, G.E Striker, S. & Klahr (Eds.), *The principles and practice of nephrology* (2nd edition) (pp. 555-564). St. Louis: Mosby Year Book.

Kaplan, B., & Batle, D. (1995). Regulation of potassium balance and metabolism. In H.R. Jacobson, G.E. Striker, & S. Klahr (Eds.), *The principles and practice of nephrology* (pp. 898-903). St. Louis: Mosby Year Book.

Llach, F. (1993c). Obstructive nephropathy. In F. Llach (Ed.), *Papper's clinical nephrology* (3rd edition) (pp. 249-264). Boston: Little, Brown and Company.

Mendyka, B.E. (1992). Fluid and electrolyte disorders caused by diuretic therapy. *AACN Clinical Issues 3,* 672-680.

Parker, K.P., & Clinton, D.R. (1992). Disorders of the kidney. In L.O. Burrell (Ed.), *Adult nursing in hospital and community settings* (pp. 1238-1308). Norwalk, CT: Appleton & Lange.

Chapter Highlights

- Patients with renal failure, both acute and chronic, may present in a variety of ways. Some have symptoms that are directly related to the kidney, such as flank pain and gross hematuria, while others may present with associated extrarenal abnormalities such as edema, hypertension, and signs of uremia.
- Chronic renal failure is the progressive, irreversible loss of renal function which occurs over varying periods of time ranging from a few months to decades. The degree of renal functional loss is usually described in terms of GFR beginning with diminished renal reserve and proceeding from renal insufficiency to chronic renal failure.
- The incidence of chronic renal failure is higher in the elderly.
- The incidence of CRF is also higher in African Americans, Native Americans, and possibly Hispanic Americans. Gender may also to be a risk factor, as both the prevalence and incidence rates of CRF are consistently higher in males than in females.
- The total estimated direct medical charges for ESRD alone, excluding the costs of care for patients with renal insufficiency, was over $8.6 billion during 1991.
- Nurses are being called upon with increasing frequency to play key roles in the management of patients with chronic renal failure. In addition, effective management of these patients requires continual collaboration, coordination, and communication between all members of the health care team.
- Conservative management of the patient with chronic renal insufficiency not yet requiring dialysis has three goals: (a) to control the rate of progression of renal disease; (b) to prevent further damage to the kidneys; and (c) to manage complications from the uremic syndrome.
- In the acute setting, fluid losses can develop from acute blood loss, fluid loss secondary to burns and vomiting/diarrhea, and increased insensible losses.
- Acute and chronic renal failure patients easily become catabolic and develop protein wasting, and dry body weight can be lost and replaced with fluid weight.
- Sodium is a major determinant of serum osmolality. It also plays an essential role in nerve conduction, acid-base balance, and numerous chemical reactions.
- As the major intracellular cation, potassium helps maintain intracellular osmolality; regulates skeletal, cardiac, and smooth muscle activity; influences acid-base balance; and participates in many intracellular enzyme reactions.
- The effects of alterations in potassium levels on neuromuscular transmission are clinically important because they are largely responsible for the most serious symptoms associated with disturbances in potassium balance: muscle weakness, potentially fatal cardiac arrhythmias, and disturbances in cardiac conduction.
- In addition to being a major constituent of bone, calcium ions are important in intracellular and enzymatic reactions and in blood coagulation. Calcium is also critical for neuromuscular transmission.
- Phosphorus is the major anion in the ICF where it functions primarily as a cofactor in many metabolic reactions.
- Clinical markers of poor protein metabolism include low serum levels of albumin, transferrin, and complements, all of which are reliable indicators of overall nutritional status.
- The development of hypertriglyceridemia is believed to be related to decreased lipoprotein lipase activity and a reduced conversion of VLDL to LDL.
- Hypertension occurs in approximately 10% to 30% of patients with ARF, 80% of those with CRF, and is usually volume dependent. However, it may be complicated by decreased renal perfusion and activation of the renin-angiotensin system, excess aldosterone secretion, increased sympathetic tone, diminished production of vasodepressor hormones, and excess release of vasoconstrictor natriuretic factors.
- Serious disturbances in cardiac rhythm may develop secondary to hyperkalemia, hypermagnesemia, hypocalcemia, and severe acidosis.
- Uremic pericarditis, an inflammation of the membrane surrounding the heart, is a condition often accompanied by the collection of varying amounts of fluid and/or blood in the pericardial sac. In most cases, the inflammation is aseptic, although some cases of bacterial and viral pericarditis have been reported.

UNIT 4

Clinical Management of the Renal Patient

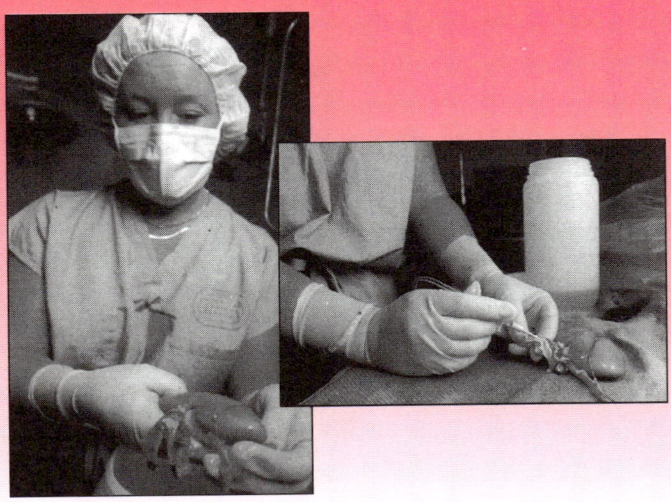

Unit Contents

Chapter 10
Psychosocial Impact of Renal Disease 269
Anita E. Molzahn, PhD, RN

Chapter 11
Nutritional Care of Renal Patients 285
Sue Dickey Roberts, MS, RD, CNSD

Chapter 12A
Pharmacology in Renal Disease 307
Terran Warren Sims, BSN, RN, CNN; Anita E. Molzahn, PhD, RN; and Robert McGory, PharmD, MS, BS

Chapter 12B
Medications in Transplant Patients 327
Karen K. Giuliano, MSN, RN, CCRN; Anita E. Molzahn, PhD, RN; and Terran Warren Sims, BSN, RN, CNN

Chapter 13
Control of Infectious Diseases in the Renal Patient 347
Janel Parker, MSN, RN, CNN; Linda Dickenson, BS, RN, CNN, CPHQ; Karen C. Wiseman, MSN, RN, CNN; Diane Alexander, MS, BSN, RN, CNN; and Eileen Peacock, MSN, RN, CNN, CIC, CPHQ

Chapter 14
Rehabilitation of the Renal Patient 403
Nancy G. Kutner, PhD

CHAPTER 10

Psychosocial Impact of Renal Disease

Anita E. Molzahn, PhD, RN

Chapter Contents

Chronic Illness 271
The Illness Trajectory of CRF 271
Stressors Associated with CRF 272
Powerlessness and Lack of Control 272
Intrusiveness 273
Restrictions Imposed by the Medical Regimen 273
Body Image 274
Sexuality and Chronic Renal Failure 274
Coping Strategies Used by Individuals with CRF 275
Social Support 275
Impact of CRF on the Family 277
Quality of Life Associated with ESRD 278
Dealing With Patients Who Have a Low Quality of Life 278
Nursing Care in Relation to Psychosocial Impact of the Illness and Treatment 279
Summary 280
References 281
Research Brief 283
Chapter Highlights 284

Psychosocial Impact of Renal Disease

Anita E. Molzahn, PhD, RN

Chronic renal failure (CRF) is a chronic illness that imposes many stressors on those affected by the illness. Those stressors and the psychosocial impact of the disease are significant, and nurses working with people who have CRF need to view the psychosocial impact as being as important as the physiological impact. The purpose of this chapter is to discuss the course or trajectory of chronic illness and CRF. Secondly, the major stressors associated with the illness, coping strategies used, impact on the family, quality of life, and nursing interventions that may be useful in caring for individuals with CRF will be discussed.

Chronic Illness

Chronic illnesses are very common; in the United States, there are 32.7 million people, or about 14% of the population, limited by at least one chronic illness (Wagner, 1996). Chronic illnesses are characterized by the long-term nature of the illness, uncertainty, a need for palliation rather than cure, complexity often involving multiple diseases/conditions, intrusiveness on the lives of individuals, need for a range of ancillary services, and cost (Strauss et al., 1984). For the most part, our health care system has been established to deal with people with acute illnesses who are treated and then return home. Chronic or long-term illnesses pose different challenges to health care professionals and individuals affected by the disease.

In chronic illness, it is important to shift the focus of care from primarily physical care, to care that considers the psychosocial impact of the illness on the daily lives of the chronically ill and their families. CRF, in particular, is a disease that poses many challenges for people affected by the illness. As discussed later in this chapter, there are numerous stressors that affect the lives of individuals with CRF and their families. The course of the illness or the illness trajectory is often difficult from both physical and psychosocial perspectives.

The Illness Trajectory of CRF

Strauss and his colleagues coined the term "illness trajectory" to refer "not only to the physiological unfolding of a sick person's disease but also to the total organization of work done over that course, plus the impact on those involved with that work and its organization" (Strauss et al., 1984, p. 64). With many chronic illnesses, there is a tendency for health and well-being to decline over time, indicating a downward trajectory. However, there are many factors that can influence an individual's illness trajectory, not the least of which are how they deal with uncertainty, how they define their illness and prognosis, and how they come to terms with their trajectory.

In one of the early studies of adaptation to dialysis, Reichsman and Levy (1972) described adaptation in three stages. The first phase was the honeymoon phase, which occurs with the initial physiological improvement brought about with dialysis. The second phase was one of disenchantment and discouragement, as clients begin to struggle with the idea of being on the machine for life. The final phase was one of long-term adaptation. However, individuals with CRF could regress or move through the stages at different times in the trajectory of their illnesses.

There has been considerable interest in the trajectory of adjustment or adaptation to dialysis. Lack of adjustment has been demonstrated by depression, suicidal tendencies, anxiety, or psychotic complications (Czackes & Kaplan De-Nour, 1976). Some studies have shown relationships among adjustment to dialysis and personality characteristics, psychiatric problems, and selected social contexts.

In addition to the challenges of dealing with a chronic illness, people who are transplant candidates experience a somewhat different trajectory. For many people, the waiting period for transplantation is unpredictable and frustrating. While there is often a feeling of excitement and euphoria around the time of transplantation, there are often frustrations that emerge with rejection episodes, side effects of immunosuppressive therapy, and complications associated with transplantation. While transplant recipients are generally stabilized within several months of the procedure, the uncertainty and anxiety regarding possible rejection remains for most people.

Discussion regarding the illness trajectory in

Table 10-1
Major stressors by treatment modality.

Hemodialysis	CAPD	Transplant
Limited physical activity	Uncertainty about the future	Uncertainty
Limited vacations	Fatigue	Risk of infections
Fluid restrictions	Frequent hospital admissions	Side effects
Fatigue	Limited physical activity	Body image
Boredom with the routine	Decreased sex drive	
Time for dialysis	Decreased income	
Decreased sex drive	Cramps	
Decreased income	Dependence on others	
Uncertainty		

CRF is often helpful to people who are anticipating or beginning treatment. However, not every individual fits the classic model or trajectory and it is important to view each client's situation as unique. People identify different things as stressful and each of us have our own coping strategies. Some of the more common stressors and coping strategies are discussed in the following paragraphs.

Stressors Associated with CRF

There is a growing body of research addressing the stressors associated with CRF treatment (see Table 10-1). People receiving either hemodialysis or CAPD frequently report losses and lifestyle changes such as physiological complications, frequent hospitalizations, decreased independence, unemployment, financial problems, fluid and diet restrictions, and decreased ability to fulfill long-range goals (Baldree, Murphy, & Powers, 1982; Fuchs & Schreiber, 1988; Gurklis & Menke, 1988). There are often role changes, loss of status, lack of control, and a frustration of basic needs such as nutrition and sexuality.

In a study of hemodialysis patients (Gurklis & Menke, 1995), participants reported 62 stressors related to being on dialysis. These stressors were organized into five major categories including: physiological stressors, psychosocial stressors, concerns about starting hemodialysis, restrictions of living with a chronic illness, and concerns about kidney transplantation. The physiological stressors include fatigue, hypotension, cramps, nausea, vomiting, decreased mobility, bone pain, etc. Psychosocial concerns included the stress of having to come for dialysis, missed activities, and the time consuming nature of dialysis therapy. In relation to restrictions of living with a chronic illness, difficulty adhering to diet and fluid restrictions, and lifestyles restricted by inadequate income were major stressors. Uncertainty also came through as a common theme, particularly in relation to the uncertainty of getting a kidney transplant and having it function.

Comparisons of stressors of hemodialysis and CAPD patients have resulted in some interesting differences. In one study (Fuchs & Schreiber, 1988), hemodialysis patients reported significantly more stress in the area of limited physical activity and limited time or places for vacations. In another study (Bihl, Ferrans, & Powers, 1988), it was found that CAPD and hemodialysis patients were similar in terms of stress levels and types of stressors. Uncertainty about the future was one of the most highly ranked stressors for both groups in this study.

After transplantation, recipients report some different stressors again. The most commonly reported stressors include: being uncertain about whether the transplant will be a success, concern about risk of infections and/or viruses, concern about the long-term side effects of antirejection drugs, and worry that changes in physical appearance will affect their social life (White, Ketefian, Starr, & Voepel-Lewis, 1990).

Some of the stressors commonly associated with CRF are discussed in the following paragraphs. They include: powerlessness and lack of control, intrusiveness, limitations in diet and fluid, body image, and changes in sexuality.

Powerlessness and Lack of Control

Many people with CRF feel that they are powerless and lack control over their destiny. Certainly, most of them are angry or frustrated by their situation, one that they obviously did not choose. However, feelings of powerlessness and helplessness escalate in the hospital when patients are subject to the routines and preferences of health care providers. Feelings of powerlessness can result in problems of communication among patients, families, and staff. Anger and frustration can escalate.

Studies have indicated that there is a relationship between feelings of helplessness and hopelessness and lack of control (Devins, Binik, Hollomby, Barre, & Guttman, 1981). Although transplantation eliminates many of the restrictions imposed by dialysis therapy, it appears that it does not necessarily result in increased perceived control. There are still many uncertainties and complications (for example, rejection) that may make transplant recipients feel as though they have little control over their situations.

Intrusiveness

In studies of stressors associated with CRF, the issue of intrusiveness of the treatment invariably is raised. Illness intrusiveness "results from the lifestyle disruptions, attributable to an illness and/or its treatment, that interfere with continued involvement in valued activities and interests" (Devins, 1994, p. 252). People with CRF often talk of their frustration with lifestyle changes, difficulty participating in activities, and lack of time. Devins (1994) argues that intrusiveness of illness is a major factor contributing to the psychosocial impact of CRF. Certainly, there are strategies that health professionals can employ to minimize the intrusiveness of therapy. For instance, in CAPD, times of exchanges can be adapted to fit a client's work (or social) schedule. Newer treatment options, such as daily nocturnal home hemodialysis may be less intrusive for some people. Flexibility on the part of health care providers and consideration of the lifestyles of individuals may reduce the intrusiveness of the illness and treatment in CRF.

Restrictions Imposed by the Medical Regimen

As noted earlier, people on dialysis find it very stressful (and probably intrusive) to restrict their diet, limit their fluids, and otherwise follow a rigid medical regimen. Not only do people with CRF require dialysis thrice weekly (or several times daily in the case of peritoneal dialysis), but they are restricted in diet and fluid intake and must take numerous medications. The implications of not following medical recommendations are very serious. Hyperkalemia and fluid overload may affect the life as well as the health of individuals. With transplant recipients, failure to take the immunosuppressive medications can result in loss of the transplanted organ due to rejection. This has been a particular concern to health care professionals working with adolescents, who often see themselves as invincible. It is not surprising, therefore, that nurses report that noncompliance is one of the major problems that they face in their clinical roles, regardless of treatment modality (Molzahn & Preisig, 1996).

What is compliance? The answer to that question is not as straightforward as might be expected. Nurses in dialysis units typically describe noncompliant patients as those people who gain more than 2 kg between dialyses, have serum potassium levels above 6 mmol/L, serum phosphate levels above 5.5 mg/dl., or those people who miss dialysis treatments or other medical appointments. However, various researchers have used different definitions of compliance behavior, and there are no agreed-upon definitions of the concept (Betts & Crotty, 1988). Similarly, people with CRF learn "what they can get away with." They learn the extent to which they can stretch the limits, in terms of what and how much they eat and drink, without requiring additional dialysis or medical therapy.

Although there is considerable variability regarding the definition of compliance in chronic renal failure, it is clear that nonadherence to the regimen is very frequent. This is the case not only with CRF; in various studies, the general rate of noncompliance is about 25% to 35% for various age groups with a variety of different health problems (Shaben, 1993). In CRF, in one report, only 20% to 30% of the sample were compliant more often than not for fluid restrictions. The comparable figure for potassium levels was between 80% and 90%, and for self-administration of phosphate binding medications, only 60% to 70% of the hemodialysis patients studied were compliant (Yanitski, 1983). Similar findings have been noted by other researchers (for example, Betts & Crotty, 1988; Blackburn, 1977; Procci, 1978). In a study of adolescents, it was found that approximately 64% of adolescents with kidney transplants did not regularly take their immunosuppressive medications (Ettenger et al., 1991). The consequences of these decisions are extremely serious because organs donated for transplants are scarce and valuable resources.

Many believe that good teaching is key to compliance. As a result, they become frustrated, when despite excellent educational programs, their patients do not follow their instructions. There have been numerous studies describing strategies to increase compliance. Some of these strategies have involved educational programs, while others have involved individualized programs. In some cases, behavioral strategies such as contracting have been employed, and yet others have involved nursing care modalities such as primary nursing (Molzahn, 1989). However, there have been mixed results. Sometimes the interventions work, and other times (more often than not), they do not.

There have been a number of models that have been proposed to address factors that could predict compliance behavior. The Health Belief Model is probably the best known model of compliance behavior (Becker, 1974; Hartman & Becker, 1978). In the model, it is hypothesized that compliance is a function of one's readiness to act, based on level of motivation, perceived susceptibility to a particular condition or its sequelae, perceived severity of the condition, and an estimate of benefits and/or barriers to compliance. Modifying and enabling variables such as age, sex, and satisfaction with care may or may not be important in enhancing compliance with prescribed regimens. For instance, using the model, individuals with CRF can perceive the sequelae of hyperkalemia and fluid overload to be very serious; if so they are more likely to be compliant. If they perceive that they are susceptible to these complications, they are more likely to comply.

Although the models of compliance behavior have been frequently used, they are not always very successful. At best, the models explain about 30% of the variance of compliance behavior. That suggests that there is much that we do not know about what makes some people follow their restrictions and others to refuse to cooperate with the treatment regimen.

The use of the term "compliance," has been questioned. Compliance denotes subservience and does not recognize that individuals choose to act in specific ways. Given that the existing models and approaches to enhancing compliance do not seem to work (at least not to any appreciable extent), it seems reasonable that the concept label and strategies to promote compliance be changed. There is a need for new approaches. Molzahn (1996) advocates use of a caring approach, encompassing principles of empowerment, health promotion, phenomenology, and multiple ways of knowing how to work with patients. If the goal of changing patient behavior (for example, following diet restrictions) remains one that is set by health professionals, it is unlikely that patients' behaviors will change. If patients decide they wish to attain particular goals, such as reducing fluid weight gain between dialyses, then the likelihood of goal attainment is greatly enhanced. Because of the serious consequences of failure to follow the prescribed regimen, health professionals are reluctant to change approaches; however, given our lack of success in this area and changing societal attitudes and perspectives (for example, consumerism, self-determination), it is time to recognize that some decisions are outside of our control.

Body Image

Another commonly reported stressor in CRF is body image. Body image refers to the mental picture or idea that people have of their bodies and body parts. Many people with CRF are not pleased with their body image. CRF affects skin coloration and texture, and often muscle wasting is evident. Dialysis therapy may affect body image as well. Some patients find the sight of AV fistulae, grafts, and peritoneal catheters objectionable, and some are concerned about the reactions of others to these external manifestations of their illnesses. After transplantation, side effects of immunosuppressive therapy, particularly Cushingoid features, weight gains, and hirsutism can be disturbing. Some people have difficulty looking at or touching their body while others make repetitive negative comments or have negative feelings about their bodies. In some situations, the body changes are temporary and can be alleviated by modification of medication dosages or cosmetic treatment. In other situations, the changes are of a more permanent nature, and individuals will need to adjust to their changed appearance.

Sexuality and Chronic Renal Failure

Closely associated with changes in body image are changes in sexual functioning. In a number of studies on sexual functioning of individuals with CRF, decreased frequency of intercourse, difficulties with erection and ejaculation, decreased sexual desire, and reduced satisfaction with the sexual relationship are common. These difficulties have been associated with increasing uremia in the predialysis period but do not seem to be improved with dialysis therapy (Binik & Mah, 1994). The causes of sexual dysfunction in men are thought to be due to diminished testosterone levels and increased prolactin production. In women, decreased libido, impaired fertility, and difficulty achieving orgasm are common. People who are transplanted typically report some improvement in sexual functioning when compared with dialysis therapy. However, they do not report going back to pre-illness levels of sexual functioning (Binik & Mah, 1994).

Sexual performance in both men and women is affected not only by physiological factors but also by anxiety, stress, depression, and the nature of the relationship with the sexual partner. There is no easy way to distinguish between organic and psychosocial causes of sexual dysfunction. With CRF, it is quite likely that both organic and psychosocial problems exist and affect each other. For instance, concerns regarding body image may decrease sexual desire, as can the changing roles associated with CRF. These factors combined with physiologic changes can lead to considerable frustration and stress regarding sexual performance.

It is important that nurses create an atmosphere of safety for clients and partners to discuss issues relating to sexual functioning. This requires sensitivity and knowledge. People are often embarrassed to discuss issues related to sex and wait for their health professionals to raise the topic. By providing patients with opportunities to discuss sexuality, nurses are more likely to uncover concerns in this area. An assessment of sexual functioning should

Table 10-2
Sexual assessment.

- Are you currently having an intimate relationship with someone?
- Are you sexually active?
- Are you having any difficulties regarding sexual performance?
- Have you noticed any changes in your sexual desire?
- Are you having difficulty reaching orgasm?
- Are you having any difficulty getting or maintaining an erection? (men)
- Are you satisfied with your sex life?

be included as part of the history and physical assessment of any CRF patient. Some sample questions are included in Table 10-2.

For any sexual problem, there are a range of possible medical, surgical, social, psychological, educational, or behavioral possibilities available. Some medications (for example, antihypertensives) are notorious for causing impotence, and a change in medication may remedy the problem (Zarifian, 1992) (see also Table 10-3). In other situations, more drastic interventions, such as penile prostheses or penile injection of vasoactive substances may be appropriate.

Many health professionals may feel that they lack knowledge and skills in this area. In some cases, referral to sex therapists or counselors may be helpful in identifying strategies for improving sexual relationships. However, support and encouragement for taking this step may be important, since many people find it difficult to discuss sexuality, and trust in health professionals is the key to successful treatment.

Coping Strategies Used by Individuals with CRF

Baldree and co-investigators (1982) outlined the most commonly reported coping methods used by 35 hemodialysis patients in their study. Some of the coping behaviors were "problem-oriented" strategies that aimed to solve the problem or handle the stressful situation. "Affective-oriented" coping methods are strategies used to manage the emotions accompanying a stressful situation. The most common coping strategies reported by the participants included: trying to maintain some control over the situation; hoping that things will get better; praying; looking at the problem objectively; worrying; and accepting the situation as it is (Baldree et al., 1982). Similarly, Gurklis and Menke (1995) described a number of categories of coping strategies. They outlined patients' rankings of the importance of various strategies, including accepting dialysis; maintaining control of one's health; maintaining a positive outlook; staying active; self-mastery; and using a support network.

Not all coping strategies are positive in nature. Depression is a common response to the multiple stressors and challenges of living with a chronic illness. In CRF, it has been particularly difficult to diagnose depression because, in the past, many of the measures of depression have actually addressed symptoms that are common to both depression and CRF. For instance, symptoms such as poor appetite, insomnia or hypersomnia; fatigue; low self-esteem; poor concentration; and feelings of hopelessness are very common among people with CRF, even when they are not clinically depressed. Nevertheless, many people on dialysis feel depressed at times (Rodin, 1994). In most people, the depression will be relatively short-lived. However, some depression is more disabling and may need psychiatric treatment. It has been estimated that depressive symptoms are reported in 25% or more of people with CRF, and one-third of these people may be suffering from a major depression, requiring treatment (Rodin, 1994). Occasionally, depression is severe enough for individuals to attempt suicide or withdraw from dialysis therapy. It is important that these people are identified early and receive appropriate treatment.

Social Support

Social support is viewed as a coping strategy by many people but it is also necessary for the health and well-being of all people. For individuals with CRF, social support is more than a coping strategy. It has been noted that absence of social support is a predisposing factor for the development of CAPD complications (Stegman & Berger, 1984), and is strongly related to quality of life (Tell et al., 1995).

In a study of hemodialysis patients, 125 of 129 participants identified at least one person upon whom they have relied for help. Most commonly, these support persons were spouses or significant

Table 10-3
Drugs associated with sexual dysfunction.

Drug Class	Decrease Libido	Cause Impotence	Inhibit Ejaculation
Hypertensive			
Methyldopa	+	+	
Guanethidine			+
Hydralazine	+		
Reserpine	+		
Propanalol	+	+	
Clonidine	+	+	
Psychiatric			
Barbiturates		+	
Tricyclic	+	+	+
Amitriptyline	+	+	+
Benzodialzipines	+	+	+
Phenothiazine		+	+
Other			
Antihistimine	+		
Clofibrinate	+		
Diphenylhydantoin	+		
Digitalis	+		
Alcohol	+	+	
Heroin	+	+	
Methadone	+		
Cocaine	+	+	

Note: From Zarifian, A.A. (1992). Sexual dysfunction in the male end stage renal disease patient. *ANNA Journal, 19,* 530. Reprinted with permission.

others, adult children, but also in fewer cases included parents, young children, and nurses. These patients received help from relatives for home management tasks such as cooking, laundry, housekeeping, and grocery shopping. Many of the participants indicated that relatives helped them follow their health regimens by reminding them about their diets and restrictions. Family and friends also offered transportation, emotional support, companionship, and financial support.

It has been hypothesized that social support for dialysis patients may fluctuate over time. For instance, O'Brien (1980) found that the quantity of the patients' interactions with family and friends increased over a 3-year period. However, the quality of those interactions decreased over time. Nurses have a role in supporting family members and friends to minimize the burdens associated with long-term caregiving.

For some people, spiritual support from God, their pastors, and/or church members was important (Gurklis & Menke, 1995). For other people, support can be obtained from peers and peer groups. Some people with CRF have expressed the sentiment that nurses do not and cannot know what "it's really like" (Molzahn, 1991). As a result, some dialysis units have established peer counseling programs, where people on dialysis are able to support and help each other. In other settings, support groups have proven to be very effective.

Impact of CRF on the Family

Family members play a critical role in the care and well-being of individuals with CRF. They provide physical care, emotional support, and instrumental support as noted earlier. However, the illness and treatment also have a major effect on family members and the family unit as a whole.

Flaherty and O'Brien (1992) studied 50 family members who were willing to discuss adaptation of families who had a member receiving dialysis therapy. They found that five family coping styles emerged from content analysis of the data. These styles were labeled: remote family style, enfolded family style, altered family style, distressed family style, and receptive family style. A remote family style was characterized by responses that suggest that the disease has not interfered with the life of the family member. In contrast, the enfolded family style was characterized by responses suggesting that the disease had strengthened the bonds among family members and that the disease had become a family affair. In the altered family style, responses suggested major changes in the family members' daily activities. The distressed family style was characterized by responses that suggest sorrow or grief regarding the disease and its impact on family life. The receptive family style indicated some degree of acceptance of the diagnosis and adjustment to it.

Although many families hope that a transplant will change their lives, transplantation is not without stresses. Concerns about the long-term side effects of immunosuppression are very common among family members; also, families have concerns about other medical conditions or complications that might arise (Voepel-Lewis, Ketefian, Starr, & White, 1990). The period of time of hospitalization after transplantation is particularly stressful as families remain very concerned about the physical well-being of recipients.

Relatively little research has examined the specific impact of CRF on the spouse or partner of the individual afflicted by the disease. There has been some research examining the perspectives of spouses as designated home hemodialysis helpers (Friesen, 1990). Some spouses were highly involved in the dialysis treatment, while others assisted only minimally. Some had very high levels of resentment regarding the dialysis treatment while others had little resentment. Friesen described the category of "joint partners" where all roles within the marriage, including those related to dialysis, were shared. These spouses described their situations as though the "abnormal becomes normal" and viewed their situations positively. However, other spouses, found dialysis to be frightening, negative, and were frustrated by the change in roles and loss of freedom. Certainly, the stress of the dialysis helper role has probably contributed to the decreasing number of people with CRF selecting home hemodialysis as the treatment modality of choice. In another study (Dunn, Lewis, Bonner & Meize-Grochowski, 1994) of spouses of CAPD patients, 21% of the spouses reported their quality of life as high, 55% reported it as moderate, and 24% perceived it to be fair to poor. The researchers noted that the quality of life of spouses was very similar to that of CAPD patients. As practitioners, we do not always recognize the very significant impact of illness on spouses/partners, and these studies should help raise our awareness of the impact of familial illness.

There has also been relatively little research addressing the impact of dialysis therapy on children who have parents with CRF. There have been indications that some children who have parents on dialysis may suffer anxiety, depression, and bodily concern (Tsaltas, 1976). In a study where eight adolescents who had parents on dialysis were compared to matched control subjects, it was found that the adolescents with a parent receiving CRF treatment demonstrated some difficulty in adjustment (Schlebusch, Naidoo, & Kallmeyer, 1983). However, in other studies, it seemed that many adolescents developed greater self-esteem and enhanced growth of identity as a result of a parents' home dialysis therapy.

There have been two studies where exploratory interviews were used to study the experiences of children whose parents were on dialysis. Beanlands (1987) conducted a grounded theory study and described three phases that children experienced: "finding out about it," "learning to live with a parent on home dialysis," and "getting sick." "Finding out about it" involved listening to parents' discussions and observing the dialysis process. It was interesting that health professionals did not play a prominent role in helping children gather more information about their parent's illness. Over time, the children and adolescents "learned to live with a parent on home dialysis." Invariably, there would be complications, such as peritonitis, which caused considerable concern for the children. This was the "getting sick" phase, after which time they had to readjust again. Uncertainty about the future and hope were themes that recurred throughout the children's experiences. Kikuchi and Molzahn (1990) also studied children who had a parent on dialysis, using a philosophical framework to define quality of life. The children generally described a very good quality of life, but discussed fear in relation to their parents' condition and treatment, and wanted carefree family vacations. In relation to fear, fear of dying, and fear of dialysis, complications (such as peritonitis and bleeding) were frequently mentioned. There was also concern that something would happen to the other (well) parent. In relation to vacations, the children and adolescents in this study expressed frustration at needing to plan vacations months in advance in order to arrange dialysis treatments in distant facilities, or the need to travel with numerous boxes of peritoneal solutions.

Two psychosocial needs identified by families as important include information and comfort (Wagner, 1996). In addition to listening to the perspectives of family members, it is essential that nurses consider the family unit to be the patient. Family members have needs for information and knowledge and needs for support and comfort in the same way that people afflicted with the illness do. Involvement of family members in the care of people with CRF can be very valuable as they provide an important protective buffer against the impact of stress. Health care providers need to pay particular attention to the frustrations and unmet needs of family members.

Much of the research in the area of psychosocial impact of CRF has not addressed culture, race, or ethnic background as variables. This body of research is based primarily on a white middle class value system. As a result, findings from many studies may not be generalizable to other ethnic groups. It is important that nurses, in their work with people of various cultures, attempt to develop an understanding of that culture and work with clients and their families in culturally relevant ways. It should be recognized that communication patterns, dress and appearance, nutrition and eating habits, time awareness, relationships, and religious beliefs are all affected by culture. As a result, our interpretations and nursing strategies may need to change with people of other cultural groups.

Quality of Life Associated with ESRD

Quality of life has often been described as a reflection of life as a whole. Some people view it as an indicator of psychological well-being. It really reflects the overall outcomes and responses to particular life situations. In health care, it is no longer satisfactory to describe the effectiveness of a treatment on the basis of morbidity and mortality alone. There have been numerous examples described in both the popular press and scientific literature that question the ethics of indiscriminately extending life. Nurses often work with people who would probably be better off not receiving treatment. As a result, quality of life has become an important variable to consider in demonstrating success of health care interventions.

Quality of life is a concept that seems to be simple, but the complexity of measuring it has stymied many researchers. There have literally been thousands of articles written over the last 30 years that debate the definitions, conceptualization, and measurement of quality of life. In terms of measurement, there have been numerous instruments that have been used to quality of life, some better than others. This makes it very difficult to draw conclusions from the research or to compare findings with other studies. Despite the difficulty that researchers have had measuring quality of life, it does seem that it is a concept that people with CRF can understand without difficulty. Quality refers to a range from very high to very low. Life is perhaps more difficult to characterize, by virtue of its breadth. However, most people, when asked to describe their quality of life seem to have no difficulty doing so.

Most of the research regarding quality of life in CRF has pertained to assessing and comparing various treatment modalities. Most researchers have reported that quality of life is highest after transplantation (for example, Evans et al., 1985; Gudex, 1995). Home therapies (for example, home hemodialysis and CAPD) tend to offer higher quality of life than hospital-based treatments (Churchill, Morgan, & Torrance, 1984). There has also been research regarding the positive effect of recombinant erythropoietin therapy on quality of life of individuals with CRF (Evans, Radner, & Manninen, 1990; Laupacis, Wong, & Churchill, 1991).

Dealing With Patients Who Have a Low Quality of Life

Most health care practitioners working with people with CRF have encountered patients who have a poor quality of life. This raises questions not only about the effectiveness of therapy, but also a range of ethical concerns. Was the individual informed of the option of no treatment? What is in the best interest of the individual? Is suffering being prolonged needlessly? Is the treatment prolonging life or extending death? Is there harm to the therapy? What are the costs (both economic and social) of therapy?

Ideally, issues relating to treating or not treating should be made before individuals become seriously ill. There has been growing interest in the use of advance directives in health care. Advance directives provide individuals with the opportunity to specify their wishes and preferences about the use of life-sustaining measures and treatment in the event of a change in condition or medical emergency. In the United States, the Patient Self-Determination Act was passed in 1990. According to this act, all adult individuals must be informed of their right to accept or refuse treatment. They must also be informed of their right to have an advance directive, and they must be asked if they have an advance directive (Colvin, Myhre, Welch, & Hammes, 1993). Health care professionals have more than a legal obligation to ask about advance directives. They have a moral obligation to provide patients with the opportunity to consider the options regarding treatment, and to provide support for and advocate their patients' decisions. Given that nurses and physicians have a long-term relationship with people with CRF, and that the morbidity and mortality rates associated with the disease and its treatment are relatively high, it is particularly important that nephrology nurses actively encourage patients and their families/friends to discuss their wishes regarding treatment.

There are a number of different advance directive documents available, developed by advocacy groups, religious organizations, lawyers, and professional associations. Mendelssohn and Singer (1994) have developed a dialysis-specific living will which has been found to be highly acceptable to people receiving dialysis therapy. It asks only about two treatment options in the event of serious health situations, specifically, dialysis and CPR. The treatment options and effectiveness are defined, as are various health situations, such as permanent coma, terminal illness, strokes (mild, moderate, and severe), and dementia (mild, moderate, and severe).

In one study (Quintana, Nevarez, Rogers, Murata, & Tzamaloukas, 1991), 146 CAPD and hemodialysis patients were asked to declare their choice regarding CPR in the event of cardiac arrest. Thirty-seven percent indicated that they would decline CPR. Predictors of refusal of CPR included severity of disability and presence of diabetes. In a Canadian study (Perry, Nicholas, Molzahn, & Dossetor, 1995), 84% of ESRD patients thought it was important to have a living will, but only 18% of those patients had actually signed an advance directive. Similarly, relatively low rates of discussions regarding advance directives, and few advance directives among ESRD patients have been reported (Mendelssohn & Singer, 1994).

There are some issues and concerns regarding the potential use of advance directives. For instance, Perry and co-authors (1995) found that 52% of the patients and relatives/friends in their study believed that major treatment decisions should be left to the physician, a perception that was not shared by physicians and nurses. It was also interesting that in many situations where physicians and nurses believed they had discussed treatment options and advance directives with patients, patients did not identify that those discussions had occurred. It is clear that nurses, physicians, clients, and their families need to have more and better communication regarding treatment choices and advance directives to ensure that inappropriate decisions and judgments are not made.

Withdrawal from dialysis treatment has become one of the most difficult issues in the care of people with CRF. It has been estimated that as many as 20% or more of deaths among people with CRF are the result of voluntary cessation of dialysis (Schwartz et al., 1994). Although many health care professionals are concerned about the legal implications of stopping dialysis, "there has never been a successful criminal prosecution for stopping life-sustaining treatment. So long as a doctor acts reasonably and in good faith to withhold or discontinue treatment with the consent of the patient or family, there is little chance of a criminal charge" (Schwartz et al., 1994, p. 265). In fact, to fail to provide the opportunity for informed consent may be illegal, as well as unethical. Nurses must be involved in individuals' request to terminate treatment; they are usually very familiar with individual patients and may know them better than do other health professionals. They are in an ideal position to provide further information to their clients as well as to support the rights of individuals to make their own choices (Motes, 1989).

Regardless of whether individuals decide to stop dialysis, or are not selected for dialysis therapy, it is possible to help renal patients die comfortably when the time comes. As nurses, we have the obligation to make the dying process as comfortable as possible. There is much that nurses working with dying CRF patients can learn from the hospice movement. Hospice care involves providing comfort to dying patients and their families, alleviating pain and symptoms, addressing spiritual needs, and providing support (Phipps, 1988). A full discussion of palliative care is beyond the scope of this chapter, but many of the principles involved in the care of people dying of cancer are also applicable in CRF.

Nursing Care in Relation to Psychosocial Impact of the Illness and Treatment

As nurses, we make many contributions to our patients and their families. However, the most important contribution we bring to the nurse-patient relationship is who we are – ourselves (i.e., "therapeutic use of self"). This means that our key role is one of developing the relationship with our patients. The development of a caring relationship is probably the major role of nurses in providing support relating to the psychosocial aspects of CRF. Through good communication, nurses develop connections with patients and their families. Nurses working with people who have CRF have the advantage of long-term relationships, enabling them to get to know their patients and families well. The caring relationship of nurses with patients is built on trust and knowledge of patients. It is through this "knowing" and connectedness with patients, that nurses are in a strong position to assist, empower, advocate for, and enhance the well-being of people in their care. As feeling, caring human beings we are able to connect with the people we care for, work with them to identify their needs, and enable them to improve their health in the broadest sense.

The role of heath care professionals in addressing the psychosocial impact of the illness and treatment is very broad and has a wide scope. In addition to the traditional roles of providing health care, conducting health assessments, investigating troublesome symptoms, giving health information, and assisting with problem solving, "showing kindness" was the most frequently identified type of emotional support that subjects in one study received from health providers (Gurklis & Menke, 1995). Health professionals give support by encouraging individuals with CRF to share feelings about health-related and personal problems, listening, and offering realistic reassurance.

CRF therapy, whether by dialysis or transplantation, involves loss of control over areas of one's life. This is extremely frustrating for many clients. Rather than considering the ways in which nurses can provide opportunities for control, it may be necessary to engage in a fundamental reshaping of the way that we work with clients. Rather than thinking about the specific choices that individuals can make (for example, when to make the bed), another approach may be to assume that clients make all decisions based on information that is provided. For instance, with respect to type of treatment modality, or living-related vs. living-unrelated transplants, patients should be provided with all the necessary information to make an informed decision.

In working with people who have CRF, nurses have tended to use a medical model for assessment. While physical assessment is a very useful skill for nurses working with people who have CRF, other approaches may elicit more information and contribute to the empowerment and decision-making of clients and their families. Hartrick, Lindsey, and Hills (1994) describe a framework for assessment of families using a health promotion framework. The framework has four components: listening to the family, participatory dialogue, recognizing patterns, and envisioning action and positive change. The emphasis is not on "what to do" but "how to do it." Partnership and action are key. This type of approach ensures that issues are addressed from the client's/family's perspective, rather than from the perspective of health care practitioners.

It seems that many nephrology nurses have relatively little contact with family members, particularly regarding the family member's own needs. It has been suggested that the designation of primary nurses for patients and their families might provide the family with more specific, personal and consistent care (Wagner, 1986). Family members play a very important role in the well-being of people with CRF, and they should not be forgotten in the process of caring for individuals.

Multidisciplinary teams and care planning are often useful the difficult problems associated with chronic illness. Nurses, physicians, social workers, and nutritionists are typically members of the renal care team. Team members bring a variety of perspectives together that are helpful to clients, families, and nurses. Some strategies work with some patients and others work with other types of people. The collective wisdom of the multidisciplinary health team is one of the major strengths of ESRD programs.

When the difficulties encountered by patients with CRF challenge the resources of the multidisciplinary team, it may be necessary to refer patients for further treatment. Like the rest of the population, people with CRF may suffer from psychopathologies that may benefit from psychiatric therapy. Medications are very useful in treating depression, schizophrenia, and anxiety. Psychotherapy and counseling may be useful and appropriate in a wide range of situations. Many renal treatment centers have developed linkages with sex therapists, who can provide several levels of therapy and counseling for sexual dysfunction.

A major role of nurses in caring for people with CRF relates to the psychosocial impact of the illness. The challenges of dealing with these issues can be much more demanding than dealing with physiological changes and complications. There are no easy solutions to the psychosocial challenges that face individuals with CRF. Nursing approaches to dealing with the implications will arise from the knowledge and relationship that nurses have with clients and their families. Referral to social workers, psychologists, or psychiatrists may be appropriate in some situations. However, such referrals do not mean that nurses no longer provide care in the realm of psychosocial issues. The role of nurses in coordinating care, acting as case managers, and facilitating rehabilitation is crucial to the well-being of patients.

Summary

In conclusion, the care of patients with CRF is both interesting and challenging given the numerous psychosocial stressors imposed by the illness and treatment. Some of these stressors include powerlessness, intrusiveness of the treatment, restrictions imposed by the regimen, changes in sexual functioning, and changes in body image. An understanding of the illness trajectory of CRF will assist patients, families, and health care professionals in anticipating possible challenges. People with CRF use a variety of coping mechanisms, but the importance of support by family and friends cannot be underestimated. It is important that nurses consider patients' families in the provision of care, so that families also understand the implications of the illness and treatment. Nurses, through their relationships with patients, are in an ideal position to work with their patients as they deal with the psychosocial impact of renal disease so that ultimately the quality of life of these patients is enhanced.

References

Baldree, K.S., Murphy, S.P., & Powers, M.J. (1982). Stress identification and coping patterns in patients on hemodialysis. *Nursing Research, 32,* 107-112.

Beanlands, H. (1987). *The experience of being a child in a family where one parent is on home dialysis.* Unpublished master's thesis, University of Toronto, Toronto, Ontario.

Becker, M.H. (1974). The Health Belief Model and sick role behavior. *Health Education Monographs, 2*(4), 409-419.

Betts, D.K., & Crotty, G.D. (1988). Response to illness and compliance of long-term hemodialysis patients. *ANNA Journal, 15,* 96-99.

Bihl, M.A., Ferrans, C.E., & Powers, M.J. (1988). Comparing stressors and quality of life of dialysis patients. *ANNA Journal, 15,* 27-37.

Binik, Y.M., & Mah, K. (1994). Sexuality and end-stage renal disease: Research and clinical recommendations. *Advances in Renal Replacement Therapy, 1,* 198-209.

Blackburn, S. (1977). Dietary compliance of chronic hemodialysis patients. *Journal of the American Dietetic Association, 70,* 31-37.

Churchill, Morgan, & Torrance (1984). Quality of life in end-stage renal disease. *Peritoneal Dialysis Bulletin, 4*(1), 20-23.

Colvin, E.R., Myhre, M.J., Welch, J., & Hammes, B.J. (1993). Moving beyond the Patient Self-Determination Act: Educating patients to be autonomous. *ANNA Journal, 20,* 564-568.

Czackes, J.W., & Kaplan De-Nour, A. (1976). *Chronic hemodialysis as a way of life.* New York: Brunner/Mazel.

Devins, G.M. (1994). Illness intrusiveness and the psychosocial impact of lifestyle disruptions in chronic life-threatening disease. *Advances in Renal Replacement Therapy, 1,* 251-263.

Devins, G.M., Binik, Y.M., Hollomby, D., Barre, P., & Guttman, R.D. (1981). Helplessness and depression in end-stage renal disease. *Journal of Abnormal Psychology, 90*(6), 531-545.

Dunn, S.A., Lewis, S.L., Bonner, P.N., & Meize-Grochowski, R. (1994). Quality of life for spouses of CAPD patients. *ANNA Journal, 21,* 237-246.

Ettenger, R.B., Rosenthal, J.T., Marik, J.L., Malekzaheh, M., Forsythe, S.B., Kainl, E.S., Salusky, I.B., & Fine, R.N. (1991). Improved cadaveric renal transplantation in children. *Pediatric Nephrology, 5,* 137-142.

Evans, R.W., Manninen, D.L., Garrison, L.P., Blagg, C.R., Gutman, R.A., Hull, A.R., & Lowrie, E.G. (1985). The quality of life of patients with end-stage renal disease. *New England Journal of Medicine, 312,* 553-559.

Evans, R.W., Rader, B., & Manninen, D.L. (1990). The quality of life of hemodialysis recipients treated with recombinant human erythropoietin. *Journal of the American Medical Association, 263,* 825-830.

Flaherty, M.J., & O'Brien, M.E. (1992). Family styles of coping in end stage renal disease. *ANNA Journal, 19,* 345-349, 366.

Friesen, D. (1990). *Spouses as designated home hemodialysis helpers.* Unpublished masters thesis, University of Alberta.

Fuchs, J., & Schreiber, M. (1988). Patients' perceptions of CAPD and hemodialysis stressors. *ANNA Journal, 15,* 282-285.

Gudex, C.M. (1995). Health-related quality of life in endstage renal failure. *Quality of Life Research, 4,* 359-366.

Gurklis, .A., & Menke, E.M. (1988). Identification of stressors and use of coping methods in chronic hemodialysis patients. *Nursing Research, 37,* 236-239, 248.

Gurklis, J.A., & Menke, E.M. (1995). Chronic hemodialysis patients' perceptions of stress, coping and social support. *ANNA Journal, 22,* 381-390.

Hartman, P.E., & Becker, M.H. (1978). Noncompliance with prescribed regimen among chronic hemodialysis patients - A method of prediction and educational diagnosis. *Dialysis and Transplantation, 7*(10), 978-987.

Hartrick, G., Lindsey, A.E., & Hills, M. (1994). Family nursing assessment: Meeting the challenge of health promotion. *Journal of Advanced Nursing, 20,* 85-91.

Kikuchi, J., & Molzahn, A.E. (1989). *Children and adolescents of parents with renal failure on dialysis: Their reported quality of life.* Unpublished manuscript, University of Alberta, Edmonton, Alberta, Canada.

Laupacis, A., Wong, C., & Churchill, D. (1991). The use of generic and specific quality of life measures in hemodialysis patients treated with erythropoietin. *Controlled Clinical Trials, 12,* 168S-179S.

Mendelssohn, D.C., & Singer, P.A. (1994). Advance directives in dialysis. *Advances in Renal Replacement Therapy, 1,* 240-250.

Molzahn, A.E. (1989). Primary nursing and compliance in a hemodialysis unit. *ANNA Journal, 16,* 167-172.

Molzahn, A.E. (1991). The reported quality of life of selected home hemodialysis patients. *ANNA Journal, 18,* 173-180.

Molzahn, A.E. (1996). Changing to a caring paradigm for teaching and learning. *ANNA Journal, 23,* 13-18.

Molzahn, A.E., & Preisig, P. (1996). Perceived problems of nephrology nurses. *ANNA Journal.* Submitted for publication.

Motes, C.E. (1989). Discontinuation of dialysis. *ANNA Journal, 16,* 413-415.

O'Brien, M.E. (1980). Hemodialysis regimen compliance and social environment: A panel analysis. *Nursing Research, 29,* 250-255.

Perry, L.D., Nicholas, D., Molzahn, A.E., & Dossetor, J.B. (1995). Attitudes of dialysis patients and caregivers regarding advance directives. *ANNA Journal, 22,* 457-464.

Phipps, W.E. (1988). The origin of hospices/hospitals. *Death Studies, 12,* 92-99.

Procci, W. (1978). Dietary abuse in maintenance hemodialysis patients. *Psychosomatics, 19,* 16-24.

Quintana, B.J., Nevarez, M., Rogers, K., Mrata, G.H., & Tzamaloukas, A.H. (1991). Reaction of patients on chronic dialysis to discussions about cardiopulmonary resuscitation. *ANNA Journal, 18,* 29-32.

Reichsman, F., & Levy, N. (1972). Problems in adaptation to maintenance hemodialysis. *Archives of Internal Medicine, 130,* 859.

Rodin, G. (1994). Depression in patients with end-stage renal disease: Psychopathology or normative response? *Advances in Renal Replacement Therapy, 1,* 219-227.

Schlebusch, L., Naidoo, N.K., & Kallmeyer, J. (1983). Psychological effects of incentre hemodialysis on the dialysands' adolescent children. *South African Medical Journal, 63,* 363-365.

Schwartz, R.D., Perry, E., Schneider, C., Burdette, T., Curtis, G., & O'Neil, M. (1994). The option to withdraw from chronic dialysis treatment. *Advances in Renal Replacement Therapy, 1,* 264-273.

Shaben, T.R. (1993). Psychosocial issues in kidney-transplanted children and adolescents: A literature review. *ANNA Journal, 20,* 663-668.

Strauss, A.L, Corbin, J., Fagerhaugh, S., Glaser, B. G., Maines, D., Suszek, B., & Wiener, C.L. (1984). *Chronic illness and the quality of life* (2nd edition). Toronto: C.V. Mosby Company.

Stegman, M.R., & Berger, A.M. (1984). Peritonitis among CAPD patients: Host, agent, and/or environment? *Peritoneal Dialysis Bulletin, 4,* 206-208.

Tell, G.S., Shumaker, S.A., Mittelmark, M.V., Russell, G., Hylander, B., & Burkart, J.M. (1995). Social support and health related quality of life in black and white dialysis patients. *ANNA Journal, 22,* 301-308.

Tsaltas, M.O. (1976). Children of home dialysis patients. *Journal of the American Medical Association, 236,* 2764-2766.

Voepel-Lewis, T., Ketefian, S., Starr, A., & White, M.J. (1990). Stress, coping and quality of life in family members of kidney transplant recipients. *ANNA Journal, 17,* 427-432.

Wagner, C.D. (1996). Family needs of chronic hemodialysis patients: A comparison of perceptions of nurses and families. *ANNA Journal, 23,* 19-27.

White, M.J., Ketefian, S., Starr, A.J., & Voepel-Lewis, T. (1990). Stress, coping and quality of life in adult kidney transplant recipients. *ANNA Journal, 17,* 421-425.

Yanitski, A.E. (1983). Compliance of the hemodialysis patient. *American Association of Nephrology Nurses and Technicians Journal,10*(2), 11-16.

Zarifian, A.A. (1992). Sexual dysfunction in the male end stage renal disease patient. *ANNA Journal, 19,* 527-532.

Readings

Artinian, B.M. (1983). Role identities of the dialysis patient. *Nephrology Nurse,* 10-14.

Burton, H.J., Kline, S.A., Lindsay, R.M., & Heidenheim, M.A. (1988). The role of support in influencing outcome of end stage renal disease. *General Hospital Psychiatry, 10,* 260-266.

Henderson, M.L. (1995). Facilitating a "good death" in patients with end stage renal disease. *ANNA Journal, 22,* 294-300.

Hilton, B.A., & Starzomski, R.C. (1994). Family decision making about living related kidney donation. *ANNA Journal, 21,* 346-354.

Kutner, N.G., Fair, P.L., & Kutner, M.H. (1985). Assessing depression and anxiety in chronic dialysis patients. *Journal of Psychosomatic Research, 29,* 23-31.

O'Brien, M.E. (1983). *The courage to survive: The life career of the chronic dialysis patient.* New York: Grune and Stratton.

Pressly, K.B. (1995). Psychosocial characteristics of CAPD patients and the occurrence of infectious complications. *ANNA Journal, 22,* 563-573.

Shaben, T.R. (1992). *The experience of the adolescent following kidney transplantation: A grounded theory.* Unpublished masters thesis, University of Alberta.

RESEARCH BRIEF

Research Utilization

There are some issues and concerns regarding the potential use of advance directives. For instance, Perry, Nicholas, Molzahn and Dossetor (1995) found that 52% of the patients and relatives/friends in their study believed that major treatment decisions should be left to the physician, a perception that was not shared by physicians and nurses. It was also interesting that in many situations where physicians and nurses believed they had discussed treatment options and advance directives with patients, patients did not identify that those discussions had occurred. It is clear that nurses, physicians, clients, and their families need to have more and better communication regarding treatment choices and advance directives to ensure that inappropriate decisions and judgments are not made.

Chapter Highlights

- Stressors related to chronic renal failure and the psychosocial impact of the disease are significant, and nurses working with people who have CRF need to view the psychosocial impact as being as important as the physiological impact.

- Chronic illnesses are very common; in the United States, there are 32.7 million people, or about 14% of the population, limited by at least one chronic illness. Chronic illnesses are characterized by the long-term nature of the illness, uncertainty, a need for palliation rather than cure, complexity often involving multiple diseases/conditions, intrusiveness on the lives of individuals, need for a range of ancillary services, and cost.

- In chronic illness, it is important to shift the focus of care from primarily physical care, to care that considers the psychosocial impact of the illness on the daily lives of the chronically ill and their families.

- There has been considerable interest in the trajectory of adjustment or adaptation to dialysis. Lack of adjustment has been demonstrated by depression, suicidal tendencies, anxiety, or psychotic complications.

- Some of the stressors commonly associated with CRF include: powerlessness and lack of control, intrusiveness, limitations in diet and fluid, body image, and changes in sexuality.

- Various researchers have used different definitions of compliance behavior, and there are no agreed-upon definitions of the concept.

- The Health Belief Model is probably the best known model of compliance behavior (Becker, 1974; Hartman & Becker, 1978). In this model, it is hypothesized that compliance is a function of one's readiness to act, based on level of motivation, perceived susceptibility to a particular condition or its sequelae, perceived severity of the condition, and an estimate of benefits and/or barriers to compliance.

- The stress of the dialysis helper role has probably contributed to the decreasing number of people with CRF selecting home hemodialysis as the treatment modality of choice.

- There has also been relatively little research addressing the impact of dialysis therapy on children who have parents with CRF. There have been indications that some children who have parents on dialysis may suffer anxiety, depression, and bodily concerns.

- In addition to listening to the perspectives of family members, it is important that nurses consider the family unit to be the patient.

- Quality of life has often been described as a reflection of life as a whole. Some people view it as an indicator of psychological well-being. It really reflects the overall outcomes and responses to a particular life situation.

- The development of a caring relationship is probably the major role of nurses in providing support relating to the psychosocial aspects of CRF.

- It is through this "knowing" and connectedness with patients, that nurses are in a strong position to assist, empower, advocate for, and enhance the well-being of people in their care. As feeling, caring human beings we are able to connect with people we care for, work with them to identify their needs, and enable them to improve their health in the broadest sense of that word.

CHAPTER 11

Nutritional Care of Renal Patients

Sue Dickey Roberts, MS, RD, CNSD

Chapter Contents

Nutritional and Renal Physiology . . . 287
Diet and Progression of Renal Failure . . . 287
Diet for Dialysis . . . 288
  Potassium . . . 288
  Sodium and Fluid . . . 288
  Phosphorus, Calcium, and Vitamin D . . . 290
  Other Vitamins and Minerals . . . 290
  Protein and Energy . . . 291
  Hyperlipidemia and Carnitine . . . 291
Nutrition and Transplant . . . 292
Nutritional Assessment . . . 292
  History . . . 292
  Anthropometric Measurements . . . 294
  Biochemical Data . . . 294
Malnutrition and Dialysis . . . 294
  Nutritional Supplementation . . . 296
  Intradialytic Parenteral Nutrition . . . 296
  Intraperitoneal Nutrition . . . 298
Patient Education . . . 299
  Cultural Diversity . . . 300
  The National Renal Diet . . . 300
  Teaching the Renal Diet . . . 301
Summary . . . 301
References . . . 301
Chapter Highlights . . . 303

Nutritional Care of Renal Patients

Sue Dickey Roberts, MS, RD, CNSD

Few conditions have the extensive effect on metabolism and nutritional status as do those which result in chronic renal failure (CRF) (Kopple, 1994; May, 1993). The failure of the kidney to maintain its normal functions results in accumulation of metabolic waste products in body fluids and abnormalities in fluid and electrolyte homeostasis, acid-base homeostasis, and renal endocrine functions. These changes impact on the body's ability to digest, absorb, and use nutrients. Patients require nutrition intervention in virtually all stages of the renal disease process and in conjunction with all treatment modalities.

Nutrition intervention in renal disease and treatment slows progression of renal failure, compensates for impaired renal function and/or limitations of treatment modalities, helps prevent or manage complications imposed by the effects on other organs, helps manage complications secondary to aberrant endocrine activities and treats or prevents malnutrition (Kopple, 1994; May, 1993). The registered dietitian (RD) serves as an integral part of the renal health care team by assessing the patient's requirements and recommending the appropriate nutrition intervention. In addition, dietitians counsel patients and their families in the diet, follow patients for compliance, and help determine additional or changing nutritional needs (American Dietetic Association, 1994). The purpose of this chapter is to provide an overview of nutritional management of renal patients, specifically those with pre-end renal insufficiency and those treated with peritoneal dialysis or hemodialysis.

Nutritional and Renal Physiology

The functional units of the kidneys are the more than 1 million nephrons within each kidney (Briggs & Schnermann, 1994). The glomerulus of the nephron selectively filters serum to remove waste products including solutes such as glucose, organic acids, and end products of metabolism while preventing the loss of large protein molecules and red blood cells (Briggs & Schnermann, 1994). Glomerular diseases frequently result in urinary excretion of protein and subsequent hypoalbuminemia. A minimum urinary volume of approximately 600 ml (obligatory fluid) is required for the excretion of the average load of solids. About two-thirds of the solute load are nitrogenous wastes, consisting mostly of urea with smaller amounts of uric acid, creatinine, and ammonia. Accumulation of these end products of protein metabolism to toxic levels is the hallmark of renal insufficiency. By limiting dietary protein, patients minimize accumulation of these products (Narins & Cortes, 1994). The proximal tubules, the loop of Henle, the distal tubules and the collecting duct of the nephron function primarily to maintain fluid and electrolyte balance and acid-base homeostasis. With renal insufficiency, patients may easily dehydrate or become fluid overloaded.

As an endocrine organ, the kidney is the chief source for renin, erythropoietin, and 1,25-dihydroxycholecalciferol (1,25$(OH)_2D_3$). The failure of the kidney to secrete these vital hormones results in the complications of hypertension, anemia, and renal osteodystrophy, respectively. Nutritional adjustments help prevent or decrease the severity of some of these complications.

Diet and Progression of Renal Failure

A diet controlled for content of protein, phosphorus, or both may retard the progression of renal insufficiency to CRF (Maroni, 1993; Narins & Cortes, 1994). Animal data show that a high protein diet increases renal blood flow and glomerular filtration rate (GFR). A low protein diet reduces intraglomerular pressure and capillary blood flow and decreases urinary protein loss, thus slowing progression to CRF (Narins & Cortes, 1994). A phosphorus-restricted diet in animals also decreased deterioration of the diseased kidney. Since reducing the phosphorus content of the diet also reduces the protein content, it is unclear which nutrient contributes the beneficial effect (Dworkin, 1994).

One nationwide study in the United States, the Modification of Diet in Renal Disease (MDRD) trial, enrolled 840 predialysis patients for intervention in diet and blood pressure. Their results indicated that the low protein diet produced a small benefit in patients with moderate renal impairment but did not significantly slow the progression if renal disease (Levey, Gassman, Hall, & Walker, 1991).

Current recommendations for CRF patients are consistent with the World Health Organization recommendations for protein intake of 0.6 g/kg body weight per day with an adequate amount from high biologic value (HBV) sources such as egg, milk, meat, fish, and poultry to meet essential amino acid (EAA) requirements (Klahr, Levey, Beck et al., 1994; Maroni, 1993).

Diet for Dialysis

The diet for dialysis compensates for lack of kidney function and dialysate losses, provides adequate nutrients for optimal health, and alleviates symptoms of uremia. The dietitian individualizes each patient's nutrition plan based on current nutritional status, the underlying disease process, and the treatment modality. Hemodialysis (HD) and peritoneal dialysis (PD), either continuous ambulatory (CAPD) or continuous cyclic (CCPD), affect nutritional status differently.

Potassium

The kidney is the primary route for excretion of potassium (Bansal, 1992). The average diet contains approximately 80-100 mEq (3-4000 mg) potassium. Hyperkalemia occurs when serum levels exceed 6.0 mmol/L (6.0 mEq/L) (Beto & Bansal, 1992). The characteristic cardiac changes can be fatal. In CRF, dialysis treatments and decreased dietary potassium prevent hyperkalemia. HD removes approximately 100-200 mmol (100-200 mEq) per treatment, but serum levels rise rapidly between treatments if intake is not curtailed (Sherman, Hwang, Bernold, & Eisinger, 1986). The recommended dietary potassium depends on residual renal function, body size, the presence of anabolism, catabolism, or infection, and the potassium content of the dialysate. Patients achieve normal predialysis serum levels with a daily intake of approximately one mEq per kilogram ideal body weight or 38-80 mmol (38-80 mEq or 1500-3000 mg) daily (American Dietetic Association, 1993; Maroni, 1993). Foods high in potassium include many fruits, vegetables, dairy products, and legumes. To help patients limit their intake of these foods, dietitians must routinely reinforce the diet parameters (Beto & Bansal, 1992).

Due to high weekly clearances, PD patients frequently do not restrict potassium but continue to maintain normal serum levels (American Dietetic Association, 1993). The dietitian works within the renal team to individualize a patient's dietary potassium instructions. Some patients easily become hypokalemic, especially in response to poor dietary intake, diarrhea, or vomiting. If increased dietary intake is unsuccessful in raising the patient's serum potassium, potassium supplements may need to be used. Other patients may become hyperkalemic in response to excessive dietary intake, particularly those who are very active, and they need to restrict their dietary potassium (Kopple & Blumenkranz, 1984).

Renal health care practitioners usually think of diet as the primary cause of hyperkalemia. However, there are a host of other conditions that may lead to high potassium levels, such as acidemia, some hormonal disturbances, and a variety of medications. Potential causes and an appropriate intervention to rule out these causes are viewed in detail by Bansal and Beto (see Table 11-1) (Bansal, 1992; Beto & Bansal, 1992).

Sodium and Fluid

Dialysis patients are unable to maintain sodium and water homeostasis and may be prone to edema, hypertension, and congestive heart failure (American Dietetic Association, 1994; Kopple, 1994). HD patients restrict their sodium and fluid intake to limit interdialytic weight gains to 0.5-1 kg (American Dietetic Association, 1994; Beto, 1995). Recommendations are individualized according to the patient's urinary losses of sodium and 24-hour urinary volume. Anephric patients receive approximately 85-90 mEq (2000 mg) sodium and 500-1000 ml fluid daily.

Some HD patients frequently gain excessive amounts of fluid between treatments due to uncontrollable thirst. Causes of excess thirst that might be seen in the HD patient include hyperglycemia, azotemia, inadequate dialysis, a high dietary intake of sucrose, and a high intake of salt. Salt is most frequently the cause as it takes only a 1% change in serum sodium to stimulate thirst. Many patients think of salt (sodium chloride) as the only source of sodium, but they may be unaware of the sodium in sources such as broth or bouillon, soy sauce, seasoning salts, convenience foods, deli foods, fast food restaurants, and preservatives for frozen, canned, or boxed food. The dietitian on the renal team works with patients to be aware of these hidden sources and to learn how to read labels where sodium content is listed. One irony in the care we provide to patients is that we frequently administer hypertonic solution or saline solution to the fluid abusers to prevent hypotension during dialysis treatment. This will trigger thirst and cause further fluid abuse between dialysis treatments.

CAPD and CCPD patients lose more sodium and fluid into the dialysate and have more continual therapy. Generally, restrictions of sodium and fluid are unnecessary (Beto, 1995; Kopple & Blumenkranz, 1984; American Dietetic Association, 1993). Patients learn to monitor for both dehydration and overhydration and the appropriate adjustments to make in their dialysis regimen. To treat fluid retention, patients infuse more concentrated dialysate solutions. Obese patients who do not want the extra glucose calories that absorbed from concentrated solutions should restrict sodium to 43-90 mEq (1000-2000 mg) (Bouma & Dwyer, 1984; Kopple & Blumenkranz, 1984).

Table 11-1
An abbreviated checklist of dietary and nondietary causes of hyperkalemia for use in evaluating chronic hyperkalemia in chronic renal failure patients. PTH, parathyroid hormone, BUN, blood urea nitrogen.

Rule out dietary causes of hyperkalemia

- Misconceptions by patient concerning unlimited intake of no-potassium foods
- Ingestion of new products and/or new varieties of fruits and vegetables
- Continuation of previous emphasis on potassium if hypertensive
- Ingestion of large amounts of licorice containing glycyrrhizic acid
- Use of ethnic-cultural traditions influencing intake, i.e., fasting, home remedies
- Document portion control is not out of control
- Consumption of nutritional supplements outside of diet parameters

Rule out nondietary causes of hyperkalemia

- Decreased gut excretion with chronic constipation
  - Consider increasing fiber in diet to promote gut motility
  - Change phosphate-binding agents to reduce constipation effect
- Check validity of laboratory values
  - Verify prior treatment postdialysis potassium
  - Rule out hemolyzed blood error
- Evaluate interaction of laboratory values
  - Check acid-base status: acidosis
    - Each 0.1 change in arterial pH may increase serum potassium by .6-1.0 mEq/L
  - Consider effect of serum glucose-insulin relationship
    - Hyperkalemia secondary to insulin deficiency particularly in diabetics
  - Elevated PTH may cause calcium-potassium intracellular shift
  - Indicators of inadequate dialysis by presence of elevated BUN or other parameters
- Review medical and treatment effects
  - Inadequacy of dialysis contributing to intradialytic accumulation of potassium
    - Type of dialysate being used, ie, high-potassium bath
    - Inefficiency of access site
    - Evaluation of continuous ambulatory peritoneal dialysis compared with hemodialysis to maximize potassium removal
  - Consider drug interactions
    - Penicillin
    - Beta-blockers
    - Angiotensin-converting enzyme inhibitors
    - Muscle relaxants
    - Nonsteroidal anti-inflammatory agents
    - Steroids
    - Over-the-counter drugs
- Presence of concomitant diseases, ie, defects of aldosterone or renin, Addisoní disease, sickle cell anemia
- Invasive therapy causing release of potassium through tissue destruction
  - Infection, chemotherapy, surgical stress
  - Catabolism, starvation, malnutrition with change in dry weight
  - Clotting, bruising, inflammation of access site or other area
- Increased activity and exercise due to use of erythropoietin to improve anemia status

Note: From Beto, J.A., & Bansal, V.K. (1992) Hyperkalemia: Evaluating dietary and nondietary etiology. *Journal of Renal Nutrition*. Philadelphia: W.B. Saunders Company. Reprinted with permission.

Phosphorus, Calcium, and Vitamin D

CRF creates a wide range of alterations in homeostasis of calcium and phosphorus and in the metabolism of vitamin D. Hyperphosphatemia and high calcium-phosphorous products lead to the development of hyperparathyroidism, bone demineralization leading to osteodystrophy, and soft tissue calcification (Massry & Kopple, 1993). Dietary intake of 12-17 mg phosphorus per kg IBW (600-1200 mg/day) helps control serum with hemodialysis (Ahmed & Kopple, 1994; Massry & Kopple, 1993). Recommendations are similar for PD patients (American Dietetic Association, 1993; Kopple & Blumenkranz, 1984). Patients must limit intake of dairy products, beef liver, chocolate, nuts, and legumes to keep dietary phosphorus to a minimum. Generally, meats and other high protein foods are also high in phosphorus. Sargent and Lowrie have estimated that in a mixed diet, patients ingest 10.13 g phosphorus for each 1 g protein (Sargent & Lowrie, 1982). Patients with higher protein needs find it difficult to achieve adequate dietary protein while maintaining very low phosphorus intakes. Having adequate protein in the diet always takes precedent over having a limited phosphorus diet.

Phosphorus binding medications need to be taken with the diet to maintain normal serum phosphorus levels of <1.94 mmol/L (6 mg/dl) (Schmitt, 1991). Most dietitians and physicians recommend calcium acetate or calcium carbonate compounds. Aluminum hydroxide agents contribute to aluminum toxicity in renal patients, and calcium citrate increases aluminum absorption. Using calcium compounds provides the added advantage of increasing calcium sources to the calcium-poor renal diet.

The final step in converting vitamin D to $1,25(OH)_2D_3$ takes place in the kidney (May, 1993). This active form of vitamin D acts at the intestines to absorb calcium into the blood stream. With CRF, the kidneys are unable to perform this function. The $1,25(OH)_2D_3$ can be provided as oral or IV calcitriol. Both suppress parathyroid hormone (PTH) secretion and decrease the severity of renal osteodystrophy (Chan, Gleim, DeVita et al., 1993; Massry & Kopple, 1993). Calcitriol should be discontinued with hyperphosphatemia or when the calcium-phosphorus product reaches 75 or greater (with each concentration expressed in mg/dl) due to precipitation and soft tissue calcification.

Other Vitamins and Minerals

Patients with renal disease are at increased risk for deficiencies of water-soluble vitamins, particularly vitamin C, folate, and pyridoxine (B_6). Causes include altered intake of foods, drug-nutrient interactions, changes in retention and excretion patterns, interference in metabolism by uremic toxins, and losses to the dialysate. High doses of vitamin C encourage the formation of oxalate stones (Beto, 1995). Supplementation should equal 60 to 100 mg. Supplementation with fat soluble vitamin A is not recommended. Studies have shown that patients develop hypervitaminosis A, which may result in bone resorption (Muth, 1991). Requirements for fat soluble vitamins E and K are thought to be similar to those of the general population (Ahmed & Kopple, 1994; American Dietetic Association, 1994). Patients need explanations as to why they take a special vitamin and instructions not to take multiple vitamins containing vitamin A or the standard form of vitamin D.

Iron metabolism plays an essential role in the anemia of CRF. Factors that contribute to anemia include failure of the kidney to secrete erythropoietin, blood loss of two to five liters per year from hemodialysis treatments, and possible binding of iron to the dialysis membrane (Amerling & Levin, 1993). Supplementation with synthetic human hormone erythropoietin (epoetin) to replace the natural hormone dramatically decreases the incidence and severity of anemia seen prior to its availability. Patients with iron deficiencies, as documented with low iron saturation or low ferritin levels, may not respond to erythropoietin. Those patients may take oral iron supplements of 250-500 milligrams ferrous sulfate, or the equivalent ferrous fumerate or glutamate (Amerling & Levin, 1993). Due to gastrointestinal (GI) intolerance, it is usually recommended that oral iron supplements be taken with meals or 1/2 hour after meals to improve tolerance. Renal patients, however, are also taking calcium-containing or aluminum-containing antacids for phosphorus binders. The antacids interact with the iron supplements in two ways: (1) by cheating the iron and preventing absorption (Mason & Boyd, 1995) and (2) by raising the pH of the stomach, causing decreased absorption. Patients should take the oral iron at least 2 hours after meals. This increases the incidence of patient noncompliance. Intramuscular or intravenous iron may be used when the patient does not tolerate or is noncompliant with oral iron. A test dose of parenteral iron should be administered before using (Amerling & Levin, 1993).

Dietary requirements for other trace elements have not been well defined (Kopple, 1994). Supplementation of the diet with 15 mg zinc per day may improve dysgeusia (abnormal tastes), poor food intake, and impaired sexual function in some uremic patients (Ahmed & Kopple, 1994; Kopple, 1994). Increased body aluminum levels have been noted when patients are dialyzing without water purification systems or with high doses of aluminum-containing antacids. Elevated serum levels have been associated with anemia, osteomalacia, and dementia. Therefore, use of aluminum-based antacids is discouraged (Schmitt, 1991).

Protein and Energy

Protein intake must meet nutritional needs and compensate for any losses. Excessive intake enhances production of nitrogenous toxins while inadequate intake promotes protein malnutrition. Amino acid and protein losses occur with dialysis requiring a higher intake than needed for healthy adults. During HD, amino acid losses may exceed 10 grams per treatment (Ahmed & Kopple, 1994; American Dietetic Association, 1994; Kopple, 1994). With CAPD and CCPD, both amino acids and albumin are lost across the peritoneal capillary membranes. Of the 4-15 grams lost daily, 50-80% is as albumin. Recommendations have been established at 1.0 to 1.4 g/kg body weight for patients on HD and 1.2-1.5 g/kg body weight for patients on CAPD and CCPD (American Dietetic Association, 1993).

Quality of protein to meet EAA requirements is also important. Two-thirds of protein should be from HBV sources to assure that minimal EAA requirements are met (American Dietetic Association, 1993; Maroni, 1993). A strict vegan (plant products only) vegetarian diet has been difficult to plan using these guidelines. Dietitians generally work with combinations of legumes and soy products (Pagenkemper, 1995). The dietitian may recommend the use of calorically dense nondairy nutritional supplements added to a patient's usual intake to enhance vegan diets and to assure that all the EAA are provided.

Energy requirements for patients undergoing maintenance HD are not well defined. Adequate energy must be supplied to prevent protein from being used for energy. This is referred to as "protein-sparing." Also, a wasting syndrome that often accompanies dialysis has been identified (Kopple, 1994). Weight maintenance may be attained with 30-35 kilocalories (kcal)/kg body weight per day for hemodialysis in most patients while 35-50 kcal/kg body weight per day will allow for weight gain (Ahmed & Kopple, 1994; Kopple, 1994).

For CAPD and CCPD patients, energy requirements are complicated by the use of dextrose as an osmotic agent in the PD fluids (Ahmed & Kopple, 1994). Total energy intake recommended should include both the oral and the dialysate content. Grodstein et al. (1981) proposed the following formula to calculate calories from absorbed dextrose:

$$Y=[(11.3\,X)-10.9] \times L \text{ dialysate} \times 3.7 \text{ kcal/g glucose}$$

where Y is the grams glucose absorbed per liter of dialysate and X is the concentration of glucose (g/L). As much as 60-80% (100-250 g) of the dialysate dextrose can be absorbed and may account for more than one-third of the patient's daily caloric needs (VonBaeyer, Gahl, Riedinger et al., 1983). It was initially thought that this extra energy source would aid the nutritionally compromised patient. However, there appears to be a spontaneous decrease in patients' intake in response to the dextrose load, precluding desired weight gains or reversals of malnutrition (Bouma & Dwyer, 1984; Grodstein, Blumenkrantz, Kopple et al., 1981). Conversely, restriction of calories for weight reduction or weight maintenance in patients who are prone to obesity is complicated with high protein needs (Bodnar, Kovach, Vidt, 1982; VonBaeyer, Gahl, Rideinger et al., 1983). In these patients, the dietitian often recommends the use of protein supplements to help replace protein losses but adding only minimal calories. The entire renal team can work together to encourage increased physical activity to prevent or help treat undesired weight gain.

Patients who have inadequate intake of protein and calories show a decrease in blood urea nitrogen (BUN), low serum proteins, particularly albumin, transferrin and prealbumin, and a low protein catabolic rate (pcr) (Acchiardo, Moore & Latour, 1983). In stable patients, the pcr reflects dietary protein intake.

Hyperlipidemia and Carnitine

Hyperlipidemia is a problem in many forms of renal disease (Appel, 1991). More patients are reported to die of coronary artery disease than of any other renal complication. Patients undergoing dialysis have increased levels of serum triglycerides, low-density lipoproteins (LDL), very low density lipoproteins (VLDL), and decreased levels of high-density lipoproteins (HDL) (Haffner, Gruber, Aldrete, 1992). These lipid abnormalities may be due to a defect or decrease in lipoprotein lipase (Wanner, Frommherz, & Horl, 1991). There is some evidence that dietary intervention can alter the lipid profile of these patients (Cattran, Steiner, Fenion, & Ampil, 1980). However, diet does not alter the underlying defect. It may be more prudent to encourage exercise, smoking cessation, and blood pressure control than to restrict dietary intake in a population already overwhelmed with diet limitations.

Carnitine supplementation has been found to be beneficial in treating those hemodialysis patients with hyperlipidemia who also have muscle fatigue associated with the treatment (Zilleruelo, Novak, Hsia et al., 1989). Carnitine, which is required for intramitochondrial transport of fatty acids, is a nitrogenous compound found primarily in muscle tissue (Feller & Rudman, 1988). Humans acquire carnitine either from endogenous biosynthesis or from the consumption of animal products and excrete it via the kidneys. Ascorbic acid, pyridoxine, niacin, and iron act as cofactors in the endogenous production. In HD patients, reduced endogenous synthesis, accelerated loss through dialysis and limited intake may combine to create a conditional essentiality of carnitine.

Studies looking at the effect of carnitine supplementation consistently demonstrate increased plasma and muscle carnitine values (Golper, Wolfson, Ahmad et al., 1990). The studies varied in the routes of carnitine supplementation, in the amounts of supplementation, and in the variables measured (muscle carnitine, free serum carnitine, or acetylcarnitine). The effects of increased carnitine levels on normalizing triglyceride levels were inconsistent. A subgroup of patients with hypertriglyceridemia appear to benefit from pharmacologic doses in the range of 600-2000 mg carnitine per day (Golper, Wolfson, Ahmad et al., 1990). In 1994 a consensus panel of the American Association of Kidney Patients concluded that for patients with carnitine deficiency, 20 mg/kg should be administered intravenously at the end of each dialysis treatment (AAKP Consensus Group, 1994).

Nutrition and Transplant

Nutritional management of the adult renal transplant patient has recently been reviewed (Pagenkemper & Foulks, 1991). The number of patients waiting to receive transplants each year far exceeds the number of donors available (The National Institute of Diabetes and Digestive and Kidney Disease, 1994). Patients have been subjected to the metabolic and nutritional consequences produced by CRF and dialysis. The posttransplantation period imposes further nutritional demands by the combined metabolic stresses of surgery and high-dose immunosuppressive therapy using corticosteroid and cyclosporine medications. Common nutritional problems include protein hypercatabolism and gluconeogenesis, obesity, steroid-induced diabetes, and hyperlipidemia (Beto, 1995; Pagenkemper & Foulks, 1991). Presurgical malnutrition, either obesity or undernutrition, has been associated with increased risk for postsurgical complications. Weight reduction should be undertaken by obese patients to decrease the surgical risk of transplant.

The immediate goal after surgery is to offset the effects of protein catabolism. Investigators have shown that positive nitrogen balance may occur when daily protein intake is 1.3 to 1.5 g/kg and the diet contains adequate calories (Pagenkemper & Foulks, 1991). It is believed that 28 to 35 kcal/kg per day are adequate. After approximately 1 month, protein can be normalized to a moderate level of about one g/kg per day with sufficient calories to attain or maintain ideal body weight. The hyperlipidemia responds to a fat content of 35% or less of total energy intake and 300 mg cholesterol or less daily.

Mineral metabolism is affected by transplantation. Calcium-phosphorus homeostasis is affected by previous renal insufficiency; glucocorticoid therapy, which acts synergistically with hyperparathyroidism; and incomplete restoration of normal renal function by the transplant (Pagenkemper & Foulks, 1991). Patients require at least 1500 mg calcium and 1200-1500 mg phosphorus intake daily. Occurrence of hyperkalemia in the acute period may occur secondary to cyclosporine therapy. Those patients require dietary potassium restrictions of 50-100 mEq (2000-4000 mg) daily. In an attempt to limit fluid retention, sodium may be limited also to 90-180 mEq (2000-4000 mg) daily in the acute postoperative phase.

Zinc status has been studied in transplant patients since candidates frequently present with abnormal zinc metabolism (Sandstead, 1980; Mahajan, Abraham, Migdal et al., 1984). In a study by Mahajan et al., patients with documented zinc deficiencies showed persistent hyperzincuria and zinc depletion until 1 year posttransplantation (Mahajan, Abraham, Migdal et al., 1984). Due to the active role zinc plays in wound healing, zinc supplements may be indicated in patients who have wound complications (American Dietetic Association, 1994).

Most studies of vitamin status in transplant patients were completed before cyclosporine was available, and patients were given higher doses of corticosteroids than is the current practice (American Dietetic Association, 1994). Those studies show that the serum levels of vitamin A decreased after surgery but remained high for more than 2 years after transplantation (Kelleher, Humphrey, Homer et al., 1983). Thus supplementation with vitamin A is not recommended. However, deficiencies in pyridoxine (vitamin B_6) and folate also persisted after transplantation. Supplementation to RDA levels is recommended (American Dietetic Association, 1994).

Nutritional Assessment

The renal dietitian assesses the patient's current nutritional status before recommending an appropriate diet. The assessment includes a medical and nutritional history, anthropometric measurements, biochemical measurements, and examination for clinical signs and symptoms of malnutrition (see Figure 11-1) (Blumenkranz, Kopple, Gutman et al., 1980).

History

The medical history focuses on preexisting illnesses, any gastrointestinal dysfunction, and current medications. The nutritional history reveals the patient's past weight history, previous diets, food intake patterns, food preferences, and the use of nutritional supplements. Family support and structure, living arrangements, type of food preparation and by whom, socio-economic status, and away-from-home dining patterns are all important factors in maintaining good dietary management

Figure 11-1
Nutrition intake evaluation. Basal energy expenditure is 1006 kcal/day based on a weight of 45.0 kg.

NUTRITION ASSESSMENT

Name:

Patient: #2215-1T

Date: 04/22/91

CASE/DATA SUMMARY
Pt. is a 74 Y/O female who has a long hx of renal insufficiency, maintained on hemodialysis for the past 4 1/2 years, and hypertension. She was hospitalized in March of this year with cardiogenic pulmonary edema, pleural effusions, and fluid overload. Pt has a hx of mild hypoxic brain damage secondary to shock with near cardiorespiratory arrest due to intraabdominal vascular hemorrhage in 1987.

Since pt's most recent hospitalization, pt has had a poor appetite and wt loss. Pt's account of food intake, reflecting 40.5 protein and 620 kcals is probably inaccurate.

Demographics
Ht= 57.5 cm (62.0 in)
Wt=45.0 kg (99.0 lb)
Age=74 years
Female
Usual wt=49.5 kg (108.0 lb)
(Done 12/18/90)
(Time=4.1 months)
Wt/Ht=54.9 kg (120.8 lb)

Anthropometrics
TSF=13.0 mm
MAC=26.0 cm
NAMC=21.9 cm
% WBC=21200/cubic mm
TTL lymph=636.0

Laboratory
Albumin=2.60 gm/dl
Trnsfrn=166.0 mg/dl
% lymph=3.0%

Clinical
Prot. intake=61.5 gm
Cal intake=1483.0 kcal
Nonprot kcal/gm NIT=126

MALNUTRITION STATUS CRITERIA

MILD	MODERATE	SEVERE
%Wt/Ht 82=(90-80%)	% Wt loss 9 (8.6-10%)	Clinical/Physical
%MAC 87 (90-80%)	Albumin 2.6 (2.1-2.9 gm%)	%TSF 54 (<60%)
	Trnsfrn 166.0 (150-179 mg%)	TTL Lymph 636 (<800)

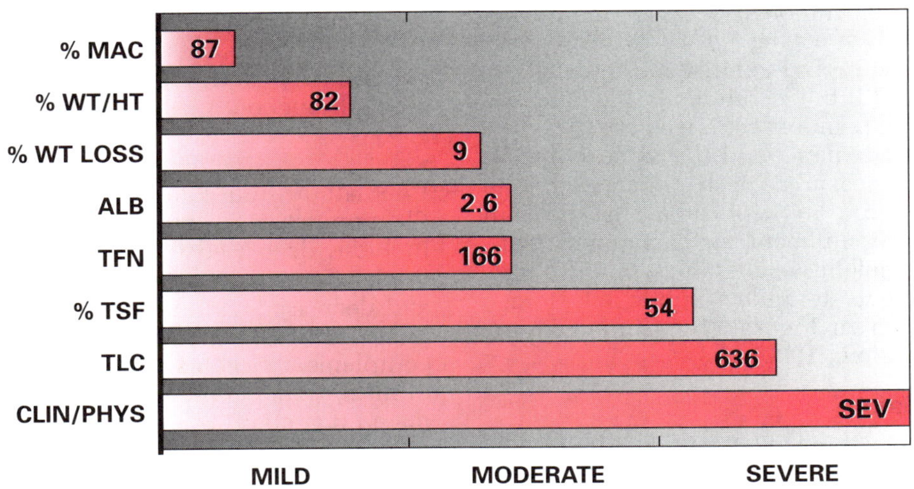

Figure 11-2
Serial measurements of a patient's triceps skinfold using a calibrated skinfold caliper while she was receiving total parenteral nutrition (TNP) before and after a surgical procedure.

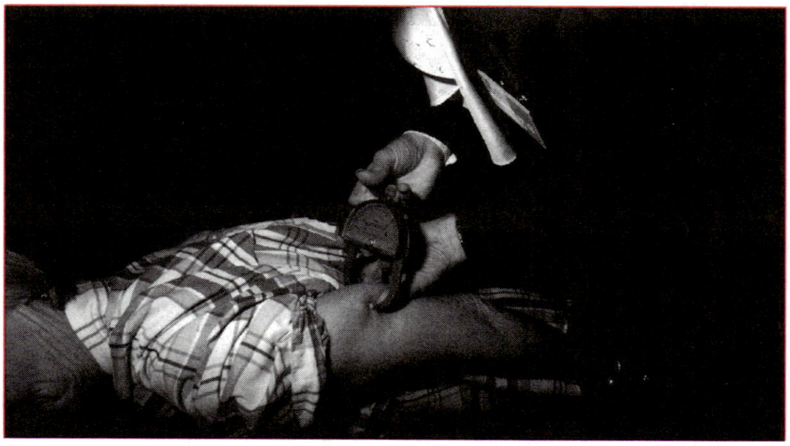

and good nutritional status.

Anthropometric Measurements

Anthropometric measurements refer to body measurements used by the nutritionist to assess skeletal reserves of muscle and fat. These may be as simple as height and weight or may involve the use of a skinfold caliper to measure subcutaneous fat stores (see Figure 11-2). The patient's height should be measured at the time of nutritional assessment. The patient's weight will be compared with the desirable weight for height and usual body weight. If the patient has lost weight, the dietitian uses the rate of loss to ascertain its severity (Blumenkranz, Kopple, Gutman et al., 1980; Grant & DeHoog, 1991).

The dietitian may use a skinfold caliper to measurement subcutaneous fat, most commonly at the midpoint between the acromial process of the scapula and the olecranon process of the elbow. Skinfold thickness must be measured in a standardized way. The reproducibility of the measurements is improved if the technique is standardized rigorously, with the same experienced observer performing all measurements and the same point on the skin being measured each time. Each site should be measured in triplicate. The dietitian compares the measurement with national standards, similar to height-weight tables, but also uses serial measurements to reflect subtle fat storage changes as shown in Figure 11-3 (Blumenkranz, Kopple, Gutman et al., 1980).

Biochemical Data

The biochemical data gives the dietitian information about the patient's nutritional status as well as disease state. Patients who are protein malnourished, or who are protein and calorie malnourished, will have depleted levels of serum proteins. Poor albumin status has been associated with increased incidence of morbidity and mortality and is, therefore, used as a primary indicator of protein status (Acchiardo, Moore & Latour, 1983; Grant & DeHoog, 1991). Levels of 35 mmol/L (3.5 g/dl) or lower are diagnostic of poor protein status. Albumin has a half-life ($t_{1/2}$) of 18-21 days. Proteins which have shorter half lives, such as transferrin with a $t_{1/2}$ of 8-10 days or with a prealbumin with a $t_{1/2}$ may be used to reflect acute changes or to detect improvements during repletion (Grant & DeHoog, 1991).

Devine et al. demonstrated that CRF patients are at greatest risk for malnutrition and weight loss at the initiation of maintenance dialytic therapy (Devine, 1994). The patient's nutritional status at that time is a good predictor of long-range nutritional status, beyond 2-3 years of therapy. Thus, a good nutritional assessment with appropriate intervention may contribute to the patient's overall well being throughout therapy.

Malnutrition and Dialysis

Malnutrition continues to plague the HD and PD populations. Evidence of wasting syndrome includes decreased relative body weight, skinfold thickness, arm muscle mass, total body nitrogen, and decreased serum concentrations of many proteins, including albumin, transferrin, and certain complement proteins. Most patients show evidence of mild to moderate malnutrition, but Kopple estimated that about 8% have evidence of severe malnutrition (Kopple, 1994). Many studies have shown that low albumin levels are associated with increased hospitalizations among dialysis patients

Figure 11-3
Measurement of a patient's triceps skinfold thickness using a calibrated skinfold caliper.

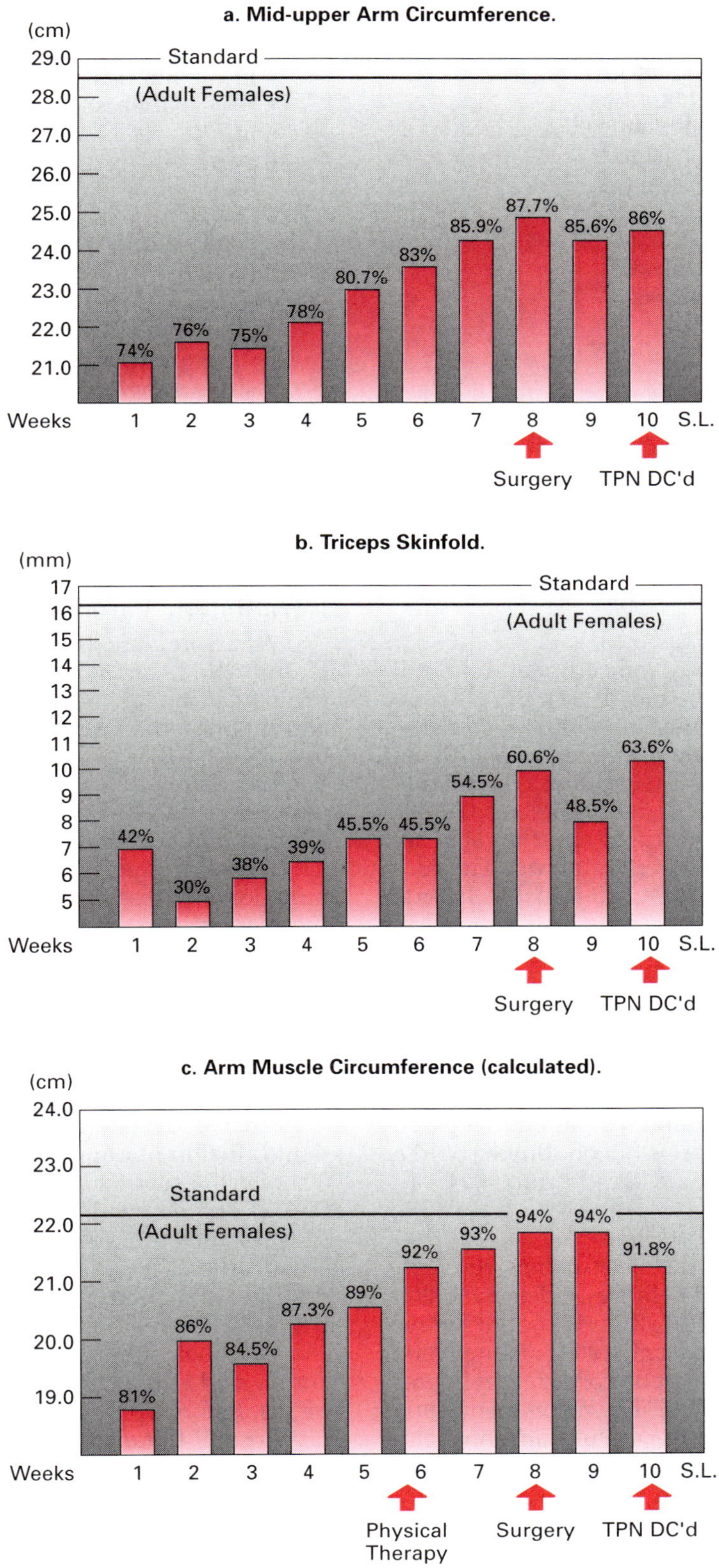

Table 11-2
Causative factors in the occurrence of malnutrition in ESRD.

I.	**Abnormal metabolic processes**
	Altered metabolism of glucose, protein and energy
	Enhanced protein catabolic rate
	Altered hormonal systems
II.	**Decreased oral intake/anorexia**
	loss of appetite, taste changes
	fatigue, anemia, sleeplessness
	pain, discomfort, early satiety
	depression, frequent hospitalizations
	uremia, inadequate dialysis
III.	**Gastrointestinal disease**
	Diarrhea or constipation
	Gastric paresis
	Medication effects
IV.	**Other**
	Nutrient losses
	Drug / nutrient interactions
	Coexistent chronic diseases

Note: Devine, 1994; Kaminski et al., 1991; Schmitt, 1991)

and increased incidences of morbidity and mortality (Acchiardo, Moore & Latour, 1983). In one study of patients in each treatment modality, Jacob et al. found the intake of protein and energy insufficient in HD patients and the intake of protein insufficient in CAPD patients (Jacob, Boyle, Wild et al., 1992).

The causes of malnutrition in the HD and CAPD population are many (Acchiardo, Moore, & Latour, 1983; Devine, 1994; Kaminski, Lowrie, Rosenblatt, & Haase, 1991). These are summarized in Table 11-2. Problems unique to the CAPD patient population predispose patients to poor nutritional states. These include abdominal distention, problems with gastric emptying, increased intraperitoneal pressure, and decreased appetite secondary to absorption of glucose from the dialysate solution. In turn, lack of appetite deprives patients of essential noncarbohydrate calories (Jacob, Boyle, Wild et al., 1992; Smathers, Moles, & Sandroni, 1992).

Nutritional Supplementation

To increase protein and energy in diets, dietitians increase the proportion of calorically dense foods in patients' diets. Frequently, this is not effective. Smathers, Moles, and Sandroni (1992) demonstrated that protein malnutrition can be corrected by aggressive nutritional intervention. They recommend serial nutrition assessments and the use of nutritional supplements to detect and treat protein malnutrition. Using calorically dense liquid supplements or modular protein powder supplements, 54% of the patients had improved serum albumin levels.

For a program to be successful, it must be easy and inexpensive for the patients. The dietitian can coordinate and facilitate this process. Some suggestions as to how this can be done are:

- Review nutritional parameters of all patients monthly and identify patients at risk.
- Educate patients on importance of nutrition in maintaining muscle and immune status.
- Give patients copies of their monthly albumin levels and weight changes.
- Work with usual food intake to increase protein and/or energy intake.
- Allow only 1 month of continued poor indicators before starting oral nutritional supplements.
- Serve as a liaison between the patients and the company providing the products by negotiating lower prices, helping to place orders, and arranging to have the product delivered without shipping charges.
- Follow the patients closely to see that they are using the supplement.
- When necessary, involve the patient's family members to assure follow-through by the patients.

Intradialytic Parenteral Nutrition (IDPN)

When oral means are unsuccessful in correcting malnutrition, more aggressive and more costly means can be taken by implementing intravenous administration of macronutrients during dialysis treatment (IDPN) (Bilbrey & Cohen, 1989; Bruno, Bagnis, Marangella et al., 1989). Studies of malnourished HD patients show an overall improvement in patient well-being when treated with IDPN. IDPN is an anabolic therapy. It repletes the patient nutritionally, creates a positive nitrogen balance in the patient, and enables the patient to restore adequate oral nutrient intake. It provides an effective alternative therapy for those HD patients who have not responded to, or are not candidates for, oral or enteral nutritional therapy and cannot tolerate the fluid load of traditional parenteral nutrition (Goldstein & Strom, 1991).

Most dialysis centers contract with an outpatient infusion pharmacy to manage IDPN. (Table 11-3 shows the suggested administration procedure for IDPN.) The nurses in the clinic infuse the formula directly into the venous drip chamber of the HD blood line. The infusion rate is determined by dividing the total IDPN solution volume by the patient's HD treatment time. Generally it will not exceed 350 ml/hr. It is common to start with 500 ml amino acid and dextrose solution for the three treatments. Before lipids are started, nurses administer a test dose. If there are no side effects, lipids may be used in the solution thereafter. Lipids increase the calorie content of the solution dramatically. Nurses should take the solution out of the refrigerator in time for it to come to room temperature (about 30

Table 11-3
Suggested administration procedure for IDPN.

1. Set up dialysis equipment per standard protocol of the clinic.
2. Set up IV pump and prime administration set and filter per pump instructions.
3. Set the transmembrane pressure (TMP) to remove the usual amount of fluid (based on the patient's weight gain) plus the amount of fluid in the parenteral nutrient solution.
4. Adjust blood level in venous drip chamber slightly higher than normal.
5. Depending upon the type of venous chamber used, the pumpset may be connected to the venous drip chamber by one of the following methods:
   a. For venous drip chambers having a pressure monitoring line, a level adjustment line and a needle injection port, connect the pumpset directly to the medication line.
   b. For venous drip chambers having a pressure monitoring line, a level adjustment line, and a needle injection port, connect the pumpset to the medication injection port using an 18 or 19 gauge needle.
   c. For venous drip chambers having only a pressure monitoring line and a level adjustment line, connect the pumpset to the level adjustment line.
      (1) If an adjustment of the venous drip chamber level is needed, temporarily clamp the venous positive pressure monitoring line.
      (2) Disconnect the line at the filter protecting the venous pressure gauge.
      (3) Attach a syringe to the line, unclamp the line and adjust the chamber to the desired level.
      (4) Reclamp the line, remove the syringe and reattach the line to the filter protecting the venous pressure monitoring gauge.
      (5) Unclamp the line and readjust the pressure limits.
6. Set the volume limit dial on the IV pump to coincide with the volume of the IDPN solution, e.g., 500 ml, 750 ml or 1000 ml.
7. Set the administration rate to deliver the entire volume over the course of the hemodialysis treatment. For example, if the solution volume is 500 ml and the dialysis treatment is to last 3 hours, the rate would be 166 ml/hr (500 ml divided by 3 hrs).
8. Once dialysis is initiated, turn on IV pump to begin nutrient infusion.
9. If lipids are prescribed, on the 4th treatment day a test dose is required. A modified test dose for the 3-in-1 formulation may be administered as follows:
   a. Set the rate at Ω the final rate.
   b. Infuse for 15 minutes.
   c. If no reaction is observed, increase infusion to the desired rate for the remainder of therapy.
   d. If an allergic reaction is observed, STOP THE INFUSION IMMEDIATELY. Notify the physician and the pharmacy. Start a lipid-free formula with the next dialysis treatment.
   e. If the patient should have an anaphylactic reaction, follow the procedures of the dialysis clinic in treating anaphylactic reactions.

Note: Copyright Option Care, Inc., 1991. Used with permission.

minutes) and check the labels for dates and names to make sure the solution is current and is being given to the appropriate patient (Nicholson, 1990).

Most patients handle the formula without difficulty. There are some side effects such as hyperglycemia, hypoglycemia, fluid overload, and a reaction to the lipids. Lipids should not be given to patients who report an egg allergy. If a reaction is going to occur, it is usually observed within the first 15-30 minutes after the test dose is administered. Symptoms observed include chest and back pain, dyspnea, dizziness, headache, nausea, and pressure over the eyes. Patients may experience wheezing, stridor, cyanosis, diaphoresis, fever, flushing,

Table 11-4
Comparison of treatments and major concerns for pre-ESRD, hemodialysis, and peritoneal dialysis patients.

	Pre-ESRD	Hemodialysis	CAPD or CCPD*
Treatment	Diet and medications	Diet and medications Hemodialysis	Diet and medications Peritoneal dialysis
Modality	Dialysis using vascular access for waste products and fluid removal	Dialysis using peritoneal membrane for waste product and fluid removal	
Duration	Indefinite	3-5 h 2-3 d/wk	3-5 exchanges 7 d/wk
Concerns	Glomerular hyperfiltration; rise in BUN*; bone disease Hypertension; glycemic control in diabetes	Amino acid loss; interdialytic electrolyte and fluid changes Bone disease; hypertension	Protein loss into dialysate; glucose absorption from dialysate Bone disease; weight gain; hyperlipidemia; glycemic control in diabetes
*CAPD, continuous ambulatory peritoneal dialysis. CCPD, continuous cyclic peritoneal dialysis. BUN, blood urea nitrogen.			

Note: From American Diatetic Association [ADA]. (1993). National renal diet: Professional guide. Chicago: Author. Reprinted with permission.

hypotension, or tachycardia. If a reaction is observed, stop the infusion immediately and alert the pharmacy (Nicholson, 1990; Powers, 1990).

Due to the high cost of IDPN and the CRF program, and with 93% of dialysis patients in the United States on the Medicare program, this therapy has been controversial. Foulks et al. suggest that IDPN (1) be reserved for malnourished patients who have not responded to intensive dietary counseling or oral supplementation and (2) be administered for a minimum of 3 months (Foulks, Goldstein, Kelly & Hunt, 1991). Current Medicare coverage dictates that patients meet the requirements for medical necessity. The policy, founded in the Medicare prosthetic device benefit, assumes that provision of parenteral nutrition administered only during dialysis would rarely be medically necessary. The nutrition assessment must show that the patient is severely malnourished, unable to absorb nutrients taken orally, and must pass the test of permanence (require treatment for a minimum of 3 months) (Medicare/Medicaid, 1990).

Intraperitoneal Nutrition (IPN)

Nutritional dialysates, or IPN, have been shown to have positive effects in PD patients. These dialysates substitute amino acids for dextrose as the osmotic agent for one or two exchanges a day. Many studies have demonstrated that amino acid-based dialysates are safe and effective. Amino acids were first infused into the peritoneum in 1968 (Goldstein & Strom, 1991). In 1982, investigators reported an 80-90% absorption of amino acids after a 6-hour dwell of a 2 liter, 2% amino acid solution. This equaled 32-36 grams of amino acids. Bruno et al, documented an increased nitrogen balance after using a 1% amino acid solution once a day for 6 months (Wise, 1993). Compatibility of medications added to IPN depend on concentration of the mixture, length of storage, contact, and existence of other additives. Those medications that can be added safely to PD solutions are also compatible

Table 11-5
General diet recommendations for renal patients.*

Treatment	Pre-ESRD	Hemodialysis	Peritoneal Dialysis
Protein (g/kg IBW)	0.6-0.8 †	1.1-1.4	1.2-1.5
Nephrotic Syndrome	0.8-1.0		
Energy (kcal/kg IBW)‡	35-40	30-35	25-35
Phosphorus (mg/kg IBW)	8-12§	≤17II	≤17II
Sodium (mg/d)	1000-3000 if necessary	2000-3000	2000-4000
Potassium (mg/kg IBW)	Typically unrestricted	approximately 40	Typically unrestricted
Fluid(mL/d)	Typically unrestricted	500-750 + daily urine output *or* 1000 mL if anuric	2000+
Calcium (kg IBW)	1200-1600	Depends on serum level	Depends on serum level

* See specific guidelines for each treatment modality.
† The upper end of this range is preferred for diabetes and malnourished patients.
‡ See guidelines for estimation energy needs based on weight and activity level on this page.
§ Whereas 5-10 mg/kg IBW is frequently cited in the scientific literature, 5 mg/kg IBW is practical only when used in conjunction with a very low protein diet supplemented with amino acids or ketoacid analogs.
II A diet that is higher in protein may make it impossible to meet the optimum phosphorous prescription.

Note: From American Diatetic Association [ADA]. (1993). National renal diet: Professional guide. Chicago: Author. Reprinted with permission.

with the IN solution. This technique may increase in use as CAPD and CCPD use are increased.

Patient Education

The renal diet, with its combination of nutritional parameters, presents a major challenge to a renal dietitian. Nutrition education and counseling are essential aspects of medical management of the renal patient. Dietitians must balance the need to limit intake of nutrients with the need to provide adequate energy and protein to maintain or restore good nutritional health (*Journal of the American Dietetic Association*, 1993). They must consider the effect of the diet on the treatment or prevention of metabolic problems associated with renal dysfunction, including osteodystrophy, anemia, hyperlipidemia, hypertension, and malnutrition. These factors, coupled with the specific nutrient requirements and limitations of the treatment modality, further complicate the renal diet. The underlying

Table 11-6
Diet instruction modules and expected patient outcome criteria.

Instruction Module	Patient Outcome Criteria
A. Kidney function and changes with failure	Increased dietary compliance
B. Protein and calories	Maintained BUN of 40-100 mg/dl Maintained Albumin of >3.8 g/dl Dry weight within desirable range
C. Potassium (K)	Serum K within a range of 3.5-6.0 mEq/L
D. Sodium and fluid	Interdialytic fluid gains of 1-2.5 kg
E. Calcium and phosphorus	Maintain serum phosphorus of <6.5 mg/dl Maintain serum calcium of 9.5-11 mg/dl Maintain desirable PTH level
F. Vitamins	Demonstrate daily renal vitamin use

disease process may also need to be considered, and the most common cause of CRF is diabetes (The National Institute of Diabetes and Digestive and Kidney Disease, 1994). Similarly, analyses of the annually compounded change in CRF incidence for the years 1986-88 versus 1989-91 show that the largest increase has been among the elderly of over 75 years of age. Also, Asian/Pacific Islanders, Native Americans, and black Americans have shown higher annualized increases than white Americans (Devine, 1994).

When faced with the complexity and many restrictions of the renal diet, patients and their families frequently have difficulty making the adjustments and experience confusion, frustration, depression, and anxiety. Nutrition practitioners play a crucial role in helping patients learn to cope with changing lifelong habits. They attempt to keep individuals' food habits as close to normal as possible, and they strive to meet their individual needs, tastes, and lifestyles.

Cultural Diversity

With a rise in the number of culturally diverse dialysis clinics, health care practitioners have had to sensitize themselves to variations in the types of food important to their patients. Many resources are available to dietitians. Dietitians in Northern California have published a guide that has information specific to eight different cultures represented in their areas: Asian, Indian, African-American, Chinese-American, Filipino-American, Japanese-American, Mexican-American, and Southeast Asian (Patel & Denny, 1988). Other dietitians have compiled information and recipe books specific to their needs, including Mexican-American, Cuban-American, Caribbean, Cajun-Creole, Jewish, Navajo, Japanese, and Chinese. Abstracts of available literature as well as information on attaining them are available elsewhere (American Dietetic Association, 1993).

The National Renal Diet

The National Renal Diet offers standardized guidelines for nutrition intervention and patient education in renal disease (Sherman, Hwang, Bernold, & Eisinger, 1986). The Renal Dietitian Dietetic group of the American Dietetic Association and the National Kidney Foundation on Renal Nutrition collaborated to develop a Professional Guide for renal nutritionists and patient education tools consisting of six brochures. Major concerns of three treatment modalities for adults and a summary of the diet recommendations are shown in Tables 11-4 and 11-5.

The patient booklets offer food lists for patients with renal insufficiency, on peritoneal dialysis, and on hemodialysis. In addition, separate calculation figures and food lists were devised for patients with diabetes receiving each treatment modality. The food groups were based on nutrient content from the United States Department of Agriculture and current data from manufacturers of brand-name products in the nutrient database compiled by Case Western Reserve University. All six diet plans were designed to be low in saturated fat but not necessarily low in total fat.

Teaching the Renal Diet

To counsel patients in making dietary adjustments, the dietitian needs to have a thorough understanding of the patient's present eating habits, needed dietary modifications, and nutritional content of foods, as well as the patient's adjustment to the process of CRF. The predialysis period is an ideal time to start counseling and educational intervention (American Dietetic Association, 1993). The process should be gradual and ongoing. Instructions should be simple and concise, teaching the diet one step at a time with built-in opportunity for patient feedback. Instruction can be broken down into modules as shown in Table 11-6 (Gentry, 1981; Moore, Ecklund, Trommeter, & Bohac, 1988). Patients should be taught the best way to cope with typical real-life situations, such as dining out, eating fast foods, and coping with holidays. Dietitians who work closely with patients teach them not only about food lists and dietary restrictions, but also about how the renal diet can help manage their disease and improve their sense of well-being (Dolecek, Olson, Caggiula, et al., 1995).

Summary

The renal diet is an integral component of the patient's overall treatment. The diet is complex, and the challenge of caring for these patients continues to grow with advances in research and technology. Guidelines of dietary modifications are available for nutrition practitioners working with this patient population (American Dietetic Association, 1993; American Dietetic Association, 1994). Limiting the intake of potassium, sodium, fluid, phosphorus, and protein is frequently the main emphasis in nutritional counseling. It is vitally important, however, for the dietitian to closely monitor patients' nutritional status and intervene as needed by the appropriate means.

Treatment of CRF patients requires an entire team of health care professionals. The dietitian is a vital component of this team. Studies show that patients have fewer complications requiring hospitalization and have improved compliance when dietitians spend more time in patient contact (minimum of 30 minutes per patient per week). The MDRD study further found that greater time is required when working with patients who have fewer years of formal education (Journal of the American Dietitian Association, 1993).

Living with chronic renal disease presents daily challenges, and the renal diet is neither simple to follow nor free of adverse side effects. Studies show that patient's compliance is poor, showing good compliance to be about 25% of patients and bad compliance about 40% (American Dietetic Association, 1994). Participation of all renal care team members is required to encourage and support patients in their struggle to survive CRF, and good communication among team members increases their effectiveness. Renal dietitians and nephrology nurses who work closely with patients to help them manage their diet, disease, and treatment and to mesh nutritional requirements with lifestyle needs offer both hope and health to persons with chronic renal failure.

References

AAKP Consensus Group. (1994). Role of L carnitine in treating renal dialysis patients. *Dialysis & Transplantation, 23,* 177-181.

Acchiardo, S.R., Moore, L.W., & Latour, P.A. (1983). Malnutrition as the main factor in morbidity and mortality in hemodialysis patients. *Kidney International, 24* (Supp. 16), S199-S203.

Ahmed, K., & Kopple, J.D. (1994). Nutritional management of renal disease. In A. Greenberg (Ed.), *Primer on kidney diseases* (pp. 287-293). Boston: Academic Press.

American Dietetic Association [ADA]. (1993). *National renal diet: Professional guide.* Chicago: American Dietetic Association.

American Dietetic Association [ADA], Renal Dietitians Dietetic Practice Group. (1994). *Nutrition care in endstage renal disease* (2nd ed.). Chicago: American Dietetic Association.

Amerling, R., & Levin, N.W. (1993). Erythropoietin update. *The Kidney, 26*(1), 18.

Anon, B. (1993). Meeting the challenge of the renal diet: A preview of the National Renal Diet educational series. *Journal of the American Dietetic Association, 93,* 637-639.

Appel, G. (1991). Lipid abnormalities in renal disease. *Kidney International, 39,* 169-183.

Bansal, V.K. (1992). Potassium metabolism in renal failure: Nondietary rationale for hyperkalemia. *Journal of Renal Nutrition, 2* (Supp. 1), 812.

Beto, J.A. (1995). Which diet for which renal failure: Making sense of the options. *Journal of the American Dietetic Association, 95,* 898-903.

Beto, J., & Bansal, V.K. (1992). Hyperkalemia: Evaluating dietary and nondietary etiology. *Journal of Renal Nutrition, 2,* 28-29.

Bilbrey, G.L., & Cohen, T.L. (1989). Identification and treatment of protein calorie malnutrition in chronic hemodialysis patients. *Dialysis & Transplantation, 18,* 669-700.

Blumenkrantz, M.J., Kopple, J.D., Gutman, R.A., Chan, Y.K., Barbour, G.L., Roberts, C., Shen, F.H., Gandhi, V.C., Tucker, C.T., Curtis, F.K., & Coburn, J.W. (1980). Methods for assessing nutritional status of patients with renal failure. *American Journal of Clinical Nutrition, 33,* 1567-1585.

Bodnar, D., Kovach, K.M., & Vidt, D. (1982). Incidence of obesity after six months on CAPD. CRN *Quarterly, 6,* 13-14.

Bouma, S.F., & Dwyer, J.T. (1984). Glucose absorption and weight change in 18 months of continuous ambulatory peritoneal dialysis. *Journal of the American Dietetic Association, 84,* 194-197.

Briggs, J.P., & Schnermann, J.B. (1994). Overview of renal function. In A. Greenberg (Ed.), *Primer on kidney diseases* (pp. 1-16). Boston: Academic Press.

Bruno, M., Bagnis, C., Marangella, M., Rovera, L., Cantaluppi, A., & Linari, F. (1989). CAPD with an amino acid dialysis solution: A long-term, crossover study. *Kidney International, 35,* 1189-1194.

Cattran, D.C., Steiner, G., Fenion, S.S.A., & Ampil, M. (1980). Dialysis hyperlipemia: Response to dietary manipulation. *Clinical Nephrology, 13,* 177-182.

Chan, R., Gleim, G.W., DeVita, M.V., Zabetakis, P.M., & Michelis,

M.F. (1993). Effects of oral vs. intravenous calcitriol on serum parathyroid hormone levels in chronic hemodialysis patients. *Dialysis & Transplantation, 22,* 736-744.

Devine, W. (1994). Review of nutritional status and diet in dialysis and renal transplant patients. *Dialysis & Transplantation, 23*(1), 3848.

Dolecek, T.A., Olson, M.B., Caggiula, A.W., Dwyer, J.T., Milas, N.C., Gillis, B.P., Hartman, J.A., & DiChiro, J.T. (1995). Registered dietitian time requirements in the Modification of Diet in Renal Disease Study. *Journal of the American Dietetic Association, 95,* 1307-1312.

Dworkin, L.D. (1994). Progression of chronic renal disease. In A. Greenberg, (Ed.), *Primer on kidney diseases* (pp. 276-281). Boston: Academic Press.

Feller, A.G., & Rudman, D. (1988). Role of carnitine ir human nutrition. *Journal of Nutrition, 118,* 541-547.

Foulks, C.J., Goldstein, D.J., Kelly, M.P., & Hunt, J.M. (1991). Indications for the use of intradialytic parenteral nutrition in the malnourished hemodialysis patient. *Journal of Renal Nutrition, 1,* 23-33.

Gentry, S.E. (1981). A modular approach to dialysis patient education. *Dialysis and Transplantation, 10,* 966-968.

Goldstein, J., & Strom, J.A. (1991). Intradialytic parenteral nutrition: Evolution and current concepts. *Journal of Renal Nutrition, 1,* 9-22.

Golper, T.A., Wolfson, M., Ahmad, S., Hirschberg, R., Kurtin, P., Datz, L.A., Nicora, R., Ashbrook, D., & Kopple, J.D. (1990). Multicenter trial of Lcarnitine in maintenance hemodialysis patients. I. Carnitine concentrations and lipid effects. *Kidney International, 38,* 904-911.

Grant, A., & DeHoog, S. (1991). Nutrition assessment and support. Seattle, WA: Authors.

Grodstein, G.P., Blumenkrantz, M.J., Kopple, J.D., Moran, J.K., & Coburn, J.W. (1981). Glucose absorption during continuous ambulatory peritoneal dialysis. *Kidney International, 19,* 564-567.

Haffner, S.M., Gruber, K.K., Aldrete, G., Morales, P.A., Stern, M.P., & Tuttle, K.R. (1991). Increased lipoprotein(a) concentrations in chronic renal failure. *Journal of the American Society of Nephrology, 3,* 1156-1162.

Heidland, A., & Kult, J. (1975). Long-term effects of essential amino acids supplementation in patients on regular dialysis treatment. *Clinical Nephrology, 3,* 234-239.

Jacob, V., Boyle, G., Wild, G., Brown, C.B., Moorhead, P.J., & El Nahas, A.M. (1992). A comparison of nutrition in hemodialysis and continuous ambulatory peritoneal dialysis patients. *Journal of Renal Nutrition, 2*(3) Suppl. 1, 13-17.

Kaminski, M.V., Lowrie, E.G., Rosenblatt, S.G., & Haase, T. (1991). Malnutrition is lethal, diagnosable, and treatable in ESRD patients. *Transplantation Proceedings, 23,* 1810-1815.

Kelleher, J., Humphrey, C.S., Homer, D., Davison, A.M., Giles, G.R., & Losowsky, M.S. (1983). Vitamin A and its transplant proteins in patients with chronic renal failure receiving maintenance haemodialysis and after renal transplantation. *Clinical Science, 65,* 619-626.

Klahr, S., Levey, A.S., Beck, G.J., Caggiula, A.W., Hunsicker, L., Kusek J.W., & Striker, G. (1994). The effects of dietary protein restriction and blood pressure control on the progression of chronic renal disease. *New England Journal of Medicine, 330,* 877-884.

Kopple, J. (1994). Nutrition, diet and the kidney. In M.E. Shils, J.A. Olson, & M. Shike (Eds.), *Modern nutrition in health and disease* (8th ed., pp. 1102-1134). Philadelphia: Lea & Febiger.

Kopple, J., & Blumenkrantz, M.V. (1984). Nutrition in adults on continual peritoneal dialysis. *Perspectives in Peritoneal Dialysis, 2*(1) 19.

Levey, A.S., Gassman, J., Hall, P.M., & Walker, W.E.G. (1991). Assessing the progression of renal disease in clinical studies: Effects of duration of followup and regression to the mean: Modification of Diet in Renal Disease (MDRD) Study Group. *Journal of the American Society of Nephrology, 1,* 1087-1094.

Mahajan, S.K., Abraham, J., Migdal, S.D., AbuHamdan, D.K., & McDonald, F.D. (1984). Effect of renal transplantation on zinc metabolism and taste acuity in uremia. *Transplantation, 38,* 599-602.

Maroni, B.J. (1993). Requirements for protein, calories, and fat in the predialysis patient. In N.A. Mason., & S.M. Boyd (1995). Drug-nutrient interactions in renal failure. *Journal of Renal Nutrition, 5*(4), 214-222.

Massry, S.G., & Kopple, J.D. (1993). Requirements for calcium, phosphorus and vitamin D. In W.E. Mitch & S. Klahr (Eds.), *Nutrition and the kidney* (2nd ed., pp. 96-113). New York: Little, Brown and Company.

May, R.C. (1993). Effect of renal insufficiency on nutrient metabolism and endocrine function. In W.E. Mitch & S. Klahr (Eds.), *Nutrition and the kidney* (2nd ed., pp. 35-60). New York: Little Brown and Company.

Medicare/Medicaid Guide 2. (1990). Provider reimbursement manual, part 1: Section 75987599Z. *Reimbursement for ESRD services and supplies.* Rockville, MD: Department of Health & Human Services.

Mitch, W.E., & Klahr, S. (Eds.). (1993). *Nutrition and the kidney* (2nd ed., pp. 185-212). Boston: Little Brown & Company.

Moore, S., Ecklund, D.K., Trommeter, C., & Bohac, C. (1988). Protocol for nutrition intervention for the adult chronic hemodialysis patient. *Contemporary Dialysis & Nephrology, 8,* 16-50.

Muth, I. (1991). Implications of hypervitaminosis A in chronic renal failure. *Journal of Renal Nutrition, 1,* 28.

Narins, R.G., & Cortes, P. (1994). The role of dietary protein restriction in progressive azotemia. *New England Journal of Medicine, 330,* 929-930.

Nicholson, S. (1990). Intradialytic parenteral nutrition: A nurse's perspective. *Contemporary Dialysis & Nephrology, 11,* 30-33.

Pagenkemper, J. (1995). Planning a vegetarian renal diet. *Journal of Renal Nutrition, 5,* 234-238.

Pagenkemper, J.J., & Foulks, C.J. (1991). Nutritional management of the adult renal transplant patient. *Journal of Renal Nutrition, 1*(3), 119124.

Patel, C., & Denny, M. (1988). *Cultural foods and renal diets for the clinical dietitian and a multilingual guide.* Concord, CA: Council on Renal Nutrition.

Powers, D. (1990). Considerations in the use of 3:1 intradialytic parenteral nutrition solutions containing long-chain triglycerides. *Contemporary Dialysis & Nephrology, 11,* 29-36.

Sandstead, H.H. (1980). Trace elements in uremia and hemodialysis. *American Journal of Clinical Nutrition, 33,* 1501-1508.

Sargent, J.A., & Lowrie, E.G. (1982). Which mathematical model to study uremic toxicity? National Cooperative Dialysis Study. *Clinical Nephrology, 17,* 303-314.

Schmitt, J. (1991). Selecting an appropriate phosphate binder. *Journal of Renal Nutrition, 1,* 38-40.

Sherman, R.A., Hwang, E.R., Bernhold, A.S., & Eisinger, R.P. (1986). Variability in potassium removal by hemodialysis. *American Journal of Nephrology, 6,* 284-288.

Smathers, J.S., Moles, K., & Sandroni, S. (1992). Strategies to improve protein intake in peritoneal dialysis patients. *Journal of Renal Nutrition, 2*(3 Suppl. 1), 33-36.

U.S. Renal Data System [USRDS]. (1994). *USRDS 1994 annual data report.* Bethesda, MD: National Institutes of Health, National Institute of Diabetes and Digestive and Kidney Disease.

Von Baeyer, H., Gahl, G.M., Riedinger, H., Borowzak, R., Averdunk, R., & Kessel, M. (1983). Adaptation of CAPD patients to continuous peritoneal energy uptake. *Kidney International, 23,* 29-34.

Wanner, C., Frommherz, K., & Horl, W.H. (1991). Hyperlipoproteinemia in chronic renal failure: Pathophysiological and therapeutic aspects. *Cardiology, 78,* 202-217.

Wise, C. (1993). Preventive nutritional intervention in peritoneal dialysis. *Contemporary Dialysis & Nephrology, 13,* 27-32.

Chapter Highlights

- Patients require nutrition intervention in virtually all stages of the renal disease process and in conjunction with all treatment modalities.
- Nutrition intervention in renal disease and treatment slows progression of renal failure, compensates for impaired renal function and/or limitations of treatment modalities, helps prevent or manage complications imposed by the effects on other organs, helps manage complications secondary to aberrant endocrine activities and treats or prevents malnutrition.
- The diet for dialysis compensates for lack of kidney function and dialysate losses, provides adequate nutrients for optimal health, and alleviates symptoms of uremia.
- If increased dietary intake is unsuccessful in raising the patient's serum potassium, potassium supplements may need to be used. Other patients may become hyperkalemic in response to excessive dietary intake, particularly those who are very active, and need to restrict their dietary potassium.
- Causes of excessive thirst that might be seen in the HD patient include hyperglycemia, azotemia, inadequate dialysis, a high dietary intake of sucrose, and a high intake of salt.
- Patients with renal disease are at increased risk for deficiencies of water-soluble vitamins, particularly vitamin C, folate, and pyridoxine.
- Patients who have inadequate intake of protein and calories show a decrease in blood urea nitrogen (BUN), low serum proteins, particularly albumin, transferrin, and prealbumin and a low protein catabolic rate (PCR). In stable patients, the pcr reflects dietary protein intake.
- Hyperlipidemia is a problem in many forms of renal disease. Patients undergoing dialysis have increased levels of serum triglycerides, low-density lipoproteins (LDL), very low density lipoproteins (VLDL), and decreased levels of high-density lipoproteins (HDL).
- In the posttransplantation period, common nutritional problems include protein hypercatabolism and gluconeogenesis, obesity, steroid-induced diabetes, and hyperlipidemia.
- The nutritional assessment includes a medical and nutritional history, anthropometric measurements, biochemical measurements, and examination for clinical signs and symptoms of malnutrition..
- IDPN is an anabolic therapy. It repletes the patient nutritionally, creates a positive nitrogen balance in the patient, and enables the patient to restore adequate oral nutrient intake. Most dialysis centers contract with an outpatient infusion pharmacy to manage the IDPN.
- Nutritional dialysates, or IPN, have been shown to have positive effects in PD patients. These dialysates substitute amino acids for dextrose as the osmotic agent for one or two exchanges a day.

CHAPTER 12

Pharmacology in Renal Disease

Terran Warren Sims, BSN, RN, CNN
Anita E. Molzahn, PhD, RN
Karen K. Giuliano, MSN, RN, CCRN
Robert McGory, PharmD, MS, BS

Chapter Contents

Chapter 12A: Pharmacologic Agents in Renal Disease

Metabolism and Elimination of Pharmacologic Agents 309
Pharmacokinetics 314
Drug-Induced Renal Disease 316
Commonly Used Drugs in Renal Failure 317
Antidiabetic Agents or Hypoglycemics 324
Cation-Exchange Resins 324
Antianemics 325
Miscellaneous Medications 326
Dialyzability of Drugs 327

Chapter 12 B: Medications in Transplant Patients

Pharmacologic Management of Patients with Solid Organ Transplant . 331
History of Immunosuppression Therapy 331
Immunosuppressive Medications Commonly Used in Transplantation . 334
New Immunosuppressants in Transplantation 339
Other Common Medications for Transplant Recipients 340
Summary 342
References and Readings 342
Chapter Highlights 345

CHAPTER 12A

Pharmacologic Agents in Renal Disease

Terran Warren Sims, BSN, RN, CNN
Anita E. Molzahn, PhD, RN
Robert McGory, PharmD, MS, BS

Chapter Contents

Metabolism and Elimination of Pharmacologic Agents 309
Absorption 311
Distribution 311
Metabolism. 312
Elimination 313
Pharmacokinetics 314
Volume of Distribution and Clearance. 314
Pharmacodynamics 315
Drug-Induced Renal Disease 316
Commonly Used Drugs in Renal Failure. 317
Diuretics. 317
Analgesics 319
Antihypertensives 319
Cardiotonics. 321
Electrolyte Supplements, Vitamin Replacements, and Phosphate Binders 321
Vitamins. 322
Antacids. 322
Histamine H_2 Receptor Antagonists 322
Stool Softeners and Cathartics. 322
Sedatives and Hypnotics 322

Chapter Contents

- Antimicrobial Agents 322
  - Miscellaneous Antibiotics 323
  - Antiviral Agents 323
  - Antituberculosis Antibiotics 324
- Antidiabetic Agents or Hypoglycemics 324
- Cation-Exchange Resins 324
- Antianemics 325
- Miscellaneous Medications 326
- Dialyzability of Drugs 327

Pharmacologic Agents in Renal Disease

Terran Warren Sims, BSN, RN, CNN
Anita E. Molzahn, PhD, RN
Robert McGory, PharmD, MS, BS

Since the kidneys are responsible for excretion of many drugs and medications, knowledge of pharmacology is essential for nurses working with patients with renal dysfunction. People with chronic renal failure, treated by either dialysis or transplantation, take numerous medications. The nurse is responsible for the safe administration of medications in hospitalized patients and for teaching dialysis patients and transplant recipients about their therapeutic regimen.

The purpose of this chapter is to describe the metabolism and elimination of pharmacologic agents, and pharmacokinetics. Drug-induced renal disease is briefly addressed. As well, the specific medications commonly used in renal failure and with transplant recipients are discussed.

Metabolism and Elimination of Pharmacologic Agents

Elaborate and complicated processes in the body have evolved to protect the body from the effects of external noxious influences. Medications are no different from any substance to which a person is exposed. To have an effect, the medication must reach the target tissue and attach to a receptor on the cell surface. Receptor stimulation will then set off a series of physiologic events that lead to the desired therapeutic effect. Unless a medication is directly infused into the bloodstream, it must be absorbed from the site of deposition. The medication must then be transported, or distributed to the target tissue, by means of cardiovascular circulation. A physiologic cleansing of foreign substances is initiated resulting in degradation of drug to a less toxic or less fat soluble form, or elimination from the body in a water soluble form via the kidneys or secretions (see Figure 12-1).

Figure 12-1
The process of normal drug activity.

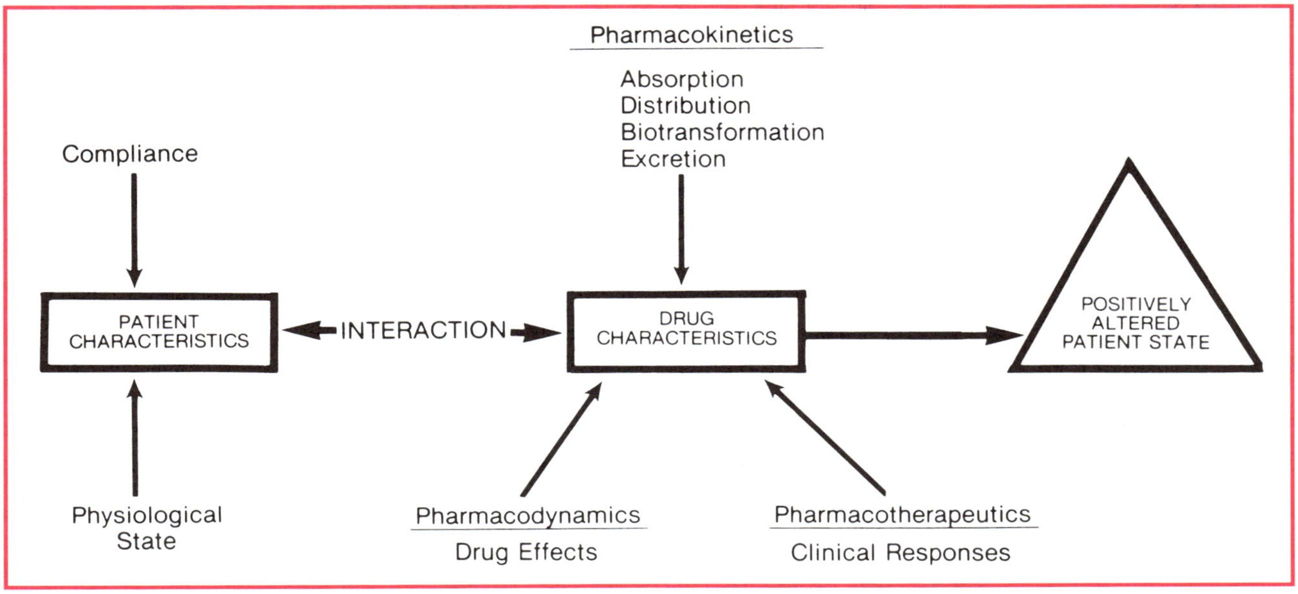

Note: From Baer, C.L. (1995). Pharmacologic aspects of renal failure. In L.E. Lancaster (Ed.), *Core curriculum for nephrology nursing* (3rd edition, p. 177). Pitman, NJ: American Nephrology Nurses' Association. Reprinted with permission.

Table 12-1
Factors affecting the rate of absorption.

Factor	Specific Properties	Effect on Absorption Rate
Physicochemical Properties	Molecular Size Large Small Degree of ionization Ionized Nonionized Lipid solubility High Low	 Decreased Increased Decreased Increased Increased Decreased
Type of Membrane Transport	Passive transport Filtration Simple diffusion Specialized transport Active Facilitated diffusion	 Dependent upon the osmotic or hydrostatic pressure gradient Dependent upon the concentration gradient Energy and carrier dependent Carrier dependent
Concentration	High Low	Increased Decreased
Dosage Form	Liquid Aqueous solution Oily solution Suspension Solid	 Increased Increased over solid forms Increased over solid forms Decreased in comparison to liquids
Route of Administration	Intravenous Intramuscular Subcutaneous Pulmonary (gases, vapors and aerosols) Oral Sublingual/buccal Rectal Topical Mucous membranes Skin	Circumvented – may have immediate effects Rapid Rapid from aqueous solutions Rapid Variable – drug dependent Rapid Variable and often incomplete Semi-rapidly More slowly
Perfusion Rate at Absorption Site	High flow rate Low flow rate	Increased Decreased
Surface Area of Absorption Site	Large surface are Small surface area	Increased Decreased

Note: From Baer, C.L. (1995). Pharmacologic aspects of renal failure. In L.E. Lancaster (Ed.), *Core curriculum for nephrology nursing* (3rd edition, p. 182). Pitman, NJ: American Nephrology Nurses' Association. Reprinted with permission.

Table 12-2
Protein binding of drugs.

Drugs that bind to:	Drugs that bind to:
Albumin	Alpha$_1$ acid glycoprotein
Carbamazepine	Bupivacaine
Diazepam	Diltiazem
Diltiazem	Dipyridamole
Etoposide	Disopyramide
Ibuprofen	Quinidine
Indomethacin	Meperidine
Lidocaine	Methadone
Meperidine	Lidocaine
Phenytoin	Propranolol
Propranolol	Verapamil
Quinidine	
Naproxen	
Valproic acid	
Verapamil	
Warfarin	

Table 12-3
Factors affecting drug distribution.

Factor	Specific Properties	Effect on Distribution
Protein Binding	High Percentage Low Percentage	Decreased Increased
Tissue Binding	High Percentage Low Percentage	Decreased Increased
Lipid Solubility	High Degree Low Degree	Increased Decreased
Polarity	Polar Nonpolar	Decreased Increased
Capillary Permeability	Increased Decreased	Increased Decreased
Volume of Body Water	Increased Decreased	Increased Decreased
Perfusion Rates	Increased Decreased	Increased Decreased
Redistribution	Increased Decreased	Increased Decreased

Note: From Baer, C.L. (1995). Pharmacologic aspects of renal failure. In L.E. Lancaster (Ed.), *Core curriculum for nephrology nursing* (3rd edition, p. 183). Pitman, NJ: American Nephrology Nurses' Association. Reprinted with permission.

Absorption

Medications administered intravenously reach the circulation immediately. However, with oral, dermal, or rectal routes of administration, absorption involves movement across cellular membranes (e.g., those lining both the absorptive surface and the blood vessel wall), and movement through intracellular spaces to reach the circulation. Local conditions can change the amount of medication that reaches the bloodstream; these conditions include pH, length of time the medication is in contact with absorptive surface, anatomic and physiologic condition of absorptive surface, and edema of the surrounding tissue. Although active and facilitated mechanisms can be present, movement of medication across surfaces is usually passive.

Oral absorption of medications can be reduced in the hospitalized patient due to physical removal by continuous or intermittent nasogastric suctioning, chemically neutralized gastrointestinal pH, altered peristalsis, villous atrophy, edematous bowel wall, and limited passage into the circulatory system because of poor perfusion of the intestines. In addition, physical medication interactions occur in the bowel lumen, hindering movement of medication through endothelial cell linings due to physical size.

Sublingual, intranasal, intramuscular, intravenous, intraventricular, intracavitary, and epidural routes of administration have been developed to enhance absorption of medications, or to administer the agent directly to the site of action. Absorption of medications from intramuscular and subcutaneous injections may be affected by changes in absorption due to decreased tissue perfusion and decreased movement through edematous tissue that may have physical distortions due to abnormal contents of fat and protein (see Table 12-1).

Distribution

Distribution of medication describes the transportation and deposition of a medication throughout the body. Very few medications can be directly administered to the site of need. Medication molecules that enter the bloodstream will be carried to their destination either in solution or attached to carrier molecules (see Table 12-2). Erythrocytes, serum proteins such as albumin, and alpha$_1$ acid glycoprotein are common carriers of drugs. Medications that are bound to carrier molecules are inactive, but binding of medication is largely reversible. Detachment of medication occurs in areas of low concentration such as the target tissue or tissue of elimination. Medications vary in their ability to bind to tissue based upon chemical con-

Table 12-4
Drugs that affect liver P450 enzyme function.

Inducers of Drug Metabolism	Inhibitors Drug Metabolism
Carbamazepine	Cimetidine
Chloral hydrate	Ciprofloxacin
Ethanol	Erythromycin
Phenobarbital	Ketoconazole
Phenylbutazone	Metoprolol
Phenytoin	Omeprazole
Rifampin	Propranolol

Table 12-5
Relation of drug metabolism to hepatic blood flow.

Flow Dependent Metabolism	Flow Independent Metabolism
Isoproterenol	Cyclosporine
Lidocaine	Diazepam
Hydrocortisone	Erythromycin
Morphine	Phenytoin
Meperidine	Theophylline
Metoprolol	Warfarin
Nitroglycerine	Propranolol
Propoxyphene	
Verapamil	

figuration and electrical charge. Chemicals may displace other chemicals if they are physically structured to better compete for attachment to the binding site on tissue or carrier molecules. Accumulation of uremic organic acids will displace acidic medications that are bound to albumin; therefore, there will be less active drug available for absorption. Basic medications are less affected by uremia.

Patients with various diseases may have impairments in their abilities to distribute medications. For example, poor perfusion of target tissue will limit the number of cells that are exposed to medication, while altered receptor binding will change the amount of medication attached to tissue. Receptors may be physically altered due to edema, malnutrition, down regulation, or the competitive binding of other drugs or toxins. Since only free drug is active, potential for medication toxicity increases when decreased binding elevates free serum concentrations of the drug, allowing tissues with functional receptors to bind more of the medication. Inflammation and loss of barrier integrity may allow medication to pass into otherwise drug-free tissue, such as cerebral spinal fluid or the peritoneal cavity. Third spacing of fluid, in clinical situations such as ascites or massive edema, may result in additional volume into which medication can diffuse (see Table 12-3), resulting in a need for higher dosage of medication to achieve therapeutic effects.

Metabolism

Medications are removed from the body through either of two major mechanisms. If the molecule is water soluble, the kidney will filter the chemical, or fluid lost through physiologic secretions will carry medication with it. If the medication is fat soluble, the medication must be altered to a water soluble form that the kidney or secretions can remove. The liver is the most prolific organ that metabolizes or detoxifies medications, but all tissue can metabolize medications to a limited extent.

The numerous enzyme systems found in hepatocytes are adept at transforming chemicals whether they are medications or cellular waste products. Detoxification occurs by denaturing the fat soluble chemical structure through reduction, demethylation, oxidation, or hydrolysis. Alternatively, the medication may be made more water soluble by attaching a polar chemical molecule such as glucuronide, sulfate, or glutathione. In renal failure, reduction and hydrolysis reactions are generally slowed, while glucouronidation, sulfated conjugation, and microsomal oxidation usually occur at a normal rate.

Enzymes are protein molecules that enhance the chemical transformation of molecules. Their effectiveness is limited by the physical environment of pH, temperature, and presence of synergistic substances called co-enzymes. Enzyme metabolism normally occurs at a defined rate. Enzymes are present in abundant concentration to allow metabolism of all molecules presented to the hepatocyte. Rarely, as in the case of alcohol or phenytoin, medication substrate will saturate the quantity of enzyme present, allowing drug accumulation to occur. Certain enzymes are inducible, which is simply a descriptive term for the synthesis of additional protein molecules. The best described example of inducible enzymes is the P450 system, which can be induced by medications such as phenobarbital and rifampin. Table 12-4 lists drugs that affect liver P450 enzyme function.

Rate of medication metabolism varies with the medication and the enzymes involved. The amount of medication metabolized may depend upon the ability of the body to deliver medication to the site of metabolism (see Table 12-5). Flow-dependent metabolism describes the ability of the liver to clear the blood of toxin so rapidly that the amount of medication metabolized can be determined principally by the rate of blood flow. Flow-dependent metabolism is synonymous with first pass effect (e.g., medication entering the circulation in the GI tract immediately passes through the liver where the majority of medication is metabolized).

Flow-independent metabolism is not influenced by blood flow. The amount of medication metabolized is limited by the inherent ability of hepatocyte detoxification. The amount of medication that can be cleared from blood will always be less than the amount of medication that is presented to the liver via blood flow.

Metabolic pathways that are influenced by blood flow are affected by diseases that reduce cardiac output or surgical revascularization that disrupts blood flow to the liver. Reduced protein binding increases the amount of free drug available for clearance and may increase the clearance of medication because the liver primarily extracts unbound medication. Hence, the patient may be at higher risk for toxicity due to elevated free concentration of drug, but the liver would also detoxify medications more rapidly. Diseases that affect hepatocyte function will also result in drug accumulation as the inherent ability to metabolize may change the relationship to one of flow-independent metabolism. Flow-independent pathways are primarily influenced by diseases that alter hepatocyte function.

Active metabolites may appear upon detoxification of parent compound. This may lead to prolonged therapeutic/toxic presence of medications such as meperidine or the benzodiazepines. In some cases, such as with the oral angiotensin enzyme inhibitor (enalapril) which has an inactive parent compound, metabolism of the drug will result in release of an active metabolite (enalaprilat). In patients with diseases such as renal failure, where metabolism or elimination are impaired, adjustments to dosage may be required to prevent drug toxicity.

Elimination

Elimination is the final pathway by which a medication or its metabolite is removed from the body. The kidney is the main organ of elimination, while the liver can concentrate medication in bile. Minor routes of medication loss are through secretions, tears, and pulmonary gas exchange.

Medication elimination is influenced by three distinct activities of the kidney. Medications may be filtered at the glomerulus, can be actively secreted into the tubules, or reabsorbed from the lumens of the proximal and distal convoluted tubule. Factors related to a medication's capacity to be filtered include: protein binding of the drug, molecular size and charge of the drug, glomerular integrity, and the number of functioning nephrons. In selected situations, these variables can be altered, such as with the use of probenecid to block the secretion of penicillins and cephalosporins, or to block the reabsorption of uric acid. Alteration of urine pH has been used to change reabsorption and secretion. Alkalinization of urine is useful in phenobarbital and salicylate overdoses to enhance urinary excretion of medication (see Figure 12-2).

Renal disease will limit the amounts of water soluble parent compound and metabolite that are removed from the blood. Diseases that affect glomerular filtration will limit the amount of excreted medication. Decreased perfusion of the kidney will reduce medication filtration, while inflammation of the glomerulus will allow large medication molecules to pass. Nephrotic syndrome is characterized by albumin loss that will carry bound medication into the urine. Changes in tubular integrity may alter secretion and reabsorption of molecules.

Secretions of body fluids through wounds, burns, or drainage of compartmentalized collections (ascites) may result in enhanced clearance of

Figure 12-2
The time course of drug actions.

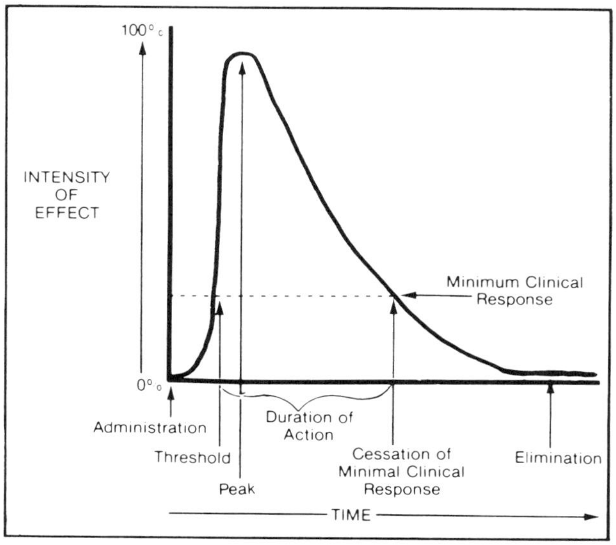

Note: From Baer, C.L. (1995). Pharmacologic aspects of renal failure. In L.E. Lancaster (Ed.), *Core curriculum for nephrology nursing* (3rd edition, p. 183). Pitman, NJ: American Nephrology Nurses' Association. Reprinted with permission.

medication from the body. Patients with reduced renal or hepatic function may need full or greater doses of medication to maintain therapeutic levels.

Extracorporeal dialysis may remove medication from the blood. As with the functioning kidney, large molecular structures (>500 daltons), fat soluble substances, and highly protein bound molecules are poorly dialyzed. The extent of removal depends upon type of dialysis, length of dialysis, and type of filter used. The size of medication molecule and extent of tissue binding establish the potential for drug removal, while the efficiency of dialysis will determine the extent of removal.

Dialysis techniques and filters have improved the removal of medication. Newer high efficiency filters will remove larger molecules such as vancomycin. Chronic veno-venous or arterial-venous dialysis continuously remove medication over days rather than hours. Care must be used to interpret dosing charts that describe removal of medications by dialysis. The majority of information is dated and may not reflect current dialysis techniques. A search of the literature or contact with the pharmaceutical or dialyzer manufacturer may be helpful in guiding drug therapy when patients are using new dialysis devices.

Successful removal of drugs by dialysis is limited to medications and drugs in the blood, both in bound and free forms. However, because of the extensive distribution of many medications into fatty tissue, the drug will rapidly redistribute from tissue stores once dialysis is stopped. In cases of phenobarbital or theophylline overdose, this brief period of dialysis may be enough to stabilize the patient before serum drug levels again rise.

Hemoperfusion with resins or activated charcoal has been successfully used to irreversibly bind water insoluble substances. It is the therapy of choice for removal of protein-bound medications.

Pharmacokinetics

Medications behave in relatively reproducible manners once they enter the body. Mathematical models have been constructed to describe the behavior of molecules for the purpose of guiding dosage changes during periods of altered absorption, distribution, metabolism, and excretion. These models are referred to as pharmacokinetics.

Medications that have a narrow therapeutic index require close monitoring to optimize dose and clinical outcome. Deterioration in function of organs of metabolism and excretion will cause medication accumulation, while fluid shifts and altered tissue binding will change the concentration of free medication in the serum. The majority of medications are either relatively safe, or minimally influenced by altered physiology. These agents can be prescribed with standard doses, or adjusted based upon population nomograms. Selected agents are either extremely toxic, or fluctuate dramatically in serum concentration with various pathologies in the body. Therapeutic drug monitoring has evolved to daily measurement of serum drug concentrations and adjustment of dosages based upon the patient status.

Medication elimination follows two basic forms. Linear elimination results when the body eliminates the same percentage of medication per unit time. The percent of medication removed is independent of the starting concentration. The amount of medication removed per unit of time will decrease as serum concentration decreases. If plotted on a log-linear graph, the serum concentration time curve will be a straight line throughout the dosing interval. Linear kinetics yield constant medication loss throughout the range of serum concentrations as well as the entire dosage interval. A percentage change in dose will yield an equivalent desired percentage change in serum concentration. Linear kinetics is also called first order kinetics.

Nonlinear elimination results when the body eliminates the same amount of medication per unit time, while the percentage of medication removed changes. This pattern is due to a saturated elimination process, usually involving an enzyme that transforms the drug molecule. A saturated enzyme is always functioning at the maximum ability. Eventually, enough medication is eliminated to unsaturate the enzymes, allowing a shift to linear kinetics previously described. The serum concentration time relationship on a log-linear graph is a curve that initially reflects slow medication loss that increases until the linear portion of the curve is achieved. Dosage adjustments are not made on a ratio and proportion relationship as with linear kinetics. Because the majority of the dosage interval is spent in the nonlinear portion of the time curve, small amounts of medication will result in larger than expected changes in serum levels. Nonlinear kinetics is also called zero order kinetics.

Volume of Distribution and Clearance

Specific parameters to consider in adjustments of drug dosage are the volume of distribution and clearance. Clearance and volume of distribution are both affected by physiologic parameters and will change as the condition of the patient changes.

The volume of distribution is the apparent space in which a medication will disperse. This space is composed of fluid compartments and tissue binding sites. Volume of distribution is influenced by fluid shifts and accumulation. Volume of distribution is 0.25 ml/kg in euvolemia, but 0.15 ml/kg in dehydration, or as great as 0.35 in fluid overload; that is, medication dosages should be reduced in dehydration, and dosage increases may be required in fluid overload. Gentamicin is sensitive to fluid shifts in the extracellular compartment. Medications with significant protein-binding can display reduced binding if receptor changes or competition for the site occurs. Medication interactions such as aspirin and warfarin, or accumulation of uremic waste products will result in higher free concentrations of drug or additional binding by tissue receptors that may not be equally effected. Phenytoin is displaced from albumin in renal failure where free drug concentration can increase from 10% to 20% and may lead to toxicity. Assay of free phenytoin levels has been recommended to better reflect dosage changes.

Clearance is the amount of blood from which medication can be removed in a defined period of time. Clearance is correlated to the function of the organ of elimination such as the liver or kidney, while volume of distribution is associated with fluid status and tissue binding efficiency.

Another pharmacokinetic parameter is the half-life, or the time required for serum concentration of a medication to fall by 50%. Half-life is the mathematical relationship that correlates volume to clearance, that is:

$$\text{half-life} = (0.693) \times \frac{(\text{volume of distribution})}{\text{clearance}}$$

When the individual parameters are determined, they are placed into standard mathematical equations to calculate the most appropriate dose to achieve the desired serum concentration. Disease processes will change parameters based upon physiologic alterations.

Artificial clearance of medication occurs with dialysis and presumably with plasmapheresis (see Table 12-6). As previously mentioned, dialysis devices will clear medication based upon type of dialysis and physical characteristics of the medication. Plasmapheresis of medication is a relatively unstudied phenomenon but the treatment will remove some fraction of drug. In limited studies, the level of clearance has been low. The small volume of serum removed or "cleansed" contains only a small portion of total medication in the body. Medications that are heavily protein bound may be removed, but the majority of drug remains distributed throughout the body in other compartments. Clinically, medications that may be affected by dialysis or plasmapheresis should be held until the end of dialysis, or an additional dose should be given at the end of the treatment. Medications with a narrow therapeutic index may be best assessed by taking a serum level upon completion of the extracorporeal procedure.

Table 12-6
Drug elimination through artificial clearance.

Dialysis	Plasmapheresis
Acyclovir	Digitoxin
Atenolol	L-thyroxine
Ceftazidime	Phenytoin
Galamine	Propranolol
Gentamicin	Salicylate
Nadolol	Tobramycin
Penicillin	
Pentazocine	
Prednisone	
Procainamide	

Pharmacodynamics

The relationship between drug concentration at the site of drug action and the physiologic response by the target tissue is called pharmacodynamics. A drug effect is produced when (a) there is a change in the physical environment of the bloodstream, through such mechanisms as albumin or bicarbonate infusion, or (b) the drug attaches to a three-dimensional receptor found on the cell membrane or on an organelle within the cell. The interaction between drug and receptor causes a change in the structure of the cell surface which may open channels in the cell membrane through which electrolytes or other molecules can pass. Receptor stimulation also activates intracellular enzymes or releases intracellular chemicals that catalyze the desired physiologic response.

For most medications, the concentration at the receptor site determines the intensity of pharmacologic outcome. A dose response curve is generated for each medication during premarketing research to establish safe dosing ranges. Medication concentration and effect are proportional at low concentrations. Patient response to increasing doses is most evident with doses in the lower end of the dosing scale. As medication effect nears maximum, the receptors become saturated, and further increases in concentration have little to no benefit. Clinically, the chance of increasing toxicity is much greater in the higher doses of a medication for the perceived benefit the patient may derive.

Medications have a characteristic course of action. A delay occurs after the administration of medication. This delay is the time required to deliver medication to the site of action, bind medication to the receptor, and alter the cellular physiology to achieve desired outcome. A maximum or peak effect occurs when accumulation of medication at the receptor site is great enough to maximally bind to the receptor. The duration of medication effect reflects the elimination of medication from the central compartment and re-equilibration of medication molecules from receptor to the central compartment. Medication effect will diminish as receptor sites are evacuated until the concentration of drug becomes subtherapeutic. Although medication will remain in the body for at least five half-lives, medication effect will not be detectable once the concentration falls below the therapeutic amount at the site of action.

Altered dynamic responsiveness is a poorly understood phenomenon. Not all patients react in the same way to equivalent doses or serum concentrations of the same drug. Differences in receptor structures, intracellular messengers, and feedback mechanisms have been proposed to account for individual differences.

Altered receptor binding is common with disease states. The three-dimensional proximity of structures of the cell membrane that define the receptor site can be altered in both design and chemical composition. Cell membranes can be physically distorted by malnourishment, edema, and inflammation. Age can also affect the chemical composition of the membrane as dietary habits as well as fat and protein content of tissue change in advancing years. Antibodies may block the receptor (insulin antibodies) or destroy the receptor site and cell. Insulin antibodies have been recognized to block the site of insulin attachment, while muromonab CD3 is a commercially available antibody specifically manufactured against the T-cell CD3 receptor to prevent recognition of foreign antigens. Down regulation, a feedback mechanism that occurs after medication exposure, may decrease the number of receptors on the cell.

Altered responsiveness to receptor stimulation is common as disease may disrupt the intracellular chemical messenger system that is activated by the receptor. Stimulation of a cell surface receptor by a drug begins a cascade of chemical events that result in the anticipated outcome. Intracellular chemicals such as electrolytes and cyclic AMP may be depleted or functionally blocked by other molecules competing for binding sites. The incidence of digoxin toxicity increases when intracellular potassium concentrations fall.

Failing physiologic reflexes may account for exaggerated or reduced pharmacologic effects, especially in the elderly. The inability of an organ system to detect or attenuate drug-induced changes could result in overwhelming drug effect and patient harm.

The metabolism and elimination of medications is clearly a complex process. Pathology in any number of areas can contribute to damage to the kidneys and drug-induced renal disease.

Drug-Induced Renal Disease

One in every five cases of acute renal failure is associated with medication toxicity while with chronic renal failure, 1% to 20% of cases are associated with drug toxicity, depending on the region of the world reporting its experience. The kidneys are uniquely susceptible to medication toxicity due to a dependence upon high blood flow for filtration, a powerful ability to concentrate substrates, a large endothelial area that comes in contact with toxic substances, and a high metabolic activity that produces intracellular toxins.

The mechanisms of medication-mediated damage are multiple. As with other causes of renal disease, pathophysiology is divided between prerenal reasons for decreased perfusion, postrenal obstruction, and intrinsic renal disease (e.g., interstitial nephritis, glomerulonephritis, or acute tubular necrosis). In addition to direct toxic effects on renal tissue, altered physiologic effects are induced by medications that change fluid and electrolyte balance (e.g., diuretics).

Renal perfusion is affected by a number of mechanisms. Medications can reduce cardiac output by inducing hypovolemia (diuretics) and causing vasodilation (antihypertensives). Afferent arteriolar vasoconstriction will reduce the perfusion of the glomerulus, while efferent vasodilation will draw blood away from the glomerulus. Both actions decrease the glomerular filtration pressures and reduce the volume of glomerular filtrate. Nonsteroidal anti-inflammatory drugs (NSAIDs) reduce the synthesis of prostaglandins, which in turn decrease the afferent blood flow in individuals with abnormal renal function. Angiotensin converting enzyme (ACE) inhibitors cause vasodilatation of the efferent arterioles decreasing glomerular filtration pressure. This induces renal dysfunction despite increased renal blood flow by increasing cardiac output through afterload reduction. Cyclosporine can cause an intense generalized intrarenal vasoconstriction that can synergistically interact with NSAIDs and ACE inhibitors.

Drug-induced acute interstitial nephritis is a hypersensitivity reaction to a medication molecule that occurs the renal interstitium. Common clinical signs and symptoms include hematuria (gross or microscopic), proteinuria, and pyuria. Occasionally, systemic manifestations of allergy, such as rash, fever, and arthralgia, are seen in interstitial nephritis. The most common diagnostic finding is the presence of eosinophils in the urine. Glomerular and vascular lesions are rarely seen in conjunction with interstitial nephritis.

Acute tubular necrosis (ATN) is a generic term that covers many different diseases with similar manifestations. Multivariate analysis of insults indicate the most frequent causes of ATN to be hypotension (74%), sepsis (31%), toxins (25%), pigmenturia (22%), and dehydration (35%). Damage may be confined to the proximal or distal convoluted tubule. Proximal tubular effects are seen most prevalently with aminoglycoside antibiotics, since the drugs can be concentrated in the renal cortex to 20 times the serum concentration. Proximal lesions can be detected by urinary appearance of enzymes found in tubular cells (N-acetylglucosaminidase and alkaline phosphatase) or impaired proximal reabsorption of the filtered protein beta2 microglobulin. Urinary magnesium and potassium losses are seen with proximal defects. Distal tubular damage is seen with platinum compounds (e.g., cisplatinum) used for cancer chemotherapy. Chronic administration disrupts the normal tubular functions and can lead to renal concentrating defects, potassium wasting, and distal renal tubular acidosis. Hydration, mannitol, and sodium loading have been used to lessen the toxic effects of drugs in the distal tubule. These treatments decrease the concentration of the medication passing through the tubule and therefore are expected to decrease the toxic effects.

Medications may precipitate in the distal tubule, but more frequently precipitate in the collecting ducts when water reabsorption concentrates the agent above its maximum solubility. When sulfonamides, methotrexate, and acyclovir precipitate, they can obstruct urine flow, leading to stasis and tubular cell death.

Antihypertensive medications may produce profound effects as limited vascular responsiveness may not temper the pressure, lowering medication actions. Sedative effects of medication may be intensified by poor cerebral perfusion or disease related neuronal dysfunction (see Table 12-7). While all medications have some side effects, some medications can induce renal disease and failure.

For many medications, there are multiple mechanisms through which renal damage can occur. For example, Amphotericin B is an intense vasoconstrictor as well as a direct nephrotoxin to the proximal and distal tubules. Radiocontrast agents may cause systemic hypotension and direct nephrotoxicity, but they can also cause obstruction through precipitation of uric acid crystals. Clinical and laboratory findings may vary dependent upon which mechanism is more prominent.

In rare instances, some medications, such as Lithium, can cause chronic renal dysfunction (as well as acute renal failure) when taken over a long period of time. Patients may present with nonspecific symptoms such as nocturia, weakness, fatigue, nausea, or vomiting. Because the disease is largely asymptomatic, the damage occurs slowly and is not clinically detectable. Patients may not present until 85% to 90% of renal function is lost. Long-term toxicity usually causes low grade inflammation and deposition of scar tissue or occlusion of blood vessels. However, most drug-induced renal diseases involve all parenchymal elements. If the medication is stopped, deterioration of renal function is usually arrested.

Analgesic nephropathy refers to the chronic interstitial nephritis that occurs as a result of long-term use of acetaminophen, aspirin, and NSAIDs. Patients with analgesic nephropathy typically have consumed large amounts of analgesics in various combinations over a period of years. Reports of chronic disease with single agents are rare. The mechanism has been suggested to be a production of toxic metabolites. Acetaminophen metabolism by the P450 enzyme system in the liver produces a toxic metabolite that is rapidly neutralized by hepatocyte stores of glutathione. Depletion of glutathione in overdose situations has been fatal due to fulminant liver failure. Chronic analgesic use apparently causes similar renal cell damage that erodes viable tissue over a long period of time. The basic lesion is papillary necrosis seemingly due to damage and occlusion of the contiguous blood vessels, leading to ischemic necrosis of the papillae. The renal tubules passing into the necrotic papillae are then blocked, leading to secondary atrophy of the overlying nephrons.

Commonly Used Drugs in Renal Failure

Despite the many factors to be considered in the metabolism and elimination of medications, particularly in patients with renal failure, there are many medications that are regularly prescribed for this population. However, use of pharmacological agents with chronic renal failure patients requires special considerations, particularly relating to dosages. Specific categories of medications will be discussed, including: diuretics; analgesics; antihypertensives; cardiotonics; calcium supplements, vitamin replacements; phosphate binders; antacids; stool softeners and cathartics; histamine H_2 receptor antagonists; sedatives and hypnotics; antimicrobial agents; hypoglycemics; cation-exchange resins; and antianemics.

Diuretics

There are numerous diuretics available for the treatment of hypertension and edema associated with renal disease. Hydrochlorthiazide is a thiazide-type diuretic that inhibits reabsorption of sodium and chloride in the distal tubule, thus promoting water loss. It is typically used as the first line of therapy to treat mild hypertension. As well, it is used to treat edema associated with congestive heart failure or edema of renal origin (e.g., nephrotic syndrome). It is seldom used or effective in patients with chronic renal failure.

Most commonly, loop diuretics (e.g., furosemide or bumetanide) are used when there is some renal insufficiency. Their action is to alter the reabsorption of water and sodium from the ascending loop of Henle (McDonald, 1980). These drugs may be given in oral doses daily, or in the hospital they may be given intravenously. In the conservative management phase when the patient is progressing toward chronic renal failure, they are used to prevent edema and hypertension. After the patient has reached chronic renal failure, loop diuretics are of little benefit. This class of diuretics is often known for its high potency and steep dose-response curve.

A group of diuretics to avoid in renal failure are

Table 12-7
The effects of renal failure on physiologic characteristics.

Physiologic Characteristics	Effect of Renal Failure	Remarks
Race, Gender and Other Genetic Factors	No effect	Hereditary genetic alterations could have caused the renal failure
Age/ Maturational State	No effect	Neonates have immature renal systems and geriatric patients have decreased function due to the aging process
Body Size	Decreased: Muscle wasting Increased: Fluid overload	Treatment of the etiology of the renal failure with steroids would increase the body fat content
Body Temperature	No effect	Uremic toxins may decrease neutrophil phagocytosis and chemotaxis making the patient more susceptible to infection
Perfusion Rates	Increased: Fluid overload Hypertension Decreased: Congestive heart failure Dysrhythmias Pericarditis Peripheral and systemic edema	
Urinary Flow Rates	Usually decreased	Could be increased in cases of nonoliguric or high output renal failure
Urinary pH	Usually increased	Varies significantly depending on the etiology and pathology of the renal failure
Nutritional State	Decreased: Anorexia, nausea and emesis Stomatitis and uremic fetor Gastritis and bleeding Dietary restrictions Hypocalcemia and impaired vitamin D metabolism	Protein wasting may occur as a result of peritoneal dialysis or catabolic processes
Activity Level	Decreased: Anemia Osteo-dystrophy	May approximate normal as the patient's tolerances increase over time
Pregnancy and Menopause	Decreased: Infertility Altered menses	May be improved through dialysis therapy
Dysfunctional Organ Systems	Increased	Renal failure has a deleterious effect on almost every body system
Psychologic Response	Altered: Decreased concentration Decreased mentation Altered perceptions	Improves with dialysis therapy
Chronology	Altered	Renal failure alters almost all metabolic and physiologic properties

Note: From Baer, C.L. (1995). Pharmacologic aspects of renal failure. In L.E. Lancaster (Ed.), *Core curriculum for nephrology nursing* (3rd edition, p. 186). Pitman, NJ: American Nephrology Nurses' Association. Reprinted with permission.

the potassium-sparing diuretics (e.g., spironolactone). Spironolactone specifically competes with aldosterone for binding to receptor sites in the tubular cells of the collecting tubule. While spironolactone is considered a weak diuretic, its primary usefulness is in the prevention or treatment of hypokalemia caused by other diuretics in individuals with relatively normal kidney function. It can also be used to augment the action of other diuretics. Spironolactone is also used as an antihypertensive agent in some cases. Hyperkalemia is a well known side effect and it is important that the nurse monitor serum potassium levels in all patients receiving the drug (McDonald, 1980). For this reason, the use of potassium sparing diuretics is contraindicated in renal failure.

All diuretics carry with them the potential complication of fluid and electrolyte imbalances and disturbances of blood chemistries. The patient should be monitored for response to the drug as well as progression toward identified goals of therapy on an ongoing basis.

Analgesics

Analgesics can be put into three classes: nonnarcotic, narcotic, and nonsteroidal antiinflammatory drugs (NSAIDs). The nonnarcotic drugs may be more frequently prescribed for chronic pain that is not alleviated through other methods. Narcotics may be administered for pain in association with a procedure or invasive intervention. Patients in the hospital for procedures or surgery may have narcotic drugs ordered, and drug dosage and frequency of administration may be affected if the patient has impaired renal function or is on dialysis.

Examples of nonnarcotic drugs include acetaminophen, phenacetin, and acetylsalicylic acid (ASA). These drugs should be given in the smallest dose that will alleviate the pain. Typically, phenacetin is not given to patients in a uremic state because it can have a negative effect on kidney function. Acetaminophen is the drug of choice for mild to moderate analgesia in patients with chronic renal failure, since it is not metabolized by the kidney. ASA is generally not prescribed for pain relief because it increases the likelihood of bleeding. However, patients on dialysis are often given small doses of ASA on a regular basis to prevent the clotting of vascular access devices.

Narcotics function to manage pain perception—to alter the pain threshold or the central nervous system's response to pain (Baer, 1990). Morphine sulfate is the drug of choice for patients with chronic renal failure who have acute pain. However, dosage and frequency of administration may need to be reduced. Codeine is also a drug of choice for pain management in that it can be used without dose adjustment in renal failure. Meperidine, however, should be avoided, particularly for long-term therapy because of the potential for build-up of meperidine metabolites that can lead to grand mal seizures. None of these narcotics are removed, to any great extent, during dialysis, so dose adjustment or supplementation is not required. However, all narcotics worsen the constipation experienced by most renal failure patients.

Nonsteroidal anti-inflammatory drugs (NSAIDs) are more readily available since they became available over the counter in 1994. It was expected that 50 million Americans would use NSAIDs intermittently or routinely in 1994. Approximately 1% of the persons exposed to NSAIDs will manifest one of several abnormalities of renal function (Whelton, Stout, Spilman & Klassen, 1990). This is of concern, since NSAIDs interfere with the production of vasodilatory prostaglandins that are secreted in an attempt to maintain renal blood flow in stress conditions (e.g., hypotension, hypovolemia). The most common side effect seen with NSAID use is the retention of sodium chloride and water, resulting in edema. NSAIDs can also cause other electrolyte abnormalities, most significantly hyperkalemia (Spilman & Whelton, 1992). Patients with renal insufficiency are at high risk for complications associated with these drugs and those who also have arthritis or other chronic inflammatory conditions should seek alternative therapy (Spilman & Whelton, 1992). Nursing assessment of the renal failure patient should include determination of the patient's use of over the counter NSAIDs.

Antihypertensives

Cardiovascular disease is the leading cause of death in patients with chronic renal failure (USRDS, 1993). Hypertension occurs in about 80% of patients with chronic renal failure (Campese & Bigazzi, 1992). An understanding of how hypertension occurs and what factors come into play helps the nurse understand management strategies. Factors associated with hypertension include retention of fluid and sodium, dysfunction of the renin-angiotensin system, increased activity of the sympathetic nervous system, changes in intracellular calcium, and reduced production of vasodilator substances by the kidneys (Ma, Greene, & Raji, 1992; Parfrey, Harnett, & Griffiths, 1990). Although many drugs can control blood pressure effectively, understanding the effects of the antihypertensive agent on the impaired kidney, as well as each drug's potential to cause new complications is essential. Antihypertensive agents that protect or improve renal function while reducing blood pressure are the most logical choice for use in patients who have renal impairment. Increased blood pressure in the presence of preexisting renal impairment continues to insult the already damaged kidney (Sandoz, 1993). On the other hand, people with narrowed blood vessels need higher than normal blood pressures to propel blood through the circulatory system and overagressive antihypertensive therapy may actually further impair renal function.

Antihypertensives are divided into several classes. In the following paragraphs, angiotensin converting enzyme inhibitors, calcium channel blockers, beta adrenergic blockers, alpha 1-receptor blockers, centrally acting alpha 2-agonists, and vasodilators are discussed.

Angiotensin-converting enzyme (ACE) inhibitors. These drugs (e.g., captopril, enalapril, benazepril) act to decrease the blood pressure by interfering with the renin-angiotensin-aldosterone system by blocking the conversion of angiotensin I, a mild vasoconstrictor, to angiotensin II, a potent vasoconstrictor. They also act to decrease sodium and water retention and peripheral resistance, and to increase plasma volume, cardiac output, and renal blood flow (Baer, 1990). ACE inhibitors also act to decrease systemic vascular resistance without affecting heart rate or cardiac output. This class of drugs would be a good choice for a patient with suspected dysfunction of the renin-angiotensin system (Weiner, 1994). Benazepril has actions similar to captopril and is effective regardless of plasma renin levels and may be used alone or in combination with other antihypertensives (Bell, 1993). In renal failure patients, the initial dose is reduced by 50% and then titrated for effect to a maximum recommended dose of 40 mg. There is no dosage reduction necessary for patients with hepatic dysfunction due to cirrhosis. It is not easily dialyzable in either hemodialysis or peritoneal dialysis (Bell, 1993).

As significant orthostatic hypotension can occur, these patients must be monitored closely when the initial doses are administered. Liver function tests should also be monitored because elevated liver enzymes and/or bilirubin, cholestatic jaundice, and hepatocellular injury have been reported. Although ACE inhibitors tend to be highly effective, they should be used with caution in patients with renal failure, since they can cause hyperkalemia, and the drug vasodilates the efferent arterioles resulting in reduced glomerular filtration. Clearly, the risks must be weighed against the potential benefits. Hemodialysis will significantly reduce the blood levels of converting enzyme inhibitors such as captopril and enalapril; therefore a careful review of blood pressure medications should be done when the blood pressure is rising during the dialysis treatment or following the treatment in a rebound fashion (Handley, 1994; Karubian, Chervu, & Campese, 1993).

Calcium channel blockers. This class of medications (e.g., diltiazem, isradipine, nifedipine, verapamil) are commonly used for their ability to inhibit movement of calcium across vascular smooth cells, which leads to coronary and peripheral vasodilation and decreased systemic vascular resistance (Weiner, 1994). Calcium channel blockers may be used alone or with thiazide-type diuretics. They are attractive for their long-acting effects and the low risk of hypotension on dialysis. In hypertensive emergencies where blood pressure can be monitored, sublingual nifedipine may be used to produce rapid results within minutes.

Caution in administration of this drug should be related to the fact that the medication may cause hypotension, peripheral edema, and bradycardia (Baer, 1990). Traditionally, calcium channel blockers are not used in patients with congestive heart failure, nor are these drugs prescribed concurrently with beta-blockers due to their negative interactions. The calcium channel blockers are also known to increase drug levels of immunosuppressive drugs such as cyclosporine and tacrolimus.

Beta adrenergic blockers. This class of antihypertensives (e.g., propranolol, acebutolol, atenolol, metoprolol, labetalol) acts to block the sympathetic stimulation of beta 1-receptors in the heart and beta 2-receptors in the bronchi, peripheral blood vessels, and pancreas (Weiner, 1994). Key factors affecting dosage relate to the fact that these agents can produce sedation, bradycardia, hypotension, and congestive failure and can mask hypoglycemia in diabetic patients (Baer, 1990). If the drug is to be discontinued, these medications should be tapered and blood pressure monitored closely.

Alpha 1-receptor blockers. This class of medications (e.g., doxazosin, prazosin, terazosin) decreases blood pressure by occupying the alpha receptors of the sympathetic nervous system and blocking the effects of epinephrine and norepinephrine at those sites. The result is vasodilation due to relaxed smooth muscle, decreased peripheral resistance, and plasma renin activity. Usually, heart rate is not affected but occasionally tachycardia may occur (Baer, 1990). As with other similar medications, alpha 1-receptor blockers can cause orthostatic hypotension and patients should be monitored for response to therapy and achievement of target blood pressure. Often the profound hypotensive side effects will pass after the first dose. Therefore, patients should be monitored closely during initial administration, particularly if it is on a hemodialysis day. Alpha 1-receptor blockers have an added benefit in men with benign prostatic hypertrophy in that they relax smooth muscle of the prostate and improve urine flow.

Centrally acting alpha 2-agonists. This class of drugs (e.g., clonidine, methyldopa) decreases blood pressure by stimulating alpha receptors in the brain, causing reduced sympathetic activity, which results in decreases in the systemic vascular resistance, heart rate, and probably cardiac output (Weiner, 1994). Alpha 2-agonists are popular because new technology enables clonidine to be administered by a slow release patch, which is changed weekly. This system, called the transdermal therapeutic system (TTS), reduces the risk of orthostatic hypotension (Weiner, 1994), and other side effects such as bradycardia, lethargy, and somnolence may be reduced. When taken orally, these medications are generally withheld prior to dialysis, and the patient is placed on a regimen where the daily dose would be after the dialysis treatment. Patients must always be slowly tapered off these medications to avoid rebound effect and hypertensive crisis.

Vasodilators. This class of medications (e.g., diazoxide, hydralazine, minoxidil, nitroprusside) are used for the effect of decreasing blood pressure by relaxing smooth muscle and therefore decreasing systemic vascular resistance (Weiner, 1994). Traditionally, these drugs are not used alone but as adjunctive therapy with another antihypertensive agent. While dose adjustments are not necessary in renal failure, the dose may be held just prior to dialysis treatments to reduce the risk of hypotension in patients for whom this is a problem during dialysis. Hemodialysis will dramatically reduce the blood levels of minoxidil; therefore, a careful review of blood pressure medications should be made when the patient's blood pressure rises during the treatment or rebound hypertension occurs after dialysis (Handley, 1994; Karubin et al., 1993).

In antihypertensive medication therapy, the nurse plays a role in both the monitoring of the regimen and advancement toward goals of therapy, but a larger role in education of the patient. Nursing interventions include monitoring blood pressure to document trends and educating the patient to do so, discussing lifestyle changes (e.g., sodium restriction, weight loss, exercise) that could positively effect blood pressure, monitoring of patient dosing routines and adherence to established regimens, and identifying factors that may affect medication effectiveness. Nurses can help the patient develop an acceptable routine for medication administration as well as decide which drugs, if any, should be held prior to dialysis. Education can also center on the need to watch for interactions between multiple antihypertensives and/or other drugs that the patient may be taking. Particularly with antihypertensives that require tapering to avoid rebound hypertension, patients should learn the importance of maintaining an adequate supply and the need to contact the physician or nurse if a prescription runs out. As with any medication administration, the nurse should monitor vital signs and patient understanding of the plan for successful therapy.

Cardiotonics

Cardiotonics (e.g., digoxin, digitoxin) are often used to manage congestive heart failure. They function to increase cardiac contractility and decrease venous pressure. At the same time, stroke volume is increased with a prolonged velocity (Baer, 1990). Digoxin has long been used for dialysis patients. However, dosage of this drug should be reduced in renal failure (usually to .125 mg daily or every other day). Monitoring of apical heart rate is important and the dose should be held if the pulse rate is too slow. In addition, serum levels of digoxin are frequently monitored to ensure that toxic levels are not reached.Traditionally, dialysate bath concentrations have been altered to increase the level of potassium for less electrolyte shifting during the treatment. Hypokalemia can potentiate the action of digoxin. This medication is not significantly removed during dialysis.

Electrolyte Supplements, Vitamin Replacements, and Phosphate Binders

Because of the many systemic effects of the disease, people with renal failure may require calcium replacement, vitamin replacement, and phosphate binders. In patients with chronic renal failure, the kidneys can no longer convert vitamin D into the active form, contributing to the development of hypocalcemia and secondary hyperparathyroidism (Peacock, 1992). Reduction of PTH has been shown to result in an improvement in renal osteodystrophy (Abbott, 1986).

Because of hypocalcemia, it is often necessary to replace calcium. There are several over the counter medications that provide needed calcium at an affordable price for renal patients (e.g., calcium carbonate or calcium acetate). Most of these preparations also serve to bind phosphate as well as supplement calcium. This results in the desired effect of reducing hyperphosphatemia, as well as increasing calcium levels. In particular, some calcium acetate preparations also serve to bind phosphorous at twice the amount of calcium carbonate, because they are better absorbed in the gut. Aluminum based phosphate binders, which were routinely used in the past, are avoided to prevent aluminum toxicity, often associated with organic brain disease (Coburn & Salusky, 1989; Mai et al., 1989). These preparations should be taken within an hour after meals to increase absorption, with the largest dose of the day taken with the largest meal. All renal patients should have their serum calcium levels, phosphate levels, and magnesium levels monitored on a regular basis. Renal failure patients should not be on other calcium additive agents simultaneously and consideration should be given to the fact that phosphate binders can interfere with the absorption of other medications.

Another important medication for people with renal failure is calcitriol, or active vitamin D. This medication helps normalize serum calcium and alkaline phosphatase levels and may help lower elevated parathyroid hormone (PTH) levels (Baker et al., 1986). Thus, calcitriol may help control and retard progression of osteitis fibrosa (Coburn, 1990; Malluche & Faugere, 1990) and alleviate the skeletal consequences of untreated bone disease (Goodman & Coburn, 1992). The medication is dispensed in both oral form and IV push to be used after dialysis.This medication must be monitored carefully, and the dose is always individualized to avoid hypercalcemia. If the serum parameters are not responding to therapy, the dose can be titrated by monitoring closely the serum calcium levels at least twice weekly. Often these patients may be treated with an alternate dialysate containing an adjusted calcium concentrate. Concurrently, appropriate phosphate binders should be used to control serum phosphate levels, and magnesium-containing products (e.g., Maalox, milk of magnesia, magnesium citrate) are not recommended because of possible hypermagnesemia. Other Vitamin D derivatives are withheld during treatment with calcitriol to avoid possible additive effects and hypercalcemia. There is a delicate balance in controlling calcium and phosphate levels. Hypercalcemia can cause life threatening cardiac arrythmias and a high calcium phosphate product (above 70) can result in metastatic calcifications.

Vitamins

All renal failure patients will need vitamin supplementation (including folic acid) due to diet restrictions, as well as dialyzability of water soluble vitamins (Baer, 1990). While patients are often encouraged to take less expensive over-the-counter preparations, there are vitamin preparations available specifically designed for renal failure patients (e.g., Nephro-vite). Since most vitamins are water soluble, it is advisable for the vitamin to be taken after dialysis for the patient to realize full therapeutic effect.

Antacids

Antacids are frequently used (e.g., Tums, sodium bicarbonate) to neutralize gastric acids. There has been an increase in the use of calcium based antacids because of the benefits of supplementing calcium at the same time. Magnesium and aluminum-based antacids are seldom used because of the risk of toxicity from these medications.

Histamine H_2 Receptor Antagonists

Renal failure patients often have gastric symptoms. Histamine H_2 receptor antagonists (e.g., ranitidine, famotidine, omeprazole) are often prescribed to offset the effects of other medication side effects or increased gastric irritation caused by renal failure. Cimetidine is a medication that often leads to mental confusion; therefore it is not recommended in renal failure. Likewise, ranitidine is usually given in a lower dose because it, too, can lead to mental confusion. Antacids can interfere with absorption of H_2 agonists if taken simultaneously. This is an area where new medications are appearing on the market annually. Each medication should be assessed initially to determine (a) whether a dose adjustment needs to be made in renal failure patients or (b) whether the medication may interfere with other medication absorption.

Stool Softeners and Cathartics

Renal patients are prone to constipation for a variety of reasons such as decreased fluid intake, constipating effect of other medications, decreased mobility, etc. Stool softeners and cathartics (e.g., docusate, methylcellulose, bisacodyl, lactulose) work in a variety of ways. There are laxatives, cathartics, stimulants, or osmotics. They work differently to meet specific patient situations. Often patients will find bowel routines that works for them and regulate these medication themselves. Cathartics and stool softeners are not removable through dialysis. For peritoneal dialysis patients, the use of a stool softener regularly is particularly important, since constipation may affect the success of the dialysis.

Sedatives and Hypnotics

Often renal patients may have trouble sleeping and request a medication to relax them and induce drowsiness. These medications (e.g., diazepam, flurazepam, lorazepam, and chloral hydrate) are prescribed only after other reasons for sleeplessness are thoroughly explored. Since any of these may cause excessive sedation in the presence of renal failure, they should be judiciously prescribed and administered. Because most of them are metabolized by the hepatic system, they are not dialyzable and, therefore not removed during a dialysis treatment. They may be more commonly seen in acute dialysis settings and used for agitation or sedation from other procedures. Chloral hydrate is rarely used because of its ability to cause excessive sedation.

Antimicrobial Agents

Antimicrobial agents are divided into several classes. Aminoglycosides, cephalosporins, penicillins, antifungal agents, antiviral agents, antituberculosis antibiotics, and tetracyclines are discussed. New antimicrobial agents are being developed regularly, with the addition of three to five new drugs monthly.

Aminoglycosides. The narrow toxic-therapeutic ratio of this class (e.g., gentamicin, tobramycin, amikacin) dictates careful management. Large cumulative doses can lead to ototoxicity and further renal impairment. Renal function should be closely monitored. Monitoring of serum levels of the drug is essential in the proper management of these agents through serum peak and trough levels. The normal peak serum level for gentamicin and tobramycin is, on average, 4.5 mg/L. Prolonged serum concentrations above 12 mg/L should be avoided and trough levels above 2 mg/L may indicate tissue accumulation. These medications are rapidly removed through dialysis and should always be given after the hemodialysis treatment (Massry & Glassock, 1989).

Cephalosporins. This class of medications has

a low toxic-therapeutic ratio. Because these medications are predominantly excreted by the kidney, the dosage needs to be adjusted in renal failure. Often these medications (e.g., cefazolin, cefaclor, cefoxitin, ceftizoxime, ceftriaxone, cefuroxime) are removed by hemodialysis. Exceptions include cefonicid, cefoperazone, and ceftriaxone (Massry & Glassock, 1989). They are well absorbed intraperitoneally, but absorption may be reduced if inflammation is present (Massry & Glassock, 1989). While these medications are effective and have few side effects, less costly penicillins should be considered before prescribing these more expensive medications.

Penicillins. Like the cephalosporins, the penicillins also have a low toxic:therapeutic ratio. The most common side effect is allergic interstitial nephritis. These medications (e.g., cloxacillin, dicloxacillin, methicillin, amoxicillin, ampicillin, mezlocillin, nafcillin, penicillin G, ticarcillin) may need dose adjustment depending on the type of dialysis treatment patients are receiving. With hemodialysis, they are usually removed; with peritoneal dialysis, they are not removed (Bennett & McCarron, 1987).

Tetracyclines. These medications (e.g., doxycycline, tetracycline, minocycline) may potentiate acidosis and raise BUN and phosphorus levels while increasing catabolism. Doxycycline is the tetracycline agent of choice in renal failure patients (Massry & Glassock, 1989). They are believed not to be removed through dialysis.

Miscellaneous Antibiotics

Erythromycin. Although only a moderate dose adjustment is necessary because of primarily nonrenal metabolism, erythromycin ototoxicity in patients with renal failure is not uncommon. Notably, the volume of distribution of this medication is doubled in dialysis (Massry & Glassock, 1989). Caution should be used in use of erythromycin in transplant recipients, since it will increase levels of cyclosporine and FK506. These drugs will require adjustment of dosage if the antibiotic is continued.

Aztreonam. The half-life of this medication is markedly increased in renal failure. Dose adjustments must be made in the face of dialysis due to its removal during treatment (Bennett & McCarron, 1987).

Vancomycin. While this medication is widely used for renal patients with infections, it must be monitored closely for toxicity through peak and trough serum levels. It can be ototoxic at serum levels >50. In renal failure, the half-life of this drug is more than 33 times the normal (Bennett & McCarron, 1987). Often a 7- to 10-day interval is used between dosages to maintain therapeutic levels while avoiding the toxic side effects. This medication is not removed during dialysis. It may be given prophylactically until culture results are known in the presence of obvious signs and symptoms of infection. In life-threatening situations, this drug may be given in conjunction with other drugs (e.g., tobramycin, gentamicin) to cover all possible organisms until culture results are known.

Antifungal agents. These medications (e.g., amphotericin B, fluconazole, miconazole, ketoconazole) are often used for fungal infections that can be life threatening for patients. Amphotericin B, given intravenously, is most commonly used. It is not dialyzable (Bennett & McCarron, 1987), requiring no dose adjustment following hemodialysis. However, it does have side effects that often require premedication prior to administration. This premedication might include acetaminophen, diphenhydramine, and hydrocortisone to inhibit the histamine effects of allergic reaction. Other side effects to watch for include renal tubular acidosis, hypokalemia, nephrogenic diabetes insipidus, and nephrotoxicity. Miconazole can cause hyponatremia. Ketoconazole is rarely used in renal failure patients, and in renal transplant patients it may interfere with cyclosporine metabolism and increase cyclosporine levels (Bennett & McCarron, 1987). If concurrent use is required, the cyclosoporine dose should be decreased and levels should be frequently monitored until the course of therapy with the antifungal agent is completed.

Antiviral Agents

Antiviral agents (e.g., acyclovir, ganciclovir sodium) are used to treat the human cytomegalovirus or CMV. Ganciclovir sodium exerts a virostatic effect on CMV. It acts by interfering with DNA synthesis both in vivo and vitro. Administered intravenously, the antiviral drug can effectively stop the CMV herpes virus from replicating in adolescents and adults. It is used to treat CMV retinitis, or in serious CMV disease, pneumonia, and gastrointestinal disease (Stevens & Roberts, 1994). It may also be used prophylactically to prevent CMV infection in transplant patients who are CMV negative and who have received a CMV positive kidney or who are CMV positive at the time of transplant. Ganciclovir has a low molecular weight, and if the patient is on dialysis, it should be given after the hemodialysis treatment is complete, as dialysis reduces plasma ganciclovir levels by about 50% (USP Convention, 1993). Ganciclovir dosage may need to be modified in the renally impaired patient because it is almost exclusively excreted unchanged in the urine. Modification may be achieved by dose reduction or prolongation of dosing interval in response to the patient's renal function tests (Stevens & Roberts, 1994). Acyclovir is an oral agent while ganciclovir can be administered intravenously. Nursing assessment of these patients should include a complete assessment, predosing laboratory work, and a complete drug and allergy history.

Antituberculosis Antibiotics

The use of antituberculosis antibiotics has increased. These medications (e.g., ethambutol, isoniazid, rifampicin) are known for side effects such as acute renal failure, decreased visual acuity, and peripheral neuritis. Both ethambutol and isoniazid must be administered following hemodialysis due to removal of these drugs during hemodialysis. Rifampicin does not need dose adjustment since it is not removed during dialysis. Serum levels of rifampin can be monitored for therapeutic doses (Bennett & McCarron, 1987).

Antidiabetic Agents or Hypoglycemics

Since diabetes is the cause of over 25% of the chronic renal failure cases, nephrology nurses need to become familiar with the actions and uses of hypoglycemic agents. This class of drugs is more closely explored in clinical application in Chapter 16 but these drugs are briefly reviewed here. Hypoglycemics (e.g., glipizide, chlorpropamide, glyburide) work to lower blood sugar by stimulating beta cells in the pancreas to release endogenous insulin. Chlorpropamide may also potentiate available antidiuretic hormone (ADH), a property not shared by other sulfonylureas. These drugs are used in the control of ketosis-resistant (maturity onset) diabetes in patients who cannot be controlled by diet alone or who do not have complications of diabetes (Giovani & Hayes, 1982).

While the second generation drugs (e.g., glipizide and glyburide) require no dose adjustment in renal failure, the others have been known to cause prolonged hypoglycemia in chronic renal failure patients and should be monitored closely (Massry & Glassock, 1989). Nurses have a role in helping the patient monitor blood sugar and other side effects. Dialysate concentrates may also be adjusted based on the patient's response to the glucose in the dialysate.

It has been demonstrated that good control of blood sugars prevents or significantly delays the progression of renal disease. Once dialysis is initiated, most diabetic patients continue regular injections of insulin. If peritoneal dialysis is selected as the treatment modality, insulin can be administered intraperitoneally. Generally, a short acting insulin is added to each exchange. Although dosages of intraperitoneal insulin may seem higher than subcutaneous requirements, it must be recognized that a significant amount of the drug adheres to the plastic bag and is not absorbed. Insulin is also used to treat acute hyperkalemia in nondiabetic as well as diabetic patients. It acts to shift potassium and sugar into the cells, temporarily reducing the extracellular potassium concentration. It is generally given with glucose solutions to prevent hypoglycemia. It should be recognized that this is a temporary treatment that should be followed by other treatments for hyperkalemia, such as dialysis or cation-exchange resins.

Cation-Exchange Resins

Cation-exchange resins (e.g., sodium polystyrene sulfonate) are used in the treatment of non-life-threatening hyperkalemia (Meyer, 1993). The mechanism of action for sodium polystyrene sulfonate involves exchanging sodium ions for potassium ions in the gut. One gram of sodium is exchanged for one milliequivalent of potassium. Cation-exchange is not completely selective to potassium, however, and small amounts of magnesium, calcium, and ammonium may also be lost (Berlyne, Janabi, & Shaw, 1966). While the slow onset of action limits the use of this medication, the medication is effective when no cardiac abnormalities are evident and the patient is otherwise asymptomatic. This medication may be administered either orally or rectally.

Since the insoluble resin is not absorbed systemically, there is no dosage adjustment required in renal failure, hepatic failure, or during dialysis. However, increased absorption of sodium could contribute to fluid volume excess and must be considered as a potential side effect of therapy (Meyer, 1993). The patient should also be monitored for cardiac effects from the sodium reabsorption as well as weight gain, edema, hypertension, hypernatremia, pulmonary edema, and worsening left ventricular failure with congestive heart failure (Berlyne et al., 1966). One key interaction that has been documented in the literature is a negative effect with magnesium hydroxide-containing antacids (Schroeder, 1969); it can reduce the resin's potassium exchange capability. The digitalized patient should be closely monitored because hypokalemia can cause digitalis toxicity (Baer, 1990).

Nursing implications center on the monitoring of maximum benefits of this therapy with minimal side effects (Meyer, 1993). The typical dose can range from 15 to 100 mg. After rectal administration, one can expect an effect within 6 hours; oral administration will result in slower and somewhat unpredictable time to action. Sorbitol is often used as a solvent for cation-exchange resins. However, caution must be used to ensure that a cleansing enema is given after rectal Kayexalate and sorbital administration since rare cases of colonic necrosis have occurred. Since the resin is not palatable, chilling the oral suspension before administration, choosing fluids that the patient likes with which to mix the powder, and assessing the need for antiemetic therapy may improve patient compliance. Monitoring the patient's bowel patterns, assessing for hypoactive bowel sounds and/or ileus before administering the resin, and determining the effectiveness of stool softeners, laxatives, or cathartics will help prevent constipation, fecal impaction, and/or bowel necrosis (Meyer, 1993).

Antianemics

Almost three-quarters of the 200,000 patients worldwide receiving dialysis are anemic, and an almost equal number of predialysis patients are anemic (Eschbach & Adamson, 1988, 1985; Humphries, 1992). Several factors lead to the development of this anemia, including decreased red blood cell survival, chronic blood loss (through blood sampling, dialysis, or gastrointestinal losses), and iron and vitamin deficiencies (folate and B12) (York, 1993). However, the most important factor is decreased erythropoietin production that results from a loss of functional renal tissue (Chandra, McVicar, & Clemons, 1988). In the past, blood transfusions were used to improve symptoms and to avoid severe tissue hypoxia that occurs in 25% to 50% of chronic renal failure patients (Eschbach & Adamson, 1988). Unfortunately, patients who receive transfusions may contact infections (such as HIV and hepatitis), develop iron overload, develop cytotoxic antibodies, and experience transfusion reactions such as flushing, urticaria, fever, and chills (Eschbach & Adamson, 1988).

A number of drugs can be used to treat anemia of renal failure. Recombinant human erythropoietin and iron supplements contribute significantly to the ultimate result of an increased hemoglobin and hematocrit.

Epoetin alfa (EPO). Until 1989, effective treatment was not available for anemia of renal failure. Following the development of recombinant human erythropoietin (EPO), studies of patients receiving EPO have demonstrated increases in hematocrit to near-normal levels, reductions in the requirement for blood transfusions, and overall improvements in quality of life (York, 1993).

This agent is indicated for the treatment of anemia associated with chronic renal failure, including patients on dialysis and not on dialysis. Prior to administration of therapy, the patient's iron stores should be evaluated, including iron, iron binding capacity, percent transferrin saturation, and serum ferritin. Transferrin percent saturation should be at least 30% and ferritin at least 300 ng/ml. If iron levels are low, oral or intravenous iron treatment should be initiated. Blood pressure should be adequately controlled before initiation of this therapy and must be closely monitored and controlled during therapy. Nondialysis patients with symptomatic anemia considered for therapy should have a hematocrit less than 30%. All patients on this therapy should have their white blood cells and red blood cell counts monitored regularly (Amgen, 1994).

The most significant side effect of EPO is hypertension. Patients with uncontrolled, serious hypertension should not be treated with EPO. Blood pressure must be controlled adequately before initiation of therapy. For patients who show a rapid increase in hematocrit (e.g., more than 4 points in any 2-week period), the dose should be reduced because of the possible association of rapid increases of hematocrit with hypertension (Amgen, 1994). Given the potential for an increased risk of seizures during the first 90 days of therapy, blood pressure and the presence of premonitory neurologic symptoms should be monitored closely. The manufacturer (in package inserts) cautions patients about driving and other potentially hazardous activities during this 90-day period. While thrombotic events are rare (0.25 events per patient year), patients with preexisting vascular disease should be monitored closely (Amgen, 1994).

Delayed or diminished response to EPO occurs in some patients. Many of the following reasons have been identified as possible causes: inability to mobilize iron stores, as demonstrated by normal ferritin levels but low transferrin saturations; underlying infectious, inflammatory, or malignant processes; occult blood loss; underlying hematologic diseases; deficiencies of folic acid or vitamin B12; hemolysis; aluminum toxicity; and osteitis fibrosa cystica (Amgen, 1994). It has also been noted in the literature that therapy with epoetin alfa results in an increase in hematocrit and a decrease in plasma volume, which could affect dialysis efficiency. In studies to date, the resulting increase in hematocrit did not appear to adversely affect dialyzer function or the efficiency of high flux dialysis. During hemodialysis, patients may require increased heparin dosing to prevent clotting of the dialyzer (Amgen, 1994).

While a variety of dosing patterns exist in clinical practice today, there are general guidelines that reflect the majority of practices with chronic renal failure patients. Starting doses in the range of 50-100 units/kg weekly have been shown to be safe and effective in increasing hematocrit and eliminating transfusion dependency in this population (Amgen, 1994). Doses may be reduced when the target hematocrit is reached or the hematocrit rises more than 4 points in any 2-week period. An acceptable target range for hematocrit is about 30% to 33% with a maximum level of 36%. This medication may be administered, based on manufacturers' recommendations, either intravenously or subcutaneously. Subcutaneous administration is typically used for patients on peritoneal dialysis.

Oral iron preparations. Iron deficiency, a common problem in chronic renal failure patients, occurs primarily as a result of gastrointestinal or procedure-related blood loss (Kirlin, 1993). Iron deficiency is a particular problem in patients receiving EPO to correct their anemia because iron is essential for the formation of red blood cells. If iron stores are insufficient, no amount of EPO will result in an increase in hematocrit (Kirlin, 1994). Virtually all patients receiving EPO will eventually require some iron supplementation. Iron deficiency has emerged as a leading cause of failure to respond to therapy (Drueke, 1990).

Oral iron supplementation is usually preferred over intravenous (IV) for initial therapy. However, there are a number of side effects of oral iron therapy that may affect whether or not the patient takes the medication. These include: constipation, diarrhea, nausea, vomiting, abdominal pain, and heartburn (Kirlin, 1993). Several strategies can be used to enhance the effectiveness of oral iron (e.g., ferrous sulfate, ferrous fumarate, ferrous gluconate). Except for those with serious iron overload, patients should start oral iron therapy before beginning EPO therapy (Van Wyck, 1989). Often ferrous sulfate, fumarate, or gluconate are used because of their relatively low cost. Kirlin (1993) suggests that less costly products that are not tolerated well and, therefore, not taken regularly are actually more expensive than ones well tolerated and taken consistently. Since a number of medications interfere with iron absorption (antacids, antiinflammatory agents, chloramphenicol, desferoxamine, penicillamine, phosphate binders, quinidine, ranitidine, sulfonamides, and tetracyclines), the nurse should closely monitor iron absorption when new drugs are prescribed for a patient (Kirlin, 1993). For patients who fail to respond to oral iron therapy, intravenous therapy may be considered, although it poses additional risks.

Iron dextran. Iron dextran is the parenteral preparation of iron that can be used to increase iron levels. If oral agents are not achieving target iron levels, this may be used as second-line drug. Iron dextran provides 50 mg of elemental iron per ml. (Schein, 1991). After injection, macrophages of the reticuloendothelial system remove iron dextran from the plasma. Ferric iron is then gradually released into the plasma, where it combines with transferrin. Transferrin transports the iron to the bone marrow to be incorporated into hemoglobin (Kirlin, 1993). Typical dosages are approximately 100 mg weekly at the end of dialysis. A test dose is recommended because of the risk of anaphylaxis. Although anaphylactic reactions, known to occur following dextran injections, are usually evident within a few minutes, it is recommended that a period of an hour or longer lapse after the test dose before the remainder of the initial dose is given (Schein, 1991). Most facilities have a standard protocol for iron dextran administration that includes a test dose before each injection. Emergency equipment and medications (e.g., diphenhydramine and hydrocortisone) should always be within reach when the test dose is administered (Krumpf & Holland, 1990). The patient should be observed for other side effects such as pruritus, hypotension, and dyspnea (Schein, 1991). Iron dextran should be diluted and administered in a 0.9% sodium chloride solution, or it can be administered slow IV push no faster than 1 ml/min or in a dilute IV piggyback over 30 minutes (Kirlin, 1993).

Miscellaneous Medications

Urokinase. This medication is a thrombolytic agent derived from human kidney cells (American Society of Hospital Pharmacists, 1994). It is a protein enzyme that acts on the endogenous fibrinolytic system, converting plasminogen to the enzyme plasmin. Plasmin degrades fibrin clots, fibrinogen, and other plasma properties. Urokinase does not activate antibody formation; therefore, an allergic reaction is rare ("Home Use of Urokinase," 1991; Northsea, 1994). Schwab and Butler (1988), who used urokinase to restore patency in double lumen subclavian and permanent jugular hemodialysis catheters, found that urokinase was a safe, efficient, cost-effective method of resolving thrombosis. In the past, catheter occlusion resulted in catheter replacement that increased risk for the patient (e.g., pneumothorax, infections), caused patient discomfort, was time consuming and costly. The use of urokinase provides an alternative to catheter replacement (Northsea, 1994).

The nurse and physician must calculate the correct dose to instill based on the lumen size of the catheter. The package insert for the catheter describes the lumen capacity. The optimal time for instillation is 30 minutes prior to withdrawal of the clot/fibrinous material. If patency is not restored, the solution should be left for another 30 minutes before checking again. If patency is restored, an additional 5 ml of blood/solution should be withdrawn and discarded from the catheter prior to use for dialysis (Northsea, 1994). It is necessary to monitor the patient for adverse reactions such as fever, bleeding, bronchospasm, skin rash, or changes in vital signs during the dialysis treatment (American Society of Hospital Pharmacists, 1994).

Hypertonic saline. Intravenous-administered hypertonic saline has long been used to alleviate side effects of severe hypotension and cramping during hemodialysis. Ideally, these symptoms should be prevented by accurate determination of dry weight, modest intradialytic fluid weight gains, and judicious fluid removal. However, despite recent advances in hemodialysis technology, intradialytic hypotension and muscle cramping still occur and adversely affect the quality of treatment (Sanderson & Katz, 1994). Symptomatic hypotension may occur in 25% to 30% of bicarbonate hemodialysis treatments (de Vires, 1990; Sturniolo et al., 1990). Intradialytic muscle cramps complicate up to 20% of treatments (Canzanello et al., 1991). Intravenous administration of hypertonic saline effectively alleviates cramps and hypotension by increasing plasma osmolality and moving fluid from the extravascular to the intravascular compartment to increase blood volume (Lancaster, 1984). It is an accepted practice in nephrology to treat both hypotension and muscle cramps with hypertonic saline; however differences of opinion exist regarding its proper use (Sanderson & Katz, 1994).

The literature does not identify a standard practice or standard dosage for hypertonic saline when treating intradialytic hypotension or muscle cramps (Sanderson & Katz, 1994). Dosages in the literature range from 45 mEq to 60 mEq IV. Cramping is usually relieved within 30 to 45 seconds (Sanderson & Katz, 1994). Sherman and coauthors (1982) completely relieved cramps 59% of the time with 60 mEq given over 1 minute. Kinet and coauthors (1982) used hypertonic saline for both prophylactic and symptomatic treatment of hypotension. Blood pressure returned to normal within 20 minutes in all cases.

While there has been concern about the potential for overadministration of hypertonic saline leading to posttreatment hypernatremia, the literature does not support this. Kinet and coauthors (1982) found no statistically significant difference in pretreatment and posttreatment sodium levels after regular administration of hypertonic saline during all 4 hours of hemodialysis treatment. Jenkins and Dreher (1975) reported that serum sodium rose and dropped within 50 seconds. Although this study was done almost 20 years ago, no other study has demonstrated the rise and fall of serum sodium after administration. Sanderson and Katz (1994) showed in their study that while a small but statistically significant amount of sodium was recovered in the dialysate, and although the majority of hypertonic saline was retained by the subject, it was clinically insignificant because there was no significant change in interdialytic weight. They concluded that hypertonic saline is safe and effective for side effects of hemodialysis without the risk of weight gains previously suspected.

Dialyzability of Drugs

Nurses should consider the dialyzability of any drug given to patients receiving dialysis therapy. Dialysis therapy may or may not significantly affect the absorption and efficacy of a medication administered to a patient with renal failure. In general, if a medication is primarily excreted by the kidney, then it is usually also dialyzable through hemodialysis. Because of the selectivity of the peritoneal clearances of many drugs, this statement does not necessarily apply to peritoneal dialysis (Baer, 1990).

The effect of hemodialysis on the half-life of a medication is a function of the following factors: the perfusion and dialysate flow rates; the dialysis membrane permeability and surface area; the molecular weight of the medication; the percent of protein binding of the medication; the lipid affinity of the drug; and the medication distribution volume (American College of Physicians, 1994; Baer, 1990; Bennett, 1986).

CHAPTER 12B

Medications in Transplant Patients

Karen K. Giuliano, MSN, RN, CCRN
Anita E. Molzahn, PhD, RN
Terran Warren Sims, BSN, RN, CNN

Chapter Contents

Pharmacologic Management of Patients with Solid Organ Transplant . 331
History of Immunosuppression Therapy 331
Immunosuppressive Medications Commonly Used in Transplantation . 334
Cyclosporine 334
Tacrolimus 336
Azathioprine 337
Steroids 337
Mycophenolate Mofetil 338
Polyclonal and Monoclonal Antibodies 338
OKT3 338
New Immunosuppressants in Transplantation 339
Cyclosporine G 339
IMM-125 339
Rapamycin 339
Brequinar 339
15-Deoxyspergualin 339
Other Common Medications for Transplant Recipients 340
Antiulcer Medication (famotidine, antacids, omeprazole, ranitidine, sucralfate) 340
Trimethoprim-Sulfamethoxazole (Bactrim) 341
Oral Antifungal Agents (clotrimazole, nystatin) 341

Chapter Contents

- Bowel Medications (docusate sodium, psyllium) 341
- Electrolyte Supplements 341
- Calcium Channel Blockers (diltiazem, verapamil, amlodipine, felodipine, isradipine, nicardipine, nifedipine). 341
- Antihypertensives 341
- Over-the-Counter Medications and Other Prescribed Medications . . . 342

Summary 342

References and Readings. 342

Chapter Highlights 345

Medications in Transplant Patients

Karen K. Giuliano, MSN, RN, CCRN
Anita E. Molzahn, PhD, RN
Terran Warren Sims, BSN, RN, CNN

Pharmacologic Management of Patients with Solid Organ Transplant

Transplantation therapy involves significant use of various immunosuppressive agents. After a brief introduction and history of transplantation and immunosuppression, the most commonly used immunosuppressive drugs (i.e., cyclosporine, azathiaprine, steroids, tacrolimus, mycophenolate mofetil, polyclonal and monoclonal antibodies, and selected other immunosuppressives) as well as other commonly prescribed medications are described.

The purpose of the immune system in humans is to protect the body from invasion by foreign pathogens. Since we are constantly in contact with microorganisms and other substances that can interfere with the normal functioning of the human body, it is essential for survival that the body be able to discriminate between substances that are its own and substances that are foreign. Once the immune system identifies a substance as foreign, the body begins the process of destroying the foreign substance. For the recipients of transplanted organs, this normally protective process is responsible for one of the greatest clinical problems in transplantation, the process of rejection. In order to prevent rejection, all transplant recipients are treated with immunosuppressive medications. However, suppression of the immune system with medications can have serious side effects. In particular, there is an increased risk of infections and malignancies with most immunosuppressive drugs. Hence, it is critical that candidates for transplants be carefully screened for malignancies prior to transplantation and monitored closely thereafter. Also, immunosuppression makes the body more susceptible to infection, many of which can be life threatening. Infections with cytomegalovirus (CMV) or Epstein Barr Virus are very serious. It is indeed a challenge to prevent these complications while suppressing the immune system enough to prevent rejection.

History of Immunosuppression Therapy

Much of the progress in the field of transplantation is related to the progress in immunosuppression therapy (see Table 12-8). This is especially true in kidney transplantation. While the surgical techniques have changed little since the 1960s, the graft survival has improved due to advances in immunosuppression. Throughout the 1960s total-body irradiation was a common method for immunosuppression. This method was successful in preventing rejection; however, it was not uncommon for the patient to die of overwhelming sepsis (Hume, Merrill, & Mill, 1955). Table 12-9 presents several of the immunosuppressive medications, along with their purpose, dose, administration, and side effects. These drugs are discussed in more detail in the following paragraphs.

Table 12-8
Landmark events in immunosuppressive therapy development.

Year	Event
1960	Glucocorticoid use for immunosuppression
1960	Antilymphocyte serum trials
1961	Azathioprine
1978	First use of cyclosporine A
1979	Muromonab CD-3 (OKT3)
1983	FDA approval of cyclosporine A
1992	Clinical trials mycophenolate mofetil (RS/Cellcept)
1993	European multi-center trail of IMM-125 (Sandoz)
1994	FDA approval FK506
1994	Clinical trials of rapamycin
1994	Phase I trials of brequinar US and Canada
1994	US and Japan trails of 15-deoxyspergualin
1994	Swedish trials for high antibody titers
1995	FDA approval mycophenolate mofetil (RS)
1995	FDA approval neoral for kidney recipients
1995	Neoral for livers in clinical trials
1995	Emlimomab trials and later removal from trials
1996	Neoral for livers approved

Steroids were first used in kidney transplantation in 1960 and were found to be useful for both preventing and treating rejection (d'Apice, 1984). In

Table 12-9
Immunosuppressive medications.

Agent	Purpose	Dose	Administration	Side Effects
Cyclosporine (Neoral/ Sandimmune@)	Maintenance Immunosuppression	Adjusted to serum drug levels; 3-4 mg/kg QD; Tablets: 25, 50, 100 mg; Liquid 100 mg/cc	IV initially, then orally; (mix in OJ or milk for solution)	Nephrotoxic Hepatotoxic Hand tremors Seizures Flushing Gingival Hyperplasia GI Distress Headaches Mild anemia Hyperkalemia Hypertension Malignancies Hirsutism
Azathioprine (Imuran)	Maintenance Immunosuppression	2-3 mg/kg QD Tablets: 50 mg	IV initially, then orally QD	Bone Marrow Suppression Anemia Thrombocytopenia Bleeding Leukopenia Hair thinning Infections GI problems Mouth Ulcers Hepatitis
FK506 (Tacrolimus)	Maintenance Immunosuppression	Adjusted to serum drug levels; Capsules 1 mg, 5 mg; IV prep-5 mg/ml	IV then orally; BID or per protocol Infections	Nephrotoxic Hypertension Neurotoxic Tremors Tingling - hands/feet Paresthesia Insomnia Headache Tinnitus Photosensitivity Sleep disturbances Mood swings
Mycopheno-late Mofetil (RS)	Maintenance Immunosuppression	1000 mg orally in split doses; Capsules 250 mg; IV prep pending release	Orally when taking POs	GI distress Neutropenia Anemia Thrombocytopenia Infections
Prednisone	Maintenance Immunosuppression	0.2 mg/kg or per protocol 20-30 mg QD	IV initially, then orally after IV taper; divided or single dose as tolerated	*Common:* Cushingoid appearance Increased appetite Obesity Na+/water retention GI distress Peptic ulcer Bruising Acne Diaphoresis Infections (opportunistic) *Less common:* Avascular joint necrosis Diabetes Cataracts Growth retardation Pancreatitis

Table 12-9
Immunosuppressive medications. (continued)

Agent	Purpose	Dose	Administration	Side Effects
Methyl-prednisolone (Solumedrol)	Induction/ Rejection therapy	15 mg/kg not > 3 days or per protocol taper	IV bolus; peripheral IV in divided doses per taper	See Prednisone
Cyclo-phosphamide (Cytoxan)	Maintenance Immunosuppression	50-75 mg QD adults	Orally QD	Leukopenia Bladder fibrosis Hematuria GI distress Thrombocytopenia
Polyclonal (ALG, ATGAM, ALS, ATS)	Induction/ Rejection therapy	15 mg/kg QD for 5-21 days	IV over 6 hours through high flow vein (TLC); premedications as in OK-3	Hypersensitivity preparations response Rash Tachycardia Dyspnea Hypotension Chills Fever Chest pain Back pain Anaphylaxis Leukopenia Thrombocytopenia Arthralgia Myalgia Fluid retention Infections (opportunistic)
Monoclonal Antibody (OKT-3)	Induction/ Rejection therapy	5 mg daily for 5-14 days	IV push via peripheral vein; Premedications per protocol: hydrocortisone, acetaminophen, diphenhydramine	*First dose:* Flu like signs & symptoms Fever Chills Tremors Nausea Vomiting Dyspnea Chest pain Wheezing Flash pulmonary edema *Long term issues:* Viral infections Lymphoma

1960-61, 6-mercaptopurine (6-MP) was used successfully, but shortly thereafter it was found that azathioprine, which is a 6-MP derivative, was a more effective immunosuppressant in kidney transplantation (Murray, Merrill, & Harrison, 1963). Starzl, Marchioro, Porter, Iwasaki, and Cerilli (1967) demonstrated that the best results came from combination therapy using azathioprine and steroids, and this was soon considered the standard of care worldwide. This regimen remained as the standard of care until the FDA approval of cyclosporine in 1982. The widespread use of cyclosporine beginning in the 1980s revolutionized immunosuppression for kidney transplant recipients and accelerated the further development of other types of solid organ transplantation. Today, most transplant recipients receive combination therapy to prevent rejection.

Immunosuppressive Medications Commonly Used in Transplantation

Cyclosporine

Cyclosporine is a potent immunosuppressant first used in clinical trials by Calne et al. (1978) in England. Throughout the next several years, clinical trials in Europe, Canada, and the United States demonstrated both the efficacy and relative safety of this drug. Cyclosporine has, by far, been the biggest clinical advancement in the care of transplant patients.

The primary action of cyclosporine is to inhibit the action of T lymphocytes. In the normal immune response, the T lymphocytes would be activated by the presence of the foreign antigens of the transplanted organ, and the process of rejection would begin. Cyclosporine interferes with the production, release, and effectiveness of both interleukin-2 (IL2) and interleukin-1 (IL1). IL-2 and IL-1 are two of the most important lymphokines (immune system hormones) that stimulate T-cell proliferation. This depressed T-cell function inhibits the activation and proliferation of cytotoxic T-cells that are responsible for actively attacking the transplanted organ during an episode of rejection (Hess, Colombani, & Esa, 1986). Because of cyclosporine's very specific mode of action, it does not interfere as greatly with the overall functioning of the immune system as some of the less specific agents. This is a very desirable quality for cyclosporine.

Cyclosporine (Sandimmune) is not well absorbed in the gut, and bile salts are required for absorption. Anything that affects GI function will affect the cyclosporine level. If patients experience diarrhea, cyclosporine absorption will be reduced and the blood level will drop, leaving the patient more vulnerable to rejection. For patients who experience constipation, cyclosporine absorption will be increased, the blood level will increase, and patients may experience cyclosporine toxicity. Because the consequences of cyclosporine dosing are so serious, very close attention should be paid to GI function, and vigilant monitoring is necessary for patients whose GI function is altered.

Neoral (cyclosporine microemulsion) was approved for patient use in 1995 by the FDA. It is an oral formulation of cyclosporine that immediately forms a microemulsion in an aqueous environment. Because it is a microemulsion, it is believed to have greater bioavailability than Sandimmune when administered orally, and hence they are not bioequivalent. In general, patients should be able to maintain adequate cyclosporine levels on a lower dose of Neoral than Sandimmune. This means higher therapeutic effects with lower doses. Because Neoral provides for better bioavailability for patients, Sandimmune will be phased out slowly over time, and patients will be converted to Neoral. Conversion protocols vary from center to center. Particular caution should be exercised during this process to avoid cyclosporine toxicity.

Unfortunately, the adverse effects of cyclosporine are many and are summarized in Table 12-10, along with other immunosuppressive medications. The most serious adverse effect is nephrotoxicity, which may be rapid or chronic. This is especially troublesome in kidney transplantation and has been shown to occur in 50%-75% of renal transplant recipients (Hamilton, Calne, & Evans, 1981; Klintman, Rigden, & Groth, 1983; Klintman, Iwatsuki, & Starzl, 1981). Nephrotoxicity is usually manifested as reduced creatinine clearance, elevated serum creatinine, increase in BUN with preserved urine volume and sodium resorption, hyperkalemia, and hypertension (Smith, 1990). Because of cyclosporine-induced nephrotoxicity, it is important to differentiate nephrotoxicity from rejection because the clinical treatments are different. A reduction in the dose of cyclosporine will successfully treat cyclosporine-induced nephrotoxicity, while antirejection regimens must be used to treat rejection. A renal biopsy is the most definitive way to distinguish between them. It is important to obtain a definitive diagnosis as soon as possible so that the appropriate treatment can be started and renal damage can be minimized.

In addition to the associated side effects with immunosuppression such as infections and malignancies, other side effects of cyclosporine include hypertension, hyperglycemia, tremors, and hyperkalemia. Gum soreness and gingival hyperplasia are also common, as is hirsutism. Parasthesias, leukopenia, diarrhea, nausea, vomiting, convulsions, and headache are less commonly reported side effects.

There are numerous drugs that are known to interact with cyclosporine. Ketoconazole, erythromycin, josamycin, corticosteroids, oral contraceptives, doxycycline, calcium channel blockers, propafenone, metoclopramide, and imipenem are known to increase the serum concentration of cyclosporine. Similar interactions are suspected with H_2 agonists, cephalosporins, thiazide diuretics, androgenic steroids, acyclovir, and warfarin. On the other hand, drugs known to decrease the serum concentration of cyclosporine include phenytoin, phenobarbitone, rifampicin, sulfadimidine, nafcillin, methidazole, carbamazepine, octreotide, and sulfinpyrazone.

Monitoring of cyclosporine levels is important to control and prevent both toxicity and graft rejection. It has been performed using whole blood, serum, and plasma, although whole blood is generally preferred because it produces more consistent and reliable results (Wenk & Follath, 1983). Currently, there are three methods available for monitoring: RIA (radioimmunoassay), HPLC (high-performance liquid chromatography), and fluorescence polarization immunoassay (FPIA) (Smith, 1990). Each test has its advantages and disadvantages, some of which are listed in Table 12-11.

Table 12-10
Comparison of side effects of immunosuppressive medications.

Side Effect	Cyclo	Azathioprine	Myco	Tacro	Steroids
Increased susceptibility to infection	Yes	Yes	Yes	Yes	Yes
Increased risk of malignancy	Yes	Yes	Yes	Yes	Yes
Nephrotoxicity	Yes	No	No	Yes	No
Hypertension	Yes	No	No	Yes	Yes
Hirsutism	Yes	No	No	Yes	Yes
Tremors/nervousness	Yes	No	No	Yes	Yes
Gingival hyperplasia	Yes	No	No	Yes	No
Hepatoxicity	Yes	Yes	Possible	Yes	No
Bone marrow suppression	No	Yes	Yes	No	No
Alopecia	No	Yes	Possible	No	No
Sensitivity to UV rays	No	Yes	Possible	No	Yes
Bone Disease	No	No	No	No	Yes
Weight gain	No	No	No	No	Yes
Hyperglycemia	Yes	No	No	Yes	Yes
Cataracts/glaucoma	No	No	No	No	Yes
Gastritis	No	No	Yes	No	Yes
Nausea	Yes	Yes	Yes	Yes	Yes
Diarrhea	Yes	No	Yes	Yes	No
Headache	Yes	No	Yes	Yes	No
Hyperkalemia	Yes	No	No	Yes	No
Hypomagnesemia	Yes	No	No	Yes	No
Muscle wasting	No	Yes	No	No	Yes
Pancreatitis	No	Yes	No	No	Yes

Note: Adapted from Sigardson-Poor & Haggerty (1990); Nursing 93 Drug Handbook; Fujisawa (1994); Roche (1995).

The HPLC method is considered to be the most accurate assessment of parent drug concentrations (Kahan, Shaw, Holt, Grevel, & Johnston, 1990), and for this reason remains the reference procedure. However, HPLC methods are very technically demanding and are not feasible for many laboratories because the level of difficulty in performing them may lead to inconsistent test results. The newest methods, specifically FPIA, use whole-blood trough concentrations with selective monoclonal antibodies. Selective antibodies measure parent compound, while nonselective antibodies measure both the parent compound and its metabolites. Selective monoclonal antibody tests seem to show promise for producing reliable test results, are easier to perform than HPLC methods, and also show a good deal of diagnostic efficacy (Kahan et al., 1990). However, because the role of metabolites is not well understood, there is still a need for using nonselective methods until it can be proven that these metabolites are of no clinical consequence (Kahan et al., 1990).

While therapeutic cyclosporine monitoring is done routinely at most transplant centers, obtained values alone are of no prognostic significance. There is tremendous individual variation from

Table 12-11
Comparison of three methods of therapeutic cyclosporine monitoring.

	RIA	HPLC	Fluorescence Polarization Immunoassay (FPIA)
Measurable Substance	Parent compound and metabolites	Parent compound only	Monoclonal tests measure only parent compound; polyclonal tests measure both parent compound and metabolites
Technical ease of test performance	Between HPLC and PF	Most difficult	Easiest
Fluid tested	Whole blood, serum, or plasma	Whole blood, serum, or plasma	Whole blood, serum, or plasma
Reliability of results	Unknown influence of metabolites	Most accurate, preferred method for clinical research studies	Selective monoclonal tests have been shown to yield similar results to HPLC

patient to patient. Most experts attribute this variation to several possible factors including differential cyclosporine susceptibility/resistance, procurement injuries, intrinsic donor diseases, variable alloimmune reactivities, and concomitant immunosuppressive therapy (Kahan et al., 1990). However, by following certain basic guidelines, the accuracy and reliability of the test can be maximized. These guidelines include consistently measuring levels in the same manner (e.g., 30 minutes before first dose of day), having a consistent amount of elapsed time between blood drawing and test performance, consistent temperature of sample, and consistent time of sample draw in relation to cyclosporine dosing regimen (most centers do trough levels). It is only when individual patient levels are reviewed within the context of the patient's clinical course that the values become useful for patient management (Kahan et al., 1990). Monitoring seems to be of the greatest clinical usefulness in the immediate posttransplant period. Its frequency can be decreased as the patient stabilizes in the months and years following transplantation (Sigardson-Poor & Haggerty, 1990).

Tacrolimus

Tacrolimus (first known as FK506 in clinical trials and then Prograf as a trade name) has very similar properties to cyclosporine. It was approved by the FDA for liver transplantation in 1994. When the clinical trials first began, it was thought that nephrotoxicity, neurotoxicity, and the tendency for hypertension would be less than cyclosporine. However, extensive clinical trials have demonstrated that tacrolimus is similar to cyclosporine with regard to those adverse effects. It does have some advantages over cyclosporine (Groth, Ohlman, Gannedahl, & Ericson, 1993). Tacrolimus has been used successfully to both prevent and treat rejection. In many early cases of rejection, the episode was reversed. Cyclosporine is able only to prevent, but not to treat a rejection episode. Patients on tacrolimus have been able to maintain lower steroid doses, which is a real advantage, as patients have fewer adverse effects from steroids. Tacrolimus used as prophylaxis in heart and liver transplant patients produced survival figures superior to patients treated with cyclosporine. Tacrolimus seems to have better efficacy in pancreas and small bowel transplant than cyclosporine (Todo et al., 1992; Tzarkis et al., 1990). In kidney transplantation, results thus far have been similar to cyclosporine (Starzl et al., 1991). Hence, clinical trials have shown that tacrolimus can be used as an effective alternative to cyclosporine, and that in some respects, it seems to be a more desirable therapy. There is some support for its value as conversion therapy for patients who fail immunosuppression with cyclosporine. Tacrolimus has shown promise as a relatively safe and effective therapy for these patients in many cases (Egawa et al., 1994).

It, too, is not without side effects. Some of the risks associated with tacrolimus therapy include renal dysfunction, gastrointestinal disturbances, neurotoxicities, hyperglycemia, hyperkalemia, and pruritis/rash. Therefore, it is important that the nurse monitor blood sugar, electrolytes, and indicators of renal function.

A number of other drugs can interact with tacrolimus to either increase or decrease action of the drug. These drugs include: itraconazole (increases levels of tacrolimus), ketoconazole (increases levels), phenytoin (decreases levels), rifampin (decreases levels), verapamil (increases levels), amphotericin B (additive or synergistic effect), carbamazepine (decreases tacrolimus levels), diltiazem (increases blood levels), erythromycin (increases blood levels), and gentamicin (additive or synergistic effects) (Peters, Fitton, Plosker, & Faulds, 1993).

Azathioprine

Azathioprine has been used successfully since the 1960s to prevent rejection. It became available for human use in 1961 after laboratory and animal experiments in the 1950s produced promising results. By 1963 its use in kidney transplantation was documented by researchers in Boston, and shortly thereafter it became the standard therapy when used concomitantly with steroids (Hamilton, 1984).

Although its precise mode of action is not well-understood, Azathioprine belongs to a drug class called antimetabolites. It interferes with both RNA and DNA synthesis, and therefore is effective in slowing the reproduction of rapidly dividing cells. In the case of transplant recipients, this is most helpful in controlling the proliferation of T-cells, which play a key role in the process of rejection. It also adversely affects the production of antibody, which is an important mechanism in the rejection process. These two actions make azathioprine an effective drug in the prevention of rejection.

The major adverse effect of azathioprine is bone marrow suppression, which can lead to leukopenia, anemia, and thrombocytopenia. For this reason, very close monitoring of bone marrow functioning must be done for patients on azathioprine therapy. This is especially true when therapy is first initiated and the patient's response is uncertain. Bone marrow depression can also be exacerbated if the patient is experiencing a concurrent episode of rejection or illness that reduces the white blood count (e.g., CMV infection, or Acyclovir treatment). A rapid decrease in the WBC, even if it has not yet dropped below 4 – 5000/mm^3 should also be taken as a likely sign of toxicity. In most cases of toxicity, a decrease in the dose of azathioprine corrects the bone marrow dysfunction.

Some drugs, most notably allopurinol, interact with azothiaprine. It should be avoided if at all possible. Alternatively, the dosage of azothiaprine must be reduced to a third or quarter of the usual dose if allopurinol therapy is continued.

Steroids

Corticosteroids are common medications that are used to treat a variety of illnesses and conditions, especially those related to inflammatory or immune-mediated responses. They have been used successfully in the prevention and treatment of rejection since the 1950s and are still an important part of antirejection therapy for most transplant recipients. However, because of the many undesirable side effects associated with the long-term use of steroids, there has been research in the area of steroid withdrawal after transplantation. The ultimate goal is the complete withdrawal of steroid therapy without causing rejection. Its use is currently limited to patients who are very stable post-transplant, and the results thus far are mixed. However, work in this area is ongoing and as other immunosuppressants are developed and put into broader use, steroid withdrawal may become a possibility for more transplant recipients.

Corticosteroids have a profound and complex effect on the overall functioning of the immune system. Corticosteroids particularly affect T-cells by altering their function and decreasing their sensitivity to antigens. The overall effect is a decrease in the cellular immune response, which is of particular importance for transplant recipients, since cell-mediated processes are so much a part of the rejection process. Steroids are also potent anti-inflammatory agents. They inhibit capillary dilatation, infiltration of leukocytes, fibrin deposition, and phagocytic activity (Bass, 1986). This anti-inflammatory response may be of ultimate importance for preserving organ function during a rejection episode by preventing irreversible organ damage from the inflammatory response (Sigardson-Poor & Haggerty, 1990).

Corticosteroids have multiple and widespread effects that vary in number and severity from individual to individual (see Table 12-10). The most worrisome adverse effect is an increased susceptibility to infection because of the overall depressive response that steroids have on immune functioning. This leaves the patient very susceptible to many different kinds of bacterial, fungal, viral, and protozoal infections that they would not normally be susceptible to. This is particularly problematic for transplant recipients because of the additive effects of all their immunosuppressants. The lifelong immunosuppressive therapy necessary for transplant recipients requires maintaining a constant and delicate balance between rejection and infection.

Other major complications of steroid therapy

include weight gain, skin changes, hirsutism, cataracts, bone disease, and diabetes. In the early posttransplant period, when steroid dosages are highest, weight gains are quite common. In addition, deposition of body fat changes and a moon face and buffalo hump are common. Thinning of the skin and acne are also commonly seen side effects. Long-term steroid therapy can result in cataract formation and avascular necrosis of the head of the femur. The latter may necessitate total hip replacements. In some patients, the steroids can induce diabetes, which may require control by insulin.

Mycophenolate Mofetil

Mycophenolate mofetil, better known in clinical trials as RS-61443, or just RS, was approved for use in humans by the FDA in 1995. Often it is recognized by the trade name Cellcept. Its immunosuppressive effects are similar to azathioprine; it is particularly effective against lymphocytes.

Mycophenolate mofetil blocks antibody formation, T and B lymphocyte proliferation, and cytoxic T-cell generation. Experimental animal models have shown its efficacy in prolonging the survival of transplanted kidneys, heart, liver, intestine, limb, small bowel, pancreas, pancreatic islets, and bone marrow. In human trials, mycophenolate mofetil was shown to be effective in reducing organ rejection when used in combination with cyclosporine and corticosteriods. In controlled clinical trials to date, patients on mycophenolate mofetil had better outcomes than patients on either placebo or azathioprine. Because of its role in inhibiting B cells and antibody formation, this drug may also have a role in the treatment of chronic rejection (Groth et al., 1993; Roche, 1995; UNOS, 1993).

The major side effects of mycophenolate mofetil include diarrhea, leukopenia, infection, sepsis, and vomiting. The diarrhea and vomiting are particularly problematic since this medication should be used in combination with cyclosporine, whose optimal absorption depends on normal GI function. However the gastrointestinal side effects of mycophenolate mofetil may be reduced by adjusting the dosage of the drug. It has been shown to have no significant nephrotoxic, neurotoxic, or hyperglycemic effects, an advantage over several of the other immunosuppressive medications (Deierhoi et al., 1993).

Polyclonal and Monoclonal Antibodies

Polyclonal antibody preparations are produced by injecting animal hosts, usually horses (although rabbits and goats have also been used), with human T-cells and then allowing the animal to produce antibodies against those T-cells. The serum is then collected and the antibodies extracted. Polyclonal preparations are not pure and contain various types of antibodies. This means that there is a variability from batch to batch that results in variable efficacy. However, polyclonal antibodies have been used successfully in the treatment of rejection. The first reported clinical trial using antilymphocyte serum (ALS) in renal transplant patients was in 1967 (Starzl et al., 1967). Since then, many trials have used polyclonal antilymphocyte antibodies either prophylactically or as a rejection treatment, and their clinical efficacy has been clearly established. In the early years, it was common for transplant centers to make their own serum. Now, the only FDA-approved product is Atgam. Minnesota Anti Lymphocyte Globulin (ALG) is no longer available as the FDA has not approved it for the commercial market.

Monoclonal antibodies are formed in a similar way, by injecting an animal host (usually a mouse) with human T-cells. The antibodies are mixed with mouse tumor cells to create a hybrid cell that can grow indefinitely in culture. This process yields a very pure mixture of identical antibody hybrid cells which are effective in the treatment of T-cell mediated rejection, and eliminates the variability in batches that is present with polyclonal preparations. The side effects include flu-like symptoms, but risk of pulmonary complications are less with monoclonal antibodies. There is a chance of allergic reaction or even anaphylaxis in patients with allergies to horses or other animals used in the drug preparation, so a pretherapy skin test should be performed.

These preparations attack and deplete circulating T-cells. This interferes with a person's ability to reject the transplanted organ. As a result, these preparations are very effective in reversing a rejection episode. Many programs also use these preparations as prophylaxis immediately after transplantation to decrease the chance of early rejection. There is some evidence that suggests that polyclonal antibody preparations are superior to monoclonal preparations for the purpose of induction therapy in the immediate postoperative period (Stratta et al., 1994).

The incidence and severity of side effects of monoclonal and polyclonal antibodies vary from preparation to preparation. Flu-like symptoms are the most common adverse effects. Fever and chills are quite common, especially with the first dose. The theory is that the massive T-cell lysis causes the release of endogenous pyrogens. Administration of acetaminophen and diphenhydramine before the first dose usually helps to ease these unpleasant side effects. (Sigardson-Poor & Haggerty, 1990).

OKT3

Muromonab CD-3 (OKT3) was the first therapeutic monoclonal antibody produced for use in humans. It was developed as a treatment for cell-mediated rejection. Since the development of OKT3 (the most common monoclonal antibody), it has been found to be successful in both removing T-cells from circulation as well as blocking their ability to recognize foreign substances.

When OKT3 is administered to a patient, it attacks the T-cells that are responsible for the rejection and usually halts the process. Although OKT3 is usually very effective as a treatment for rejection, it has several undesirable side effects associated with its use. The patient usually experiences a severe flu-like reaction with the administration of the first few doses. While this reaction is generally not life threatening, it is very frightening and uncomfortable for patients. However, in some patients, this reaction is so severe that the patient is unable to tolerate OKT3 therapy. Some patients do experience flash pulmonary edema with the initial dose administration, and this can be life threatening if not treated immediately and appropriately. A preadministration assessment of fluid status, including weight and chest x-ray to assure that fluid overload is not present, can usually prevent this severe complication. Because OKT3 is recognized as foreign antigen, patients may develop antibodies against the drug once it has been used, so it is not always possible to repeat the course of therapy. However, now this seems like a lesser risk than was initially anticipated. Jaffers et al. (1986) reported that 75% of patients treated with OKT3 developed antibodies after one course of treatment. Shields (1987) reported a 40% incidence of antibody development, and Stratta et al. (1994) reported only a 6% incidence of antibody development. Clearly these results represent a wide variance in antibody development rates. Concomitant drug therapy and other possible contributing factors must be studied further before a more consistent incidence of antibody development can be determined. Furthermore, patients can be tested for antibody formation prior to a second course of therapy.

In summary, cyclosporine, azathiaprine, corticosteroids, tacrolimus, and monoclonal antibodies are the key immunosuppressants used in transplant therapy today. However, the complication of rejection has not been overcome, and research is continuing to identify new immunosuppressive agents that reduce complications, particularly the risk of infection.

New Immunosuppressants in Transplantation

There are many new promising antirejection medications being developed. While cyclosporine has made long term graft survival a reality, there is still the need for better and more selective immunosuppressive agents. Some of the newer agents that are discussed in the following paragraphs include Cyclosporine G, IMM-125, rapamycin, brequinar, and 15-deoxyspergualin.

Cyclosporine G

Several years ago Sandoz developed a new cyclosporine that seemed to be less nephrotoxic than cyclosporine A, called cyclosporine G. It seems that both immunosuppressive and nephrotoxic properties are about the same. In addition, some studies have found an increase in liver enzymes, indicating a greater degree of hepatotoxicity than cyclosporine A. While animal studies have supported this, human trials so far have not. Human trials are continuing with close monitoring, although results do not seem to support much advantage (Ohlman et al., 1992).

IMM-125

In 1991, Sandoz presented another cyclosporine analogue named IMM-125. While the immunosuppressive qualities appear to be similar, both nephrotoxicity and hepatoxicity seem to be less with equivalent doses in animal models. Ongoing human clinical trials will reveal whether IMM-125 offers similar immunosuppressive qualities with a wider margin of safety (Groth et al., 1993; Hiestand, Graber, Hurtenbach, Hermann, & Cammisuli, 1993).

Rapamycin

Rapamycin's mode of action differs from cyclosporine in that it blocks the effect of IL-2 (cyclosporine and tacrolimus inhibit its production). This is important because that property allows it to be used in conjunction with cyclosporine or FK 506. Rapamycin does not appear to be nephrotoxic at therapeutic doses (DiJoseph, Mihatsch, & Sehgal, 1994). It appears to be most effective in antibody-mediated rejection and is also able to reverse an acute rejection episode (Morris, 1993). GI side effects have been observed in animals (possibly due to vasculitis) and have sometimes been quite severe (Groth et al., 1993). Human clinical trials are currently ongoing in the United States and Europe.

Brequinar

Animal experiments have demonstrated that brequinar has similar immunosuppressive effects to RS-61443. Brequinar inhibits both T and B cell proliferation and is most effective in antibody-mediated rejection (Morris, 1993). The most consistent side effects noted so far have been bone marrow depression and GI disturbances. Human clinical trials are currently ongoing in the United States and Canada.

15-Deoxyspergualin

Derived from a bacterium found in Japan, 15-deoxyspergualin was originally developed for cancer therapy but was also discovered to have an immunosuppressive effect. It works by inhibiting the formation of antibodies in both allograft and xenograft transplantation. While the exact mechanism is unknown, it works by somehow inhibiting both T and B cells and can be given only parenterally. It has been used in Japan to treat rejection in

Table 12-12
Common problems and OTC medications.

Problem	Nonpharmacologic Treatment	OTC Medications
Constipation	Increase fluids in diet Increase fiber foods` Increase exercise	Metamucil Fiber-con Senekot Ex-lax
Diarrhea	Increase fluids to prevent dehydration Stop Colace (if taking) Avoid foods that cause bowel irritation	Donnagel Kaopectate
Headache, muscle aches, or pains	Decrease or stop activities that cause these symptoms	Aspirin Tylenol AVOID Ibuprofen (Advil, Motrin, Nuprin)
Sinus congestion, allergies, cold, cough	Rest	Actifed Sudafed Benadryl Dristan Nyquil Robitussin Theraflu Vick's Cold Formula 44

Note: From University of Virginia, unpublished data, 1995. Reprinted with permission.

kidney transplant patients with promising results. It appears to be most effective in the later stages of rejection, which makes it viable as rescue therapy for rejection. Side effects include bone marrow depression and some mild GI problems. In the United States, a study is in progress administering it prophylactically to renal transplant patients. In Sweden, the drug is being used in a treatment protocol for patients with high antibody titers (Groth et al., 1993; UNOS, 1993).

It is hoped that these and other new drugs will provide better options for more effective immune control after transplantation. There seems to be much promise for these medications because many of them have different modes of action than the existing immunosuppressants. It is likely that combination therapy will continue to be the best option to maximize benefits and minimize side effects with some of these newer agents. However, the risk of unwanted secondary infection and increased risk of malignancy still exists with all agents currently being tested.

Other Common Medications for Transplant Recipients

Because of the many adverse effects of immunosuppressive medications, there are several other (nonimmunosuppressive) medications that transplant recipients usually receive. Although specific regimens will vary from center to center and from patient to patient, some of the medications that are commonly prescribed in the posttransplant period are: antiulcer medication, trimethoprim-sulfamethoxazole, oral antifungal agents, bowel medications, electrolyte supplements, calcium channel blockers, antihypertensives, and over the counter medications. These medications are briefly discussed in the following paragraphs.

Antiulcer Medication (famotidine, antacids, omeprazole, ranitidine, and sucralfate)

Steroids tend to cause a gastric irritation which can lead to peptic ulcers if left untreated. Patients are especially prone to serious gastric disturbances in the immediate postoperative phase when their steroid doses are highest, their physiologic stress is also high, and their normal dietary habits are interrupted. For these reasons, most centers use ulcer prophylaxis as part of the posttransplant medication management.

Trimethoprim-Sulfamethoxazole (Bactrim)

Trimethoprim-sulfamethoxazole is a combination antibiotic that may be used prophylactically in the posttransplant period to protect transplant recipients from opportunistic infections, especially pneumocystic carinii pneumonia. While protocols differ from center to center, it is usually given daily in the initial period after transplant when the doses of immunosuppressants are highest, and then gradually decreased and may be continued for 6 to 12 months after transplantation. If a patient is allergic to sulfonamides, alternative therapies such as dapsone or pentamidine inhalations may be substituted.

Oral Antifungal Agents (clotrimazole, nystatin)

Fungal infections of the mouth and throat are very common in transplant recipients, especially in the immediate posttransplant period. Prophylaxis using antifungal agents is a very important part of posttransplant management to prevent and control these fungal infections. Fungal infections are not usually serious initially, but if left untreated, these infections can spread rapidly, be extremely uncomfortable, and even fatal for transplant patients.

Bowel Medications (docusate sodium, psyllium)

Because oral cyclosporine and tacrolimus are absorbed through the GI tract, maintaining normal bowel function is an important part of posttransplant care. If patients experience diarrhea, their cyclosporine or tacrolimus levels can drop, and this places the patient at risk for rejection. Conversely, if patients become constipated, their cyclosporine or tacrolimus levels can rise and put the patient at risk for drug toxicity. Medications that promote normal bowel function are an important part of posttransplant care when they are needed. The actions of other medications on bowel functioning should also be considered; for instance, Cellcept and magnesium hydroxide can cause diarrhea. However, even when patients are not using medications to help them maintain normal bowel function, they should be encouraged to keep bowel movements regular primarily through diet and exercise.

Electrolyte Supplements (sodium bicarbonate, calcium, magnesium, potassium, phosphorus)

Because of fluid and electrolyte imbalances are common in the posttransplant period, any combination of electrolyte supplements may be appropriate and necessary for optimal patient management. Preoperative conditions, the stress of surgery and hospitalization, abnormal dietary intake, abnormal activity patterns, medications, and other factors contribute to electrolyte imbalances after transplant. Patients should have their electrolyte status closely monitored and replacement initiated as appropriate. It is important to recognize that sodium bicarbonate is commonly needed in patients receiving pancreas/kidney transplants. However, high dosages of sodium bicarbonate can interfere with the absorption of tacrolimus (FK506).

Calcium Channel Blockers (diltiazem, verapamil, amlodipine, felodipine, isradipine, nicardipine, nifedipine)

Calcium channel blockers interact with cyclosporine to increase the blood levels (Johannsen, 1993). Calcium channel blockers may be given in small doses for the purpose of decreasing the patient's need for cyclosporine. Because cyclosporine is so expensive, the concomitant use of calcium channel blockers may be a more cost-effective way to maintain adequate cyclosporine levels in some patients. Since these medications also lower blood pressure, this therapy is particularly useful for patients who are hypertensive in the posttransplant period (Donwerth, 1994).

Calcium channel blockers may also increase the blood levels of FK506. Because the pharmacology of tacrolimus is similar to cyclosporine, it is likely to have similar interactions with other medications. However, few drug interaction studies have been carried out (Fujisawa, 1994).

Antihypertensives

Hypertension is a very common problem in the renal posttransplant population. It has been estimated that 28%-75% of renal transplant recipients develop persistent hypertension (Cohen et al., 1984). Although the exact cause has not been proven, there are several possible reasons for persistent hypertension in the posttransplant period. Cyclosporine and tacrolimus have a known vasoconstrictive effect on renal vasculature. Cyclosporine and steroids promote salt and water retention. Renal artery stenosis may be a contributing cause. The patient's native kidneys may hypersecrete renin, and grafts from hypertensive donors may cause hypertension in the recipients (Mimran, Mourad, & Ribstein, 1990). Persistent hypertension is a significant problem for many patients in the posttransplant period, and it must be treated aggressively if the long-term complications, including damage to the transplanted kidney, are to be avoided. A number of antihypertensive medications are used in the posttransplant period to control the patient's blood pressure. Many of these agents have been described earlier in this chapter. Calcium channel blockers seem to be most effective in treating persistent hypertension in the posttransplant period (Donwerth, 1994).

Over-the-Counter Medications and Other Prescribed Medications

Because of the many medications that transplant patients must take, patients should always check with the transplant team before taking any over-the-counter medications, or medications prescribed by other health care providers. Cyclosporine and probably tacrolimus both have interactional effects with many medications, including common antibiotics such as erythromycin. Some medications can potentially affect a patient's cyclosporine or tacrolimus level, putting them at risk for either toxicity or rejection. Please refer to Table 12-12 for a list of common problems and recommended over the counter medications which are usually safe to treat those problems.

Summary

To accurately assess a patient's response to medication therapy, nurses must have a comprehensive knowledge of the medications they are administering to patients with renal failure or patients who have received transplants. The patient with renal disease is exposed to a variety of drugs with a multitude of toxicities and interactions. Because the perfect medication has yet to be discovered, the nurse must be aware of the toxicities that accompany each medication and carefully monitor the patient for side effects. Selection of the most appropriate medication for the clinical situation should be based upon a particular mechanism of action or avoidance of a toxicity. Medications should always be monitored for effectiveness and appearance of side effects. With the complicated renal patient, the expected outcome is not always achieved through normal prescribing patterns and must often be tailored to the patient's kidney function and renal replacement therapy.

Nurses have an important role to play in patient education and ensuring compliance with medication therapy. The basis of the nursing process outlines for us the role specifically: assessment of interventions, planning for desired outcomes, interventions to achieve outcomes, and evaluation of those interventions. This is nursing's role when caring for renal patients who are on any type of medication therapy. While only a few nurses (nurse practitioners) possess prescriptive authority, the nurse plays a large role in assessing patient responses to therapy and compliance with a regimen. Nurses working with the patient and physician to design a medication regimen that is acceptable to both clinicians and patients can increase the likelihood that the patient will take the medications as prescribed.

The nurse administering the medication has the need to understand the pharmacology and pharmacokinetics of that medication before administering it. In renal disease, this is especially relevant as the medication dose may be altered to accommodate renal insufficiency, renal failure, and renal replacement therapy. If a patient is assuming responsibility for his or her own medication dosing and regimen, the nurse can positively influence this process through teaching and continued assessment of the patient's ability and willingness to correctly take the medication. The nephrology nurse plays a significant role in drug administration and education of patients regarding their medications. Successful prevention and treatment of renal insufficiency and renal failure is contingent on the proper management of medications taken by renal failure patients both before and after transplantation.

References and Readings

Abbott Laboratories. (1986). *Calcijex: Calcitriol injection.* Chicago: Abbott Laboratories Renal Care.

American Society of Hospital Pharmacists, Inc. (1994). *American hospital formulary services: Drug information*, 944.

Amgen, Inc. (1994). *EPOGEN: Epoetin alfa for injection.* Thousand Oaks, CA: Author.

Baer, C.L. (1995). Pharmacologic aspects of renal failure. In L.E. Lancaster (Ed.), *Core curriculum for nephrology nursing* (3rd edition, pp. 177-183). Pitman, NJ: American Nephrology Nurses' Association..

Baer, C.L. (1990). The pharmacological aspects of renal failure. In L.E. Lancaster (Ed.), *Core curriculum for nephrology nursing* (2nd edition) (pp.167-194). Pitman, NJ: American Nephrology Nurses' Association.

Baker, L.R., et al. (1986). *Clinical Nephrology, 26*, 185-191.

Bass, M. (1986). Common complications of immunosuppression in the renal transplant patient. *ANNA Journal, 13*, 196-199.

Bell, J. (1993). Benazepril: A new ACE inhibitor. *ANNA Journal, 20*, 187-188.

Bennett, W.M. (1986). *Drugs in renal disease* (2nd edition). New York: Churchill Livingstone.

Bennett, W.M., & McCarron, D.A. (1987). *Pharmacology of renal disease and hypertension.* New York: Churchill Livingstone.

Berlyne, G.M., Janabi, K., & Shaw, A.B. (1966). Dangers of resonium A in the treatment of hyperkalemia in renal failure. *Lancet, 1*, 167-169.

Calne, R.Y., White, D.J.G., Thiru, S., Evans., D.B., McMaster, P., Dunn, D.C., Craddock, G.N., Pentlow, B.D., & Roles, K. (1978). Cyclosporine A in patients receiving renal allografts from cadaveric donors. *Lancet, 2*, 1323-1327.

Campese, V.M., & Bigazzi, R. (1992). Hypertension in chronic renal failure, dialysis, and transplantation. In R.J. Glassrock (Ed.), *Current therapy in nephrology and hypertension* (3rd edition) (pp.391-405). St. Louis, MO: Mosby-Year Book.

Canzanello, V.J., Hylander-Rossner, B., Sands, R.E., Morgan, T.M., Jordan, J., & Burkart, J.M. (1991). Comparison of 50% dextrose water, 25% mannitol, and 23.5% saline for the treatment of hemodialysis-associated muscle cramps. *Transactions of the American Society of Artificial Organs, 37*, 649-652.

Chandra, M., McVicar, M., & Clemons, G.K. (1988). Pathogenesis of the anemia of chronic renal failure: The role of erythropoietin. *Advances in Pediatrics, 35*, 361-389.

Coburn, J.W. (1990). Use of oral and parenteral calcitriol in the treatment of renal osteodystrophy. *Kidney International, 38*, 54-61.

Coburn, J.W., & Salusky, I.B. (1989). Control of serum phosphorus in uremia. *New England Journal of Medicine, 320*, 1140-1141.

Cohen, D.J., Loertscher, R., Rubin, M.F., Tilney, N.L., Carpenter, C.B., & Strom, T.B. (1984). Cyclosporine: A new immunosuppressive agent for organ transplantation. *Annals of Internal Medicine, 101*(5), 667-682.

d'Apice, A.J.F. (1984). Non-specific immunosuppression: Azathioprine and steroids. In P.J. Morris (Ed.), *Kidney transplantation: Principles and practice* (2nd edition) (pp. 239-259). Orlando, FL: Grune & Stratton.

Deierhoi, M.H., Kauffman, R.S., Hudson, S.L., Barber, W.H., Curtis, J.J., Julian, B.A., Gaston, R.S., Laskow, D.A., & Diethelm, A.G. (1993). Experience with mycophenolate mofetil (RS61443) in renal transplantation at a single center. *Annals of Surgery, 217*, 476-484.

deVires, P.M. (1990). Fluid balance during haemodialysis and haemofiltration: The effect of dialysate sodium. *Nephrology, Dialysis and Transplantation* (Supp. 1), 158-161.

DiJoseph, J.F., Mihatsch, M.J., & Sehgal, S.N. (1994). Renal effects of rapamycin in the spontaneously hypertensive rat. *Transplant International, 7*(2), 83-88.

Donwerth, J.J. (1994). Nursing overview: Reduction of posttransplant hypertension. *Dialysis and Transplantation, 23*(8), 456-461.

Drueke, T.B. (1990). Resistance to recombinant human erythropoietin in hemodialysis patients. *American Journal of Nephrology, 10*(Supp. 2), 34-39.

Drug prescribing in renal failure. (1994). Philadelphia: American College of Physicians.

Egawa, H., Esquivel, C.O., So, S.K., Cox, K., Concepcion, W., & Lawrence, L. (1994). FK506 conversion therapy in pediatric liver transplantation. *Transplantation, 57*(8), 1169-1173.

Eschbach, J.W., & Adamson, J.W. (1988). Modern aspects of the pathophysiology of renal anemia. *Contributions to Nephrology, 66*, 63-70.

Eschbach, J.W., & Adamson, J.W. (1985). Anemia of end-stage renal disease (ESRD) (Editorial). *Kidney International, 28*, 1-5.

Fujisawa USA. (1994). *Prograf: A new option for liver transplant immunosuppression.* Deerfield, IL: Author.

Giovani, L.E., & Hayes, J.E. (1982). *Drugs and nursing implications.* Norwalk, CT: Appleton-Century-Crofts.

Goodman, W.G., & Coburn, J.W. (1992). *Annual Review of Medications, 43*, 227-237.

Groth, C.G., Ohlman, S., Gannedahl, & Ericson, B.G. (1993). New immunosuppressive drugs in transplantation. *Transplantation Proceedings, 25*(4), 2681-2683.

Hamilton, D. (1984). Kidney transplantation: A history. In P.J. Morris (Ed.), *Kidney transplantation: Principles and practice* (2nd edition) (pp. 1-13). Orlando, FL: Grune & Stratton.

Hamilton, D.V., Calne, R.Y., & Evans, D.B. (1981). Effect of cyclosporine A on renal function. *Lancet, 1*, 1218-1219.

Handley J. (1994). Rebound hypertension during hemodialysis. *ANNA Journal, 21*, 279.

Hess, A.D., Colombani, P.M., & Esa, A. (1986). Cyclosporine: Immunobiologic aspects in transplantation. In G.M. Williams, J.F. Burdick, & K. Solez (Eds.), *Kidney transplant rejection: Diagnosis and treatment* (pp. 353-382). New York: Marcel Dekker.

Hiestand, P.C., Graber, M., Hurtenbach, U., Herrmann, P., & Cammisuli, S. (1993). New cyclosporine derivative SDZ IMM 125: In vitro and in vivo pharmacologic effects and toxicologic evaluation. *Transplantation Proceedings, 25*(1), 691-692.

Home use of urokinase prevents central line problems. (1991). *Hospital Home Health, 8*(4), 41-44.

Hume, D.M., Merrill, J.P., & Mill, B.F. (1955). Experiences with renal homotransplantation in the human: Report of nine cases. *Journal of Clinical Investigation, 334*, 327.

Humphries, J.E. (1992). Anemia of renal failure: Use of erythropoietin. *Medical Clinics of North America, 76*, 711-725.

Jaffers, G.J., Fuller, T.C., Cosimi, A.B., Russel, P.S., Winn, H.J., & Colvin, R.B. (1986). Monoclonal antibody therapy: Anti-idiotypic and non anti-idiotypic antibodies to OKT3 arising despite intense immunosuppression. *Transplantation, 41*, 572-578.

Jenkins, P.G., & Dreher, W.H. (1975). Dialysis-induced muscle cramps: Treatment with hypertonic saline and theory as to etiology. *Transactions of the American Society of Artificial Organs, 21*, 479-482.

Johannsen, J.M. (1993). Update: Guidelines for treating hypertension. *American Journal of Nursing, 93*(3), 42-49.

Kahan, B.D., Shaw, L.M., Holt, D., Grevel, J., & Johnston, A. (1990). Consensus document: Hawk's Cay meeting on therapeutic drug monitoring of cyclosporine. *Clinical Chemistry, 36*(8), 1510-1514.

Karubian, F., Chervu, I., & Campese, V. (1993). Hypertension in chronic dialysis patients. In A. Nissenson & R.N. Fine (Eds.), *Dialysis therapy* (pp. 243-252). Philadelphia: Hanley & Belfus.

Kinet, J.P., Soyeur, D., Balland, N., Saint-Remy, M., Colligon, P., & Gordon, J.P. (1982). Hemodynamic study of hypotension during hemodialysis. *Kidney International, 21*, 868-876.

Kirlin, L.E. (1993). Case management of the anemic patient: Epoetin alfa – Focus on iron supplementation. *ANNA Journal, 20*, 678-681.

Klintman, G., Rigden, O., & Groth, G.G. (1983). Clinical and laboratory signs of nephrotoxicity and rejection in cyclosporine-treated renal allograft recipients. *Transplantation Proceedings, 15*, 2815-2820.

Klintman, G., Iwatsuki, S., & Starzl, T.E. (1981). Nephrotoxicity of cyclosporine A in liver and kidney transplant patients. *Lancet, 1*, 470-471.

Krumpf, V.J., & Holland, E.G. (1990). Parenteral iron dextran therapy. DICP, *The Annals of Pharmacotherapy, 24*, 162-166.

Lancaster, L.E. (1984). *The patient with end stage renal disease.* New York: John Wiley & Sons.

Ma, K.W., Greene, E.L., & Raji, L. (1992). Cardiovascular risk factors in chronic renal failure and hemodialysis populations. *American Journal of Kidney Disease, 19*, 505-513.

Mai, M.L., Emmett, M., Sheikh, M.S., Santa Ana, C.A., Schiller, L., & Fordtran, J.S. (1989). Calcium acetate, an effective phosphorous binder in patients with renal failure. *Kidney International, 36*, 690-695.

Malluche, H.H., & Faugere, M.C. (1990). *Kidney International, 38*, 48-53.

Massry, S.A., & Glassock, R.J. (1989). *Textbook of nephrology,* (pp. 1450-1457). Baltimore: Williams & Wilkins.

McDonald, F.D. (1980). *Progress in clinical kidney disease and hypertension.* New York: Thieme-Stratton Inc.

Meyer I. (1993). Sodium polystyrene sulfonate: A cation exchange resin used in treating hyperkalemia. *ANNA Journal, 20*, 93-95.

Mimran, A., Mourad, G., & Ribstein, J. (1990). Is renal transplantation useful for understanding the pathogenesis of hypertension? *Advances in Nephrology, 19*, 53-67.

Morris, R.E. (1993). New small molecule immunosuppressants for transplantation: Review of essential concepts. *Journal of Heart and Lung Transplantation, 12*(6) Pt 2, S275-86.

Murray, J.E., Merrill, J.P., & Harrison, J.H. (1963). Prolonged survival of human kidney homografts by immunosuppressive drug therapy. *New England Journal of Medicine, 268*, 1315.

Northsea C. (1994). Using Urokinase to restore patency in double lumen catheters. *ANNA Journal, 21*, 261-264.

Nursing '93 drug handbook. (1993). Springhouse, PA: Springhouse Corporation.

Ohlman, S., Lindholm, A., & Gabel, H., et al. (1992). *Transplant International, 5* (Supp. 1), 464.

Parfrey, P.S., Harnett, J.D., & Griffiths, S.M., et al. (1990). The clinical course of left ventricular hypertrophy on survival in dialysis patients. *Nephron, 55*, 114-120.

Peacock, E. (1992). Calcitriol injection for the management of renal osteodystrophy. *ANNA Journal, 19*, 575-577.

Peters, D.H., Fitton, A., Plosker, G.L., & Faulds, D. (1993). Tacrolimus: A review of its pharmacology and therapeutic potential in hepatic and renal transplantation. *Drug*

Evaluation 46(4), 746-794.

Roche Labs. (1995). *Package insert for Cellcept, Mycophenolate Mofetil capsules.* Nutley, NJ: Author.

Sanderson, N.A., & Katz, M.A. (1994). The fate of hypertonic saline administered during hemodialysis. *ANNA Journal, 21,* 162-169.

Sandoz Pharmaceuticals Corporation. (1993). *Hypertension in patients who have special safety concerns: Patients who have renal impairment.* East Hanover, NJ: Sandoz USA.

Schein Pharmaceuticals, Inc. (1991). *InFeD, Iron dextran injection, USP.* Roslyn, NY: Author.

Schroeder, E.T. (1969). Alkalosis resulting from combined administration of a "non-systemic" antacid and a cation-exchange resin. *Gastroenterology, 56,* 868-874.

Schwab, S., & Butler, G. (1988). Prospective evaluation of a dacron cuffed hemodialysis catheter for prolonged use. *American Journal of Kidney Disease, 6*(2), 166-169.

Sherman, R.A., Goodling, K.A., & Eisinger, R.P. (1982). Acute therapy of hemodialysis-related muscle cramps. *American Journal of Kidney Disease, 2,* 287-288.

Shields, CF III. (1987, March). Reuse of monoclonal antibodies. In *Monoclonal antibodies in transplantation: State of the art.* Symposium conducted at Montefiore Hospital, New York, NY.

Sigardson-Poor, K.M., & Haggerty, L.M. (1990). *Nursing care of the transplant recipient.* Philadelphia: W.B. Saunders Company.

Smith, S. (Ed). (1990). *Tissue and organ transplantation. Implications for nursing practice.* St. Louis, MO: C.V. Mosby Company.

Spilman, P., & Whelton A. (1992). Nonsteroidal anti-inflammatory drugs: Effects on kidney function and implications for nursing care. *ANNA Journal, 19,* 19-25.

Starzl, T., Marchioro, T.L., Porter, K.A., Iwasaki, Y., & Cerilli G.J. (1967). The use of heterologous antilymphoid agents in canine renal and liver homotransplantation and in human renal homotransplantation. *Surgery, Gynecology, & Obstetrics, 124,* 301-318.

Starzl, T., Todo, S., & Thompson, A., et al. (Eds.). (1991). *Transplant Proceedings, 23*(6).

Stevens, C., & Roberts, W.B. (1994). Ganciclovir: Treatment of cytomegalovirus in immunocompromised individuals. *ANNA Journal, 21,* 204-205.

Stratta, R.J., Taylor, R.J., Lowell, J.A., Bynon, J.S., Cattral, M.S., Frisbie, K., Miller, S., & Brennan, D.C. (1994). OKT3 induction in 100 consecutive pancreas transplants. *Transplantation Proceedings, 26*(2), 546-547.

Sturniolo, A., Costanzi, S., Barbera, G., Ruffini, M.P., Passalacqua, S., Fulignati, P., & Splendiani, G. (1990). Computerised monitoring of sodium and fluid during haemodialysis. *Nephrology, Dialysis and Transplantation* (Supp. 1), 162-164.

Todo, S., Tzarkis, A.G., Abu-Elmagd, K., et al. (1992). *Annals of Surgery, 216,* 223.

Tzarkis, A.G., Ricordi, C., Alejandro, R., et al. (1990). *Lancet, 336,* 402.

United Network for Organ Sharing (UNOS). (1993). *United Network for Organ Sharing annual report.* Richmond, VA: Author.

United States Renal Data System. (USRDS). (1993). *1993 annual report.* Bethesda, MD: Author.

United States Pharmacopeial (USP) Convention, Inc. (1993). *USP DI: Drug information for the health care professional* (13th edition) (pp.1449-1453). Rockville, MD: Author.

University of Virginia Health Sciences Center (1995). *Solid organ transplant patient teaching manual.* (Unpublished manual).

Van Wyck, D.B. (1989). The challenge of iron deficiency during rHuEPO therapy. *Seminars in Dialysis, 2,* 135-136.

Weiner, J. (1994). Antihypertensive therapy in dialysis patients. *Nephrology Nursing Today, 4,* 1-8.

Wenk, M., & Follath, F. (1983). Temperature dependency of apparent cyclosporine A concentrations in plasma. *Clinical Chemistry, 29,* 1965.

Whelton, A., Stout, R., Spilman, P., & Klassen, D. (1990). Renal effects of ibuprofen, piroxicam, and sulindac in patients with asymptomatic renal failure: A prospective randomized, crossover comparison. *Annals of Internal Medicine, 112,* 568-576.

York, S. (1993). Current perspectives: Iron management during therapy with recombinant human erythropoietin. *ANNA Journal, 20,* 645-650.

Chapter 12A Highlights

- Medications are no different from any substance to which a person is exposed. To have an effect, the medication must reach the target tissue and attach to a receptor on the cell surface. Receptor stimulation will then set off a series of physiologic events that lead to the desired therapeutic effect.
- Sublingual, intranasal, intramuscular, intravenous, intraventricular, intracavitary, and epidural routes of administration have been developed to enhance absorption of medications, or to administer the agent directly to the site of action. Absorption of medications from intramuscular and subcutaneous injections may be affected by changes in absorption due to decreased tissue perfusion and decreased movement through edematous tissue that may have physical distortions due to abnormal contents of fat and protein.
- Medications are removed from the body through either of two major mechanisms. If the molecule is water soluble, the kidney will filter the chemical, or fluid lost through physiologic secretions will carry medication with it. If the medication is fat soluble, the medication must be altered to a water soluble form that the kidney or secretions can remove.
- Elimination is the final pathway by which a medication or its metabolite is removed from the body. The kidney is the main organ of elimination, while the liver can concentrate medication in bile. Minor routes of medication loss are through secretions, tears, and pulmonary gas exchange.
- Medications behave in relatively reproducible manners once they enter the body. Mathematical models have been constructed to describe the behavior of molecules for the purpose of guiding dosage changes during periods of altered absorption, distribution, metabolism, and excretion. These models are referred to as pharmacokinetics.
- Specific parameters to consider in adjustments of drug dosage are the volume of distribution and clearance. Clearance and volume of distribution are both affected by physiologic parameters and will change as the condition of the patient changes.
- The relationship between drug concentration at the site of drug action and the physiologic response by the target tissue is called pharmacodynamics. A drug effect is produced when (a) there is a change in the physical environment of the bloodstream, through such mechanisms as albumin or bicarbonate infusion, or (b) the drug attaches to a three-dimensional receptor found on the cell membrane or on an organelle within the cell.
- One in every five cases of acute renal failure is associated with medication toxicity while with chronic renal failure, 1% to 20% of cases are associated with drug toxicity, depending on the region of the world reporting its experience.
- Despite the many factors to be considered in the metabolism and elimination of medications, particularly in patients with renal failure, there are many medications that are regularly prescribed for this population. However, use of pharmacological agents with chronic renal failure patients requires special considerations, particularly relating to dosages.
- There are numerous diuretics available for the treatment of hypertension and edema associated with renal disease. Hydrochlorthiazide is a thiazide-type diuretic that inhibits reabsorption of sodium and chloride in the distal tubule, thus promoting water loss. . . Most commonly, loop diuretics (e.g., furosemide or bumetanide) are used when there is some renal insufficiency.
- Analgesics can be put into three classes: nonnarcotic, narcotic, and nonsteroidal antiinflammatory drugs (NSAIDs). The nonnarcotic drugs may be more frequently prescribed for chronic pain that is not alleviated through other methods. Narcotics may be administered for pain in association with a procedure or invasive intervention.
- Cardiovascular disease is the leading cause of death in patients with chronic renal failure (USRDS, 1993). Hypertension occurs in about 80% of patients with chronic renal failure (Campese & Bigazzi, 1992). An understanding of how hypertension occurs and what factors come into play helps the nurse understand management strategies.

Chapter 12B Highlights

- The purpose of the immune system in humans is to protect the body from invasion by foreign pathogens. Since we are constantly in contact with microorganisms and other substances that can interfere with the normal functioning of the human body, it is essential for survival that the body be able to discriminate between substances that are its own and substances that are foreign. Once the immune system identifies a substance as foreign, the body begins the process of destroying the foreign substance.

- Much of the progress in the field of transplantation is related to the progress in immunosuppression therapy (see Table 12-8). This is especially true in kidney transplantation. While the surgical techniques have changed little since the 1960s, the graft survival has improved due to advances in immunosuppression.

- Cyclosporine is a potent immunosuppressant first used in clinical trials by Calne et al. (1978) in England. Throughout the next several years, clinical trials in Europe, Canada, and the United States demonstrated both the efficacy and relative safety of this drug. Cyclosporine has, by far, been the biggest clinical advancement in the care of transplant patients.

- Unfortunately, the adverse effects of cyclosporine are many and are summarized in Table 12-10, along with other immunosuppressive medications. The most serious adverse effect is nephrotoxicity, which may be rapid or chronic. This is especially troublesome in kidney transplantation and has been shown to occur in 50%-75% of renal transplant recipients (Hamilton, Calne, & Evans, 1981; Klintman, Rigden, & Groth, 1983; Klintman, Iwatsuki, & Starzl, 1981).

- Tacrolimus (first known as FK506 in clinical trials and then Prograf as a trade name) has very similar properties to cyclosporine. It was approved by the FDA for liver transplantation in 1994. It does have some advantages over cyclosporine (Groth, Ohlman, Gannedahl, & Ericson, 1993). Tacrolimus has been used successfully to both prevent and treat rejection. In many early cases of rejection, the episode was reversed. Cyclosporine is able only to prevent, but not to treat a rejection episode.

- Although its precise mode of action is not well-understood, Azathioprine belongs to a drug class called antimetabolites. It interferes with both RNA and DNA synthesis, and therefore is effective in slowing the reproduction of rapidly dividing cells. In the case of transplant recipients, this is most helpful in controlling the proliferation of T-cells, which play a key role in the process of rejection.

- Because of the many undesirable side effects associated with the long-term use of steroids, there has been research in the area of steroid withdrawal after transplantation. The ultimate goal is the complete withdrawal of steroid therapy without causing rejection. Its use is currently limited to patients who are very stable posttransplant, and the results thus far are mixed.

- In human trials, mycophenolate mofetil was shown to be effective in reducing organ rejection when used in combination with cyclosporine and corticosteriods. In controlled clinical trials to date, patients on mycophenolate mofetil had better outcomes than patients on either placebo or azathioprine. Because of its role in inhibiting B cells and antibody formation, this drug may also have a role in the treatment of chronic rejection (Groth et al., 1993; Roche, 1995; UNOS, 1993).

- Polyclonal antibody preparations are produced by injecting animal hosts, usually horses (although rabbits and goats have also been used), with human T-cells and then allowing the animal to produce antibodies against those T-cells. The serum is then collected and the antibodies extracted.

- Monoclonal antibodies are also formed by injecting an animal host (usually a mouse) with human T-cells. The antibodies are mixed with mouse tumor cells to create a hybrid cell that can grow indefinitely in culture. This process yields a very pure mixture of identical antibody hybrid cells which are effective in the treatment of T-cell mediated rejection and eliminates the variability in batches that are present with polyclonal preparations.

CHAPTER 13

Control of Infectious Diseases In the Renal Patient

Janel Parker, MSN, RN, CNN
Linda Dickenson, BS, RN, CNN, CPHQ
Karen C. Wiseman, MSN, RN, CNN
Diane Alexander, MS, BSN, RN, CNN
Eileen Peacock, MSN, RN, CNN, CIC, CPHQ

Chapter Contents

An Overview of Epidemiology 350
The Natural History of Disease and Levels of Prevention 350
Epidemiological Methods 351
Epidemiology and the Nurse 352
Hepatitis 353
Hepatitis A 353
Hepatitis B 355
Hepatitis C 359
Hepatitis D 361
Hepatitis E 362
Human Immunodeficiency Virus and Acquired Immune Deficiency Syndrome 362
Epidemiology 363
Pathophysiology 363
HIV Infection 363
Incubation Period 363
Clinical Manifestations 363

Chapter Contents

Opportunistic Infections 364
Transmission 364
Test to Determine HIV Infection 365
Vaccine 365
Treatment 365
Risk to Health Care Workers 366
Tuberculosis: An Old Disease With a New Face 367
Etiology 367
Pathophysiology 368
Multidrug-Resistant TB 369
Signs and Symptoms of TB 369
BCG Vaccine 369
Screening Methods for TB 370
Diagnosis of TB 373
Drug Therapy for TB 374
Infection Control Strategies 378
Screening 378
Surveillance 378
OSHA's Bloodborne Pathogens Regulations 379
Nursing Management of Patients With Infectious Diseases 381
Nursing Management of Exposure to Bloodborne Pathogens 382
Nursing Management Specific to the Hepatitis Patient 383
Nursing Management Specific to the HIV/AIDS Patient 383
Nursing Management of Patients With TB 384
Major Drug-Resistant Organisms 389
MRSA and VRE: History/Epidemiology/High Risk Groups 390
Infection Control Strategies 391
Prudent Vancomycin Use 392
The Renal Community 393
Summary 395
References/Readings 395
Chapter Highlights 401

Control of Infectious Diseases In the Renal Patient

Janel Parker, MSN, RN, CNN
Linda Dickenson, BS, RN, CNN, CPHQ
Karen C. Wiseman, MSN, RN, CNN
Diane Alexander, MS, BSN, RN, CNN
Eileen Peacock, MSN, RN, CNN, CIC, CPHQ

Editor's Note: Two sections in this chapter were reprinted with permission from various sources. We extend our appreciation to the authors and publishers of the following sections for their contributions to this chapter:

The section, "Nursing Management of Patients with TB," is reprinted from the article "Tuberculosis: An Old Disease with a New Face," from the December 1995 issue of ANNA Journal, volume 22, number 6, pages 541-553., published by the American Nephrology Nurses' Association.

The section, "Major Drug-Resistant Organisms, is reprinted with permission from the following sources:

Alexander, D., & Peacock, E. (1997, October). Part 1. Drug resistant organisms and their implications for the outpatient dialysis setting. Nephrology News & Issues, 11(10), 27-34. Publisher: Nephrology News & Issues, Inc.

Peacock, E., & Alexander, D. (1997). Part II. Control of drug resistant organisms in the outpatient dialysis unit. Nephrology News & Issues, 11(11), 30-33. Publisher: Nephrology News & Issues, Inc.

Patients receiving chronic dialysis treatments and organ transplants have a compromised immune system and co-morbidities that make them more susceptible to infectious diseases both in the hospital and in the community (Favero, Alter, & Bland, 1992; Schlatter & McNatt, 1995).

Prior to the 20th century, epidemic diseases spread rapidly among a population weakened by starvation. Poor sanitation, poverty, and overcrowding facilitated the survival and spread of disease organisms. Lack of hygiene led to high mortality from simple wound infections, postpartal infection, and infections of infancy (Valanis, 1992). During the latter half of the 19th century and the beginning of the 20th century, major advances in environmental sanitation, immunization, and antibiotic therapy, resulted in control of many serious and frequently fatal infections.

During the early days of the End Stage Renal Disease (ESRD) program, patients and staff were among the highest risk groups for hepatitis B infection after male homosexuals and injecting drug abusers. In 1977, the Centers for Disease Control (CDC) published guidelines for controlling bloodborne infections and these recommendations were immediately implemented by the dialysis community. The incidence of hepatitis B virus (HBV) decreased 10 fold before the hepatitis B vaccine became available in 1982 (Favero, 1996).

During the 1980s, the guidelines for controlling bloodborne infections were stated in a document titled "Universal Precautions" and these same recommendations were also effective in controlling human immunodeficiency virus (HIV) transmission in dialysis settings. Currently, in the United States, there has not been one report of HIV transmission from patient to patient in dialysis centers. However, there have been several reports of patient-to-patient transmission of HIV infection in developing countries that were all due to breeches in infection control practices. There has been one documented case of a dialysis staff member becoming infected after a percutaneous exposure to an HIV-infected patient. The patient was known to be infected and was being dialyzed in isolation (Favero, 1996).

The clearest mode of infection by the hepatitis C virus (HCV) is percutaneous transmission with contaminated blood (Bader, 1995). Although the transmission rate is high in transplant recipients (Mayo Clinic Update, 1993), it has been demonstrated in this decade that HCV can be controlled in dialysis centers with good practices.

In 1994, the Centers for Disease Control (Favero, 1996) investigated outbreaks of HBV in five dialysis units that were associated with significant deficiencies in implementing the infection control guidelines that were published by the CDC in 1977 and had virtually eradicated HBV as a clinical problem in dialysis units.

The presence of a large immunosuppressed population, due to the acquired immune deficiency syndrome (AIDS) epidemic and organ transplant patients, and the penalty for the random use of antibiotics was realized in the health care community in

Table 13-1
Levels of prevention.

PERIOD	STAGE	PREVENTATIVE MEASURE	INTERVENTION
Prepathogenesis	Susceptibility	Primary prevention	Health promotion & protective measures
	Adaptation	Primary prevention	
Pathogenesis	Presymptomatic disease Early Pathogenesis Clinical Recognition of Disease/Early Symptoms	Secondary prevention	Early diagnosis/treatment
	Clinical Disease	Tertiary prevention	Treatment/rehabilitation

Note: Adapted from Valanis, B. (1992). Epidemiology in nursing and health care (2nd ed.). Norwalk, CT: Appleton & Lange.

the 1990s. The emergence of new strains of antibiotic-resistant organisms and the potential for tuberculosis bacillus and HCV to reach epidemic proportions places the health and safety of renal patients and nephrology nurses at risk (Gallagher, 1995).

The purposes of this chapter are to: (a) present an overview of infectious diseases and the disease process associated with dialysis and organ transplant patients; and (b) explore the methodologies for prevention and control of infectious diseases in the renal community by use of an epidemiologic framework.

An Overview of Epidemiology

Epidemiology is a science of "the study of the distribution of states of health and the determinants of deviations from health populations" (Valanis, 1992). Epidemiology is based on two fundamental assumptions: (a) that human disease does not occur at random and (b) that human disease has causal and preventative factors that can be identified through systematic investigations of different populations or subgroups of individuals within a population in different places or different times (Hennekens & Buring, 1987).

The Natural History of Disease and Levels of Prevention

Occurrence of disease in humans is not a single event but rather, a process occurring over a period of time. This is referred to as the natural history of disease. The process involves the interaction of three factors: the causative agent(s), a susceptible host (human), and the environment. The natural history of disease is divided into two periods, prepathogenesis and pathogenesis. Each of these periods is further subdivided into two stages. The stages in prepathogenesis are susceptibility and adaptation. Stages in pathogenesis are early pathogenesis and clinical disease. Levels of prevention describe how the occurrences at each stage can be utilized as a basis for determining interventions. A brief overview of these concepts is presented below (see Table 13-1).

Prepathogenesis. In the first stage of prepathogenesis, a foundation has been laid for susceptibility. Although the disease has not developed, factors that render the host resistant to the agent are present. Examples are patients with HBV (factor whose presence causes disease) or with impaired antigen-antibody response (factor whose absence causes disease) (Dayton & Lancaster, 1995). Exposure of a host to an agent occurs at this time. Either adaptation is successful and no disease occurs or the physiological responses are unsuccessful and in the case of infectious agents, exposure is followed by an incubation period that is usually short, lasting from hours to months.

Pathogenesis. The first stage of pathogenesis is early pathogenesis or presymptomatic disease. The patient has no visible signs or symptoms indicating the disease process has begun. The physiological changes that have begun to occur are referred to as subclinical because the changes are only detectable by sophisticated laboratory tests. These laboratory tests are often used for screening to ascertain the early presence of disease in high-risk populations.

The last stage in the process of the natural history of disease is the clinical disease. At this stage, adequate physiological and functional changes have occurred to produce symptoms that are experienced by the patient or identified by the clinician during examination (Valanis, 1992). It is at this point in the disease process that classification schemes are used for varying degrees of disease severity, such as hepatitis B: acute-icteric, anicteric, and subclinical; and chronic-persistent, lobular, and chronic active (Bader, 1995).

Pathological change becomes less reversible as the disease evolves over time. The ultimate goal of intervention strategies is to stop or reverse the disease process as early as possible to prevent further damage. Three levels of intervention consistent with the stages of natural disease history have been identified as primary, secondary, and tertiary prevention (Valanis, 1992; Hennekens & Buring, 1987).

Primary prevention attempts to separate the agent and the host or to eliminate or reduce host susceptibility. These objectives are accomplished by general health promotion and protection against specific agents, for example, use of immunizations against hepatitis and removal of harmful agents from the environment.

The goal of secondary prevention is to diagnose and treat presymptomatic infectious diseases. Screening is the most common type of secondary prevention and can often detect physiological indicators of disease before the patient is symptomatic. If cure of the disease is not possible then secondary prevention attempts to slow its progression, prevent complications, and limit chronic disabilities.

Tertiary prevention pertains to those persons in the middle to late stages of the clinical disease. The goal of tertiary prevention is to limit any disabilities resulting from pathologic changes and to begin the process of rehabilitation by maximizing a patient's remaining capabilities (Hennekens & Buring, 1987; Valanis, 1992).

Epidemiological Methods

Epidemiology is an organized, sequential process of investigation that begins with descriptive research, moves to analytical studies, and finally experimental studies. In this section, a brief synopsis of the design strategies in epidemiologic research is presented. It is beyond the scope of this chapter to discuss the design and conduct of each type of epidemiological study and therefore, the study designs have only been identified within the appropriate context.

Descriptive epidemiology is the report of the general characteristics of the distribution of a disease, in relation to person, place, and time. Descriptive studies, recorded as disease rates, are primarily useful for the formulation of hypotheses that can be tested using an analytic study design and in planning for health care utilization and resource allocation. There are three main types of descriptive epidemiologic studies: (a) the correlational study that uses data from an entire population to compare disease frequencies between different groups during the same time period or in the same population at different points in time; (b) the case report, which is a detailed profile by one or more clinicians of a single patient and can be expanded into a case series, which describes characteristics of a number of patients with a given disease; and (c) the cross-sectional survey in which the status of a patient with respect to the presence or absence of both exposure and disease is assessed at the same point in time (Hennekens & Buring, 1987).

Analytic epidemiology tests the hypotheses formulated from descriptive studies and determines whether or not the risk of disease is different for individuals exposed or not exposed to a particular factor. There are two types of analytic studies: observational and intervention.

Observational analytic epidemiology focuses on relationships between factors or events and disease frequency or level, based on aggregate data for entire populations; presence or absence of the disease and the etiological factor for patients are not established. There are two types of observational analytic investigation:

1. The case-control study can be defined as a study that begins with the identification of persons with the disease and a suitable comparison (control) group of persons without the disease. It then compares the proportions of persons with regard to the frequency of the hypothesized causal attribute.
2. The cohort study (*prospective*, which looks forward from an exposure to an outcome, or *retrospective*, which looks backward from a disease to a possible cause) is a study in which a designated group of persons are classified on the basis of presence or absence to a particular factor and followed over a period of time.

Intervention analytic epidemiology studies are often referred to as clinical trials. The distinguishing feature of a clinical trial is that patients are enrolled on the basis of their exposure status and the treatments are allocated by the investigators at random. During these studies, patients are followed to determine whether they develop the disease.

Intervention studies are usually categorized as therapeutic or preventive. Therapeutic or secondary prevention clinical trials are conducted among patients with a particular disease to determine the ability of an agent or procedure to alleviate symptoms, prevent recurrence, or lessen the risk of death from that disease. A preventive or primary prevention clinical trial evaluates if an agent or procedure reduces the risk of developing disease among individuals free from that disease condition at enrollment (Hennekens & Buring, 1987; Valanis, 1992). When issues of ethics, feasibility, and cost are addressed, the randomized clinical trial or experimental design presents the strongest and most direct epidemiologic evidence on which to base a decision regarding the presence of a cause-effect relationship between a specific factor and the

Table 13-2
Viruses that cause a specific type of hepatitis.

	Hepatitis A	Hepatitis B	Hepatitis C	Hepatitis D	Hepatitis E
Etiology	Hepatitis A virus (HAV)	Hepatitis B virus (HBV)	Hepatitis C virus (HCV)	Hepatitis D virus (HDV)	Hepatitis E virus (HEV)
Viral type	Small RNA virus	DNA virus	RNA virus	Delta virus, defective RNA; requires the presence of HBV to replicate	RNA virus-like particle
Transmission	Fecal-oral route; contaminated food, water	Contact with blood, transplanted organs, saliva, semen, sexual activity	Contact with blood	Same as HBV	Fecal-oral route; predominantly water
Incubation period	15-50 days	40-80 days	2-21 weeks	2-10 weeks	2-9 weeks
Risk of chronic liver disease	low	high	high	high	Nonexistent
Vaccine available	Havrix	Recombivax HB Energix-B	None available	None available	None available

occurrence of a particular disease.

The goal of intervention studies is to provide a definitive positive result on which policy can be formulated or a dependable and informative null finding that can permit a redistribution of resources (Hennekens & Buring 1987).

In epidemiology, no presentation would be complete without a discussion of rates as measures of events. Mortality and morbidity rates are a special interest within themselves. Again the scope of this chapter does not permit an in-depth discussion but only a brief presentation of the rates most commonly used in the care of patients with renal disease.

Mortality rate. This is defined as an estimation of the proportion of the population that dies during a specific time period (Hennekens & Buring, 1987). Mortality rates can be adjusted for age, sex, or ethnic group.

$$\frac{\text{No. of deaths from renal disease in place in year}}{\text{No. of total deaths from all causes in place, in year}} \times 100 = \text{Percent of deaths due to renal disease.}$$

Morbidity rate. Morbidity rates are a measure of frequency in which there is any departure from a state of physiological or psychological well-being (Last, 1988). The most commonly used morbidity rates are incidence and prevalence.

Incidence rates are the measure of all new disease cases occurring in a population at risk over a specified period of time.

$$\frac{\text{Number of new cases in a specified period}}{\text{Average population at risk at midpoint in time}} \times 10^n$$

Prevalence rates are the number of instances of a given disease in a given population at a designated time. (Prevalence rates when unspecified usually mean point prevalence as opposed to period prevalence).

$$\frac{\text{No. of existing cases in place at a specified point in time}}{\text{No. of persons in place at midpoint in a year}}$$

Incidence and prevalence rates give very different pictures of a disease status of a population. Two diseases with similar incidence rates will have very different prevalence rates, if one disease is chronic and one disease is acute. Mortality and recovery rates also have an impact on prevalence rates (Valanis, 1992; Hennekens & Buring, 1987).

Epidemiology and the Nurse

The focus of care for a nurse or other health care clinician is the health and well-being of the individual patient. Clinical practice evolves from the concept of patient care. Epidemiology focuses on the health of the group to which an individual is a member. The clinical description of a disease differs from its epidemiological description in so far as the former relates to an individual patient whereas the latter describes a group of individuals similarly affected. The epidemiologist must single out, in terms of probabilities, averages, and means, those characteristics that are significantly more common in the diseased population (Valanis, 1992).

Epidemiological information is invaluable to the health care professional in predicting illness in individual patients, and these professionals are essential in providing the required data to identify patterns of disease occurrence and progression. Patterns of symptoms often cluster in a particular age group, geographical area, or time period. Recognition of such patterns is the first step in learning what causes a particular disease (Valanis, 1992, p. 8). Nursing assessments rely on epidemiological information to determine appropriate intervention and optimal therapy. Early detection of a disease improves prognosis and identification of risk factors may enhance the determination of populations at risk (Valanis, 1992; Hennekens & Buring, 1987). Broad descriptive and clinical disease categories include several different factors. Variations in the statistical distribution of these factors and the natural history of a disease make it possible to distinguish elements of one disease from another disease. A cluster analysis of signs and symptoms by disease, time and/or place may be used to identify syndromes in a population.

Epidemiological investigations originated in response to infectious diseases in Europe in the nineteenth century. As changes in the environment have modified the natural history of many infectious diseases, man-made factors have changed the susceptibility of the human host; for example, with the medical management of organ transplantation, immunosuppressive drugs have altered the resistance of the host and patients receiving dialysis treatments are rendered vulnerable to direct transmission of infectious diseases (Hennekens & Buring, 1987).

There are a variety of infectious diseases caused by specific infectious agents. Our discussion will be limited to the diseases most prevalent in the ESRD population. The infectious diseases most prevalent in ESRD patients are caused by three types of infectious agents, specifically: (a) tuberculosis bacterium, (b) HIV and hepatitis viruses, and (c) drug-resistant organisms, such as methicillin-resistant staphylococcus aureus and vancomycin-resistant enterococci.

Hepatitis

Hepatitis may be defined as an inflammation of the liver, usually a result of a viral infection, but sometimes from toxic agents (Spraycar, 1995). Symptoms of hepatitis commonly include fatigue, low-grade fever, muscle and/or joint pain, anorexia, and sometimes jaundice (Jackson & McPherson, 1991; Bader, 1995). Many people infected with hepatitis are not aware of their disease state because the symptoms are absent or too mild to seek medical attention. Occasionally patients with an acute illness will have fulminant disease, and the mortality rate for these patients is high. Most individuals recover uneventfully, however, for some persons affected with the hepatitis B virus (HBV) and hepatitis C virus (HCV), a chronic carrier state develops that may persist for a lifetime. The outcomes of a chronic carrier state differ among individuals, including cirrhosis, hepatocellular carcinoma, and hepatic failure (Jackson & McPherson, 1991; Stein, 1993).

Five viruses have now been identified that each cause a specific type of hepatitis (see Table 13-2). Hepatitis A is an acute, usually self-limited illness. Prophylaxis with immune globulin is effective in household and sexual contacts of infected patients. Hepatitis B has both acute and chronic forms. Treatment trials for chronic hepatitis B with interferon alfa-2b have shown some promise. Hepatitis C is the name now given to non-A non-B hepatitis. Interferon alfa-2b has been approved for treatment of chronic hepatitis C. Hepatitis D occurs only in patients with hepatitis B. The only treatment for hepatitis D is prevention of hepatitis B. Hepatitis E is seen after natural disasters in developing regions around the world. No chronic form has been reported (Kools, 1992).

Hepatitis A

Hepatitis A (HAV) is an acute, self-limited disease caused by a small RNA picornavirus.

Incubation period. The virus has a short incubation period, usually about 15 to 50 days with 28 days as the average (Spraycar, 1995). HAV infection has a fluctuating clinical course in which symptoms are very much age dependent.

Symptoms. Children tend to exhibit symptoms such as nausea and vomiting, diarrhea, and fever or influenza type illness while adults are generally jaundice, malaise, and complain of muscular pain (Bader, 1995).

Laboratory findings. Laboratory findings include elevated aminotransferase (SGOT) and alkaline phosphatase (SGPT) values. Leukopenia is common and occasionally the value is less than 5,000/mm^3 (normal values: Leukocytes total cell count 4,800-10,800/uL; SGOT 5-40 u/L; SGPT 7-56 u/L) (Spraycar, 1995; Bader, 1995).

Diagnosis. Illness due to hepatitis A is diag-

Figure 13-1
Structure of HBV

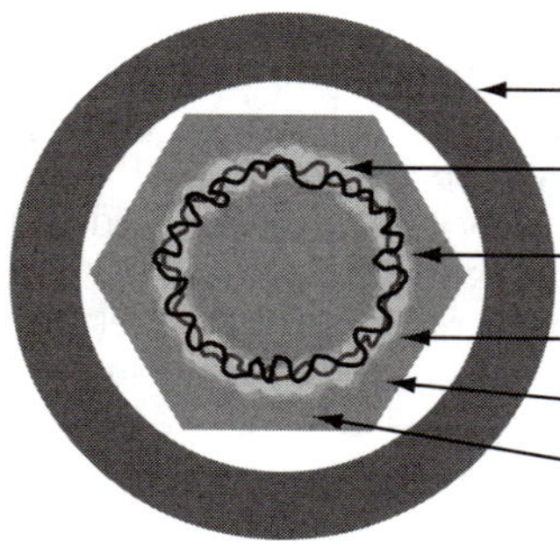

nosed by detection in the blood of an IgM antibody to hepatitis A. The sensitivity of the IgM antibody is 100%, or there are no false negative results. When hepatitis A is active, the IgM test will always be positive (Hoofnagle, 1989). The IgM antibody value is intended to become negative approximately 3 months after the onset of disease and can rarely be detected for as long as 18 months (Decker et al., 1981; Kao, Aschcavai, & Redeker, 1984). The IgG antibody evolves after the acute illness and represents HAV immunity. There is no chronic form of HAV (Storch et al., 1982) and the development of fulminant hepatitis is extremely rare (Bader, 1995).

Mode of transmission. The principal modes of transmission of the HAV is fecal contamination and oral ingestion. Transmission is facilitated by poor sanitation and personal hygiene, and sexual or intrahousehold contact. Common source outbreaks are contaminated water and food, often the result of infected food handlers. A viral shedding in the stool is a result from the passage of the virus into bile. HAV particles appear at least 5 days before the onset of symptoms and disappear when the aminotransferase levels are the highest (Kiyasu & Caldwell, 1993; Dienstag, 1983).

There are two uncommon clinical manifestations with hepatitis A. A small number of adults may develop a cholestatic illness with elevations of alkaline phosphatase, gamma-glutamyl transferase, and total bilirubin. This unusual form may persist for several months and may be associated with pruritus, but is usually self-limited. Another uncommon manifestation is an acute relapse several weeks after the time of resolution. The relapse is often more cholestatic than the initial round of hepatitis A and is occasionally associated with arthritis, vasculitis, and cryoglobulinemia (Inman et al., 1986).

Epidemiology of prevention and treatment. Historically, epidemics of hepatitis A have been a major problem in the military. American soldiers with acute hepatitis missed 6 to 8 weeks of duty (Bancroft & Lemon, 1984; Hoke et al., 1992). Day care centers, restaurants, and sporadic cases in travelers often cause large numbers of hepatitis A cases (Shapiro et al., 1992; Hadler et al., 1980). A 1991 CDC study showed an increase in HAV infections among homosexual men, reflecting a fecal-oral contamination (CDC, 1992). While it is possible to transmit HAV by injection, it is more likely that drugs are contaminated at the cultivation site or from person to person transfer under poor hygienic conditions (CDC, 1988).

Immune serum globulin (ISG) administered to close contacts of infected individuals within 2 weeks of exposure has a 90% protective rate. Dose response studies show that 0.02 ml/kg is the optimal level (Masterson et al., 1991). Before visiting developing countries, travelers can protect themselves by obtaining an injection of immune globulin containing antibodies against HAV; one injection available from a physician or health department may provide protection for 3 to 4 months (Stein, 1993). The use of ISG does not result in serum antibody levels detectable by available immunoassay methods (Lemon, 1985).

Havrix®, the inactivated hepatitis A vaccine, is indicated for active immunization of persons $\geq$ 2 years of age against disease caused by HAV. Havrix® is supplied in single-dose vials or single dose prefilled syringes. The vaccine has been generally well tolerated. The most frequently reported adverse reaction in clinical trials was injection-site soreness (56% of adults; 15% of children); headache (14% adults; less than 5% of children) (SmithKline Beecham Biologicals, 1996). The typical dose of Havrix® vaccine for adults is 720 ELISA units in 1 cm^3 of volume. Several studies indicate that 95.7% of adults seroconvert 1 month after a single dose (anti-HAV titer is 304 mIU/ml). A second dose after 1 month increases the seroconversion rate to 99.8% (anti-HAV titer is 517 mIU/ml). The titers of vaccine-induced antibody are 25 times higher than those observed following the administration of ISG (Tilzey et al., 1992). Protective antibody levels exist 1 to 2 years with a two-dose regimen. A booster dose given at 6 or 12 months will provide an antibody level greater than 10 mIU/ml for 6 to 7 years (Wiedermann et al., 1992). The booster given at 12 months results in higher antibody titers than the booster given at 6 months. Whether or not immunity exists beyond detectable antibody levels is still questionable (Bader, 1995).

Nursing care of patients with acute hepatitis includes measurement of HAV IgM and HAV IgG antibody titers. The patient should be evaluated for the severity of the disease by monitoring prothrombin time and mental status. If these are normal, the patient may be monitored as an outpatient. Secondary cases may be prevented by avoiding sexual relations for at least 1 week and administering immune serum globulin to close contacts. Nurses should provide the following recommendations to patients: activity and bedrest as tolerated; emphasis on high caloric intake in the morning when appetite is best; no alcohol consumption for a minimum of 1 year; discontinuation of all possible medications until patient has recovered; avoidance of elective surgery; and meticulous handwashing. All cases of hepatitis A should be reported to the health department (Bader, 1995).

Hepatitis B

Hepatitis B (HB) is a disease caused by hepatitis B virus (HBV), a DNA virus and member of the family Hepadnoviridae. Hepatitis B is a virus containing both double-stranded and single-stranded DNA (Bader, 1995). The component parts of the virus are listed in Figure 13-1. The hepatitis B surface antigen (HBsAg) is a nonreplicating part of the virus that is produced in large quantities. Antibody to the surface antigen is called surface antibody (anti-Hbs). These antibodies will appear 2 to 3 months after the onset of symptoms. Generally, anti-Hbs and HBsAg are exclusive of each other, and the anti-HBs confers immunity and convalescence.

The Dane particle has an interior core antigen (HBcAg), which is detected in liver tissue but not in serum; therefore, there is no serological test for it. Antibodies to the core antigen are called core antibodies (anti-HBc) and appear together in the IgM class (anti-HBc-IgM), during acute hepatitis B (usually about 4 to 6 months) (Jackson & McPherson, 1991), and the IgG class (anti-HBc-IgG), during convalescence or chronic infection. The anti-HBc does not confer immunity.

The hepatitis E antigen (HBeAg) is part of the interior core antigen or HBcAG. It appears simultaneously with the HBsAg and denotes viral replication. Viral status refers to the degree of viral replication. Hepatitis B carriers who are also HBeAg positive are likely to be more infectious than those who are HBeAg negative or antibody to HBeAg (anti-HBe) positive. The antibody to HBeAg indicates that viral replication is at a low level, but it does not confer immunity (Bader, 1995; Jackson & McPherson, 1991).

Incubation period. The incubation period for HBV is approximately 40 to 80 days (Spraycar, 1995). A common misunderstanding is to equate acute or chronic hepatitis B with jaundice. Only a small amount of patients actually become jaundice and anicteric patients tend to have fewer symptoms and a lower mortality rate but are more likely to advance to a chronic carrier state.

Symptoms. Symptoms that are common in icteric hepatitis B patients are: anorexia, nausea, weakness, epigastric discomfort, vomiting, diarrhea, malaise, right upper quadrant pain, and urticaria. Symptoms common in anicteric hepatitis B patients are: anorexia, nausea, vomiting, malaise, and right upper quadrant pain. The list of symptoms for hepatitis B are similar to the symptoms identified for hepatitis A. However, the severity of the illness, prodromal period, extrahepatic symptoms, and increased bedrest requirements are more pronounced in patients affected by hepatitis B virus (Bader, 1995).

Laboratory findings. Laboratory findings include an elevated aminotransferase level ranging from 1,000 to 4,000 IU/liter (SGOT = 5-40 IU/L) and an elevated total bilirubin in icteric patients usually 340 mol/L (normal total bilirubin range values equal 3-22 mol/L) (Wilkenson et al., 1978; Seeff, 1990).

Clinical course. In most patients diagnosed with HBV, the HBsAg will disappear within 4 months after the onset of symptoms. The median time of HBsAg clearance is 7 weeks after symptoms begin. The severity of the hepatitis, as measured by the degree of bilirubin elevation, roughly correlates with the duration of HBsAg positivity (Hoofnagle, Seeff, & Bales, 1978). In < 3% of patients infected with HBV, the disease progresses to subacute hepatic necrosis. Subacute hepatic necrosis can be correlated with hepatitis B patients > 40 years of age, drug addicts, and those patients experiencing an insidious onset of anicteric hepatitis B. During a 4 to 12-week time period, jaundice increases and coagulation factors deteriorate. Signs of the development of portal hypertension, such as ascites, peripheral edema, and splenomegaly may appear (Bader, 1995).

In < 1% of patients with acute hepatitis B, fulminant hepatitis or fulminant hepatic failure will occur (Kiyasu & Caldwell, 1993). Viral hepatitis accounts for up to 72% of all cases (Lee, 1993). Fulminate hepatitis is defined as an altered mental status (i.e., hepatic encephalopathy) and coagulopathy occurring within 8 weeks of the onset of symptoms referable to the liver in those previously well (Fingerote & Bain, 1993; Lee, 1996; Bader, 1995). Signs of fulminant hepatitis include: bacterial and fungal infections (Lee, 1996); hypoglycemia (Sherlock & Dooley, 1993); bleeding from gastric mucosal lesions (Martin & Maddrey, 1990); and hepatic encephalopathy with cerebral edema, gastrointestinal hemorrhage, electrolyte disturbances, and hypoxemia (Martin & Maddrey, 1990).

In 5% of patients with acute hepatitis B, a chronic carrier state develops. Chronic infection with HBV may be defined as HBsAg remaining in a host for more than 6 months (Kools, 1992). Important factors that influence the development of a chronic carrier state are: the age of the patient when infected; gender; the form of expression of the acute disease; and the immune status of the infected host (Seeff & Koff, 1986). The carrier state can be divided into two types: chronic active hepatitis (CAH) and chronic persistent hepatitis (CPH).

Table 13-3
Recommended doses of yeast-recombinant hepatitis B vaccine.

GROUP	DOSE (mcg)	(ml)	Intervals
Recombivax HB			
Children (Ages 11-19 years)	5	(0.5)	3
Adults > 20 years	10	(1.0)	3
Dialysis and other immunocompromised patients	40	(1.0)*	3
Energix B			
Children (Ages 11-19 years)	20	(1.0)	3
Adults > 20 years	20	(1.0)	3
Dialysis and other immunocompromised patients	40	(2.0)**	4

* Special formulation
** Two 1.0 ml doses administered at one site, in a four dose schedule at 0, 1, 2, and 6 months
Note: Adapted from Bader, T. (1995). *Viral hepatitis*. Seattle, WA: Hogrefe & Huber Publications.

Chronic active hepatitis is diagnosed by significant fibrosis and erosion of the portal triad limiting plate by mononuclear cells progressing to liver disease (Spraycar, 1995); it occurs in approximately one-quarter of the chronic carriers. Cirrhosis develops in 50% of these adult patients (Bader, 1995). Chronic persistent hepatitis is a type of chronic hepatitis B in which the patient is asymptomatic and little if any histological damage occurs (Spraycar, 1995).

Age at the time of infection is the greatest determinant on the development of chronicity (90% of neonates, 20% of children, 1-5% of adults). Infected males are 1.6% more likely to become a carrier when compared to females (Sampliner, 1979). Chronic hepatitis B occurs more often in anicteric than in icteric patients (Redeker, 1975). The development of chronic hepatitis B in dialysis units is an excellent example of the result caused by differences in immune status. Dialysis patients have a mild illness and develop a chronic carrier state at a rate of 40%-90% (Robinson, 1990); whereas, dialysis staff develop icteric hepatitis that resolves completely in most instances (Seeff & Koff, 1986; Bader, 1995). Although the Black and Oriental population have a higher rate of chronic hepatitis B, it is still not clear whether race or ethnic origin predispose these populations to a chronic carrier state (Seeff, Ishak, & Gerber, 1991).

The majority of chronic carriers are asymptomatic and will not develop chronic liver disease (Bader, 1995). The clinical outcome of approximately one-fourth of hepatitis B carriers is progressive liver failure and cirrhosis develops in 50% of these adult patients. Cirrhosis rarely occurs in children (Bader, 1995). The causes of death for cirrhotic hepatitis B carriers, in order of frequency, are: hepatocellular carcinoma, liver failure, and upper gastrointestinal bleeding (DeJongh, Jansen, & Deman, 1992).

Special topics. In 10%-20% of all chronic carriers, co-expression of HBsAg and anti-HBs represents the presence of an unusual type of antibody (Tsang et al., 1986). Whether this pattern results from a mutation in the surface antigen or a dual subtype infection is unknown. Such patients are thought to progress clinically like other chronic carriers (Kiyasu & Caldwell, 1993). The HBeAg negative, HBsAg positive, and anti-HBe phase of chronic hepatitis B is not always a stable one. Reactivation of the *e* antigen can occur, and the signs and symptoms are similar to that of the onset of acute viral hepatitis (Bader, 1995). Chemotherapeutic agents associated with malignancies (Seeff & Koff, 1986; Flowers, Heathcote, & Wanless, 1990), immunosuppression associated with organ transplantation, and withdrawal of corticosteriods (Seeff & Koff, 1986) have caused reactivation.

Mode of transmission. Hepatitis B is spread by parental and per mucosal/percutaneous routes. In the United States and other western countries, hepatitis B is transmitted primarily by infusion of infected blood or blood products, use of contaminated needles and surgical instruments, and sexual contacts (Kiyasu & Caldwell, 1993; Spraycar, 1995). There is little doubt why dialysis units were once considered high-risk areas.

In areas of high HBV endemicity, mother-infant transmission, in particular at the time of birth, is the most common mode of HBV acquisition in the world (Kiyasu & Caldwell, 1993). The HBV is present in all body secretions, including saliva, tears, semen, vaginal secretions, and breast milk. Only feces are considered to have insignificant amount of HBV present (Villarejos, Visona, & Guiterrez, 1974).

The strongest factor in determining the risk of transmission of HBV in percutaneous or nonpercutaneous exposure is the presence or absence of the HBeAg. Mothers who are HBeAg positive at delivery transmit the infection to their infants about 90% of the time while mothers who are HbsAg positive and anti-HBe positive will transmit HBV to their untreated infants about 10% of the time (Bader, 1995). Needlestick injuries from known HBsAg donors follow a similar pattern. When the donor is HBeAg positive, the recipient has a 20% chance of becoming infected with the HBV compared with a 1% infection rate from a HBsAg positive and HBeAg negative donors (Millman, Eisenstein, & Blumberg, 1984).

Health care workers with acute or chronic hepatitis rarely infect patients. However, more than 10,000 health care workers are estimated to become infected with HBV every year (Bader, 1995). Family members of persons with acute hepatitis or chronic carriers are considered high risk individuals.

Occasionally arthritic symptoms appear in the late incubation period of hepatitis B. The arthritic symptoms usually disappear in 3 to 7 days or with the onset of jaundice. No deformity or joint destruction occurs (Bader, 1995).

Dermatologic manifestations are varied and occur infrequently. Urticaria is the most common but angioedema, palpable purpura, erythema nodosum, erythema multiform, and lichen planus may also develop (Weiss et al., 1978; McElguan, 1983).

Epidemiology of prevention and treatment. Hepatitis B virus infection is a global problem. The Centers for Disease Control estimates that HBV infects up to 12,000 health care workers annually, and 300 of these workers die each year. Over 300 million chronic carriers of HBV exist each year and 1.5 million of these carriers reside in the United States. An estimated 200,000 to 300,000 acute hepatitis B infections occur annually in the United States. The risk of hepatitis B infection is 100 times that of HIV infection after a contaminated needlestick (Goldsmith, 1990).

The first hepatitis B vaccine (Hepavax®) used in the United States was derived from plasma donors and produced anti-HBs in 95% of the vaccinated subjects (Szmuness, Stevens, & Zang, 1981). The production of this vaccine was discontinued due to increased costs for AIDS testing (Bader, 1986). Vaccines are now produced by recombinant DNA technology and use synthetic HBsAg. Two yeast recombinant vaccines are now available: Recombivax-HB® (Merck, Sharper, and Dohme) and Engerix® (Smith-Kline Biologicals). Both doses are given in a three-dose series. The recommended dose for dialysis and other immunocompromised patients is more than double the usual adult dosage (see Table 13-3). The hepatitis B vaccine has been evaluated more than any other vaccine in the history of health care services. Over 4 million adults and at least that many children have received the vaccine worldwide (Bader, 1995). The only side effect noted on occasion is tenderness at the injection site. The hesitancy in vaccinating all populations – not only high-risk groups – is the cost of the vaccination, which usually averages over $100 for the three-dose regimen.

Protection against hepatitis B infection is complete for persons who develop antibody response after the vaccination; however, between 30% and 50% of persons who develop adequate antibody after three doses will no longer maintain detectable antibody titers after 7 years. Immunity appears to continue, and there are currently no recommendations from CDC for routine booster doses at specific intervals (Jackson & McPherson, 1991). About 5% of the healthy adult population fail to develop adequate levels of anti-HBs with three injections of the vaccine. The primary reason for nonresponse appears to be under genetic control. A major histocompatibility complex haplotype (HLA-B8, SCO1, DR3) has been identified and acts as a recessive trait (Bader, 1995). Obesity, immunocompromised, gluteal injection, and over 60 years of age are factors that are associated with poor vaccine response (CDC, 1991).

Hyperimmune hepatitis B immunoglobulin (HBIG) is a plasma-derived product containing a high titer of anti-HBs. Prior to the use of hepatitis B vaccines, HBIG was the only treatment available for postexposure prophylaxis (see Table 13-4). HBIG now appears to be most effective when given in

Table 13-4
Postexposure prophylaxis: Recommendations for hepatitis B prophylaxis following percutaneous or permucosal exposure.

	Treatment when source is found to be:		
Exposed person	**HBsAG-positive**	**HBsAG-negative**	**Source not tested or unknown**
Unvaccinated	HBIG x 1* and initiate HB vaccine	Initiate HB vaccine	Initiate HB vaccine
Previously vaccinated known responder	Test exposed for anti-HBs 1) If adequate, ‡ no treatment 2) If inadequate, HB vaccine booster dose	No treatment	No treatment
Known nonresponder	HBIG x 2 or HBIG x 1 + 1 dose	No treatment	If known high-risk source, may treat as if source were HBsAG-positive HB vaccine
Response unknown	Test exposed for anti-HBs 1) If inadequate, ‡ HBIG x 1 + HB vaccine booster dose 2) If adequate, no treatment	No treatment	Test exposed for anti-HBs 1) If adequate, ‡ HB vaccine booster booster dose 2) If adequate, no treatment

* HBIG dose 0.06 ml/kg IM
‡ Adequate anti-HBs is ≥ 10 SRU by RIA or positive by EIA

conjunction with hepatitis B vaccine. A regimen of two doses of HBIG (one given after exposure and one a month later) combined with hepatitis B vaccine given at the same time (different injection sites are recommended) has shown to be about 75% effective in preventing hepatitis B. Fully immunized individuals do not need HBIG (Jackson & McPherson, 1991; Bader, 1995). In addition, there is no evidence that HIV can be transmitted by HBIG (CDC, 1990; Seeff, 1990).

Antiviral therapy for chronic hepatitis B is directed toward patients with active hepatitis and viral replication, preferably before cirrhosis and significant liver damage occur. Elimination of chronic hepatitis B is possible in only a small amount of patients. The goal of alfa-interferon therapy is to suppress the virus and cause a remission of the associated liver disease (Dusheiko & Zuckerman, 1993).

HBV is considered suppressed or eliminated and the carrier state terminated when HBsAg is no longer detectable. This goal is usually not realized after initial alfa-interferon therapy. However, most patients who become HBeAg negative and HBV-DNA negative will eventually eliminate HBsAg (Korenman, Baker, & Waggoner, 1994). Thus, it is as important to monitor HBeAg and HBV-DNA outcomes as it is HBsAg results (Bader, 1995).

The recommended doses for treatment of chronic hepatitis B is 5 million units daily or 10 million units three times per week. Adverse effects of alfa-interferon are common and occur in a dose-related manner. Alfa-interferon must be administered parenterally and the subcutaneous route appears most convenient for patients (Jackson & McPherson, 1991; Bader, 1995; Kiyasu & Caldwell, 1993).

Adverse reactions to alfa-interferon appear after the first few doses or after 1 to 2 weeks. The initial symptoms are mild "influenza-like" symptoms, such as: fever, headache, chills, fatigue, and muscle pain. Later symptoms include diarrhea, anorexia, nausea, depression, irritability, and alopecia (Bader, 1995). Myelosuppression, bacterial infections, and the development of autoantibodies occur in some degree to the majority of HBV patients treated with alfa-interferon. Myelosuppression can be life-threatening if a patient already has decreased hematological values before therapy. Bacterial infections are a serious side effect to those patients who have compromised immunity, and antibiotics should be initiated early (Renault & Hoofnagle, 1989). The development of autoantibodies, with or without autoimmune disease, occurs in approximately one-half of patients treated with alfa-interferon (Mayet, Hess, & Gerken, 1989). The results can be so severe (i.e., autoantibodies to the thyroid [Renault & Hoofnagle, 1989], systemic lupus erythematosus, pernicious anemia, vasculitis, autoimmune thrombocytopenia, and polyarthropathy [Perrillo, 1993]), that alfa-interferon should be used with prudence, if at all in patients with a preexisting auto immune disorder (Bader, 1995; Dusheiko & Zuckerman, 1993).

Although patients receiving liver transplants for fulminant hepatitis appear to do well, patients receiving transplants for chronic hepatitis B have a poor response (Todo et al., 1991). The recurrence of HBV is almost pervasive (Starzl, Demetris, & Van Thiel, 1989), and often leads to accelerated liver disease, such as cirrhosis and hepatocellular carcinoma. Although interferon appears to be safe after transplantation, this therapy has not demonstrated significant results in preventing or treating HBV infection (Wright, Hollander, & Kim, 1991; Bader, 1995; Kiyasu & Caldwell, 1993).

The best treatment for hepatitis B viral infection is prevention. For acute hepatitis B, the patient should perform activities and bedrest as tolerated, emphasize calories in the morning when the appetite is better, abstain from alcohol for at least 1 year, discontinue all medications possible, avoid elective surgery, and report the case to the local health department. For chronic hepatitis B, the patient's place in the course of the disease should be defined to stage the amount of current liver damage and determine the potential for progression to cirrhosis. If the patient's serum albumin level is normal, ALT level is normal or slightly elevated, and the patient is asymptomatic, no liver biopsy is indicated. Otherwise the patient's viral status, age, and host response can be valuable information in predicting the patient's prognosis and response to alpha-interferon treatment. Members of the patient's household should be vaccinated and the patient should be evaluated to rule out hepatitis C and D. The patient should never drink alcohol or use tobacco products, avoid corticosteriods and chemotherapeutic agents to prevent reactivation, and receive the influenza vaccine every year and the pneumococcal vaccine once (Bader, 1995; Stein, 1993).

Hepatitis C

Hepatitis C virus (HCV) can be defined as the principal reason (> 90%) for non-A non-B posttransfusion hepatitis, caused by a single-stranded RNA virus that is classified as a separate genus in the Flaviridae family (Spraycar, 1995; Medin et al., 1993). Since the early 1970s, it has been apparent that the majority of posttransfusion hepatitis is caused by a virus other than hepatitis A or B. Epidemiologic studies have established that this virus was relatively common and infectious (Soloway, 1990). In the absence of specific and sensitive immunologic tests, this form of viral hepatitis was designated non-A non-B and a diagnosis of exclusion became necessary (Alter et al., 1982).

Diagnosis. In 1989, Michael Houghton and his colleagues at the Centers for Disease Control and the Chiron Corporation reported the cloning of part of a genome, which they designated the hepatitis C virus. Expression of the corresponding HCV cDNA in yeast made it possible to develop a serologic test that detects antibody against the protein. This immunoassay was licensed in May 1990 (Choo et al., 1989; Kuo, Choo, & Alter, 1989). Several limitations of this first generation assay (enzyme-linked immunosorbent assay-1) (EIA-1) led to the development of a more sensitive and specific second-generation assay (EIA-2). The second generation assay identifies HCV as the etiologic agent in approximately 20%-30% more cases and within a 6 to 8-week period after the onset of hepatitis as opposed to 4 to 6 months with the first generation assays (Aach, Hirschman, & Holland, 1992). A supplemental test approved by the Food and Drug Administration (FDA) in 1993, Recombinant immunoblot assay-II (RIBA-II), uses a different methodology to test for the same antigens as EIA-II.

The approach to diagnosis depends on the risk factors associated with the patient population being evaluated (Bader, 1995). In patient populations with low-risk factors, normal ALT levels, or alcoholic liver disease, every EIA-II should be supplemented with a RIBA-II assay. RIBA-II assay testing increases the specificity of EIA-II results but not the sensitivity. With this testing only about a 30% false positive rate exists. In high-risk populations, if the patient has a clear risk factor for hepatitis C supplemental testing is not necessary and false positive results rarely occur (Bader, 1995). High-risk populations include: hemophiliacs, IV drug abusers, transplanted organ recipients, and health care workers. The role of household, sexual, and maternal-infant transmission has not been completely evaluated but data suggests that infection occurs on only rare occasions.

The principal reason for difficulty in identifying a marker for this virus is its very low concentration in the serum. In contrast to hepatitis B, where the concentration of virus is 1 to 10 million infective particles per ml of serum, only 1 to 10 virions per ml of hepatitis C may be present (Bader, 1995).

The screening of blood donors for hepatitis C has greatly reduced, though not eliminated, the number of new hepatitis C infections among transfusion recipients. Transfusions now account for about 4% of new hepatitis C infections. Approximately 30% of patients have a history of IV drug use: 2% are health care workers (0.2% dialysis staff) and 1-1.2% are dialysis patients (Stein, 1993; Niu et al., 1993). Blood transfusions screened by EIA-2 have an infectivity rate of 0.03% per unit or 1 in 3,000 units will transmit posttransfusion hepatitis (Bader, 1995).

Mode of transmission. The primary mode of HCV transmission continues to be percutaneous infection with contaminated blood. An explanation for the continued reoccurrence may be donors who test negative for all sensitive assays (Sugitani, Inchauspe, & Shindo, 1992) and/or the presence of another virus with the proposed designation of hepatitis F (Lancet, 1990).

Incubation period. Non-A, non-B hepatitis has a mean incubation period of 7.8 weeks. The range is

Table 13-5
Control of hepatitis C in hemodialysis centers.

- Patients who are positive for hepatitis C antibody or who have a diagnosis of non-A, non-B hepatitis do not have to be isolated or dialyzed separately on dedicated machines.
- They can participate in dialyzer reuse programs.
- Infection control strategies should emphasize basic barrier precautions, commonly referred to as "Universal Precautions."

2-26 weeks but 80%-90% of cases occur within 5-12 weeks after transfusion (Dienstag, 1983).

Symptoms/laboratory findings/clinical course. Most patients with acute HCV are asymptomatic. Hepatitis C has an approximately 50% incidence of progression to a chronic carrier state (Aach et al., 1992). Hepatitis C is defined as a chronic infection after being present for 6 to 12 months. Chronic carriers of HCV are often asymptomatic and discovered incidentally.

The most common symptom of 102 patients referred to the liver unit was fatigue and only 18% of patients gave a history of hepatitis or jaundice (Merican, Sherlock, & McIntyre, 1993). Other laboratory findings may include hypoalbumenia, increased alanine aminotransferase (ALT), AST/ALT ratio (< 1 for noncirrhotic disease and >1 for cirrhosis) (Williams & Hoofnagle, 1988), and platelet count (< 140,000 cells cc^3) abnormalities. All of these values need to be evaluated as a total picture; dependence on any one parameter may be misleading (Bader, 1995).

The same staging in liver biopsies is used in chronic hepatitis B and C (see hepatitis B, Clinical Course). Chronic persistent hepatitis is usually considered to be a nonprogressive entity and chronic active hepatitis is considered a severe form that progresses to more severe forms and usually cirrhosis (Bader, 1995).

The most frequent complication of HCV infection is hepatocellular carcinoma with ranges of 51% to 94% (Takeda, Nagafuchi, & Tashiro, 1992; Kiyosawa, Sodeyama, & Tanaka, 1990). Almost all cases of hepatocellular carcinoma occur with cirrhosis, which is unlike hepatitis B where hepatocellular carcinoma may occur without cirrhosis being present (Takeda et al., 1992; Gerber, Shieh, & Shim, 1992; Faranati et al., 1992). Other complications of HCV infection include essential mixed cryoglobulinemia, porphyria cutanea tarda, and lichen planus (Bader, 1995).

Special topics. Little data are available regarding hepatitis C in the pediatric population. Current information suggests that the pathology and natural history of HCV infection in children appears similar to that of the adult population (Maggiore & DeGiacoma, 1992; Bortolotti et al., 1992; Resti et al., 1992). No growth retardation is apparent in pediatric patients with hepatitis C and no other major age-related differences in the course or outcome have been noted (Bader, 1995).

The prevalence of EIA-2 or RIBA positive results in patients with chronic renal failure or undergoing kidney transplantation ranges from 4.2% to 27% (Holzberger et al., 1992; Getzug et al., 1990). Hepatitis C virus positivity has been correlated with the number of blood transfusions and length of time on dialysis (Chan et al., 1993; Neves & Amorim, 1992). It is difficult to separate the two factors since these risk factors are correlated. However, two trends will assist in explaining the risk relationship between dialysis and hepatitis C infection: (a) the decrease of HCV infectivity via blood transfusions, and (b) the use of erythropoietin to maintain hematocrit levels (Bader, 1995).

Data are not available to suggest hemodialysis as a risk factor for HCV infection. Currently, the CDC does not recommend that dialysis of HCV-positive patients be performed in an isolated room or on a dedicated machine; only, that the universal precautions established in the early 1980s be implemented (Favero, 1996; Moyer, 1991) (see Table 13-5).

Two major studies have indicated that HCV does not affect the survival of the patient or the transplanted organ for over 10 years (Pol et al., 1992; Ynares, Johnson, & Kerlin, 1993). However, to date there is no systematic data as to whether alfa-interferon can be used to treat renal transplant patients with hepatitis C. The principle concern of using alfa-interferon is producing organ rejection.

The presence of HIV infection seems to worsen hepatitis C in some patients (Martin et al., 1989; Watson et al., 1992). The incidence of rapidly progressive liver disease is uncertain but clearly occurs in a minority (Martin et al., 1989; Eyster et al., 1993). HCV viremia probably increases after the onset of HIV infection (Wright et al., 1992). It is not known in cases with a sustained normalization of ALT after alfa-interferon treatment whether this will actually result in an increased life expectancy since HIV infection persists (Marriott et al., 1993; Bader, 1995). At the present time, it is essentially unknown if HCV has a deleterious effect on HIV disease.

Epidemiology of prevention and treatment. Donor blood screening for non-A, non-B hepatitis has greatly reduced the occurrence of transfusion-related hepatitis C. Although the utilization of gamma globulin (ISG) has demonstrated some reduction in the incidence of transfusion associated non-A, non-B hepatitis (Sanchez-Quijara, Pineda, & Lissen, 1988; Kuhns, Prince, & Brotman, 1976;

Knodell et al., 1976), Bader (1995) does not recommend its use for prevention of hepatitis C. The difference in the effectiveness of ISG is most likely related to the timing of gamma globulin injections. In the trials where ISG proved effective, ISG was given prior to the blood products, and in the two trials where ISG proved ineffective, the ISG was started after the transfusions were received.

Hepatitis may be defined as a chronic infection after being present in the blood stream for 6 months. Although hepatitis C appears to have a benign natural history, after several decades of infection, greater than 20% of patients may develop cirrhosis over several decades and HCV is so prevalent that it has become the most common indication for liver transplant in the United States (Bader, 1995). Since hepatitis C does not appear to cause progressive disease in a majority of carriers, liver biopsy and alfa interferon treatment should be based on the identification of patient parameters that would indicate progressive liver disease in those patients who have not yet decompensated from complications of the disease. These parameters are: fatigue, the degree of ALT abnormality (>5X/normal or above 200 IU/L), whether serum albumin level is within normal limits, and platelet count is $\geq$ 70,000/mm^3.

Alfa interferon was first reported effective for the treatment of chronic non-A non-B hepatitis in 1986 (Hoofnagle et al., 1986). Subsequent randomized, controlled trials have proven the effectiveness of alfa-interferon treatment at a dose of 3 million units (MU) three times weekly for 6 months for chronic HCV infection (Tine et al., 1991). The dose can be administered subcutaneously or intramuscularly. To some degree, the probability of response is both time dependent and dose related. A meta-analysis of randomized controlled interferon trials suggests that approximately 50% of patients normalize their AST (aspartate aminotransferase, formerly SGOT) while on treatment. However, 50% of the responding patients relapse after treatment, leaving only 20%-25% of patients with a sustained response after treatment (Tine et al., 1991). Increasing the dose of alfa-interferon to 5-7.5 MU or lengthening the time of treatment to 12-26 months does not appear to improve the rate of sustained remission (Colombo et al., 1991; Metreau et al., 1991; Saez-Royuela et al., 1991; Reichard et al., 1994). See hepatitis B, Treatment for discussion of the side effects of alfa interferon.

Transplantation of the liver for end stage liver disease caused by HCV is an appropriate treatment. Unfortunately, transplantation does not cure the infection. Approximately 93% of patients transplanted for liver disease due to HCV develop recurrent infection in the new liver (Lake et al., 1993). Eligibility for transplantation, therefore, depends on the severity of associated diseases rather than on the presence or absence of HCV.

Figure 13-2
Structure of a delta virus.

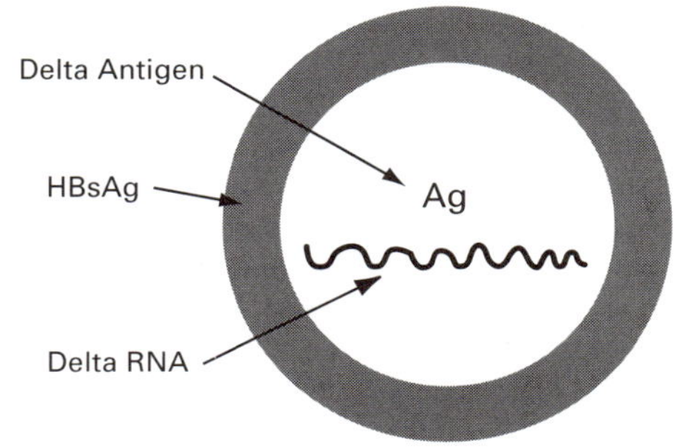

Hepatitis D

Hepatitis D virus (HDV), initially described in southern Italy by Rizzetto and co- workers in 1977, is an RNA virus that requires the presence of HBV infection. It has a complex interaction with HBV but generally worsens the prognosis of patients infected with HBV (Kiyasu & Caldwell, 1993).

Clinical course. HDV and HBV may be acquired at the same time as a coinfection, or HDV infection can be imposed on a chronic carrier of HBV as a superinfection. The clinical expression, incidence of fulminant hepatitis, and chronic carrier rate differ between coinfection and superinfection (Bader, 1995).

Coinfection seldom leads to a chronic carrier state of either HBV or HDV. The chronic carriers in this situation occur in approximately 2.4%-4.7% of patients. Superinfection with HDV leads to a chronic carrier state more than 90% of the time (Polish et al., 1993; Hoofnagle, 1989). Over 60% of patients with chronic HDV will develop cirrhosis (Kiyasu & Caldwell, 1993). Most cases of chronic HDV are thought to result from acute superinfection.

Diagnosis. The only available assay for diagnosis of HDV infection is a blocking RIA test for total antibody (anti-HD) to delta antigen. Anti-HD measures both IgG and IgM antibodies. HDAg occurs in low titer and is short lived (less than a week) in acute infections (Hoofnagle, 1989).

Anti-HD levels will disappear in 1 to 2 years when the acute infection resolves. Chronic delta infection is simple to diagnose since anti-HD levels will be persistently high (Bader, 1995).

Mode of transmission. Sources of infections for delta virus are intravenous drug use, homosexuality, blood transfusions, and heterosexual contact (DeCock et al., 1986). Figure 13-2 shows the structure of a delta virus. Mode of transmission is identical to hepatitis B since HDV is dependent on HBV for survival.

Epidemiology of prevention and treatment. For unknown reasons, geographical location or ethnic

Table 13-6
A brief history of AIDS.

1981:	Centers for Disease Control report first cases
1982:	Disease is named AIDS. Congress allocates 5.6 million for research.
1984:	Scientists isolate human immunodeficiency virus believed to cause AIDS.
1985:	Actor Rock Hudson dies from AIDS. Screening of blood banks for HIV begins.
1986:	Surgeon General urges AIDS education, condom utilization.
1987:	AZT approved as first drug for treatment of AIDS: Congress adds HIV to list of diseases that prevent immigrants from entering U.S.
1988:	Federal AIDS funding approximately $1 billion.
1990:	First case of health-care worker transmitting AIDS to patient. Teen-age AIDS patient, Ryan White, once isolated and rejected, dies. Congress acts to prevent discrimination against people with AIDS.
1991:	White House delays decision to allow immigrants with HIV to enter U.S. About 1 million Americans are infected with HIV; 126,000 have died (CDC, 1997a).
1995:	FDA approves a new class of drugs called protease inhibitors
1996:	FDA approves a home-use blood test for HIV and a test that uses a treated cotton pad to collect an oral specimen from between the cheek and gum. Home testing is promoted.

background affects the severity of hepatitis D. In Northern Europe, the United States, and Italy, over 90% of cases result in liver disease; while in Rhodes, Greece and the Samoan Islands in the Pacific Ocean, the majority of HDV-infected subjects are asymptomatic and healthy (Rizzetto, 1993).

Alfa-interferon has not been approved for treatment of delta hepatitis in the United States. The trials have been disappointing since improvements in aminotransferase relapsed uniformly after cessation of therapy (Hoofnagle & DiBisceglie, 1993). Liver transplantation may be considered but HDV infection recurs in the majority of patients following transplantation (Kiyasu & Caldwell, 1993).

Hepatitis E

Hepatitis E is an enterally transmitted RNA virus that causes an illness similar to HAV.

Clinical features. Hepatitis E causes a clinical picture of a benign disease very similar to that of hepatitis A. There is no recognized chronic form. Fulminant cases are rare with the exception of infection during pregnancy, where severe illness is common (Kiyasu & Caldwell, 1993).

Diagnosis. Immune election microscopy (IEM) has been the only reliable means of identifying both HEV antigen and antibody (Sherlock & Dooley, 1993).

Incubation period. The incubation period of hepatitis E ranges from 2 to 9 weeks with a mean of 6 weeks (Purcell & Ticehurst, 1988).

Modes of transmission. Contaminated water is the best understood mode of transmission.

Epidemiology of prevention and treatment. Hepatitis E infection occurs in the settings of epidemics (mainly Asia, Africa, and Mexico) (Stein, 1993; Jackson & McPherson, 1991) and sporadic cases in endemic areas. Cases that occur in nonendemic areas are imported by travel (Bader, 1995). At the current time, prophylactic gammaglobulin has not decreased the number of cases and the severity of the disease (Joshi, Babu, & Sarin, 1985; Purcell & Shikata, 1991). General treatment measures are as outlined for hepatitis A.

Human Immunodeficiency Virus and Acquired Immune Deficiency Syndrome

Rarely in the history of mankind has a disease spread at the rate of the human immunodeficiency virus (HIV) (see Table 13-6). HIV causes immunosuppression of the host individual and the development of acquired immune deficiency syndrome (AIDS) (Clavel, Mansinho, & Charmaret, 1987). First identified in 1981, by 1987 it was the leading cause of death among U.S. men between the ages of 25 and 44. The virus has become pandemic. In 1986, a second human immunodeficiency virion, HIV-2, was identified. HIV-2 is a subtype of HIV-1 found in West Africa although it has been reported in other countries including the U.S. The HIV-2 virus affects the body in a manner similar to the HIV-1 virus. However, it appears to be less destructive to the immune system and slower growing than HIV-1. The strains of virus that have caused the worldwide pandemic have been designated the group M viruses. Another strain designated group O has been identified in individuals in West and Central Africa. The group O viruses have a different genetic configuration than the group M viruses. As of this writing, only one individual in the United States has been identified as having group O virus (Centers for Disease Control and Prevention [CDC], 1996a).

The first person to die from AIDS in the United States was a 15-year-old boy, diagnosed with several sexually transmitted diseases and admitted to St. Louis City Hospital in 1968 (Freeman, 1991). Blood and tissue samples were preserved since the cause of his death was not clearly understood. A serum specimen was later tested and found positive for HIV-1.

One theory of origin is that the virus originated in Africa in monkeys and was transmitted to man through bites, scratches, or eating infected monkeys. The spread of the virus is attributed to an increase in international travel and the sexual revolution of the 60s and 70s (Freeman, 1991).

Epidemiology

HIV infection affects individuals from all socioeconomic and age levels. The Joint United Nations Programme on HIV/AIDS reported that an estimated 22.6 million people worldwide are infected with HIV. Of these, 21.8 million are adults and 830,000 are children (less than 13 years of age). Women are becoming increasingly affected by HIV. Approximately 42% of the 21.8 million adults living with HIV/Aids are women (CDC, 1997a). Cumulative AIDS cases reported to the Public Health Service of the United States through June 30, 1997, totaled 612,078 (CDC, 1997a). The total number of deaths attributed to AIDS through June 10, 1997, is 379,348 – including 374,656 adults and 4,692 children. From 1995 to 1996, the number of cases reported increased by 11% (CDC, 1997d). Concurrently the number of deaths attributed to AIDS decreased by 19% from 1995 to 1996. This is due in part to the increase in new antiviral therapies affecting patient survival. During 1996, an estimated 56,730 persons were diagnosed with AIDS opportunistic infections and 38,780 deaths were attributed to AIDS opportunistic infections (CDC 1997d). Despite the decrease in the number of deaths, AIDS opportunistic infections remain the leading cause of death among persons ages 25-44 years.

Pathophysiology

The HIV virus infects cells of the human body by inserting RNA into body cells. HIV binds to the CD4+ antigen receptor site on the helper T-lymphocyte cell or other cells that have a CD4+ antigen receptor site. A CD4+ T-cell is a white blood cell that regulates the production of antibodies to fight invading viruses or bacteria. After it binds to the CD4+ T-cell, HIV injects its RNA strands into the T-cell. HIV is a retro virus that uses an enzyme, reverse transcriptase, to reverse the flow of genetic information from the virus to the body cells. This allows the virus to reproduce a DNA copy of its RNA strand, which is necessary for it to replicate and reproduce. When the virus fuses onto the CD4+ T-cell, it dominates the cell and begins to replicate the cell. The CD4+ T-cells are then producing new AIDS viruses that circulate and produce more copies. Antibodies to HIV produced in the body are unable to inactivate the AIDS virus. In HIV infection the CD8 T-cells or suppressor T-cells are normal or slightly elevated, which is a reversal of the normal T-cell helper to suppressor ratio (McCance & Huether, 1994).

HIV Infection

HIV infection begins when the virus attaches to the CD4+ antigen on the T-cell and fuses. The virus injects the core protein and two strands of RNA into the cell. The virus is uncoated and the RNA is released into the cell cytoplasm. The virus migrates to the nucleus of the cell and is integrated into the cell DNA. It remains latent or activates a copy of its RNA. The new RNA is translated into new virons that bud from the cell. This process may take place slowly or so rapidly that the cell is ruptured and destroyed (McCance & Huether, 1994). HIV also infects the central nervous system resulting in AIDS dementia complex in the late stages of the disease.

Women with AIDS have different health problems than men. They become sicker and die faster than men with AIDS. Most women with AIDS are poor, malnourished, receive public assistance, and maintain poor health care, contributing to the higher mortality rates. Women with AIDS are more likely to have gynecological problems as opportunistic infections (McCance & Huether, 1994).

Incubation Period

The incubation period begins when the person develops antibodies to HIV and is completed when the person is diagnosed with full-blown AIDS. Usual incubation period is 7-10 years. After infection with the virus antibodies in the body develop within a month or two. However, some people do not develop antibodies until 6 to 14 months after infection. In the late stages of the disease, HIV antibodies may be negative because of a deficient immune system. The period between infection and the appearance of antibodies is called the window period (CDC, 1996d). The individual may not have detectable antibodies but the virus is growing and the individual may be infectious within 2 weeks after infection (CDC, 1996d).

Acute retro viral syndrome occasionally occurs in people shortly after exposure to HIV. Acute retro viral syndrome presents with relatively mild symptoms such as night sweats, swollen lymph glands, diarrhea, or fatigue. The virus can remain in the person's body for as long as 10 years before symptoms appear. The body is fighting the virus that is replicating and destroying the body's defense system. When the number of CD4+ T-cells is less than 200 (normal is 1000), the body can no longer fend off invasive pathogens and opportunistic infections occur.

Clinical Manifestations

HIV-infected individuals usually go to the health provider with one common symptom, recurrent infections. Early symptoms include fevers, night sweats, swollen glands, rashes, fatigue, weight loss, confusion, persistent headaches, deteriorating vision, persistent dry cough, shortness of breath, oral thrush, dry mouth, sore throat, painful swallowing, watery diarrhea, and rectal bleeding (McCance & Huether, 1994). Ten percent of all people with AIDS suffer neurological complaints as their first symptom (Scherer, 1990). AIDS is characterized by severe symptoms and an increase in infections and malignancies. Some patients with HIV have wasting syndrome. Symptoms include major weight loss, chronic diarrhea, weakness, and constant or intermittent fevers for at least 30 days. This is considered an AIDS defining illness. Due to the suppressed immune system, the HIV infected individual is vulnerable to food-borne illnesses (Food & Drug Administration [FDA], 1997).

Opportunistic Infections

Opportunistic infections are infections that take advantage of the body's immune-compromised state. Bacterial, fungal, and viral infections all pose serious threats to individuals who are severely immunosuppressed, that is, have a CD4+ T-cell count less than 200 cells/uL (CDC, 1997e). Pneumocystis carinii pneumonia (PCP), toxoplasmic encephalitis, mycobacterium tuberculosis, and mycobacterium avium complex, and fungal infections such as cryptosporidiosis and microsporidiosis are common among severely immunosuppressed individuals. The bacterial infections that are common in the community, but potentially deadly to severely immunosuppressed individuals include: streptococcus pneumonia, haemophilus influenzae, and bacterial enteric infections such as listeriosis. In addition, Herpes simplex virus, varicella-zoster virus, cytomegalovirus, and human papillomavirus are dangerous to immunosuppressed individuals. In 1995 the Public Health Service published guidelines for treatment of opportunistic infections. These recommendations were updated in June 1997 (CDC, 1997e). In the United States in 1996, there was a decline in the incidence of AIDS opportunistic infections. This represents the first year AIDS opportunistic infections did not increase (CDC, 1997d).

Transmission

HIV is found in the blood, semen, and vaginal secretions of an infected individual. Sexual contact, needle sharing among IV drug abusers, and intrauterine transmission between mother and newborn infant are the most common routes of transmission. Early in the identification of HIV, homosexual activity was attributed as the major route of transmission. However, heterosexual AIDS cases are increasing at 15% - 20% per year. HIV-positive mothers can transmit HIV to the fetus as early as the eighth week of gestation. Perinatal transmission accounts for most HIV infections among children (CDC, 1994b). HIV is currently the seventh leading cause of death in children ages 1 to 4 years in the United States and the fourth leading cause of death in women age 25-44. Sharing contaminated needles continues to be a source of infection among IV drug abusers.

Blood transfusions have been screened for HIV-1 virus since March, 1985 and for HIV-2 since June, 1992 (CDC, 1996d). Of the 100,000 blood donations tested in 1993, only 6 tested positive for HIV. It is estimated that of the 450,000 to 660,000 blood donations yearly, only 1 is positive for HIV but not detected by available screening methods (CDC, 1996c). Between 1985 and September 1997, only 35 cases of AIDS by blood transfusion in the United States were documented. The FDA recommended all donated blood be screened for HIV-1 p24 antigen in 1995. This is expected to reduce the number of otherwise undetected infectious donations by approximately 25% per year (CDC, 1996d). The test for p24 antigen can detect HIV earlier than antibody testing for HIV. The p24 antigen is the core structural protein of HIV. It is detectable 2-3 weeks after infection with HIV when the person is highly infectious. On the average, the p24 antigen is detected 6 days earlier than HIV antibodies. When antibodies are detected the p24 antigen is no longer detectable. The reliability of the test is reportedly 99.95%. Testing for p24 would decrease the window period for detecting donors recently infected, but not yet HIV antibody positive (CDC, 1997c). The p24 test is not recommended for routine diagnosis of HIV infection because the estimated time of detection of p24 antigen to detection of HIV antibodies is only 6 days and not all recently infected persons have detectable levels of p24 antigen (CDC, 1996d). In addition to plasma testing, donors are interviewed for high risk behaviors and persons with questionable high risk behaviors are excluded from donating blood.

The number of organ transplants has increased over the last several years. Reports of HIV transmission following transplant of organs such as the kidney, liver, heart, pancreas, bone, and skin led to the development of guidelines for the procurement and transplantation of organs (CDC, 1994b). Several federal agencies' guidelines, state agencies' guidelines, and voluntary industry standards have significantly decreased the risk of infection with HIV following organ transplant. The Public Health Service requires all organs, tissues, and blood intended to be used for transplant to be tested for HIV-1 and HIV-2. In addition to laboratory test the donor is interviewed if possible for high risk behaviors. Behavior/history exclusionary criteria have been published by the Public Health Service (CDC, 1994a).

HIV is less transmissible than Hepatitis B in occupational settings and does not warrant strict isolation measures required for Hepatitis B. Strict isolation measures are required for treating Hepatitis B positive individuals in the occupation setting because Hepatitis B is readily transmissible through contact with contaminated surfaces. However, the HIV viron level is less concentrated in the blood than Hepatitis B viron level. And the HIV viron does not survive on environmental surfaces (CDC, 1989). In the ESRD setting, HIV may be transmitted only through percutaneous inoculation (i.e., needle stick) or contact of HIV infected blood or body fluid with an open wound, nonintact skin, or mucous membrane (CDC, 1989). Blood is the single most important source of HIV in the workplace setting (see Table 13-7).

Table 13-7
Risk of HIV infection.

- 0.3% all types of percutaneous exposure.
- > 0.3% with deep injury, visible blood on device causing injury, or source patient died from AIDS within past 60 days.
- 0.1% mucous membrane exposure.
- <0.1% skin exposure.

Test to Determine HIV Infection

The FDA licensed tests for HIV-1 antibody detection in 1985. In 1991, a test to identify HIV-1 and HIV-2 simultaneously was licensed. If the test results for HIV-1 and HIV-2 are repeatedly reactive, an additional test is necessary to confirm the diagnosis of HIV. Results of a positive test may only be given when a confirmatory test such as the western blot test or immunofluorescence (IFA) is done (CDC, 1992).

In the ELISA (enzyme-linked immunosorbent assay) also called the EIA, a plastic bead coated with dead HIV is exposed to the subject's serum for an hour. If the subject has been exposed to HIV the antibodies in the serum will stick to the bead. The bead is then placed in a chemical that turns yellow if antibodies are present. The total time for the test is about 3 hours. False negative results may be reported if the person has been infected but has not yet formed antibodies to HIV.

The Western blot test is used to confirm the diagnosis of HIV infection after two positive ELISA results. The Western blot can tell the difference between the HIV antibody and other antibodies that react to the ELISA. It is more expensive and time consuming and is, therefore, used as a confirmatory test. Used in combination with the ELISA, repeatedly reactive results are considered 99% accurate (CDC, 1992).

After an individual has been diagnosed as HIV antibody positive, the CD4+ T-cell count is monitored every 3-6 months. The measurement of CD4+ T-cell count is used to make decisions regarding initiation of prophylactic treatment for opportunistic infections and to monitor the efficacy of antiviral therapy (CDC, 1997c). The viral load, or amount of HIV virus in the blood, is also monitored and used to guide treatment decisions. As the disease progresses the viral load increases. Testing for viral load measures the amount of HIV RNA in one milliliter (ml) of blood. Three tests are available for determining viral load. The polymerase chain reaction (PCR) test was approved by the FDA for testing viral load, and reports are listed as copies per milliliter of plasma. The branched chain DNA assay (bDNA) is also utilized and reports results in units per milliliter of plasma. The NASBA or nucleic acid sequence-based amplification test also reports in units per milliliter of plasma. The same type of test should be used to follow an infected client. Current recommendations are for two different tests 2 to 3 weeks apart to establish a baseline. The test is repeated every 3 to 6 months or 4 to 6 weeks after initiation of therapy. Due to the expense of the test, more frequent testing should be reviewed for necessity. The test should not be conducted after immunizations for 3 to 4 weeks. A recent infection may alter the accuracy of the results. Changes are reported as log changes. A one-log increase equals a 10-fold increase in the viral load. A one-log decrease equals a ten-fold decrease in the viral load. A change of less than one half a log is insignificant. In fact, it may not be important if the load tripled or decreased by one half. A second viral load test should be performed before a change in therapy is considered (CDC, 1997a).

Vaccine

There is no vaccine available for HIV. HIV is a retro virus which enables it to enter cells and hide from the immune system. Also, the virus is always changing so it confuses the immune system by changing some of its parts. To be effective a vaccine must recognize all the parts of the virus. As many as 40 variants of the virus have been identified from one individual during progression of the disease (McCance & Huether, 1994). HIV also hides in the brain where antibodies are unable to reach. The virus disables the immune system, making elimination of the virus itself difficult.

Treatment

There are two approaches to treatment of HIV infection and AIDS: restoration of immune function and prevention of viral replication. Unfortunately, attempts at restoration of immune function have not been successful. Several medications have been tried to inhibit the replication of the virus. Some success at slowing the progression of the disease has been achieved, although no agent has been able to eradicate the virus. Thus, the HIV infected individual may have to take antiviral medications for

Table 13-8
AZT or ZVD.

• Shown to decrease seroconversions by 79%.
• Must be initiated promptly within 1-2 hours after exposure.
• May not be effective if when started later than 24-36 hours.

the rest of his/her life (McCance & Huether, 1994).

The approaches to control the virus are aimed at interrupting the replication cycle of the virus. HIV is subject to attack by drugs at several stages. Dideoxynucleosides prevent reverse transcription of viral RNA into viral DNA. Antisense oligonucleotides block the translation of mRNA into viral proteins. Interferon prevents the virus from budding from the cell and spreading (McCance & Huether, 1994). A protease inhibitor blocks an enzyme called protease that is vital to the final stages of HIV's replication (CDC, 1996c). Protease inhibitors are the second generation of treatment drugs produced to treat HIV infection. The first generation of treatment drugs were the reverse transcriptase inhibitors. A non-nucleoside reverse transcriptase inhibitor, Delavirdine mesylate (DLV), or Rescriptor®, was approved for treatment of HIV infection in 1997. Research into antiviral drugs continues. Most recent medications used for treatment of HIV include zidovudine, lamivudine, and indinavir (CDC, 1997a).

Azidothymidine (AZT) was the first drug approved for treating HIV. It works by sabotaging the virus' attempt to reproduce itself. However, it does not work perfectly, and HIV eventually spawns mutant strains that resist the medication. AZT or zidovudine is now marketed as ZVD, or Retrovir, by Burroughs Wellcome of Research Triangle Park, NC. ZVD cannot cure HIV but may slow the progression of the disease. It works by stopping production of reverse transcriptase. It is only effective for a limited amount of time, as little as 6 months, because of the decline in the virus' ability to resist the medication. Taking ZVD early in the disease may reduce the ability of the virus to produce resistance against the medication. Zidovudine has usually been well tolerated when taken as recommended. The most common side effects include nausea, vomiting, diarrhea, tiredness, and headaches (CDC, 1996c).

Lamivudine (3TC), or Epivir™, is added to ZVD for use against ZVD resistant types of virus. Used in combination with ZVD, it has been shown to be effective in slowing the progression of HIV infection. The side effects include nausea, vomiting, and diarrhea. In rare instances, pancreatitis has been diagnosed as a side effect of 3TC (see Table 13-8).

Indinavir sulfate (IDV), or Crixivan®, also called MK-639, is a protease inhibitor added for the highest risk exposures. This potent antiviral drug is safe when taken for a short period of time. The side effects include jaundice and kidney stones, although these side effects are rare when IDV is taken for less than 1 month.

Didanosine (ddI), a nucleoside analog, marketed as VIDEX® and as Dideoxyinosine, is similar to AZT. Zalcitabine (ddC), also called Dideoxycytidine or HIVID®, and Stavudine (d4T) or Zerit, are other nucleoside analogs used for treating HIV. Nucleoside analogs block a protein active in the early reproduction cycle of the virus but the virus quickly develops resistance to their effect.

The potent three drug combination of ZVD, 3TC, and IDV, first used in 1996, continues to suppress the virus in many patients at all stages of the disease. Viral suppression is most likely in patients who are relatively healthy and have not had years of less effective treatment (CDC, 1997a).

Other medications are used for treatment of opportunistic infections. Aerosolized pentamidine and TMP-SMX are used to prevent Pneumocystic carinii. Acyclovir, marketed by Burroughs Wellcome as Zovirax, is used for treating herpes infections. Recombinant human alpha interferon, marketed as INTRON by Schering Plough in Madison, NJ and as Roferon A by Hoffman LeRoche of Nutley, NJ, is used for treatment of Kaposi's sarcoma (FDA, 1997).

Risk to Health Care Workers

The health care worker may become exposed to HIV through needle sticks and cuts with other sharp instruments, through exposure of the eye, nose, and mouth (mucous membranes), or through open skin lesions with an infected person's blood (CDC, 1987). The risk of infection varies with the type of exposure and factors such as the amount of blood involved in the exposure, the client's viral load or amount of virus in the blood, and post-exposure treatment steps. The risk of HIV infection after percutaneous exposure increases with a larger volume of blood and a higher titer of HIV in the source individual's blood (Cardo et al., 1997). HIV is not as transmissible as Hepatitis B. One milliliter of blood may contain 100 million particles of Hepatitis B virus but only a few hundred to 10,000 particles of HIV.

The first reported case of a health care provider becoming infected was in 1986. An emergency room nurse became infected after holding gauze over an open bleeding wound. As of the end of 1997, 52 health care workers had been diagnosed as HIV positive as a result of occupational exposure. Twenty-four have developed AIDS. One hundred-eleven possible cases of occupationally acquired HIV infection have been reported among health care workers in the United States (CDC, 1997a). Exposure can be prevented by following recommended procedures for prevention such as Universal Precautions.

Nurses are the most commonly exposed health care providers. Most exposures are the result of needle sticks. The risk of HIV infection after a needle stick or cut exposure is low, but it is not zero. The average risk of infection after a needle stick/cut exposure to HIV infected blood is 0.3% or 1 in 300 (CDC Internet, 1997). The risk of infection after exposure to the mucous membranes of the eye, nose, and mouth is estimated to be on average 0.1% or 1 in 1,000. The risk of infection is increased if the exposure involves a larger volume of blood or if the source individual has a high viral count in the blood. Source clients near death with AIDS usually have a higher amount of HIV in their blood (Cardo et al., 1997).

Health care providers that are exposed to the blood of an HIV positive client should wash the area immediately with soap and water. If the exposure was the result of a splash to a mucous membrane the area should be flushed with water. Eyes should be irrigated with clean water, saline, or sterile irrigants. Report the exposure to your supervisor promptly (CDC, 1989). Your employer should have a control plan in place for post-exposure treatment. As of this writing, post-exposure treatment with zidovudine and other antiviral drugs may prevent infection with HIV. However, the efficacy of these agents used for post-exposure prophylaxis to HIV has not been consistent. The risk of long-term (i.e., delayed) toxicity for healthy persons not infected with HIV is not known (CDC, 1996 a, b)

The decision to treat with medications should be based on the type and circumstances of exposure. Side effects of the medications prescribed may outweigh the risk of infection (CDC, 1997a). Treatment following an exposure with a source individual with low viral load may not warrant the side effects associated with the drugs. Treatment with zidovudine may be recommended for exposures involving a large amount of blood from a source individual with a high viral load. In one study, the use of ZVD after exposure reduced the risk of infection by 81% (Henderson, 1997). Currently, treatment with zidovudine is recommended to be instituted promptly, preferably within 1-2 hours after exposure. (CDC, 1997a). The exposed health care worker should be tested for HIV immediately after the exposure for a baseline result. Follow-up HIV testing at 6 weeks, 12 weeks, and 6 months is recommended and should be available for all workers.

Tuberculosis: An Old Disease With a New Face

After decades of declining incidence, tuberculosis (TB) is once again becoming a major health concern in the United States. Considering the disease on the verge of eradication, health departments, social agencies and medical professionals decreased the time, money and effort spent on controlling and eliminating TB. The presence of a large immunosuppressed population, due in part to the AIDS epidemic, and the indiscriminate use of antibiotics, have contributed to the resurgence of TB. Not only is TB back, but in many places it is back with a vengeance. Multidrug resistant strains of TB are emerging that are resistant to many of the drugs commonly used to treat TB. TB is of interest in chronic dialysis settings because chronic renal failure (CRF) and diabetes mellitus are identified as risk factors that increase the risk of developing clinical TB once a person is infected with the tuberculosis bacillus.

Etiology

Tuberculosis is caused by the tubercle bacillus Mycobacterium tuberculosis, a gram-positive, acid-fast organism. Acid-fast refers to the fact that Mycobacteria do not lose their color in acid after staining. Unfortunately, this is not a specific diagnostic indicator for TB, since some acid-fast bacilli are not M. tuberculosis. There are approximately 30 members of the genus Mycobacterium, only a few of which cause disease in humans (Daniel, 1987).

TB is spread primarily by respiratory means. Although the disease can involve any organ, the lungs provide the primary route for infection. Whenever persons with active pulmonary or laryngeal TB speak, sing, talk, cough or sneeze, thousands of tiny respiratory droplets are released into the air. The smallest of these droplets (known as droplet nuclei) dry and remain airborne for indefinite periods of time and may contain one to several mycobacteria. Larger particles fall to the floor or other surfaces and are not sources of airborne transmission of the disease (Protic & Hardy, 1993; Riley & Nardell, 1993). Droplet nuclei are approximately 1 to 5 microns in size and are the most dangerous particles, because they are small enough to be readily inhaled by susceptible hosts and deposited into alveoli in the lungs. The upper respiratory tract is highly resistant to infection with TB, while infectious particles that enter the lower portions of the lungs will readily survive and multiply. Even a single droplet nuclei containing an infectious TB particle is enough to cause infection in a susceptible host (Lindberg, 1993; Riley & Nardell, 1993).

The number of bacilli exhaled by most infected patients is not large, although patients with cavitary disease, or laryngeal or endobronchial TB may be highly contagious. Infectiousness generally coincides with the numbers of infectious organisms in sputum, the extent of the pulmonary disease and the frequency of coughing. When presented to a host with a functional immune system, M. tuberculosis is a highly infectious but not highly virulent organism, so repeated, prolonged exposure is usually necessary for infection to occur. However, when the immune system is defective, it appears that infection can progress to active disease after short exposure times to small numbers of organisms (Daniel, 1987; Protic & Hardy, 1993).

Pathophysiology

While similar in many ways to other bacteria, there are some characteristics peculiar to M. tuberculosis that are important to remember when caring for patients infected with TB. The first difference is the slow rate of reproduction of the bacilli when compared to other bacteria. Escherichia coli, a common pathogen, normally divide every 20-30 minutes and produce visible colonies after an overnight incubation period. M. tuberculosis has a mean doubling time of 12-24 hours and may require weeks of growth to produce a visible colony. This is significant because it can delay identification and diagnosis of the organism. In some cases (particularly when infection with drug resistant strains is suspected) this slow growth can also delay drug-susceptibility tests, which may delay appropriate drug therapy.

Another unusual characteristic of M. tuberculosis is the structure of its cell wall. The cell wall contains an outer layer of fatty acids and waxes that are toxic to host cells and tissues and that make the bacilli hydrophobic (insoluble in water). This layer contributes to its slow growth rate and also serves to protect the organism from many antimicrobial agents. In addition, the layer prevents the body's macrophages (cells that ingest foreign matter) from being able to completely destroy all of the invading bacilli. Since M. tuberculosis is able to remain viable within macrophages, it has an enhanced ability to remain inaccessible to several antitubercular drugs (Protic & Hardy, 1993). This is one reason why drug therapy for TB is prolonged.

Once an individual inhales tubercle bacilli into the alveoli, how the body reacts to the presence of the bacilli depends in part on the susceptibility of that person, how many particles were inhaled, and how virulent the organisms are. The lung tissue responds to the presence of the bacilli with inflammation, and the body's normal defense mechanisms attempt to eliminate the invader. Inflammation may lead to the development of nodules called primary tubercles. As cells gather around the tubercle the outer portion becomes fibrosed, which leads to decreased blood flow and nutrition to the tubercle center. As the center becomes necrotic, the outer fibrosis acts to wall off the area of infection. This necrotic tissue becomes soft and cheesy in consistency, a process called caseation. Over time, this material may become either calcified or liquefied (liquefaction necrosis). At times the person infected with TB may cough up some of the liquefied material, leaving a hole or cavity in the lung tissue. On x-rays, these cavities are visible and are termed cavitary disease, which is suggestive of TB. Lymph nodes in the hilar region of the lung may be involved as they filter drainage from infected areas (Daniel, 1987; Phipps & Daly, 1983).

If the host has a competent immune system, further multiplication and spread of the organisms are halted, usually within 2-10 weeks of the initial infection. Alveolar macrophages, which ingest bacilli present in the alveoli of the lungs, spread throughout the host's body. However, viable bacilli remain in the host's macrophages in a dormant or resting state, and reactivation of the disease is possible at a later time. These people are considered to have TB infection or latent TB. Even though they have TB infection, they have no signs or symptoms of the disease and are not capable of transmitting TB to others at this point, although they will demonstrate a positive reaction to a purified protein derivative (PPD) skin test. Persons with latent TB have approximately a 10% risk during their lifetime of developing active (infectious and symptomatic) TB, with the greatest risk occurring within the first 2 years after infection. It is currently estimated that 10 to 15 million persons in this country are already infected with TB, and 90% of the new cases being reported are in this previously infected group (CDC, 1994a; Protic & Hardy, 1993).

When the host's defenses are inadequate and unable to check the spread of the bacilli, the person is said to have active TB disease. In this case, the individual would demonstrate clinical symptoms of TB and would be capable of spreading the infection to others. Many of the new cases of TB being seen now are in older persons who were infected decades ago, and the disease emerges when the host's immune system is weakened and no longer able to contain the infection. Rates of TB, are also increased in racial and ethnic minorities who have other risk factors for TB, such as birth in a country with high prevalence rates of TB, and in individuals with HIV infection, low socioeconomic status, and/or exposure in congregate settings (for example, prisons and shelters) (CDC, 1994a).

The HIV epidemic has played a key role in the resurgence of TB. HIV-positive patients with defective immune systems have a much higher risk of developing active clinical disease after the initial infection, or of developing disease subsequent to earlier infection. There is also evidence to suggest that HIV-positive patients may have a shorter time interval between disease exposure and the development of active clinical disease. It also appears that at present, HIV-infected persons have a 10%- 40% TB infection rate, while patients with full-blown acquired immunodeficiency syndrome (AIDS) have a TB incidence rate of almost 500 times that of the general population. In many instances, the diagnosis of TB is made before HIV is detected (Jo, 1993).

Multidrug-Resistant TB

Another cause for alarm is the increased incidence of TB that is resistant to at least two of the first-line drugs used to successfully treat TB. In the past drug resistance was commonly the result of inappropriate or inadequate treatment of TB, but it appears now that multidrug resistant TB (MDR-TB) is also being spread among patients by direct exposure, particularly in locations with many HIV-infected patients (Casey, 1993). Before the onset of the AIDS epidemic, drug resistance was most often seen in immigrants from countries in which TB is endemic. In these countries, anti-tubercular drugs are often available over the counter so patients may take only one drug, which they discontinue when symptoms subside. In situations like this where treatment is inadequate, only the most susceptible organisms are eliminated. In this situation, where single drug therapy is employed for an insufficient length of time or when dosing schedules are erratic, the development of resistant strains will be encouraged. This type of resistance is known as secondary or acquired drug resistance.

Primary drug resistance occurs when only a few of the organisms present have an inherent resistance to one or more of the most commonly used antitubercular drugs. In this situation, drug resistance is a random event that occurs apart from any drug therapy.

To prevent the emergence of drug-resistant strains of TB, certain principles of drug therapy must be applied consistently to patients treated for TB. Appropriate drug regimens must contain several different drugs to which the organism is susceptible, and the dosing schedule must maintain sufficient drug concentrations at infection sites to inhibit or kill the organisms present. Drug regimens must also be continued long enough to ensure that all organisms are eliminated, usually a period of several months (Protic & Hardy, 1993). Specific drug therapy for resistant strains of TB will depend on whether the organism is resistant to one or more of the drugs commonly used to treat TB. Some organisms are resistant to only one drug, while others show resistance to multiple drugs. Prior to the AIDS epidemic, it was uncommon to see cases of MDR-TB in the U.S., with most cases seen in immigrants from countries with endemic TB where insufficient treatment is common (Jo, 1993).

In the past, two and three drug regimens were considered sufficient for treating TB since drug-resistant organisms were rare (primary isoniazid resistance rates in most of the U.S. were less than 4%). In areas where community rates of primary isoniazid resistance remain less than 4%, initial drug regimens of fewer than four drugs may still be acceptable, but it is crucial to continually monitor drug susceptibility patterns for each community to ensure that initial therapy will be likely to eliminate the strains of TB organisms commonly encountered in that community (American Thoracic Society, 1994).

Signs and Symptoms of TB

Pulmonary TB should be suspected in persons who complain of fevers, chills, night sweats, fatigue, weight loss, decreased appetite, chest pain, prolonged and productive coughing (longer than 3 weeks duration), or hemoptysis. While these symptoms can be due to numerous factors, they are the classic symptoms of TB. Whenever patients present with any of these complaints they should be viewed with suspicion for TB until that diagnosis is ruled out. If the disease presents at an extrapulmonary site, the symptoms will depend on the body sites/systems affected; risk factors for TB must always be considered when evaluating an ill person who may have been exposed to the disease (CDC, 1994a).

While extrapulmonary TB occurs more often in persons with HIV, pulmonary TB is still the most common form of TB in all persons, including those with HIV. While HIV-negative patients have a 10% rate of extrapulmonary TB, patients with full-blown AIDS have a 70% rate of TB at sites other than the lung, and patients with HIV whose immune systems are not as impaired have a 24%-45% rate of extrapulmonary TB. Patients with HIV and extrapulmonary TB most often demonstrate lymphadenitis (inflammation of lymph nodes) and miliary disease (formation of tubercles throughout body organs due to dissemination of the bacilli through the bloodstream). These patients may complain of tender lymph nodes, fever, fatigue and weight loss. Persons with extrapulmonary TB are not usually considered infectious unless they have an open abscess or draining lesion (Jo, 1993). Anyone who is suspected of having TB must be immediately placed in isolation and be referred for further evaluation, which should consist of a physical examination, a Mantoux tuberculin skin test, a chest x-ray, and sputum smears and cultures.

BCG Vaccine

In many countries where TB is endemic, bacillus Calmette-Guerin (BCG) vaccine is used in an effort to provide immunity to TB. It is not normally used in this country because of the low risk of infection and the lack of consistent evidence supporting its efficacy in preventing disease. BCG contains attenuated tubercle bacilli unable to produce disease. Eight major trials of the vaccine have demonstrated effective rates from 0-76%, with no explanations for the wide range of results (CDC, 1994a). One trial conducted in South India did not demonstrate a protective effect from the vaccine, even

Table 13-9
Medical conditions that increase the risk of developing TB disease once infection has occurred.

- HIV infection
- Substance abuse (especially drug injection)
- Silicosis
- Recent infection with TB (within the past 2 years)
- Abnormal chest x-ray, which suggests previous TB (in a person who received inadequate or no treatment)
- Diabetes mellitus
- Prolonged corticosteroid therapy or other immunosuppressive therapy
- Hematologic and reticuloendothelial diseases (for example, leukemia, Hodgkin's disease)
- End stage renal disease
- Intestinal bypass or gastrectomy
- Chronic malabsorption syndromes
- Cancer of the head and neck
- Being > 10% below ideal body weight

Note: From Centers for Disease Control. (1994). *Core curriculum on tuberculosis*. Atlanta, GA: Author.

though two of what were believed to be the most potent strains available were used. There is evidence from a variety of other studies that BCG vaccine may provide some protection to infants and young children against the more serious forms of TB, although that protection does not appear to apply to adults (American Thoracic Society, 1994). It is interesting to consider that even if BCG vaccine had proven ability to prevent disease, its efficacy in the U.S. at the present time would be limited because the majority of TB cases now presenting are the results of persons infected previously.

Even though there is no clear evidence supporting the effectiveness of the BCG vaccine, many countries where TB is endemic still use the vaccine, especially for infants. One disadvantage to using BCG is that it often leads to positive PPD skin test results in vaccinated individuals, which lessens the effectiveness of the skin test as a screening tool. There is currently no way to detect the difference between a positive reaction due to vaccination and a positive reaction due to TB infection. However, in persons vaccinated with BCG, the probability that positive skin tests are due to TB infection increases:

1. as the size of the skin test reactions increase,
2. as the length of time between vaccinations and skin testing increases,
3. when patients were in contact with persons who have infectious TB disease,
4. when there are positive family histories of TB,
5. when chest x-rays show evidence of previous TB, or
6. when patients are from countries where TB is common.

In most situations, a history of BCG vaccination does not alter the guidelines for interpreting skin test results. Current CDC recommendations are that persons vaccinated with BCG who demonstrate any of the previously listed risk factors for TB and who have positive skin tests be evaluated for TB. Once active TB has been ruled out, these persons may require preventive therapy. It cannot be overemphasized that BCG vaccination can never be assumed to be the cause of a positive skin test (CDC, 1994a).

Because of the lack of clear data demonstrating the efficacy of BCG, and the fact that use of BCG may interfere with future skin test results, the use of BCG is recommended in only a few limited situations:

1. For infants and children with negative tuberculin skin tests who are at high risk of intimate and/or prolonged exposure to persistently ineffectively or untreated persons with infectious pulmonary TB; who cannot be protected or removed from exposure to infectious persons; and who cannot be placed on long-term preventive therapies. Infants and children should also be given BCG if they are continually exposed to persons with infectious TB that is resistant to both isoniazid (INH) and rifampin.
2. For use in skin-test negative infants and children in areas in which the rate of new infections exceeds 1% per year and for whom normal surveillance and treatment programs are impractical or unfeasible (such as groups without regular access to health care; those for whom this health care would be socially or culturally unacceptable; or those groups who have demonstrated an inability to effectively use existing accessible care).

Vaccinations should be administered following the instructions provided in package labeling. Newborns should be vaccinated with one-half the usual dose. Immunosuppression (such as from HIV or immunosuppressive drug therapy) is a contraindication to the use of BCG (American Thoracic Society, 1994). Although no effects on the fetus have been observed as a result of BCG, it is not recommended that pregnant women be given the vaccine (CDC, 1994a).

Screening Methods for TB

Risk factors. Screening tests done in the U.S. are used to identify infected persons who need preventive therapy to prevent progression to active disease, and as a part of the work-up of persons with signs or symptoms of active disease. It is recommended that screening be done in groups with disease and infection rates in excess of those found in the general population. Institutional screening is recommended for staff of all health care facilities and residents of long-term care institutions where TB cases are identified or where those populations have a high incidence of TB disease and infection. Centers for Disease Control and Prevention (CDC, 1994a) guidelines currently recommend that all health care facilities establish a TB screening program for their health care workers. The Occupational Safety and Health Administration (OSHA) now mandates that employers develop and follow TB screening and control programs for personnel (Domin, 1993). This should be done to determine whether the health care worker is infected with TB and to determine if TB is being transmitted within the facility.

To adequately assess the risk for exposure to TB within any facility or setting, it is important to be aware of the known risk factors associated with TB. Identified risk factors that increase the risk of a person developing clinically active TB after being infected are listed in Table 13-9. Although TB can occur within any population or group, certain subpopulations have been identified that have a higher-than-average risk for TB. These groups are listed in Table 13-10. Knowing exposure risks helps employers and caregivers design plans to minimize or prevent exposure to TB.

Groups and individuals who should be screened. Proper interpretation of test results and appropriate follow-up and care are necessary components of any screening program. Screening usually consists of the Mantoux purified protein derivative (PPD) skin test. OSHA now mandates that all health care facilities, nursing homes, drug rehabilitation centers, homeless shelters, and prisons develop and implement controls to protect workers and employees from TB (Domin, 1993). Current CDC (1994a) guidelines have listed groups that should be screened with tuberculin skin tests, and these are found in Table 13-11.

Included in these groups who should be screened are those persons who have medical conditions that increase their risk of progression to clinical disease once TB infection has occurred. Nephrology nurses should note that CRF is a risk factor for the progression of TB infection to disease, and many CRF patients may have additional risk factors as well (such as diabetes, substance abuse, or corticosteroid therapy). CDC (1994a) recommends that tuberculin skin test screening be done in high-risk groups, which includes patients with CRF.

TB skin testing. At the present time, tuberculin skin testing is the only means available to demonstrate whether or not a person has been infected with TB. It is important to remember that skin testing is valuable only as a screening test and is not appropriate for use as a diagnostic tool. The test is based on the body's immune responses; a person infected with TB will demonstrate a cell-mediated or delayed hypersensitivity reaction when given the PPD test because of antibodies they have formed in response to the TB infection. PPD testing uses a highly purified product that contains protein from actual tubercle bacilli. In North America, a standard intermediate-strength dose of 5 tuberculin units of PPD is used for skin-testing purposes. Multiple-puncture methods of skin testing are convenient but not appropriate because of decreased specificity.

The Mantoux test provides the most accurate results. Using a tuberculin syringe, 0.1 ml containing 5 units of PPD is injected intradermally with the

Table 13-10
Populations with a high prevalence of TB infection.

- Close contacts of infectious tuberculosis cases
- Foreign-born persons from high-prevalence countries (Asia, Africa, Latin America)
- Medically underserved, low-income populations, including high-risk racial and ethnic groups
- The elderly

Note: From Centers for Disease Control. (1994). *Core curriculum on tuberculosis*. Atlanta, GA: Author.

Table 13-11
Groups to screen with a tuberculin skin test.

- Persons with HIV infection
- Close contacts of infectious tuberculosis cases
- Persons with medical conditions that increase the risk of TB (see Table 13-9)
- Foreign-born persons from high prevalence countries
- Low-income populations, including high-risk minorities
- Alcoholics and intravenous drug users
- Residents of long-term care facilities (including prisons and nursing homes)
- Populations identified locally as being at increased risk for TB, such as health care workers in some areas/settings

Note: From Centers for Disease Control. (1994). *Core curriculum on tuberculosis*. Atlanta, GA: Author.

Table 13-12
Classification of TB skin test results.

An induration of 5 mm or more is considered a positive reaction in the following persons:	An induration of 10 mm or more is considered positive in the following persons:	An induration of 15 mm is considered positive for persons who do not have any risk factors for TB.
• HIV infected persons or persons suspected of having HIV • Close contacts of a person with infectious TB • Persons with abnormal chest x-rays • Persons who inject drugs and whose HIV status is unknown	• Foreign-born persons • HIV-negative persons who inject drugs • Medically underserved, low-income populations • Residents of long-term care facilities • Locally identified high-prevalence groups (for example, migrant farm workers or homeless persons) • Children 4 years old without any other risk factors	

Note: From Centers for Disease Control. (1994). *Core curriculum on tuberculosis.* Atlanta, GA: Author.

needle bevel facing up, usually in the skin of the inner forearm. When properly applied, the injection should produce a pale, sharply raised wheal just underneath the skin surface that is 6 to 10 mm in diameter. If the injection is made too deeply into the tissues, results would be suspect because a reaction may be too deep to palpate and assess properly. If the injection is too shallow, not enough of the PPD may have been delivered to properly elicit a response. The reaction should be read and documented by designated, trained personnel 48 to 72 hours after the injection. Patient or health care worker self-reading and reporting of skin test results should not be accepted (CDC, 1994a).

When recording skin test results, the terms positive and negative are no longer considered appropriate. Instead, results should be recorded as the number of millimeters of induration (hardness) at the largest diameter of the induration present. This should be measured perpendicularly to the long axis of the forearm at the injection site. All reactions, even those classified as nonreactive, should be recorded in millimeters (such as 0 mm of induration). The area of induration should be assessed by gently palpating the site. Redness or erythema are not diagnostic criteria and should not be used to interpret test results. Interpretation of skin tests results are based on risk factors of the person being tested. Table 13-12 provides current CDC (1994a) criteria for evaluating and classifying skin test reactions in different individuals.

It is possible that some persons may demonstrate false-positive results to the tuberculin skin test. These false-positive reactions could be due to infections with mycobacteria other than M. tuberculosis or due to immunization with BCG. False-negative results are also a problem that can occur for several reasons. Persons recently infected with TB may not demonstrate a positive skin test because it takes approximately 2 to 10 weeks after the initial infection to mount an immune response. For this reason, persons exposed to infectious TB should have an immediate skin test to determine their baseline status and then be retested 10 to 12 weeks later to determine if infection has occurred.

Another reason for false-negative readings is related to the time period that has elapsed since the initial infection. In some persons, the ability to react to skin tests may wane over time. When given a skin test years after the initial infection, they may at first manifest a negative reaction. However, the skin test acts as a stimulant to the immune system and the person will demonstrate a positive reaction to subsequent skin tests. This type of reaction is termed the booster phenomenon, and it is useful when trying to distinguish between old and newly acquired infections. In some settings, persons who have an initial negative test are given another test 1 to 3 weeks later. If the reaction to the second test is positive, it is probably a boosted reaction, meaning that the person is infected but the infection probably occurred a long time ago. If both skin tests are initially negative, then any subsequent positive skin tests would more likely be due to recent infection with TB, a process termed conversion. Two-step testing is especially useful in settings where persons are going to be tested at periodic intervals, such as health care workers or nursing home residents.

An increasingly common cause for false-negative skin tests results is anergy, the inability of the body to react to skin tests because of immunosuppression. HIV is becoming a more common cause of anergy, although it can be caused by other medical conditions, such as viral or bacterial infections, chronic renal failure, corticosteroids, chemotherapy, stress or age. It is estimated that 1 in 10 persons infected with TB is both anergic and asymptomatic (Lavin & Haidorfer, 1993). One way to test for anergy is to administer two delayed-type hypersensitivity antigens, such as tetanus toxoid, mumps, or Candida by the Mantoux technique when the PPD is administered. These antigens are used because most adults will have developed antibodies to them either through exposure, disease, or vaccination. If the person fails to respond to these antigens, including the PPD, then it is very likely that the person is anergic and the PPD results are suspect at best.

Diagnosis of TB

Anyone who demonstrates symptoms of TB must be referred immediately for further medical care and follow-up, which should include a thorough medical history, physical exam, Mantoux tuberculin skin test, chest x-ray, and sputum smear and culture (or smears and cultures from the affected site in extrapulmonary TB, if possible). The health department must be notified within 24 hours of any suspected or confirmed cases of TB. As was mentioned earlier, patients should be assessed for any risk factors that could increase the risk of acquiring TB or that may increase the risk of progression to active disease. Demographic factors, such as country of origin, age, ethnic or racial factors, occupation or living conditions, should be evaluated in this assessment. While physical examination does not definitively diagnose or confirm TB, it can provide valuable information regarding the patient's current health status and other factors that may determine the prescribed treatment regimen.

Chest x-rays are also important when evaluating persons with TB symptoms, although radiologic findings are not diagnostic of TB. The usual x-ray view obtained is the posterior-anterior view, although other views (such as lateral or lordotic) may be necessary. In some instances it may be necessary to obtain CT scans or other studies for evaluation. In pulmonary TB, the abnormalities seen usually occur in the apical and posterior segments of the upper lobe or in the upper segments of the lower lobe (CDC, 1994a). Parenchymal changes demonstrated by x-rays and commonly associated with TB include cavitation, parenchymal infiltration and air-space consolidation (such as with endobronchial spread of TB), miliary nodules and pleural effusion (Schluger & Rom, 1994). However, lesions may be evident anywhere in the lung fields and may have markedly different appearances between patients, especially if they have HIV or are immunosuppressed due to other causes (CDC, 1994a). Persons with AIDS and TB tend to demonstrate more atypical chest x-ray features, such as predominantly lower lobe infiltrates, miliary patterns, mediastinal and/or hilar lymphadenopathy, and an absence of cavitary disease. On the other hand, persons with AIDS and TB may present with normal chest x-rays in 10% of this population, even when sputum cultures are positive (Jo, 1993).

At the present time, sputum cultures are the only means available to definitively diagnose TB. Anyone suspected of having pulmonary or laryngeal TB should produce three sputum specimens on three different days, preferably early morning specimens. To ensure that patients are able to properly provide sputum samples (not saliva or mucous from the nose and throat), health care workers should coach and directly supervise them in obtaining at least the first specimens. For persons unable to cough up an adequate sample, aerosol induction can be used to stimulate them to cough up sputum. Induced sputum samples are usually watery and resemble saliva, so it is crucial that this specimen be labeled "INDUCED" so lab personnel do not discard it due to its appearance. In other cases bronchoscopy may be required to obtain the necessary samples. Gastric aspiration is sometimes useful in obtaining swallowed sputum specimens, particularly in infants and young children unable to cough up sputum (CDC, 1994a).

Whenever patients are attempting to provide specimens, hazardous aerosols may be produced. All appropriate infection control measures must be taken to prevent any persons in close proximity from becoming infected. These infection control measures are beyond the scope of this article and are discussed in references listed at the end of the article. This would include procedures such as coughing to obtain specimens, sputum induction using aerosol treatments, bronchoscopy, or any other required diagnostic procedures (Domin, 1993).

Although TB is primarily a pulmonary disease, it must be remembered that TB can affect almost any site in the body. When the patient presents with extrapulmonary TB, specimens obtained will depend on the organs or tissues affected and can include urine, cerebrospinal fluid, pleural fluid, pus, or tissue samples. Tissue samples should be placed in saline solution, not formalin, and must be delivered to the laboratory immediately (CDC, 1994a).

Smears can determine within 24 hours whether or not the infection is caused by acid-fast bacilli (AFB), but cannot distinguish between infections caused by M. tuberculosis or other mycobacteria. Complicating the diagnosis is the fact that many patients with TB have negative AFB smears. For this reason, cultures are necessary to provide a definitive diagnosis and determine drug susceptibility patterns of the infecting organism, and should be done on all specimens regardless of smear results. Since traditional methods of isolating the organism have taken anywhere from 6-12 weeks, many clinicians begin treatment for TB with only a presumptive diagnosis based on x-ray results, clinical signs and symptoms, and smear results.

A more rapid means of organism identification has now been developed that uses a liquid, broth-based culture medium and automated radiometric techniques (the BACTEC system). Using this method, culture results may be available in as little as 2 weeks. Tests using nucleic acid probes in addition to BACTEC systems can provide even more rapid identification of organisms (Schluger & Rom, 1994).

Tests using polymerase chain reaction (PCR) techniques are being developed that may eventually provide the means to identify the organism directly from the clinical specimen and that theoretically could detect even a single organism in a specimen. The PCR assay is still considered an experimental technique because of the cost involved, the technical expertise required to perform the test and the varying results obtained in clinical settings. It appears that PCR or a similar procedure may have use in the future as a tool for rapid detection of antibiotic drug resistance. A procedure known as restriction fragment length polymorphism (RFLP) has been developed that can fingerprint specific strains of M. tuberculosis. This test may eventually be used to identify outbreaks and transmission patterns (CDC, 1994a; Schluger & Rom, 1994).

Follow-up bacteriologic testing should be done at least monthly to determine if patients are still contagious and to evaluate their clinical response to therapy. All initial isolates should be subjected to drug susceptibility testing, and these tests should be repeated on patients who do not respond clinically to therapy or who continue to have positive cultures after 2 months of therapy. To curtail the spread or further development of drug resistant strains, it is imperative to identify drug resistance early and implement appropriate and effective treatment. CDC (1994a) has identified groups of people who are at increased risk of drug resistance, and they include:

- those with a history of previous treatment with TB medications,
- contacts of persons known to have drug-resistant TB,
- foreign-born persons from areas where there is a high incidence of drug-resistant TB (such as Asia, Latin America, Africa),
- residents of geographic areas in the U.S. where the prevalence of isoniazid-resistant TB is documented to be 4% or greater,
- persons whose smears or cultures remain positive after 2 months of therapy with TB drugs.

Drug Therapy for TB

Treatment for TB currently falls into three categories: preventive therapy, treatment of active disease, and treatment for drug-resistant strains. Regardless of the reason for treatment, there are certain basic principles that apply to any drug regimen: the appropriate drugs must be given at proper dosage intervals and for a length of time sufficient to eliminate all organisms. Lack of adequate follow-through with the prescribed drug regimen is one of the main reasons for the current resurgence of TB and the increase of drug-resistant strains.

Preventive therapy. Preventive therapy is prescribed for persons infected with TB (but who do not have active, clinical disease) in order to prevent progression to active disease at some later date. Certain groups, as outlined in Table 13-6, have a high risk of developing TB disease after infection occurs. When prescribing preventive therapy, clinicians must consider the risk of developing TB and the potential risk of INH toxicity. Before preventive therapy is initiated, clinicians should (a) rule out the possibility of TB disease, (b) determine if the patient has a history of treatment for TB infection or disease, (c) assess for any contraindications to administering INH (such as previous INH-associated hepatic injury; reactions to INH, for example, drug fever, rash or arthritis; or acute or unstable liver disease of any cause), and (d) determine whether the patient is at high risk for adverse reactions to INH. INH is normally used alone for preventive therapy, and current CDC (1994a) guidelines recommend daily doses of 300 mg in adults (and 10-15 mg/kg body weight for children, not to exceed 300 mg) for 6 to 12 months. In settings where compliance to daily doses is questionable or unlikely, current data suggest that twice-weekly doses of INH of 15 mg/kg may be effective in preventing TB disease in adults and children. Persons infected with HIV or who are immunosuppressed for other reasons should receive a full 12 months of therapy (American Thoracic Society, 1994). Some persons with positive skin tests may not be candidates for preventive therapy; these groups would include: (a) persons at high risk for adverse effects due to INH therapy, (b) persons who cannot tolerate INH, (c) persons likely to be infected with drug-resistant strains of TB, or (d) persons who are highly unlikely to complete a full course of preventive therapy (such as homeless persons or migrant farm workers).

These persons should be thoroughly educated about TB infection and disease and instructed to seek medical care immediately if they develop any signs or symptoms of the disease. Although there are instances where alternative therapies may be necessary, there is no clinical data to document clinical efficacy of any drug other than INH as a preventive therapy.

Persons receiving preventive therapy should be seen for follow-up on at least a monthly basis. Each patient should be evaluated for:

- Adherence to the prescribed treatment regimen (including pill counts and/or urine tests to determine if INH metabolites are present).
- Symptoms of hepatitis, such as nausea, loss of appetite, vomiting, persistently dark urine, yellowish skin, malaise, unexplained elevated temperature for more than 3 days, or abdominal tenderness, especially in the right upper quadrant.
- Symptoms of neurotoxicity, such as paresthesias of the hands or feet.

Persons with increased risk of hepatotoxicity due to INH should have a serum glutamic-oxaloacetic transaminase (SGOT or AST) drawn just prior to the start of therapy and monthly thereafter. Persons at increased risk of hepatotoxicity include those who: (a) are age 35 or older, (b) use other medications that may cause interactions, (c) use alcohol daily, (d) have chronic liver disease, (e) use intravenous drugs, (f) are pregnant, or (g) have discontinued use of INH in the past due to adverse effects. It should be noted that having a positive hepatitis B surface antigen is not necessarily a contraindication to preventive therapy with INH. There is some evidence to suggest that Black and Hispanic women may be at increased risk for fatal hepatitis associated with use of INH. Approximately 10%-20% of persons taking INH will demonstrate mild increases in liver enzymes, which tend to resolve even with continuance of INH therapy. Discontinuation of INH should be considered only if liver enzyme measurements exceed three to five times the upper limit of normal or if the patient reports symptoms of adverse reactions.

Peripheral neuropathy is associated with the use of INH; administration of pyridoxine (10-15 mg/day) has been shown to prevent INH induced neuropathy, especially in persons predisposed to neuropathy due to other disease states (e.g., diabetes, uremia, alcoholism and malnutrition) (American Thoracic Society, 1994).

Treatment of TB disease. There are four basic principles that underlie any treatment regimen prescribed for active TB disease. They are:

1. Provide the safest, most effective therapy in the shortest period of time possible.
2. Always use multiple drugs to which the organisms are susceptible.
3. Never add a single drug to a failing regimen.
4. Ensure that the patient adheres fully to the treatment regimen.

CDC (1994a) currently recommends an initial drug regimen that includes at least four drugs: INH, rifampin, pyrazinamide, and either ethambutol or streptomycin. When INH resistance is known to be less than 4% for a certain region, a three-drug regimen (INH, rifampin, and pyrazinamide) may be adequate as an initial treatment regimen. The rationale behind multidrug therapy is to prevent emergence of resistant strains. Patients are usually most infectious before the diagnosis is made and before treatment is initiated, so it is imperative that drug therapy be started immediately, even before the diagnosis of TB is confirmed. Initial therapy will in part be determined by the patient's risk factors, clinical symptoms and medical history, and by the characteristics of TB found in that particular community (for example, numbers of cases overall, prevalence of drug-resistant strains, and predominance of high-risk populations). Once culture and drug sensitivity results are determined, the drug regimen can be tailored to the specific characteristics of the infective organisms.

Patient adherence to the treatment regimen is the major determinant to the outcome of treatment. Since treatment for TB requires numerous drugs to be taken for prolonged periods, and since many people with TB are those whose socioeconomic status provides numerous barriers to treatment, compliance with the treatment regimen is the first and primary goal of all health care providers. No drug therapy will work if it does not enter the patient's body. Careful coordination of all available community health resources with patients is necessary to ensure compliance with therapy. Directly observed therapy (DOT) is an option that has been used successfully in some settings and must be used with any intermittent treatment schedule. When DOT is used, a designated health care team member, family member, or other designated responsible person observes the patient actually ingesting the medication. For those individuals who self-administer their antitubercular drugs, there are some fixed-dose combinations of drugs that may enhance patient adherence and reduce the risk of inappropriate monotherapy. In the U.S., the Food and Drug Administration has licensed fixed-dose combinations of INH and rifampin (Rifamate®) and also combinations of INH, rifampin and pyrazinamide (Rifater®) (CDC, 1994a).

Treatment of pulmonary TB. The duration of therapy depends on the drugs used, culture and drug susceptibility test results, and the patient's clinical response to therapy. There are treatment regimens that can be used for either 6 or 9 months, and these are referred to as short-course therapies. Most persons with untreated pulmonary TB can be adequately treated using either the 6 or 9-month regimen, although the 6-month course is preferred. INH and rifampin must be included in all drug regimens lasting 9 months or less, and all 6 month courses must contain INH, rifampin, and at least initially, pyrazinamide. The major adverse reactions associated with the first-line drugs commonly used to treat TB, adjustments necessary for ESRD

Table 13-13
Information on first-line TB drugs.

Drug and Route	Major Adverse Reactions	Recommended Monitoring	Considerations for Patients with CRF
Isoniazid (PO, IM)	Hepatic enzyme elevations; hepatitis; peripheral neuropathy; mild CNS effects; interactions with phenytoin	Baseline measurements of hepatic enzymes. Repeat studies if: - baseline results are abnormal - patient at high risk for adverse reactions - patient has symptoms of adverse reactions	Removed by both peritoneal and hemodialysis. Minor dosage adjustments may be required for patients with severe renal impairments. On hemodialysis days, give dose after dialysis treatment
Rifampin (PO, IV)	GI upset; rash; drug interactions; hepatitis; bleeding problems; flu-like symptoms.	Baseline CBC, hepatic enzymes Repeat studies if: - baseline results are abnormal - patient has symptoms of adverse reactions	Plasma concentrations not appreciably affected by peritoneal or hemodialysis.
Pyrazinamide (PO)	Hepatitis; rash; GI upset; joint aches; hyperuricemia; gout (rare).	Baseline uric acid, hepatic enzymes Repeat studies if: - baseline results are abnormal - patient has symptoms of adverse reactions	Use with caution in patients with renal failure or diabetes.
Ethambutol (PO)	Optic neuritis	Baseline and monthly tests: - visual acuity - color vision	Removed by peritoneal dialysis. Removed to a lesser extent by hemodialysis; on hemodialysis days, give dose after treatment. Longer dosage intervals and lower drug doses with renal failure.
Streptomycin (IM)	Ototoxicity; renal toxicity	Baseline and repeat as needed: - hearing - renal function studies	Dosages for renal failure patients should be based on serum drug levels. Give half of normal dose after hemodialysis treatment. Removed by peritoneal and hemodialysis.

Note: Adapted from:
Centers for Disease Control. (1994a). *Core curriculum on tuberculosis*. Atlanta, GA: Author.
Lentino, J., & Leehey, D. (1994). Infections. In J. Daugirdas & T. Ing (Eds.), *Handbook of Dialysis* (2nd ed.) (pp. 469-490). Boston: Little, Brown and Company.

patients, and monitoring parameters are listed in Table 13-13.

Adults with positive smears or cultures should have a 6-month course that begins with INH, rifampin, and pyrazinamide for the first 2 months. Until drug susceptibility of the organism is known, the first 2 months of therapy should also include either ethambutol or streptomycin, unless it is certain that there is little chance of drug resistance. If the organism is susceptible to INH and rifampin, the remaining 4 months of treatment should consist of these two drugs. For patients unable to take pyrazinamide, it is acceptable to use a 9-month regimen of INH and rifampin; this regimen should include either ethambutol or streptomycin until drug sensitivities are known or there is known to be little chance of drug resistance.

Adults with negative smears and cultures may follow a 4-month course of INH and rifampin, combined with pyrazinamide for the first 2 months, when the risk of drug resistance is judged to be low. Although 4-month courses of drug therapy have generally demonstrated unacceptably high relapse rates, in this particular population the success rates of 4-month therapy are high (American Thoracic Society, 1994). If the patient has any risk factors for drug-resistance, or lives in an area with a prevalence of drug-resistant TB that is 4% or greater, then the drug regimen should contain four drugs (INH, rifampin, pyrazinamide, and either ethambutol or streptomycin) for the full 4-month course.

As mentioned previously, DOT is required with any intermittent dosage schedule, in which drugs are administered 2-3 times weekly instead of daily. Intermittent therapies are not appropriate for patients who self-administer their own drugs.

TB and HIV. Recommendations for the duration of TB treatment for persons also infected with HIV are the same as for non-HIV infected persons. However, HIV patients must be closely followed to assess clinical and bacteriological responses to treatment, since the prevalence of drug resistance in this population is higher. These patients also require close follow-up because they seem to have a higher incidence of adverse effects caused by antitubercular drug therapy (American Thoracic Society, 1994). Treatment periods should be lengthened if the clinical response is slow or suboptimal in any way. Adherence to the treatment regimen is especially critical in this population, and the CDC strongly recommends DOT for this group (CDC, 1994a).

Extrapulmonary TB. In most situations, drug regimens to treat pulmonary TB are also adequate for treating TB at sites other than the lungs, however, children or infants with miliary TB, bone or joint TB, or TB meningitis should complete a minimum of 12 months of drug therapy. Surgery may at times be required to obtain specimens for diagnosis or to relieve cardiac compression (from constrictive pericarditis) or spinal cord compression (resulting from tubercular erosion of vertebrae). Cardiac constriction, resulting from tuberculous pericarditis, may be prevented by the use of corticosteroids, which may also decrease neurologic sequelae of TB meningitis, especially when administered early in the course of the disease. The type of follow-up to assessments to determine the response to therapy will depend on the site of the infection and its accessibility (American Thoracic Society, 1994).

Drug-resistant TB. Drug-resistance of the infecting organism may not be known until several weeks after the initiation of drug therapy. When the organism is resistant to INH, if the patient was begun on an initial four drug regimen, then INH should be discontinued and the other three drugs continued for 6 months. TB known to be resistant to INH only may be alternatively treated for 12 months with rifampin and ethambutol. If the patient is on the previously mentioned 9 month regimen, INH should be discontinued when INH resistance is documented. If ethambutol was included in the initial drug regimen, a 12-month course of drug therapy with both ethambutol and rifampin should be completed. If ethambutol was not used initially, INH should be stopped, susceptibility tests should be repeated, and two new drugs, such as ethambutol and pyrazinamide, should be added. Further alterations in the drug regimen should then be made based upon results from susceptibility tests (American Thoracic Society, 1994; CDC, 1994a).

MDR-TB (TB that is resistant to at least INH and rifampin) presents a major treatment dilemma. These patients require prolonged treatment regimens based on their medical history and drug-susceptibility studies. Many times these organisms are also resistant to other first-line drugs, such as ethambutol and streptomycin. Clinicians unfamiliar with the treatment of MDR-TB are strongly urged to consult experts in the care of these patients. These patients frequently require treatment with several second-line drugs, which are less effective and can cause serious adverse effects, so close and continuous monitoring throughout the treatment period is mandatory when treating MDR-TB. Since there have been documented cases of MDR-TB being spread by direct contact, and since these strains are so difficult to treat, it is imperative that appropriate treatment be started as soon as possible and that adherence to treatment be ensured by whatever means are necessary.

Infectivity. Infectiousness of a patient with TB is directly related to the number of tubercle bacilli released into the air whenever that person coughs, talks, sings or sneezes. Most patients are considered infectious if they are coughing, undergoing cough-inducing or aerosol-generating procedures or if they have sputum smears that demonstrate the presence of acid-fast bacilli and at the same time are not receiving therapy, have just started therapy, or have a poor clinical or bacteriologic response to therapy. Infectiousness may persist for weeks or even months in patients with drug-resistant TB. Once effective therapy is begun, patients are no longer considered infectious as long as they meet all of the following criteria: (a) they have been receiving adequate drug therapy for 2 to 3 weeks, (b) they demonstrate a favorable clinical response to therapy, and (c) consecutive sputum smears collected on three separate days are negative (CDC, 1994a).

Infection Control Strategies

Infection control strategies in the renal community consist of guidelines for the prevention and treatment of pyrogenic reactions and infections with bloodborne pathogens. These strategies must be considered in the presence of a large immunosuppressed population. Since the inception of dialysis, the Centers for Disease Control and Prevention (CDC) has collaborated with specific organizations to develop and implement standards that enhance the protection of renal patients and the safety of nursing care delivered.

The CDC and the Association for the Advancement of Medical Instrumentation (AAMI) published bacteriology guidelines/standards to control bacterial and endotoxin contamination at key points in the dialysis system. In addition, the standards promoted safe and effective water treatment and the importance of frequent disinfecting in preventing pyrogenic reactions. The practice of dialyzer reuse has been approved by the federal government and the Public Health Service (PHS). In 1986, the PHS subsumed the AAMI standards for reusing hemodialyzers (AAMI, 1986) and recommended these as PHS guidance to HCFA, which in turn made them conditions for participation in Medicare/Medicaid (see Chapter 19).

Since the inception of dialysis centers, patients and staff members have been among the highest-risk groups for hepatitis B infections after male homosexuals and injecting drug abusers (Favero, 1996). In 1977, the CDC published a set of guidelines for preventing the spread of hepatitis B in the hemodialysis setting (CDC, 1977). The guidelines recommended serologic and disease surveillance of patients and staff for hepatitis B surface antigen. Disinfection of surfaces and specific cleaning practices were recommended. Also, all patients who were positive should be dialyzed in a separate area with dedicated machines and staff (Favero et al.,1992; Favero, 1996).

The advent of AIDS in the early 1980s brought about the publication of "Universal Precautions" (Favero, 1989). Universal precautions are the same strategies for controlling bloodborne infections that have been used by the dialysis community since 1977. Although there was an initial period of frenzy, the dialysis community demonstrated that HIV transmission could be controlled in dialysis centers by using these same procedures.

The 1990s brought new infection control problems with the advent of hepatitis C, but it too can be controlled by maintaining good infection control practices with an emphasis on basic barrier precautions. In 1994, the CDC investigated outbreaks of hepatitis B in five dialysis centers and determined that the outbreaks were associated with significant deficiencies in carrying out the long-recommended infection control strategies originally published in 1977 (Favero, 1996). The presence of a large immunosuppressed population due in part to the AIDS pandemic and the transplanted population, and the indiscriminate use of antibiotics have contributed to a need to reemphasize basic infection control strategies.

Screening

Recommended screening tests for early detection in the general population and high-risk groups applicable to the renal community are: blood pressure measurements for hypertension in the general population (see Chapter 8); urine testing for glucose for diabetes mellitus in patients with a family history of diabetes, gestational diabetes, and circulatory dysfunctions (see Chapters 8 and 16); and a tuberculin test for TB in patients with a positive TB family member, and children and elderly living in high prevalence areas (Valanis, 1992).

It is beyond the scope of this chapter to discuss the various types, characteristics, criteria, and practice guidelines for the implementation screening programs. However, it is important to note that the concept of screening is not as straightforward as it may appear. In this decade of limited fiscal resources for health care, screening programs must be objectively evaluated. There are risks and costs associated with screening and subsequent diagnostic procedures that must be weighed against the benefit of screening. The feasibility of the screening program, the types of diseases that are most suitable for screening, as well as factors that need to be considered in the evaluation of the program, the validity of the test itself, and whether its implementation actually achieves a reduction in morbidity and mortality from the disease must be considered (Hennekens & Buring, 1987). The same epidemiologic principles and methods that apply to primary prevention of diseases apply to the evaluation of screening programs as a means for secondary prevention of disease (Valanis, 1992) or disease control in populations.

Surveillance

Surveillance can be defined as "the collection, collation, analysis, and dissemination of data; a type of observational study that involves continuous monitoring of disease occurrence within a population" (Spraycar, 1995; CDC, 1990). The four major functions of surveillance can further be defined as the *collection* of relevant data for a specified population and geographic area; *collation* of the data into meaningful arrangements; *analysis* of the data; and regular *dissemination* of the data and interpretations to those in disease control programs.

The main objective of disease surveillance is to determine the extent of infections and the risk of disease transmission so control measures can be applied effectively and efficiently (CDC, 1990). The immediate use of surveillance data is to initiate disease control efforts. The primary application of surveillance systems is for the determination of long-term trends and patterns in disease occurrence at the local, state, and national levels. Data provide the foundation to define endemic and epidemic activity, evaluate intervention efforts of clinicians or public health officials, and evaluate the effect of social and political activity on the occurrence of disease (Thacker et al., 1983; CDC, 1990).

The Centers for Disease Control and Prevention has been conducting surveillance of hemodialysis-associated hepatitis since the early 1970s. From 1972 to 1974, CDC reported that the incidence of hepatitis B among patients and staff had increased by more than 100% to 6.2% and 5.2%, respectively. Because hepatitis B virus (HBV) infection was recognized as an increasing problem in hemodialysis centers, CDC issued recommendations for the control and prevention of this disease. These early surveys were based on only a 50% to 65% response rate of centers listed in the National Dialysis Registry. In an effort to obtain a higher response rate, CDC initiated a cooperative program with HCFA in 1976 that provided for a questionnaire from CDC to be included in HCFA's annual facility survey. As a result, the response rates to the CDC questionnaire have increased to an average of 90%.

Since 1982, the CDC survey, "National Surveillance of Dialysis-Associated Diseases in the United States," has been distributed annually. Other hemodialysis and associated diseases and practices not related to hepatitis have been included over the years, and the questionnaire is continually updated and revised to consider new clinical practices such as those associated with HIV infection and policies for routine testing, serologic testing, management, and vaccination utilization for hepatitis. Incidence of hepatitis non-A non-B among staff and patients, and procedures for cleaning and disinfecting equipment and disposables are examples of data collected. The objectives of the ongoing program of national surveillance of dialysis-associated diseases are to determine the frequency with which these diseases occur over time, what factors might be associated with the occurrences of the diseases, and what effect various control measures have in preventing transmission of disease in the hemodialysis environment (Tokars, Alter & Favero, 1993).

OSHA's Bloodborne Pathogens Regulations

OSHA's Bloodborne Pathogens Regulations (OSHA, 1989) set forth procedures for protection of workers who are exposed to blood or other potentially infectious materials.

The targeted diseases include HIV and HBV. Other bloodborne diseases include syphilis, malaria, babesiosis, brucellosis, leptospirosis, arboviral infections, relapsing fever, creutzfelt-jakob, and human T-lymphotrope virus Type I viral hemorrhagic fever.

This exposure control plan differs from traditional infection control rules by placing emphasis on the employer's responsibility for protecting health-care workers and staff from dangerous bloodborne diseases. Traditional infection control measures are directed at the prevention and management of general infection in and among patients. OSHA's regulations focus on identifying health-care workers at various degrees of risk to reduce the risk of infection by bloodborne pathogens.

The Infection Control Program (ICP) is the core element used to reduce worker risk by minimizing or eliminating employee exposure to bloodborne pathogens.

Exposure control components include:

1. Exposure determination;
2. Information and training of employee hazard communication;
3. Universal precautions, engineering and work practice controls;
4. Personal protective equipment;
5. Hepatitis B vaccination and post-exposure follow-up;
6. Labels and biohazard signs;
7. Housekeeping;
8. Laundry practices; and
9. Recordkeeping.

Exposure determination. The employer must identify all employees who are directly exposed or whose jobs have the likelihood of exposure to blood or other potentially infectious materials that have been recognized by the Centers for Disease Control (CDC) as directly linked to the transmission of HBV and/or HIV:

1. Blood;
2. Blood products; and
3. Peritoneal fluid.

The exposure determination must be made without regard to the use of personal protective equipment.

Information and training of staff. All staff with exposure to blood or other potentially infectious materials must participate in a training and education program provided at no cost to the employee. Training must be provided at the time of initial assignment, and once a year thereafter.

Universal precautions/engineering controls/

work practice controls. Universal precautions refer to a method of infection control in which all human blood and other potentially infectious materials are treated as if known to be infectious with HIV or HBV. Universal precautions do not apply to feces, nasal secretions, sputum, sweat, tears, urine, or vomitus unless they contain visible blood.

Universal precautions must be implemented during actions designated as having an increased risk to the employee. Actions designated as an increased risk include, but are not limited to the following:

1. Initiation/termination of the hemodialysis treatment, or a CAPD exchange.
2. A break in the dialysis system, such as a clotted dialyzer, an IV medication given at a location other than the IV port, changing a transducer filter, and drawing lab work.
3. Open skin wounds of a staff member, i.e., skin breakdown on an exposed area.
4. Emergency situations such as a code or seizure activity where there is an increased chance of a line becoming disconnected or a needle dislodged.
5. Patient known to exhibit unacceptable behavior, such as scratching exposed sores, pulling needles out, and otherwise exposing staff to the potential for splattering with blood or body fluids.

Universal precautions include, but are not limited to the following:

1. Hands must always be washed even when gloves have been worn. If hands come in contact with blood or body fluids, they must be washed immediately with soap and water.
2. Gloves must be worn when contact with blood or body fluids is anticipated, or if breaks in skin are present.
3. Breaks in skin should be covered with a clean Band-Aid before gloving.
4. Impervious gowns or plastic aprons must be worn in the patient care area during times of increased risk.
5. Masks and protective eye goggles with side shields or a face shield must be worn if aerosolation or splattering is likely to occur as with cannulation, and the initiation and termination of dialysis.
6. Resuscitation bags, mouth pieces, or other ventilation devices must be strategically located and available for use in areas where the need for resuscitation is predictable.
7. Sharp objects must be handled in such a manner as to prevent accidental cuts or punctures. Used needles should not be bent, broken, recapped or unnecessarily handled.
8. Sharps must be discarded intact immediately after use, into a puncture resistant needle disposal container, which must be readily accessible.
   (a) Report any sharps containers that are mounted too high or otherwise not easily accessible.
9. External machine parts and surfaces, hemostats, clamps and patient chairs must be decontaminated per facility procedure immediately after every treatment. A 1:10 to 1:100 solution of household bleach is effective in destroying the HIV and HBV viruses on external surfaces.
10. Blood spills must be cleaned up promptly with a disinfectant solution such as a 1:10 bleach solution.

Universal precautions include measures to avoid ingestion of bloodborne pathogens:

1. Eating, drinking, smoking, application of cosmetics or lip balm and handling contact lenses are prohibited in work areas where there is a reasonable likelihood of occupational exposure, such as the patient care area.
2. Food and drink must not be kept in refrigerators or freezers, or on shelves, cabinets, counter tops or bench tops where blood or other potentially infectious materials are present.

Blood specimens must be considered biohazardous and procedures must be followed when collecting and packaging biological specimens of blood or other potentially infectious materials:

1. Proper collection devices must be used. Gloves must be worn.
2. Do not use mouth pipetting or suctioning.
3. Use safeguards against splashing, and generation of droplets.
4. Secure the specimen in an approved leakproof puncture-resistant container.
5. Seal the container immediately in the area in which the sample was obtained.
6. Clean obvious soiling from the outside of the container using detergent germicide. Properly mark container using detergent germicide. Properly mark or color code the container if not pre-coded. If the source person has a known infection, comply with state or local laws regarding color-coding.
7. Refrigerator used for storing blood must be marked with an orange or red biohazard label.
8. If leakage occurs or if there is any question about the integrity of the primary container, the container must be placed in a second approved container, which must also be color-coded or labeled.

Pregnant health-care workers are not known to be at greater risk of contracting HBV or HIV infection than health-care workers who are not pregnant, however, if a health-care worker develops HBV or HIV infection during pregnancy, the infant is at risk of infection resulting from perinatal transmission.

Availability and accessibility of personal protective equipment (PPE) and engineering controls.

1. PPE is specialized clothing or equipment used by staff to protect themselves from direct exposure to blood or other potentially infectious materials.
2. Engineering control is the use of available technology and devices to isolate or remove hazards from the worker.
3. Engineering controls should be used in preference to other control methods to eliminate or minimize staff exposure to blood or body fluids.
4. PPE and engineering controls must be available at all times.

Hepatitis B vaccination for staff at risk for occupational exposure to HBV. Prior to assignment of an employee to a job that has been classified as involving a risk of occupational exposure to blood borne pathogens, the employee shall be advised of this risk and counseled by a physician regarding current U.S. Public Health Service recommendations regarding HBV vaccination. The staff must be offered a test to determine his/her current vaccination or immunity status at no cost to the employee. Staff must receive the vaccination series at no costs during normal working hours, prior to or not later than 10 working days after assignment to the job.

Management of percutaneous exposure to blood and other infectious body fluids. Following a report of an exposure incident, the staff member must be provided with a confidential evaluation.

Cleaning of potentially contaminated work areas and handling of infectious waste. Tags that comply with 29 CFR 1910.145 (f) (Bloodborne Pathogen Regulations) must be used to identify the presence of an actual or potential biological hazard.

1. Tags must contain the word "*BIOHAZARD*" or the biologic hazard symbol.
2. Tags or labels must be an integral part of the container or affixed as close to their respective hazard by string, wire, or unintentional removal.
3. Red bags or red containers may be substituted for labels on containers of infectious waste.
4. Labels must be affixed to refrigerators and freezers containing blood or other potentially infectious material and other containers used to store, transport, or ship blood or other potentially infectious materials.
   (a) Individual vials of blood or other potentially infectious materials that are placed in a labeled container (zip-lock bag and color-coded box) during storage, transport, shipment or disposal are exempt from the labeling requirement.

Laundry practices. Laundry practices include the following:

1. Laundry that is contaminated with blood or other potentially infectious materials or that may contain contaminated needles or sharps must be treated as if it were HBV/HIV infectious.
   (a) Handled as little as possible with a minimum of agitation.
   (b) Must be placed and transported in bags that are labeled or color-coded and would prevent seepage if such a potential exists.
   (c) Bagged at the location where it was used and must not be sorted or rinsed in patient areas.
   (d) PPE must be provided to the employees at no cost. If PPE is not disposable and requires laundering, the employer must provide this service at no cost to the employee.

Record-keeping requirements. Recordkeeping requirements under the Bloodborne Pathogens regulations facilitate tracking each worker's reported exposure incident.

1. Needlestick injuries must be included on the OSHA 200 occupational injury and illness log, along with medical treatment such as gamma globulin, hepatitis B immune globulin, or hepatitis B vaccine is prescribed and administered by licensed medical personnel.
2. HBV and HIV infections must be recorded on the OSHA 200 log if the illness can be traced back to an injury or other exposure incident.
3. The health care professional's written opinion, medical records, incident report, etc. must be maintained for at least the duration of employment plus 30 years.

Nursing Management of Patients With Infectious Diseases

A primary nursing consideration in the care of patients with infectious diseases is the understanding that the patient and family have of the disease process and the means to control it. Nephrology nurses maintain an advantageous position in making this assessment, since they usually are in frequent contact with dialysis or transplant patients and often have the opportunity to visit the patient's home and see how family members interact with the patient.

Nephrology nurses should also assess for the reaction of others to the patient's diagnosis of infectious disease. In some cultural groups, there may be a stigma associated with the diagnosis of an infectious disease, and patients may be blamed for the illness or labeled as "unclean." Simple, thorough, and repeated explanations of the basic pathology of and treatment for infectious diseases may allay the fear and suspicion that others have about infectious disease. Patients may go through periods of depression or denial, and may become discouraged after periods of isolation and feeling unwell, which is compounded when others respond negatively out of fear or ignorance. It is crucial that contacts of patients understand clearly the difference between infectiousness and noninfectiousness, and their risk of exposure to the disease in each situation. Contacts of infectious patients will require follow-up and evaluation, and possibly drug therapy for disease prevention or treatment. It is possible that some of these contacts may demonstrate feelings of anger or hostility, blaming patients for their infection, adverse reactions to drug therapy, or time missed from work or school if the contact is found to be infectious. Nephrology nurses must carefully evaluate the responses that others have towards patients and the diagnosis, and should work towards increasing knowledge and understanding of all the consequences associated with a diagnosis of an infectious disease.

Special attention should be devoted to patients who refuse treatment or are noncompliant with treatment. Often it is necessary for nurses to work with these patients, demonstrating patience, understanding, and flexibility in trying new approaches to ensure compliance with treatment. It is useful to make a written contract with patients, clearly stating benefits or services that they may obtain by continued adherence to the treatment regimen. In most cases, nurses support the right of any competent patient to refuse treatment. However, when treating patients with infectious diseases the obligation to protect the community must be considered before the individual patient's rights (Wiseman, 1995).

Emphasis on the control and treatment of infectious diseases is today a greater part of the scope of nephrology nursing practice than ever before. The dialysis population is aging and presenting with more risk factors. Patients who are immunosuppressed by medications or disease are increasing at unprecedented rates, and society is facing the challenge of increased homelessness and poverty. Nephrology nurses are obligated to know the most current information available regarding prevention and treatment option for patients and their families. State and local health departments and the CDC are all excellent resources for clinicians needing the most current data available regarding hepatitis, HIV/AIDS, and TB and the methods to control and treat it (Wiseman, 1995; Elrod, 1996).

If a patient acquires an infectious disease, infection precautions are needed. In 1995, CDC drafted new guidelines for isolation precautions. The 1995 draft guidelines contain two levels of precautions: (a) Standard Precautions, which are designed for the care of all patients in the hospitals regardless of their diagnosis or presumed infection status; and (b) Transmission-Based Precautions, which are used for patients known to be or suspected of being infected with epidemiologically important pathogens that can be transmitted by airborne or droplet transmission or by contact with dry skin or contaminated surfaces.

The 1995 Standard Precaution system synthesizes the major features of Universal Precautions and Body Substances Isolation. Standard Precautions apply to blood, all body fluids, secretions, and excretions regardless of whether they contain visible blood, nonintact skin, and mucous membranes. Standard Precautions are designed to reduce the risk of transmission of microorganisms from both recognized and unrecognized sources of infection in hospitals.

Transmission-Based Precautions are designed for patients diagnosed or suspected to be infected with highly transmissible or epidemiologically important pathogens for which additional precautions beyond Standard Precautions are needed to interrupt transmission in hospitals. The three types of Transmission-Based Precautions include airborne precautions, droplet precautions, and contact precautions. They may be combined together for diseases that have multiple routes of transmission. When used either by themselves or in combination, these precautions are used in addition to Standard Precautions (Lynch et al., 1990; Lewis, 1996 a,b). All hospitals and outpatient care centers are encouraged to review and consider adoption of Standard Precautions and Transmission-Based Precautions.

Nursing Management of Exposure to Bloodborne Pathogens

The OSHA policy on preventing occupational transmission of bloodborne pathogens (including universal precautions) was revised in 1992. The basis of universal precautions is the assumption that blood and body fluids of all patients may be infectious, and that measures to protect against exposure must be preserved at all times. The ruling mandated that employers provide at-risk employees with appropriate personal protective equipment (PPE). The nephrology nurse should minimize or eliminate exposure to infectious material. When this is not possible, gloves, clothing (gowns, aprons, shoe covers, hats, hoods), and facial protection (masks, shields, glasses, and goggles) must be used.

Housekeeping in renal care centers removes soil and waste on a regular basis and prevents the accumulation and concentration of potentially infectious material in the patient-staff environment and thus, maintains an environment that is conducive to quality patient care. A hemodialysis unit can be compared to a surgical suite more appropriately than a patient's hospital room because of the requirement for aseptic access to the patient's blood supply. Disposable items should be discarded in bags strong enough to contain the weight and possible fluid leakage. Sharp instruments must be placed in puncture-proof containers. Nondisposable items should be treated as potentially infectious. Adequate disinfec-

Table 13-14
Recommendations for hepatitis B serologic surveillance in chronic hemodialysis centers.

	Frequency of HBsAg Screening		Frequency of anti-HBs Screening	
Vaccination and Serologic Status	**Patients**	**Staff**	**Patients**	**Staff**
Unvaccinated				
Susceptible	Monthly	Semiannually	Semiannually	Semiannually
HBsAg Carrier	Annually	Annually	None	None
Anti-HBs-positive*	None	None	Annually	None
Vaccines				
Anti-HBs-positive*	None	None	Annually	None
Low Level or no anti-HBs	Monthly	Semiannually	Semiannually	Semiannually

HBsAg = hepatitis B surface antigen; anti-HBs = antibody to HBsAg.
* At least 10 miU/mL (milli international units) or at least 10 SRUs by RIA or positive by EIA.

tion and proper sterilization methods should be implemented (Favero et al., 1992; Mayfield, 1993; Oakley, 1994).

Nursing Management Specific to the Hepatitis Patient

There is no specific treatment or therapy for hepatitis (Hoofnagle, 1994). Goals for nursing care include provisions of rest, assisting the patient in obtaining optimal nutrition, and special precautions while caring for the patient to prevent self-contamination and spread of the virus (see Table 13-14). Bed rest should be initiated immediately because it decreases the metabolic demands on the liver and promotes liver cell regeneration. The nurse can assist the patient in planning necessary activities to ensure adequate rest. Medications to help the patient relax or sleep may not be ordered because most require clearance by the liver, which is impaired during the acute phase of the disease.

A priority for nursing is the nutritional status of the patient. Loss of appetite, nausea, and vomiting may persist for weeks. A high carbohydrate diet is usually recommended, and fatty and greasy foods should be avoided. Administration of antiemetics may be helpful, but all hepatotoxic drugs should be avoided. Small, frequent meals are easier to tolerate.

Special precautions should be implemented for renal failure patients. Blood samples must be labeled. Hemodialysis patients who are HBsAg positive should be dialyzed in a separate room on equipment designated only for HBsAg patients. Anti-HBsAg positive patients may undergo dialysis in the same area as HBsAg positive patients, or with seronegative patients. Staff members in dialysis units should not care for HBsAG negative and HBsAg positive patients in the same shift. Although there is no evidence that patients or staff in centers that reuse hemodialyzers are at a greater risk of acquiring HBV infection (Alter, Favero, Miller, Coleman, & Bland, 1988; Alter et al., 1990; Favero, Deane, Leger, & Sosin, 1981), the CDC believes that the HBsAg patients should not participate in the reuse program. The handling of dialyzers during reprocessing procedures may place staff members at a greater risk for HBV infection.

It is not necessary for patients who are positive for HCV or non-A, non-B hepatitis to be dialyzed in separate areas or on designated equipment. Nephrology nurses can prevent the transmission of HCV by implementing standard universal precautions. In addition, these patients can also participate in reuse programs.

Screening for HDV would be warranted, when there are patients who are known to be infected with HDV or there appears to be evidence of transmission of HDV in a renal center. Patients who are infected with HDV should be separated from all other dialysis patients, including those who are HBsAg positive. They should be dialyzed in separate areas on designated machines and barrier precautions should be utilized (Favero et al., 1992).

Nursing Management Specific to the HIV/AIDS Patient

The CDC emphasizes the need to consider all patients as potentially infected with HIV or other bloodborne pathogens, and to adhere rigorously to infection control precautions for minimizing the risk of exposure to blood and body fluids of all patients. The efficiency of transmission of HIV is significantly less than that of HBV, presumably

Table 13-15
Opportunistic infections in AIDS patients.

Bacterial
Mycobacterium Tuberculosis (TB)
Salmonella
Fungal
Candida albicans
Cryptococcus neoformans
Coccidioidomycosis
Viral
Herpes Simplex Virus (HSV type 1 and type 2)
Cytomegalovirus (CMV)
Progressive multifocal leukoencephalopathy (PML)
Protozoal
Pneumocystic carinii
Toxoplasma gondii
Cryptosporidium
Isospora belli

because of the significant difference of the amount of infectious virus circulating in the blood of infected individuals. Therefore, patients with HIV infection can be treated with either hemodialysis or peritoneal dialysis, and they need not be isolated from other patients either in separate rooms or on designated machines (Favero et al., 1992; Favero, 1996; Favero, 1989). Routine testing of dialysis patients or staff members for anti-HIV for purposes of infection control is not necessary. Anti-HIV testing for purposes of patient management, medication, and other reasons may be necessary (Favero, 1989).

HIV disease progression can be delayed by promoting a healthy immune system and encouraging the following behaviors:

- Nutritional changes that promote lean body mass, increase weight, and assure appropriate levels of vitamins and micronutrients;
- Cessation of smoking, drug use, and alcohol intake;
- Regular exercise;
- Stress reduction;
- Minimum exposure to infectious agents; and
- Psychosocial counseling and support groups.

The patient should be educated regarding his/her prognosis and recognition of clinical manifestations that may indicate progression of HIV to ensure that prompt medical attention is initiated. The patient should be given as much information as needed to make decisions about health care. Common opportunistic infections in AIDS patients are found in Table 13-15.

Early manifestation that need to be reported include unexplained weight loss, night sweats, diarrhea, persistent fever, swollen lymph nodes, oral hairy leukoplakia, oral candidiasis, and persistent vaginal yeast infections.

Nursing care becomes more complicated as the patient's immune system deteriorates and new problems rise to compound existing difficulties. The focus shifts to quality of life issues and caring rather than on cure issues (see Chapter 10). When opportunistic diseases develop, intensive nursing intervention is required. Nursing care includes monitoring the respiratory status, administering medications and oxygen, positioning the patient to facilitate breathing, guiding relaxation exercises to decrease anxiety, promoting nutritional support, and conserving energy to decrease oxygen demand. In the final stages of HIV infection and AIDS, diarrhea, wasting syndrome, and AIDS-dementia complex (ADC) are common (Bradley-Springer, 1995).

Nephrology nurses are experienced in providing support to improve the quality and quantity of patients' lives with chronic illnesses. They are in a unique position to provide psychosocial support to HIV/AIDS patients with chronic renal failure. Nephrology nurses are prepared to assist the patient and family to cope with stress, dependence, social isolation and the imminent decisions regarding initiation and/or continuation of treatments (Bradley-Springer, 1995).

Nursing Management of Patients With TB

Prevention of TB is preferred to treatment of the disease. Techniques developed to prevent the progression of TB infection to disease should be the primary goal of all caregivers. Since ESRD patients have been identified as a population at risk, prudence dictates that a screening program in this population would help to eliminate progression to active disease in this group. Nephrology nurses in chronic hemodialysis settings are in an ideal position to administer TB skin tests to determine which patients are infected, since they usually see the patients several times a week. The ideal situation would be to administer skin tests to patients who dialyze 3 times a week just before the weekend. For example, a patient who dialyzes Mondays, Wednesdays and Fridays could have a skin test administered on Friday, and the nurse could read it on the following Monday, approximately 72 hours after administration. The results would then be documented in the patient's permanent medical record.

Since immunosuppression is known to be associated with chronic renal failure, consideration should be given to administration of other antigens along with the PPD to assist nurses in determining whether or not anergy may interfere with interpretation of skin test results. Nephrology nurses caring for home dialysis patients should individualize the plan for reading skin test results based on each patient's situation. Any nursing personnel with responsibilities for administering or interpreting skin test results must be thoroughly trained to properly perform these procedures. Health department personnel or home health nurses may be able to assist with reading skin tests in home patients unable to return to the clinic to have the tests read. Before beginning any skin testing in dialysis units, the staff must be prepared to answer any questions patients may have about the skin tests, as well as being prepared for possible positive results from the skin tests. Clinicians should be prepared to evaluate, isolate, educate, and refer any patients who demonstrate positive skin test results. Written literature, which is easily obtained from the health department or CDC, should be available for all patients before and after skin testing is begun.

The major obstacle health care workers face when caring for patients with TB is that of patient compliance. In all chronic illnesses, including chronic renal failure, compliance is an issue requiring constant attention. Couple the difficulty of managing the treatment regimen imposed by renal failure with the long-term and sometimes complicated treatment regimen required for TB, and the situation can become very complex and overwhelming.

Although primary care physicians frequently care for patients with TB, the health department has the ultimate responsibility for ensuring that TB is not spread to others. Laws in every state require reporting to the local health department of all new or suspected cases of TB, and labs should promptly report all positive TB cultures and smears, as well as all results of drug susceptibility tests. Early reporting is crucial to controlling outbreaks of TB, and it gives caregivers access to resources that the health department can provide (such as assistance with case management and contact investigations). Public health nurses or community outreach workers are available through health departments to help patients adhere to and complete prescribed treatment regimens. In many cases, health department personnel who share the same cultural, linguistic, and ethnic background as the patients they serve are available to work with the patients to address and overcome treatment obstacles.

Unfortunately, the socioeconomic conditions that predispose many to becoming infected with TB also preclude adherence to the treatment regimen. Poverty, homelessness, substance abuse, and lack of accessible medical care are issues that must be addressed as aggressively as the drug regimen. Directly observed therapy is a must for patients who have a history of nonadherence to a TB treatment regimen or who are at high risk for being treatment failures (such as the homeless, mentally ill or substance abusers), who repeatedly miss follow-up appointments, or who are on any type of intermittent therapy. Some health departments employ personnel who go to patients' homes or other mutually-agreed upon places to administer medications. Other programs offer free meals, babysitting services, food coupons or small gifts as incentives to comply with the treatment regimen, and in areas where drug abuse is a close corollary to TB, methadone treatments are combined with TB treatments (Casey, 1993; Jo, 1993).

All patients should be assessed for compliance to therapy with every contact with the health care system. Pill counts and random urine tests may be used to determine if medications are actually being taken. Thorough record-keeping is mandatory to ensure that all clinic visits and provision of medications are noted and that the proper health department personnel are promptly notified when problems are identified. Nephrology nurses are in ideal positions to provide care and follow-up to ESRD patients with TB because of the frequency of contact dictated by the treatment regimen for chronic renal failure. If patients receive incenter hemodialysis treatments 3 times per week, nephrology nurses caring for these patients could provide DOT (under the oversight of the physician and health department) and follow-up closely for any adverse effects of treatment or other problems patients are experiencing related to TB therapy. Dialysis clinics also have social workers available who are already familiar with patients' social and economic situations and who the patients already know and trust to some degree. Social workers have an important role in working with the health department and social services agencies to assist in coordinating benefits and social support for ESRD patients who require treatment for TB. Home patients are usually seen in the clinic on a monthly basis, providing these patients with another point of contact with the health care system for follow-up care and assessments.

Any patient with any baseline abnormalities should have close follow-up to ensure that there is no worsening of the patient's clinical status. If the patient reports or demonstrates any symptoms of drug toxicity or adverse drug reactions, then appropriate lab testing and follow-up are necessary to ensure that the patient is on the safest drug regimen possible. An additional result of adverse or unpleasant effects of drug therapy is that it increases the chance that patients will omit doses of the offending medication or quit taking it entirely. Since patients being treated for TB disease will be on multidrug therapy, the risk is that patients may not know which drug is causing the problem and may therefore quit taking all of them. To prevent this from happening, nurses working with these patients must ensure that they understand each medication that is prescribed, the proper dose and times to take it, and any possible side effects of each one. Patients should be taught what symptoms to watch for, which ones must be reported, and who it must be reported to. To help ensure compliance with the treatment regimens, patients should know who to contact and how to contact them whenever problems are encountered, whether it is to report undesirable drug reactions or to get assistance with housing or child care. Whenever possible, friends and family should be included in teaching sessions.

When caring for ESRD patients with TB, nephrology nurses must be aware of possible interactions that TB medications may have with the other medications patients are taking. Some of the drugs commonly used to treat TB are known to have numerous interactions with other drugs, so close and continuous evaluation of every medication the patient takes is necessary to provide the safest drug regimen possible. Nephrology nurses must also be aware of the dialyzability of antitubercular drugs and alter the dosing schedule when appropriate (see Table 13-16). Some drugs will require time or dosage alterations based on the dialysis regimen, while others may require no adjustments at all.

Patient and family education is crucial to successful outcomes. Providing specific written instructions to patients and families may help to ensure that all persons in the home understand the care plan and can work with patients to ensure compliance to the prescribed treatment regimen. To protect family members and co-workers or other close contacts, they must understand the principles of disease transmission and control. As long as patients require isolation, whether in acute health care settings or home settings, family or other support is crucial to ensuring that patients are compliant with infection control (isolation) measures. For the family or significant others to support patients through these crises, the family must understand the reasons for infection control measures and treatment regimens. Investigation and screening of all close contacts of infectious patients are done as soon as the case is reported to the health department.

In inpatient settings, anyone suspected of having TB is placed in TB isolation rooms, which have negative pressure relative to other rooms in the facility (air flows into the room whenever the door is opened). The door to these rooms must remain closed and traffic into and out of the rooms kept to a minimum, and patients should be instructed to ask health care personnel to bring them anything that they need that is not in the room. Patients should be taught to cover their nose and mouth with disposable tissues whenever they cough or sneeze. If a tissue is not handy, their hand will serve to stop the spread of droplet nuclei, but should then be washed immediately.

Before discharge it is also important to assess for any situations that might make it difficult, if not impossible, for patients to comply with treatment (such as homelessness, lack of money for food and drugs, or lack of family or social support). These issues must be addressed before patients can be released back into the community. As long as patients are considered infectious, they must not go to work or school. Education of school officials and employers is often necessary to ensure that they understand the reasons for patients' activity restrictions; the risks that they personally may have resulting from contact with TB patients; and the follow-up, evaluations, and therapy that associates of patients may require. When care of TB patients is coordinated among all health care and social support agencies (acute care nurses and clinicians, health department personnel, and social services workers), the chances of positive treatment outcomes for TB patients are increased.

In outpatient settings, persons suspected of having TB should be immediately moved to an area away from other patients, and a thorough evaluation should be done as soon as possible. Patients should be given a surgical mask and instructed to wear it at all times until they can be placed in an appropriate TB isolation room. They should also be instructed to cover their nose and mouth with disposable tissues whenever they cough or sneeze to decrease the numbers of infectious droplet nuclei dispersed into the air.

Patients with infectious TB may be discharged home after starting drug therapy. This is still an accepted practice in many cases because once treatment has been started, persons with TB are much less likely to transmit disease than persons not receiving therapy. However, patients with MDR-TB may remain hospitalized and in isolation for longer periods, because they may remain infectious for weeks or even months. These patients are also more likely to experience treatment failure or relapse. Before discharge, however, it is important to assess the exposure that family members may have received, evaluate whether any persons in the home fall into any of the high-risk categories previously listed, and whether any of these persons demonstrate any signs or symptoms of TB.

Patients isolated in home settings will require much physical and emotional support from families or significant others, so it is imperative that caregivers assess whether or not this kind of support will be available to patients after discharge. It may be that some of these contacts will need preventive therapy. Patients are asked by health department personnel to list all other persons they have had close contact with, such as co-workers or friends.

Once home, there are several steps that patients can take to protect others in the home. Taking the prescribed medications, at the proper times and in the prescribed doses is the primary means of preventing the spread of TB to others. This is a responsibility that can be shared with patients, families or significant others. It must be stressed repeatedly

Table 13-16a
Drug regimens for adults and adolescents — Prophylaxis for first episode of opportunistic disease in HIV-infected adults and adolescents.

	Preventive regimens	
Pathogen	**First choice**	**Alternatives**
I. Strongly recommended as standard of care *Pneumocystic carinii*	Trimethoprim-sulfamethoxazole (TMP-SMZ), 1 DS po q.d.; TMP-SMZ, 1 SS po q.d.	TMP-SMZ, 1 DS po t.i.w.; dapsone, 50 mg po b.i.d. or 100 mg po q.d.; dapsone, 50 mg po q.d. plus pyrimethamine, 50 mg po q.w. plus leucovorin, 25 mg po q.w.; dapsone, 200 mg po plus pyrimethamine, 75 mg po plus leucovorin, 26 mg po q.w.; aerosolized pentamidine, 300 mg q.m. via Respirgard II™ nebulizer
Mycobacterium tuberculosis Isoniazid-sensitive	Isoniazid, 300 mg po plus pyridoxine, 50 mg po q.d. x 12 mo or isoniazid, 900 mg po plus pyridoxine, 50 mg po b.i.w. x 12 mo	Rifampin, 600 mg po q.d. x 12 mo
Isoniazid-resistant	Rifampin, 600 mg po q.d. x 12 mo	Rifabutin, 300 mg po q.d. x 12 mo
Multidrug- (isoniazid and rifampin) resistant	Choice of drugs requires consultation with public health authorities	None
Toxoplasma gondii	TMP-SMZ, 1 DS po q.d.	TMP-SMZ, 1 SS po q.d.; dapson, 50 mg po q.d. plus pyrimethamine, 50 mg po q.w. plus leucovorin, 25 mg po q.w.
Mycobacterium avium complex	Clarithromycin, 500 mg po b.i.d. or azithromycin, 1,200 mg po q.w.	Rifabutin, 30 mg po q.d.; azithromycin, 1,200 mg po q.w. plus rifabutin, 300 mg po q.d.
Streptococcus pneumoniae	Pneumococcal vaccine, 0.5 mL im x 1 (CD4+ $\geq$/200 mcL; CD4+ <200/mcL)	None
Varicella zoster virus (VZV)	Varicella zoster immune globulin (VZIG), 5 vials (1.25 mL each) im, administered $\leq$96 h after exposure, ideally within 48 h	Acyclovir, 800 mg po q.d. x 5 for 3 weeks
II. Generally recommended Hepatitis B virus	Energix B®, 20 mcg im x 3; or Recombivax HB®, 10 mcg im x 3	None
Influenza virus	Whole or split virus, 0.5 mL im/yr	Rimantadine, 100 mg po b.i.d. or amantadin, 100 mg po b.i.d.
III. Not recommended for most patients; indicated for use only in unusual circumstances Candida species	Fluconazole, 100-200 mg po q.d.	
Bacteria	Granulocyte-colony-stimulating factor (G-CSF), 5-10 mcg/kg sc q.d. x 2-4 w or granulocyte-macrophage colony-stimulating factor (GM-CSF), 250 mcg/m^2 iv over 2 h q.d. x 2-4 w	
Cryptococcus neoformans	Fluconazole, 100-200 mg po q.d.	Itraconazole, 200 mg po q.d.
Histoplasma capsulatum	Itraconazole, 200 mg po q.d.	None
Cytomegalovirus (CMV)	Oral ganciclovir, 1 g po t.i.d.	None

Table 13-16b
Drug regimens for adults and adolescents — Prophylaxis for recurrence of opportunistic disease (after chemotherapy for acute disease) in HIV-infected adults and adolescents.

	Preventive regimens	
Pathogen	**First choice**	**Alternatives**
I. Recommended for life as standards of care		
Pneumocystis carinii	Trimethoprim-sulfamethoxazole (TMP-SMZ), 1 DS po q.d.; TMP-SMZ 1 SS po q.d.	TMP-SMZ, 1 DS po t.i.w.; dapsone, 50 mg po b.i.d. or 100 mg po q.d.; dapsone, 50 mg po q.d. plus pyrimethamine, 50 mg po q.w. plus leucovorin, 25 mg po q.w.; dapsone, 200 mg po plus pyrimethamine, 75 mg po plus leucovorin 25 mg po q.w.; aerosolized pentamidine, 300 mg q.m. via Respirgard II™ nebulizer
Toxoplasma gondii	Sulfadiazine 500-1000 mg po q.i.d. plus pyrimethamine 25-75 mg po q.d. plus leucovorin 10 mg po q.d.	Clindamycin, 300-450 mg po q 6-8 h plus pyrimethamine, 25-75 mg po q.d. plus leucovorin, 10-25 mg po q.d.-q.i.d.
Mycobacterium avium complex	Clarithromycine, 500 mg po b.i.d. plus one or more of the following: ethambutol, 15 mg/kg po q.d.; rifabutin, 300 mg po q.d.	Azithromycin, 500 mg po q.d. plus one or more of the following: ethambutol, 15 mg/kg po q.d.; rifabutin, 300 mg po q.d.
Cytomegalovirus	Ganciclovir, 5-6 mg/kg iv 5-7 days/wk or 1,000 mg po t.i.d.; or foscarnet, 90-120 mg/kg iv q.d.; or cidofovir, 5 mg/kg iv q.o.q.; or (for retinitis) ganciclovir sustained-release implant q 6-9 months	
Cryptococcus neoformans	Fluconazole, 200 mg po q.d.	Ampotericin B, 0.6-1.0 mg/kg iv q.w.-t.i.w.; itroconazone, 200 mg po q.d.
Histoplasma capsulatum	Itraconazole, 200 mg po b.i.d.	Ampotericin B, 1.0 mg/kg iv q.w.; fluconazole, 400 mg po q.d.
Coccidioides immitis	Fluconazole, 400 mg po q.d.	Ampotericin B, 1.0 mg/kg iv q.w.; itroconazole, 200 mg po b.i.d.
Salmonella special (non-typhi)	Ciprofloxacin, 500 mg po b.i.d. for several months	None
II. Recommended only if subsequent episodes are frequent or severe		
Herpes simplex virus	Acyclovir, 200 mg po t.i.d. or 400 mg po b.i.d.	
Candida (oral, vaginal, or esophageal)	Fluconazole, 100-200 mg po q.d.	Ketoconazole, 200 mg po q.d.; itroconazole, 200 mg po q.d.

Adapted from: Centers for Disease Control. (June 25, 1997). *Morbidity & Mortality Weekly Report.*

that all medications must be taken for the full treatment time, even when patients no longer feel ill. The reasons for prolonged periods of drug therapy must be continually reinforced with patients and families. Patients should be instructed to continue to cover their noses and mouths with disposable tissues any time they cough or sneeze. These tissues should be placed in a closed paper sack and discarded. Patients should not return to school or work and they should avoid close contact with others until it is determined that they cannot infect others. While contagious, patients should stay in a separate room, away from others, and they should eat, sleep, and remain in that room as much as possible. Whenever patients leave their designated room, they should wear a surgical mask over their nose and mouth. If it is not too cold outside, patients' windows should be left open.

Placing a fan in the window to blow air from the room to the outside atmosphere helps to decrease the number of TB bacilli floating in the room air, which decreases the risk of others becoming infected. Sunlight kills TB bacilli, and any organisms that the sun doesn't eliminate will be dispersed in the outside air and are unlikely to infect others. Once it is determined that patients are noninfectious, they can resume a normal life-style, and can return to school or work as their physical condition permits (CDC, 1994b).

It is important to assess the understanding that patients and families have of the disease process. Going into the home to see how family members and others interact with patients will give nurses clues as to whether or not there is an appropriate understanding of the disease process and means to control it. Since TB is not spread by fomite or surface contact, there is no need to use disposable dishes, or to do excessive surface cleaning of bathrooms, walls, floors, or other surfaces or objects.

Nurses should also assess for the reaction of others to the patient's diagnosis of TB. Particularly in some cultural groups, there may be stigma associated with the diagnosis of TB, and patients may be blamed for the illness or labeled as being unclean. Simple, thorough, and repeated explanations of the basic pathology of and treatment for TB may allay the fear and suspicion that others have about TB. Patients may go through periods of depression or denial, and may become discouraged after periods of isolation and feeling unwell, which is compounded when others respond negatively out of fear or ignorance. It is crucial that contacts of patients understand clearly the difference between infectiousness and noninfectiousness, and their risk of contracting TB in each of those situations. Contacts of infectious patients will require follow-up and evaluation, and possibly drug therapy for disease prevention or treatment. It is possible that some of these contacts may demonstrate feelings of anger or hostility, blaming patients for their infection, adverse reactions to drug therapy, or time missed from work or school if the contact is found to be infectious. Nurses must carefully evaluate the responses that others have towards patients and the diagnosis, and should work towards increasing knowledge and understanding of all the consequences associated with a diagnosis of TB.

Special attention should be devoted to patients who refuse treatment or are noncompliant with treatment. Many times nurses work with these patients, demonstrating patience, understanding, and flexibility in trying new approaches to ensure compliance with treatment. It may be useful to make a contract with patients, clearly stating benefits or services that they may obtain by continued adherence to the treatment regimen.

Before the advent of effective drug therapy to treat TB, patients with the disease were effectively quarantined in sanatoriums. Treatment consisted of rest, proper nutrition, and plenty of exposure to fresh air and sunshine. As effective antibiotics were developed to treat TB, the need for sanatoriums declined and most were closed by the late 1960s. Consideration of a return to quarantine as a means to ensure proper treatment for some TB patients may be appropriate. Today TB is reemerging, primarily in populations experiencing homelessness, poverty and substance abuse. The same conditions that predispose people to infection with TB also block access and adherence to effective treatment. MDR-TB enhances the threat that the public now faces from TB, and talk is once again returning to consideration of quarantine, possibly in the form of sanatoriums, as an option for those persons who either cannot or will not complete a treatment regimen. For homeless, transient (such as migrant farm workers), incompetent persons, or others with no social, emotional or financial support, sanatoriums may provide the structure these people need to complete therapy while protecting others in the community.

Major Drug-Resistant Organisms

The development of pathogens resistant to antimicrobial agents is rapidly becoming a serious concern. In fact, antibiotic resistance is widely acknowledged to be one of the most pressing medical problems facing the world today (PSL Consulting, 1995). According to a report released by the World Health Organization (WHO), drug-resistant strains of microbes have evaded common treatments for tuberculosis (TB), malaria, cholera, and pneumonia (Brown, 1996). New or increasing drug resistance has also been seen in organisms that cause gonorrhea, middle ear infections, diarrheal disease, and hospital acquired infections.

In the U.S. alone, 13,300 hospitalized patients died in 1992 due to drug-resistant bacterial infections. The incidence of rapidly growing antibiotic resistance is further evidenced by a 150% increase in drug resistant pneumococci between 1987 and 1994 and a 20 fold increase between 1989 and 1993 in hospital acquired vancomycin resistant enterococci (VRE) (PSL Consulting, 1995).

It is common knowledge among the health care community that methicillin-resistant Staphylococcus aureus (MRSA) has become a significant nosocomial or hospital acquired pathogen in the U.S. MRSA isolates were first reported in the 1960s. By the mid-1970s, MRSA was recognized as a significant clinical problem in both Europe and the U.S. (Kluytmans, 1996).

Today, 160 antibiotics, all based on a few basic chemical structures, are on the market (Brown, 1997). Resistance to all the different kinds of antibiotics has been observed in organisms of all different species (Medical Sciences Bulletin, 1996). Resistance develops when bacteria find new ways to disarm these antibiotics. Bacteria may be capable of changing their cell walls to keep drugs out, crossbreed with related species and transferring resistance from one bacteria to another, and produce enzymes to destroy or inactivate the drugs (Coastal, 1997). For example, one mechanism responsible for the resistance of Staphylococcus aureus (S. aureus) to B-lactam antimicrobial agents (penicillins) is the production of B lactamases. The B lactamases were responsible for the development of widespread resistance to penicillin and led to the development of the B-lactamase-resistant anti-staphylococcal penicillin such as methicillin (Mulligan et al., 1993).

Treating patients who have resistant organisms often requires both prolonged hospitalization and the use of expensive alternative antimicrobial drugs. New drugs to combat drug-resistant pathogens are being developed but will not be commercially available for some time. In the U.S., prolonged hospitalization and the use of more expensive antimicrobial agents have increased the cost of treating resistant infections, which is estimated to range from $100 million to $30 billion per year (CDC[a], 1996).

MRSA and VRE: History/Epidemiology/ High Risk Groups

Pathogens acquiring resistance to antimicrobial agents is not a new phenomenon. Penicillin resistance first was seen in 1940 in a strain of E coli. In 1944, just four years after the large scale production of penicillin, the first penicillin-resistant strain of S. aureus was reported in Europe (Medical Sciences Bulletin, 1996). Just shortly after the introduction of methicillin in the mid-1960s, 20%-40% of S. aureus isolates in Europe were resistant to methicillin. Due to cross-resistance between methicillin and other B-lactam antibiotics and its association with resistance to other classes of antibiotics, the term MRSA became synonymous with multi-resistant S. aureus (Kluytmans, 1996). The first U.S. outbreak of MRSA was reported in 1968, with 3%-5% of strains reported as being resistant to methicillin. By 1970, modern strains of MRSA were showing resistance to multiple antimicrobial agents and by 1994, anywhere from 18% to 29% of strains of S. aureus were reported as multiple drug resistant (Thornsberry, 1994; Vandenbroucke-Grauls, 1994; Kluytmans, 1996).

A growing concern is the rapid increase of vancomycin resistance in certain bacteria. As previously noted, this increase is most evident when examining the incidence of infection and colonization with VRE reported by hospitals in the past 5 years.

From 1989 through 1993, the percentage of nosocomial enterococcal infections reported to the CDC National Nosocomial Infections Surveillance (NNIS) system that were resistant to vancomycin increased from 0.3% to 7.9%. Though the increase was due mainly to a 34-fold increase in infections due to VRE in intensive care units, a trend towards increased vancomycin resistance was also noted in non-ICU patients as well (*Federal Register,* 1994).

The increase in VRE poses several problems, including the lack of effective antimicrobial(s) for therapy of infections due to VRE. Most VRE are also resistant to other drugs, for example, aminoglycoside and ampicillin, which were previously used to treat infections due to VRE. Another dilemma is the possibility that the vancomycin-resistance genes present in VRE may be transferred to other gram-positive microorganisms such as S. aureus (*Federal Register*, 1994).

Because vancomycin attacks a fundamental point in cell-wall construction of the bacteria, some experts had predicted that resistance to vancomycin might never be seen. However, some types of bacteria have acquired a set of genes that eliminate and replace the portion of cell wall to which vancomycin normally binds (Lauerman, 1997). Just recently, the Associated Press (1997) reported a case of a Michigan peritoneal dialysis patient developing a rare strain of S. aureus with an intermediate level of resistance to vancomycin.

Several factors have contributed to the development of drug-resistant organisms. The administration of antibiotics can foster and even promote drug resistance by destroying the susceptible organisms and allowing the drug-resistant organisms to survive (Coastal, 1994). Appropriate, as well as inappropriate, antibiotic use may increase the rate at which bacteria develop mutations that render them resistant to antibiotics (Medical Sciences Bulletin, 1996). Patient noncompliance or non-adherence to the prescribed antibiotic regimen contributes to the emergence of resistant strains. The use of antibiotics in veterinary medicine, animal husbandry, and agriculture is another factor thought to contribute to resistance (Medical Sciences Bulletin, 1996). For example, almost 50% of the antibiotics in use in the U.S. are used on animals. It is not uncommon for antibiotics to be used on livestock to increase weight gain in cattle and pigs (Lauerman, 1997).

Certain patient populations may be more at risk of acquiring drug-resistant organisms such as MRSA and VRE. Both MRSA and VRE may cause infections in patients who are critically ill, those with severe underlying diseases or immunosuppression, such as ICU patients, oncology and transplant patients, those who have had intra-abdominal or cardiothoracic surgical procedures; those with indwelling urinary or central venous catheters; those who have frequent hospitalization or prolonged hospital stays, and those being treated with multiple antibiotics and those receiving prolonged steroid therapy. HIV positive patients, nursing home patients, and the elderly are also at increased risk of acquiring drug-resistant organisms (CDC[b], 1995).

Infection Control Strategies

Methicillin-resistant staphylococcus aureus (MRSA). In order for infection control strategies to be effective they must be practical, based on the disease/organism epidemiology, mode of transmission, and the needs of the patient, such as the environment or settings where the patient is receiving care. For example, the recommendations for preventing the spread of vancomycin resistance that were published in a 1995 Morbidity and Mortality Weekly Report (CDC[b], 1995), apply only to acute care hospitals, and not to nursing homes and outpatient facilities.

Adaptations of such recommendations for application in the outpatient dialysis setting should be well thought out, based on factual data, and decided by individual unit policy (Mid Atlantic Renal Coalition, 1996; CDC[b], 1995).

The principal mode of MRSA transmission within an institution is from patient to patient via the transiently colonized hands of personnel who acquire the organism after direct patient contact or after handling contaminated materials. Although personnel who are chronic carriers have been implicated in nosocomial transmission, such occurrences are uncommon (Mulligan et al., 1993).

Transmission via the inanimate environment may be important for special populations such as those in burn or intensive care units where extensive environmental MRSA contamination occurs. Whereas environmental contamination may be common, but not contribute to transmission in a different type of health care setting (Mulligan et al., 1993).

Airborne transmission of MRSA may be important for patients with tracheotomies who are unable to handle their secretions. However, air samples are rarely positive in most investigations, although burn units appear to be an exception (Mulligan et al., 1993).

With an understanding of this organism's mode of transmission, the standard infection control precautions recommended by the CDC, and followed in outpatient dialysis settings should provide protection against the spread of MRSA. "Standard Precautions" require that all patients be cared for as though they may be infected. Standard Precautions combine the major features of universal precautions, which are aimed at reducing the risk of transmitting bloodborne pathogens and body-substance isolation, which reduces the risk of transmitting pathogens from moist body fluids and substances.

The CDC's Standard Precautions include:

- Washing hands after touching blood, body fluids, excretions, and contaminated items, even when wearing gloves.

  Hands must also be washed after gloves are removed, between tasks, and between procedures on the same patient to prevent cross contamination of different body sites.
- Wearing gloves when touching blood, body fluids, excretions, and contaminated items. Gloves should be donned before touching mucous membranes and nonintact skin, and should be removed promptly after use.
- Wearing a mask and eye protection or face shield. Facial protection is worn in order to protect the mucous membranes of the eyes, nose, and mouth during procedures that are likely to cause splashing or spraying of body fluids.
- Wearing a gown or apron for protection of skin and soiling of clothing during procedures and patient-care activities when contamination with blood/body fluids or moist body substance is likely.
- Handling patient-care equipment that is soiled with body fluids and excretions in a manner that prevents skin exposures and contamination of clothing.
- Making sure reusable equipment is not used for the care of other patients until it has been properly cleaned and disinfected. (American Health Consultants, 1997).

If MRSA is judged by a hospital infection control program to be of special clinical or epidemiological significance then additional precautions, such as contact precautions, should be considered.

These precautions include:

- Placing the patient in a private room. When a private room is not available, cohort the patient in an area with a patient(s) who has active infection with MRSA, but with no other infection.
- Wearing gloves when entering the room. During the course of providing care for a patient, change gloves after having contact with infective material that may contain high concentrations of microorganisms (fecal material and wound drainage). Remove gloves before leaving the patient's room and wash hands immediately with an antimicrobial agent.
- Wearing a gown when entering the room if it is anticipated that the health care provider's clothing will have substantial contact with the patient, environmental surfaces or items in the patient's room, or if the patient is incontinent, or has diarrhea, an ileostomy, a colostomy, or wound drainage not contained by a dressing.
- Ensuring that patient-care items, equipment, and frequently touched surfaces are cleaned after use.
- When possible, dedicate the use of noncritical

patient-care equipment and items such as a stethoscope or sphygmomanometer, to a single patient to avoid sharing between patients. If use of common equipment or items is unavoidable, then the equipment must be adequately cleaned and disinfected before use with another patient (CDC, 1996[c], document #370105).

Vancomycin-resistant enterococci (VRE). Enterococci are part of the normal flora of the gastrointestinal and female genital tracts. Because of this, most infections with these microorganisms have been attributed to sources within the patient. However, recent reports indicate that enterococci, including VRE, can spread by direct patient-to-patient contact or indirectly via transient carriage on hands of personnel or contaminated environmental surfaces and patient-care equipment (National Kidney Foundation, 1996). VRE viability on environmental surfaces is high, though VRE virulence and infectivity is low (Mid Atlantic Renal Coalition, 1996).

As previously mentioned, the recommendations for preventing the spread of vancomycin resistance were published in *Infection Control and Hospital Epidemiology* (1995; volume 16, 105-115 and the *MMWR* (1995, *44* [RR-12]) and apply only to acute care hospitals. Reprints are available from the National Technical Information Service. Current infection control recommendations are based on limited data regarding the epidemiology of VRE. It is possible that as new data become available, recommendations may be revised (CDC, 1997[c]; document #370105).

Infection control strategies for VRE in the outpatient dialysis setting are similar to those that may be used for MRSA. However, in addition to the standard precautions previously described, patients with VRE who have a draining wound not contained by dressings, who have diarrhea or are incontinent, who have poor hygiene or are confused and are handling their dressings, etc. should be dialyzed in a separate room or area. Additional precautions such as the contact precautions, also previously described, should be utilized. It is important to dedicate the use of noncritical items, such as a stethoscope or sphygmomanometer, to a single patient or group of patients who are infected with or are carriers of VRE. If such devices are to be used on other patients, adequate cleaning and disinfecting must first take place. There is no evidence that VRE is more resistant to routinely used hospital disinfectants. It is important to ensure that routine procedures for cleaning and disinfection of medical devices and environmental surfaces are followed carefully (CDC, 1997[c], document #370105).

Prudent Vancomycin Use

Since vancomycin use has been reported consistently as a risk factor for VRE and may increase the possibility of the emergence of vancomycin-resistant S. aureus (VRSA) and/or vancomycin-resistant Staphylococcus epidermidis, the CDC recommends the following guidelines be considered for prudent vancomycin use.

A. Situations in which the use of vancomycin is appropriate or acceptable:

1. For treatment of serious infections due to beta-lactam (penicillins) resistant gram-positive microorganisms. Clinicians should be aware that vancomycin may be less rapidly bactericidal than beta-lactam agents for beta-lactam susceptible staphylococci.
2. For treatment of infections due to gram-positive microorganisms in patients with serious allergies to beta-lactam antimicrobials.
3. When antibiotic-associated colitis (AAC) fails to respond to metronidazole (Flagyl) therapy or if AAC is severe and potentially life-threatening.
4. Prophylaxis, as recommended by the American Heart Association, for endocarditis following certain procedures in patients at high risk for endocarditis.
5. Prophylaxis for surgical procedures involving implantation of prosthetic materials or devices at institutions with a high rate of infections due to MRSA or methicillin-resistant Staphylococcus epidermidis (S. epidermidis). A single dose administered immediately before surgery is sufficient unless the procedure lasts more than six hours, in which case repeat the dose. Prophylaxis should be discontinued after a maximum of two doses.

B. Situations in which the use of vancomycin should be discouraged:

1. Routine surgical prophylaxis;
2. Empiric antimicrobial therapy for a febrile neutropenic patient, unless there is strong evidence at the outset that the patient is infected by gram-positive microorganisms (e.g., inflamed exit site of central venous catheter), and the prevalence of infections due to B-lactam-resistant gram-positive microorganisms (e.g., MRSA) in the facility is substantial;
3. Treatment in response to a single blood culture positive for coagulase-negative staphylococcus, if other blood cultures drawn in the same time frame are negative, i.e., if contamination of the blood culture is likely. Because contamination of blood cultures with skin flora, e.g., S. epidermidis, may cause vancomycin to be inappropriately administered to patients, phlebotomists and other personnel who obtain blood cultures should be properly trained to minimize microbial contamination of specimens;
4. Continued empiric use for presumed infections in patients whose cultures are negative for beta-

lactam-resistant gram-positive microorganisms;
5. Systemic or local prophylaxis for infection or colonization of indwelling central or peripheral intravascular catheters or vascular grafts;
6. Selective decontamination of the digestive tract;
7. Eradication of MRSA colonization;
8. Primary treatment of AAC; and
9. Routine prophylaxis for patients on continuous ambulatory peritoneal dialysis. (As printed in: "Centers for Disease Control and Prevention: Preventing the Spread of Vancomycin Resistance -Report from the Hospital Infection Control Practices Advisory Committee").

The Renal Community

Significance for the renal setting. Infections are a significant cause of morbidity and mortality in dialysis and transplant patients. Long-term chronic illness such as end-stage renal disease may render patients more susceptible to infection. The changing demographics of the ESRD population contributes to this problem. More and more patients with varying degrees of immunosuppression such as those who are elderly, diabetic, HIV positive, or have AIDS, are receiving chronic dialysis.

Changes in the renal setting may also play a part as more patients are receiving treatment in long-term care settings or chronic care facilities that may serve as a reservoir for pathogens introduction such as MRSA, into other settings. MRSA has been endemic in long-term facilities for some time. However, MRSA infection rates are increasing in long-term care facilities. Not unlike dialysis facilities, long-term care facilities are now providing care to patients with an increasing number of comorbidities and complications that require more antibiotic use (Muder, 1997). As the complexity of medical care for these patients increases, there is a concomitant use of indwelling lines such as central venous catheters, which in turn places patients at further risk for infection.

Control of drug-resistant organisms in the outpatient dialysis unit. As a result of resistant mechanisms developed by bacteria, many antibiotics formerly resistant to bacterial pathogens are no longer effective. There are numerous reports in the literature of a simple infection turning into a life-threatening condition because of a lack of antibiotic efficacy (Medical Sciences Bulletin, 1996). About two million of the 20 million people hospitalized each year in the United States become infected with bacterial pathogens during the course of hospitalization. Up to 1.2 million of those infections are due to drug-resistant organisms such as Salmonella, meningococci, multidrug-resistant tuberculosis, microbacterium, methicillin resistant Staphylococcus aureus (MRSA), and vancomycin-resistant enterococcus (VRE) (Coastal, 1997).

MRSA has become a prevalent nosocomial pathogen in the United States. In one study, Steinberg et al. (1996) found that from 1990 to 1993, MRSA was the causative organism for 73 (32%) of 230 nosocomial S. aureus bacteremias compared with one (1.54%) of 65 bacteremias during an earlier 3-year period between 1980 and 1983. In addition, infection is a significant cause of morbidity and mortality in patients on hemodialysis, with S. aureus being the most frequently isolated pathogen. Just recently, a Michigan peritoneal dialysis patient who had been treated with multiple courses of intraperitoneal and intravenous vancomycin was diagnosed as having peritonitis due to the first U.S. case of S. aureus isolate with intermediate resistance to vancomycin (VISA). This case, along with the development of a second U.S. case of VISA in a New Jersey resident, justifies the concern that a S. aureus strain with full resistance to vancomycin may eventually emerge (CDC, 1997).

Enterococci have also become important nosocomial pathogens in many hospitals in the United States within the past few years. Antibiotics that were once the main treatment of enterococci, including the penicillins, aminoglycosides, and vancomycin, are no longer effective in many instances when resistant enterococci are encountered (Flores et al., 1996). The development of vancomycin-resistant enterococci is in part thought to be related to the increased use of vancomycin for the treatment of MRSA, as well as other gram-positive organisms that are beta-lactam-resistant (Flores et al., 1996). One study conducted in 1994 demonstrated an 18% prevalence of VRE among dialysis patients in a free-standing inner city dialysis facility. The prevalence of VRE among dialysis patients in a hospital-based inner city facility was 28% (Ramos et al., 1994; Mid-Atlantic Renal Coalition, 1996).

Prevention strategies: MRSA. In addition to the infection control strategies, including standard precautions and contact precautions when justified, as well as recommendations regarding prudent vancomycin use, clinicians should be aware of other measures to curtail the proliferation and spread of drug- resistant organisms.

Despite the availability of CDC recommendations regarding surveillance culturing, the dissemination of confusing and conflicting information on this topic is not uncommon. Though many healthy adults are persistently or intermittently colonized (harbor the bacteria without infection) with methicillin-susceptible S. aureus (MSSA) (Doebbeling, 1994), methicillin-resistant S. aureus (MRSA) colonization of health care workers has been considered uncommon. A rate of 2% has been found, although higher rates have also been reported (Mulligan, 1993).

Health care workers have been more commonly identified as a link for transmission of MRSA between colonized or infected patients. The main mode of this transmission is via hands which become contaminated by contact with an infected or colonized patient; contact with colonized or infected body sites of the personnel themselves, or contact with environmental surfaces contaminated with body fluids containing MRSA (CDC fax service, document #370105; Mulligan, 1993). Obviously, good hand washing remains a vital, important infection control measure.

Routine surveillance culturing of all staff is not recommended. Per the recommendations of the Centers for Disease Control and Prevention (CDC fax service, document #370105) "unless the objective of the health care facility is to eradicate all MRSA carriage and treat all personnel who are MRSA carriers whether or not they disseminate MRSA, it may be prudent to culture only personnel who are implicated in MRSA transmission based on epidemiological data. MRSA-carrier personnel who are epidemiologically linked to transmission should be removed from direct patient care until treatment of the MRSA carrier state is successful. If the health care institution elects to culture all personnel to identify MRSA carriers, surveillance cultures need to be done frequently and it is likely that staff members colonized by MRSA who are not linked to transmission and/or who may not be MRSA disseminators will be identified, subjected to treatment, and/or removed from patient contact unnecessarily. Because of the high cost associated with repeated surveillance cultures and the potential of repeated culturing to result in serious consequences to health care workers, health care institutions should weigh the advantages and the adverse effects of routinely culturing personnel before doing so."

Treatment of staff members in order to eradicate colonization has been controversial (Jewell, 1996). Indications for attempting to eliminate carriage of MRSA are usually either to halt an outbreak or to prevent recurrent infections in an individual. Treatment for eradication of the carrier state is often thought not to be cost effective with endemic colonization or non-outbreaks. There is also concern that attempts to eradicate colonization could possibly lead to the emergence of new resistance (Mulligan, 1993). Eradication of the carrier state may, however, be indicated in an outbreak situation in which it is likely that one carrier is responsible for the spread of MRSA (Mulligan, 1993).

Studies also show that staphylococcal infections in colonized patients are often due to the staphylococcal strain responsible for colonization. Eradication of colonization to prevent recurrent infections due to endogenous origins has been shown to decrease S. aureus infections (Edmond, Wenzel, & Pasculle, 1996).

Calcium mupirocin ointment has been found to eradicate nasal colonization with MRSA in both adult patients and health care workers. Several studies report a significant decrease in S. aureus colonization and a lower incidence of related infections in dialysis patients without the emergence of nasal mupirocin resistance (Holton, 1991; Boelaert et al., 1991; Boelaert et al., 1993; Boelaert et al., 1995; Mupirocin Study Group, 1996).

Intravascular devices such as long-term indwelling catheters have become an important cause of hospital acquired S. aureus bacteremias including those due to MRSA. Steinberg (1996) and colleagues report that out of 230 bacteremias being examined, 128 or (56%) were associated with the use of intravascular devices. Measures to reduce the incidence of catheter-related infections include judicious use of intravascular devices, not to overuse the devices for sake of convenience, as well as taking meticulous care when inserting and maintaining the devices. Whenever possible, physicians should consider using indwelling catheters coated with antiseptics, known to lower the incidence of catheter-related infections (Steinberg et al., 1996). Central venous catheters coated with chlorhexidine and silver sulfadiazine have been reported to decrease infection rates by as much as 80% (Maki, 1997).

Prevention strategies: VRE. Vancomycin-resistant enterococci were first described in the U.S. in the late 1980s. The National Nosocomial Infectious Surveillance System (NNISS) of the CDC provides national data on nosocomial infections. Prevalence of resistance to vancomycin is reported to vary by site of infection with approximately 7.8% of enterococcal isolates from intra-abdominal infections being resistant to vancomycin, 4.1% for skin, and 3.8% for blood isolates. The NNISS reports VRE occurring in nine of 33 reporting states with the highest number in New York, Pennsylvania, and Maryland. Teaching hospitals had significantly more cases of VRE than non-teaching hospitals (Flores, 1996; CDC, 1995).

Most VRE outbreaks involve primarily ICU or hematology-oncology patients. In these populations, risk factors for VRE colonization or infection are severity of illness, underlying disease, and antimicrobial exposure (particularly to vancomycin). Outbreaks caused by a single strain are easier to control and eliminate than outbreaks involving multiple strains.

The CDC recommendations for preventing the spread of vancomycin resistance that were published in *Infection Control and Hospital Epidemiology* (1995; *16*, 105-115) and *MMWR* (1995; *44* [RR-12]) apply only to acute care hospitals, not to nursing homes and outpatient facilities. Adaptations of such recommendations in the outpatient dialysis setting should be well thought out, based on factual epidemiological data, and decided by the individual unit (Mid-Atlantic Renal Coalition, 1996; CDC, 1995). Current infection control recommendations are based on limited data regarding the epidemiology of VRE. It is possible that as new data become available, recommendations may be revised (CDC document #370105).

In addition to the infection control measures reviewed earlier, the CDC Hospital Infection Control Practices Advisory Committee regarding VRE emphasizes that controlling the spread of vancomycin-resistance can only be achieved if each of the following elements is addressed:

1. Prudent vancomycin use by clinicians.
2. Education of staff regarding the problem of vancomycin resistance.
3. Early detection and prompt reporting of vancomycin resistance in enterococci and other gram-positive microorganisms by the facility laboratory.
4. Implementation of appropriate infection control measures to prevent person-to-person transmission of VRE.

Routine surveillance culturing for VRE in the outpatient dialysis facility is thought not to be necessary due to the associated cost of repeat culturing and the improbability of eradicating the carrier state (Mid-Atlantic Renal Coalition, 1996). Surveillance culturing is recommended if there is an increased number of cases with VRE infection or if there is a clustering of cases on shift/room/day suggesting the need for epidemiological investigation (Mid-Atlantic Renal Coalition, 1996). Typing of VRE organisms is required in order to determine isolated single strains from the spread of a single strain (CDC, 1995; Mid Atlantic Renal Coalition, 1996).

The dialysis facility's Infection Control Committee or Quality Assurance/Quality Improvement Committee should document and monitor all patients with VRE or MRSA infection and/or colonization. It is also recommended that the lab used by the facility test the organism for resistance to multiple antibiotics including vancomycin. Upon transfer, the facility should notify the accepting facility of infection status. Conversely, dialysis facilities should request recent infection/carrier status upon receiving a patient transferring from another facility or hospital (Mid Atlantic Renal Coalition, 1996; CDC, 1995).

A sound inservice/education program is vitally important to preventing the spread of drug- resistant organisms. The educational program should consist of all clinical staff including students (if any) and physicians. Infection control procedures, the epidemiology of MRSA and VRE, and its impact on outcomes and cost should be reviewed annually and on an as-needed basis. The monitoring of staff adherence to infection control procedures should take place frequently as part of the facility Quality Assurance/Quality Improvement Program.

Summary

The prevention and treatment of infectious diseases in dialysis and transplant patients is a formidable challenge for nephrology nurses. In an already immunosuppressed population, this may be impossible. Therefore, nephrology nursing practice must be guided by a clear understanding of epidemiological principles to define infectious disease occurrence in order to develop and implement control measures.

The implementation of Universal Precautions consisting of standard barrier precautions to prevent infection transmission, routine serologic testing of all patients and staff members for HBsAg and anti-HBs, providing positive HBsAg patients with separate areas and dedicated equipment, and not including HBsAg positive patients in reuse programs are the responsibilities of nephrology nurses. As part of the surveillance system, written documentation of laboratory tests results and disinfection/sterilization procedures should be maintained.

The importance of constant vigilance and continual patient assessment for the onset of symptoms related to the infectious disease process cannot be over emphasized. Well-educated nephrology nurses can assess the underlying mechanisms for fever, inflammatory response, and clinical deterioration that can best facilitate an appropriate course of therapy and minimize the consequences of the disease.

References/Readings

Aach, R., Hirschman, S., Holland, P. (1992, August 15). The ABCs of viral hepatitis. *Patient Care*, pp. 34-38.

Alexander, D., & Peacock, E. (1997). Part I. Drug resistant organisms and their implications for the outpatient dialysis setting. *Nephrology News & Issues, 11*(10), 27-34.

Alter, M., Favero, M., Miller, J., Coleman, P., & Bland, L. (1988). Reuse of hemodialyzers. Results of nationwide surveillance for adverse effects. *Journal of the American Medical Association, 260,* 2073.

Alter, M., Favero, M., Moyer, L., Miller, J., & Bland, L. (1990). National surveillance of dialysis-associated diseases in the United States, 1988. *Transcript of the American Association of Artificial and Internal Organs, 36,* 107-118.

Alter, M., Gerety, R., Smallwood, L., Sampliner, R., Deinhardt, F., Tabor, E., Frosner, G., & Matanoski, G. (1982). Sporadic non-A, non-B hepatitis: Frequency and epidemiology in an urban United States population. *Journal of Infectious Disease, 145,* 886-893.

American Thoracic Society. (1994). Treatment of tuberculosis and tuberculosis infection in adults and children. *American Journal of Respiratory and Critical Care Medicine, 149,* 1359-1374.

Association for the Advancement of Medical Instrumentation. (1986). *Recommended practice for reuse of hemodialyzers.* Arlington, VA: Author.

Association for the Advancement of Medical Instrumentation. (1981). *American National Standard for Hemodialysis Systems.* Arlington, VA: Author.

Bader, T. (1995). *Viral hepatitis: Practical evaluation and treatment.* Seattle, WA: Hogrefe & Huber Publishers.

Bader, T. (1986). A protocol for needle-stick injuries. *Emergency Medicine, 18,* 36-43.

Bancroft, W., & Lemon, S. (1984). Hepatitis A from a military perspective. In R. Gerety (Ed.), *Hepatitis A* (pp. 81-100). Orlando: Academic Press.

Binney, P. (1994). Barrier method. *Nursing Times, 90*(38), 69-72.

Bortolotti, F., Vajro, P., & Cadrobbi, P., et al. (1992). Cryptogenic chronic liver disease and hepatitis C virus infection in children. *Journal of Hepatology, 15,* 73-76.

Bradley-Springer, L. (1995). The human immunodeficiency virus and nephrology nursing: Implications for infected clients. *ANNA Journal, 22*(6), 557-562, 617.

Cardo, D.M., Culver, D.H., Ciesielski, C.A, Srivastava, P.U., Marcus, R., Abiteboul, D., Heptonstall, J., Ippolito, G., Lot, F., McKibben, P.S., & Bell, D.M. (1997). A case control study of HIV seroconversion in health care workers after percutaneous exposure. *New England Journal of Medicine, 337,* 1585-90.

Casey, K. (1993). Fighting MDR-TB. *RN, 56,* 26-30.

Centers for Disease Control and Prevention (CDC). (1997a). *Occupational exposure to HIV, Information for health care workers* [On-line]. Available: http://www.cdc.gov.

Centers for Disease Control and Prevention (CDC). (1997b). Performance evaluation programs for determining HIV-1 viral loads, testing for HIV p24 antigen, and identifying Mycobacterium tuberculosis using nucleic acid amplification tests. *Morbidity and Mortality Weekly Report, 46,* (No. 7) 155.

Centers for Disease Control and Prevention (CDC). (1997c). 1997 revised guidelines for performing CD4+ T-cell determinations in persons infected with human immunodeficiency virus (HIV). *Morbidity and Mortality Weekly Report, 46,* (No. RR-2) 1.

Centers for Disease Control and Prevention (CDC). (1997d). Update: Trends in AIDS incidence - United States, 1996. *Morbidity and Mortality Weekly Report, 46,* (No. 37) 861-866.

Centers for Disease Control and Prevention (CDC). (1997e). 1997 USPHS/IDSA guidelines for the prevention of opportunistic infections in persons infected with human immunodeficiency virus. *Morbidity and Mortality Weekly Report, 46,* (No. RR-12) 1-30.

Centers for Disease Control and Prevention (CDC). (1997f). *Methicillan-resistant staphylococcus aureus/VRE.* Hospital Infections Program, CDC Fax Information Service. Document #370105.

Centers for Disease Control and Prevention (CDC). (1996a). Identification of HIV-1 group O infection - Los Angeles County, California, 1996. *Morbidity and Mortality Weekly Report, 45,* (No. 26) 561-563.

Centers for Disease Control and Prevention (CDC). (1996b). Update: Provisional public health service recommendations for chemoprophylaxis after occupational exposure to HIV. *Morbidity and Mortality Weekly Report, 45,* (No. 22) 468-472.

Centers for Disease Control and Prevention (CDC). (1996c). Update: Provisional public health service recommendations for chemoprophylaxis after occupational exposure to HIV. *Morbidity and Mortality Weekly Report, 45,* 468-472.

Centers for Disease Control and Prevention (CDC). (1996d). U.S. Public health service guidelines for testing and counseling blood and plasma donors for human immunodeficiency virus type 1 antigen. *Morbidity and Mortality Weekly Report, 45,* (No. RR-2) 1-4.

Centers for Disease Control and Prevention (CDC). (1994a). Guidelines for preventing transmission of human immunodeficiency virus through transplantation of human tissue and organs. *Morbidity and Mortality Weekly Report, 43,* (No. RR-8) 1-13.

Centers for Disease Control. (CDC) (1994a). *Core curriculum on tuberculosis - What the clinician should know* (3rd ed.). Atlanta, GA: Author.

Centers for Disease Control. (CDC). (1994b). *Questions and answers about TB.* [Patient Education Booklet]. Atlanta, GA: Author.

Centers for Disease Control and Prevention (CDC). (1994b). Recommendations of the U.S. Public Health Service task force on the use of zidovudine to reduce perinatal transmission of human immunodeficiency virus. *Morbidity and Mortality Weekly Report, 43,* (No. RR-11) 1.

Centers for Disease Control and Prevention (CDC). (1992). Testing for antibodies to human immunodeficiency virus type 2 in the United States. *Morbidity and Mortality Weekly Report, 41,* (No. RR-12) 1-7.

Centers for Disease Control. (1991). Hepatitis B virus: A comprehensive strategy for eliminating transmission in the United States through universal childhood vaccination. *Morbidity & Mortality Weekly Report, 40*(r-13).

Centers for Disease Control. (1990). *Principles of epidemiology: Disease surveillance* (Self- study course 3030-G: Manual 5). Atlanta, GA: Author.

Centers for Disease Control. (1990). Protection against viral hepatitis: Recommendations of the Immunization Practices Advisory Committee (ACIP). *Morbidity & Mortality Weekly Report, 39*(S-2).

Centers for Disease Control and Prevention (CDC). (1989). Guidelines for prevention of transmission of human immunodeficiency virus and hepatitis B virus to health care and public safety workers. *Morbidity and Mortality Weekly Report, 38,* (No. S-6) 4-5

Centers for Disease Control. (1988). Hepatitis A among drug users. *Morbidity & Mortality Weekly Report, 37,* 297-300.

Centers for Disease Control (CDC). (1977, November). Control measures for hepatitis B in dialysis centers. In *Viral hepatitis investigation and control series.* Atlanta: Author.

Chan, T., Lok, A., & Cheng, I. et al. (1993). A prospective study of hepatitis C virus infection among renal transplant recipients. *Gastroenterology, 104,* 862-868.

Choo, Q-L., Kuo, G., Weiner, A., Overby, L., Bradley, D., & Houghton, M. (1989). Isolation of a cDNA clone derived from a bloodborne non-A, non-B viral hepatitis genome. *Science, 244,* 359.

Clavel, F., Mansinho, K., Chamaret, S. (1987). Human immunodeficiency virus type 2 infection associated with AIDS in West Africa. *New England Journal of Medicine, 316,* 1180-1185.

Colombo, M., Rumi, M., & Marcelli, R., et al. (1991). Randomized controlled trial of recombinant alfa in patients with chronic hepatitis C. *Hepatology, 14,* 73(abstract).

Daniel, T. (1987). Tuberculosis. In E. Braunwald, K. Isselbacher, R. Petersdorf, J. Wilson, J. Martin, & A. Fauci, (Eds.), *Harrison's principles of internal medicine* (11th ed.) (pp. 625 -633). New York: McGraw-Hill Book Company.

Davis, G., Balart, L., & Schiff, E., et al. (1989). Treatment of chronic hepatitis C with recombinant interferon alpha. A multi-centered randomized, controlled trial. *New England Journal of Medicine, 321,* 1501-1506.

Dayton, K.D., & Lancaster, L.E. (1995). The immune system in patients with renal failure — Part 1: Review of immune function. *ANNA Journal, 22*(6), 523-529.

Dayton, K.D., & Lancaster, L.E. (1995). The immune system in patients with renal failure — Part 2: Effects of renal failure and its treatment on the immune system and assessment of immune system function. *ANNA Journal, 22*(6), 530-537, 572.

Decker, R., Kosakowski, S., Vanderbilt, A., et al. (1981). Diagnosis of acute hepatitis A by HAVAB-M, a direct radioimmuno-assay for IgM anti-HAV. *American Journal of Clinical Pathology, 76,* 140-147.

DeCock, K., Govindarajan, S., & Chin. K., & Redeker, A. (1986). Delta hepatitis in the Los Angeles area: A report of 126 cases. *Annals of Internal Medicine, 105,* 108-114.

DeJongh, F., Janssen, H., & DeMan, R. (1992). Survival and prognostic indicators in hepatitis B surface antigen-positive cirrhosis of the liver. *Gastoenterology, 103,* 1630-1635.

Dienstag, J. (1983). Non-A, non-B hepatitis. Recognition, epidemiology, and clinical features. *Gastroenterology, 85,* 439-462.

Domin, M. (1993). The new face of tuberculosis: Preventing nosocomial transmission in health care facilities. In Plant technology & safety management series: *Controlling occu-*

pational exposure to tuberculosis. Oakbrook Terrace, IL: Joint Commission on Accreditation of Healthcare Organizations.

Dusheiko, G., & Zuckerman, A. (1993, July). Treatment of chronic viral hepatitis. *Journal of Antimicrobial Chemotherapy, 32*(suppl A), 107-120.

Elrod, R. (1996). Nursing role in management of problems of the liver, biliary tract, and pancreas. In S.M. Lewis, I.C.Collier, & M.M. Heitkemper (Eds.), *Medical-surgical nursing: assessment and management of clinical problems* (pp.1258-1308). St. Louis, MO: Mosby Year Book, Inc.

Eyster, M., Fried, M., & Di-Bisceglie, A. et al. (1993). HCV-RNA in hemophiliacs with antibody to hepatitis C virus: Relationship to HIV infection and liver failure. *International AIDS Conference,* Berlin (abstract).

Favero, M. (1996). Infection control. *Dialysis & Transplantation, 25*(10), 699-702.

Favero, M., Alter, M., & Bland, L. (1992). Dialysis-associated infections and their control. In J. Bennett & P. Brachman (Eds.), *Hospital infections* (3rd Edition) (pp. 375-403). Boston: Little, Brown & Company.

Favero, M. (1989). Precautions for dialysing Human Immunodeficiency Virus-Infected Patients. In P. Monkhouse (Ed.) *Aspects of Renal Care,* 3, pp.55-61. London:Balliere Tindall.

Favero, M. (1984). Epidemiology of hepatitis viruses. *Viral hepatitis and liver disease* (pp. 433- 437). (ISBN 0-8089-1678-5). Orlando, FL: Grune & Stratton.

Favero, M., Deane, N., Leger, R. & Sosin, A. (1981). Effect of multiple use of dialyzers on hepatitis B incidence in patients and staff. *Journal of the American Medical Association, 245,* 166.

Fingerote, R., & Bain, V. (1993). Fulminant hepatic failure. *American Journal of Gastroenterology, 88,* 1000-1010.

Flowers, M., Heathcote, J., Wanless, I. (1990). Fulminant hepatitis as a consequence of reactivation of hepatitis B virus infection after discontinuation of low-dose methotrexate therapy. *Annals of Internal Medicine, 112,* 381-382.

Food and Drug Administration (FDA). (1997). FDA approved drugs for HIV and AIDS-related conditions [On line]. Available: http://www.hivatis.org/fdachrt.html

Freeman, G. (1991). *Common sense about AIDS - The educational resource.* Atlanta, GA: American Health Consultants.

Gallagher, N. (1995). Monograph on infectious diseases revisits earlier nephrology nursing practice issues (President's Message). *ANNA Journal, 22*(6), 519.

Gerber, M. Shieh, Y., & Shim, K. (1992). Detection of replicative hepatitis C virus sequences in hepatocellular carcinoma. *American Journal of Pathology, 141,* 1271-1277.

Getzug, T., Brezina, M., & Lindsay, K., et al. (1990). Hepatitis C virus antibody in hemodialysis patients: comparison of prevalence using first and second generation assays. *Hepatology, 12,* 845 (abstract).

Goldsmith, M. (1990). Even in perspective, HIV specter haunts health care workers most. *Journal of the American Medical Association, 263,* 2413-2420.

Hadler, S., Webster, H., & Erben, J., et al. (1980). Hepatitis A in day-care centers. *New England Journal of Medicine, 302,*1222-1227.

Henderson, D.K. (1997). Postexposure treatment of HIV – taking some risk for safety's sake. *New England Journal of Medicine, 337*(21), Editorial.

Hennekens, C. & Buring, J. (1987). *Epidemiology in medicine.* Boston: Little, Brown, and Company.

Hoke, C., Binn, L., & Egan, J., et al. (1992). Hepatitis A in the U.S. Army: Epidemiology and vaccine development. *Vaccine, 10*(Suppl 1), S75-S80.

Holzberger, G., Seidl, S., & Peschke, B., et al. (1992). Second generation anti-HCV test: Seroprevalence in hemodialysis and blood donors. *Transplant Proceedings, 24,* 2648-2649.

Hoofnagle, J. (1994). Therapy of acute and chronic viral hepatitis. *Advances of Internal Medicine, 15*(241).

Hoofnagle, J., & DiBisceglie, A. (1993). Therapy of chronic delta hepatitis: an overview. In S. Hadziyannis, J. Taylor, & F. Bonino (Eds.), *Hepatitis delta virus: Molecular biology, pathogenesis, and clinical aspects* (pp. 337-343). New York: Wiley-Liss.

Hoofnagle, J. (1989). Delta hepatitis and the hepatitis delta virus. In L. Seeff & J. Lewis (Eds.), *Current perspectives in hepatology* (pp. 47-62). New York: Plenum Press.

Hoofnagle, J. (Presentation, October 29, 1989). Serologic diagnosis of acute and chronic hepatitis. *American Association for Study of Liver Disease,* pp. 187-190.

Hoofnagle, J., Mullen K., & Jones, D. et al. (1986). Treatment of chronic non-A, non-B hepatitis with recombinant human alpha-interferon. A preliminary report. *New England Journal of Medicine, 315,* 1575-1578.

Hoofnagle, J., Seeff, L., & Bales, Z. (1978). Serologic responses in hepatitis B. In G. Vyas, S. Cohen, R. & Schmid, (Eds.), *Viral hepatitis* (pp. 219-242). Philadelphia: Franklin Institute.

Inman, R., Hodge, M., Johnston, M., Wright, J., & Heathcote, J. (1986). Arthritis, vasculitis, and cryoglobulinemia associated with relapsing hepatitis A virus infection. *Annals of Internal Medicine, 105,* 700-703.

Jackson, M. (1992). Infection prevention and control. *Critical Care Nursing Clinics of North America, 4*(3), 401-409.

Jackson, M., & McPherson, D. (1991). Hepatitis A through E – Current and future trends. *Today's OR Nurse,* 7-12.

Jo, H. (1993). Assessment and management of persons coinfected with tuberculosis and human immunodeficiency virus. *Nurse Practitioner, 18,* 42-49.

Joshi, Y., Babu, S., & Sarin, S. (1985). Immunoprophylaxis of epidemic non-A, non-B hepatitis. *Indian Journal of Medical Research, 81,* 18-19.

Kao, H., Ashcavai, M., & Redeker, A. (1984). The persistence of hepatitis A IgM antibody after acute clinical hepatitis A. *Hepatology, 4,* 933-936.

Kiyasu, P., & Caldwell, S. (1993). Diagnosis and treatment of the major hepatotropic viruses. *The American Journal of the Medical Sciences, 306*(4), 248-261.

Kiyosawa, K., Sodeyama, T., & Tanaka, E., et al. (1990). Interrelationship of blood transfusions, non-A, non-B hepatitis and hepatocellular carcinoma: Analysis by detection of antibody to hepatitis C virus. *Hepatology, 12,* 671-675.

Knodell, R., Conrad, M., & Ginsberg, A. et al. (1976). Efficacy of prophylactic gamma-globulin in preventing non-A, non-B post-transfusion hepatitis. *Lancet, 1,* 557-561.

Kools, A. (1992). Hepatitis A, B, C, D, and E: Update on testing and treatment. *Postgraduate Medicine, 91*(3), 109-114.

Korenman, J., Baker, B., Waggoner, J. (1991). Long-term remission of chronic hepatitis B after Alpha-interferon therapy. *Annals of Internal Medicine, 114,* 629-634.

Krumberger, J. (1993). Gastointestinal disorders. In M. Kinney, D. Packa, & S. Dunbar (Eds.), *AACN'S clinical reference for critical-care nursing* (3rd Edition) (pp. 1141-1185). St. Louis: Mosby Year Book, Inc.

Kubic, M. (1997). Federal Drug Administration. *New ways to prevent and treat AIDS* [On line]. Available: http://www.fda.gov/fdac/features/1997/197-aids.html.

Kuhns, W., Prince, A., & Brotman, B. (1976). A clinical and laboratory evaluation of immune serum globulin from donors with a history of hepatitis: Attempted prevention of post-transfusion hepatitis. *American Journal of Medical Science, 272,* 255-261.

Kuo, G., Choo, Q., Alter, H. (1989). An assay for circulating antibodies to a major etiologic virus of human non-A, non-B hepatitis. *Science, 244,* 362-364.

Lake, J., Wright, T., Ferrell, L., & et al. (1993). Hepatitis C and B in liver transplantation. *Transplantation Proceedings, 25,* 2006-2009.

Lavin, J., & Haidorfer, C. (1993). Anergy testing - A vital weapon. *RN, 56,* 31-32.

Lee, W. (1996). Acute liver failure. *New England Journal of Medicine, 329,* 1862-1872.

Lemon S. (1985). Type A viral hepatitis: new developments in an old disease. *New England Journal of Medicine, 313,* 1059-1067.

Lentino, J., & Leehey, D. (1994). Infections. In J. Daugirdas & T. Ing (Eds.), *Handbook of Dialysis* (2nd ed.) (pp. 469-490). Boston: Little, Brown and Company.

Lewis, S. (1996a). Nursing role in management of cell injury and inflammation. In S.M. Lewis, I.C. Collier, & M.M. Heitkemper (Eds.), *Medical-surgical nursing: Assessment and management of clinical problems* (4th edition) (pp.181-206). St. Louis: Mosby Year Book, Inc.

Lewis, S. (1996b). Nursing role in management of human immunodeficiency virus infection. In S.M. Lewis, I.C. Collier, & M.M. Heitkemper (Eds.), *Medical-surgical nursing: assessment and management of clinical problems* (4th edition) (pp. 235-260). St. Louis, MO: Mosby Year Book, Inc.

Lindberg, P. (1993). Improving hospital ventilation systems for tuberculosis infection control. In Plant technology & safety management series: *Controlling occupational exposure to tuberculosis.* Oakbrook Terrace, IL: Joint Commission on Accreditation of Healthcare Organizations.

Lynch, P., Cummings, J., & Roberts, P. et al. (1990). Implementing and evaluating a system of generic infection precautions: Body substance isolation. *American Journal of Infection Control, 18*(1), 1-12.

Maggiore, G. & DeGiacoma, C. (1992). Chronic viral hepatitis in children. *Archives Virology Supplement, 4,* 259-262.

Marriott, E., Nauns, S., & del Romero, J., et al. (1993). Treatment with recombinant alpha-interferon on chronic hepatitis C in anti-HIV positive patients. *Journal of Medical Virology, 40,* 107-111.

Martin, P., & Maddrey, W. (1990). Fulminant hepatic failure. *Practical Gastroenterology, 14,* 50-59.

Martin, P., DiBisceglie, A., & Kasaianides, C. et al. (1989). Rapidly progressive non-A, non-B hepatitis in patients with human immunodeficiency virus infection. *Gastroenterology, 97,* 1559- 1561.

Maruyama, T., Iino, S., Koike, K. (1993). Serology of acute exacerbation in chronic hepatitis B virus infection. *Gastroenterology, 105,* 1141-1151.

Masterson, R., Strike, P., & Teltmar, R. (1991). Hepatitis A immunity and travel history. *Journal of Infection,* 23, 321-326.

Mayet, W., Hess, G., & Gerken, G. (1989). Treatment of chronic type B hepatitis with recombinant alpha-interferon includes autoantibodies not specific for autoimmune chronic hepatitis. *Hepatology, 10,* 24-28.

McCance, K.L., & Huether, S.E. (1994). Alterations in immunity and inflammation. In S. Schrefer (Ed.), *Pathophysiology: The biologic basis for disease in adults and children* (pp. 288- 294). St. Louis, MO: Mosby-Year Book, Inc.

McElguan, P. (1983). Dermatologic manifestations of hepatitis B virus infection. *Journal of the American* Academy of *Dermatology, 8,* 539-548.

Medin, C., Allander, T., & Roll, M., et al. (1993). Seroconversion to hepatitis C virus in dialysis patients: A retrospective and prospective study. *Nephron, 65,* 40-45.

Merican, I., Sherlock, S., & McIntyre, N. (1993). Clinical, biochemical, and histological features in 102 patients with chronic hepatitis C virus infection. *Quarterly Journal of Medicine, 86,* 119-125.

Metreau, J., Calmus, Y., & Poupon, AR., et al. (1991). Twelve-month treatment, compared to 6-month treatment, does not improve the efficacy of alpha-interferon in NANB chronic active hepatitis. *Hepatology,* 14, 72(abstract).

Mid Atlantic Renal Coalition. (1996, December). *Reducing the spread of vancomycin-resistant enterococcus in the dialysis setting.*

Millman, I., Eisenstein, S., & Blumberg, B., (Eds). (1984). *Hepatitis B: The virus, the disease, and the vaccine.* New York: Plenum Press.

National Kidney Foundation (1996). *What you should know about infectious diseases: A guide for renal facilities.*

Neves, P., & Amorim, J. (1992). Should patients with hepatitis C virus antibodies in chronic hemodialysis be isolated? *American Journal of Kidney Disease, 20,* 422.

Niu, M., Coleman, P., & Alter, M. (1993). Multicenter study of hepatitis C virus infection in chronic hemodialysis center staff members. *American Journal of Kidney Diseases, 22*(4), 568-573.

Occupational Safety and Health Agency & Centers for Infectious Diseases Centers for Disease Control. (1989). *Guidelines for prevention of transmission of human immunodeficiency virus and hepatitis B virus to health care and public safety workers* (GPO # 017-033-004422-1). Washington, DC: Author.

Peacock, E. (1993). *Certification review guide.* Pitman, NJ: American Nephrology Nurses' Association.

Peacock, E., & Alexander, D. (1997). Part II. Control of drug resistant organisms in the outpatient dialysis unit. *Nephrology News & Issues, 11*(11), 30-33.

Perillo, R. (1993). Interferon in the management of chronic hepatitis B. *Digest of Disciplinary Science, 38,* 577-593.

Phipps, W. & Daly, B. (1983). Problems of the lower airway. In W. Phipps, B. Long, & N. Woods, (Eds.), *Medical-surgical nursing: Concepts and clinical practice* (2nd. ed.) (pp. 1297-1307). St. Louis: C.V. Mosby Company.

Pol, S., Legendre, C., & Saltiel, C., et al. (1992). Hepatitis C virus in kidney recipients. *Journal of Hepatology, 15,* 202-206.

Polish, L., Gallagher, M., & Fields, H. et al. (1993). Delta hepatitis: Molecular biology and clinical and epidemiological features. *Clinical Microbiology Review, 6,* 211-229.

Protic, J., & Hardy, D. (1993). Resurgence of tuberculosis and emergence of multidrug-resistant strains: Implications for healthcare personnel. In Plant technology & safety management series: *Controlling occupational exposure to tuberculosis.* Oakbrook Terrace, IL: Joint Commission on Accreditation of Healthcare Organizations.

Purcell, R., & Shikata, T. (1991). General discussion on hepatitis E. In T. Shikata, R. Purcell, T. Uchida (Eds.), *Viral hepatitis C, D, and E.* (pp. 379-387). New York: Excerpta Medica.

Purcell, R., & Ticehurst, J. (1988). Enterically transmitted non-A, non-B hepatitis: Epidemiology and clinical characteristics. In A. Zuckerman (Ed.), *Viral hepatitis and liver disease* (pp. 131-137). New York: Alan Liss.

Redeker, A. (1975). Viral hepatitis: Clinical aspects. *American Journal of Medical Science, 270,* 9-16.

Reichard, O., Foberg, U., & Fryden, A., et al. (1994). High sustained response rate and clearance of viremia in chronic hepatitis C after treatment with interferon-alpha 2b for 60 weeks.

Renault, P., & Hoofnagle, J. (1989). Side effects of alpha-interferon. *Seminars in Liver Disease,* 9, 273-277.

Resti, M., Azzari, C., & Rossi, M. et al. (1992). Hepatitis C virus antibodies in long-term follow-up of beta-thalassaemic children with acute and chronic non-A, non-B hepatitis. *European Journal of Pediatrics, 151,* 573-576.

Riley, R., & Nardell, E. (1993). Controlling transmission of tuberculosis in health care facilities: Ventilation, filtration and ultraviolet air disinfection. In Plant technology & safety management series: *Controlling occupational exposure to tuberculosis.* Oakbrook Terrace, IL: Joint Commission on Accreditation of Healthcare Organizations.

Rizzetto, M. (1993). Hepatitis delta virus disease: An overview. In S. Hadziyannis, J. Taylor, & F. Bonino (Eds.), *Hepatitis delta virus: Molecular biology, pathogenesis, and clinical aspects* (pp. 425-430). New York: Wiley-Liss.

Robinson, W. (1990). Biology of human hepatitis viruses. In D. Zakim & T. Boyer (Eds.), *Hepatology: A textbook of liver disease.* Philadelphia: WB Saunders Company.

Saez-Royuela, F., Porres, J., & Morero, A., et al. (1991). High doses of recombinant alpha- interferon or gamma interferon for chronic hepatitis C: A randomized controlled trial. *Hepatology, 13,* 327-331.

Sampliner, R. (1979). The duration of hepatitis B surface antigenemia. *Archives of Internal Medicine, 139,* 145-146.

Sanchez-Quijara, A., Pineda, J., & Lissen, E. (1988). Prevention of post-transfusion non-A, non- B hepatitis by non-specific immunoglobulin in heart surgery patients. *Lancet, 1,* 1245-1249.

Scherer, P. (1990, January). How AIDS attacks the brain. *American Journal of Nursing, 90,* 46- 53.

Schlatter, S., & McNatt, G.E. (1995). Risk of community infections in transplant patients: A literature review. *ANNA Journal, 22*(6), 590-595, 630.

Schluger, N., & Rom, W. (1994). Current approaches to the diagnosis of active pulmonary tuberculosis. *American Journal of Respiratory and Critical Care Medicine, 149,* 264-267.

Seeff, L., Ishak, K., & Gerber, M. (1991). Unresolved clinical issues and histopathologic and immunologic aspects of chronic active hepatitis B and C. In S. Lemon & H. Margolis (Eds.), *Viral hepatitis and liver disease. Proceedings of the 1990 International Symposium on Viral Hepatitis and Liver Disease: Contemporary issues and future prospects* (pp. 805-813). Baltimore: Williams & Wilkins.

Seeff, L., & Koff, R. (1986). Evolving concepts of the clinical and serologic consequences of hepatitis B infection. *Seminars in Liver Disease, 6,* 11-22.

Shapiro, C., Coleman, P., McQuillan, G., et al. (1992). Epidemiology of hepatitis A: seroepidemiology and risk groups in the USA. *Vaccine,* 10(Suppl 1), S59-S62.

Spraycar, M. (Ed.). (1995). *Stedman's medical dictionary* (26th ed.). Baltimore: Williams & Wilkins.

Starzl, T., Demetris, A., & Van Thiel, D. (1989). Liver Transplantation. *New England Journal of Medicine, 321,* 1092-1099.

Stein, R. (1993, June). The ABCs of hepatitis. *American Health, 12*(5), 65-69.

Storch, G., Bodicky, C., & Parker, M. (1982). Use of conventional and IgM-specific radioimmunoassays for anti-hepatitis A. *American Journal of Medicine, 73,* 663-668.

Streiner, D., Norman, G., & Munroe Blum, H. (1989). *Epidemiology PDQ.* Toronto: B.C. Decker, Inc.

Sugitani, M., Inchauspe, G., & Shindo, M. (1992). Sensitivity of serological assays to identify blood donors with hepatitis C viremia. *Lancet, 339,* 1018-1019.

Szmuness, W., Stevens, C., & Zang, E. (1981). A controlled clinical trial of the efficacy of the hepatitis B vaccine: A final report. *Hepatology, 1,* 377-385.

Takeda, S. Nagafuchi, Y., & Tashiro, H. (1992). Anti-hepatitis C virus status in hepatocellular carcinoma and the influence on clinicopathological findings and operative results. *British Journal of Medicine, 79,* 1195-1198.

Thacker, S., Keewhan, C., Brackman, P. (1983). The surveillance of infectious diseases. *Journal of the American Medical Association, 249*(9), 1181-1185.

The A to F of viral hepatitis (Editorial). (1990). *Lancet, 336,* 1158-1160.

Tilzey, A., Palmer, S., & Barrow, S., et al. (1992). Effects of hepatitis A vaccination schedules on immune response. *Vaccine, 10*(Suppl 1), S121-123.

Tine, F., Margrin, S., & Craxi, A., et al. (1991). Interferon for non-A, non-B chronic hepatitis. A meta-analysis of randomized clinical trials. *Journal of Hepatology, 13,* 192-199.

Tokars, J., Alter, M., & Favero, M. (1993). National surveillance of dialysis-associated diseases in the U.S., 1990. *American Society of Artificial and Internal Organs Journal, 39*(1), 71-80.

Tsang, T., Blei, A., O'Reilly, D., & Decker, R. (1986). Clinical significance of concurrent hepatitis B surface antigen and antibody positivity. *Digest of Disease Science, 31,* 620-624.

Valanis, B. (1992). *Epidemiology in nursing and health care.* Norwalk, CT: Appleton & Lange.

Villarejos, V., Visona, K., Gutierrez, A. (1974). Role of saliva, urine, and feces in the transmission of type B hepatitis. *New England Journal of Medicine, 291,* 1375-1378.

Watson, H., Zhang, L., & Simmonds, P., et al. (1992, July 19-24). Hepatitis C virus load increases with time after HIV infection. *International Conference on AIDS,* 195 (abstract No. PoB 3629).

Weiss, T., Tsai, C., & Baldassare, A., et al. (1978). Skin lesions in viral hepatitis. *American Journal of Medicine, 64,* 269-273.

Wiedermann, G., Ambrosch, F., & Andre, F., et al. (1992). Persistent of vaccine-induced antibody to hepatitis A virus. *Vaccine,* 10 (Suppl 1), S129-131.

Wilkinson, S., Davies, M., et al. (1978). Renal failure in otherwise uncomplicated acute viral hepatitis. *British Medicine Journal, 2,* 338-341.

Williams, A., & Hoofnagle, J. (1988). Ratio of serum aspartate to alanine aminotransferase in chronic hepatitis. *Gastroenterology, 95,* 734-739.

Wiseman, K. (1995). Tuberculosis: An old disease with a new face. *American Nephrology Nurses Association Journal, 22*(6), 541-553.

Wright, T., Hollander, H., & Kim, M. (1992). Hepatitis C viremia in human immunodeficiency virus infected patients with and without AIDS. *Hepatology,* 16, 70(abstract).

Ynares, C., Johnson, H., & Kerlin, T. (1993). Impact of pretransplant hepatitis C antibody status upon long-term patient and renal allograft survival: A 5 and 10-year follow-up. *Transplant Proceedings, 25,* 1466-1468.

References/Readings for Major Drug-Resistant Organisms

Associated Press. (1997, August 22). Latest germ enters U.S.; Strain of Staph bacteria resists drug of last resort.

Boelaert, J.R., De Baere, Y.A., & Geernaert, M.A., et al. (1991). The use of nasal mupirocin ointment to prevent Staphylococcus aureus bacteremias in hemodialysis patients: An analysis of cost-effectiveness. *Journal of Hospital Infections, 19*(suppl B), 41-46.

Boelaert, J.R., Van Landuyt, H.W., & Godard, C.A., et al. (1993). Nasal mupirocin ointment decreases the incidence of Staphylococcus aureus bacteremias in hemodialysis patients. *Nephrology, Dialysis and Transplantation, 8*(3), 235-239.

Boelaert, J.R., Van Landuyt, H.W., & De Baere, Y.A., et al. (1995). *Nasal mupirocin decreases the incidence of Staphylococcus aureus bacteremia in hemodialysis: A five-year study.* 35th ICAAC, San Francisco J122. Abstract.

Brown, K.S. (1996, June). Pharmaceutical and biotech firms taking on drug-resistant microbes. *The Scientist, 10*(12), 1, 8-9.

Centers for Disease Control (CDC). (1995). Recommendations for preventing the spread of vancomycin resistance. *Morbidity & Mortality Weekly Report, 44,* No. RR-12.

Centers for Disease Control. (CDC). (1997). Update: Staphylococcus aureus with reduced susceptibility to vancomycin – United States. *Morbidity & Mortality Weekly Report.*

Centers for Disease Control. (CDC [A]). (1996). Defining the public health impact of drug-resistant streptococcus pneumoniae: Report of a working group. *Morbidity & Mortality Weekly Report, 45,* No. RR-1.

Centers for Disease Control (CDC [B]). (1995). Recommendations for preventing the spread of vancomycin resistance. *Morbidity & Mortality Weekly Report, 44,* No. RR-12.

Centers for Disease Control (CDC [c]). (1997). *Methicillin-resistant staphylococcus aureus/VRE, hospital infections program.* Atlanta, GA: CDC Fax Information Service, Document No. 370105.

Coastal (1997). *Drug-resistant organisms: A clinical approach.*

Doebbeling, B. (1994). Nasal and hand carriage of Staphylococcus aureus in healthcare workers. *Journal of Chemotherapy, VI,* Supplement N.2 (11-17).

Edmond, M., Wenzel, R., & Pasculle, W. (1996). Vancomycin-resistant Staphylococcus aureus: Perceptions on measured need for control. *Annals of Internal Medicine, 124,* 329-334.

Federal Register. (1994). Centers for Disease Control and Prevention, Preventing the spread of vancomycin resistance – Report from the Hospital Infection Control Practices Advisory Committee. Comment Period & Public Meeting. Notice, 59(4), 25758-25763.

Five quick tips to prevent MRSA infection: Home care education management. (1997). *American Health Consultants, 2*(2), 17-32.

Flores R., Haley, J., & Ross, T. (1996). Infections in oncology: Vancomycin-resistant enterococci: Approach to treatment and control. *Cancer Control Journal, 3*(1).

Holton, D.L., Nicolle, L.E., & Diley D. et al. (1991). Efficacy of mupirocin nasal ointment in eradicating Staphylococcus aureus nasal carriage in chronic hemodialysis patients. *Journal of Hospital Infections, 17,* 133-137.

Jewell, M. (1996). Cost containment using an outcome-based best practice model for the management of MRSA. *Journal of Chemotherapy, 6,* Supplement n.2.

Kluytmans, J.A. (1996). Global Epidemiology of methicillin-resistant staphylococcus. *Nasal Carriage of Staphylococcus Aureus: The Key to Preventing Staphylococcal Disease.*

Lauerman, J.F. (1997). Drug-resistant bugs. *Harvard Magazine,* Microsoft Internet Explorer.

Maki, D. (1997, October). New study proves effectiveness of antimicrobial catheters. *Nephrology News & Issues,* p. 33.

Medical Sciences Bulletin. (1997). *Novel antibiotics in trial against drug-resistant bacteria, 18*(9), 4.

Mid-Atlantic Renal Coalition. (1996, December). *Reducing the spread of vancomycin resistant enterococcus in the dialysis setting.*

Muder, R.R. (1997). MRSA in long-term care facilities. *Staph News.* SmithKline Beecham Pharmaceuticals, *2*(3).

Mulligan, M.E., Murray-Leisure, K., Ribner, B.S. Standiford, H.C., John, J.F., Korvick, J.A., Kauffman, C.A., & Yu, V. (1993). Methicillin-resistant Staphylococcus aureus: A consensus review of the microbiology, pathogenesis, and epidemiology with implications for prevention and management. *American Journal of Medicine, 94,* 313-327.

National Kidney Foundation. (1996). *What your should know about infectious diseases: A guide for renal facilities.*

PSL Consulting Group, Inc. (1995). *New class of antibiotics shows promise in drug-resistant diseases.* Webmaster@pslgroup.com.

Ramos, E., Light. P.D. Morris G.J., Polish, L., Schwalbe, R.S., Spar, B., & Thomas, R. (1994). *Clinical and epidemiological features of vancomycin resistant enterococcus (VRE) bacteremia in a dialysis center.* Baltimore: University of Maryland.

Steinberg, J.P. Clark, J.P.P., & Hackman, B.O. (1996). Nosocomial and community-acquired Staphylococcus aureus bacteremias from 1980 to 1993: Impact of intravascular devices and methicillin resistance. *Clinical Infectious Diseases, 23,* 255-259.

The Mupirocin Study Group. (1996). Nasal mupirocin prevents Staphylococcus aureus exit-site infection during peritoneal dialysis. *Journal of the American Society of Nephrology, 7*(11), 2403-2408.

Thornsberry C (1994). Epidemiology of Staphylococcal infections – A USA perspective. *Journal of Chemotherapy, VI,* Supplement n.2.

Vandenbroucke-Grauls C. (1994). Epidemiology of Staphylococcal infections – A European Perspective. *Journal of Chemotherapy, Vol. VI,* Supplement n.2.

Chapter Highlights

- Epidemiology is an organized, sequential process of investigation that begins with descriptive research, moves to analytical studies, and finally experimental studies.

- Epidemiology is based on two fundamental assumptions: (a) that human disease does not occur at random and (b) that human disease has causal and preventative factors that can be identified through systematic investigations of different populations or subgroups of individuals within a population in different places or different times.

- There are three main types of descriptive epidemiologic studies: (a) the correlational study that uses data from an entire population to compare disease frequencies between different groups during the same time period or in the same population at different points in time; (b) the case report, which is a detailed profile by one or more clinicians of a single patient and can be expanded into a case series, which describes characteristics of a number of patients with a given disease; and (c) the cross-sectional survey in which the status of a patient with respect to the presence or absence of both exposure and disease is assessed at the same point in time.

- The infectious diseases most prevalent in ESRD patients are caused by three types of infectious agents, specifically, (a) tuberculosis bacterium; (b) HIV and hepatitis viruses; and (c) drug-resistant organisms such as MRSA and VRE.

- Five viruses (A, B, C, D, E) have now been identified that each cause a specific type of hepatitis.

- Hepatitis may be defined as a chronic infection after being present in the blood stream for 6 months.

- During the early days of the End Stage Renal Disease (ESRD) Program, patients and staff were among the highest risk groups for hepatitis B infection after male homosexuals and injecting drug abusers.

- In the ESRD setting HIV may be transmitted only through percutaneous inoculation (i.e., needlestick) or contact of HIV infected blood or body fluid with an open wound, nonintact skin, or mucous membrane.

- The incubation period begins when the person develops antibodies to HIV and ends when the person is diagnosed with full-blown AIDS. Usual incubation period is 7-10 years.

- Michael Houghton and his colleagues at the Centers for Disease Control and the Chiron Corporation reported the cloning of part of a genome which they designated the hepatitis C virus.

- Despite the decrease in the number of deaths, AIDS opportunistic infections remain the leading cause of death among persons ages 25-44 years.

- There are two approaches to treatment of HIV infection and AIDS: restoration of immune function and prevention of viral replication.

- The presence of a large immunosuppressed population, due to the acquired immune deficiency syndrome (AIDS) epidemic and organ transplant patients, and the penalty for the random use of antibiotics was realized in the health care community in the 1990s.

- TB is of interest in chronic dialysis settings because chronic renal failure (CRF) and diabetes mellitus are identified as risk factors that increase the risk of developing clinical TB once a person is infected with the tuberculosis bacillus.

- MDR-TB (TB that is resistant to at least INH and rifampin) presents a major treatment dilemma. These patients require prolonged treatment regimens based on their medical history and drug-susceptibility studies. Many times these organisms are also resistant to other first-line drugs, such as ethambutol and streptomycin.

- Since the inception of dialysis, the Centers for Disease Control and Prevention (CDC) has collaborated with specific organizations to develop and implement standards that enhance the protection of renal patients and the safety of nursing care delivered.

- When the host's defenses are inadequate and unable to check the spread of the bacilli, the person is said to have active TB disease. In this case, the individual would demonstrate clinical symptoms of TB and would be capable of spreading the infection to others.

Chapter Highlights (continued)

- Universal precautions are the same strategies for controlling bloodborne infections that have been used by the dialysis community since 1977.

- The basis of universal precautions is the assumption that blood and body fluids of all patients may be infectious, and that measures to protect against exposure must be preserved at all times.

- There are risks and costs associated with screening and subsequent diagnostic procedures that must be weighed against the benefit of screening.

- The four major functions of surveillance can further be defined as the *collection* of relevant data for a specified population and geographic area; *collation* of the data into meaningful arrangements; *analysis* of the data; and regular *dissemination* of the data and interpretations to those in disease control programs.

- Emphasis on the control and treatment of infectious diseases is today a greater part of the scope of nephrology nursing practice than ever before.

CHAPTER 14

Rehabilitation of the Renal Patient

Nancy G. Kutner, PhD

Chapter Contents

Historical Perspective .405
Defining Rehabilitation .406
The Rehabilitation Process and Disability Classification .407
A Conceptual Model of the Rehabilitation Process .407
Domains of Science and the Medical Rehabilitation Process .408
Physical, Psychosocial, and Vocational Issues in Renal Rehabilitation .410
Physical Issues .410
Psychosocial Issues .412
Vocational Issues .412
Special Populations in Renal Rehabilitation .413
ESRD Treatment Modality and Rehabilitation .415
The Diabetic Patient .416
The Pediatric Patient .416
The Geriatric Patient .417
Outcomes Assessment: Relevance for Renal Rehabilitation .421
Evaluation as a Process to Improve Medical Practice .421
Specification and Measurement of Health Outcomes .422
Utility of a Comprehensive Health Outcomes Database for ESRD .423
Rehabilitation Research Needs .424
Whole Body System Response .424
Behavioral Adaptation .424
Management, Assessment, and Epidemiology .425
Treatment Effectiveness .425
Summary .425
References .426
Chapter Highlights .430

Rehabilitation of the Renal Patient

Nancy G. Kutner, PhD

Rehabilitation is the goal of renal replacement therapy for stable patients. It requires a total plan of care that incorporates physical, psychosocial, and vocational objectives. Patient-specific goals are outlined as early as possible, and progress toward those goals is continually reassessed. Functional status and well-being outcomes, which are traditional rehabilitation indicators, provide crucial markers of the effectiveness of renal patients' care. Enlarging the knowledge base in the field of rehabilitation and improving clinical practice in ESRD are closely linked activities.

This chapter seeks to familiarize readers with some of the basic principles of the field of rehabilitation and to suggest ways that these principles can be applied to care of chronic renal patients. Five areas are addressed: (a) concepts central to the medical rehabilitation process and medical rehabilitation research; (b) physical, psychosocial, and vocational issues in renal rehabilitation; (c) selected dimensions for targeting renal rehabilitation protocols; (d) outcomes assessment relevant to renal rehabilitation; and (e) research needs in rehabilitation, including renal rehabilitation.

The chapter begins with an overview of the concepts and vocabulary used by the National Center for Medical Rehabilitation Research (NCMRR), the focus of rehabilitation investigations within the National Institutes of Health (NIH). The Institute of Medicine Committee to study the ESRD Program noted that because "the challenges of ESRD are apt to be encountered elsewhere," "the issue of rehabilitation...should be examined in the context of all chronic disease patients" (Rettig & Levinsky, 1991, p. 156). Rehabilitation issues that exist for individuals with ESRD parallel many of the concerns shared by other individuals who are living with a chronic condition or disorder.

Historical Perspective

Rehabilitation was the promise on which the ESRD Program was founded. The Congressional leaders who supported enactment of Public Law 92-603, the amendment to the Social Security Bill that established the End Stage Renal Disease (ESRD) Program of Medicare, did so on the belief that virtually all renal patients could carry on active, productive lives. They had been persuaded that 40% of dialysis patients could immediately return to work after starting treatment and that the remaining 60% would return with retraining. The ESRD Program was seen as a way to relieve the personal financial burden of dependence on expensive medical technology, allowing patients to concentrate on pursuing their work, family, and other life goals.

Less than 10 years after the ESRD Program began, evidence emerged that questioned the program's promise of rehabilitation. The Inspector General's Office conducted a service delivery assessment of the ESRD Program in 1980, obtaining data from 225 patients in 14 dialysis facilities that were "carefully chosen to mirror the diversity reflected in that larger universe." The Inspector General's survey found that only 25% of patients who had been working full-time continued to work after kidney failure, and the report concluded that "the ESRD Program tends to foster dependence much more than to minimize it...This situation is unfortunate, first of all, from a quality of care standpoint...Secondly, the dependency-generating mode of operation is unfortunate from a cost standpoint" (Office of Service Delivery Assessment [OSDA], 1980). The next year, the *New England Journal of Medicine* published a study by Gutman, Stead and Robinson (1981) that reported data from a survey of 2,481 patients in 18 dialysis facilities primarily located in the Southeast. The findings indicated that over half of diabetic ESRD patients, as well as approximately 20% of nondiabetic patients, were unable to care for themselves completely. Among patients most likely to be employed — nondiabetic men 21-59 years old — 39% were employed. These data sounded an alarm that a large proportion of dialysis patients might not be rehabilitatable in terms of self-care or employment, and continuation of federal funding for dialysis was questioned in the media (Kolata, 1980; "Reagan's Ax," 1981).

In 1981-1982, an ESRD Rehabilitation Task Force was convened by the Health Care Financing Administration (HCFA). The Task Force recommended changes in reimbursement and disability policies to encourage patients' increased return to work and outlined the components of promising model rehabilitation programs. However, except for the support they provided for the eventual establishment of the United States Renal Data System (USRDS), the Task Force recommendations received little attention. The USRDS was created in 1988 and provides an important source of data about ESRD patients' mortality and treatment modality experience, but it is not the clinical information system called for by the Rehabilitation Task Force and does not routinely collect rehabilitation-relevant data on variables such as patients' educational or employment status.

The 1986 Omnibus Budget Reconciliation Act mandated "that the maximum number of patients who are suitable candidates for vocational rehabilitation services be given access to such services and encouraged to return to gainful employment," but no specific guidelines to accomplish these objectives have ever been formulated.

In early 1994, the media again questioned the value of maintaining patients on dialysis (such as, Associated Press, 1994), following the publication in the *Journal of the American Medical Association (JAMA)* of a paper describing "dismal" rehabilitation in a sample of 104 dialysis patients ages 65+ (Ifudu et al., 1994a). The authors of the *JAMA* paper reinforced their allegations of "dismal" rehabilitation in a second paper, describing disappointing functional status and employment outcomes in a sample of 430 patients ages 21-92 years (Ifudu et al., 1994b).

Just as the Rehabilitation Task Force was organized by HCFA in 1981, following the OSDA and Gutman reports, there were efforts on the national level in 1994 to provide a constructive response to rehabilitation issues in the ESRD Program. A multidisciplinary group of renal patients, providers, policy specialists, researchers, and the Life Options Rehabilitation Advisory Council became active, and a National Workshop on Barriers to Rehabilitation of Persons with ESRD was organized by the National Kidney and Urologic Diseases Advisory Board (A historic gathering, 1994). At the same time, the need for outcomes assessment and evaluation of medical effectiveness was being stressed in virtually all areas of health care.

For the most part, the approach to rehabilitation since the beginning of the ESRD Program has been to arrange specific services for patients, for example, a physical therapy consult or referral to a vocational rehabilitation counselor, on a largely ad hoc basis. The Institute of Medicine Committee for the Study of the Medicare ESRD Program concluded that both kidney transplant and dialysis patients generally lack the rehabilitation services they need (Rettig & Levinsky, 1991). Data collected in the National Kidney Dialysis and Kidney Transplantation Study (NKDKTS) indicated that approximately half of the patients represented in that study had received *no* rehabilitation services (Evans, Manninen, Garrison, & Hart, 1983). Additional studies have shown that relatively few renal patients report receiving vocational rehabilitation services (OSDA, 1980; Kutner, Brogan, & Fielding, 1991). Transplanted patients report receiving more services than do dialysis patients, but even the majority of patients with kidney transplants seem to lack access to services to assist them posttransplant with issues regarding immunosuppressive regimen, nutrition, psychosocial concerns, and vocational objectives (McKevitt & Norwood, 1993). Moreover, receiving isolated services is unlikely to promote successful rehabilitation. A coordinated plan must exist; "the essence of the rehabilitation process is that all its parts be integrated" (Chyatte, 1979b, p. 29).

Improving the level of rehabilitation among ESRD patients requires care-providers to move beyond emphasizing survival as the main element of ESRD care, to promoting functional outcomes and well-being for stable patients. Ironically, one of the recommendations of the Inspector General's report in 1980 was to "broaden the assessment process through which care plans are developed" (OSDA, 1980). Promoting functional gains extends beyond facilitating patients' *adjustment* to their disease status and treatment regimens. Targeted clinical protocols must be developed and implemented with renal patients, as they are with cardiac patients, in order to reduce risk factors for increased disability and to restore and maintain patients' functional status. When all members of the treatment team adopt this perspective on the goal of renal therapy, a major step toward improved rehabilitation occurs.

Defining Rehabilitation

Rehabilitation begins with an evaluation process to identify problems that need solutions, followed by a program of positive action and follow-up with feedback (Chyatte, 1979b). These steps closely parallel the assessment, planning, implementation, and evaluation components of the nursing process (Robinson, 1993), and nephrology nurses should therefore be natural rehabilitation catalysts. Dr. Samuel Chyatte, a physiatrist and a dialysis patient himself, wrote, "I learned long ago that an experienced nurse can be a great source of medical and supervisory wisdom" who frequently challenges the physician to "look as if he's on the ball" (Chyatte, 1979a, p.95).

Rehabilitation can be defined as a process that mobilizes an individual's residual capacity for optimal function in his or her usual environment (Lippman, 1985). This definition does not preclude the possibility that rehabilitation accomplishes a return to premorbid functioning, but it seems to be a more useful definition for individuals who are likely to have one or more chronic conditions and/or may be elderly. The concepts included in the definition — *process, mobilizes, residual capac-*

ity, optimal function, usual environment — all represent significant elements of rehabilitation.

The "ideal rehabilitation opportunity" has been described as "a coordinated program of medical treatment, education, counseling, and dietary and exercise regimens designed to maximize...vocational potential, functional status, and quality of life" (Life Options, 1994, p.2). Five main outcome goals for patients with kidney failure include:

- enhanced fitness to improve physical functioning;
- increased control over the effects of kidney disease and dialysis;
- improved understanding about adaptation and options for living well with dialysis;
- employment for those who are able to work; and
- resumption of activities enjoyed prior to dialysis.

Enhanced rehabilitation opportunity for renal patients requires interdisciplinary, comprehensive care planning to coordinate services that begin, whenever possible, pre-ESRD treatment. As Dr. Chyatte noted, it is the integration of all the parts of the rehabilitation process into a system that has been most notably neglected (Chyatte, 1979b). The focus of the rehabilitation system should be the individual's opportunity for optimal functioning across multiple domains. Functional outcomes are, therefore, key indicators of the quality of care that patients receive.

The Rehabilitation Process and Disability Classification

The primary source of information about the epidemiology of disability in the United States is the National Health Interview Survey (NHIS), which identifies causes of activity-related disability. Survey respondents are asked about limitation of major activity due to any health condition, physical or mental. Major activity is defined as ordinary play for children under 5 years of age, attending school for persons 5-17 years of age, working or keeping house for persons 18-69 years of age, and capacity for independent living for persons aged 70 and older. For individuals aged 70 and older, "unable" to perform major activity means needs assistance in performing activities of daily living (ADL); "limited in kind or amount of major activity" means needs assistance only in performing instrumental activities of daily living (IADL). Based on recent NHIS data, about 14% of people in the U.S., of all ages, living outside of institutions, are limited in activities considered normal for their age group (Verbrugge, 1989; Zola, 1993).

It is estimated that about one-third (32%) of reported disability in the U.S. is due to chronic disease. Other primary sources of disability are mobility limitations (38%), sensory limitations (8%), and intellectual limitations (7%); a miscellaneous "other" disability category comprises the remaining 15% (NCMRR, 1993, p.22). Many individuals with a specific chronic disease such as ESRD may experience limitations representative of several disability categories, which illustrates the difficulty of generating precise disability statistics. In addition, variation in the severity of individuals' limitations and in the presence of co-morbidity further complicates the picture. It is clear, however, that chronic disease is a major contributor to disability in this country.

A Conceptual Model of the Rehabilitation Process

The NCMRR recommends a systems approach in order to understand the complexities involved

Figure 14-1
The rehabilitation process: A systems approach.

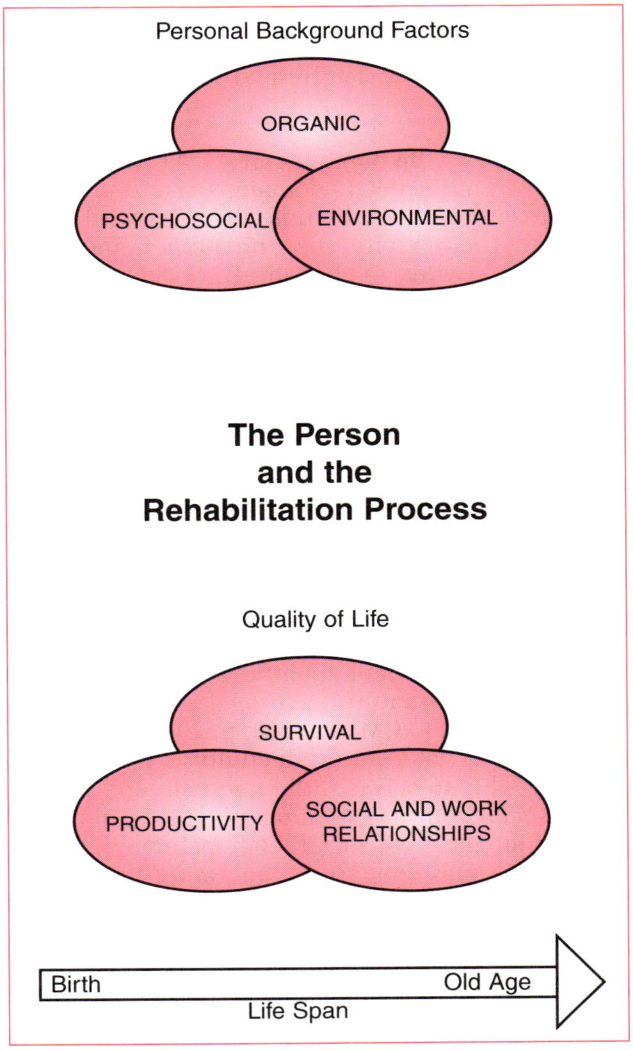

for each individual undergoing rehabilitation (see Figure 14-1). Bidirectional arrows in Figure 14-1 reflect the complexities, feedback loops, and integrating aspects of the process. The individual is viewed as the primary focus of this model. Each person brings unique personal background factors to the rehabilitation process that shape that individual's response to a given situation. In addition, both the person and the rehabilitation process are affected by the health care environment and the larger society.

Personal background factors. Three categories of personal background factors are emphasized: organic, psychosocial, and environmental. *Organic factors* shape a particular individual's reaction to disability onset and that individual's capacity for daily functioning; these factors include characteristics such as endurance, strength, general health status, and genetic predisposition to certain disorders. *Psychosocial factors* might be described as internal "enabling resources" that the individual brings to life situations (Patrick & Erickson, 1993), for example self-reliance, problem-solving, social skills, and ability to cope with stress. Finally, *environmental factors* are resources available externally to the individual, such as family and interpersonal support, income, transportation, and health care access.

Quality of life domains. In the NCMRR model, the quality of life (QOL) domains that are shaped by the process of rehabilitation are survival, broadly defined; productivity, also broadly defined; and social and work relationships. *Survival* issues include not just staying alive, but also preventing complications, maintaining capacity for mobility, and maintaining control of the usual tasks of daily living. Productivity, broadly defined, has especially strong emphasis as a desired outcome:

> The outcomes of the medical rehabilitation process are strategies, products, and treatments which enhance the probability that people with disabilities will participate in society. Activities that enhance productivity and give a sense of purpose and enjoyment to life must be possible; these may include employment, education, recreation, family, and community involvement. This participation should provide meaning and dignity to life so that people with disability have a reason to live, not merely to exist (NCMRR, 1993, p. 29).

Closely related to productivity is the outcome of being able to successfully maintain and manage one's *social and work relationships* — development and maintenance of social relationships with family, friends, and co-workers; and ability to manage finances, and personal and work life.

Life span issues. Life span issues, represented horizontally at the bottom of Figure 14-1, are viewed as modifying both personal background factors and potential QOL outcomes. Intervention strategies, life activities, and QOL outcomes will vary according to the individual's age. An individual's place in the developmental cycle shapes the disability experience and the requirements of an effective rehabilitation process. For example, an initial impairment may be complicated by succeeding impairments across the life span. Potential variations in function across time are important considerations in building a conceptual model of rehabilitation.

Domains of Science and the Medical Rehabilitation Process

The NCMRR specifies five domains of science relevant for rehabilitation research: pathophysiology, impairment, functional limitation, disability, and societal limitation. These domains reflect the range of problems involved in the recovery, restoration, and maintenance of function in persons with disabilities. The system builds on the classification approach presented in the Institute of Medicine report, *Disability in America* (Pope & Tarlov, 1991), with the addition of the concept of societal limitation and the stipulation that progression from one conceptual domain to another is not always sequential or unidirectional.

Table 14-1 includes examples provided by the NCMRR of issues within the five domains that can affect rehabilitation for adults with spinal cord injury or multiple sclerosis, or for a child born with cerebral palsy; readers will be able to think of parallel examples of rehabilitation issues for adults or children with chronic renal failure.

Dialysis and transplantation assist in replacing impaired organ function that is lost due to chronic renal disease (pathophysiology), but multiple organ system effects of chronic renal failure can contribute to residual impairment and to functional limitation. Additional potential sources of impairment, functional limitation, and/or disability for ESRD patients are concurrent disease (for example, diabetes) and chronic conditions (for example, the aging process). Finally, ESRD patients encounter societal limitation if they are restricted because of social policy or other barriers (structural or attitudinal) in fulfilling roles or gaining access to services and opportunities associated with full participation in society. The terms impairment, functional limitation, disability, and handicap (societal limitations) tend to be used interchangeably in everyday discussions, but rehabilitation specialists view these terms as representing conceptually important distinctions.

The classification system in Table 14-1 portrays the diversity and breadth of activities that are essential for rehabilitation. Rehabilitation must address a broad spectrum of issues: biological phenomena at the fundamental levels of tissue, cellular, and molecular events; the impairment of organs or body parts; the functioning of organ systems; individuals' response to a reduction or loss of func-

Table 14-1 — Domains of science relevant to medical rehabilitation research.

Pathophysiology	Impairment	Functional Limitation	Disability	Society Limitation
Interruption of or interference with normal physiological and developmental processes or structure.	Loss and/or abnormality of cognitive, emotional, physiological, or anatomical structure or function; including all losses or abnormalities, not just those attributable to the initial pathophysiology.	Restriction or lack of ability to perform an action in the manner or within a range consistent with the purpose of an organ or organ system.	Inability or limitation in performing tasks, activities, and roles to levels expected within physical and social contexts.	Restriction, attributable to social policy or barriers (structural or attitudinal), which limits fulfillment of roles or denies access to services and opportunities that are associated with full participation in society.
		Level of Impact		
Cell & Tissues	*Organs & Organ Systems*	*Function of Organ & Organ Systems*	*Individual*	*Society*
Structural or functional	Structural or functional	Action or activity performance of organ or organ system.	Task performance by person in physical and social contexts.	Societal attributes relevant to individuals with disability.
		Examples		
1. Adult with high spinal cord damage. Traumatic injury to cells and tracts within the cervical spinal cord.	Primary damage to central nervous system and autonomic nervous system, secondary effects on lungs, bladder, bowel.	Absent, or limited, movement of legs and/or arms. Limited ability to cough. Dysfunction of bowel and bladder.	Bodily functions require more time and assistance. Change in job status. Unable to perform previous hobbies and recreational activities.	Difficulties in finding employment. Health insurer will not pay to assistive device or purchase of van. Lack of involvement in social activities due to public buildings and facilities being inaccessible.
2. Child with cerebral palsy — present at birth. Abnormal development of or perinatal injury to the central nervous system.	Excess muscle contraction, excess reflex activity, poor control of balance and posture.	Slow and inefficient movements. Difficulty with reaching, grasping, and walking. Difficulties with activities of daily living such as eating, dressing, and hygiene.	Lacks independence in mobility. Not independent with family or peers. Requires assistance for school and recreational activities.	Lack of full integration in school activities. Lack of health insurer coverage for payment of powered wheelchair.
3. Adult with multiple sclerosis. Demyelination of centra nervous system axons.	Decreased control of movement and balance. Hearing and visual difficulties. Symptoms fluctuated across time.	Difficulty in walking. Unable to type or write. Blurred vision. Hard of hearing.	At times, may lack independence in mobility; at other times, may be nearfully independent in mobility. May need corrective lenses or be legally blind.	Employer may not be accommodating to progressive or fluctuating course of multiple symptoms. May be unable to afford personal assistant for activities of daily living.

Modified from work initially developed by the Institute of Medicine and published in *Disability in America*, 1991.

tion; and the interactions of individuals with their physical, social, and societal environment. The focus of rehabilitation is the individual, the site at which all of these issues intersect. Effective rehabilitation depends not only on maximum restoration of functioning of affected organs and the individual, but also on the restoration of the individual's maximum functioning within society (NCMRR, 1993).

Physical, Psychosocial, and Vocational Issues in Renal Rehabilitation

Physical Issues

The skills of rehabilitation medicine specialists (physiatrists) have not been widely applied in the care of renal patients. A basic physiatric approach to the patient, as outlined by Cardenas (1989), begins with a history of present illness, current function (which can be anything from walking to working), and — in the case of an inpatient consultation — prehospitalization function and prehospitalization living situation. The history and assessment of function are followed by the physical examination. If the history reveals a disability, the physical examination serves not only to assess impairments and functional limitations, but also to determine residual strengths upon which to build in an effort to reestablish functional skills (Chyatte, 1979b; Stolov, 1984).

The physical examination includes not only the traditional examination but also a detailed neurologic and musculoskeletal exam with manual muscle testing and range of motion assessment, a mental status examination, and a functional neuromuscular examination (testing, for example, standing balance and ambulation). By "functional examination," the physiatrist means the translation of objective neurologic, musculoskeletal, and mental status examinations into performance. The examination measures the patient's skill in executing ADLs at a given point in time. This provides a point from which improvement can occur through treatment, even when the basic disease process cannot be changed (Stolov, 1984).

Problems, goals, and initial treatment are defined based on the physical examination. Problems may range from generalized weakness secondary to decreased activity, deconditioning, and unemployment, to total dependence in mobility and ADLs. Goals may range from general conditioning to comprehensive rehabilitation. Examples of initial treatment prescriptions are bracing or application of prosthesis and gait training, strengthening and range of motion exercises, ADL training, general conditioning exercises, and referral for psychological or vocational counseling (Cardenas, 1989). Finally, an adequate maintenance program must be determined so that functional gains, once made, are not progressively lost (Kottke, Stillwell, & Lehmann, 1984).

While evaluation by a physiatrist may not be routinely available to renal patients, renal professionals can ensure that appropriate exercise and physical conditioning are a routine part of renal patients' care. The appropriate role of exercise training in management of renal patients will be more clearly defined through research on the interaction between exercise training and patients' receipt of Epoetin alfa (Painter & Moore, 1994). Although a number of studies have shown improvements in renal failure patients' perceived functional ability and QOL in association with receipt of Epoetin therapy (Levin, 1992), renal patients' exercise tolerance tends to remain limited. However, even low-risk, low-impact exercise programs can improve patients' general conditioning and energy levels, as well as their feelings of well-being and control over their health (for example, Jagusch & Butchart, 1985; Underwood, Cardenas, & Kutner, 1985).

Exercise is a generic health-promotion intervention with demonstrated physiological and psychosocial benefits for persons of all ages and for persons who have various health problems and disabilities (Vallbona & Baker, 1984; Fletcher, 1988; Stamford, 1988). Exercise can benefit the musculoskeletal and the cardiovascular systems in a variety of ways. In addition, people who exercise regularly are less likely to report anxiety, depressive symptoms, or feelings of stress (Springer, 1990), and they may report an enhanced sense of control over the body and over life (Sobie & Lewis, 1989). Increased physical activity and fitness is listed at the top of the priority areas found in the health promotion/disease prevention agenda known as "Healthy People 2000" (Mason & McGinnis, 1990).

The benefits of exercise for ESRD patients are discussed in a number of studies (Goldberg, Hagberg, Delmez, Florman, & Harter, 1979; Goldberg et al., 1983; Hagberg et al., 1983; Painter & Zimmerman, 1986; Painter et al., 1986; Painter, 1988). With exercise training, ESRD patients show improvement in exercise capacity, lipid metabolism, glucose metabolism, hypertension, and hematologic effects. The contribution of exercise to stress management and improved sense of well-being in ESRD patients has also been demonstrated in a number of studies (for example, Carney et al., 1983; Boettcher, 1989; Brunier & Graydon, 1993).

Renal patients tend to have low tolerances for exercise stemming from the multi-system effects of kidney failure and from muscle changes (Painter & Zimmerman, 1986; Diesel, Noakes, Swanepoel, & Lambert, 1990; Painter & Moore, 1994). Patients are more likely to be physically active if they receive direct encouragement from dialysis staff (Newmann, 1983; Painter, 1993). Painter and Carlson (1994) stress that nurses can have a tremendous impact on patients' involvement in efforts to improve physical functioning, because their expectations, encouragement, and support significantly influence patients' efforts in this area. Four steps are outlined by Painter and Carlson (1994) for dialysis staff to follow. Step 1 is recommended as a standard; the additional steps should be incorporated whenever possible:

Step 1: Incorporate exercise into the patient care plan. This process starts with adding the following question to the routine patient assessment: What are you doing for regular exercise? The question signals the patient that regular physical activity, like medications and dialysis, is an important part of treatment. When exercise is viewed as something "extra but not essential" or is simply not mentioned at all, patients are unlikely to consider it important and probably will not do it.

It is helpful to give patients basic information on the benefits of regular exercise, what they should and can do, and how to get started. Useful resources are the patient pamphlet *Fitness for Life after Kidney Failure*, available from the National Kidney Foundation; and *Pep Up Your Life*, available from the American Association of Retired Persons.

Step 2: Automatically refer patients for physical therapy. Physical therapy for dialysis patients is covered by Medicare Part B. Visits may be limited to eight sessions in some cases; but for ambulatory patients and those whose physical function is good, this number is probably enough to educate them on what they need to do independently to increase strength and endurance. Extensions for coverage can be obtained for patients who need more intensive physical therapy, as long as there is a documented need for continued services and the patient is progressing toward the goals established by the physical therapist.

Step 3: Develop contacts with community programs for referral of patients. These might include programs at the YMCA, Jewish Community Centers, senior citizens' centers, local recreation programs, or cardiac rehabilitation programs. Activities appropriate for many dialysis patients include low-impact aerobics, water exercise or swimming, yoga, and low-level strengthening programs.

In addition to community programs, dialysis staff or a group of patients may want to organize a regular walking club. Patients could meet weekly at a park or 3 days a week at the dialysis center before treatment. Patients can participate at the level they choose, and such an activity encourages socializing and peer support.

Motivation is an integral part of any exercise program. Staff can use motivational strategies in the center to encourage patients who are exercising independently at home or in a community program. Motivational strategies might include using charts to track the amount of time spent in participation, the distance walked or cycled, or the number of exercise sessions attended. Charts should be updated weekly and placed in a visible location to help motivate other patients to start their own programs. A state map on which patients recorded the distance they walked for exercise was a useful motivational strategy in a project involving older dialysis patients (Ennis & Miko, 1988).

The President's Council on Physical Fitness also provides a way to promote exercise participation. In this program, individuals record their activity on sheets provided by the Council. When they achieve a certain goal, they send in their records and receive a patch and certificate of achievement.

Step 4: Develop an incenter program. Providing the opportunity for patients to exercise at their treatment center represents strong staff commitment to the value of this activity. Stationary exercise bicycles may be used before or during patients' dialysis treatment. This type of program has been successfully implemented in several centers: An exercise physiologist gets patients started, advises staff members on their role, and facilitates the continuation of the program as a part of the treatment, with cooperation from patients and staff. An incenter program featuring dance-like movements performed to music was successfully implemented by Jagusch and Butchart (1985). A video demonstrating chair exercises performed during hemodialysis treatment is available (Southeastern Kidney Council [SKC], 1992).

If staff members decide that an incenter program is desirable, they should understand that there are no fixed guidelines for such a program. They may want to start with their most stable patients until staff, physicians, and patients are comfortable with the intervention. Consultation with a physical therapist or an exercise physiologist is suggested when initiating an incenter program.

It is very important to select exercise that fits a patient's needs. In patients who are not candidates for aerobic exercise, simple exercises such as stretching can increase muscle flexibility and enhance feelings of doing something to promote own health. Painter and Carlson (1994) suggest that patients who are nonambulatory or have difficulty walking, who have severe muscle wasting, or who are severely deconditioned would probably benefit most from an automatic referral to physical therapy for muscle strengthening, gait training, and help with ambulation. Patients with significant cardiac involvement may qualify for cardiac rehabilitation programs for exercise conditioning. Fully ambulatory patients who have minimal comorbidity could be given information to enable them to exercise independently at home or in a community-based program. Whatever the patient's specific needs, information about the value of exercise, along with ongoing encouragement and reinforcement for this health-promotion behavior, are essential components of a rehabilitation plan.

Psychosocial Issues

Another chapter in this unit deals specifically with the psychosocial impact of renal disease, and the special case of psychosocial outcomes in elderly patients is discussed in the next section of this chapter.

Psychosocial measures (for example, measures of well-being, mood, distress) tap an outcome area that is a complex product of personality and coping styles, as well as health status and disease experience. Individuals appear to differ in ability to withstand stress, an aspect of demonstrating resilience, which in turn is identified by Patrick and Erickson (1993) as a domain of the opportunity concept of health-related QOL. In addition, people's assessments of well-being are made within contexts that are salient to them — for example, relative to other people my age, relative to other people in my community, etc. — and may therefore not seem consistent with the individual's situation as viewed by an external observer. For example, Evans et al. (1985) reported an average level of life satisfaction among ESRD patients that was not significantly different from the general population. However, it is clinically important to consider potentially manipulatable factors (for example, activity/exercise, self-care participation, treatment modality, enabling resources in the patient's social environment) that may affect patients' subjective well-being, and to monitor potential change over time in patients' subjective well-being. The NCMRR notes that although the central purpose of this new agency is to "incorporate medical rehabilitation into the mainstream of medicine...this does not mean that the psychosocial aspect should be de-emphasized. On the contrary, these two aspects are intimately related..." (NCMRR, 1993, p.27)

It appears that multi-item, generic indexes measuring *function* (how people are functioning within their lives) and multi-item, generic indexes measuring *feeling* (how people feel about their lives) are often weakly correlated (Deniston, Carpentier-Alting, Kneisley, Hawthorne, & Port 1989). For example, based on interviews with 742 ESRD patients in Michigan, Deniston et al. (1989) found a weak correlation (.28) between responses to the physical performance dimension of the Sickness Impact Profile (Bergner, Bobbitt, Carter, & Gilson, 1981) and responses to the Affect Balance Scale (Bradburn, 1969), which measures mood during the past week. Similarly, Kutner (1994a) found a relatively weak correlation (.39) between older dialysis patients' scores on a functional impairment index that assessed ADL performance and mobility (House, 1989-90) and these patients' scores on a widely used depression index (Radloff, 1977). Stronger associations may exist between measures of physical symptoms and affect or emotion measures that are disease-specific, that is, known to be closely linked with a particular disease, than among more generic measures of function and psychosocial status. For example, in a trial investigating effects associated with dialysis patients' use of erythropoietin (EPO), fatigue and other physical symptom components of a disease-specific instrument (a "Kidney Disease Questionnaire") were moderately to highly correlated with the depression, frustration, and relationship components of that same instrument (Laupacis, Wong, Churchill, & The Canadian Erythropoietin Study Group, 1991). A better understanding is needed of how specific comorbid conditions and physical symptoms associated with chronic renal failure relate to patients' functional status and psychosocial well-being.

Ongoing encouragement and education provided by staff is likely to be among the most important strategies for promoting psychosocial well-being among renal patients (Life Options, 1994). Patients benefit from receiving continuing messages about what they *can,* rather than what they *cannot*, do (for example, Painter, 1993).

Vocational Issues

While employment is only one aspect of rehabilitation, being employed carries important potential self-esteem and social rewards for individuals. In addition, a higher percentage of employed patients reflects a more positive overall image of the ESRD Program to the larger society. Dialysis patients' retreat from participation in the labor force increases net costs to society (Garner & Dardis, 1987; Rettig & Levinsky, 1991). There is an official expectation on the part of the federal government that more ESRD patients should be employed. The 1986 Omnibus Budget Reconciliation Act (OBRA-1986-PL 99-509, § 9335 [h]) mandated that "the maximum number of patients who are suitable candidates for vocational rehabilitation services be given access to such services and encouraged to return to gainful employment."

Cross-sectional surveys consistently indicate that no more than about 20% of working-age patients on dialysis are formally employed (Kutner & Brogan, 1985; Curtin, Oberley, & Friedman, 1994). Data for an incident cohort analyzed in a Special Study and summarized in the USRDS 1991 Annual Data Report (p. 9) showed that 55% of ESRD patients were in the labor force the year before onset, a figure that dropped to 44% at the onset of ESRD. Based on the data from this special study, patients who were employed 1 year prior to ESRD onset and were still employed at ESRD onset were significantly more likely to have had at least some college education, be in a professional occupation, have had medical insurance before start of ESRD, *not* to have diabetes as a cause of their renal failure or a history of diabetes, and *not* to have cardiovascular comorbid conditions (Kutner 1994c).

Recent studies indicate that there is a group of patients who are not currently working who acknowledge that they are able to work and would like to work. This group may include 20%-30% of patients ages 18-59 who are not currently employed (Kutner, Brogan, & Fielding, 1991; Curtin et al., 1994). There has long been anecdotal evidence that some dialysis patients who are not formally employed do engage in activities for which they receive money, that is, work "off the books" (Neff, Slifkin, & Eiser, 1981). Vocational incentives for those who have the potential to work must be identified (Domoto, 1994). It is reasonable to believe that it is possible to increase the number of employed ESRD patients, if appropriate candidates are identified and supported in their efforts to enter the job market.

A vocational rehabilitation workgroup was convened during a National Workshop on Barriers to Rehabilitation of Persons with End Stage Renal Disease and Chronic Urinary Incontinence, organized by the National Kidney and Urologic Diseases Advisory Board (NKUDAB) in 1994. The workgroup identified the following factors as being especially significant barriers that discourage renal patients from labor market participation:

- inflexible treatment scheduling in dialysis units;
- treatment providers who discourage employment;
- inadequate readiness on the part of renal clients to access vocational rehabilitation (VR) services;
- lack of advocacy for ESRD clients in job placement; and
- fear of benefits loss with return to work.

The first four of these barriers can be markedly altered by changes in renal care providers' outlook on the importance of encouraging employment among patients who believe that they are able to work. Candidates who have employment potential should be screened for referral to VR specialists, with follow-up contacts to furnish additional information and to monitor candidates' progress. This requires ongoing cooperation between VR service providers and renal care staff, and both must take responsibility to strengthen these linkages.

Whenever possible, there should be cooperative efforts focused on early intervention to restructure job requirements *before* workers withdraw from employment. Most dialysis and transplant patients who are employed are individuals who never stopped working (Friedman & Rogers, 1988; McKevitt & Norwood, 1993). Rasgon et al. (1993) compared employment outcomes for 45 ESRD patients who received a predialysis orientation program and 57 ESRD patients who did not receive such a program. All patients were started on incenter dialysis. Their mean age was 50. The educational levels of the two groups were not significantly different, and they did not differ significantly in presence of diabetes or in pretreatment functional status as measured by the Karnofsky Scale (Karnofsky & Burchenal, 1949). The predialysis intervention consisted of physician referral to a licensed clinical social worker prior to the start of dialysis therapy; social worker assessment of patient and significant others; patient education and counseling regarding treatment options, adjustment to chronic illness, and maintaining predialysis activities; orientation to the dialysis unit; and follow-up by the entire renal care team. Compared to patients who did not receive the intervention, a significantly higher percentage of patients who received the intervention continued working after beginning dialysis, and the difference was even more pronounced when only patients in blue-collar jobs were compared. Individuals in lower socioeconomic status jobs are especially likely to leave the labor market when they start ESRD treatment, and the effect of early intervention on job retention in this study is impressive.

The fifth barrier listed by the NKUDAB workgroup, fear of jeopardizing the security provided by disability income and related benefits, is not specific to renal patients. This barrier affects individuals with many disabilities and must be addressed within the broad system of welfare reform. However, even the existing system of disability benefits allows patients to test their ability to function in a paid employment situation, and renal care providers can furnish information to patients about the options available to them (see Table 14-2).

Special Populations in Renal Rehabilitation

Rehabilitation protocols can be targeted to the needs of special populations of patients. The field of cardiac rehabilitation provides a good example. Exercise training protocols for cardiac patients take into consideration the patient's type of drug therapy, type of cardiac disease (for example, heart failure, peripheral vascular disease), comorbid disease or conditions (for example, diabetes mellitus, musculoskeletal deficiencies), and age. Activity guidelines are recommended for classes of cardiac patients who demonstrate specified profiles with respect to type of therapy, primary disease, comorbidity, and age (Fletcher, 1992). Given the prevalence of cardiovascular comorbidity among renal patients, cardiac rehabilitation protocols may prove useful in the development of activity guidelines that can be recommended for classes or categories of renal patients.

Renal rehabilitation service protocols can be developed to address the needs of patient categories such as: treatment modality groups, the diabetic patient, pediatric patient, and the geriatric patient. Separate chapters in this text also address the care of patients in relation to these categories.

Table 14-2
A desktop guide to Social Security and SSI work incentives.

Special rules make it possible for people with disabilities receiving Social Security or Supplemental Security Income (SSI) to work and still receive monthly cash payments and Medicare or Medicaid. Social Security calls these rules "work incentives." Some rules are different for Social Security and SSI beneficiaries. Following are the rules that apply under each program. For more copies or additional materials on work incentives, contact any Social Security office.

Social Security

Trial Work Period — A nine-month period, not necessarily consecutive during, which the earnings of a Social Security beneficiary who is blind or disabled will not affect his or her benefit. (The nine months of work must occur within a 60-month period.)

Extended Period of Eligibility — For at least three years after a successful trial work period, a Social Security beneficiary who is blind or disabled may receive a disability check for any month that his/her earnings are below the substantial gainful activity level (in 1994, $500 for people who are disabled, $930 for people who are blind).

Continuation of Medicare — If Social Security disability payments stop because a person has earnings at or above the substantial gainful activity level, but the person is still disabled, Medicare can continue for at least 39 months after the trial work period. After that, the person can buy Medicare coverage by paying a monthly premium.

Recovery During Vocational Rehabilitation — If a person recovers while participating in a vocational rehabilitation program that is likely to lead to becoming self-supporting, benefits may continue until the program ends.

Special Rules For Persons Who Are Blind — Several special rules apply to working beneficiaries who are blind. For example, they can earn up to $930 before their benefits are affected. Ask at the Social Security office for details on work incentives for beneficiaries who are blind.

Supplemental Security Income (SSI)

Continuation of SSI — Working SSI recipients who are blind or disabled may continue to receive payments until countable income exceeds SSI limits.

Continuation of Medicaid Eligibility — Medicaid may continue for SSI recipients who are blind or disabled and earn over the SSI limits, if they cannot afford similar medical care and depend on Medicaid in order to work.

Plan for Achieving Self-Support — An SSI recipient who is blind or disabled may set aside income and resources for up to 48 months toward an approved plan for achieving self-support (PASS).

Impairment-Related Work Expenses — Certain expenses for things a person with a disability needs because of his/her impairment in order to work may be deducted when counting earnings to determine if a person is eligible and to figure the payment amount. For working persons who are blind, the work expenses need not be related to the impairment.

Recovery During Vocational Rehabilitation — If a person recovers while participating in a vocational rehabilitation program that is likely to lead to becoming self-supporting, benefits may continue until the program ends.

Sheltered Workshop Payments — Pay received in a sheltered workshop is treated as earned income, regardless of whether it is considered wages for other purposes. This enables Social Security to exclude more of the sheltered workshop employee's earnings when computing his/her SSI payment.

Students With Disabilities — Tuition, books, and other expenses related to getting an education may not be counted as income for recipients who go to school or are in a training program.

U.S. Department of Health and Human Services

Social Security Administration

SSA Publication No. 005-11002

January 1994

ICN 480240

ESRD Treatment Modality and Rehabilitation

Better rehabilitation and (QOL) outcomes for renal patients are attributed to treatment by transplantation as compared to treatment by dialysis (for example, Evans et al., 1985; Simmons & Abress, 1990), and renal transplantation is therefore considered the treatment of choice for patients with chronic renal failure (Suthanthiran & Strom, 1994). Although kidney transplantation can restore medical health in ways that chronic dialysis cannot, receipt of a kidney transplant does not automatically accomplish optimal rehabilitation. A number of physiological system alterations and behavioral changes are common to end-stage patients who undergo transplantation and require immunosuppressive regimens. Posttransplant immunosuppressive regimens are potentially associated with alteration in metabolism, leading to weight gain; hyperlipidemia, or steroid-induced diabetes; alteration in stability of connective tissue; muscle weakness and pain; and hypertension. In addition, depression is frequently observed both pre- and posttransplant; mood swings are common in patients on immunosuppressive regimens, especially in the first year posttransplant. These behavioral problems significantly affect patients' social functioning and vocational rehabilitation potential. Rehabilitation-oriented interventions in the pretransplant phase, the acute phase, and the long-term posttransplant phase could significantly improve patients' functional capacity and related QOL (Kutner, 1993).

Rehabilitation can be incorporated into an extended plan of medical management of the transplant patient. For example:

1. **Pretransplant**
   - exercise training to improve maximal oxygen update and exercise tolerance
   - education regarding immunological therapy and potential side effects
2. **Acute phase**
   - minimizing sensory deprivation
   - minimizing physical deconditioning
   - prevention of unnecessary complications: contractures, skin problems
3. **Posttransplant**
   - appropriate exercise training to improve exercise capacity and promote wellness (suggested guidelines for "Fitness for Life After Transplant" are available from Painter, 1992)
   - continued education regarding medication administration, interpreting lab values, and blood monitoring
   - psychosocial support services to optimize familial and societal functioning

Among dialysis patients, better functional status and QOL outcomes are attributed to treatment by home hemodialysis (HHD), continuous ambulatory peritoneal dialysis (CAPD), and continuous cycling peritoneal dialysis (CCPD) than to treatment by incenter, full care hemodialysis (HD) (for example, Evans et al., 1985; Kutner, Brogan & Kutner, 1986; Wolcott & Nissenson, 1988). However, the case-mix of patients selected into these therapies differs, which means that outcomes may reflect differential patient selection rather than modality effects. Simmons and Abress (1990, pp. 205, 207), who investigated QOL issues for 766 prevalent ESRD patients, concluded that "the ideal way to control for case-mix factors and to study issues of causality would involve a longitudinal study in which patients were followed over time, and baseline pretreatment values would be compared with later states of quality of life...With more knowledge about the personal characteristics of the patients and the aspects of the therapy responsible for success, changes and recommendations for therapeutic choice could be made with more confidence."

More information is needed about what therapies work best for which patients, at which stages of their lives (Scribner, 1987). For example, one study conducted in the Southeast suggested that older white patients may have better QOL outcomes on CAPD or CCPD, while older African-American patients may have better QOL outcomes on incenter HD — perhaps as a function of differential social support available to these patient groups (Kutner, Fielding & Brogan, 1993b).

Regardless of their particular treatment modality, patients are *suppliers*, as well as consumers, of the care process. Kurtin (1991, p.19) noted that "although the patient is the ultimate 'consumer' of the efforts of the staff, it may be useful to reexamine and expand the patient's role in the process of care. Chronic dialysis requires a great deal of patient compliance; however, little attention has been paid to the patient as a 'supplier' of care within the dialysis unit...When viewed in this way...dialysis is no longer something done to a patient, but a process in which the patient actively participates."

The relationship of treatment modality to rehabilitation and QOL outcomes may depend to a large extent on the patient's level of self-care participation. Self-care activities can be encouraged within all treatment groups, including patients on incenter HD treatment. In a unit that successfully emphasizes training for self-care, staff are likely to be surprised when patients who are initially considered unmotivated, learn dialysis procedures and develop self-confidence. Staff must learn to allow patients to work out minor problems, rather than stepping in immediately to help. A contractual relationship should be established between patients and providers, emphasizing patients' responsibilities as technicians and the staff's roles of teacher and consultant (Spooner, 1985).

In a sample of 349 dialysis patients aged 60+ who were studied in Georgia, patients who were participating either in a form of home dialysis or in self-care activities at the dialysis facility had a significantly greater sense of control over their future health ($p < 0.05$) than patients who were receiving full care in the dialysis facility (Kutner, Cardenas & Bower, 1992). Among younger patients as well, patients who have a dominant role in their own care are more likely to feel that they can influence their own health status and are less likely to attribute their health status to chance or to the actions of powerful others (Kutner & Brogan, 1985). Patients who elect to carry out self-care activities may already have a stronger feeling of control over their health at the outset. Thus, these data may reflect a selection bias, and outcomes associated with self-care should be prospectively studied in an incident sample of dialysis patients. However, self-care is considered a fundamental element in medical rehabilitation (Keith, 1984).

The Diabetic Patient

More severe forms of peripheral neuropathy may be seen in diabetic patients, with resulting ambulation and/or hand function problems. Paresis of the dorsiflexors and evertors of the ankle and toe extensors produce foot-drop and steppage gait, which are seldom reversible in diabetic patients. If weakness in borderline and footdrop is barely apparent, simply reducing the shoe weight may improve functioning. If paresis is more pronounced, ankle-foot orthoses with dorsiflexion assist may be added to a lightweight shoe. For distal sensory and motor deficits that affect hand function, an activity of daily living review by an occupational therapist is indicated. Range of motion and mild strengthening exercises for hand and forearm may be beneficial.

Diabetic patients may also be subject to amyotrophy that produces proximal weakness in contrast to the distal weakness of peripheral neuropathy. Because hips, trunk, and shoulders may be affected, mobility can be impaired and rising from a seated position may become difficult. As with distal weakness, mild strengthening and range of motion exercises are indicated. Vigorous exercise is contraindicated because it can produce an overfatigued muscle that requires prolonged recovery and, if extreme, may irreparably damage the weakened muscle. Amyotrophy, more than peripheral neuropathy, is the cause of muscle pain and cramps. These symptoms can be relieved by applying heat and small doses of muscle relaxants (Chyatte, 1979b).

It is essential that diabetic patients receive a carefully individualized exercise prescription, in order to avoid potential hazards such as the musculoskeletal and soft-tissue injuries described above or complications from foot injuries. However, properly prescribed exercise has many potential benefits for diabetic patients, including lowering blood pressure and improving blood lipid profile and energy level (Fletcher, 1992, pp.193-194).

The Pediatric Patient

While there are unique challenges associated with pediatric rehabilitation, there may be an advantage that is frequently not present with older patients — the opportunity for early education and intervention. Pediatric patients are usually referred before renal therapy is actually started, and teaching can be accomplished gradually over the course of many visits.

Because children and young adults are in the process of negotiating important developmental stages in their lives, the term "habilitation," rather than "rehabilitation," may more accurately summarize the goals for this special population (Pediatric Renal Rehabilitation, 1994). Each stage of the young patient's development — infant, preschooler, early school age, adolescence — requires a reevaluation of the individual's needs and treatment. However, the objective in providing renal replacement therapy to pediatric patients is the same as the objective in providing renal replacement therapy to any patient, that is, to maximize the individual's functioning. With younger patients, maximizing age-appropriate functioning is the specific objective.

Optimal functioning for pediatric patients requires optimal functioning in the whole family unit. Despite a child's chronic illness, it is important to promote normalcy within the household. Parents must avoid tendencies to over-protect the child by setting limits and defining the behavior they expect. Needs of the child's siblings must also be acknowledged. In school settings, teachers should be encouraged to have the same expectations of the child as they do of other children. Camp and recreation programs for children with chronic illness offer a "reality test" by providing a setting in which children can safely participate in a range of physical activities that can convince them they are quite capable of being active (McRae, Mullins, Moncrief, & Moncrief, 1988; Page & Pearson, 1990). In short, avoiding the mind set of disability is essential in caring for pediatric patients.

Striving for normalcy is not easy, however; all family members are likely to need support. Parent support groups help to raise optimism about the potential for skill-building, an enhanced lifestyle for pediatric patients, and for their futures as adults. The summer camp experience for pediatric patients provides an opportunity to bond with peers going through similar life challenges.

As with all renal patients, a crucial element of habilitation/rehabilitation for pediatric patients is physical activity and exercise. Specific physical benefits are denser bones and stronger muscles; feeling better physically and an improved body image are likely to be additional benefits. Standard strength testing is used with patients at the University of Wisconsin Children's Hospital to jump-start exercise participation; "Kids can see that they are not all that weak to begin with and that they can become stronger fairly quickly" (Friedman, quoted in Pediatric Renal Rehabilitation, 1994, pp. 3-4). This testing is the basis for prescribing specific individualized strength-building programs. Strength tests are then repeated at each visit so that children can see and measure their own progress, building self-esteem, as well as strength and endurance.

Again, as with all patients, providing information and promoting involvement in their own care should be encouraged. At the Fairfax Hospital for Children-Kidney Center in Virginia, pediatric patients are required to attend all of the team conferences held regarding their care. "Parental attendance is not enough; if kids are there as well, they are more likely to be active participants as opposed to victims" (Ruley, quoted in Pediatric Renal Rehabilitation, 1994, p.5).

For younger pediatric patients, the emphasis is on assuring that individuals can stay in school, continue to achieve at their grade levels academically, and have the opportunity to participate in school activities. For young adults, that is, individuals who are post-high school to late 20s, issues of independence and vocational goals become principal concerns (Thompson, 1990). Young adults who developed chronic renal failure as children often have significantly impaired stature and underdeveloped secondary sex characteristics. Body-image and feelings are affected by disease and treatment experiences such as rapid fluid shifts, required medications, and diet/fluid restrictions. Normal adolescent concern about physical appearance is heightened and is likely to continue into young adulthood. Patients may report peer rejection, or they may fear peer rejection and avoid social contacts with peers. They may continue living with their parents rather than living independently, resulting in a prolonged, ambivalent dependence that is characteristic of adolescence. All of these factors make it difficult for young adult patients to develop a stable sense of self and goals for life (Klein & Simmons, 1977; Magrab & Jacobstein, 1984; Klaskin, 1984).

If the special developmental needs of young people who experience kidney failure early in life can be addressed, these young people are good candidates for vocational development. They can be encouraged to pursue college or technical training that will increase their employability, and it may be possible to influence their thinking about the future before they slip into a permanent nonemployment mode with reliance on the disability system. Programs developed to promote the developmental/vocational habilitation of young renal clients have been very successful. Components of two such model programs, *Springboard* and *Forward Bound*, are summarized in Table 14-3.

The Geriatric Patient

Renal care providers are aware that some elderly patients would be better served *not* to be started on dialysis, but they also know many elderly dialysis patients do well for months or years. In the first case, many would agree that the patients' rehabilitation prospects are dismal. In the second case, however, the patients' rehabilitation prospects are promising. What does the term rehabilitation mean in the case of older patients on chronic dialysis? How can it be meaningfully assessed? Are there important sources of variation in rehabilitation outcomes among older patients?

A 1994 paper published in the *Journal of the American Medical Association* (Ifudu et al., 1994a) stirred extensive discussion with its allegation that geriatric HD patients are characterized by "dismal rehabilitation" (Blagg & Fitts, 1994; Stanton, Andary, & Goldberg, 1994; Chertow, Owen, & Lazarus, 1994; Kutner, 1994b; Lundin, 1994). The study, which was based on interviews with 104 patients aged 65 or older in Brooklyn, New York, alleged that these patients tended to lead "a marginal existence, not participating in family, home, church, or social activities." The research highlighted important issues surrounding functional outcomes on chronic dialysis for patients of all ages, especially the need to: (a) systematically measure and monitor dialysis patients' physical functional status and (b) address as early as possible, and certainly from the outset of treatment, factors that contribute to patients' deconditioning and inactivity (Blagg & Fitts, 1994).

The authors of the Brooklyn study of geriatric patients on HD suggested that rehabilitation means "a return to preillness function" (Ifudu et al., 1994a, p.32). While this is certainly one definition of rehabilitation found in the literature, returning to preillness function is difficult for any patient with a chronic illness. It is also difficult for individuals experiencing physiologic and systemic changes related to aging. For older dialysis patients, functional change is likely to reflect the compounded effects of chronic illness and aging (Brody & Ruff, 1986). As suggested above, a much more realistic rehabilitation objective is to mobilize individuals' residual capacity for optimal function (Lippmann, 1985).

Assessment of functioning is the cornerstone of rehabilitation, pointing to areas of deficiency for which individualized therapy and rehabilitation regimens can be devised (Branch & Meyers, 1987). Information about restricted activity days, bed disability days, self-care ability, and mobility limitations is especially important in monitoring older patients. Geriatric assessment tools, including performance-based measures such as the Physical Performance Test developed by Reuben and Siu (1990), can provide useful data. Table 14-4 outlines

Table 14-3
Model programs developed for young adults with kidney disease.

Springboard (NKF-GA, Inc.)	Forward Bound (NKF-MS, Inc.)
4 weekend retreats (Friday afternoon-Sunday noon) held at different locations across the state for young persons 19-30	3 weekend sessions (Saturday morning-Sunday noon) held at a centrally located group camp setting (in a state park) for young adults 18-37
Weekend #1: Team building, assertiveness training, exercise	Weekend #1: "Tapping into Your Personal Power": Personality styles and communication patterns
Weekend #2: Personal development, dressing and etiquette, dating and sexuality issues, independence and relationships with parents	Weekend #2: "Tapping into Your Vocational Power": Social Security benefits, employment potential, vocational opportunities
Weekend #3: Values clarification, career exploration, job interviewing skills	Weekend #3: "Tapping into Your Relationship Power": Conflict management, communication skills, sexuality issues
Weekend #4: Goal setting, decision-making, "graduation"	

Both programs: Completion of short-term assignments between sessions and participation in follow-up, reunion/refresher weekend retreats

Table 14-4
Comprehensive geriatric assessment.

Dimensions/Domains	Examples of Measures
Physical	Current medications; vision and hearing status; need for assistive devices
Mental	Folstein Mini-Mental State Exam*
Social	Marital status; persons lived with; frequency of visiting/communicating with friends, relatives
Emotional	Philadelphia Geriatric Center Morale Scale*
Economic	Income; health insurance
Functional	Katz Index of Activities of Daily Living*; PGC Instrumental Activities of Daily Living*; Barthel Index*
Environmental	Independent/congregate living situation; transportation access

*For these and other available measures, see R.A. Kane & R. L. Kane. (1988). Assessing the elderly: A practical guide to measurement. Lexington, MA: D.C. Health.

the dimensions of comprehensive geriatric assessment and provides examples of geriatric assessment measures.

All older persons undergoing dialysis do not have the same experience, and it is important to analyze factors that are related to this differential experience. In general, black patients live longer and do better on dialysis than do white patients (Eggers, 1990; Gordon, 1990), but there has been little specific attention to race differences in outcomes among older patients. The National Institute on Aging (NIA) and the National Institute on Diabetes, Digestive and Kidney Diseases (NIDDK) funded a longitudinal study of older (60+) dialysis patients and a control group of age-matched peers not on dialysis (Kutner, Brogan, Fielding, & Hall, 1991; Kutner, Fielding, & Brogan, 1993a). The two samples were purposely selected to facilitate comparison of older blacks and older whites. Baseline interviews with 349 older dialysis patients and 354 older persons not on dialysis indicated that when carefully compared with a comparable group of similar-age peers, older persons on dialysis did in fact report lower QOL. However, a lowered QOL effect was much more evident for older white patients than for older black patients on dialysis. Data for older patients studied in Brooklyn, New York, showed a similar pattern. Among nondiabetic older dialysis patients in the New York sample, white patients had significantly higher functional status (based on a modified Karnofsky scale) 2 years prior to starting dialysis than did black patients. At the time of the study, however, the functional status scores reported by whites and blacks were not significantly different (Ifudu et al., 1994a), indicating that the functional losses associated with becoming a dialysis patient were apparently greater for white patients than for black patients.

In the study supported by NIA/NIDDK, baseline data indicated that older patients' race, along with cardiovascular comorbidity and educational level, significantly influenced patients' reported QOL (Kutner et al., 1993b). Older black patients in the sample were less likely than older white patients to experience dialysis-related physical complications. It has been speculated that blacks may be more likely than whites to die of "competing risks" before reaching kidney failure, so that black persons who begin chronic maintenance dialysis therapy may for this reason constitute a physically hardier group (U.S. Renal Data System, 1992). Eggers (1990) has suggested that "unmeasured severity differences" exist between black and white dialysis patients of all ages.

Longitudinal studies can help to identify contributors to development of poor functional status and QOL in dialysis patients (old and young, black and white), and how these outcomes can be prevented (Blagg & Fitts, 1994). While severe impairment is likely to be quickly recognized by clinicians, moderate impairments in elderly patients are less likely to be identified. In a study of medical inpatients aged 70 and older, Pinholt et al. (1987) found that physicians and nurses correctly identified severe impairment on the basis of clinical judgment, but that the sensitivity of their clinical judgment was poor in detecting moderate impairment in the areas of mental status, vision, and nutrition. Comprehensive functional assessment can detect moderate impairments that can be remediated through early intervention.

Attention to functional deficits can make an important difference even in elderly patients. A Japanese group recently reported that their patients aged 65 and older at the start of HD who had impaired ADLs showed a significant improvement after 2.2 months of participation in a rehabilitation program designed to increase ability to stand and walk unaided (Asai et al., 1993). This study illustrates the utility of evaluating elderly dialysis patients' functional status by means of a standardized instrument and determining the relation of specific disorders to patients' functional status scores. The investigators' evaluation of elderly (71.7 $\pm$ 4.3 years) patients' functional status, and determination of disorders contributing to these outcomes, indicated a need for patients to participate in exercises designed to help them stand and walk without assistance. After 2.2 months of participation in this rehabilitation program, patients' functional status was reevaluated and the majority showed significant improvement in functional status as measured by the Barthel index (a standardized functional status measure). Identifying patients' areas of functional deficit and determining what comorbid factors are related to these deficits provides valuable guidelines for targeting rehabilitation programs capable of improving patients' functioning.

It is likely that "patients...are often not too excited by the prospect of a long-slow course of rehabilitation...Rehabilitation requires the cooperation of the patient, and it is hard work. For many elderly patients, rehabilitation may be the most demanding physical work they have ever faced" (Campion, 1990). However, geriatric rehabilitation has been shown to stand up to the most rigorous type of controlled evaluation of effectiveness. For example, Applegate et al. (1990) found that functionally impaired elderly patients (mean age = 79) who were recovering from acute medical or surgical illnesses and received care in a specialized geriatric rehabilitation unit had significantly more improvement in basic self-care activities and a reduced risk of subsequent nursing home placement than did similar patients who received usual care. Beneficial effects were greater for patients who were at moderate risk, as opposed to high risk, of nursing home placement.

More studies are needed on the effectiveness,

including the cost-effectiveness, of geriatric rehabilitation (Campion, 1990), and this certainly should include geriatric patients placed on chronic dialysis. Strategies are needed to maintain physical function in elderly renal patients who require hospitalization and are subsequently returned to a regimen of outpatient dialysis. Repetitive use of the sensory and motor nerves and synapses associated with movement, as well as the use of the muscles themselves, help prevent loss of movement, speed, strength, and balance (Daleiden & Lewis, 1990). Sensory impairment and muscle atrophy tend to characterize geriatric patients who have poor circulation and cardiovascular insufficiency. Specific exercises can be prescribed to strengthen muscles and increase circulation (see Irwin and Zadai's [1990] recommended evaluation and training programs for the elderly person with possible cardiopulmonary complications). Asking patients to maintain a daily activity log helps to monitor progress and simultaneously encourages patients to accept a long-term commitment to exercise and physical activity (Johnson, Searles, & McNamara, 1993).

The addition of renal failure and chronic dialysis treatment to already existing physical and psychosocial problems associated with aging might be expected to produce "a devastating cumulative effect" (Auer, 1986). Renal failure and dialysis treatment present potential psychological stressors, and aging itself is potentially linked to psychological stressors, for example, bereavement, social isolation, loss of social status and social roles following retirement, and cognitive losses.

A number of investigators have compared older and younger patients on chronic dialysis, using varying definitions to group patients into these two categories. With only a few exceptions, studies that have compared psychosocial outcomes in older and younger patients suggest that outcomes for older patients are at least as good, and perhaps better than, psychosocial outcomes observed in younger patients. The added lifetime that older patients gain on dialysis seems to be satisfying. As noted by Nissenson, Diaz-Buxo, Adcock, & Nelms (1990), elderly patients are likely to require more social and other support services than do younger patients, and receiving these services may be an important contributor to the well-being they report.

Increased understanding of the relation of aging to psychosocial issues in chronic renal failure requires research that is both methodologically sound and theoretically informed. Many studies have used relatively small, convenience samples of patients rather than scientifically selected samples that are large enough to provide sufficient power for statistical analyses. Age criteria for categorizing patients into "older" and "younger" groups has varied among investigators, and the categorization has not necessarily been based on any socially significant independent criteria such as average age of retirement in a given society. However, there are likely to be important differences among individuals of any given chronologic age. Rather than comparing psychosocial outcomes of patients who are grouped into arbitrary age categories, therefore, it is useful to treat age as a continuous variable, and to investigate not only direct effects of age on psychosocial outcomes but also potential interaction effects of age with other variables.

Research using indepth personal interviews with elderly patients, along with selected standardized instruments that assess psychosocial well-being, has suggested that fewer physical problems on dialysis tend to be correlated with a better overall psychological outlook among patients (Kutner & Brogan, 1990). However, there is also evidence that adjustment problems may be more pronounced among patients who were especially active before their kidney failure and among those who must cope not only with their own adjustment to dialysis but also with family relationship problems. Patrick and Erickson (1993) have called attention to the significance of opportunity in shaping individuals' perception of their health-related QOL. Psychosocial measures tap an outcome area that is a complex product of perceived opportunities available to individuals and of individual personality and coping styles, as well as a product of health status and disease experience.

Despite its increasing relation to ESRD and to chronic illness in general, aging remains a relatively neglected area of study. It is generally assumed that older persons with a chronic illness are simultaneously challenged both by the burdens of that illness and by the aging process. However, we lack a model for "normal aging" and therefore lack clear expectations about problems associated with aging (Gibbons, 1990). The Institute of Medicine Committee that evaluated the ESRD Program of Medicare in the U.S. explicitly rejected chronological age as a criterion for patient acceptance to treatment, because age does not measure the ability of the individual to benefit from treatment. Rather than age, the committee emphasized that "comorbidities — at any age — are the primary determinants of quality of life and of survival" (Rettig & Levinsky, 1991, p. 53).

The clinical challenge is to identify factors that contribute to compromised functioning in dialysis patients, regardless of age, and to recognize and respond to patients' needs for targeted supportive services. The social context in which most dialysis patients receive treatment can potentially compensate for losses associated with both chronic renal failure and aging if dialysis staff have sufficient time and patience to address issues impacting the psychological well-being of their elderly patients (Auer, 1986). As a group, elderly renal patients seem to evidence less psychological dysfunction and a greater capacity to handle a variety of important stressors than do younger patients (Kline, Barton, & Akhtar, 1986). Data from a series of studies indicate that, despite a higher frequency of morbidity and mortality with the dialysis procedure, greater prevalence of heart disease, and more frequent hospitalization, elderly dialysis patients can derive satisfaction from life. "It is this relative optimism among elderly dialysis patients that encourages the continued search for improvements in the dialysis procedure and in the prevention and treatment of comorbid conditions" (Henrich, 1990), so that opportunity for rehabilitation and psychosocial well-being can be maximized in the care of older patients undergoing chronic renal replacement therapy.

Outcomes Assessment: Relevance for Renal Rehabilitation

In medical rehabilitation research generally, including renal rehabilitation research, measurement tools to assess the effectiveness of interventions are not well developed. Refining these tools is an important prerequisite to assembling a useful system of rehabilitation management.

> ...Until a measurement system is developed that can integrate the findings of many different outcomes in the context of the whole person with a disability, scientific investigations in the field of medical rehabilitation will remain isolated snapshots of specific effects of a limited number of variables and how they affect one aspect of the life of a person with a disability...(NCMRR, 1993, p. 48)

Evaluation as a Process to Improve Medical Practice

Promoting effective health care and developing better information for patients and health care providers about the effectiveness of particular health services are goals that should benefit all participants in health care (Roper, Winkenwerder, Hackbarth, & Krakauer, 1988).

To promote these goals, a science of health care evaluation is developing, patterned after industrial quality management science (IQMS). IQMS is also referred to as continuous quality improvement (CQI) and total quality management (TQM). Three activities are generally emphasized as central to this quality management approach: (a) efforts to better understand the "customer" (in this case, the patient); (b) efforts to mold the culture of the organization, through effective leadership, to foster joy, pride, collaboration, and scientific thinking; and (c) efforts to continuously increase knowledge of and control over variation in the processes of work through the widespread use of scientific methods of data collection and analysis and action on data (Blumenthal, 1993).

While it is acknowledged that IQMS may not be equally applicable to all the important clinical situations that health-providers face, it may help to turn data into usable information more quickly and efficiently. Thus, collection of outcomes data using well-validated measures is a prominent component of the effectiveness initiative. Appropriate outcomes for assessment include patients' functional status, well-being, and satisfaction, as well as morbidity and mortality. Functional status data provide important markers of ESRD patients' rehabilitation status and potential.

An Effectiveness Initiative was proposed in 1988 by HCFA "to bring the resources of Medicare to bear on the question of what works in the practice of medicine" (Heithoff, Lohr, & Rettig, 1990). A closely related effort is the Outcomes Research Program authorized by Congress in 1987 and administered by the National Center for Health Services Research (renamed the Agency for Health Care Policy and Research [AHCPR] in 1989).

Outcomes research and effectiveness research are conceptually similar. In 1989, the Department of Health and Human Services announced that it was including the HCFA Effectiveness Initiative in a comprehensive outcomes and effectiveness research program. The evolution of this DHHS program "has made it clear that improving patient outcomes is a unifying, primary objective and that identifying additional issues for further research is also important" (Heithoff et al., 1990). In addition to its responsibility for health services research, including outcomes research and technology assessment, AHCPR has the responsibility of developing medical practice guidelines. The congressional view is that such guidelines represent the practical application of outcomes and effectiveness research to the practice of medicine.

The initiative to improve health care quality in the ESRD Program is part of HCFA's Health Care Quality Improvement Initiative (HCQII). HCQII is a broad-based effort to provide information and feedback to health care providers to use in improving care for Medicare beneficiaries. The HCQII is implemented through peer review organizations' (PROs), use of explicit, nationally uniform criteria to examine patterns of care and outcomes, and to identify "persistent differences between the observed and the achievable in both care and outcomes..." (Jencks & Wilensky, 1992). A major goal of HCQII is "to use practice guidelines to define a set of objectives around which HCFA, PROs, hospitals, and physicians can work together" (Jencks & Wilensky, 1992). HCFA believes that providers will be more willing to change practice when concepts are backed up with specific information on how individual providers' practices and outcomes conform to those in the community.

Table 14-5
Examples of patient-assessed generic outcome measures in ESRD studies.

Functioning	Well-Being*
Sickness Impact Profile Deniston et al. (1989); Harris et al. (1993); Hart & Evans (1987); Julius et al. (1989); Laupacis et al. (1991).	Overall Life Satisfaction Deniston et al. (1989); Evans (1991); Kutner, Brogan, & Fielding (1991); Parfrey et al. (1989); Simmons & Abress (1990).
ADL Index (1989)	Psychological Affect Deniston et al. (1989); Evans et al. (1985); Evans (1991); Parfrey et al. (1989); Deniston et al. (1989); Simmons & Abress (1990).
Functional Impairment Index Kutner, Brogan, & Fielding (1991)	Index of Well-Being Deniston et al. (1989); Evans et al. (1985); Evans (1991); Parfrey et al. (1989); Simmons & Abress (1990).
Self-rated Activity Limitation Due to Health Kutner, Brogan, & Fielding (1991)	Affect Balance Deniston et al. (1989); Kutner, Brogan, & Fielding (1991).
Self-rated Health Status Kutner, Brogan, & Kutner (1986); Kutner, Brogan, & Fielding (1991).	General Well-Being Index Deniston et al. (1989)
Self-rated Ability to Work Evans et al. (1985); Evans (1991); Kutner et al. (1991).	Illness Intrusiveness Devins, et al. (1993)
Symptom Checklist (SCL)-90-R Beck et al. (1991)	

* Standardized depression and anxiety measures have also been included in a number of studies.

Functioning and Well-Being
Medical Outcomes Study Short-Form 36 (MOS SF-36) Kurtin et al. (1992); Meyer et al. (1992).
Function Status Profile Classification and Quality of Well-Being Scale Beck et al. (1991)
Time Trade Off Churchill et al. (1991); Laupacis et al. (1991).

Specification and Measurement of Health Outcomes

Strategies for health outcomes assessment are beginning to be applied to patients with chronic health conditions. These strategies can provide a framework for defining and collecting outcomes data that are important for a better understanding of the variables related to rehabilitation of ESRD patients. Major dimensions of health outcomes include:

- Mortality,
- Morbidity and impairment (long-term clinical status), and
- Health status/functional outcome/health-related QOL.

Mortality (death) may be treated as all-cause mortality, or cause of death may itself be an outcome for analysis.

Morbidity and impairment are outcomes of chronic diseases and conditions, for which many standardized clinical measures exist (blood pressure, hematocrit, tumor size, ventricular function, visual acuity, etc.) (Patrick & Erickson, 1993).

The remaining category of health outcomes, that is, health status/functional outcome/health-related QOL, represent what individuals are able to do and how individuals perceive their overall health and related feelings of well-being. Useful discussions of these health outcome concepts are found in Ware (1990) and Patrick (1990). Functional outcome and functional status include disability assessment and refer to behavioral dysfunctions due to health. Functional status measures use a standard external to individuals, such as usual role activity, walking at a certain rate, or customary self-care behaviors. These outcomes in themselves can serve as indicators of rehabilitation status or may predict other rehabilitation outcomes such as employment.

Selection of specific assessment tools to measure health status/functional outcome/health-related QOL outcomes requires consideration of several measurement issues:

- Is information most usefully collected with performance-based measures, with patient-reports, with health provider-reports, or with some combination of these?
- Is information desired in a generic format, allowing comparison to patients with other diseases or conditions for whom the same assessment tools are used; or is information desired that is disease- or condition-specific, that is, uniquely relevant to the condition being assessed (for example, hemodialysis access or peritoneal access issues); or is a combination of generic and disease-specific assessments useful? See Table 14-5 for examples of generic instruments that have been applied in studying ESRD patients and Table 14-6 for examples of ESRD-specific instruments.

Utility of a Comprehensive Health Outcomes Database for ESRD

Providers need to place patients in a larger context in order to compare different patients' experience over time and to evaluate the effects of various forms of treatment. Health outcomes assessment furnishes a means for systematically assessing, tracking, and analyzing health outcomes that are important to patients. When patient characteristics (age, race, gender, etc.) and treatment facility characteristics (for example, size, profit status, urban/rural, etc.) are incorporated in the data system, the effects of care can be tracked not only for individual patients but also for aggregations of patients, allowing analysis of outcomes by patient demographics or diagnosis, treatment modality, provider group, cost, and many other variables.

Appropriately analyzed, an epidemiologically sound database can furnish information that will assist in managing cases and selecting therapies, including efforts to improve patients' functional status. Such a database therefore has utility as an ongoing clinical information system, as well as for research investigations. Moreover, "policy research tends to rely on available national data, and cur-

Table 14-6
Examples of ESRD-specific patient-assessed outcome measures.

Scales and Indexes

Symptom Scale
Parfrey et al. (1989)

Affect Scale
Parfrey et al. (1989)

Kidney Disease Questionnaire (KDQ)
Laupacis, Muirhead, Keown, & Wong (1992)

Quality of Life (QLI-Dialysis Index
Ferrans & Powers (1992)

Hemodialysis Quality-of-Life (HQL) Questionnaire
Churchill et al. (1991)

Hemodialysis Stressor Scale
Baldree, Murphy, & Powers (1982)

Fatigue
Cardenas & Kutner (1982); Chyatte (1979b); Kutner, Brogan, & Kutner (1986); Kutner, Fielding, & Brogan (1993a, 1993b).

Symptom and Problem Lists

Patient Symptom Form
Beck et al. (1991)

Disease- or treatment-related complaints
Chyatte (1979b); Kutner, Fielding, & Brogan (1993a).

Symptoms/Problems during past month
Hoe, Evans, & Elworth (1984)

Hemodialysis access problems
Kutner, Brogan, & Kutner (1986); Kutner, Fielding, & Brogan (1993b).

Peritoneal dialysis problems
Kutner, Brogan, & Kutner (1986); Kutner, Fielding, & Brogan (1993b).

Single-item and Summary Measures

Time required to "recover" after HD treatment
Kutner, Fielding, & Brogan (1993a)

Satisfaction with dialysis treatment modality
Kutner, Fielding, & Brogan (1993a, 1993b)

Therapy satisfactory summary
Simmons & Abress (1990)

rently these data provide limited information about health status. The Effectiveness Initiative will be successful only if it motivates data collection and methods that incorporate a broad spectrum of health outcomes..." (Patrick, 1990).

HCQII in the ESRD Program represents ongoing statistical surveillance of variations in processes of care and the ways that patterns of care vary from what is believed to be effective; and variations in outcomes of care to determine what is effective care and to identify remediable sources of poor outcomes. HCFA has said that it will link existing databases for the development of ESRD quality assurance and oversight systems. Information about ESRD patients' health status, functional outcome, and health-related QOL will be needed in these databases. A comprehensive database must also incorporate detailed information about morbidity and impairment in order to analyze sources of variation in health-related QOL outcomes. This information is essential in order to determine what levels of functioning characterize ESRD patients, the relation of functional outcome to patient characteristics, what remediable sources may be related to poor functional outcomes, and what interventions should be tested.

Rehabilitation Research Needs

Understanding of alteration in functional abilities as a consequence of disease is a primary focus of medical rehabilitation research. Individuals' behavioral responses to physical impairment and functional change can be investigated in a wide variety of clinical and applied studies. The societal impact, both positive and negative, of how persons with disabilities adjust to the demands of culture (for example, family, work, support systems) and to environmental barriers frames the outcome success or failure of medical rehabilitation programs.

Studies of adaptation to functional loss can be conducted by researchers from a wide variety of scientific disciplines, such as specialists in physical and rehabilitation medicine (physiatry), neurology, pediatrics, urology, orthopedics, neurosurgery, nursing, physical therapy, occupational therapy, rehabilitation psychology, sociology, epidemiology, and other related health professionals. Interdisciplinary as well as intradisciplinary, research is needed.

Several research initiatives that the NCMRR wishes to promote represent important areas for research with renal patients. These initiatives include

- body systems response to lost function;
- behavioral adaptation to functional loss;
- outcome measurement systems to track functional change over time in different domains; and
- treatment intervention effectiveness in restoring function (NICHD, 1992).

Whole Body System Response

Disability should be examined at multiple levels. For example, chronic pain may result from the complex interaction of musculoskeletal and neurologic pain syndromes. Disorders of one organ system may cause serious dysfunction in other organs, as well as in the whole organism. Studies of the combined effects of pathophysiology on multiple organ systems may explain overall changes in individuals' functioning more adequately than do single system studies. In turn, a cross-domain approach may better explain an individual's response to functional loss. Issues affecting whole body system response are especially likely to be relevant when individuals who incur a disorder are also experiencing the aging process.

Examples of research opportunity for improving whole body system response include:

- Studying the mechanisms of pain following disease. Identify and enhance the adaptive mechanisms that the human body develops in response to chronic pain.
- Studying long-term effects of kidney transplantation, especially multiple organ effects, behavioral changes, vocational, and social effects.

Behavioral Adaptation

The principal objective of research on behavioral adaptation is to better understand how to facilitate the process of positive adjustment to functional limitations. Behavioral adaptation research requires coordinating information from studies of a variety of individual responses to physical and/or psychological disability, as well as responses to societal limitations. Individual profiles can be developed to describe the course of functional loss and differential effectiveness of treatment interventions addressing recovery of function. Individuals can then be compared to those with similar functional loss, as well as to people without disability.

Examples of research opportunities for improving behavioral adaptation include:

- Identifying primary and secondary behavioral factors that influence adjustment to, and prevention of, the disabling process across the life span;
- Identifying factors that enable persons with disabilities to perform self-care;
- Identifying coping strategies and support mechanisms, including service provision and family education, that promote individuals' successful adjustment and community integration;
- Identifying the special coping methods needed for disabilities with fluctuating and/or unpredictable symptomatology;
- Identifying strategies that contribute to optimal function, including psychological factors, social integration, and employment;

- Identifying and characterizing behavioral and psychological factors that influence a person's willingness to cooperate with prescribed treatment approaches;
- Identifying methods to enhance the functional capabilities of individuals who experience pain secondary to illness; and
- Identifying strategies to enhance the functional capabilities of individuals with impaired sexual function secondary to illness, and programs to promote maintenance of stable, loving relationships.

Measurement, Assessment, and Epidemiology

Scientifically-based outcome measures are needed in order to adequately evaluate rehabilitation practice. Investigators can develop new measurement tools, develop standardized research protocols, provide expertise for transformation of existing data bases, collect data, and provide guidance to national surveys. This work is essential for the final priority area, that is, assessment of differential treatment effectiveness.

Examples of research opportunities in measurement, assessment, and epidemiology include:

- Developing precise quantitative measures of impairment, with particular emphasis on disability and societal limitation;
- Developing core rehabilitation outcome measures. Key variables of human performance must be identified, especially those relating to outcomes of adaptation and environmental interaction. Disease- or condition-specific supplementary measures should be developed and evaluated to complement generic measures;
- Investigating the sensitivity of subjective well-being measures (or developing new, standardized measures) for assessing effects of rehabilitation interventions;
- Identifying antecedent and comorbidity risk factors (for example, substance abuse, risk-taking behaviors) that contribute to or influence the disabling process;
- Developing and testing theoretical models of the determinants and course of the disabling process: (a) factors that influence the relationships among pathophysiology, impairment, functional and societal limitation, and disability; (b) relationships between disorders and interventions; and (c) factors predictive of recovery and adaptation; and
- Investigating patterns and models of care delivery, in order to better understand variations in rehabilitation outcomes and encourage needed policy changes. Information should be gathered on access, sources of payment, costs, location, type of facility, length of treatment, and involvement of service providers.

Treatment Effectiveness

Outcome/effectiveness studies must include balanced input from representatives of the rehabilitation team. Factors that should be studied in relation to the primary underlying disease or impairment include comorbidity, nutrition, substance abuse, and psychological status. Data should be collected on outcomes related to occupational and vocational activities, productivity, social interaction, and performance of societal roles. The short- and long-term efficacy of treatment must be evaluated. Multisite, collaborative studies are advocated.

Examples of research opportunities in treatment effectiveness include:

- Studying the development, prevention, and amelioration of secondary conditions associated with disabilities, such as depression and sexual dysfunction;
- Studying how interactions among biological, psychological, sociological, and environmental factors contribute to the onset and amelioration of impairments, functional limitations, disabilities, and secondary conditions;
- Identifying factors that may modify the relationships among pathophysiology, impairments, functional and societal limitations, and disabilities;
- Investigating patterns and models of health care and their effect on outcomes of rehabilitation; and
- Conducting longitudinal studies that track the progress of people with disabilities during rehabilitation and postrehabilitation.

Summary

National attention has focused intermittently on promoting renal failure patients' rehabilitation, but there has been no sustained momentum within the ESRD Program to support progress toward rehabilitation goals (Vachon, 1992a, 1992b). The move to apply a quality management approach in health services delivery may furnish the impetus that is needed for a sustained effort. Quality improvement emphasizes interdisciplinary team effort and the continuous monitoring of progress toward specified goals. These principles are highly compatible with elements of the rehabilitation process. The first step in rehabilitation is evaluation, in order to identify problems needing solution. A program of positive action can then be pursued. Follow-up evaluation, with feedback to participants in the rehabilitation process, should be ongoing (Chyatte, 1979b).

The rehabilitation process is most usefully conceptualized by a systems approach, which recognizes the interrelation of personal background factors shaping the individuals' unique rehabilitation needs, as well as their response to care, components of the rehabilitation process, and functional status and health-related QOL outcomes. In addition, varying developmental influences are related to individuals' particular location in the life span over time and further shape the dynamic context within which the rehabilitation process occurs.

Restoration and maintenance of function in persons with a chronic disorder such as renal failure require attention to five domains of science: pathophysiology, impairment, functional limitation, disability, and societal limitation. Physiological system changes characteristic of renal failure (for example, anemia, increased risk of atherosclerotic changes and subsequent cardiac event, and osteoporotic changes) are a natural focus for secondary prevention of disability. The five domains simultaneously identify discrete foci for rehabilitation research and provide a conceptual framework for classifying problems that are addressed by the process of rehabilitation.

Rehabilitation is frequently viewed as having three principal dimensions — physical, psychosocial, and vocational — in terms of the disabled individual's needs and concerns. These dimensions, like all aspects of rehabilitation, must also be viewed as interrelated. The 1993 NIH Consensus Development Conference on Morbidity and Mortality of Dialysis concluded that "exercise and physical training can add to physical well-being and should...be initiated at the beginning of dialysis, or in the predialysis period" (Morbidity and Mortality, 1993, p. 23). The Conference Consensus Statement also stressed the need for early assessment and intervention to maximize patients' psychosocial functioning, and studies consistently underscore the importance of early intervention to promote job retention among renal patients.

ESRD treatment modality groups can be viewed as ESRD populations with distinct rehabilitation needs; however, the importance of "ensuring patients' understanding and positive participation in their care" (Morbidity and Mortality, 1993, p. 23) should be emphasized for all patients. Diabetic patients and pediatric patients represent special populations with respect to rehabilitation needs, but there should be valuable opportunities for early intervention in these two groups. Among geriatric patients, another special population, existing tools for geriatric assessment can help to jump-start the process of measuring outcomes.

The opportunities for increased insight into quality patient care derived from rehabilitation research are virtually endless. While nutrition instruction is a first step in facilitating patient understanding of nutritional needs and restrictions, and referral to a vocational rehabilitation resource is one step in securing vocational planning services, "the long-term impact or outcome of ongoing monitoring, educational, and counseling services has...received little attention thus far" (McKevitt & Norwood, 1993, p. 36). Nephrology nursing brings expertise in the ongoing assessment of patient outcomes and should be the source of many needed rehabilitation research investigations.

Rehabilitation is not an "extra" aspect of care for renal patients, something to be incorporated when time and resources permit. It must be the *objective* of renal patients' plan of care. Nephrology nurses are crucial team leaders in the development and implementation of this plan. Rehabilitation strategies that restore and maintain patients' functional status and reduce their risk factors for increased disability — whether physical, psychosocial, or vocational — represent secondary prevention. Rehabilitation, viewed as secondary prevention of disability, is both cost-effective and essential for promoting patients' optimal functioning and well-being.

References

A historic gathering: NKUDAB workshop. (1994). *Renal Rehabilitation Report, 2(3)*, 7-8.

Applegate, W.B., Miller, S.T., Graney, M.J., Elam, J.T., Burns, R., & Akins, D.E. (1990). A randomized, controlled trial of a geriatric assessment unit in a community rehabilitation hospital. *New England Journal of Medicine, 322*, 1572-1578.

Asai, K., Kawahara, H., Takenaka, R., Toriyama, T., Hori, R., Takahashi, H., & Yoshimine, N. (1993). Hemodialysis and the elderly patient: Retrospective analysis of morbidity and mortality. *Geriatric Nephrology and Urology, 3*, 139-144.

Associated Press. (1994). Quality of life may be "dismal" for older kidney patients. *Atlanta Constitution, January 5*, B2.

Auer, J. (1986). Psychological aspects of elderly renal patients. *Aspects of Renal Care, 1*, 200-208.

Baldree, K., Murphy, S., & Powers, M. (1982). Stress identification and coping patterns in patients on hemodialysis. *Nursing Research, 31*, 107-112.

Beck, G.J., Berg, R.L., Coggins, C.H., Gassman, J.J., Hunsicker, L.G., Schluchter, M.D., & Williams, G.W. (1991). Design and statistical issues of the modification of diet in renal disease trial. *Controlled Clinical Trials, 12*, 566-586.

Bergner, M., Bobbitt, R.A., Carter, W.B., & Gilson, B.S. (1981). The Sickness Impact Profile: Development and final revision of a health status measure. *Medical Care, 19*, 787-805.

Blagg, C.R., & Fitts, S.S. (1994). Dialysis, old age, and rehabilitation. *JAMA, 271*, 67-68.

Blumenthal, D. (1993). Total quality management and physicians' clinical decisions. *JAMA, 269*, 2775-2778.

Boettcher, S.W. (1989). Exercise during dialysis. In N.G. Kutner, D.D. Cardenas, & J.D. Bower (Eds.), *Maximizing rehabilitation in chronic renal disease* (pp. 87-90). New York: PMA.

Bradburn, N.M. (1969). *The structure of psychological well-being.* Chicago: Aldine.

Branch, L.G., & Meyers, A.R. (1987). Assessing physical function in the elderly. *Clinics in Geriatric Medicine, 3*, 29-51.

Brody, S.J., & Ruff, G.E. (1986). Preface. In S.J. Brody, & G.E. Ruff (Eds.), *Aging and rehabilitation: Advances in the state of the art* (pp. xiii-xviii). New York: Springer.

Brunier, G.M., & Graydon, J. (1993). The influence of physical activity on fatigue in patients with ESRD on hemodialysis. *ANNA Journal, 20*, 457-461.

Campion, E.W. (1990). Geriatrics and rehabilitation: Awkward partners. *The Gerontologist, 30*, 707-709.

Cardenas, D.D. (1989). Contributions of the rehabilitation medicine specialist. In N.G. Kutner, D.D. Cardenas, & J.D. Bower (Eds.), *Maximizing rehabilitation in chronic renal disease* (pp 71-78). New York: PMA.

Cardenas, D.D., & Kutner N.G. (1982). The problem of fatigue in dialysis patients. *Nephron, 30*, 336-340.

Carney, R.M., McKevitt, P.M., Goldberg, A.P., Hagberg, J., Delmez, J., Harter, H.R. (1983). Psychological effects of exercise training in hemodialysis patients. *Nephron, 33*, 179-181.

Chertow, G.M., Owen, W.F., & Lazarus, J.M. (1994). Outcomes of older patients receiving chronic dialysis. *JAMA, 272*, 274.

Churchill, D.N., Wallace, J.E., Ludwin, D., Beecroft, M.L., & Taylor, D.W. (1991). A comparison of evaluative indices of quality of life and cognitive function in hemodialysis patients. *Controlled Clinical Trials 12*, 159S-167S.

Chyatte, S.B. (1979a). *On borrowed time: Living with hemodialysis.* Oradell NJ: Medical Economics.

Chyatte S.B. (1979b). Rehabilitation medicine in chronic renal failure. In S.B. Chyatte (Ed.), *Rehabilitation in chronic renal failure* (pp. 28-45). Baltimore: Williams & Wilkins.

Curtin, R.B., Oberley, E., & Friedman, A.L. (1994). Rehabilitation/Reemployment of ESRD patients on EPOGEN® therapy. Madison, WI: Unpublished study.

Daleiden, S., & Lewis, C.B. (1990). Clinical implications of neurologic changes during the aging process. In C.B. Lewis (Ed.), *Aging: The health care challenge* (2nd ed.) (pp.162-180). Philadelphia: F.A. Davis.

Deniston, O.L., Carpentier-Alting, P., Kneisley, J., Hawthorne, V.M., & Port, F.K. (1989). Assessment of quality of life in end-stage renal disease. *Health Services Research, 24*, 555-578.

Devins, G.M., Edworthy, S.M., Seland, T.P., Klein, G.M., Paul, L.C., & Mandin, H. (1993). Differences in illness intrusiveness across rheumatoid arthritis, end-stage renal disease, and multiple sclerosis. *Journal of Nervous and Mental Disease, 181*, 377-381.

Diesel, W., Noakes, T.D., Swanepoel, C., & Lambert, M. (1990). Isokinetic muscle strength predicts maximum exercise tolerance in renal patients on hemodialysis. *American Journal of Kidney Diseases, 16*, 109-114.

Domoto, D.T. (1994). Rehabilitation of the end-stage renal disease patient: Are the right questions being asked? *American Journal of Kidney Diseases, 23*, 467-468.

Eggers, P.W. (1990). Mortality rates among dialysis patients in Medicare's End-Stage Renal Disease Program. *American Journal of Kidney Diseases, 15*, 414-421.

Ennis, J., & Miko, P.S. (1988). *"Learning a new you through recreation and community involvement"* (Videotape). Atlanta GA: National Kidney Foundation of Georgia, Inc.

Evans, R.W. (1991). Recombinant human erythropoietin and the quality of life of end-stage renal disease patients: A comparative analysis. *American Journal of Kidney Diseases, 18* (suppl 1), 62-70 .

Evans, R.W., Manninen, D.L., Garrison, L.P., & Hart, L.G. (1983). The use of rehabilitation services by patients with chronic renal failure: Results from the National Kidney Dialysis and Kidney Transplantation Study. *AANNT Journal, 10(6)*, 19-25.

Evans, R.W., Manninen, D.L., Garrison, L.P., Jr., Hart, L.G., Blagg, C.R., Gutman, R.A., Hull, A.R., & Lowrie, E.G. (1985). The quality of life of patients with end-stage renal disease. *New England Journal of Medicine, 312*, 553-559.

Ferrans, C.E., & Powers, M.J. (1992). Psychometric assessment of the Quality of Life Index. *Research in Nursing and Health 15*, 29-38.

Fletcher, G.F. (1992). Current status of cardiac rehabilitation. *Current Problems in Cardiology, 17(3)*, 147-203.

Fletcher, G F. (Ed.). (1988). *Exercise in the practice of medicine.* (2nd edition). Mount Kisco, NY: Futura.

Friedman, N., & Rogers, T.F. (1988). Dialysis and the world of work. *Contemporary Dialysis & Nephrology 9*, 16, 18-19.

Garner, T.I., & Dardis, R. (1987). Cost-effectiveness analysis of end-stage renal disease treatments. *Medical Care, 25*, 25-34.

Gibbons, A. (1990). Gerontology research comes of age. *Science, 250*, 622-625.

Goldberg, A.P., Geltman, E.M., Hagberg, J.M., Gavin, J.R., Delmez, J.A., Carney, R.M., Naumowicz, A., Oldfield, M.H., & Harter, H.R. (1983). Therapeutic benefits of exercise training for hemodialysis patients. *Kidney International, 24(Supp. 16)*, S303-S309.

Goldberg, A.P., Hagberg, J.M., Delmez, J.A., Florman, R.W., & Harter, H.R. (1979). Effects of exercise on coronary risk factors in hemodialysis patients. *Proceedings of the Clinical Dialysis and Transplantation Forum, 9*, 39-43.

Gordon, D. (1990). Racial differences in ESRD. *Dialysis & Transplantation, 19*, 114-116.

Gutman, R.A., Stead, W.W., & Robinson, R.R. (1981). Physical activity and employment status of patients on maintenance dialysis. *New England Journal of Medicine, 304*, 309-313.

Hagberg, J.M., Goldberg, A.P., Eshani, A., Heath, G.W., Delmez, J.A., & Harter, H.R. (1983). Exercise training improves hypertension in hemodialysis patients. *American Journal of Nephrology, 3*, 209-212.

Harris, L.E., Luft, F.C., Rudy, D.W., & Tierney, W.M. (1993). Clinical correlates of functional status in patients with chronic renal insufficiency. *American Journal of Kidney Diseases, 21*, 161-166.

Hart, L.G., & Evans, R.W. (1987). The functional status of ESRD patients as measured by the Sickness Impact Profile. *Journal of Chronic Diseases, 40(Supp. 1)*, 117S-130S.

Heithoff, K.A., Lohr, K.N., & Rettig, R.A. (1990). Genesis of the Effectiveness Initiative and IOM's role. In K.A. Heithoff, & K.N. Lohr (Eds.), *Effectiveness and outcomes in health care* (pp.3-7). Washington, DC: National Academy Press.

Henrich, W.L. (1990). Dialysis considerations in the elderly patient. *American Journal of Kidney Diseases, 16*, 339-341.

Hoe, M.M., Evans, R.W., & Elworth, J.T. (1984). *National Kidney Dialysis and Kidney Transplantation Study: A summary of results.* Baltimore: Health Care Financing Administration.

House, J.S. (1989-90). *Americans' changing lives: Wave I, 1986 (ICPSR 9267).* Ann Arbor: University of Michigan, Institute for Social Research.

Ifudu, O., Mayers, J., Matthew, J., Tan, C.C., Cambridge, A., & Friedman, E.A. (1994a). Dismal rehabilitation in geriatric inner-city hemodialysis patients. *JAMA, 271*, 29-33.

Ifudu, O., Paul, H., Mayers, J.D., Cohen, L.S., Brezsnyak, W.F., Herman, A.I., Avram, M.M., & Friedman, E.A. (1994b). Pervasive failed rehabilitation in center-based maintenance hemodialysis patients. *American Journal of Kidney Diseases, 23*, 394-400.

Irwin, S.C., & Zadai, C.C. (1990). Cardiopulmonary rehabilitation of the geriatric patient. In C.B. Lewis (Ed.), *Aging: The health care challenge* (2nd ed.) (pp.181-211). Philadelphia: F.A. Davis.

Jagusch, W., & Butchart, B. (1985). A conducted exercise program for the ESRD patient at an outpatient dialysis center. *Dialysis & Transplantation, 14*, 467-468, 471.

Jencks, S.F., & Wilensky, G.R. (1992). The Health Care Quality Improvement Initiative: A new approach to quality assurance in Medicare. *JAMA, 268*, 900-903.

Johnson, J.H., Searles, L.B., & McNamara, S. (1993). In-home geriatric rehabilitation: Improving strength and function. *Topics in Geriatric Rehabilitation, 8*, 51-64.

Karnofsky, D.A., & Burchenal, J.H. (1949). The clinical evaluation of chemotherapeutic agents in cancer. In C.M. MacLeod (Ed.), *Evaluation of chemotherapeutic agents* (pp. 191-205). New York: Columbia.

Keith, R.B. (1984). Functional assessment measures in medical rehabilitation: Current status. *Archives of Physical Medicine & Rehabilitation, 65*, 74-78.

Klaskin, M. (1984). Psychosocial implications of children and adolescents on CAPD. *Dialysis & Transplantation, 13(5)*, 304, 306-308, 310.

Klein, S.D., & Simmons, R.G. (1977). The psychosocial impact of chronic kidney disease on children. In R.G. Simmons, S.D. Klein, & R.L. Simmons (Eds.), *Gift of life: The social and psychological impact of organ transplantation* (pp.89-118). New York: John Wiley and Sons.

Kline, S.A., Burton, H.J., & Akhtar, M. (1986). The elderly patient on dialysis—psychosocial considerations. In D.G. Oreopoulos (Ed.), *Geriatric nephrology* (pp. 183-201). Boston: Martinus Nijhoff.

Kolata, G.B. (1980). Dialysis after nearly a decade. *Science, 208*, 473-474, 476.

Kottke, C.J., Stillwell, G.K., & Lehmann, J.F., Eds. (1984). *Krusen's handbook of physical medicine and rehabilitation* (3rd ed.). Philadelphia: W.B. Saunders Company.

Kurtin, P.S. (1991). Measuring quality: Patients as consumers, suppliers. *Nephrology News & Issues, 5(10)*, 19, 25.

Kurtin, P.S., Davies, A.R., Meyer, K.B., DiGiacomo, J.M., & Kantz, M.E. (1992). Patient-based health status measures in outpatient dialysis: Early experiences in developing an outcomes assessment program. *Medical Care, 30*, MS136-MS149.

Kutner, N.G. (1993). Rehabilitation revisited. *Transplantation Proceedings, 25*, 2506-2507.

Kutner, N.G. (1994a). Assessing ESRD patients' functioning and well-being: Measurement approaches and implications for clinical practice. *American Journal of Kidney Diseases, 24*, 321-333.

Kutner, N.G. (1994b). Outcomes of older patients receiving chronic dialysis. *JAMA, 272*, 274-275.

Kutner, N.G. (1994c, March 8). *Rehabilitation data, United States Renal Data System: Labor force participation pre- and post-ESRD onset.* Presented at the National Workshop on Barriers to Rehabilitation of Persons with ESRD or Chronic Urinary Incontinence, Bethesda, MD.

Kutner, N.G., & Brogan, D. (1985). Disability labeling versus rehabilitation rhetoric for the chronically ill: A case study in policy contradictions. *Journal of Applied Behavioral Science, 21*, 169-183.

Kutner, N.G., & Brogan, D. (1990). Expectations and psychological needs of elderly dialysis patients. *International Journal of Aging and Human Development, 31*, 239-249.

Kutner, N.G., Brogan, D., & Fielding, B. (1991). Employment status and ability to work among working-age chronic dialysis patients. *American Journal of Nephrology, 11*, 334-340.

Kutner, N.G., Brogan, D., Fielding, B., & Hall, W.D. (1991). Older renal dialysis patients and quality of life. *Dialysis & Transplantation, 20*, 171-175.

Kutner, N.G., Brogan, D., & Kutner, M.H. (1986). End-stage renal disease treatment modality and patients' quality of life: Longitudinal assessment. *American Journal of Nephrology, 6*, 396-402.

Kutner, N.G., Cardenas, D.D., & Bower, J.D. (1992). Rehabilitation, aging and chronic renal disease. *American Journal of Physical Medicine & Rehabilitation, 71*, 97-101.

Kutner, N.G., Fielding, B., & Brogan, D. (1993a). Changes over time in older dialysis patients' self-assessed quality of life. *Geriatric Nephrology and Urology, 3*, 145-150.

Kutner, N.G., Fielding, B., & Brogan, D. (1993b). Quality of life for elderly dialysis patients: Effects of race and mode of dialysis. In D.G. Oreopoulos, M.F. Michelis, & S. Herschorn (Eds.), *Nephrology and urology in the aged patient* (pp. 263-276). Boston: Kluwer Publishers.

Laupacis, A., Muirhead, N., Keown, P, & Wong, C. (1992). A disease-specific questionnaire for assessing quality of life in patients on hemodialysis. *Nephron, 60*, 302-306.

Laupacis, A., Wong, C., Churchill, D., & The Canadian Erythropoietin Study Group. (1991). The use of generic and specific quality-of-life measures in hemodialysis patients treated with erythropoietin. *Controlled Clinical Trials, 12*, 168S-179S.

Levin, N.W. (1992). Quality of life and hematocrit level. *American Journal of Kidney Diseases, 20 (suppl 1)*, 16-20.

Life Options Rehabilitation Advisory Council. (1994). *Renal rehabilitation: Bridging the barriers.* Madison WI: Medical Education Institute, Inc.

Lippman, H.I. (1985). The role of rehabilitation medicine in the care of the geriatric patient. *The Einstein Quarterly Journal of Biology and Medicine, 3*, 164-167.

Lundin, A.P. (1994). Outcomes of older patients receiving chronic dialysis. *JAMA, 272*, 275.

Magrab, P., & Jacobstein, D. (1984). Adolescents coping with renal disease and hemodialysis. *Dialysis & Transplantation, 13(3)*, 151-152, 155.

Mason, J. O., & McGinnis, J.M. (1990). 'Healthy People 2000': An overview of the national health promotion and disease prevention objectives. *Public Health Reports, 105*, 441-446.

McKevitt, P.M., & Norwood, K. (1993). Availability of services to transplant recipients. *Dialysis & Transplantation, 22*, 27-28, 32-33, 36.

McRae, C., Mullins, C., Moncrief, B., & Moncrief, J. (1988). Summer camp: A positive effect on children with chronic illnesses. *Contemporary Dialysis & Nephrology, 9(8)*, 25-27.

Morbidity and mortality of dialysis. (1993, November 1-3). *NIH Consensus Statement, 11(2)*, 1-33.

National Center for Medical Rehabilitation Research. (NCMRR). (1993). *Research plan for the National Center for Medical Rehabilitation Research* (NIH Publication No. 93-3509). Bethesda MD: National Institute of Child Health and Human Development, National Institutes of Health.

National Institute of Child Health and Human Development (NICHD). (1992). Medical rehabilitation research. *NIH guide for grants and contracts, 21(7)*, part 2, 17-22.

Neff, M.S., Slifkin, R.F., & Eiser, A.R. (1981). Status of patients on maintenance dialysis. *New England Journal of Medicine, 305*, 646.

Newmann, J. (1983). A patient's perspective on patient-staff interaction. In N.G. Levy (Ed.), *Psychonephrology II: Psychological problems in kidney failure and their treatment* (pp.43-52). New York: Plenum Press.

Nissenson, A.R., Diaz-Buxo, J.A., Adcock, A., & Nelms, M. (1990). Peritoneal dialysis in the geriatric patient. *American Journal of Kidney Diseases, 16*, 335-338.

Office of Service Delivery Assessment. (OSDA). (1980). *The End Stage Renal Disease Program: A service delivery assessment.* Boston: U.S. Department of Health and Human Services.

Page, C.J., & Pearson, J. (1990). Creating therapeutic camp and recreation programs for children with chronic illness and disabilities. *Pediatrician, 17*, 297-307.

Painter, P. (1993). Exercise expectations: Are ESRD patients receiving mixed messages? *Contemporary Dialysis & Nephrology, 14(5)*, 17, 21-22.

Painter, P. (1992). *Fitness for life after transplant.* Unpublished manuscript.

Painter, P. (1988). Exercise in end stage renal disease. *Exercise and Sports Sciences Reviews, 16*, 305-339.

Painter, P., & Carlson L. (1994). Case study of the anemic patient: Epoetin alfa—Focus on exercise. *ANNA Journal, 21*, 304-307.

Painter, P., & Moore, G.E. (1994). The impact of recombinant human erythropoietin on exercise capacity in hemodialysis patients. *Advances in Renal Replacement Therapy, 1*, 55-65.

Painter, P., Nelson-Worel, J.N., Hill, M.M., Thornbery, D.R., Shelp, W.R., Harrington, A.R., & Weinstein, A.B. (1986). Effects of exercise training during hemodialysis. *Nephron, 43*, 87-92.

Painter, P., & Zimmerman, S.W. (1986). Exercise in end-stage renal disease. *American Journal of Kidney Diseases, 7*, 386-394.

Parfrey, P., Vavasour, H., Bullock, M., Henry, S., Harnett, J.D., & Gault, M.H. (1989). Development of a health questionnaire specific for end-stage renal disease. *Nephron, 52*, 20-28.

Patrick, D.L. (1990). Assessing health-related quality of life outcomes. In K.A. Heithoff, & K.N. Lohr (Eds.), *Effectiveness and outcomes in health care* (pp. 137-151). Washington, DC: National Academy Press.

Patrick, D.L., & Erickson, P. (1993). *Health status and health policy: Allocating resources to health care.* New York: Oxford Press.

Pediatric renal rehabilitation: Views from the experts. (1994). *Renal Rehabilitation Report, 2(3)*, 1-6.

Pinholt, E.M., Kroenke, K., Hanley, J.F., Kussman, M.J., Twyman,

P.L., & Carpenter, J.L. (1987). Functional assessment of the elderly: A comparison of standard instruments with clinical judgment. *Archives of Internal Medicine, 147*, 484-488.

Pope, A.M., & Tarlov, A.R. (Eds.) (1991). *Disability in America.* Washington, DC: National Academy Press.

Radloff, L.S. (1977). The CES-D Scale: A new self-report depression scale for research in the general population. *Applied Psychological Measurement, 1*, 385-401.

Rasgon, S., Schwankovsky, L., James-Rogers, A., Widrow, L., Glick, J., & Butts, E. (1993). An intervention for employment maintenance among blue-collar workers with end-stage renal disease. *American Journal of Kidney Diseases, 22*, 403-412.

Reagan's ax hovers over federal funding for dialysis. (1981, May 28). *Atlanta Journal,* p, B6.

Rettig, R.A., & Levinsky, N.G. (1991). *Kidney failure and the federal government.* Washington, DC: National Academy Press.

Reuben, D, & Siu, A. (1990). An objective measure of physical function of elderly outpatients. *Journal of the American Geriatrics Society, 38*, 1105-1112.

Robinson, J. (1993). From theory to practice: Putting the pieces together. In *Collaborative care planning: A patient-centered approach: Selected topics from the American Nephrology Nurses' Association's 24th National Symposium* (pp.14-25). Laurel, MD: Adverceutics, Inc.

Roper, W.L., Winkenwerder, W., Hackbarth, G.M., & Krakauer, H. (1988). Effectiveness in health care: An initiative to evaluate and improve medical practice. *New England Journal of Medicine, 319*, 1197-1202.

Scribner, B. (1987, May 15). *ESRD: Past, present, and future.* Presented at the National Kidney Foundation Second Annual Nephrology Potpourri, Tulsa OK.

Simmons, R.G., & Abress, L. (1990). Quality-of-life issues for end-stage renal disease patients. *American Journal of Kidney Diseases, 15*, 201-208.

Sobie, T., & Lewis, C. (1989). Quantification of functional capacity in the elderly—A modified industrial approach. *Clinical Management, 9(5)*, 24-28.

Southeastern Kidney Council (SKC), Inc. (1992). *"Dialysis workout"* (Videotape). Atlanta GA: Emory University Department of Rehabilitation Medicine.

Spooner, G.R. (1985). Self-care as a mechanism for maximum rehabilitation of the chronic renal disease patient. In N.G. Kutner, D.D. Cardenas, & J.D. Bower (Eds.), *Rehabilitation and the chronic renal disease patient* (pp. 53-59). New York: SP Medical.

Springer, I. (1990). A new miracle cure: It's called exercise—You ought to try it. *AARP Bulletin, 31(11)*, 2, 10.

Stamford, B.A. (1988). Exercise and the elderly. *Exercise and Sports Sciences Reviews, 16*, 241-379.

Stanton, D.F., Andary, M.T., & Goldberg, G. (1994). Outcomes of older patients receiving chronic dialysis. *JAMA, 272*, 274.

Stolov, W.C. (1984). Evaluation of the patient. In C.J. Kottke, G.K. Stillwell, & J.F. Lehmann (Eds.), *Krusen's handbook of physical medicine and rehabilitation* (3rd ed.). Philadelphia: W.B. Saunders Company.

Suthanthiran, M., & Strom, T.B. (1994). Medical progress: Renal transplantation. *New England Journal of Medicine, 331*, 365-376.

Thompson, C.E. (1990). Transition of the disabled adolescent to adulthood. *Pediatrician, 17*, 308-313.

U.S. Renal Data System. (1991). *USRDS 1991 annual data report.* Bethesda, MD: The National Institutes of Health, National Institute of Diabetes and Digestive and Kidney Diseases.

U.S. Renal Data System. (1992). *USRDS 1992 annual data report.* Bethesda, MD: The National Institutes of Health, National Institute of Diabetes and Digestive and Kidney Diseases.

Underwood, H.C., Cardenas, D.D., & Kutner, N.G. (1985). Effects of low-risk exercise therapy for chronic dialysis patients. *Dialysis & Transplantation, 14*, 688-690, 694-695.

Vachon, R.A. (1992a). Rehab: Should we just give up? *Nephrology News & Issues, 6(7)*, 25, 29-30, 45.

Vachon, R.A. (1992b). Part II. Rehabilitation of the renal patient: Should we just give up? *Nephrology News & Issues, 6(8)*, 22-23.

Vallbona, C., & Baker, S.B. (1984). Physical fitness prospects in the elderly. *Archives of Physical Medicine and Rehabilitation, 65*, 194-200.

Verbrugge, L.M. (1989). Gender, aging, and health. In K.S. Markides (Ed.), *Aging and health: Perspectives on gender, race, ethnicity, and class* (pp.23-78). Newbury Park CA: Sage Publications.

Ware, J.E., Jr. (1990). Measuring patient function and well-being: Some lessons from the Medical Outcomes Study. In K.A. Heithoff, & K.N. Lohr (Eds.), *Effectiveness and outcomes in health care* (pp 107-119). Washington DC: National Academy Press.

Wolcott, D., & Nissenson, A.R. (1988). Quality of life in chronic dialysis patients: A critical comparison of continuous ambulatory peritoneal dialysis (CAPD) and hemodialysis. *American Journal of Kidney Diseases, 11*, 402-412.

Zola, I.K. (1993). Disability statistics, what we count and what it tells us. *Journal of Disability Policy Studies, 4(2)*, 9-39.

Readings

Julius, M., Hawthorne, V.M., Carpentier-Alting, P., Kneisley, J., Wolfe, R.A., & Port, F.K. (1989). Independence in activities of daily living for end-stage renal disease patients: Biomedical and demographic correlates. *American Journal of Kidney Diseases, 13*, 61-69.

Meyer, K.B., Kurtin, P.S., DeOreo, P.B., Kaufman, A.M., Levin, N.W., & Davies, A.R. (1992, November). *Health-related quality of life (HRQL) and clinical variables in hemodialysis patients* (abstract). Presented at annual meeting of the American Society of Nephrology, Baltimore, MD.

Spitzer, W.O., Dobson, A.J., Hall, J., Chesterman, E., Levi, J., Shepherd, R., Battista, R.N., & Catchlove, B.R. (1981). Measuring the quality of life of cancer patients: A concise QL-index for use by physicians. *Journal of Chronic Diseases, 34*, 585-597.

Ware, J.E., Jr., & Sherbourne, C.D. (1992). The MOS 36-item short-form health survey (SF-36). *Medical Care, 30*, 473-483.

Chapter Highlights

- Rehabilitation was the promise on which the ESRD Program was founded.
- Less than 10 years after the ESRD Program began, evidence emerged that questioned the program's promise of rehabilitation.
- The approach to rehabilitation since the beginning of the ESRD Program has been to arrange specific services for patients, for example, a physical therapy consult or referral to a vocational rehabilitation counselor, on a largely ad hoc basis.
- Receiving isolated services is unlikely to promote successful rehabilitation. A coordinated plan must exist; "the essence of the rehabilitation process is that all its parts be integrated" (Chyatte, 1979b, p. 29).
- Improving the level of rehabilitation among ESRD patients requires care-providers to move beyond emphasizing survival as the main element of ESRD care, to promoting functional outcomes and well-being for stable patients.
- Targeted clinical protocols must be developed and implemented with renal patients, as they are with cardiac patients, in order to reduce risk factors for increased disability and to restore and maintain patients' functional status. When all members of the treatment team adopt this perspective on the goal of renal therapy, a major step toward improved rehabilitation occurs.
- Rehabilitation begins with an evaluation process to identify problems that need solutions, followed by a program of positive action and follow-up with feedback. These steps closely parallel the assessment, planning, implementation, and evaluation components of the nursing process, and the nephrology nurse should therefore be a natural rehabilitation catalyst.
- Rehabilitation can be defined as a process that mobilizes an individual's residual capacity for optimal function in his or her usual environment.
- Rehabilitation must address a broad spectrum of issues — biological phenomena at the fundamental levels of tissue, cellular, and molecular events; the impairment of an organ or body part; the functioning of organ systems; the individual's response to a reduction or loss of function; and the interactions of the individual with his or her physical, social, and societal environment. The focus of rehabilitation is the individual, the site at which all of these issues intersect. Effective rehabilitation depends not only on maximum restoration of functioning of affected organs and of the individual, but also on the restoration of the individual's maximum functioning within society (NCMMR, 1993).
- While employment is only one aspect of rehabilitation, being employed carries important potential self-esteem and social rewards for an individual.
- Candidates who have employment potential should be screened for referral to vocational rehabilitation (VR) specialists, with follow-up contacts to furnish additional information and to monitor candidates' progress. This requires ongoing cooperation between VR service providers and renal care staff, and both must take responsibility to strengthen these linkages.
- Given the prevalence of cardiovascular comorbidity among renal patients, cardiac rehabilitation protocols may prove useful in the development of activity guidelines that can be recommended for classes or categories of renal patients.
- Collection of outcomes data using well-validated measures is a prominent component of the effectiveness initiative. Appropriate outcomes for assessment include patients' functional status, well-being, and satisfaction, as well as morbidity and mortality. Functional status data provide important markers of ESRD patients' rehabilitation status and potential.
- Health outcomes assessment furnishes a means for systematically assessing, tracking, and analyzing health outcomes that are important to patients.
- Appropriately analyzed, an epidemiologically sound database can furnish information that will assist in managing cases and selecting therapies, including efforts to improve patients' functional status.
- The principal objective of research on behavioral adaptation is to better understand how to facilitate the process of positive adjustment to functional limitations.

Chapter Highlights (continued)

- Scientifically-based outcome measures are needed in order to adequately evaluate rehabilitation practice. Investigators can develop new measurement tools, develop standardized research protocols, provide expertise for transformation of existing data bases, collect data, and provide guidance to national surveys.
- Outcome/effectiveness studies must include balanced input from representatives of the rehabilitation team. Factors that should be studied in relation to the primary underlying disease or impairment include comorbidity, nutrition, substance abuse, and psychological status. Data should be collected on outcomes related to occupational and vocational activities, productivity, social interaction, and performance of societal roles.
- The rehabilitation process is most usefully conceptualized by a systems approach, which recognizes the interrelation of personal background factors shaping the individual's unique rehabilitation needs, as well as his/her response to care, components of the rehabilitation process, and functional status and health-related quality of life outcomes.

UNIT 5

Special Patient Populations

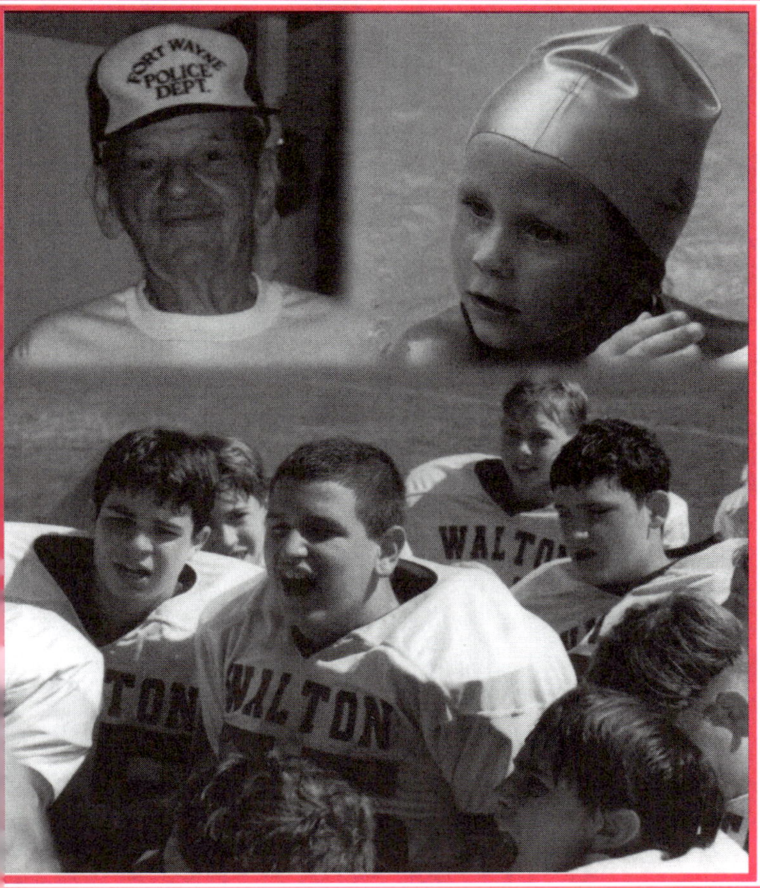

Unit Contents

Chapter 15
The Pediatric Patient 435
Cyrena M. Gilman, MN, RN, CNN, and Annette C. Frauman, PhD, RN, FAAN

Chapter 16
The Diabetic Patient 465
Marta R. Taylor, MSN, RN, NP, CNN

Chapter 17
The Geriatric Patient 481
Terran Mathers, MSN, BA, RN, CNN

CHAPTER 15

The Pediatric Patient

Cyrena Gilman, MN, RN, CNN
Annette C. Frauman, PhD, RN, FAAN

Chapter Contents

Philosophy of Pediatric Renal Nursing 437
Brief History of Pediatric Nephrology Care 437
Epidemiological Data 439
Etiologies of Renal Failure In Children 439
Congenital 439
Acquired 440
Effects of Renal Failure on Children 440
Cardiovascular 440
Cutaneous 440
Gastrointestinal 440
Genitourinary 441
Hematologic 441
Metabolic 441
Neuromuscular 441
Respiratory 441
Skeletal 441
Immune 442
Growth and Development 442
Treatment Modalities 444
Hemodialysis 444
Peritoneal Dialysis 450
Continuous Renal Replacement Therapies 453
Measuring Adequacy of Dialysis in Children 455
Transplantation 455

Chapter Contents

Specific Nursing Interventions 456
- Nutrition 456
- Pharmacologic Concerns 456
- Therapeutic Environment 457

Normal Life 458
- Family Relationships 458
- Psychosocial Care of Patient and Family 459
- Play 459
- School 460
- Special Occasions 460

Programs Assisting the Family 461
- Financial 461
- Information Sources 461

Care for Children with Chronic Renal Failure in Other Countries. 462

Summary 462

References 462

Chapter Highlights. 464

The Pediatric Patient

Cyrena Gilman, MN, RN, CNN
Annette C. Frauman, PhD, RN, FAAN

This chapter will present an overview of care of the child with chronic renal failure. No attempt will be made to repeat information that is identical to that for adult patients. The age range to be covered will include children from birth to 21 years. Necessarily, a great deal of emphasis will be placed on the families of the children, since that is the context in which the children live their lives, and often nurses provide care by working with parents in addition to patients. A philosophy about the care of children is an essential component of the pediatric nephrology nursing approach. The following philosophical assumptions guide this chapter.

Philosophy of Pediatric Renal Nursing

Children with renal failure should be thought of as essentially normal children who happen to have a physical illness requiring ongoing treatment. Renal failure, its symptoms, and the side effects of treatment present many impediments to attaining a normal lifestyle. Each of the treatment modalities commonly used for children with chronic renal failure imposes time constraints and limitations that detract from their ability to attend school and play as other, healthy, children do. Children in renal failure and their families need as much normality in their lives as possible. Health care providers and family members should treat children in renal failure with the same expectations as those for healthy children of similar developmental levels, and providers should expect developmentally congruent behaviors from these children. They need to participate in their own treatment regimen, and should have the same limits and expectations imposed on behavior as do peers and other children in the family. Children with chronic illness should not be indulged or treated specially based solely on having the illness, or treated as a "poor thing" (Gilman & Frauman, 1979). Children who are frequently referred to as a "poor thing," verbally or in other ways, will soon come to believe it. They will not progress developmentally, will not become adequately socialized, and will not be prepared to become functional adults, whether sick or well at that stage of life. In order to avoid becoming a "poor thing," children must be encouraged to be as independent as possible for their particular developmental levels.

Brief History of Pediatric Nephrology Care

At one time, conservative management was the only modality available to children with chronic renal failure. As the degree of kidney failure began to exceed the physician's ability to control it with diet and medications, the family was told to prepare for the child's death. The death was often slow and agonizing, balancing slow starvation against the toxic build-up of metabolites in the bloodstream and body tissues. Infrequently, when the cause of renal failure was thought to be potentially reversible, intermittent peritoneal dialysis (IPD) was tried for brief periods, perhaps 36 to 72 hours, usually in the intensive care unit (ICU). At times, only one series was done; other times IPD was tried on an ongoing basis. When prolonged treatment was tried, the peritoneal trocar was removed after the stay in the ICU, and the child sent home for 3 to 5 days, until the next IPD session. The children were kept alive, but the widely varying serum chemistries, and frequent admissions to the ICU for painfully invasive procedures effectively prevented any semblance of normality in their lives. If renal function did not return, the treatment was discontinued.

Then in the mid-to-late 1960s, a few centers began to attempt hemodialysis of children, usually adolescents, as a last resort to preventing death. Unfortunately, equipment and supplies were available only in adult sizes. A number of children died as a result of being attached to an extracorporeal circuit that was too large for their circulating blood volumes. In 1971, Dr. Kjellstrand and co-investigators at the University of Minnesota figured out that anyone could spare 10% of their circulating blood volume for an extracorporeal circuit without untoward sequelae. About that time, vendors began making smaller hemodialyzers and bloodlines to accommodate pediatric patients with chronic renal failure. Still, chronic hemodialysis did not permit a normal lifestyle. Diets were severely restricted in protein, sodium, potassium and fluid intake. For access, most children had external arteriovenous shunts that were frequently problematic. Often the entire access limb required immobilization. Wide swings in blood pressure during treatments due to inexact ultrafiltration techniques, frequent episodes of nausea and vomiting (some children vomited *every* dialysis treatment), frequent fevers during treatments, and anemia requiring blood transfusions every 2 to 4 weeks were facts of life. Stunted emotional and physical growth were common; children who were transplanted were often unable to adjust to normal life in school and at home.

Although the peritoneum was used as a successful delivery system for rehydrating infants as early as 1918, it was not employed for renal therapy until 1948-1949. The technique used then in two different centers was what is now called "peritoneal lavage," but it was successful in treating acute renal failure. However, the technique was thought to be too costly and labor-intensive to pursue. Further developments were not made until the later 1950s, but, again, the focus was on the treatment of acute renal failure in children (Alexander, 1994).

In 1960, Dr. Harold McDonald at the University of Michigan developed a program for teaching patients to do peritoneal dialysis (PD) on themselves either in the hospital or at home. His work to develop procedures for inserting peritoneal catheters with a trocar, and to develop automated delivery systems for peritoneal dialysate helped further the care of younger patients (McBride, 1984). However, it was Moncrief and Popovich's development of continuous ambulatory peritoneal dialysis (CAPD) in 1976 that resulted in the widespread successful use of PD for treating pediatric patients with chronic renal failure. It was first used on a child in Toronto in 1978. The high degree of biochemical control, liberalized diet, freedom from needle punctures and disequilibrium syndrome, and ability to perform treatments at home resulted in very normal lifestyles for children receiving this therapy (Alexander, 1994).

The vascular anastomosis techniques used in kidney transplantation were perfected in the early 1900s. However, the earliest xenographic transplants from pigs, goats and apes failed. The "biologic barrier" to such transplants was recognized by Carrel in 1914, but progress in overcoming the barrier was extremely slow (Alexander, 1990).

In 1953, a boy whose solitary kidney was destroyed in a motor vehicle accident received a kidney from his mother. However, after 22 days of function, the graft suddenly failed, probably due to rejection. The first renal transplant surgery between identical twins was done in 1954. The tenth such transplant involved 12-year-old identical twin sisters, and has become the longest surviving pediatric transplant. Both sisters are still alive and well with normal renal function (Alexander, 1990).

During the late 1950s, total body irradiation was attempted to prevent rejection, followed by the development of first 6-mercaptopurine, then the less-toxic azathioprine in the early 1960s. Combining azathioprine and prednisone brought long-term graft survival for living-related donor kidneys. In the 1970s, there was increased use of cadaver kidneys due to improved tissue typing, pretransplant donor and recipient screening, cadaver harvest, and kidney preservation techniques. The advent of cyclosporine in the 1980s markedly improved cadaver graft survival rates (Alexander, 1990).

Even before many of the improvements in transplantation were perfected, a working kidney transplant was the goal for pediatric patients with chronic renal failure (Alexander, 1990). There are two major problems with pediatric transplantation: first, it is a relatively rare procedure due to the small number of patients requiring transplantation

Table 15-1 United States Renal Data System data.

Prevalence Rates by Age+

Ages	Number
0-4 years	14
5-9 years	30
10-14 years	53
15-19 years	111

+ per million population

*Combined Incidence Rates for Years 1989-1991 (Incidence by Age and Race)**

Ages	Number
0-9	6
10-14	10
15-19	22

Race	Number
Whites	10
Blacks	17
Asian/PI	9
Native American	14

* per million population

Note: From United States Renal Data System. (1993). *United States Renal Data System 1993 annual data report* (NIH Publication No. 93-3176). Bethesda, MD: U.S. Government Printing Office.

(a very busy center will do only 15-25 patients a year); second, most advances in transplantation procedures are designed for and tested on adult patients. They are often then applied to children without specific research into their validity for pediatric patients (Alexander, 1990).

In fact, throughout history, the newer technologies and treatments modalities usually have been created for and perfected on adult patients first. Only then are they adapted for application to pediatric patients. It would appear that this trend will continue in the future because it is more cost effective to develop and implement new procedures and equipment for the larger adult population.

Epidemiological Data

In 1990, 899 children between the ages of birth and 19 were admitted to services in the chronic renal failure program of Medicare. This corresponds to a rate of more than 1 in 100,000 U.S. children, a rate that has remained constant since the 1980s (United States Renal Data System [USRDS], 1993). There is increased reported incidence by age (see Table 15-1). Males have higher incidence rates among children in all four age groups. The overall incidence rate is 11 per million U.S. population (see Table 15-1) (USRDS, 1993).

Treatment modalities for children differ sharply by age. PD is the preferred modality of treatment in the first year of renal replacement therapy for children under age 5, with slightly more than half receiving some form of PD (Held et al., 1991). Mortality rates were highest in this age group. For children ages 5-9, 40% were receiving PD after 6 months of treatment, and by the end of the first year, more than half had a functioning transplant. After 6 months of treatment, 41% of children 10-14 had a functioning transplant, and 25% were receiving hemodialysis. Fifty percent of children 15-19, the largest group of pediatric chronic renal failure patients, were receiving treatment with hemodialysis, but after the first 9 months of chronic renal failure, transplantation became the predominant mode of treatment (Held et al., 1991).

Etiologies of Renal Failure in Children

The etiologies of renal failure are quite different in children than in adults. For example, diabetes and hypertension, two major causes of renal failure in adults, are rarely causes of renal failure in children. Less than 6% of pediatric cases reported in 1987-1990 list diabetes and hypertension as primary diagnosis, in contrast to more than 60% of adult patients (USRDS, 1993). Diabetes does occur in children, but the degree of damage necessary to result in renal failure usually takes more than 20 years to evolve, by which time the child has become an adult. Only 1.4% of children with chronic renal failure have diabetes as a primary cause, and the median age of onset for those children is 18 (USRDS, 1993). Serious renal disease in children may result in hypertension, but essential hypertension is rarely seen in children. The most frequent cause of chronic renal failure in children is glomerulonephritis (37.6% of all reported cases), followed by congenital/other hereditary diseases (19.1%) (USRDS, 1993). Blacks are overrepresented among children whose primary cause of renal failure is hypertension, lupus nephropathy, primary glomerulonephritis, or sickle cell disease. Whites have higher percentages of chronic renal failure caused by cystic kidney disease, hemolytic uremic syndrome, and congenital/hereditary conditions. Males predominate among pediatric patients, especially among those with obstructive conditions and other congenital/hereditary conditions (USRDS, 1993).

Most frequently, chronic renal failure that has its onset between birth and age 5 is due to congenital disease. That which occurs between ages 6 and 10 is most often a result of urological defects, and after age 12, glomerulonephritis is the most frequent cause of chronic renal failure in children.

Congenital

Malformations of the urinary tract are extremely common, probably related to the complex embryology of the kidney and urinary tract. The human kidney is first detectable in the fifth gestational week. It is initially composed of a small epithelial bud surrounded by undifferentiated mesenchymal stem cells. The bud is a branch from the mesonephric or Wolffian duct, and forms the collecting ducts and ureters. Interactions between various cell types and the surrounding matrices stimulate each cell lineage to differentiate, resulting ultimately in a nephric unit, with collecting ducts connected to distal tubules and the glomerular epithelium. The vasculature surrounds all the cells, and forms loops within the glomerulus (Ekbaum, 1994). The primitive urogenital sinus develops primarily into the bladder; the superior section shrinks and becomes a solid fibrous cord, connecting the bladder to the umbilicus. In males, the prostatic and membranous urethra and the penile urethra are formed from the inferior portion of the urogenital sinus; it forms a small portion of the urethra and vestibule in the female (Clarren, 1994). While the mechanisms resulting in malformations are not well understood, research is increasingly identifying the biochemical processes involved, which will result in information beyond description and speculation (Clarren, 1994).

Renal agenesis can occur from failure in formation of the metanephros or the ureteric bud, while duplications arise from very early duplications in the ureteric bud. Numerous conditions have been identified that have renal anomalies as a component, including VATER syndrome, MURCS association, and many others. Obstructive uropathy may be associated with dysgenesis, or damage may occur because of back pressure of urine and/or resulting infections of the urinary tract. Obstructions may occur at any point along the urinary tract, from the meatus to the renal pelvis. These may be formed of abnormal structures, misplaced vessels, or valves where there should be none. Abnormal innervation to the ureters such as that seen in prune-belly syndrome and other cases of obstructive uropathy, slows or causes cessation of the normal peristalsis of the ureter, resulting in an obstruction just as an ileus, or nonfunctioning bowel, causes GI obstruction. More than 90% of the time, the cause of renal system anomalies is not known (Clarren, 1994). Other congenital syndromes cause renal failure through abnormalities of the glomerulus, including Alport's syndrome, nail-patella syndrome, Fabry disease, and Charcot-Marie-Tooth syndrome. Inherited errors of metabolism, such as cystinosis, and oxalosis can cause renal failure in children and infants. Congenital nephrotic syndrome, especially the Finnish type, is also a cause of renal failure in infants and children.

Acquired

Glomerulonephritis of various types can often be effectively treated. At other times, glomerular disease progresses to renal failure and it is a major cause of renal failure in infants and children, accounting for 37.6% of cases. Many cases of acute glomerulonephritis in children follow infection with an organism, including group A betahemolytic streptococci, viruses including varicella, Epstein-Barr, rubeola, and cytomegalovirus. Often, the precipitating organism is not identified. Pathology of the glomerulus results from infiltration of the tissues with antibodies, resulting in enlargement of the glomeruli and obliteration of capillary lumens. The degree of luminal obliteration correlates with decreased glomerular filtration rates. In some children, especially those with initially severe disease, progression to renal failure occurs, though often slowly. Other types of glomerulonephritis cause damage to the glomerulus and the basement membrane, with progression to renal failure in some cases. A congenital form of polycystic disease does occur in children, and other diseases such as collagen vascular diseases, malignancies, and hemoglobinopathies may cause renal failure in children just as they do in adults. Hemolytic uremic syndrome causes acute renal failure in children, with resulting damage that may or may not be permanent. In this disease, microthrombi are formed in the kidneys and other organs resulting in ischemia. Cortical necrosis of the kidney may be seen and is associated with an unfavorable prognosis (Frishberg, Obrig, & Kaplan, 1994).

Effects of Renal Failure on Children

Most of the effects of renal failure on both children and adults were noted and described prior to the widespread availability of dialysis and transplantation. Many of these effects are well controlled by treatment, and some are not often seen. Some of the effects of renal failure on children and adults are identical; others are markedly different due in part to children's unique metabolic state resulting from growth, their height-to-weight ratio, and their increased percentage of body water.

Cardiovascular

The cardiovascular effects of renal failure in children are similar to those seen in adults, including hypertension, which can result in retinopathy and encephalopathy if unchecked; circulatory overload; edema; congestive heart failure; pericarditis; and arrhythmias. Hypertension in children with chronic renal failure is usually caused by extracellular volume expansion and is controlled by ultrafiltration (Solhaug, Adelman, & Chan, 1992). Children also may have marked left ventricular hypertrophy with considerable lateral displacement of the point of maximum impulse (PMI) (Morris, Skinner, Wren, Hunter, & Coulthard, 1993). Children do not have the co- or preexisting cardiovascular disease so common in adults. Children may erroneously be thought to have congestive heart failure when their function is normal, as S_3 heart sounds are normally audible in children because of their thin chest walls.

Cutaneous

The cutaneous effects of chronic renal failure on children are quite obvious upon even cursory observation. Even while receiving erythropoietin, the overall appearance is relatively pale or sallow. Accumulation of urinary pigments in the skin may occur, just as they do in the adult. The skin is somewhat less likely to be dry or scaly in younger children with chronic renal failure, and itching is less likely to occur than in adults. As in adults, when dialysis is discontinued or not possible, urea may be deposited on the skin as sweat evaporates. The resulting crystal formations resemble frost, and are thus called uremic frost. Bruising is sometimes noted in children with chronic renal failure. This is due to the capillary fragility resulting from chronic renal failure, and is a sequela of most of the treatment modalities requiring heparinization.

Gastrointestinal

Children with chronic renal failure are likely to suffer frequently from nausea and anorexia, sometimes progressing to vomiting. The anorexia may be due in part to changes in taste, particularly a constant metallic aftertaste. In addition, they are also increasingly prone to infections of the GI tract as well as GI bleeds. Children who have an infection of the urinary tract often experience nausea and vomiting, in contrast to the symptoms of frequency, urgency, and pain commonly seen in adults.

Genitourinary

Children with chronic renal failure are much more likely to have high output renal failure than are adults. In these children, fluid is removed by the kidney(s), but the urine specific gravity is extremely low, and other substances are poorly excreted at best. Serum BUN, creatinine and electrolyte levels may resemble those of oliguric or anuric patients. Usually, the ability of children with chronic renal failure to concentrate their urine is greatly impaired and they may have a fixed urinary specific gravity with a total inability to respond to fluctuations in fluid status. Children, especially those with nephrotic syndrome, can have extremely high urine proteins, to the point that the urine will jell if refrigerated.

Female adolescents with chronic renal failure may experience amenorrhea and anovulation even after the onset of puberty, which is often greatly delayed. They may not have a corresponding loss of libido, however, and may have difficulty with vaginal lubrication and painful intercourse, just as adults with renal failure do. Similarly, males have delayed puberty, and may suffer from impotence and sterility. However, the adolescent sex drive is powerful, and loss of libido and sterility should not be depended on to inhibit either male or female adolescents. Despite decreased likelihood of pregnancy, sexually active adolescents with chronic renal failure need to use birth control measures. Choosing an appropriate method may not be easy, because of the need to balance safety and efficacy. Barrier methods (diaphragm, condom) are safest, but may not be well accepted by adolescents, and are likely to be ineffective due to sporadic use. Intrauterine devices are contraindicated, and hormonal contraceptive methods may not be well tolerated. Additionally, because of their suppressed immune system, sexually transmitted diseases (STDs) are particularly hazardous for adolescents with chronic renal failure. They should be given information about preventive measures before they become sexually active.

Hematologic

Like adults, anemia is a problem for children with chronic renal failure, though this problem has been considerably diminished with the advent of recombinant erythropoietin. Hemolysis is also a problem, particularly for children on hemodialysis. Children who are posttransplantation and receiving azathioprine should be carefully monitored for its effects on bone marrow function, including diminished thrombocytes, erythrocytes, and leukocytes.

Metabolic

Children with chronic renal failure are more likely than adults to experience metabolic acidosis. However, the other metabolic effects of chronic renal failure, including azotemia, hyperkalemia, sodium retention or wasting, hypermagnesemia, hyperuricemia, protein intolerance, and lipid abnormalities, are similar.

Neuromuscular

Neuromuscular effects of chronic renal failure on children are also similar to those seen in adults. However, problems with growth and development are particularly problematic. Fatigability, muscle wasting, and lethargy greatly interfere with the developmental drive of children and with their ability to perform new skills and tasks. Other neuromuscular effects are discussed in the section on growth and development.

Respiratory

Respiratory effects of chronic renal failure in children are similar to those in adults. Because of their smaller size, however, a relatively small amount of excess fluid may result in pulmonary edema.

Skeletal

The effects of chronic renal failure on bone in children is devastating, and include abnormalities of metabolism such as hypocalcemia, hyperphosphatemia, and hyperparathyroidism. Renal osteodystrophy is common, along with pathologic fractures due to demineralized bone. Calcium salts may be deposited in soft tissue (around joints, in blood vessels, heart, lungs, conjunctiva).

A particularly devastating effect of long-term renal failure and dialysis is the deposition of beta-2 microglobulin in the soft tissues and bones. As in adults, the longer one is on dialysis and exposed to elevated levels of beta-2 microglobulin; the more likely one is to have this type of amyloidosis. If a pediatric patient rejects several transplants at a young age and faces the remainder of life on some type of dialysis, development of beta-2 microglobulin bone disease is inevitable (McCarthy, Williams & Johnson, 1994).

McCarthy et al. (1994) found that CAPD patients are less likely to develop beta-2 microglobulin disease than are hemodialysis patients, and patients hemodialyzed against high-flux synthetic membranes have a lower incidence than those dialyzed against cellulose acetate membranes. The progression of amyloid deposition is delayed with synthetic membrane hemodialysis, but not prevented. The researchers found that most patients will begin to develop the syndrome after 4 or 5 years of therapy; when the number of "beta-2 microglobulin months" (the serum beta-2 microglobulin level times the number of months of dialysis) exceeds 1500, the disease will definitely be present. Only natural kidney function, whether from native kidneys or a transplant, can avoid this devastating problem.

Immune

Children with chronic renal failure, like adults, have long been noted to have decreased resistance with an increased incidence of bacterial, viral, and fungal infections. Uremic patients also have a much-higher incidence of malignancies than the normal population (Benfield & Michael, 1992).

In a study of children receiving CAPD, significantly lower serum IgG levels were found than in the controls, but all levels were in the normal range. Additionally, these children had essentially normal responses to vaccinations with live vaccine for measles, mumps and rubella (Hisano et al., 1991).

Uremic patients have normal to slightly elevated granulocyte counts, but the migration and chemotaxic function of these cells is usually slightly abnormal. Phagocytosis, on the other hand, is typically normal (Benfield & Michael, 1992).

Numerous investigators have found widely varying results in studying the number and function of lymphocytes in uremic patients. Although normal levels of IgG, IgA, and IgM are found in uremic patients, seroconversion and antibody titer formation are usually impaired. Impaired T-cell function, increased suppressor cell activity, intrinsic monocyte/macrophage dysfunction, and abnormal production of interleukin-2 have been demonstrated in uremic patients, but are difficult to reproduce in animals with experimentally-induced uremia. Uremic patients also have been noted to have thymic atrophy at autopsy (Benfield & Michael, 1992).

The vitamin and mineral deficits associated with the malnutrition present in most uremic patients have serious effects on the immune system. Some kidney diseases are treated with long-term immunosuppressive medication before end stage renal failure is reached. Thus the impaired immune system function found in uremic patients is most likely influenced by many factors, not the uremic condition alone (Benfield & Michael, 1992).

Although their suppressed immune systems may not respond as well, that is, create as high a level of antibody titre or have that titre last as long, children with chronic renal failure need to have the same immunizations as their healthy peers on approximately the same schedule. Whether or not to immunize all children with chronic renal failure against Hepatitis B is still under discussion in some circles. However, the issue seems to concern financing the widespread use of this expensive immunization, rather than its efficacy or desirability.

Growth and Development

Children with chronic renal failure have the same developmental needs as healthy children. They may need additional assistance from parents, health care providers, educators, and others to achieve their maximum potential at each of the developmental stages. Certainly prevention of developmental problems is preferred to intervention after they have occurred. The focus needs to be positive: enhance what the child can do, encourage progress, and deemphasize deficits or handicaps.

In this society, children are usually approached based on the age they appear to be. For the child with short stature or delayed puberty due to chronic renal failure, this is inappropriate. In order to help the child with chronic renal failure achieve as normal a life as possible, the pediatric nephrology nurse must first determine exactly what developmental level the child has attained. In determining this, the whole child must be observed. The child's behavior; relationships with family, friends and peers; fine and gross motor coordination; and coping mechanisms all help establish what his/her developmental levels in those domains are. In addition, the child's abilities compared with other children of chronological age, as well as likes and dislikes, must also be considered.

Children with chronic renal failure go through the same developmental stages that other children do. However, the rate at which they progress through the stages is often markedly delayed, and not necessarily consistent across developmental domains. Generalized psychological assessment tools for younger children (birth to 6 years), such as the Denver Developmental Screening Test, the Goodenough Draw-A-Man test, and the Brazelton Scale for Infant Development can help in establishing a developmental level. The Vineland Adaptive Behavior Scales can be used clinically to determine which social and adaptive skills the child possesses, and by implication, which ones need to be worked on next. It is an excellent idea to have testing conducted by a child psychologist, using global measures such as the Bayley and the Weschler Intelligence Scale for Children (WISC). The evaluation should also include tests of neuropsychological function such as Raven's Progressive Matrices, the Beery Developmental Test of Visuomotor Integration, and tests of vigilance, auditory memory and reaction time, since these have been shown to be affected by chronic renal failure (Fennell et al., 1990). These tests will provide an indepth examination of the child's developmental attainments, which can be used in patient education or in assisting the child and family to obtain appropriate school placement. If a clinical or developmental psychologist is not available on the team caring for the child, their services may sometimes be obtained through the school system, a nearby university's psychology department, or a child psychiatry facility.

Physical growth and sexual maturation. Physical growth failure is perhaps the most pervasive developmental issue for children with chronic renal failure. Despite numerous studies, the mechanisms of growth failure are still not well understood. Nutrition; metabolic acidosis; fluid and electrolyte disturbances, especially calcium and phosphorus; medications used in treatment, especially corticosteroids; and decreased production and use of hormones have all been implicated in growth failure (Mehls, Blum, Schaefer, Tonshoff, & Scharer, 1992). Probably all of these factors, and perhaps others, are influential, but how each or the combination result in growth failure is not known. In reading and interpreting studies of growth in children with chronic renal failure, it is difficult to compare studies, since a variety of measures such as growth velocity, change in percentile, and bone age are used.

In general, the earlier the onset of renal failure, and the longer its duration, the more severe growth deficiencies will be. Height reductions are most profoundly affected in infancy and adolescence, the periods in which growth is most rapid. Once growth potential is lost in these time periods, it will probably never be regained (Mehls et al., 1992). Children with renal disease often have a relatively normal growth curve, but usually remain well below the 3rd percentile of normal parameters. Additionally, adult height is usually reduced.

A number of studies have addressed the impact of treatment strategies on growth. Growth is usually improved after successful renal transplantation, but the amount of additional growth is related to the remaining growth potential, the immunosuppressive regimen, and the pubertal status of the recipient (Harmon & Jabs, 1992). Growth is most enhanced after transplantation in younger children who are receiving alternate day steroids. Early studies indicated that growth was improved on CAPD, as compared to hemodialysis, but other studies have not confirmed this result.

In the early days of hemodialysis of children, an improvement in growth was seen over that on conservative management. In retrospect, it is clear that this was related to the extremely poor nutritional status of children treated by extreme dietary restrictions during conservative management. Treatment with hemodialysis permitted a more liberal diet, and better nutrition. Currently, no improvement in growth is seen in children on hemodialysis (Mehls et al., 1992).

Puberty, with its rapid growth and maturation of secondary sex characteristics, is often delayed and its intensity diminished. In a 1990 study, Scharer noted that puberty was delayed in their subjects by an average of 2.5 years, and that the growth attainment in the prepubertal growth spurt was significantly impaired. Other studies have noted diminished estrogen and testosterone levels in pubertal children with chronic renal failure.

Use of human growth hormone has become a standard treatment for children with chronic renal failure. Prior to the development of synthetic human growth hormone, children with chronic renal failure did not meet the criteria for cadaveric hormone use — a documented hormonal deficiency. Children with chronic renal failure have normal or elevated levels of the hormone, but are apparently not able to use their natural supply. Administration of additional hormone does enhance growth as demonstrated by numerous studies (Benfield, Parker, Waldo, Overstreet, & Kohaut; 1993; Fine et al., 1994; Koch et al., 1989).

Cognitive development. The effects of chronic renal failure on cognitive development of infants has been the subject of a number of studies. These studies have primarily evaluated the efficacy of various treatment modalities in preventing detrimental effects of chronic renal failure on neurological development. Polinsky, Kaiser, and Stover (1987) concluded from a review of 15 of these studies that chronic renal failure most consistently affected gross motor and language development. Development of infants is improved after renal transplantation, with studies showing improvement on a variety of measures, including the DDST, the Bayley, and the Revised Yale Developmental Schedule. However, neonates with chronic renal failure continue to have developmental delays even after transplantation.

Studies of the effects of chronic renal failure on cognitive development in older children have used both global measure of intelligence (for example, Stanford-Binet, WISC-R) as well as specific neuropsychological measures such as tests of vigilance, auditory memory, and reaction time. Associations have been found between age at onset of chronic renal failure, length of time in renal failure, treatment method, and a variety of measures of cognitive development (Crittenden, Holliday, Piel, & Potter, 1985; Fennell et al., 1990; Rasbury, Fennell, Fennell, & Morris, 1986). Based on their body of work, Fennell and colleagues (1990) have advanced the hypothesis that renal failure affects cognitive development in two ways: one that influences the acquisition of new skills, and is less likely to improve after successful transplantation, and another affects attention, speed of processing, and modulation of responses. This latter effect seems to be dependent on abnormal blood chemistries, and is thus more susceptible to improvement after successful transplantation (Fennell et al., 1990).

School attendance in children with chronic renal failure has received some attention, mostly in children who have received successful transplantation. Studies of these children are optimistic: Fine et al. reported in 1978 that of 54 transplant recipients old enough to finish high school, only 3 failed to graduate. In 1991, Morel and colleagues reported that of 9 transplant recipients of school age, all were attending; of 48 older than high school age, 93% had graduated, and 60% had attended college or technical training. Few studies have reported school attendance on children receiving hemodialysis or PD. A German study reported a high school completion rate of 14% (Rosenkranz, Bonzel & Bulla, 1992), while a European Dialysis and Transplant Association (EDTA) study reports that of 617 adult subjects receiving renal replacement therapy as children, 41% did not complete school and only 58% were employed (Ehrich et al., 1992).

Psychosocial development. The effects of chronic renal failure on psychosocial development are not as devastating as once feared. Children with chronic renal failure seem to be quite resilient psychologically, especially those with successful renal transplants. Children treated at home with either hemodialysis or PD fare better than those on incenter treatment. Psychosocial adjustment is better for those with transplants than for those on either mode of dialysis. Most studies of children with chronic renal failure as they approach adulthood have found few problems except in the areas of growth failure, and the formation and maintenance of intimate relationships (Beck, Nethercut, Crittenden, & Hewins, 1986; Morel et al., 1991).

Table 15-2
Approximate blood volume by age.

Age	Total Blood Volume
Premature infants	90-105 ml/kg
Term newborns	78-86 ml/kg
> 1 month	78 ml/kg
> 1 year	74-82 ml/kg
Adult	68-88 ml/kg

Note: From Johnson, K.B. (Ed.). (1993). *The Harriet Lane Handbook* (13th ed.). St. Louis: C.V. Mosby Company.

Treatment Modalities

Hemodialysis

Techniques. The hallmark of pediatric hemodialysis is the requirement that only 10% or less of the child's circulating blood volume can be in the extracorporeal circuit. One calculates circulating blood volume based on the ml of blood per kilogram of body weight found in the patient's age group (see Table 15-2). Although there is a wide variation in volumes between the age groups, most pediatric dialysis centers multiply the child's weight in kilograms by 70-80 ml. The kidney and bloodlines which will not exceed 10% of that total are selected. Generally speaking, the lower the factor, the lower the allowable extracorporeal volume, and the safer the hemodialysis system.

In the early days of pediatric hemodialysis, parallel plate dialyzers were the only ones available. If a parallel plate dialyzer was selected, one needed to be observant for membrane compliance, a situation in which more blood is compartmentalized in the dialyzer as the blood pump speed and, therefore, the blood pressure within the lines and dialyzer increases. For example, the Cobe-Gambro-Hospal 0.23 m2 Dialyzer (formerly known as the Gambro Mini-minor kidney) had a blood volume of 20 ml at 100 mmHg of transmembrane pressure (TMP), but for each additional 100 mm of TMP, another 6 ml of blood was sequestered in the kidney. When dialyzing an infant, an additional 3 ml in the extracorporeal circuit can make the difference between normotensive and hypovolemic shock.

Recently, production of pediatric parallel plate dialyzers has been discontinued. Although there are several pediatric hollow fiber kidneys on the market, none are truly suitable for children smaller than 10 kg. Due to the small number of pediatric patients on hemodialysis, many companies are considering discontinuing production of other pediatric size hemodialysis products.

Hemodialyzers are selected for pediatric patients based on extracorporeal blood volume, their rate of solute removal or efficiency, and their ultrafiltration rate. All types of dialyzer membranes (cuprophan, cellulose acetate, polyacrylonitrile, polymethylmethacrylate, and polysulfone) have been used on pediatric patients, as have the many different configurations of dialyzers (coils, flat plates, hemicapillary, and hollow fiber). Each type of dialyzer has different permeability to larger solutes and different ultrafiltration coefficients, which are the prime factors to be considered in making the choice (Gruskin, Baluarte, & Dabbagh, 1992).

Dialyzer first-use reactions are reported to be more common in patients who are less than 30 years old. The incidence is approximately 3 to 4 episodes per 100 new dialyzers. The symptoms can be major, such as dyspnea, localized, or generalized itching and/or burning sensations, angioedema, runny nose and eyes, abdominal cramps, or hives. Minor symptoms, such as mild back or chest pain, hypotension, nausea and vomiting, or muscle cramps, are also possible. Using a different dialyzer with a different membrane type, or different mode of sterilization may be necessary. Predialysis antihistamine administration may also decrease symptoms (Gruskin et al., 1992). Reuse of dialyzers is sometimes recommended to prevent this reaction, but most pediatric dialysis units do not have the facility arrangements, equipment or staffing to successfully perform reuse. In addition, the small numbers of pediatric patients on hemodialysis tend to make reuse less of a cost benefit.

Smaller artificial kidneys provide lower clearances of blood urea nitrogen (BUN) and creatinine, and much lower ultrafiltration rates. In the current age of volumetric hemodialysis machines, that is not so critical as it was when fluid removal was based solely on the transmembrane pressure and the kidney's *in vitro* ultrafiltration rate.

In the early days of pediatric hemodialysis, one multiplied the TMP by the *in vitro* ultrafiltration rate to calculate the amount of fluid to be removed

Figure 15-1
Figuring clearances and blood pump speeds.

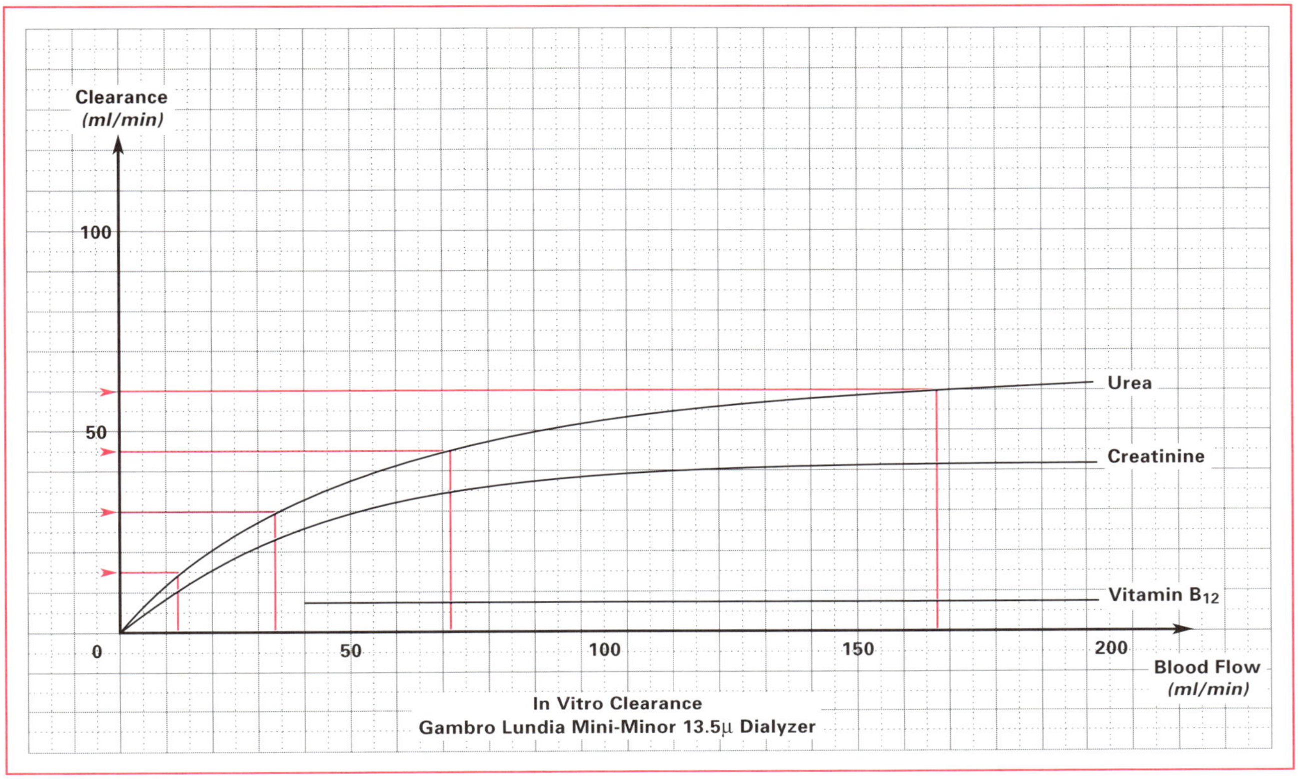

Note: From "In Vitro Clearance Gambro Lundia Mini-Minor 13.5 Micron Dialyzer" by Gambro AB, date unknown.

in 1 hour (see Table 15-3). Multiplying that number by the number of hours of treatment yielded the total amount of fluid to be removed. The reverse calculation, desired fluid removal divided by the hours of treatment, divided by the *in vitro* ultrafiltration rate yielded the TMP to be set on the machine. Unfortunately, this was only an approximate number, and there would always be some variation between desired and actual fluid removal. Due to their exacting fluid removal, modern volumetric machines are the best to use for pediatric patients.

Central hemodialysis delivery systems, which mix and pipe the same dialysate to many different hemodialysis stations in a center, are almost never used for pediatric patients. Each child requires an individualized treatment plan. It is unlikely that a pediatric center will have many hemodialysis patients, and far less likely that several will require the same dialysate formulations (Gruskin et al., 1992).

The blood flow rates in pediatric dialysis units are always individualized. Similar to extracorporeal volume, the flow rates are based on the pediatric dialysis patient's weight. Although not a difficult calculation, the pediatric nephrologist is the one to prescribe blood flow rate.

In order to calculate blood flow rates correctly, a clearance chart for the dialyzer must be available (see Figure 15-1). Clearance tables will not work; the information must be in graph form. The patient's weight in kilograms is multiplied by 1.0, 2.0, 3.0, and, for the long-term patient, by 4.0. These figures are located on the "Clearance rate in ml/minute," or Y-axis of the chart. A line is then drawn to the right until it intersects the BUN clearance curve. The line then is extended straight down to the "Blood flow in ml/minute," or X-axis, where the correct blood pump speed will be noted for a 1.0 ml clearance, a 2.0 ml clearance, a 3.0 ml clearance, or a 4.0 ml clearance.

Patients with very high serum BUNs (> 100 mg/dl) and creatinines (> 8.0 mg/dl) will start out with very low clearance rates in order to prevent side effects during the first few dialysis sessions. When their serum chemistries are closer to normal at the beginning of a session, the clearance rate can be increased. If a child weighed 15 kg, clearances on the graph y-axis would be 1.0 ml = 15, 2.0 ml = 30, 3.0 ml = 45, and 4.0 ml = 60. The child would be treated with a pump speed of 13 ml/min for the first treatment, 34 ml/min for the second and possibly third treatments, and 72 ml/min for subsequent

Table 15-3
Calculating Fluid Removal on Hemodialysis

A. Calculating the amount of fluid that will be removed during a treatment:

TMP X UFR = the amount of fluid to be removed in 1 hour X hours of treatment = approximate total fluid that will be removed during the entire treatment

B. Calculating the dialysate pressure to be set on a nonvolumetric machine:

total fluid desired to be removed during the treatment / hours of treatment = amount of fluid to be removed during 1 hour / UFR = TMP needed to remove desired amount of fluid - venous pressure = dialysate pressure to be set on the machine

TMP = transmembrane pressure (venous blood line pressure, measured at the venous drip chamber, + dialysate pressure, both expressed in millimeters of mercury)

UFR = *in vitro* ultrafiltration rate for the dialyzer, expressed in ml/hour. The manufacturer provides this number.

treatments (see Figure 15-1). If the child became a chronic hemodialysis patient, a pump speed of 167 ml/min might be required to give the patient maximum clearances, and to increase the potential for growth by allowing for maximum dietary intake.

In the early days of pediatric hemodialysis, a bicarbonate dialysate was used. However, difficulties with bacterial contamination of this dialysate caused all patients, adult and pediatric alike, to be switched to acetate baths. If a pediatric patient has essentially normal liver function, this is usually not a problem. Some children are sensitive to the acetate, however, and will develop impressive nausea and vomiting if treated with an acetate bath.

The correction of the bacterial growth problem has allowed most pediatric centers to return to using a bicarbonate dialysate. This provides for a much gentler, less-stressful treatment, and is absolutely essential in the child with compromised liver function.

All dialysate used on pediatric patients should contain dextrose. Children receive extra calories for energy from a high dextrose bath, and also have fewer side effects. The dextrose level should be in the 200-250 mg% range.

Continuous monitoring of the patient's weight with metabolic weight scales during a hemodialysis treatment is another hallmark of pediatric dialysis. It is critical for hemodialysis of infants (those less than 12 kg), and highly recommended for children weighing less than 20 kg. Even with accurate fluid removal provided by volumetric hemodialysis machines, membrane compliance (sequestering additional blood in the parallel plate dialyzer as the transmembrane pressure increases) is still a possibility. Metabolic scales may detect the start of this condition before the patient's blood pressure reflects it.

When a small child is to be hemodialyzed on metabolic scales, an exacting technique is required. Initially, all of the supplies, such as bed linens, diapers, clothing changes, toys, and creative materials, must be placed on the bed prior to the child. The weight of the bed and supplies is then calibrated to zero. Once the child is placed on the bed, the monitor will read only the weight of the child. The metabolic scales' accuracy may be verified by weighing the child on a standard scale prior to placement on the bed.

Immediately after the hemodialysis treatment has begun, the monitor will show an increased value due to the weight of the bloodlines running to the child. The weight monitor should be readjusted to reflect just the starting weight of the child.

All lines running onto the bed must be double taped, first to the bed rail, then to any stable piece of equipment next to the bed to avoid a dampening effect on the weight readings due to the pull of the lines. Keeping the line slack between both pieces of tape is essential. Otherwise, as the bed raises or lowers even slightly on the scale, the bloodline could drag on the bed rail and thus change the weight reading. For infants, the overhead heater may be used; for older children it might be the dialysis machine itself. If the second piece of equipment is on wheels, it may be necessary to lock the wheels and then tape the equipment to the floor to ensure that it is not moved at all during the treatment (Kjellstrand et al., 1971).

In the early days of pediatric dialysis, the weight scales registered change with a needle indicator on a scale. To ensure the greatest possible accuracy, gram weights were added to the bed to keep the indicator at zero. One totalled the gram weight values to know how much fluid had been removed from the child (Kjellstrand et al., 1971). The more modern weight scales with digital readouts have deleted the need to use gram weights. However, it is difficult to get an accurate scale that will give readings to two decimal places, and yet stand up to the rigors of life in a pediatric dialysis unit.

Volumetric machines would seem to obviate the need for metabolic weight monitoring during hemodialysis, but when dialyzing a very small child or infant, every available indicator of the patient's condition must be used. This allows the nursing staff to detect and prevent potential problems, rather than deal with the consequences.

Heparinization of the pediatric renal patient on hemodialysis is much different than for the adult. An initial bolus of heparin is given based on the patient's weight, usually 5 U/kg for patients weighing less than 25 kg, or 3 U/kg for patients weighing more than 25 U/kg. Then a continuous infusion of heparin, which can be full strength (1000 U/ml) or diluted (500 U/ml, 100 U/ml, or even 50 U/ml) depending on the child's weight as well, is administered over the entire treatment. The rate of the infusion starts out at 30 U/kg/hr for patients under 25 kg, up to 1000 U/hr for those over 25 kg. The rate is adjusted in order to keep the activated clotting times (ACTs) of blood taken from the venous blood tubing between 180 and 200 seconds. For "tight" heparinization, the clotting times should be kept at no more than 25% above the baseline or preheparinization value. The heparin infusion is usually maintained throughout the treatment for children with subclavian or femoral catheter blood vessel access. It is often discontinued 30-60 minutes before completion of the treatment for children with arteriovenous fistulae.

ACTs are done frequently on the acute patient or the new chronic patient to ascertain the child's heparin needs. Although they remain basically the same, these needs tend to fluctuate much more during subsequent treatments than they do in adult patients. As a result, even long-term chronic hemodialysis patients need ACTs performed at least once or twice per treatment. Infection or exposure to cigarette smoke, whether in the home environment or if the child takes up smoking, will markedly increase the child's heparin requirements. Children with acute renal failure may need higher doses of heparin at first since they have not had renal failure long enough for the normal clotting factors to be affected. Children being dialyzed or hemoperfused for drug overdoses or poisonings definitely will need more heparin than a child of similar size in renal failure.

In an effort to decrease the amount of time required for each adult hemodialysis treatment, high-flux and high-efficiency hemodialysis modalities were developed. More permeable hemodialyzer membranes and volumetric ultrafiltration control delivery systems have been crucial to this progress.

High-flux dialysis uses a membrane that is permeable to solutes with a wide range of molecular weights, including the relatively heavy beta-2 microglobulin. High-efficiency dialyzers have membranes permeable to solutes in the low to middle molecular weight range; the upper limit is usually a molecular weight of 5000 (Keen & Gotch, 1991).

In addition to rapid solute removal, the high-flux and high-efficiency membranes also move fluid rapidly. High-flux dialyzers ultrafiltrate 10-60 ml/hour times the TMP; and high-efficiency dialyzers, 5-15 ml/hour times the TMP. Precise volumetric control of ultrafiltrate is required to prevent rapid dehydration of the patient or back filtration of dialysate across the membrane when low ultrafiltration pressures are used (Keen & Gotch, 1991).

Increased blood flow rates of 300-500 ml/min and increased dialysate flow rates of 1000 ml/min or more are required to maintain an optimal diffusion gradient with countercurrent flow through the dialyzer (Keen & Gotch, 1991).

Although children have a smaller volume of distribution, they receive the same clearance of solutes as adults do, which leads to a much greater overall mass transfer of solutes. Furthermore, they achieve maximum clearance levels of solutes at relatively low blood flow speeds. It might be argued then, that children receive high-efficiency dialysis all the time (Harmon & Jabs, 1994).

Shortened hemodialysis treatment time is not appropriate for children. The very rapid blood flows required cannot be obtained from pediatric patients' access, and a short time on dialysis is not sufficient for meeting pediatric metabolic needs. Short-time dialysis does not provide adequate clearances to allow growth, or sufficient time for complete middle molecule clearance. The usual pediatric hemodialysis schedule is a 4-hour treatment three times a week, unless severe fluid overload or metabolic problems, such as hyperkalemia, call for a longer treatment. Five or 6-hour treatments may be required occasionally. For home hemodialysis patients, 3 hours every other day is an option that may be adequate, however, it results in only 21 hours on the machine every 2 weeks, vs. 24 hours every 2 weeks with the usual schedule.

In order to control beta-2 microglobulin buildup in pediatric patients who are going to require long-term hemodialysis, the use of high-flux hemodialyzers may be required. Beta-2 microglobulin is removed by natural kidney function, removed partially by PD, and minimally removed by standard hemodialyzers. High-flux dialyzers will slow the rate of buildup, but will not prevent amyloid deposition altogether. Neither will these synthetic membrane dialyzers remove beta-2 microglobulin already accumulated in the patient's body, so they will not cure bone disease or other side effects of that accumulation (McCarthy et al., 1994).

Access issues. Blood vessel access issues are, in some ways, the same for children as for adults. In the early days of pediatric hemodialysis, external shunts and AV fistulae were the most common accesses. Gradually, the use of single lumen subclavian catheters and single-needle dialysis became more common for acute hemodialysis. The development and rapid improvements in dual-lumen subclavian catheters caused their increased use in children because they allow more efficient hemodialysis.

Some centers use permanent subclavian catheters as the only access for pediatric patients on chronic hemodialysis. The catheters offer needleless therapy, a real plus for young children with tiny veins or for those with a needle phobia.

Diligent sterile technique during attachment and detachment from hemodialysis, and exacting exit site care both in the dialysis unit and at home can result in long-term catheter function. One center had used a 3-minute povidone iodine scrub followed by a 3-minute soak of the arterial and venous catheter limbs at the start and finish of treatments. However, a fairly high catheter infection rate caused the staff to change to a 5-minute scrub and a 5-minute soak before putting a child on or taking her off dialysis. The catheter infection rate is almost zero now, and one patient had the same subclavian catheter for almost 6 years.

Although a viable long-term access for pediatric patients, subclavian catheters can be problematic. Their function is much more likely to be positional in children than in adults. Pediatric patients with subclavian catheters often have to be coaxed into assuming and holding unusual positions throughout a treatment to ensure adequate blood flow for the procedure. This is a particularly difficult task if the child is a toddler whose coping mechanism is movement.

After a hemodialysis treatment, subclavian catheter lumens are flushed with sterile normal saline, a sterile cap is applied, and the lumen is either flushed with a heparin solution (50, 100, or 500 u/ml, depending on the patient's weight), or straight 1000 u/ml heparin is instilled in the lumen. It is important that the pediatric dialysis unit staff know the exact volume of each lumen of the catheter as one should only instill that amount of heparin plus 0.1-0.2 ml more to ensure the entire lumen is heparinized.

Generally the children who are admitted to the hospital will receive flushes with dilute heparin every 6 to 12 hours, depending on the frequency of using their subclavian access for blood samples or medication administration. It is best if such use can be avoided, as repeated access increases the likelihood of infection. Sometimes there is just no way to avoid using the subclavian.

Children who are outpatients should not have to use heparin flushes at home because of increased likelihood of bleeding due to excessive heparinization, and of infection secondary to contamination. Some pediatric centers have found that instilling undiluted heparin at the end of a hemodialysis treatment will keep most subclavian catheters patent until the beginning of the next treatment. The heparin will be withdrawn from the catheter prior to the next hemodialysis treatment in order to prevent overheparinization. After each treatment, the catheter's exit site is cleaned and a sterile dressing is applied to the exit site. The dressing and the external catheter limbs are held in place with a transparent plastic dressing, such as Tegaderm® or Op-site®.

In spite of careful heparinization, catheters can clot. If a partial clot or fibrin collection forms, it can sometimes be cleared by using urokinase in the catheter. The children call it "Drano® for catheters," and it can be that effective.

Children with subclavian catheters should not take showers, swim, or engage in activities likely to bump or pull on their catheters or exit sites. In addition, keeping cool enough to prevent perspiration from dislodging the sterile dressing is important, particularly in summer. Although they seem intricate, these precautions enhance long-term catheter function.

Acute and chronic dual-lumen hemodialysis catheters are the most prevalent pediatric accesses. However, some chronic hemodialysis patients are unable to tolerate the lifestyle changes necessary to keep a subclavian catheter functioning well long term. Children can have arteriovenous (AV) fistulae created from natural veins, or with polytetrafluoroethylene (PTFE) grafts if their own veins are too small. Once hemostasis is achieved at the end of a treatment, and bandaids applied, the children are free to do most activities. Traumatizing or lacerating the fistula is to be avoided, but water sports and showers are permissible.

AV fistulae can have the same malfunctions in children as in adults: clotting, insufficient flow, infection, and steal syndrome. A complication of AV access unique to children is that the limb with the fistula may grow more slowly than the contralateral limb. Because of their small veins, it is also easier to compromise circulation in children and possibly cause the loss of the limb distal to the fistula.

Some children may experience repeated vascular access problems and may eventually lose all possible access sites. The long-term implications of this problem are greater in the pediatric patient who may have 50 or 60 years of hemodialysis ther-

Table 15-4
Pediatric hemodialysis complications.

Patient problems
- hyperkalemia
- hypocalcemia
- hypernatremia
- fluid overload
  - pulmonary edema
  - hypertension
  - edema
- muscle cramps
- fever

Minor emergencies
- hypertension
- hypotension
- blood leaks from the dialyzer, tubing or access
- machine malfunctions
- allergic reaction to initiation of dialysis

Major emergencies
- air embolism
- cardiac arrest
- seizures
- spontaneous bleeding
- disequilibrium syndrome

apy ahead of him, than in the adult patient with only 10 or 20 years of additional life expectancy.

One of the issues that makes pediatric dialysis much more expensive than adult dialysis is the high staff-to-patient ratio that is required to safely hemodialyze children. A child who weighs more than 25 kg and is physiologically and psychologically stable on hemodialysis, probably needs no more attention than an adult. However, if physiological or psychological problems occur, that child may need a 1:2, or possibly even 1:1 staff-to-patient ratio. Children who weigh between 12 kg and 25 kg definitely require 1:1 staffing, and those weighing less than 12 kg may require 2:1 staffing.

Children should be desensitized to prepare for hemodialysis therapy whenever possible (Gilman & Frauman, 1982). Children who need hemodialysis acutely, and who are very young or have not been prepared for the treatment, must be entertained and encouraged to remain in one place during the treatment. The very uncooperative child can be sedated, but children should never be restrained during a hemodialysis treatment.

Hemodialysis of the acutely ill neonate is extremely labor intensive. Two RNs skilled in neonatal hemodialysis, or one RN and one technician, along with the pediatric nephrologist, must be in the room throughout the hemodialysis session. A neonatologist, nurses from the neonatal ICU, and possibly a respiratory therapist, will also need to care for the infant whether the dialysis is done in the neonatal ICU or in the pediatric dialysis unit. Constant observation and instantaneous response to correct physiological changes are vital to a successful treatment outcome. Neonates often show minimal signs or symptoms of physiologic change before their vital signs vary. Crying, yawning, a change in facial expression, or in color of skin or mucous membranes may indicate an adverse reaction is about to occur (Topor, 1981). While not all of these professionals will be needed at any one time, instant accessibility to their expertise may be required at unpredictable moments.

Complications. The complications that arise in pediatric hemodialysis patients are essentially the same as for adult patients. The main difference with children is that their smaller size and metabolic sensitivity make such complications much more likely to occur. There are three categories of complications: patient problems, minor emergencies, and major emergencies (see Table 15-4).

As with adult patients, prevention is preferable to correction for any of these complications. The pediatric patient will require close observation and frequent assessment; blood pressures are usually taken once every 15 to 20 minutes. Children weighing less than 12 kg need a blood pressure taken every 5 minutes on acute dialysis. Neonates receiving hemodialysis may need one taken every minute.

Incenter vs. home hemodialysis. Acute hemodialysis and chronic hemodialysis of the pediatric patient who weighs less than 25 kg should be done in a unit staffed and equipped to handle pediatric hemodialysis. However, for the child who will be on hemodialysis for the foreseeable future, and who is larger than 25 kg, home hemodialysis is a reasonable option.

Whether or not a family succeeds with home hemodialysis depends on their interest in accomplishing this treatment goal, their ability to learn the procedures, and the support they receive from their dialysis center. A complete training program that teaches sterile technique, machine function, trouble shooting, and minor machine maintenance, as well as basic hemodialysis operations, and monitoring and adjustment skills is required. Many pediatric dialysis centers find that they have very few home hemodialysis candidates. In that instance, referring the pediatric patient to a well-established home hemodialysis program in an adult dialysis center is very appropriate, instead of formulating a program for just one or two patients in the pediatric center. Physiologically, if the child is large enough to dialyze safely at home, he/she is large enough to dialyze safely in an adult unit.

Peritoneal Dialysis

There are many different techniques to use in performing PD. Intermittent peritoneal dialysis (IPD), continuous ambulatory peritoneal dialysis (CAPD), and continuous cycling peritoneal dialysis (CCPD), which is sometimes called automated peritoneal dialysis (APD), are the ones routinely used with pediatric patients.

Techniques. *Intermittent peritoneal dialysis* (IPD) is commonly used for the acutely ill renal failure patient who requires frequent (every 1 to 2 hour) exchanges, and thus uses large volumes of fluid each day. Most patients on IPD are dialyzed in the pediatric intensive care unit, are usually quite ill, and require constant nursing interventions in addition to their hourly PD exchanges. Fluctuations in their serum chemistries often require frequent adjustments to the composition of their peritoneal dialysate.

The main disadvantage to IPD is that it is done with an open system, one that has air vents and other openings that permit bacteria on dust motes and droplet nuclei to enter the system in spite of careful nursing techniques. This, combined with the frequent breaks in the system required by the recurring changes of fluid bags, increases the likelihood of developing peritonitis. A child on IPD much longer than 4 to 5 days will almost certainly develop peritonitis. Many centers will try to convert the pediatric IPD patient to a closed CAPD system as quickly as possible after the patient's condition stabilizes to forestall the development of peritonitis.

Continuous ambulatory peritoneal dialysis (CAPD) is a description of the method of performing this PD therapy, not a description of the patient who uses it. Just like the elderly diabetic with bilateral below-the-knee amputations, the infant who has not yet learned to walk can be very appropriately dialyzed with CAPD.

CAPD provides the opportunity for the most normal lifestyle for the pediatric dialysis patient who will not be transplanted in the foreseeable future. Being on CAPD requires few, if any, dietary restrictions, and generally fewer medications than other renal replacement therapies. Children on CAPD who are doing well generally come to clinic only once a month, so they can remain in school almost full time.

The usual CAPD prescription is an exchange volume of 30-50 ml/kg body weight given three to five times a day, depending on the child's residual renal function and catabolic rate. As is true with adult patients, the higher the percentage of dextrose in the PD solution, the more fluid removed. Children use the standard 1.5%, 2.5% and 4.25% solutions, but their exact prescription varies with individual eating habits, residual renal function, blood pressure, and fluid status.

There are many different types of commercial systems available to deliver PD fluid to the patient. Some involve keeping the bag that contained the peritoneal dialysate on the solution transfer set attached to the Tenckhoff catheter until after the used fluid is drained out of the peritoneal cavity. In that instance, the child will store the empty bag in a jeans pocket, a fanny pack or other carrying device. Creative families have devised many different alternatives (see Figures 15-2a through 15-2d). Other systems allow the patient to disconnect from the original dialysate container, keeping only a short transfer set attached until time for the next exchange. Several vendors offer mechanical devices to assist in performing the exchange quickly and accurately.

Each PD vendor offers several different types of systems, and each vendor attempts to make their systems user-friendly and resistant to user error. Almost any system can be adapted for the pediatric patient. The center must choose a vendor based on the quality of patient support services, reliability of supply sterility, supply availability, and cost-effectiveness.

The major disadvantage of CAPD is that it is unremitting. The exchanges must be done four times a day every day for as long as the child is receiving that therapy. Unlike some adult patients who are only required to do exchanges on 6 days out of 7, children need all the exchanges they can get in order to optimize growth.

Some families adapt well to this requirement and treat CAPD as just another general body maintenance procedure, like taking a shower or brushing teeth. Other families find the relentless responsibility very tiring, and look for different ways to lighten the burden. This might involve additional caretakers, such as extended family members or family friends, being trained to do CAPD in order to relieve the parent. Usually the adult CAPD patient and one other helper are trained to do CAPD. A pediatric patient with divorced and remarried parents and a busy lifestyle may need up to six people trained to provide care.

Children dialyzed on CAPD do very well. They grow, have the maximum possible time in school, have about the same energy level as their well peers, and enjoy diets with few restrictions. The children's serum chemistries remain in an acceptable range, and they generally feel good. As a result, many pediatric centers recommend CAPD as the dialysis treatment of choice for their pediatric patients.

Automated peritoneal dialysis (APD), or *continuous cycling peritoneal dialysis* (CCPD), operates on the same principles as CAPD. However, a machine is used to infuse the proper amount of dialysate, time the dwell period, and drain the dialysate from the body. The machines are designed

Figure 15-2
Ways to Carry PD Bags When Baxter PD System III Is Used

Photos courtesy of Riley Hospital for Children, Indianapolis, IN.

Figure 15-2a
In an ammunition pouch purchased at an Army-Navy Surplus store.

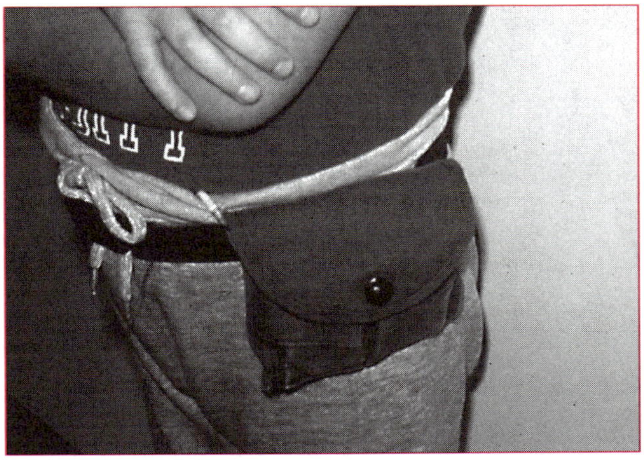

Figure 15-2b
In a child-sized over-the-shoulder purse.

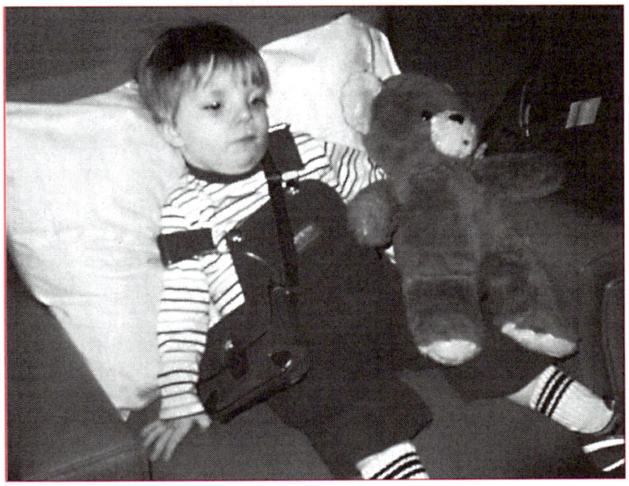

Figure 15-2c
Wrapped around child's body and held in place with wide ACE bandage.

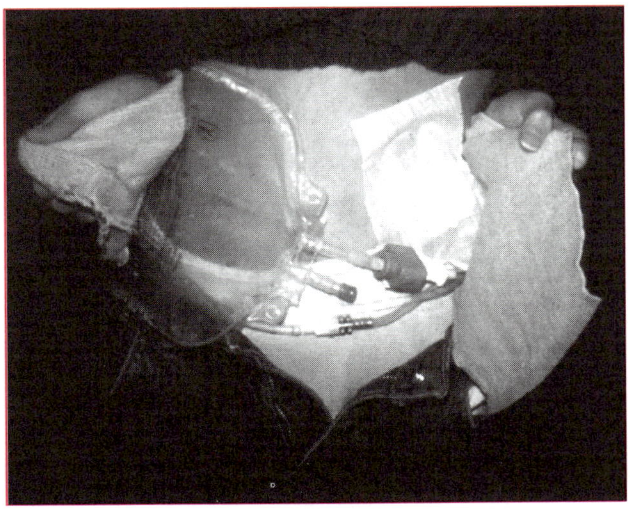

Figure 15-2d
Same child with ACE bandage fastened. DO NOT use safety pins!

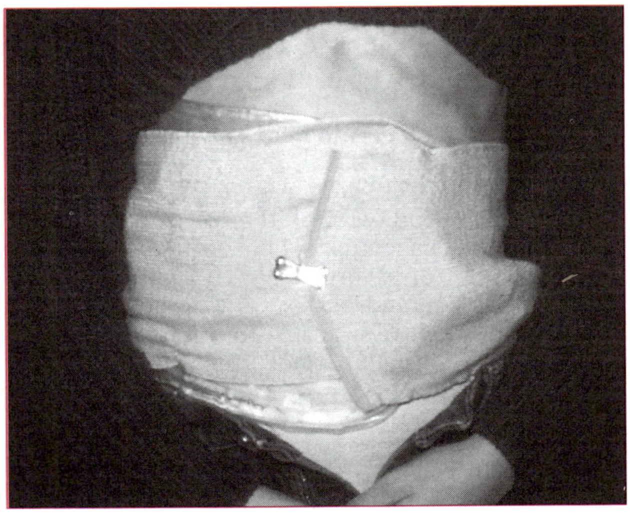

to alarm if any of these procedures are not occurring properly or completely. The exchanges are done while the child is attached to the machine for 10 to 12 hours each night.

Many pediatric dialysis centers routinely start each child in chronic renal failure on CCPD because they feel the weight of parental responsibility in performing CAPD dialysis exchanges is excessive. Other centers use CCPD for temporary or permanent parental respite. It is more expensive than CAPD but provides a viable alternative.

Children who develop recurrent hernias when walking around with CAPD fluid in their abdomen should be switched to CCPD. An 8-year old with encopresis on CAPD was totally continent when changed to CCPD. In addition to fewer demands on family caregivers, CCPD requires fewer breaks in the closed PD system, and thus decreases the likelihood of contamination. Children with frequent bouts of peritonitis on CAPD may have fewer episodes on CCPD.

The main disadvantage of CCPD is that clearances are decreased as dialysis takes place only during a 10 to 12-hour period, instead of throughout the entire day. As a result, more fluid volume per day is required to get enough dialysis, which, in addition to the tubing sets and drain bags as well as machine rental or purchase price, results in a higher cost than CAPD. Often pediatric patients on CCPD run higher serum creatinines than children on CAPD, or than they did on CAPD. Sometimes an overday dwell, or an additional exchange during the day may be needed to control the creatinine.

An important consideration in doing CCPD is that the child not feel isolated from the family during the exchange time. Children whose cycler is kept in their bedroom, and who are old enough not to be asleep during the entire procedure, will hate the whole experience if the rest of the family spends the evening gathered in the family room (Hislop & Lansing, 1983).

Families who are able to switch back and forth between CAPD and CCPD will be the most successful on CCPD. On a regular school night, doing CCPD at home is very appropriate. However, if the family wants to go to grandmother's for the weekend, it may be too much of a hassle to arrange to have a cycler moved for such a short time period. In that instance, the family can switch to CAPD for the weekend, and feel free to travel without compromising the child's therapy (Hislop & Lansing, 1983).

Access issues. Access for each type of PD is achieved with a Tenckhoff catheter. The choice of straight or curly, of one cuff or two, varies from center to center. A nonfunctioning Tenckhoff catheter is extremely frustrating for patients, family and caregivers. As with adults, poor positioning of the catheter, constipation, fibrin, omentum, and adhesions from past abdominal surgeries have all been known to interfere with catheter function. Some children are hypersensitive to the catheter, and get eosinophilia at the exit site or in the peritoneal cavity.

Figure 15-3
Infant's Tenckhoff catheter exit site located well away from the diaper area.

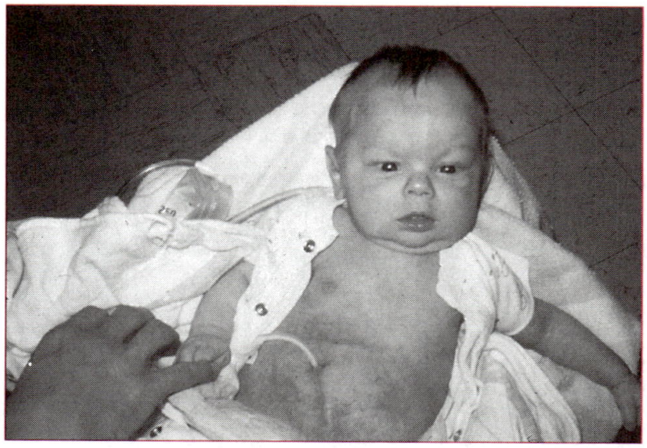

Photo courtesy of Riley Hospital for Children, Indianapolis, IN.

Children, particularly those not yet toilet trained, have a high risk of exit site and tunnel infections. For those still wearing diapers, a long subcutaneous tunnel with the exit site well away from the diaper area is strongly recommended (see Figure 15-3).

The exit site care procedure varies with each institution. Some are absolutely adamant about sterile technique and insist dressings be worn over the exit site at all times. Other units just ask the patient to wash the exit site with Betadine during the daily shower, and tape the transfer set to the abdominal skin to prevent pulling on the Tenckhoff at the exit site.

Complications. Children on PD run similar risks of complications as adults do. Exit site infections are more prevalent in children still wearing diapers, but for the toilet-trained child they may be no more frequent than in the adult population. Tunnel infections are usually secondary to exit site infections. These infections can progress to peritonitis, or peritonitis can be the result of contaminations during the exchange procedure.

Breaks in the closed system, rather than poor exchange technique, are more often the cause of contamination. Children have been known to bite holes in the tubing or bag (teething babies are notorious chewers), stick needles through the solution transfer set, play tug-of-war with the dog using the solution transfer set, pull the tubing off the Tenckhoff when jumping out of a tree, or pull the spike out of a bag due to walking away while a parent is performing an exchange. Parents, too, can cause contaminations. One mother, who was holding her baby while cooking dinner, melted the solution transfer set when it rubbed on a stove burner. In short, if there is a way to cause a break in the system, someone will do it sooner or later.

Frequent episodes of peritonitis can cause the peritoneal membrane to thicken, thus reducing ultrafiltration and solute movement efficiency. Membrane failure, which can be defined as insufficient ultrafiltration with or without abdominal adhesions or decreased peritoneal surface area, may be severe enough to require a patient change from PD to hemodialysis (Andreoli et al., 1993). Some children with ultrafiltration failure may need to be hemodialyzed intermittently (once or twice a week) for fluid removal while being maintained on PD.

Peritonitis caused by alpha streptococci or *Pseudomonas aeruginosa* leads to membrane failure more often than that caused by other bacteria. In addition, patients treated with PD for a long time will develop membrane failure, possibly due to damaging effects of prolonged exposure to hypertonic glucose. Decreased membrane function can begin as early as 24 months after initiation of PD. The exact duration of treatment before total membrane failure varies with individuals. It is further difficult to define as more children are transplanted than are peritoneally dialyzed for lengthy time periods (Andreoli et al., 1993).

A final complication of PD is family burnout. The continuous requirement for treatment interventions in the home, including daily PD exchanges, concomitant tube feedings, injections of erythropoietin and/or growth hormone, and medication administration, put a great burden on home caregivers (Rigden, 1994). Treatment demands along with the high stress level of modern society, such as two-income families, child care requirements, and the financial and social burdens of rearing a child with renal failure, can quickly lead to mental, physical, and emotional exhaustion. If the caregiver is a single parent, or perceives that few supportive resources are available, the progression to depletion will be much quicker. Pediatric renal nurses must be alert for signs of burnout and help families develop coping mechanisms or obtain respite to prevent serious side effects, such as poor exchange technique or cessation of dialysis altogether.

Incenter vs. home PD. The purpose of CAPD or CCPD is that it can be done in the home to maximize normality for the patient and family. Incenter PD would be too intermittent if done every 3 to 5 days as in the past. It would not promote wellness as the child's serum chemistries would be too far out of the normal range, and diet and fluid intake too restricted to permit growth. If incenter PD were to be done daily, the child would have to reside in the hospital, which would be a totally abnormal lifestyle.

Continuous Renal Replacement Therapies

Techniques. Continuous renal replacement therapies (CRRT) are relatively recent additions to the list of treatment modalities being used on children. There are several forms of CRRT. Those used on children most frequently include continuous arteriovenous hemofiltration (CAVH), continuous arteriovenous hemodiafiltration (CAVHD), continuous venovenous hemofiltration (CVVH), and continuous venovenous hemodiafiltration (CVVHD). Slow continuous ultrafiltration (SCUF) and therapeutic plasma exchange (TPE) are also available, but are infrequently used in the pediatric renal failure patient population. Consequently they will not be discussed here.

While some centers have almost totally replaced acute hemodialysis in children with some form of CRRT, other centers use it only on the most critically ill patients — those who would be unlikely to survive the stress of intermittent hemodialysis treatments. Naturally, the center's choice in this matter is directly reflected in its survival statistics. Those using CRRT for almost all acute renal failure episodes have very good outcome statistics. Centers using CRRT only for ventilated patients in the pediatric intensive care unit with several major organ systems in failure in addition to the kidneys, naturally have fewer successful outcomes.

The same volume considerations in pediatric hemodialysis apply to the extracorporeal circuit in any of the CRRTs. No more than 10% of the child's circulating blood volume can be in the extracorporeal circuit at any one time. Blood prime may be required if the commercial set-up is not within the patient's 10% limit.

CAVH. CAVH provides the critically ill and hemodynamically unstable patient with safe, effective therapy through slow, continuous fluid and solute removal (Stapleton & Wright, 1992). The system has a built-in feedback loop: if the patient's blood pressure drops, the rate of ultrafiltration will automatically decrease (Macias, Mueller, Scarim, Robinson, & Rudy, 1991). Along with improved fluid and electrolyte balance, CAVH also provides improved myocardial contractility in children with postoperative decreased cardiac output. Better pulmonary gas exchange, decreased CVP, and reduced afterload with few changes in the mean arterial pressure (MAP) are additional benefits (Suddaby, Bell & Murphy, 1990; Zobel et al., 1991)

CAVH for children is set up in the same manner as it is on adult patients. Just as in adults, a child must have an MAP of 60 mmHg and sufficient cardiac function to push the blood through the extracorporeal circuit in order for CAVH to be successful. Both an arterial and a venous access is required, because it is the pressure differential that permits blood flow through the circuit and causes the filter to remove fluid from the circuit. Finding an arterial access with sufficient flow, particularly in the very small patient, is an extremely difficult task. In addition, the severely ill pediatric patient, especially the severely ill infant, is unlikely to be able to maintain an MAP sufficient to ensure adequate CAVH function.

In the early days of CAVH, some units compensated for this lack of cardiac function by splicing a blood pump segment into the system and running the pump at a very low speed (2 to 5 ml per minute) to assist the flow through the circuit (Bell, 1988). Eventually this technique evolved into CVVH.

In some adult units, CAVH filtrate is allowed to flow out by gravity, and replacement fluid inflow rate is increased or decreased to match the rate of outflow. Pediatric patients must have the filtrate rate regulated by an IV pump or flow controller. This prevents too much fluid coming off too quickly, thus getting ahead of the replacement fluid rate, and causing hypotension or shock.

Heparinization of the CAVH circuit attached to the pediatric patient is based, at least at the outset, on the patient's weight. An initial bolus of 20-40 u/kg is given, followed by a slow infusion of 10 u/kg/hr. The goal is to maintain the patient's activated clotting time (ACT) between 180-220 seconds, in order to prevent clotting within the circuit. Because the flow rate within the circuit may be slow, or may fluctuate, a higher level of heparinization may be required.

CVVH. CVVH offers the advantage of a blood pump to provide flow through the extracorporeal circuit and maintain system function. This means that an arterial access is not required, and the patient's MAP is not an issue. However, having a blood pump in the circuit makes it very easy to entrain air in the system, thus requiring a venous drip chamber and foam detector to be added to the circuit. Hemodialysis bloodlines are used as they have enough length and all the required attachments. However, the longer length of hemodialysis bloodlines increases the risk that the extracorporeal volume will exceed the 10% limit on smaller children. Blood prime of the circuit will be necessary in that event.

Heparin is infused through the saline-Y along with both replacement fluids and any required saline boluses. The built-in heparin administration line is then available for use as a pressure monitoring line, and is hooked up to the cardiac monitor via an arterial pressure monitoring set-up.

Heparinization during CVVH can be a little tighter than that for CAVH as the flow though the filter is easily maintained by the blood pump. A bolus of 20 u/kg is given when attaching the patient to a new system, which is followed by a continuous infusion of 20 u/kg/hr. The infusion is usually adjusted to keep the ACTs between 180-200 seconds, but they may be allowed to drop as low as 160 in children with bleeding tendencies. The infusion is generally diluted to 50 or 100 u/ml so that small amounts of heparin are infused via higher flow rates on the IV pumps. This results in greater dose accuracy and better mixing in the system than if very small amounts of fluid were used.

Figure 15-4
Continuous venovenous hemodiafiltration (CVVHD) in the newborn intensive care unit. Dialysate system is on the IV stand on the right.

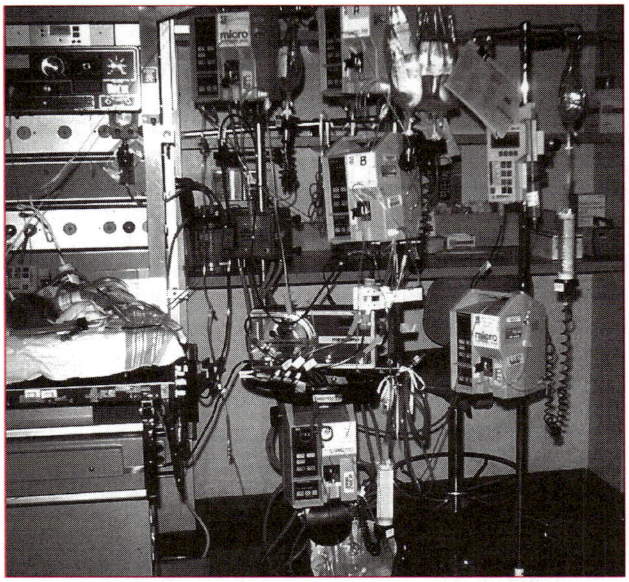

Photo courtesy of Riley Hospital for Children, Indianapolis, IN.

Hemodiafiltration. If CAVH or CVVH is not able to provide enough solute removal to control a patient's catabolic state, CAVHD or CVVHD can be begun. In hemodiafiltration, dialysate, usually sterile 1.5% dextrose peritoneal dialysate is pumped into the filter countercurrent to the blood flow (see Figure 15-4). The ultrafiltrate pump must be set high enough to withdraw the volume of dialysate plus the required volume of fluid to be removed. The dialysate works in the same manner as it does in hemodialysis to increase solute removal via osmosis (Jenkins, Harrison, Jackson, & Funk, 1991).

The dialysate used in CAVHD or CVVHD must be sterile because of the large pores in the filter membranes that would permit bacteria to travel across into the patient's blood. Septicemia would result if the dialysate used were only clean, as it is in hemodialysis.

The rate of the dialysate flow is guided by the rates available on the pump used to remove both the filtrate and used dialysate from the filter. There are few IV pumps available that can exceed 1000 ml/hour, so dialysate flow cannot exceed half that rate unless more than one pump is used on the outflow port.

Access issues. As in all treatments involving extracorporeal circulation, blood vessel access is the biggest problem. CAVH requires use of femoral or umbilical arteries, and some type of vein. It should be noted that standard thick-walled umbilical catheters do not permit adequate blood flow for CAVH, but thin-wall catheters will prevent mechanical obstruction and stasis.

The blood pump in CVVH permits the use of dual-lumen catheters in a subclavian or femoral vein in larger children. Either the acute or chronic type catheter may be used. In the past, Mauer and Lynch (1976) found that umbilical catheters worked well for neonatal hemodialysis, but more recent investigators have found that umbilical vessels do not permit sufficient blood flow for CVVH on neonates. They recommend, instead, the use of 6.5 or 7 French dual lumen catheters placed in the femoral or subclavian vein (Bell, 1988; Thompson et al., 1991). Internal jugular veins have also been used for access on very small babies.

Complications. Both CAVH and CVVH can present many complications. CAVH system function is dependent on the arterial pressure the patient's ventricle can generate. Decreased MAP, ultrafiltrate changes, or clotting problems in the system or filter will result in decreased blood flow through the filter and less-effective therapy. Air embolism is a particular problem in CAVH. Air bubbles in the system will quickly enter the patient with the usual complications.

CVVH presents the unique problem of continued ultrafiltration even if the patient becomes hypotensive. The blood pump in the circuit also increases the risk of drawing air into the system. The foam detector on the venous drip chamber should prevent air embolism to the patient.

Patients receiving treatment from either modality run the risk of infection, or bleeding due to heparinization or coagulopathies. In addition, there can be clotting in filter or circuit due to low flow or underheparinization. Blood loss can occur from the circuit if system parts separate, or the patient may bleed due to over-heparinization. Incorrect fluid replacements will lead to electrolyte imbalance, hypotension if too much fluid is removed, or hypertension if not enough fluid is removed. Circulation to a limb distal to access point may also be impaired, resulting in ischemic damage.

Measuring Adequacy of Dialysis in Children

Normalized whole body clearance of urea is widely used in adult hemodialysis patients to assess adequacy of dialysis. If the patient's dietary protein intake is adequate, a Kt/V value of 1.0 or more is considered to indicate sufficient dialysis. Because of their higher nutritional needs and metabolic requirements by weight, children require higher urea clearances than do adults. A greater postdialysis disequilibrium between intracellular fluid (ICF) and extracellular fluid (ECF) urea concentrations in children may skew the results if an immediate postdialysis blood sample were used as it is in adult patients. When Kt/V is calculated in pediatric hemodialysis, the postdialysis blood sample should be drawn 1 hour after the treatment is finished to allow full equilibration between ICF and ECF urea concentrations (Evans, Smye & Brocklebank, 1992).

Unfortunately, no studies have been done to determine that a Kt/V of 1.0 or greater will guarantee adequate dialysis and desired clinical outcomes in children. Studies of adequacy measurements in children receiving PD are only just beginning. It will be several years before valid results will be available to permit formulation of recommendations for pediatric adequacy guidelines.

Transplantation

Transplantation is, for the most part, the treatment goal for all children with chronic renal failure. In the past, it was the only long-term goal. Currently, there is some speculation about the advisability of delaying transplantation and maintaining a child on long-term PD while administering synthetic growth hormone in order to achieve maximum stature prior to transplant. Transplanting children as quickly as possible is still the treatment of choice. Some centers support preemptive transplants before dialysis is necessary. Unlike adults, who may decide to continue dialysis indefinitely or who may not be offered transplantation due to advanced age, long-term dialysis is used for children only when transplantation is not available. Living related donor transplants are more likely in children than adults, because two biological parents who are genetically a 50% match for the child are often available, even eager, to donate a kidney. Siblings over age 18 can also donate. Each sibling stands a 25% chance of matching four antigens, a 50% chance of matching only two antigens, and a 25% chance of matching no antigens.

It is feasible to transplant an adult organ into a small child, but fluid shifts and maintaining an adequate blood pressure to perfuse the kidney may be a problem initially. In addition, mechanical difficulties, such as crimped arteries or kinked ureters can arise if the kidney is too large for the child. The transplant surgeon will make the determination about using an adult kidney.

The immune suppressive regimen in children is similar to that in adults, with the exception of attempting to move to alternate day steroids as quickly as possible because of the adverse effects of steroids on growth.

Specific Nursing Interventions

The purpose of nursing intervention for the child and family is to attain independence from health care providers, normality in lifestyle and optimal emotional, physical, mental and social development. Children and their parents must be an integral part of the care given. Prevention of problems is always to be preferred to intervening after the problem has occurred or worsened.

Nutrition

Nutritional needs of children with chronic renal failure are complex and require a great deal of attention from a multidisciplinary team of renal health care providers. Physicians are adept at determining the metabolic needs of children with chronic renal failure, dietitians are knowledgeable about determining the food and fluid intake that will meet those needs, but nurses and parents must implement a dietary plan that the child will actually consume. Most children need encouragement to eat enough nutrients and calories, but a few may need to be on restrictive diets. In that event, children must be prevented from eating the wrong things, and encouraged to eat enough for energy and growth.

An additional consideration is the need to cope with school cafeterias, restaurants, birthday parties, and sleepovers, while maintaining the child's dietary regimen. This needs to be done with sensitivity, perhaps allowing the child mild indiscretions, compensating either with dialysis or with greater restrictions during another part of the day. Often restaurants, theme parks, and other facilities will be happy to provide a nutritional analysis of the foods available; they need only to be asked. All parents and all children who are old enough to be making choices about food, need to be aware of exactly what dietary restrictions or requirements are necessary, and be taught to read food labels so that they can meet those needs. With the advent of mandatory food labels, specifying the amounts of protein, sodium, potassium and other nutrients present, this task has become easier.

The major difference in renal dietary regimens for children is their need for sufficient nutrients, especially calories, for growth; these must be superimposed on the requirements and restrictions inherent in a renal failure diet. Pure carbohydrates and pure fats are used for this purpose, since these have little effect on renal function. Supplementing with polycose and other sugars, sometimes with the addition of concentrated medium-chain triglyceride (MCT) oils, is often necessary to provide adequate calories for growth. These substances may cause digestive problems such as poor absorption or diarrhea, and adjustments must be made accordingly. Additionally in very small children or infants, nasogastric (NG), gastrostomy, or other tube feeding techniques may be needed to ensure adequate intake. Feeding by mouth is obviously preferable, but anorexia is common in chronically ill children. Severely anorexic teenagers may also have to be treated with tube feeding regimens.

Children treated with hemodialysis have restrictions on intake similar to those of adults. However, what they eat, what they prefer to eat, and when and where they eat may differ widely. Protein restrictions are poorly tolerated by children, especially those who have begun to eat meat. It is very difficult for a parent, especially when others are present, to refuse a crying child one more bite of chicken or hamburger. Just like other children of similar ages, children with renal failure may develop strong attractions (fads) or aversions to certain foods. However, maintaining optimal nutrition is critical to enhancing growth and development. Helping parents and children come to agreement on how the dietary regimen will be handled will be most effective in resolving these issues.

Children receiving PD have fewer dietary restrictions than children on hemodialysis. They may actually require higher than normal amounts of protein because of losses from the peritoneal cavity. Nutrition may be adversely affected, at least initially, by the feeling of fullness induced by the dialysate in the abdominal cavity.

Nutrition after transplantation resembles that for healthy children. Again, the emphasis is on optimal nutrition. Steroid use may cause a great increase in appetite with resulting undesirable weight gain in some children. Additionally, sodium and fluid retention may be a problem for some children. As the steroid dosage is decreased to an alternate day regimen, these problems are likely to resolve.

Pharmacologic Concerns

Children with chronic renal failure receive most of the same medications as adults do. However, medication dosages for children are *always* calculated on the basis of milligrams of medication per kilogram of body weight per day. Dosages are then divided as appropriate for the drug. When growth occurs, doses must be recalculated on a timely basis.

Tables indicating proper dosages are found in a variety of pediatric texts, and must be used every time a new medication is given. As in adults, consideration must be given to the route of excretion of the drug, and modified when the route is via the kidneys. Dialyzability of drugs is also a consideration, just as it is in adults. In addition, children may metabolize certain drugs differently than do adults, and a pediatric reference text should be consulted when giving drugs to children. Children are often less able to articulate symptoms resulting from drug side-effects; they must be observed carefully, and questioned in terms they understand.

One medication given much more frequently to children is Shohl's solution or bicitra. This is an acidic preparation, which metabolizes to alkaline, and buffers the metabolic acidosis so common in children. Both Shohl's solution and bicitra are preparations of sodium citrate and citric acid, with 1 mEq of acid per cc of solution. These medications are usually locally prepared by a pharmacist, and modifications can thus be made if necessary.

The actions, side effects, and risks of medications are the same in children as in adults. There are only two real differences in medicating children. First, ensure that the dosage is appropriate in mg/kg of body weight for the size of the child. Second, it may be necessary to come up with different administration techniques to coax the uncooperative child to actually take the medicine. Oral medications are often vomited, especially when the child is in renal failure. The nurse may need to find little tricks to prevent this outcome, or just to readminister the dose. For example, pills may be crushed between two spoons and mixed with ice cream, jelly, or honey. Some medications come in both pill or liquid forms. Be careful when mixing medications in food that the volume of food is not too great for the child to consume.

Therapeutic Environment

Florence Nightingale, the fundamental nursing theorist, was the first to note how important a therapeutic milieu was to promote healing. She wrote that ventilation, food, light, cleanliness, noise level, and variety were important considerations in the care of the sick. She also noted that children "...are affected by the same things, but much more quickly and seriously, viz., by want of fresh air, of proper warmth, want of cleanliness...by startling noises...by dullness and by want of light" (Nightingale, 1859, p. 72).

In addition to ensuring that a pediatric renal unit is clean, light, airy, and reasonably quiet, decorations must be planned keeping in mind the viewpoints of the children who will be the patients. The actual needs and preferences of the children should be considered, not just the adults' ideas of their areas of interest (Thompson & Stanford, 1981). Most pediatric renal units serve a wide range of ages, so providing age-appropriate decor can be a real challenge. The staff may need to decorate different parts of the unit with materials appropriate for each of the age groups coming to the unit.

One should keep in mind that younger children are very concrete, and pictures, posters or murals of cartoons or other characters with missing or broken body parts will be very disturbing to them. Young children may assume that dialysis leads to the loss of body parts in that instance (Frauman & Gilman, 1989). Furthermore, some murals that look innocuous to an adult may be more frightening than entertaining for the very young child.

Older children are at least bored, or even insulted if the decor is focused on too young a theme. In addition, too young a focus can demean children's very real concerns about their serious illness, or imply denial that they experience pain or sadness about their disease (Hardgrove, 1980).

The ultimate goal in a pediatric renal unit is to "create a sense of caring, of gentleness, of beauty, of reassurance" (Hardgrove, 1980, p. 68). The use of color, carefully selected posters and murals, and, above all, the children's artwork can lead to a cheerful therapeutic environment. Hanging children's artwork makes them feel valued, as well as in control of their environment. Holiday decorations made by the children and used repeatedly enhance their feelings of being valued, and also give a sense of continuity in the unit. It also helps the staff remember the children who made the decorations, and who may have been transplanted, recovered function, graduated to an adult dialysis unit, or died.

Patient safety must be a prime consideration when planning a pediatric renal unit. Space, lighting, electrical outlets' location and relationship to the emergency generator, location of electrical cords running to machines, handwashing facilities and hoppers for waste disposal, isolation capabilities for infectious patients, and washable walls and flooring must be carefully planned (Frauman & Gilman, 1989). The unit floor plan must be designed to maximize nursing care, prevent falls, and limit children's access to sharp instruments and hazardous chemicals.

Furniture in the pediatric renal unit must be appropriate for the various sizes of children served, yet allow staff to give care without intractable back pain. Tables and chairs, cribs, beds, and hemodialysis chairs must accommodate all sizes of children to be cared for. If small toilet facilities are not feasible, portable potty chairs or seat adapters for adult-size toilets must be available (Frauman & Gilman, 1989).

Play materials differentiate the pediatric renal unit from an adult unit. There must be appropriate materials for all ages of children served, but this does not mean that they must be complicated or expensive. Creative materials such as watercolors, scented markers, crayons and paper, or clay are particularly good choices. Books, puzzles, board games, card games, bubble makers, stacking toys and other items for quiet play are also useful. Television, videotapes, and computer games are good diversions that help time pass quickly, but they must not be allowed to take the place of interpersonal interactions with staff members or other children. Water play, finger painting, and tempera painting on easels are fun and creative, though messy (Frauman & Gilman, 1989). Cover-ups need to be handy to preserve clothing and contain messes.

Making appropriate decorations for each of the holidays, even made-up holidays like the dialysis unit's birthday, help to relieve monotony, and provide an opportunity for creativity and fun. The decorations made by patients and staff are almost always preferable. Flour and salt sculpting dough, paper for chains or cutouts, and paint are inexpensive materials to use for these projects. Bulletin boards, chalk boards, or the door into the unit can be decorated in holiday themes. Even the windows can be painted with washable paint to complete the decor (Frauman & Gilman, 1989).

The physical facilities, equipment and supplies alone are not enough to ensure that the pediatric renal unit provides a therapeutic environment. Child and family-oriented care provided by a multidisciplinary staff with an attitude oriented to children is the most crucial element (Frauman & Gilman, 1989). Promoting normality in parent-child interactions, encouraging the child's participation in his/her care to the greatest possible extent, and incorporating siblings in the therapy are vital steps in that care.

Normal Life

Family Relationships

Children with complex physical problems often come from families with complex problems as well. Family relationships do not always conform to societal expectations, and they are not always what they seem on the surface. As there are many possible configurations for families, it is best to let the members define the scope of their particular family group (Frauman & Gilman, 1990; Gilman & Frauman, 1979). Careful assessment is necessary through both interviews and observations.

Children frequently live with a single parent, almost always the mother, putting a tremendous burden on one person to provide for all of the child's needs. If this parent is employed, she provides most or all of the family's income and health insurance coverage as well. Providing full-time care at home to the child with chronic renal failure is not an option. Clearly, help must come from somewhere. Enlisting the services of the social worker to obtain assistance with child care, enhance extended family support, and work with church and neighborhood groups, who then become in effect an extended family, may all be necessary. Often, older siblings become surrogate parents, which may lead to problems, especially during adolescence. Sometimes, the single parent may have to stop working and accept public assistance in order to provide the needed care for the child with chronic renal failure and siblings. Any single parent caring for a child with chronic renal failure will need exceptional assistance and support.

Step-parent families, and families in which the mother has a live-in boyfriend, are increasingly common. The male figure's relationship with the child may range anywhere from virtually indistinguishable from that of a biological parent to nonexistent. Often families are reluctant to share information about the relationship, and feel inquiries are intrusive. Except in an urgent situation, it is probably best to assess the relationship over time, and through observation as much as through direct questioning.

Direct questions may cover a wide range of issues. For example, does the step-parent (or surrogate) bring the child to clinic or treatments? Does he or she participate in the care of the child or attempt to learn about the child's care? Does the person touch or hold the child? Is he or she patient with inevitable tears, or is the person angry and demanding of the child much of the time? The answers to these questions can provide valuable clues as to the nature of the relationship. Even if a step-parent or other companion is in the household, if the relationship with the child is strained or nonexistent, the parent will require support similar to that needed by a single parent.

Grandparents should neither be ignored, nor expected to act as surrogate parents by the health care team. Ascertaining the relationships between grandparents, parents, and grandchildren is necessary, just as in assessing other family relationships. Grandparents who seem very involved in a crisis situation, may not be able to maintain their support because of illnesses of their own, or living some distance away. Routing information to grandparents through the parents is ideal, but this may not be possible when the parents are very young, poorly educated, or when the supply of bad news seems overwhelming. Grandparents' questions should be answered without betraying family confidences. Grandparents should also be involved in family teaching to the degree comfortable for them, the parents and the child. A grandparent innocently handing a banana to a child on potassium restrictions can be a dangerous situation. Other extended family members may also have very close ties to the child with chronic renal failure, and thus must be considered by the nurse in planning care.

Siblings of the child with chronic renal failure are often not directly available to health team members for assessment or intervention. Helping parents to provide adequate care for the siblings, without feeling constantly guilty, or neglecting the other children, can be difficult. Again, enlisting aid from all those available to provide support is necessary. It may be helpful to bring the sibling(s) in to clinic or to the treatment facility to demystify what is happening to the child with chronic renal failure.

Psychosocial Care of Patient and Family

In caring for the child with chronic renal failure and his family, it is crucial to focus on keeping life as normal as possible for the entire family. The impact of chronic renal failure on the family unit can be devastating physically, psychologically, socially and educationally (Frauman & Gilman, 1985). Upon receiving the diagnosis of chronic renal failure, the family will begin the grief process, which mourns the change in the child's health as well as the loss of a normal healthy child. Families come to realize that "...life...will never be the same again" (Dracopoulos & Weatherly, 1983, p. 141). The resulting anger, fear and frustration can last a long time. In fact, pain often recurs as siblings and peers achieve normal developmental milestones. Family members are reminded that the child with chronic renal failure may not reach these milestones, or may not reach them as easily; the child will always be different. When the child understands that chronic means forever, he or she may develop behavior problems. These problems along with the treatment demands, disruption of work, altered family life and relationships, and financial considerations leave all family members feeling overburdened and out of control (Dracopoulos & Weatherly, 1983).

In beginning to assist pediatric chronic renal failure patients and their families, nephrology nurses must ensure that they are presented with all possible treatment options, and given assistance in making a truly informed choice. Nephrology nurses must be sure that they have clear explanations of the goals and problems attached to each treatment modality (Rigden, 1994). Participation in formulating the treatment plan gives the family maximum control of the situation.

Children must also participate in planning and give their consent for treatment at a developmentally appropriate level (Gilman & Frauman, 1982). They should participate in their treatment, or at least cooperate while someone else performs it. Parents will learn to care for the child initially, but should gradually decrease their participation as the child matures and is able to take increasing responsibility for self-care. Remember, parents naturally have a hard time trusting anyone, even their child, to do the required care as well as they have themselves over the years (Frauman & Gilman, 1985).

In coping with chronic renal failure, the family should avoid centering itself around the sick child. This is not a normal situation, and will predictably lead to sibling resentment, fears, and guilt. Furthermore, family members should avoid personifying the child as the illness and parent(s) as the successful treatment. Thus undesired outcomes will not be equated with parenting failure (Dracopoulos & Weatherly, 1983).

Family members should be encouraged to expect the child with chronic renal failure to make progress toward developmental milestones, in the normal chronological order, if not at the usual ages. Making adaptations to assist the child's progress may be necessary. However, mastering self-care skills, going to school, participating in extracurricular activities as well as activities of daily living, finishing school, and progressing to employment are normal goals for all children. Working on these achievements helps family members to keep a perspective on the illness, to view the child as normal, and improves everyone's self-esteem (Frauman & Gilman, 1985, 1990; Gilman & Frauman, 1979). Expecting the child with chronic renal failure to assume the same kinds of household responsibilities that their healthy siblings do goes a long way toward decreasing anger and conflicts.

The nephrology nurse's goal should be to enhance the family's ability to care for the child, without being intrusive or fostering dependence. Suggestions should be carefully phrased, and interventions made in a nonjudgmental manner so that the family does not feel criticized, even by implication (Frauman & Gilman, 1990). One begins by identifying family strengths and weaknesses, and the type and extent of support they are likely to require from the pediatric nephrology team (Rigden, 1994). It may be difficult to recognize the need for emotional support, as some families try to garner caregiver approval, or to appear competent by hiding their stress from caregivers (Frauman & Gilman, 1990).

Anticipatory guidance should be offered at the critical events in the child's illness such as diagnosis, starting dialysis, or transplantation. At each of these events, the nurse will teach family members about how to care for the child; and explain everything that will be done, including how it works, how it feels, and why it is necessary in a manner appropriate to the child's and family's level of understanding (Gilman & Frauman, 1979).

Nurses should identify expected issues or problems at each of the critical events, and help all family members deal with them. They can also help the family find effective coping mechanisms. Fostering and maintaining extended family relationships and friendships is helpful. Calling upon the family's past successes in dealing with problems is particularly effective. Facilitating networking with families of other children with chronic renal failure can enhance coping skills. Promoting open, honest two-way communication between caregivers and family is crucial to success with these interventions (Frauman & Gilman, 1985, 1990; Gilman & Frauman, 1979; Rigden, 1994).

Play

Play is a very convenient intervention strategy when providing nursing care to children with chronic renal failure. Play can be used for assessment, patient teaching, and providing some much-needed pleasure to the child.

It is often difficult to gauge the emotional status of children receiving treatment for chronic renal failure. Small children, especially, have difficulty identifying and articulating their feelings of fear, anger, and frustration. Projective techniques using play, stories, and drawings can help nurses to understand what the child is perceiving and feeling, making them thus able to intervene more appropriately (Gilman & Frauman, 1987).

Play activities can also be used to facilitate physical assessment. Drawing pictures on tongue blades, allowing children to explore equipment and examine parents or the nurse may make assessments less threatening, particularly when a child is first ill. Children will reciprocally play with the nurse during the assessment, such as during contests to determine who can open their mouth the widest. Having a focus for the child's eyes, such as a favorite toy or an adult doing something silly, will greatly facilitate eye examinations even in a very small child (Gilman & Frauman, 1987).

Teaching techniques based in play are probably the most effective methods that can be used with children. Even a child who can read a brochure or booklet will learn better through play demonstrations and games. Providing pleasure for the child is a goal of therapeutic play that should not get lost in the intense care necessary for these children.

School

School placement is a critical necessity for children with chronic renal failure. However, schools are often reluctant to have such children attend. Despite their misgivings, though, schools are required to provide education services for children with chronic renal failure and other chronic disorders. Federal legislation, including PL 94-142, PL 99-457, and the Individuals with Disabilities Education Act (IDEA), requires that all children receive an appropriate education in the least-restrictive environment. Children with chronic conditions are considered to be at risk for developmental disabilities, and may be eligible for services from birth to 5 years for that reason. Despite a variety of federal, state, and local case finding initiatives, parents may need to be quite assertive in securing these services for their child with chronic renal failure.

In addition, parents of children with chronic renal failure are often only offered services in handicapped classes or in homebound instruction. These may not be appropriate placements for an individual child. Appropriate placement should be determined on the basis of a thorough psychological evaluation, and discussions with health care providers, parents, the child, and professional educators.

Decreased expectations of accomplishment for children with chronic renal failure may lead to diminished performance. Since the majority of children with renal failure survive to adulthood, they have the same need to develop independence as do other children; part of that independence is the ability to support oneself through meaningful employment. This is impossible without an adequate education. Such a concern may seem far-fetched when thinking about a 3-year-old, or an 8-year-old who doesn't have much energy, but all too soon the child becomes an adult without the needed knowledge and skills.

In addition, children with chronic renal failure need the social interaction preschool and school activities afford. Isolation from other children is not only lonely, but may affect self-esteem and retard development of social and adaptive behaviors. Often parents and children discover a number of skills previously unidentified, and sources of pleasurable activity not before tried. School placement is an absolute necessity for children with chronic renal failure, as necessary for future life as renal replacement therapy.

Special Occasions

Birthday parties, their own and those of other children, are a part of normal life for most children. Children with chronic renal failure need to have those same opportunities. For the child's own party, having refreshments, activities, and other aspects of the party as much like their peers as possible, is important. If serving hamburgers and french fries or pizza is the norm, then that must be done. If the child with chronic renal failure is on a restricted diet, smaller amounts, or food cooked without salt can be provided unobtrusively. Going on an outing can be planned to follow a rest period if the child tires easily.

Travel is possible for children with chronic renal failure, but it requires considerable advance planning. For a child on dialysis, referral to another facility in the area to be visited is a necessity. The child on hemodialysis will need to be treated in the facility, and the child on PD will require services should there be a crisis with supplies or equipment, or should peritonitis develop. The facility should preferably be a pediatric unit: most are accustomed to dealing with transient patients, especially those near frequent child tourist spots such as Disney or other theme parks, or national parks. Care of equipment and medications should be planned for. Some equipment is very sensitive to movement, and many medications lose their efficacy in a hot car. If the child tires easily, flying or making short trips in the car may be needed. Sometimes sleeping while traveling prevents the child with chronic renal failure from arriving at a greatly desired destination in an extremely fatigued state.

Camp is a normal activity for most children, and children with chronic renal failure are no exception. There are a number of special camps around the country designed exclusively for children with chronic renal failure. Camp facilities may include hemodialysis stations, PD exchange clean rooms, and medication dispensing areas. Alternatively, arrangements may be made with a nearby facility for dialysis treatments. Usually these camps accept children receiving all modalities of treatment, including conservative management. Ideally, the emphasis is usually on having fun, and providing respite for parents rather than the pursuit of a therapeutic goal such as patient teaching. Children with chronic renal failure, especially those with a functioning transplant, may elect to attend a camp primarily for healthy children, such as scout camp or a religious camp. In that case, informing everyone of the child's status and having locally available facilities for care is imperative.

Programs Assisting the Family

Financial

Medicare. Ever since Congress passed PL 92-603 in 1972, the chronic renal failure program of Medicare has covered anyone under age 65 if they have renal or kidney failure. Thus, children with chronic renal failure can indeed qualify for Medicare. Of course, it is highly unlikely that a child could meet the quarters-of-work requirement, so either one or both of the parents' work histories can be used (Oberley, Schatell, & Sacksteder, 1992).

Medicaid. If neither parent has sufficient work quarters to qualify for Medicare, a real likelihood with teenage parents of an infant with chronic renal failure, a family with a limited income may well qualify for Medicaid. This program is administered differently in each of the states, but essentially it is designed to pay for medical expenses for persons unable to fund their own medical care. The extent of the coverage and the application process also varies from state to state; the pediatric dialysis unit social worker should be able to guide patients' families concerning local procedures. If a family exceeds the income levels to qualify for Medicaid, exceptions may be made if a high percentage of the family's income is spent on medical costs; the family should be encouraged to explore this possibility (Oberley et al., 1992).

Supplemental Security Income (SSI). This federal program supports aged, disabled, or blind individuals with limited income and assets (including cash, land, personal property, and life insurance). The monthly payments can be a temporary measure until the patient qualifies for Social Security Disability, an unlikely event for the pediatric patient, or can be a permanent source of income. One applies for this program at the local Social Security Office (Oberley et al., 1992).

Handicapped Children's Assistance. This program will have different names, application procedures, and coverage in different states. Crippled Children's Assistance and Children with Special Health Care Needs are two examples. Generally, these programs help with the medical expenses arising from catastrophic diseases, and may provide other services as well.

Private support. Local agencies, communities and/or states may have private funds available to help specific beneficiaries, such as pediatric renal failure patients. These funds often arise in aid of a particular patient and then continue as a memorial to that patient. Churches or community groups may offer short or long-term financial aid to a family (Dracopoulos & Weatherly, 1983). Some families even choose to start such a fund for themselves, but should be warned that excessive fund-raising may affect their qualification for governmental assistance programs, or programs funded by other sources.

Method I vs Method II Payments. Families who will be performing dialysis at home are required to sign HCFA form 382-U4 when a child has reached chronic renal failure, and is certified by the physician on HCFA Form 2728. It is purely up to the family whether to select Method I or Method II for payments. However, most families are completely overwhelmed with the diagnosis of chronic renal failure, and with their new responsibility to learn to care for the child at home. They frequently turn to the dialysis center staff for guidance in making this decision. One may reassure them that the net effect on the family of the choice of Method I or Method II is probably not very different. The backup support and care they receive from the dialysis center is the same. The kind of bills that will show up in their mailbox is the same. The major distinction is that they will be required to contact the vendor to arrange for supply delivery if they select Method II. For intelligent or medically sophisticated families, this is not a daunting concept. Those new to the medical system will probably find it much easier to select Method I and let the center do the supply procurement work.

Should the family become unhappy with their Method selection, it is always possible to change. However, the window opens for change only once each year on January 1. The center should get the paperwork signed and sent in mid-December, so beginning the new Method at the first of the new year is not problematic.

Information Sources

When first presented with the diagnosis that their child will be in chronic renal failure, most families are overwhelmed. For many the next step is to gather as much information as they can find. The pediatric dialysis unit will have information about the specific treatment modality selected for the child, as well as how their unit functions in general. For information about kidney disease, all treatment modalities available, and sources of both financial and psychosocial assistance, parents may contact their local chapter of the National Kidney Foundation and the American Kidney Fund, or their local chronic renal failure Network office (Tri-State Renal Network, 1991).

The National Institute of Diabetes and Digestive and Kidney Disease (NIDDK), part of the National Institutes of Health, also has booklets, fact sheets, information packets, catalogs and guides available at minimal prices. In addition, it offers comprehensive lists of professional-level articles available by treatment modality, as well as a newsletter, *KU Notes,* describing the latest developments and information available about kidney and urologic disease.

As with most chronic illnesses, there is a real lack of instructional material available at a level appropriate for younger children. Several organizations and pediatric dialysis centers have identified this problem, and are working on developing material at reading levels appropriate for preschool, school-age, and teenage patients.

Care for Children with Chronic Renal Failure in Other Countries

Care for children with chronic renal failure is not markedly different in countries other than the United States. Acceptance rate per million child population for treatment of chronic renal failure differs widely by country, ranging from 0 in countries including Iceland, Ireland, and Morocco, to 12 and 18 in Finland and Cyprus. This can be compared with an overall acceptance rate of 4.6 for the EDTA community (Broyer et al. 1993). Transplantation is the preferred treatment modality throughout Europe, Australia, and Japan (Broyer et al., 1993; Hisano et al., 1991; Hodson et al., 1990), but PD and hemodialysis are also frequently used. Similar problems with treatment and rehabilitation are reported, and outcomes are largely similar. However, unlike the adult population, children with chronic renal failure less than 15 years old in the U.S. are more likely to survive than their counterparts in either Europe or Japan (Held et al., 1990).

Summary

Care for children with chronic renal failure is a complex but rewarding nursing task. The pediatric nephrology patient is not just a tiny adult, but a member of a special patient population with unique requirements. Children differ markedly from adults in their physiological responses to chronic renal failure, and treatment regimens differ considerably. Furthermore, the child with renal failure is not a discreet entity, but part of a family unit.

In order to provide successful care, the pediatric nephrology nurse must recognize the total impact of renal failure on the child and all family members, and plan to meet the needs of everyone in the family. Careful attention must be given to growth and development issues, nutrition, psychosocial support, and educational achievement, in addition to the special techniques required for performing successful renal replacement therapies on pediatric patients. Development of the child needs to be considered continually in every aspect of care, and adaptations must be made as the child develops. Because the child with chronic renal failure has a much-longer total remaining life span than the adult chronic renal failure patient, the pediatric nephrology nurse's work has a far-reaching impact.

References

Alexander, S.R. (1990). Controversies in pediatric renal transplantation. *American Kidney Fund Letter, 7*(2), 5-21.

Alexander, S.R. (1994). Peritoneal dialysis. In M.A. Holliday, T.M. Barratt, & E.D. Avner (Eds.), *Pediatric nephrology* (3rd ed.) (pp. 1339-1353). Baltimore: Williams & Wilkins.

Andreoli, S.P., Langefeld, C.D., Stadler, S., Smith, P., Sears, A., & West, K. (1993). Risks of peritoneal membrane failure in children undergoing long-term peritoneal dialysis. *Pediatric Nephrology, 7*, 543-547.

Beck, A.L., Nethercut, G.E., Crittenden, M.R., & Hewins, J. (1986). Visibility of handicap, self-concept, and social maturity among young adult survivors of end-stage renal disease. *Developmental and Behavioral Pediatrics, 7*, 93-96.

Bell, S.B. (1988). CAVH in pediatrics: Meeting the challenge. *ANNA Journal, 15*(1), 25-26.

Benfield, M., & Michael, A. F. (1992). Immunology of uremia. In C.M. Edelmann (Ed.), *Pediatric kidney disease* (2nd ed.) (pp. 783-790). Boston: Little, Brown and Company.

Benfield, M., Parker, K.L., Waldo, F.B., Overstreet, S.L., & Kohaut, E.C. (1993). Treatment of growth failure in children after renal transplantation. *Transplantation, 55*, 305-308.

Broyer, M., Chantler, C., Donckerwolke, R., Ehrich, J.H.H., Rizzoni, G., & Scharer, K. (1993). The paediatric registry of the European Dialysis and Transplant Association: 20 years experience. *Pediatric Nephrology, 7*, 758-768.

Clarren, S.K. (1994). Malformations of the renal system. In M.A. Holliday, T.M. Barratt, & E.D. Avner (Eds.), *Pediatric nephrology* (3rd ed.) (pp. 491-514). Baltimore: Williams & Wilkins.

Crittenden, M.R., Holliday, M.A., Piel, C.F., & Potter, D.E. (1985). Intellectual development of children with renal insufficiency and end stage disease. *International Journal of Pediatric Nephrology, 6*, 275-280.

Dracopoulos, D.T., & Weatherly, J.B. (1983). Chronic renal failure: The effects on the entire family. *Issues in Comprehensive Pediatric Nursing, 6*, 141-146.

Ehrich, J.H., Rizzoni, G., Broyer, M., Brunner, F.P., Brynger, H., Fassbinder, W., Geerlings, W., Selwood, N.H., Tufveson, G., & Wing, A.J. (1992). *Nephrology Dialysis and Transplantation, 7*, 579-586.

Ekbaum, P. (1994). Embryology and prenatal development. In M.A. Holliday, T.M. Barratt, & E.D. Avner (Eds.), *Pediatric nephrology* (3rd ed.) (pp. 2-20). Baltimore: Williams & Wilkins.

Evans, J.H.C., Smye, S.W., & Brocklebank, J.T. (1992). Mathematical modelling of haemodialysis in children. *Pediatric Nephrology, 6*(4), 343-353.

Fennell, R.S., Fennell, E.B., Carter, R.L., Mings, E.L., Klausner, A.B., & Hurst, J.R. (1990). A longitudinal study of the cognitive function of children with renal failure. *Child Nephrology and Urology, 10*, 199-204.

Fine, R.N., Malekzadeh, M.H., Pennisis, A.J., Ettenger, R.B., Uittenbogaart, C., & Korsch, B.M. (1978). Long-term results of renal transplantation in children. *Pediatrics, 61*, 641-650.

Fine, R.N., Koch, V.H., Boechat, M.I., Lippe, B.H., Nelson, P.A., Fine, S.E., & Sherman, B.M. (1994). Growth after recombinant human growth hormone treatment in children with chronic renal failure: Report of a multicenter randomized double-blind placebo controlled study. *Journal of Pediatrics, 124*, 374-382.

Frauman, A.C., & Gilman, C.M. (1990). Care of the family of the child with end stage renal disease. *ANNA Journal, 17*(5), 383-386, 401.

Frauman, A.C., & Gilman, C.M. (1989). Creating a therapeutic environment in a pediatric renal unit. *ANNA Journal, 16*(1), 20-22, 26.

Frauman, A.C., & Gilman, C.M. (1985). "Normal life" - A goal for the child with chronic renal failure. *ANNA Journal, 12*(3), 192-195.

Frishberg, Y., Obrig, T.G., & Kaplan, B.S. (1994). Hemolytic uremic syndrome. In M. A. Holliday, T.M. Barratt, & E.D. Avner (Eds.), *Pediatric nephrology* (3rd ed.) (pp. 871-889). Baltimore: Williams & Wilkins.

Gambro, A.B. (date unknown). *In vitro clearance Gambro Lundia Mini-minor 13.5 micron dialyzer.* (Graph). Lund, Sweden: Author.

Gilman, C.M., & Frauman, A.C. (1982). Dialysis desensitization: Preparation of the very young child for chronic hemodialysis. *Dialysis and Transplantation, 11*(8), 660-661.

Gilman, C.M., & Frauman, A.C. (1979). Psychosocial care of the child in renal failure. *AANNT Journal, 6*(3), 143-148.

Gilman, C.M., & Frauman, A.C. (1987). Use of play with the child with chronic illness. *AANNT Journal, 14*(4), 259-261.

Gruskin, A.B., Baluarte, H.J., & Dabbagh, S. (1992). Hemodialysis and peritoneal dialysis. In C.M. Edelmann (Ed.), *Pediatric kidney disease* (2nd ed.) (pp. 827-916). Boston: Little, Brown and Company.

Hardgrove, C. (1980). Children respond to therapeutic art. *Hospitals, 54*, 67-69.

Harmon, W.E., & Jabs, K. (1992). Factors affecting growth after renal transplantation. *Journal of the American Society of Nephrology, 2*, S295-S303.

Harmon, W.E., & Jabs, K. (1994). Hemodialysis. In M.A. Holliday, T.M. Barratt, & E.D. Avner (Eds.) *Pediatric nephrology* (3rd ed.) (pp. 1354-1372). Baltimore: Williams & Wilkins.

Held, P.J., Brunner, F., Odaka, M., Garcia, J.R., Port, F.K., & Gaylin, D.S. (1990). Five-year survival for end-stage renal disease patients in the United States, Europe, and Japan, 1982-1987. *American Journal of Kidney Disease, 15*, 451-457.

Held, P.J., Turenne, M.N., Liska, D.W., Zobel, D.L., Alexander, S.R., & Jones, D. (1991). In P. Terasaki (Ed.), *Clinical transplants.* Los Angeles: UCLA Tissue Typing Laboratory.

Hisano, S., Miyazaki, C., Hatae, K., Kaku, Y., Yamane, I., Ueda, K., & Okamua, S. (1991). Immune status of children on continuous ambulatory peritoneal dialysis. *Pediatric Nephrology, 6*, 179-181.

Hislop, S., & Lansing, L. (1983). A comparison of pediatric home peritoneal dialysis modalities: The family point of view. *AANNT Journal, 11*(10), 22-23, 53.

Hodson, E.M., Knight, J.F., Sheil, A.G.R., Roy, L.P., Harris, J.P., Rogers, J.R., Stephen, M.S., Boulas, J., Thompson, J.F., & May, J. (1990). End-stage renal failure in children: 16 years' experience at one Australian center. *Medical Journal of Australia, 152*, 245-250.

Jenkins, R.D., Harrison, H.L., Jackson, E.C., & Funk, J.E. (1991). Continuous renal replacement in infants and toddlers. *Contributions to Nephrology, 93*, 245-249.

Johnson, K.B. (Ed.). (1993). *The Harriet Lane handbook* (13th ed.). St. Louis: C.V. Mosby Company.

Keen, M.L., & Gotch, F.A. (1991). Dialyzers and delivery systems. In M.G. Cogan, & P. Schoenfeld (Eds.), *Introduction to dialysis* (2nd ed.) (pp. 1-44). New York: Churchill Livingstone.

Kjellstrand, C.M., Shideman, J.R., Santiago, E.A., Mauer, S.M., Simmons, R.L., & Buselmeier, T.J. (1971). Technical advances in hemodialysis of very small pediatric patients. *Proceedings of the Dialysis and Transplant Forum*, 124-132.

Koch, V.H., Lippe, B.M., Nelson, P.A., Boechat, M.I., Sherman, M.M., & Fine, R. (1989). Accelerated growth after recombinant human growth hormone treatment of children with chronic renal failure. *Journal of Pediatrics, 115*, 365-371.

Macias, W.L., Mueller, B.A., Scarim, S.K., Robinson, M., & Rudy, D.W. (1991). Continuous venovenous hemofiltration: An alternative to continuous arteriovenous hemofiltration and hemodiafiltration in acute renal failure. *American Journal of Kidney Diseases, 18*(4), 451-458.

Mauer, S.M., & Lynch, R.E. (1976). Hemodialysis techniques for infants and children. *Pediatric Clinics of North America, 23*(4), 843-856.

McBride, P. (1984) The development of hemo- and peritoneal dialysis. In A.R. Nissenson, R.N. Fine, & D.E. Gentile (Eds.), *Clinical dialysis* (pp. 1-26). Norwalk, CT: Appleton-Century-Crofts.

McCarthy, J.T., Williams, A.W., & Johnson, W.J. (1994). Serum beta-2 microglobulin concentration in dialysis patients: Importance of intrinsic renal function. *Journal of Laboratory and Clinical Medicine, 123*(4), 495-505.

Mehls, O., Blum, W.F., Schaefer, F., Tonshoff, B., & Scharer, K. (1992). Growth failure in renal disease. *Bailliere's Clinical Endocrinology and Metabolism, 6*, 665-685.

Morel, P., Almond, P.S., Matas, A.J., Gillingham, K.J., Chau, C., Brown, A., Kashan, C. E., Mauer, S.M., Chavers, B., Nevins, T.E., Dunn, D.L., Sutherland, D.E.R., Payne, W.D., & Najarian, J.S. (1991). Long-term quality of life after kidney transplantation in childhood. *Transplantation, 52*, 47-53.

Morris, K.P., Skinner, J.R., Wren, C., Hunter, S., & Coulthard, M.G. (1993). Cardiac abnormalities in end stage renal failure and anemia. *Archives of Disease in Childhood, 68*, 637-643.

Nightingale, F. (1859). *Notes on nursing: What it is and what it is not.* London: Harrison Publishing.

Oberley, E.T., Schatell, D., & Sacksteder, P. (1992). *Employment, insurance and finance - facts and resources for the dialysis patient.* Madison, WI: Medical Media Publishing.

Polinsky, M.S., Kaiser, B.A., & Stover, J.B. (1987). Neurologic development of children with severe chronic renal failure from infancy. *Pediatric Nephrology, 1*, 157-165.

Rasbury, W., Fennell, R.S., Fennell, E.B., & Morris, M. (1986). Cognitive functioning of children with end stage renal disease pre- and post-dialysis session. *International Journal of Pediatric Nephrology, 7*, 45- 50.

Rigden, S. (1994). Planning therapy. In M.A. Holliday, T.M. Barratt, & E.D. Avner (Eds.), *Pediatric nephrology* (3rd ed.) (pp. 1419-1422). Baltimore: Williams & Wilkins.

Rosenkranz, J., Bonzel, K.E., & Bulla, M. (1992). Psychosocial adaptation of children and adolescents with chronic renal failure. *Pediatric Nephrology, 6*, 459-463.

Scharer, K. (1990). Growth and development of children with chronic renal failure. *Acta Paediatrica Scandinavia, 366*, S90-S92.

Solhaug, M.J., Adelman, R.D., & Chan, J.C.M. (1992). Hypertension in the child with chronic renal insufficiency or undergoing dialysis. *Child Nephrology and Urology, 12*, 133-138.

Stapleton, S., & Wright, J. (1992). Continuous arteriovenous hemofiltration: An alternative dialysis therapy in neonates. *Neonatal Network, 11*(4), 17-25.

Suddaby, E.C., Bell, S.B., & Murphy, K.J. (1990). Continuous hemofiltration in infants and children. *Pediatric Nursing, 16*(1), 79-82.

Thompson, G.N., Butt, W.W., Shann, F.A., Kirby, D.M., Henning, R.D. , Howells, D.W., & Osborne, A. (1991). Continuous venovenous hemofiltration in the management of acute decompensation in inborn errors of metabolism. *The Journal of Pediatrics, 118*(6), 879-884.

Thompson, R.H., & Stanford, G. (1981). *Child life in hospitals.* Springfield, IL: Charles C. Thomas.

Topor, M. (1981). Chronic renal disease in children. *Nursing Clinics of North America, 16*(3), 587-597.

Tri-State Renal Network, Inc. (1991). *Living with kidney disease: A patient manual.* Indianapolis, IN: Author.

United States Renal Data System. (1993). *United States Renal Data System 1993 annual data report* (NIH Publication No. 93-3176). Bethesda, MD: U.S. Government Printing Office.

Zobel, G., Stein, J.I., Kuttnig, M., Beitzke, A., Metzler, H., & Rigler, B. (1991). Continuous extracorporeal fluid removal in children with low cardiac output after cardiac operations. *The Journal of Thoracic and Cardiovascular Surgery, 101*(4), 593-597.

Chapter Highlights

- There are two major problems with pediatric transplantation: First, it is a relatively rare procedure due to the small number of patients requiring transplantation (a very busy center will do only 15-25 patients per year); second, most advances in transplantation procedures are designed for and tested on adult patients.

- Less than 6% of pediatric cases reported in 1987-1990 list diabetes and hypertension as primary diagnosis, in contrast to more than 60% of adult patients (United States Renal Data System, 1993).

- The most frequent cause of chronic renal failure in children is glomerulonephritis (37.6% of all reported cases), followed by congenital/other hereditary diseases (19.1%) (United States Renal Data System, 1993).

- Children with chronic renal failure have the same developmental needs as healthy children. They may need additional assistance from parents, health care providers, educators, and others to achieve their maximum potential at each of the developmental stages.

- Children with chronic renal failure go through the same developmental stages that other children do. However, the rate at which they progress through the stages is often markedly delayed, and not necessarily consistent across developmental domains.

- Physical growth failure is perhaps the most pervasive developmental issue for children with chronic renal failure.

- Nutrition; metabolic acidosis; fluid and electrolyte disturbances, especially calcium and phosphorus; medications used in treatment, especially corticosteroids; and decreased production and use of hormones have all been implicated in growth failure (Mehls, Blum, Schaefer, Tonshoff, & Scharer, 1992).

- The hallmark of pediatric hemodialysis is the requirement that only 10% or less of the child's circulating blood volume can be in the extracorporeal circuit.

- Play materials differentiate the pediatric renal unit from an adult unit. There must be appropriate materials for all ages of children served..

- The physical facilities, equipment, and supplies alone are not enough to ensure that the pediatric renal unit provides a therapeutic environment. Child and family-oriented care provided by a multidisciplinary staff with an attitude oriented to children is the most crucial element (Frauman & Gilman, 1989).

- School placement is an absolute necessity for children with chronic renal failure; it is as necessary for future life as renal replacement therapy.

CHAPTER 16

The Diabetic Patient

Marta R. Taylor, MSN, RN, NP, CNN

Chapter Contents

Forms of DM and History of Disease 467
Screening for Diabetes 468
Structural and Functional Abnormalities in Diabetic Nephropathy . . . 468
Diagnosis of Diabetic Nephropathy 469
Clinical History 469
Physical Examination 469
Laboratory Tests 469
Clinical Features of Established Diabetic Nephropathy 470
Management of Established Diabetic Nephropathy 471
Control of Blood Glucose Levels 471
Control of Blood Pressure 471
Use of ACE Inhibitors 471
Protein Restriction 471
Patient Education 471
Extrarenal Disease 471
Microangiopathy 472
Macroangiopathy 472
Interference with Pregnancy 472
Acute Metabolic Complications 472
Renal Replacement Therapy 472
Patient Assessment 472
Medical Assessment 472

Chapter Contents

Social-Family Issues 473
Hemodialysis 474
Peritoneal Dialysis 475
Transplantation 476
Role of Nephrology Nurses 477
Summary 477
References 478
Chapter Highlights 479

The Diabetic Patient

Marta R. Taylor, MSN, RN, NP, CNN

Diabetes mellitus (DM) is a chronic illness that produces serious deleterious effects in several organ systems in the body. The changes in the kidney, known as diabetic nephropathy, now account for over one-third of the patients entering the End Stage Renal Disease (ESRD) program. This number continues to grow annually with no indication of a reversal of this trend. Among this group there is a higher percentage of females than males. Native Americans experience this disease at a rate almost twice that found in the white or black population. Not unlike other disease entities, there is a large percentage of patients who are older than 65.

The many complications caused by the disease and the increasing number of patients affected consume a great deal of financial resources. Beyond the dollar cost is the high morbidity and mortality found in patients suffering from diabetes. After 5 years on dialysis, only 17.6% of the patients with diabetes mellitus can expect to be alive as compared to over 80% for those with the diagnosis of glomerulonephritis (United States Renal Data System [USRDS], 1993). The purpose of this chapter is to present an overview of DM and diabetes nephropathy, and to review the special needs of the complicated daily care of individuals with DM.

Forms of DM and History of Disease

DM exists in two forms that have been differentiated by the American Diabetes Association (ADA) as follows.

- *Type I* - Patients are dependent on insulin due to the inability of islet cells in the pancreas to produce insulin. The disease is aptly known as insulin-dependent diabetes mellitus (IDDM). This type of DM may be associated with specific HLA types with a predisposition to viral insulitis or autoimmune phenomena. Type I may occur at any age and in the most common manifestation of the disease in youth, and once was commonly called "juvenile diabetes." These patients are more prone to ketosis because of their lack of insulin.
- *Type II* - Patients may produce insulin, but in insufficient amounts, or the body may be resistant to the insulin produced. This type of diabetes is referred to as noninsulin-dependent (NIDDM). Many patients with DM or NIDDM are overweight. The disease may also be seen in families as an autosomal genetic trait. Insulin may be required for glucose control particularly during stress (ADA, 1995).

The physiological changes leading to diabetic nephropathy begin with the onset of the disease. Although knowledge of the natural course of the disease comes from research on the patients with IDDM, it appears that the findings are present in the NIDDM patient too. The course of the disease has been delineated into five stages, which assists in understanding the diagnosis and treatment of the disease.

- *Stage I* - At the onset of DM, there is an increase in kidney size with a resultant increase in glomerular volume and glomerular filtration rate. Albumin is usually not found in the urine. The changes in the kidney may be stabilized or resolve with strict glycemic control.
- *Stage II* - This stage evolves over the next 3-7 years. The urinary dipstick remains negative for proteinuria. Albuminuria will be present only if marked hyperglycemia or hypertension occurs. The glomerular filtration rate remains normal or higher. A renal biopsy would reveal glomerular hypertrophy and capillary basement membrane thickening.
- *Stage III* - The early stage of nephropathy begins with the onset of microalbuminuria. Microalbuminuria is defined as an urinary albumin excretion level, which until recently was detectable only by radioimmunoassay or other sensitive laboratory assays. The development of a dipstick for microalbuminuria may make detection easier. The amount of microalbuminuria may be a predictor of advancement to the next stages on diabetes. This stage typically begins after approximately 7 years of diabetes.
- *Stage IV* - This stage is depicted by persistent dipstick-positive proteinuria indicating greater than 300 mg/day. The glomerular filtration rate is no longer elevated, and blood pressure has begun to rise. Diabetic retinopathy is also present. This stage normally occurs 15 to 18 years after the onset of the disease. Patients should be referred to a nephrologist at this time.

- *Stage V* - This stage is characterized by the development of progressive renal insufficiency leading to chronic renal failure (CRF). Patients may present with severe hypertension, nephrotic-range proteinuria (greater than 3.5 gm/day), and hyperlipidemia as evidence of their advanced diabetic nephropathy. This stage usually is found after 25 years of diabetes (Hirsch, 1994; Mauer, Mogensen, & Kjellstrand, 1993).

Recent research has indicated that the progression of the disease in all of these stages can be slowed and perhaps prevented with intensive therapy aimed at better glucose control (The Diabetes Control and Complications Trial Research Group, 1993; The Diabetes Control and Complications [DCCT] Research Group, 1995). Implementation of this type of therapy requires that the patient receive extensive continuing education, which is a vital part of the nephrology nurse's roles.

Screening for Diabetes

Preventing or delaying the onset of diabetic nephropathy and other end organ damage by diabetes depends on early detection and management of the disease. The ADA has developed guidelines for the screening of the general population in hopes of identifying individuals without symptoms that meet the criteria for DM. Diabetes screening done in physicians' offices or in community settings should have as their primary goal to identify individuals with more than one diabetes risk factor. These factors are found in Table 16-1.

In screening programs, these risk factors may be identified by means of a written or verbal questionnaire. Individuals with more than one risk factor should be referred to a physician for evaluation and testing. Individuals indicating that they have any of the symptoms of diabetes should also be referred to a physician for appropriate evaluation. These symptoms most commonly include excessive thirst, excessive hunger, and excessive urination. The screening test of choice is the fasting plasma glucose test, however random plasma glucose measurements may also provide some useful information (ADA, 1995).

After the diagnosis of DM has been made, the patient should be followed closely by the nephrology team and diabetologists. The Diabetes Control and Complications Trial (DCCT) demonstrated that intensive therapy with close monitoring and control of blood sugar can delay and slow the progression of diabetic nephropathy as well as retinopathy and neuropathy. This type of therapy requires self-monitoring of glucose by the patient at least four times a day and administration of insulin three or more times daily. The dosage of insulin is determined by the self-glucose monitoring results, the dietary intake, and anticipated exercise. The goals of therapy are:

- Fasting glucose levels between 70 and 120 mg /dl
- Postpreprandial blood glucose levels of less than 180 mg/dl.
- Glycosylated hemoglobin (Hgb A1c) within normal range measured monthly

Patients visited their care providers monthly and were in contact with them more frequently by telephone to review and adjust their regimes (DCCT Research Group, 1993; DCCT, 1995). This intensive therapy has spurred the need for a specialized nurse known as a Certified Diabetes Educator who must meet predetermined educational requirements and satisfactorily complete a certification examination.

Beyond the studies listed above, the ADA also recommends the following tests be monitored frequently:

- fasting lipid profiles;
- serum creatinine levels;
- urinalysis for glucose, ketones, and protein;
- microalbuminuria determination (ADA, 1995).

Structural and Functional Abnormalities in Diabetic Nephropathy

Structural changes in the kidney correlate with the stages of progression of diabetic nephropathy. In Stage I or at the onset of diabetes, there is glomerular hypertrophy resulting in an enlargement of the kidney itself. The structure of the glomerulus appears to be normal. This enlargement of the glomerulus produces hyperfiltration, which produces an increase in glomerular filtration rate. Microalbuminuria may be present but can be eliminated by insulin therapy and glucose control.

As the disease progresses to Stage II, a renal biopsy would reveal increasing thickness of the basement membrane of the glomerulus. The mesangium or glomerular stalk also enlarges. This may be considered a silent stage as the urinary albumin excretion may be normal in spite of changes occurring in the structure of the kidney. Stress such as exercise or poor glycemic control may produce an increase in urinary albumin excretion. The glomerular filtration rate may remain within normal range but is decreased from Stage I.

Stage III of the disease begins the overt changes that places a patient at high risk for diabetic nephropathy. There is persistent microalbuminuria, which progresses through this stage of the disease. The mesangium continues to expand. There is sclerosis of some glomeruli and hypertrophy of the remaining ones. By the end of this stage, there is a decline in glomerular filtration rate.

Stage IV DM indicates further expansion of the mesangium, which causes a reduction in the filtration surface of the glomerulus. This proliferation of mesangial cells causes pressure on the vascular supply to the glomerulus, impeding blood flow.

The microalbuminuria of the earlier stages now progresses to proteinuria. These changes produce a greater decrease in the glomerular filtration rate.

Stage V changes include further proliferation of the mesangium, producing scarring and closure of the remaining glomeruli. These nodular glomerularsclerotic lesions are called the hallmarks of diabetic nephropathy and were originally described by Kimmestiel and Wilson (Mauer et al., 1993; Hostetter, 1991).

Diagnosis of Diabetic Nephropathy

The diagnosis of diabetic nephropathy must be based upon the clinical history and physical examination of the patient. The laboratory examinations will confirm the presence and stage of diabetic nephropathy.

Clinical History

The clinical history should include the following elements:

- *Family history of DM* – There is a strong family tendency particularly in Type II diabetes.
- *Onset of DM* – Changes in the kidney tend to occur at certain intervals after the time of diagnosis or onset of symptoms.
- *Therapeutic management for hyperglycemia* – An insulin requirement and history of glycemic control are also predictors of the stages of the disease process.
- *Other organ involvement, i.e. retinopathy, cardiac myopathy* – Organ involvement tends to follow set time frames with nephropathy appearing or present concurrently with retinopathy.
- *Peripheral vascular involvement* – The presence of peripheral vascular disease is a predictor of additional complications associated with treatment for CRF.
- *Hypertension* – The presence of high blood pressure suggests increased risk for diabetic nephropathy.

Physical Examination

Health care providers examining the patient will be particularly interested in the following findings.

- *Eye ground changes on fundascopic examination* – Microaneurysms appear as cherry-red spots, which change to waxy spots as they thrombose and fuse together. Edema, hemorrhages, and arteriolar and venous changes may also be present. Cotton wool spots, which are gray-white microinfarcts in the superficial retinal layers, are characteristic. These changes are known as nonproliferative retinopathy. An ominous sign is the proliferative changes of neovascularization and fibrosis of the retina, which may progress to create a vascular connective tissue mass over the retina leading to blindness (Robbins & Cotran, 1979). The presence of arteriovenous nicking and silver or copper wire arterioles indicate changes caused by long-standing hypertension (Bates, 1983).
- *Presence of high blood pressure* – If present, therapeutic measures should be instigated in an attempt to slow the progression of the disease and protect other organs.
- *Diminished peripheral pulses* – These are an indication of peripheral vascular involvement.
- *Unsteady gait, inability to walk* – This is an indication of peripheral neuropathy or central nervous system involvement.
- *Loss of muscle mass* – Loss of muscle mass is an indication of malnutrition or of poor glycemic control.

Laboratory Tests

Several tests are available to help clinicians determine the stage of DM as well as ascertain abnormalities that might respond to therapy.

Urine tests. Urine tests for diagnostic use include: urinalysis, creatine clearance, timed collections, 24-hour collections, overnight urine collections, protein excretion, and microalbumin excretion.

- *Urinalysis* – The urinalysis is often performed. The albumin is measured by dipstick. The glucose dipstick reading may not be of value if renal disease has progressed to the kidneys since it no is longer able to filter glucose appropriately or a change in the renal threshold for sugar has occurred. Urine sediment is microscopically examined for red blood cell casts and other abnormalities such as crystals. The findings of these may indicate the presence of glomerulonephritis or other diseases that may influence the decline in renal function. A clean catch specimen is not necessary for this examination but an early morning specimen is preferred as the urine will be more concentrated at that time.
- *Creatinine clearance* – The measurement of creatinine cleared by the kidney during a set period of time provides a determination that is roughly equivalent to the glomerular filtration rate. The test is performed by measuring the amount of creatinine found in a predetermined amount of urine. The serum creatinine must be obtained at the time of the urine collection.

The formula for computing the creatinine clearance is:

$$\text{Creatinine clearance} = \frac{\text{Urine creatinine} \times \text{Volume} \times \text{Time}}{\text{Plasma creatinine}}$$

The values for creatinine in the formula must be

in mg/dl and the volume of urine in cubic centimeters. The time is the length of the collection in minutes.

An estimated creatinine clearance may be obtained by the following formula when a urine creatinine is not available.

$$\text{For Males - Creatinine clearance} = \frac{(140\text{-patient age}) \times \text{weight in kg}}{72 \times \text{Plasma creatinine}}$$

For Females - Multiply the result by 0.85 (Aronoff & Abel, 1990).

- *Timed collections* – The urine is collected for a specific length of time and this time is used in the formula to compute the excretion value. These examinations are very reliable if patients can void completely and follow the instructions precisely. Complete voiding may be a problem in patients with a degree of diabetic nephropathy.
- *24-hour urine collection* – These collections have been standard renal function testing throughout the years. Patients are instructed to discard the first morning specimen and collect all urine through the night and the first voiding of the next day. The creatinine is quantitated, and the serum creatinine is used in the mathematical formula to determine the creatinine clearance. Patients may find it difficult to keep a complete collection for a variety of reasons. Nephrology nurses should impress its importance on patients, however, for incomplete collections may distort the interpretation of the test values.
- *Overnight urine collections* – The specimen is collected much like the 24-hour specimen. Patients are told to void immediately before going to bed. These samples are discarded and the time recorded. Any urine passed during the night should be collected as well as the first specimen immediately after arising. The time should also be noted when the first morning voiding occurs. This type of specimen usually results in a complete collection of urine.
- *Protein excretion* – The presence or absence and amount of protein excreted in the urine is an important parameter in the evaluation of the progression of diabetic nephropathy. The simplest procedure is dipstick of a random urine sample. Clinicians performing this procedure must take care to perform the test correctly using a fresh dipstick and waiting the required amount of time before reading test strips. The quantitative measurement and excretion of protein can be determined by the same tests as described above for the measurement of creatinine.
- *Microalbumin excretion* – The measurement of microalbumin is of great importance in predicting the development of nephropathy. Until recently these measurements were made by sophisticated evaluations using radio- or chemico immunoassays. The advent of the microalbumin dipstick has increased the availability of this measurement and should promote the earlier detection of microalbumin abnormality. Earlier detection of microalbumin in patients with DM will lead to sooner intervention and a delay in the progression of diabetic nephropathy.

Hematology tests. Several hematology tests exist that are available to clinicians. These include: creatinine, blood urea nitrogen (BUN), and BUN/creatine ratio.

- *Creatinine* – Creatinine is a breakdown product of muscle tissue. The normal value is 0.7 - 1.5 mg/dl. The creatinine of patients with diabetes who have lost muscle mass is often lower than their level of renal function would indicate. For instance, the normal serum creatinine for nondiabetic patients with 25% of renal function remaining should be around 4 mg/dl; in diabetic patients, the serum creatinine for 25% of renal function may be lower depending on the amount of muscle mass lost.
- *Blood urea nitrogen (BUN)* – BUN is a measurement of the amount of protein breakdown in the blood. The normal value is 5-22 mg/dl. This amount rises as renal function decreases. The BUN may be spuriously low in the late stages of diabetic nephropathy, reflecting a large amount of protein loss in the urine.
- *BUN/creatinine ratio* – The normal ratio is in the area of 15:1. A BUN risen out of proportion to the creatinine level may indicate dehydration, gastrointestinal bleeding, malnutrition, or a spuriously low creatinine. A BUN level decreased in proportion to the serum creatinine suggests low protein intake, high protein loss, overhydration, or severe liver failure (Epstein, 1992).

Clinical Features of Established Diabetic Nephropathy

The progression of diabetic nephropathy is marked by an increase in the amount of urinary protein, a rise in BUN and serum creatinine, and a decrease in glomerular filtration rate as measured by the creatinine clearance. As has been noted, by the time patients reach Stage III in the progression of the disease microalbumin may be found in as small amounts as 30 mg/24 hours. Clinically, patients may present with a rise in blood pressure at this time. By the time Stage IV occurs, overt clinical diabetic nephropathy is present. The GFR pro-

Table 16-1
Factors That Put Individuals at Greater Risk for Diabetes

- Native American, Hispanic, Black race
- Family history of diabetes mellitus
- Obesity
- Age greater than 40 years
- Previously identified impaired glucose tolerance
- Hypertension
- Hyperlipidemia
- History of gestational diabetes mellitus in women.

Note: Individuals with more than one risk factor should be referred to a physician for evaluation and testing.

gressively declines as indicated by a decrease in creatinine clearance and a rise in serum creatinine and blood urea nitrogen. Proteinuria increases usually over 300 mg/24 hr. Stage V is the final stage of diabetic nephropathy with rapid decline of the GFR and a loss of up to 3% of kidney function per month. Hyperlipidemia is usually present. Patients may experience vision problems and diabetic retinopathy may be found. It is not uncommon for weight loss and muscle wasting to occur. Patients usually start dialysis when the serum creatinine is around 6 mgm/dl (Dunfee, 1995).

Because chronic renal failure usually occurs into the second decade of the disease, patients may have already experienced many of the physical complications caused by diabetes. Patients may have already lost one or more limbs, or developed vision impairment, heart disease, GI enteropathies, and/or infections. Being presented with a new regime and the need for dialysis or transplantation may challenge their coping skills; patients may also experience depression, anger, or withdrawal (Carosella, 1993). Nurses must be aware of these feelings and provide support and referral to social workers or psychologists if indicated.

Management of Established Diabetic Nephropathy

Until recently, there were few therapeutic interventions available to treat patients once diabetic nephropathy was present. Comprehensive and conclusive research is now available that has given practitioners guidelines for interventions to slow the progression of this disease (Hirsch, 1994; Carella, Gossain, & Rovner, 1994). These include control of glucose, control of blood pressure, use of angiotensin-converting-enzyme (ACE) inhibitors, protein restriction, and patient education.

Control of Blood Glucose Levels

Control of glucose remains the primary intervention for preventing and decreasing the progression of end organ disease. Patients should be taught home glucose monitoring and adjustment of insulin. The development of short and long-acting insulins has facilitated control of blood glucose. Some patients have benefited from insulin pumps. An insulin pump is a wearable device that delivers preprogrammed amounts of insulin to patients through an established access, thus eliminating the need for injections and assuring the administration of the correct dosage.

Control of Blood Pressure

The deleterious effects of high blood pressure on the kidney have long been known. Studies have shown even more beneficial effects of blood pressure control in the diabetic patient (Marken, 1994). Blood pressure control has been shown to decrease microalbuminuria. The large arsenal of hypertension drug therapy has made it easier to find a regime that controls blood pressure with limited side effects, and among these agents are the ACE inhibitors and calcium channel blocker drugs. Betablockers should be avoided because of their masking of hypoglycemia symptoms.

Use of ACE Inhibitors

ACE inhibitors have been shown to protect against deterioration in renal function in normotensive DM patients. Research suggests that these drugs lowers glomerular intracapillary pressure while preserving renal plasma flow, resulting in a decrease in proteinuria. For this reason many diabetic patients are being started on these drugs early in the course of their disease (Lewis, Lawrence, Hunsicker, Bain, & Rohde, 1993; Marken, 1994; Parving, Rossing, Hommel, & Smidt, 1995).

Protein Restriction

Restricting protein has also shown some therapeutic benefits both in laboratory animals and in human research studies. The ADA recommends a daily protein intake of 0.8 gm/kg of protein intake for all patients with diabetes. This is almost half of the protein found in a typical American diet (ADA, 1995).

Patient Education

Patient education is recognized as a major component in the successful management of DM and a major role of the nurse. As the patient's education of DM progresses, preparation and management for ESRD therapy must be included.

Extrarenal Disease

The kidney is not the only organ affected by DM. Retinopathy, cardiac myopathy, and peripheral vascular disease are often present with long-term DM. These extrarenal diseases, which include microangiopathy, macroangiopathy, interference with reproduction and sexuality, and acute metabolic complications, may be summarized as follows.

Microangiopathy

Microangiopathy is a thickening of the capillaries and arterioles accompanied with increased accumulation of glycoprotein. With hyperglycemia there is an increased rate of formation of basement membrane cells. This vascular complication produces the following changes:

- *Retinopathy* - microaneurysms that appear in retinal arterioles causing hemorrhages, neovascularization, and retinal scars leading to blindness.
- *Peripheral neuropathy* - an inflammation or degeneration of the peripheral nerves producing pain, parasthesias, muscle weakness, and atrophy.
- Autonomic nervous system neuropathy - degeneration of autonomic nerves causing diarrhea, delayed gastric emptying, impotence, and postural hypotension.
- Effects in muscle tissue causing cardiomyopathy

Macroangiopathy

The histopathological characteristics of atherosclerosis are present in this disease. It is manifested in the following conditions:

- Vascular occlusion probably due to the accumulation of sorbitol in the vascular intima leading to intermittent claudication and gangrene of the extremities.
- Abnormalities in blood coagulation.
- Hyperlipoproteinuria

(Price & Wilson, 1982)

Interference with Pregnancy

Interference with pregnancy is also a possible extrarenal disease. When this occurs, there is an increased incidence of spontaneous abortions, intrauterine fetal death, large fetal size, and premature infants in diabetic women.

Acute Metabolic Complications

Acute metabolic complications may arise, and include ketoacidosis and hypoglycemia. Ketoacidosis results from insulin insufficiency leading to hyperglycemia, decreased lipogenesis, and the production of ketone bodies. Patients may become hypotensive and develop shock, which can lead to coma and death.

Hypoglycemia usually results from a change in insulin requirements. The need for insulin may be reduced if patients modify their diet, lose weight, or increase exercise. As renal function deteriorates, the insulin requirement may also be reduced due to the impaired clearance of insulin by the kidney. Patients may assume that their DM is improving rather than acknowledging that their renal function is decreasing (Price & Wilson, 1982).

Renal Replacement Therapy

Renal replacement therapy for diabetic patients remains a challenge in spite of new knowledge and technology. Diabetic patients experience more cardiovascular disease and infection than their nondiabetic counterparts. These diseases are the main contributors to the increased rate of mortality and morbidity in the diabetic population receiving renal replacement therapy. The options for treatment of CRF in diabetic patients are the same as those in the rest of the ESRD population. Controversy remains as to which type of therapy is the most desirable (Williams, 1995). Table 16-2 summarizes advantages and disadvantages of each modality of therapy in the diabetic population.

Patient Assessment

Similar to other patients beginning renal replacement therapy, the diabetic patient may be confused, angry, depressed, or in a state of denial. These emotional needs must be considered by the care provider who is evaluating the patient. The patient and family must be taught regarding the advantages and disadvantages of the various modalities so that they may make an informed decision. Unfortunately, their emotional state may make learning and evaluation difficult. However, frequent sessions using a variety of approaches should improve their understanding of the disease and the therapy involved.

Medical Assessment

Medical assessment should include cardiovascular assessment, peripheral vascular assessment, evaluation of retinopathy, evaluation of neuropathy, checking for the presence of hypertension, and the state of blood glucose control.

The presence or progression of this disease suggests that peritoneal dialysis would be a better choice of therapy. Transplantation tends to be less successful and be contraindicated in patients with cardiovascular disease. Severe peripheral vascular disease may make arteriovascular access difficult or impossible, suggesting the need for peritoneal therapy. Decreased vision may impair patients' ability to independently perform their care. Although hemodialysis would appear to be the choice, many blind diabetics have successfully managed peritoneal dialysis with the assistance of special technological devices, however, often a partner is needed. Impaired manual dexterity may make the peritoneal dialysis procedure difficult. Often special assist devices and/or a partner may make peritoneal dialysis a viable option.

Table 16-2
Advantages and Disadvantages of Each Modality of Therapy in the Diabetic Population

Modality	Advantages	Disadvantages
Hemodialysis	Very efficient	Patients with cardiac disease at more risk
	Close medical supervision	Arteriovenous access problematic with risk of hand ischemia
	No loss of protein	High incidence of hypotension
		Hyperkalemia
		Unstable blood glucose levels
CAPD	Less cardiovascular stress	Peritonitis, catheter-related infections similar to nondiabetic patients.
	No arteriovenous access needed	Loss of protein to dialysate
	Liberalization of diet	Inconvenient schedule if partner is required.
	Serum potassium better controlled	
	Slower progression of neuropathy	
	Intraperitoneal insulin may aid in glucose control.	
	Fluid overload less likely	
CCPD	Less cardiovascular stress	Less risk of peritonitis
	No arteriovascular access	Loss of protein to dialysate
	Good control of serum potassium	Easier for self-care
Renal Transplant	Increased patient well being	Patients with cardiovascular disease at greater risk of death
	Slower progression of neuropathy	Hypertension
	Decreased cost to Medicare	Increased peripheral vascular disease (Tzamaloukas, 1994; Reddi & Camerini-Davalos, 1990; Miller, Sigala, & Upham, 1990).

High blood pressure will have a deleterious effect in any mode of therapy. It can be more difficult to control and present a very serious problem in transplant patients as some immunosuppressive drugs tend to raise blood pressure. High blood pressure will also have a deleterious effect on the transplanted kidney. A history of poor control would indicate an increased risk for the complications listed above. Poor control may also be a reflection of the patient's ability to participate in self-care.

Social-Family Issues

Chronic renal failure affects the family on several levels. The various components, including psychological issues, economic pressures, availability of assistance in the home, indications for therapy, and contraindications for renal replacement therapy, are summarized here.

Patients and their families are faced with many lifestyle changes that require a great deal of coping skills. Among these are moving from interdependence to dependence, change in role, change in body image, and the fear of complications or dying.

Moving from interdependence-dependence is an important issue. Although diabetic patients have been living with the ramifications of DM for years, the onset of renal failure presents additional complications. Dependence on a machine for life often produces ambivalent feelings in patients. Impaired vision or motor skills may also increase dependent behavior. A change in role may also be a factor. Patients may find it difficult to remain employed, and a role change occurs from family provider to dependent family members for physical necessities. A change in body image is a psychological consideration as well. The presence of an arteriovenous fistula or conduit or the installation of a peritoneal catheter may be distressful to patients.

Long-term diabetic patients may also have fears of complications or even death, and see the initiation of renal replacement therapy as the beginning of the end. Patients should be encouraged to talk about their feelings.

Although programs such as Medicare and Medicaid help considerably with the cost of therapy, certain expenses must still be borne by patients. These may present at the same time that income has been reduced or discontinued. Patients should be referred to social workers for assistance with these issues.

Several activities of daily living and requirements related to therapy may be beyond the capability of patients. The social worker will often arrange transportation to the center or clinic for therapy and seek out availability for preparations of meals meeting dietary requirements.

Indications for therapy. For all patients the decision to begin renal replacement therapy is based on clinical symptoms and laboratory evaluation. Nondiabetic patients are usually initiated on dialysis when the creatinine clearance drops to 8-10 ml/min for the average 70-kg male patient. The current practice to initiate dialysis for diabetic patients at a higher level of creatinine clearance, approximately 10-15 ml/min or a serum creatinine of 5-6 ml/dl. This earlier initiation is often necessary for several reasons, including: (a) improved control of blood pressure; (b) earlier onset of uremic symptoms at higher levels of creatinine clearance; and (c) rapid decline of renal function after the diagnosis of diabetic nephropathy has been made.

Contraindications for renal replacement therapy. The severe complications of DM along with those of CRF may influence patients to decide that the risks and complications of continued therapy outweigh the benefit of prolonging life. This decision is often made by those patients whose quality of life has been severely compromised by their disease. Patients who are mentally competent and well-informed about the therapy have the right to make this decision and in this situation, dialysis is contraindicated. Whenever possible, this decision should be made when patients are neither depressed nor under the stress of an acute illness or life-threatening situation. However, patients' right to refuse therapy should be honored and conservative care provided to alleviate unnecessary pain and suffering. Another absolute contraindication to therapy is extrarenal disease that in the opinion of the patient and/or physician has diminished the quality of life to such a degree that dialysis or transplantation would only prolong suffering and postpone death. Again the wishes of patients or guardians should be honored.

A contraindication for therapy is a severe handicap or disability in infants who would have difficulty in adjusting even to a sheltered existence. Another relative contraindication is mentally impaired patients who cannot comprehend the benefits of therapy. These individuals may see the restrictions required for adequate therapy as punishment and endure undue suffering. A patient's physical deterioration or quality of life may change their perspective. If the changes render therapy more of a burden than a benefit, patients should be allowed to discontinue therapy. Care providers must remember that renal replacement therapy is a life-saving measure. As such, there is no legal or moral reasons that patients cannot elect to refuse or discontinue therapy (Miller, Sigala, & Upham, 1990).

Hemodialysis

For many years, hemodialysis was not offered to patients with DM because of poor outcomes. The advent of new technology and a better understanding of the disease has made hemodialysis an option in care. There are still many problems in management.

One of the first presenting problems is the establishment of an arteriovenous access. The high incidence of peripheral vascular disease in diabetic patients often makes creation of an adequate access difficult. The use of a synthetic graft may be more beneficial than a native arteriovenous fistula, but it too is less successful than in nondiabetic patients.

Regulation of blood glucose levels is difficult on hemodialysis. Hypoglycemia becomes problematic particularly if patients do not eat before initiation of hemodialysis, or are dialyzed against a dialysate bath that does not contain glucose. The risk of hypoglycemia is increased in malnourished patients with depleted glycogen stores. Patients with malabsorption problems may also experience hypoglycemia. The use of beta-blocker medications can also impair glycogenolysis and thus can lead to hypoglycemic problems.

Diabetic patients' diet are not significantly different than those prescribed for nondiabetic patients. Diets should contain enough calories to prevent wasting and should not contain concentrated sweets. Potassium restriction is a serious departure from the diabetic diet and must be stressed in patient education. Perhaps most importantly is the assurance of eating at regular meal times. Patients whose hemodialysis schedule overlaps these times should be encouraged to bring food with them to eat before or after the dialysis procedure. Hyperglycemia may also occur and be asymptomatic in dialysis patients. Occasionally thirst, weight gain, and even pulmonary edema may be indications of this hyperglycemia. Diabetic ketoacidosis may occur and may be accompanied by severe hyperkalemia.

Patients should have their blood glucose monitored at each dialysis and taught to perform home glucose testing. If hyperglycemia does occur, it should be managed with insulin administration. The traditional administration of large amounts of fluid is contraindicated and unnecessary.

Insulin therapy. Normally, uremic patients with NIDDM experience a reduction of insulin secretion by the beta cells of the pancreas coupled with a reduced responsiveness of tissue to insulin. There is a decrease in the rate of catabolism, resulting in the prolongation of insulin half-life in the circulation. For these reasons and because of variations in dietary intake, food absorption, and changes in dialytic therapy, tight control of glucose concentrations are difficult to manage.

A goal of fasting blood sugar less than 140 mg/dl and a postprandial of less than 200 mg/dl are reasonable parameters in this population. These levels should protect patients from hypoglycemia. The optimal insulin regime for patients on hemodialysis usually requires administration of long-acting insulin at two separate times during the day and by supplementing with regular insulin for meals as needed. Nurses administering insulin to patients on dialysis should be aware of the drugs' duration of action. If the insulin is going to reach its peak at the end of dialysis, food should be available to prevent patients from becoming hypoglycemic (Tzamaloukas, 1994).

Hypertension and peripheral vascular disease. Hypertension is frequently a problem in diabetic patients on hemodialysis. It is important to control hypertension if cardiovascular and retinal deterioration are to be retarded or prevented. Diabetic patients who are volume sensitive can control hypertension with sodium restriction and adequate fluid removal. If medications are required, calcium channel blockers or vasodilators are usually the first drugs of choice. Beta-blockers should be avoided because of the risk of masking hypoglycemic symptoms. Angiotensin-converting-enzyme (ACE) inhibitors must be used carefully because of their tendency to cause hyperkalemia (Tzamaloukas, 1994). The newer angiotensin receptor blocker drugs may also be useful and have fewer side effects, including hyperkalemia (Cozaar Product Description, 1995). Fluid management may be difficult as hyperglycemia contributes to thirst and thus volume overload.

Prognosis. Diabetic patients continue to experience increased mortality and morbidity when compared to nondiabetic patients, but more efficient hemodialysis and better control of serum glucose levels may change this prognosis. Hemodialysis is the second choice of therapies for patients who cannot or choose not to perform peritoneal dialysis. Peritoneal dialysis should not be the preferred method for patients with severe peripheral or cardiovascular disease.

Patient/family education. Education on diabetes and nephropathy should begin with the first visit to the nephrologist and be comprehensive in nature. Social workers and dietitians should also be involved with patients in developing a plan of care. Hemodialysis affects the whole family and produces many changes in lifestyle. If these are not addressed from the beginning, serious problems can occur.

Peritoneal Dialysis

The advantages of chronic peritoneal dialysis have been outlined in this chapter. Patients who prefer a more active lifestyle will usually choose this modality. Others may choose this method because of the unavailability of hemodialysis units in close proximity and the inability to perform home hemodialysis. There are some areas in the world where the water supply is inadequate for hemodialysis and peritoneal dialysis becomes a necessity.

Peritoneal dialysis produces less strain on the cardiovascular system and should always be considered for patients with these conditions. Patients with compromised lung function or lumbar, sacral problems may find it impossible to tolerate the required 2 liters of fluid in the abdomen. Peritoneal dialysis may be impossible if patients have had multiple abdominal surgeries or other conditions that have left the peritoneal membrane scarred and impermeable.

Infection of the catheter site and peritonitis remain the most common complications with this modality. It is imperative that participants in this procedure be able to follow directions and adhere to technique. If patients have problems in visual acuity, a partner may be required to assist in the procedure. Since the procedure must be done 4-5 times every day, this becomes stressful for partners. All of these factors should be considered when assessing patients for continuous peritoneal dialysis. The management of diabetics on peritoneal dialysis should address the concerns such as diet, insulin therapy, prognosis, and patient/family education.

Diet. Protein intake for continuous ambulatory peritoneal dialysis (CAPD) patients should be around 1.2 gm/km body weight per day. This is not always achieved and patients may become malnourished. The 500-600 calories a day provided by the glucose in the peritoneal solution may have a protein sparing component and serve to protect patients from malnutrition. Potassium is also lost in the peritoneal fluid so the potassium intake can usually be liberalized to 3-4 gms per day. The continuous aspect of peritoneal dialysis lends itself to better control of fluid removal, liberalizing the fluid restriction. Impaired gastric motility may also contribute to malnutrition.

Insulin therapy. Some patients have benefited

from the procedure of providing insulin through the peritoneal solution, thus eliminating the need for subcutaneous injection. If this method is employed, the total daily dose of insulin added to the peritoneal solution must be 2-3 times the usual subcutaneous dosage. This is necessary since variable amounts of insulin are absorbed by the dialysis solution container and the tubing. There has been a reported increase in peritonitis in some patients and consequently loss in the efficiency of the peritoneal dialysis. Subcutaneous insulin may also be used in these patients in much the same manner as in chronic hemodialysis patients (Tzamaloukas, 1994).

Prognosis. It does not appear that there is a significant difference in mortality and morbidity between diabetic patients on CAPD and hemodialysis. The greater freedom provided by CAPD should produce a better quality of life. However, some find that the frequent exchanges and adherence to aseptic technique required by CAPD produces more stress than hemodialysis treatments.

Patient/family education. Education should focus on the need for exactness in the procedure. There is no margin of error in peritoneal dialysis. The self-directed approach may cause conflict among family members who also want to participate in the care. Nurses must be aware of these types of conflicts and provide counseling and intervention as the need arises.

Transplantation

In choosing transplantation the same indications and contraindications must be considered as applying to the general ESRD population. Diabetic patients without significant cardiovascular disease have demonstrated an improved outcome with a kidney transplant as compared to hemodialysis, especially the elderly (Badsonna et al., 1992; Khauli et al., 1986). Controversy remains over the benefits of transplantation to diabetic patients with cardiovascular disease with Williams (1995) reporting a better survival for transplantation than dialysis in diabetic patients. Other researchers have noted several risk factors that predict a more unfavorable outcome in transplant candidates with DM. These are: (a) poor glycemic control; (b) coronary artery disease; (c) other vascular disease; (d) vision loss; (e) autonomic, peripheral neuropathy; (f) bladder dysfunction; and (g) fractures (Williams, 1995). All of these conditions should be evaluated before transplantation and corrected if possible.

There appears to be no greater loss of graft in the immediate postoperative period for diabetic patients although management is more difficult. Diabetic patients have difficulty with wound healing and an increase in the risk of incisional infections. Serum glucose levels are difficult to manage with patients being at risk for both hyperglycemia and hypoglycemia. Potassium may also be difficult to control. Programs that transplant large numbers of diabetic patients have developed considerable skill in managing this perioperative period. Problems with glucose and potassium control usually continue into the postoperative period. Patients may be disappointed that their diet must still be restricted. Education and close monitoring become essential if patients are to do well (Williams, 1995).

Chronic complications. HTN is the most common problem in long-term transplant survivors with DM. This condition must be adequately treated or it will increase the risk of vascular disease and graft rejection. Coronary artery disease, if not present before transplantation, can occur posttransplantation and patients should be encouraged to make the necessary lifestyle changes that reduce the risk of developing this condition (Luke, 1987).

Williams (1995), in an extensive review of studies in the management of transplant recipients found that diabetic patients often experience many changes. Retinopathy appeared to remain stable and neuropathy appeared less progressive than in diabetic patients receiving hemodialysis or peritoneal dialysis. Neither did diabetic transplant recipients experience greater serous infections than nondiabetic patients. However, peripheral vascular complications produced a higher rate of surgical amputations, and urologic complications were seen twice as frequently. Increased bone disease leading to weakness and fractures causing greater immobility was a severe problem for diabetic transplant recipients (Williams, 1995).

Prognosis. Long-term survival for diabetic transplant recipients appears to be greater than survival on chronic dialysis. The younger age and generally healthier status of transplant recipients may play some role in statistics. Success also varies from one transplant center to another with large programs having the best results. As in chronic dialysis, diabetics have increased morbidity and mortality when compared to nondiabetic patients (Williams, 1995).

Patient/family education. Patients tend to view transplantation as a miracle cure. It is important to be realistic and explain the need for medication, diet restrictions, and other aspects of kidney transplantation. Economic concerns should be addressed as the cost of immunosuppressive therapy is great and may not be totally covered by insurance programs. It is helpful to have written or video materials available for patients to refer to. These materials should be placed on audiotape for the visually impaired. Patients should visit the transplant programs and meet with other diabetic transplant recipients. Posttransplantation, patients must learn careful glucose management as well as the care of the kidney transplant. The management of diabetes requires constant attention on the part of patients and their families.

Kidney-pancreas transplant. The combined kidney-pancreas transplantation is performed with the hope of eliminating the need for dialysis as well as insulin therapy, and to reverse or arrest the secondary complications of diabetes such as nephropathy in the transplanted kidney, peripheral and autonomic neuropathy, and retinopathy. In the past decade, kidney-pancreas transplant has moved out of the realm of experimental procedures to a viable option for some patients. Complications and mortality remain higher than in renal transplant patients. Pancreas transplants are technically more difficult, which may have some bearing on the poorer success rate (Solinger & Geffner, 1994; Manske, Wang, & Thomas, 1995). Typical complications from kidney-pancreas transplant are as follows: infection, pancreatitis, and surgical complications (Ozaki et al., 1992).

Because of the increased risk, combined kidney-pancreas transplantation is recommended for young patients with no history of congestive heart failure and for those whom hypoglycemia is life-threatening (Ozaki et al., 1992). Because patients must remain on immunosuppressive drugs, questions have been raised as to the benefit of this procedure. Long-term studies are evaluating whether the benefit of slowing the progression of diabetes outweighs the risks of immunosuppressive therapy. In spite of increased morbidity and mortality, individuals with a successful transplants indicate a better quality of life (Milde, Hart, & Zehr, 1992).

Patient/family education. Patients who are to be evaluated for a combined procedure should be sent to a center that has considerable experience in this type of procedure. The risks and benefits should be carefully explained. Transplant programs include nurse specialists who have developed detailed teaching programs for transplant candidates.

Kidney-islet cell transplantation. Although this procedure is relatively new in modern day medicine, it was actually first performed in 1894 (Soon-Shiong & Lanza, 1990). A large number of islet cells are required for transplantation and there is difficulty in isolating a sufficient number from a single adult pancreas donor (Solinger & Geffner, 1994). This shortage has limited its application to those who require a renal transplant. There are several indications and criteria for this procedure which include:

- chronic renal failure with the need for a renal transplant;
- indication that the islet cells of the patient's pancreas are not functioning adequately;
- history of compliance with previous medical management; and
- low panel reactive antibodies (Soon-Shiong & Lanza, 1990).

After donor cells have been harvested and prepared from a donor kidney, they are infused into the portal vein of recipients. It is hoped that the cells will revascularize within the portal vein and function normally within weeks to a few months. The major complication is rejection, which appears more frequently in this procedure than in any other transplant procedure. Postoperatively, patients must be monitored closely for signs of hyperglycemia or hypoglycemia. Nursing measures should be implemented to minimize the risk of infection.

Patient education. Patients who elect this procedure require definitive teaching, including the management of their blood glucose, the signs and symptoms of rejection, and the avoidance of infection. The transplantation of islet cells is a minor surgical procedure when compared to a total pancreas transplant. Unfortunately, the results thus far have not been encouraging as few if any patients have remained insulin free. It is hoped that with improved islet cell preparation and more research, it will become a viable choice for patients (Budinger & Donnelly, 1994).

Role of Nephrology Nurses

Nephrology nurses, social workers, and dietitians from the early days of renal replacement therapy have recognized the need to function as a multidisciplinary team. The complex care of diabetic patients demands the services of well-educated nurses. Nurses provide day to day clinical care, which results in more successful outcomes for patients. Patient and family education become increasingly important if diabetic patients are to succeed with renal replacement therapy. The teaching of glucose monitoring, dietary management, medication regime, and support and counseling for psychological and social problems are within the domain of nephrology nurses.

As the diabetic and elderly population on dialysis continues to increase, the role of nurses will continue to expand. Unfortunately, in recent times, as these demands have increased, the number of available personnel has decreased. Nurses will need to identify patient outcomes and cost-effective means for achieving this for so many patients.

Summary

DM remains a disease with high mortality and even higher morbidity. The increasing age of the general population coupled with the trend toward obesity may continue to increase the numbers entering Medicare's ESRD Program. Early detection of the disease and better management may slow its progression and perhaps prevent some of the cardiovascular complications that interfere with the effectiveness of renal replacement therapy. Better technology and more effective medications may bring longer lives with a better quality of life to DM patients. Further research in the area of pancreas and islet cell transplants may increase the benefits of these procedures. Researchers continue to explore the progression of DM. Currently, available research findings confirm the importance of intensive therapy in preventing and decreasing DM complications. To improve the outcomes of diabetic patients, nurses will need to possess a knowledge of clinical care to assist DM patients and the challenges they bring with chronic renal failure.

References

American Diabetes Association (ADA). (1995). Clinical practice recommendations. *Diabetes Care 18*(1), 5-15.

Aronoff, G.R., & Abel, S.R. (1990). Practical guidelines for drug dosing in patients with renal impairment. In R.W. Schrier (Ed.), *Manual of nephrology* (p. 189). Boston: Little, Brown & Company.

Badsonna, G., Matas, A.J., & Najarian, J.S. (1992). Kidney transplantation in diabetic patients: The University of Minnesota experience. *Kidney International, 42*(Supp. 38), S-193-S-196.

Bates, B. (1983). *A guide to physical examination* (Third Edition) (pp. 194-111). Philadelphia: J.B. Lippincott Company.

Budinger, J.M., & Donnelly, S.S. (1994). Nursing care protocols for the kidney/islet cell transplant recipient. *ANNA Journal, 21*(2), 123-128.

Carella, M.J., Gossain, V.V., & Rovner, D.R. (1994). Early diabetic nephropathy: Emerging treatment options. *Archives of Internal Medicine, 154,* 625-630.

Carosella, J. (1993). Reexperiencing loss: Diagnosis of end-stage renal disease in diabetic patients. *Dialysis & Transplantation 72*(12), 723-732.

Cozaar, Product Description. (1995). West Point, PA: Merck & Company, Inc.

The Diabetes Control and Complications Trial Research Group. (1993). The effect of intensive treatment of diabetes on the development and progression of long-term complications in insulin-dependent diabetes mellitus. *The New England Journal of Medicine,* 329(14), 977-986.

The Diabetes Control and Complications (DCCT) Research Group. (1995). Effect of intensive therapy on the development and progression of diabetic nephropathy in the Diabetes Control and Complication Trial. *Kidney International, 47,* 1703-1720.

Dunfee, T.P. (1995, May 15). The changing management of diabetic nephropathy. *Hospital Practice,* pp.45-55.

Epstein, M. (1992). Assessment of the patient with renal disease. In *The Kidney: A Handbook* (p. 6). Sandoz Pharmaceuticals.

Hirsch, I.B. (1994). Current concepts in diabetic nephropathy. *Clinical Diabetes,* pp. 8-12.

Hostetter, T.H. (1991). Diabetic nephropathy. In B.M. Brenner and F.C. Rector (Ed.), *The kidney* (Fourth Edition), (pp.1695-1726). Philadelphia: W.B. Saunders Company.

Khauli, R.B., Steinmuller, D.R., Novick, A.C., Buszta, C., Goormastic, M., Nakamoto, S., Vidt, D., Magnusson, M., Paganini, E., & Schreiber, M. (1986). A critical look at survival of diabetics with end-stage renal disease, transplantation versus dialysis therapy. *Transplantation, 41*(5), 598-602.

Lewis, E.J., Lawrence, G., Hunsicker, M.D., Bain, R.P., & Rohde, R.D. (1993). The effect of angiotensin converting-enzyme on diabetic nephropathy. *New England Journal of Medicine, 329,* 1456-1462.

Luke R.G. (1987). Hypertension in renal transplant recipients. *Kidney International, 3,* 1024-1037.

Manske, C.L., Wang, Y., & Thomas, W. (1995). Mortality of cadaveric kidney transplantation versus combined kidney-pancreas transplantation in diabetic patients. *Lancet, 346,* 1658-1661.

Marken, C.E. (1994). The use of antihypertensive agents in the management of patients with diabetic nephropathy. *Dialysis & Transplantation, 23*(3), 116-124.

Mauer, S.M., Mogensen, C.E., & Kjellstrand, C.M. (1993). Diabetic nephropathy. In R.W. Schrier & C. Gottschalk (Eds.), *Diseases of the kidney* (pp. 2173-2175). Boston: Little, Brown, and Company.

Milde, F.K., Hart, L.K., & Zehr, P.S. (1992). Quality of life of pancreatic transplant recipients. *Diabetes Care, 15*(11), 1459-1463.

Miller, R.B., Sigala, J.F., & Upham, A.T. (1990). The patient with chronic azotemia, with emphasis on chronic renal failure. In R.W. Schrier, (Ed.), *Manual of Nephrology Diagnosis and Therapy,* (Third edition) (pp. 147-188). Boston: Little, Brown & Co.

Ozaki, C.F., Stratta, R.S., Taylor, R.J., Langnas, A.N., Bynon, J.S., & Shaw, B.W. (1992). Surgical complications in solitary pancreas and combined pancreas-kidney transplantation. *The American Journal of Surgery, 164,* 546-551.

Parving, H.H., Rossing, P., Hommel, E., & Smidt, L.M. (1995). Angio-converting enzyme inhibition in diabetic nephropathy: Ten years' experience. *American Journal of Kidney Disease, 26*(1), 99-107.

Price, S.A., & Wilson, L.M. (1982). Glucose metabolism and diabetes mellitus. In *Pathophysiology clinical concepts of disease processes* (Second edition) (pp. 722-727). New York: McGraw-Hill.

Reddi, A.S., & Camerini-Davalos. (1990). Diabetic nephropathy an update. *Archives of Internal Medicine, 150,* 31-43.

Robbins, S.L., & Cotran, R.S. (1979). *Pathologic basis of disease* (Second edition) (pp. 327-343). Philadelphia: W.B. Saunders Company.

Solinger, H.S., & Geffner, S.R. (1994). Pancreas transplantation. *Surgical Clinics of North America, 75*(5), 1183-1195.

Soon-Shiong, P., & Lanza, R.P. (1990). Pancreas and islet cell transplantation. *Transplantation, 87*(8), 133-140.

Tzamaloukas, A.H. (1994). Diabetes. In *Handbook of dialysis* (pp. 422-432). Boston: Little, Brown and Company.

U.S. Renal Data System (1993, March). *USRDS 1993 annual data report* (pp. 19-52). Bethesda, MD: Institute of Diabetes and Digestive and Kidney Diseases.

Williams, M. (1995). Principal discussant: Management of the diabetic transplant recipient. *Kidney International, 48,* 1660-1674.

Suggested Readings

Bretzel, R.G., Hering, B.J., & Federlin, K. (1989). Islet transplantation in diabetes mellitus. *Diabetes and the Kidney, 73,* 217-228.

Hirschl, M.M., Heinz, G., Sunder-Plassman, G., & Derfler,K. (1992). Renal replacement therapy in type 2 diabetic patients: 10 years experience. *American Journal of Kidney Disease, 20*(6), 564-568.

Chapter Highlights

- The changes in the kidney known as diabetic nephropathy now account for over one-third of the patients entering an end stage renal disease (ESRD) program.
- Earlier detection of microalbumin in known diabetics will lead to sooner intervention and a delay in the progression of diabetic nephropathy.
- Preventing or delaying the onset of diabetic nephropathy and other end organ damage by diabetes depends on early detection and management of the disease.
- Individuals indicating that they have any of the symptoms of diabetes should also be referred to a physician for appropriate evaluation. These symptoms most commonly include excessive thirst, excessive hunger, and excessive urination.
- The Diabetes Control and Complications Trial (DCCT) demonstrated that intensive therapy with close monitoring and control of blood sugar can delay and slow the progression of diabetic nephropathy as well as retinopathy and neuropathy. This has spurred the need for a specialized nurse known as a Certified Diabetes Educator.
- The progression of diabetic nephropathy is marked by an increase in the amount of urinary protein, a rise in BUN and serum creatinine, and a decrease in glomerular filtration rate as measured by the creatinine clearance.
- Chronic renal failure usually occurs into the second decade of the disease. The patient may have already experienced many of the physical complications caused by diabetes.
- Comprehensive or conclusive research is now available that has given practitioners guidelines for interventions to slow the progression of this disease.
- The large arsenal of drug therapy for hypertension has made it easier to find a regime that controls blood pressure with limited side effects; among these agents are the ACE inhibitors and calcium channel blocker drugs. Beta-blockers should be avoided because of their masking of hypoglycemia symptoms.
- ACE inhibitors have been shown to protect against deterioration in renal function in normotensive patients. Research suggests that the drug lowers glomerular intracapillary pressure while preserving renal plasma flow resulting in a decrease in proteinuria. For this reason many diabetics are being started on this drug early in the course of their disease.
- Ketoacidosis results from insulin insufficiency resulting in hyperglycemia, decreased lipogenesis, and the production of ketone bodies. Patients may become hypotensive and develop shock, which can lead to coma and death.
- Hypoglycemia usually is a result of a change in insulin requirements. The need for insulin may be reduced if patients modify their diet, lose weight, or increase exercise. As renal function deteriorates, the insulin requirement may also be reduced due to the impaired clearance of insulin by the kidney. Patients may assume that their DM is improving rather than acknowledging that their renal function is decreasing.
- Diabetic patients experience more cardiovascular disease and infection than their nondiabetic counterparts. These diseases are the main contributors to the increased rate of mortality and morbidity in the diabetic population receiving renal replacement therapy.
- There does not appear to be a significant difference in mortality and morbidity between CAPD and hemodialysis procedures in diabetic patients.
- There appears to be no greater loss of graft in the immediate postoperative period for diabetic patients, although management is more difficult.
- In the past decade, kidney-pancreas transplant has moved out of the realm of experimental procedures to a viable option for some patients.
- Patient and family education become increasingly important if diabetic patients are to succeed with renal replacement therapy.

CHAPTER 17

The Geriatric Patient

Terran R. Mathers, MSN, BA, RN, CNN

Chapter Contents

Aging in Perspective 483
Demographics 483
Chronic Illness and Aging 483
Incidence and Prevalence of Renal Disease. 483
Nursing Home Placement 484
Holistic Care 484
Goal of Medical Treatment 484
Relevant Issues Facing Elderly Nephrology Patients 484
Functional/Physiological Changes 484
Psychosocial Challenges and Realities 488
Comprehensive Nursing Assessment and Interventions 491
Nursing Strategies/Adaptations 492
Assessment Tools and Interventions 492
Renal Replacement Therapies. 495
Hemodialysis 495
Peritoneal Dialysis 496
Transplantation 497
Who Makes the Choice? 497
Nutritional Issues of Adequacy 497
Physiological Considerations 497
Psychosocial Considerations 498
Environmental Considerations. 498
Pathological Considerations 498
Addressing Nutritional Issues 498

Chapter Contents

Drug Therapy 498
- Pharmacodynamics 499
- Pharmacokinetics. 499
- Compliance Issues 499
- Nursing Interventions 500

Education - Adaptation for Life's Changes 501
- Elderly CRF Patients 501
- Environmental Conditions 501
- Instructional Systems Design 501
- Educational Outcomes 502

Ethical Aspects of Care 502
- Allocation of Resources 503
- Quality of Life 503
- Autonomy and Decision Making 503
- Death and Dying 504

Rehabilitation and Elderly Patients 504
- Components of Elderly Rehabilitation 505
- Considerations for Implementation 506

Caregivers 506

Gerontological Research 506
- Methodological Considerations 507
- Ethical Issues 507
- Future Implications 507

Summary 507

References 509

Chapter Highlights. 513

The Geriatric Patient

Terran R. Mathers, MSN, BA, RN, CNN

Aging in Perspective

Caring for the elderly is different from that of the younger population when considering that changes occur because of the aging process itself, the numerous diseases that tend to occur within this cohort, and the problems one encounters because of the treatment received (Kane, Ouslander, & Abrass, 1994). These changes often coexist and are interrelated. This is the main reason why it is often difficult to diagnose specific diseases. Changes occurring with normal aging have been viewed in the past as gradual. However, longitudinal research, which follows the same individuals over a period of time, indicates that this may not be so (Svanborg, Bergstrom, & Mellstrom, 1982). Due to demographic projections, more studies are being conducted on the elderly population than before. Therefore, nurses need to be aware of any current findings and be ready to adjust assessments, plans, interventions, and evaluations to facilitate quality patient care. The usual way to categorize elderly adults, that is, those over 65 years of age, is as follows: young-old (65-74 years), middle-old (75-84 years), and old-old (85 years and older) (Miller, 1995, p. 15). The purpose of this chapter is to provide an overview of the elderly chronic renal failure (CRF) patient and describe nursing care that will promote maximal health, comfort, and independence.

Demographics

The number of individuals over the age of 65 has increased as well as the proportion of this group to the total population. It is predicted that these numbers will continue to increase to the extent that this population will outnumber all others, particularly during the years of 2010 and 2030. It is during this time that the baby boomer generation will reach 65 years of age. Individuals are living longer for several reasons: emphasis on health promotion, prevention of and technological advances providing treatment for cardiovascular conditions, control of infectious diseases, and improvements in maternal care during pregnancy and child care immediately after and during early childhood (Miller, 1995, p. 5). Other demographic characteristics of the elderly population are summarized in Table 17-1.

Chronic Illness and Aging

Chronic illness can be defined as the "irreversible presence, accumulation, or latency of disease states or impairments that involve the total human environment for supportive care and self-care, maintenance of function and prevention of further disability" (Lubkin, 1990, p. 6). Eighty percent of those elderly individuals aged 65 years and older have been identified as having as least one chronic illness (U.S. Senate Special Committee on Aging, 1991). That is, they have a condition which has at least one of the following characteristics: it is permanent, leaves a disability, is caused by a pathological condition that is nonreversible, requires rehabilitative training, and/or requires long-term supervision and care (Dimond & Jones, 1983). This may be due (particularly the prevalence) to the increased mortality rate of this population. It is hoped that continued research for the elderly will potentially decrease those needing to initiate dialysis.

Incidence and Prevalence of Renal Disease

The median age of a new patient initiating CRF therapy is 63, according to the 1996 United States Renal Data System (USRDS) reflecting 1993 data (USRDS, 1996). However, the rate of incidence and prevalence currently decreases somewhat with the 65-74 age groups of patients when compared with the others (USRDS, 1996).

Vascular diseases tend to be the predominating cause of CRF for the elderly population (Mignon, Michel, Mentre, & Viron, 1993). Studies in this area are ongoing as researchers try to determine appropriate prevention and treatment of these diseases. Research in the area of diabetes, one of the other known causes of CRF in the general CRF adult population, including the elderly, is expected to demonstrate methods to prevent diabetic nephropathy. Continued attempts to improve conservative management, particularly in the areas of nutrition and pharmacological agents should demonstrate improvement of CRF prevention, or at least slow the rate of progression. Schreiner (1990) addresses treatable causes of renal failure in the elderly as being those of obstruction, hypertension, diabetes, drug interactions, and carcinomas, with obstruction as that "in the forefront of our considerations" (p. 360).

Table 17-1
Demographics highlighting an aging population.

	Males	**Females**
Life Expectancy	15.6 (over 65) years	18.9 (over 65) years
Marital Status		
Married	77%	43%
Widowed	13%	47%
Single (Never Married)	5%	4%
Divorced	5%	6%
Living Arrangements		
Lives with spouse	75%	41%
Lives with other relatives	6%	17%
Lives alone or with nonrelatives	19%	42%
Median Income	$16,484	$9,355
House Owners	86%[a]	67%[a]
Employed in Labor Force	17%	9%

Note: Adapted from The American Association of Retired Persons and USDHHS Administration on Aging, *A Profile of Older Americans* (1996), whose information is based on data from the U.S. Bureau of the Census.

[a] Older male householders and married couples were more likely to be owners (86%) than were female householders (67%).

Nursing Home Placement

Currently only 5% of the elderly reside in nursing homes (AARP, 1996). As the general population gets progressively older this percentage is expected to increase, thus increasing the number of elderly CRF patients that will be in nursing homes. Although Anderson, Kraus, and Sturgeon (1993) found that there was a lower incidence of nursing home placements in their specific Network, they and others (Schleifer, 1990) believe that this is due to reasons such as: transportation, finances, and reluctance of nursing homes to accept these individuals with CRF.

Holistic Care

It must be kept in mind that to care for the nephrology patient means to care for the whole person, referred to as holistic care in the realm of nursing. The geriatric care provided encompasses more than the physical person. There must also be inclusion of the psychological, social, spiritual, and familial aspects (Brodeur, 1990).

Goal of Medical Treatment

The general goal of treatment of a geriatric nephrology patient should be the maintenance of health status at an optimal level of functioning. How this is accomplished is dependent on the individual patient and that patient's condition at various points of treatment. Amount and types of medical treatment will fluctuate based on the decision-making of the multidisciplinary team in collaboration with the patient as an active participant in the process. Therapeutic communication with the patient concerning the provision of nephrology care will facilitate patient autonomy and decision making as discussed in the ethics section of this chapter.

Relevant Issues Facing Elderly Nephrology Patients

Physiological/Functional Changes

The physiological and pathophysiological changes that occur with aging affect both internal and external structures in the human body (see Table 17-2). This may bring about adaptive responses needed to achieve even the smallest of activities of daily living, depending on the severity of the physiological change. Because of the uniqueness of each person, there is no typical model on which one can assume as their future bodily existence. However, the health care professional can assess for those changes known to occur most often among the elderly and integrate this knowledge with appropriate accommodations into an effective plan of care. For the elderly nephrology patient, a change in other areas of the body can affect the overall biological, psychological, and sociological functioning of that individual. Responses made to general assessments, communication with health care professionals, and educational interventions can be profoundly affected. The following sections address those areas of specific significance to nephrology health care providers when caring for elderly patients. Other physiological changes that occur with aging are presented in an array of books that are specifically written on the biology of aging. The purpose of this chapter, a condensed overview of these changes is presented.

Sensory. The five senses of hearing, vision, smell, taste, and touch have been found to be affected more by the aging process, more in some individuals than others. Those of hearing and vision can alter the way an individual perceives and comprehends information presented, while that of smell and taste can affect the nutritional status. Alterations in touch can interfere with manipulation and safety.

Auditory deficiencies can occur from changes within air and/or bone conduction. The former results in difficulty with clarity of sounds, specifically with the discrimination of high-pitched sounds, while the latter causes diminished amplification of speech that is of normal loudness (Coyne & Hojlo, 1985). Causes for impairment may be attributed to nerve cell degeneration; noise exposure in one's previous workplace causing damage; head injury or strokes; medications; and a disruption of blood flow to the inner aspect of the ear due to disease processes, including kidney disease and hereditary tendencies (AARP, 1984). Consequences of hearing loss among the elderly population may include inhibition of verbal communication and contact with others, contributing to loneliness and self-esteem disturbance (Chen, 1994). Any changes in hearing can have an effect on what is being understood by the patient, ultimately affecting patient care.

Normal physiological changes that occur within the eyes can cause functional changes that bring with it the difficulty in recognizing or seeing persons, places, and things. Some of the changes include: color perception (making it difficult to discriminate between greens and blues), a decrease in peripheral vision, depth perception, response to change in lighting, refraction that affects the focusing on objects that are close (presbyopia), and an increased sensitivity to glare (AARP, 1986; Miller, 1995). All of these can have an affect on the care given elderly persons, including education, rehabilitation, and even as research participants.

The sense of smell can serve several purposes for an elderly person: safety (to detect gas leaks or smoke), association with pleasant events of the past (cinnamon and Mom's pumpkin pie), and maintenance of nutritional status (stimulation of salivation and hunger) (Yurick, Spier, Robb, & Ebert, 1989). Any deficiency in smell is a cause for concern for the elderly person, especially if they live alone.

Taste and the nutritional status of an individual can be affected by those factors indicated in this chapter's discussion of the nutritional issues of adequacy. The renal patient often has difficulty adhering to a special diet, but it is of even more concern for the elderly nephrology patient who has other issues that may play a significant role in nutritional status.

As an individual ages, there is a decreased tactile sensation. That is, the skin does not sense as readily the pressure or changes in the degree of temperature of something placed upon it, whether it be the hands, the arms, the legs, the buttocks, or other areas of the body. This is a cause for concern for elderly people for they may not be able to determine water temperature, sense when they have a firm grasp of something, or feel the pressure being exerted upon parts of the body, thereby causing breakdowns. In the case of the renal dialysis patient, decreased recognition of touch may cause a breakdown of the skin when in a chair for long periods of time during a hemodialysis treatment. Another consideration would be for the peritoneal dialysis patient may not be able to connect the tubing for treatment because of decreased touch sensitivity necessary for complete manual dexterity.

Cardiovascular system. Research in the area of cardiovascular functioning of the aging has been a controversial issue. Current studies contradict earlier findings, which reported a decline in this system due to the aging process. However, because of the increased number of diseases as one grows older, it has been difficult to determine if cardiovascular changes are disease-related rather than due to aging alone. Technological advancement is now allowing researchers to determine those older individuals who are disease free so that studies may be conducted to determine the affect that the aging process alone has on cardiovascular functioning. Controlling for other variables including a person's lifestyle (i.e. smoking, nutrition, stress) and cultural influence can also affect research outcomes (Miller, 1995).

Cardiac complications are considered to be the leading cause of death in those patients with CRF (USRDS, 1996). According to Ismail, Hakim, Oreopoulos, and Patrikarea (1993), older age in a dialysis patient can be considered a risk factor for left ventricular hypertrophy, dilated cardiomyopathy, and ischemic heart disease. The impact of heart disease has been demonstrated in small studies conducted on patients ages 65 and older receiving dialytic therapy. Survival rate is noted to be shorter when results are compared with the general dialysis population (Alpert, 1995). With this in mind, and using the information provided in the first paragraph, it becomes clear that nursing care needs to be individualized with regards to cardiovascular functioning. Awareness of the signs and symptoms,

Table 17-2
Expected changes related to the aging process.

Understanding normal age-related changes is the foundation to understanding health and disease in older people. The following section highlights changes within each organ system that are known to decline with age.

Skin and connective tissue

- Loss of dermal thickness produces transparent, thin skin appearance.
- In the epidermis, melanocytes' (pigment-producing cells) number and activity decrease, making skin more sensitive to ultraviolet sunlight.
- Progressive loss of melanocytes in hair bulbs and decreased number of hair follicles result in greying and thinning of hair.
- Decrease in epidermis turnover contributes to slower wound healing.
- Sebaceous and sweat glands decrease in number, size, and function, therefore producing less oil and sweat.
- Decreased vascular bed and responsiveness (and sweating) predispose older people to hypothermia and hyperthermia.
- Decreased vitamin D3 production and decreased exposure to sunlight may contribute to osteoporosis and osteomalacia.

Nervous System

- Moderate cortical atrophy.
- Loss of neurons in the neocortex, substantia nigra, and limbic system.
- Lipofuscin pigment accumulates primarily in glial tissues.
- Certain neurotransmitters decline.
- Binding sites for dopamine and serotonin decrease.
- Peripheral nerve fibers decrease in number and size.
  - Motor and sensory nerve conduction decreases.
  - A decrease in vibratory sensation in feet and ankles may occur.

Special senses

Vision

- Atrophy of periorbital tissue may cause upper and lower lids to droop.
- Visual activity may decrease due to changes in the retina or neural components.
- Loss of accommodation causes hyperopia.
- Nuclear sclerosis causes myopia.
- Decreased tear secretion may cause dryness of eyes.

Hearing

- Pure tone loss is greater at high frequencies than at low frequencies.
- Pitch discrimination declines primarily at very high and low frequencies.
- Speech discrimination declines and is worsened with background noise.

Smell

- Olfaction declines, causing poor detection and discrimination by the eighth decade.

Oral

- A reduction in the integrity of epithelial and connective tissue causes a thinning of the oral mucosa and affects bone pulpal tissues.
  - Blood supply is decreased.
  - Nerve innervation is compromised.
  - Tissue quality is modified.
  - Calcifitic tissue changes occur.
- A compositional change in the nature of saliva.
  - Altered sodium levels.
  - Increase in potassium.
  - Decrease in secretory proteins.
- A reduction in taste perception.
  - Increase in threshold potentials for salt and bitter tastes.
- Structural changes to the teeth.
  - Erosion.
  - Abrasion.
  - Attrition.
- Gingival recession.
  - Alveolar dehiscence.
  - Compromised spatial position of teeth.

Cardiovascular

- Conducting system loses cells and fibers and becomes infiltrated with fat.
- Heart rate at rest and achievable maximum declines [maximum HR = (220-age)].
- Increase in stroke volume (S.V.) compensates for lower heart rate (H.R.) and maintaining cardiac output (C.O.) [C.O. = H.R. x S.V.].
- Intrinsic contractile function declines.
- Vascular compliance decreases due to changes in the vessel walls with intima cellular proliferation and fibrosis and media elastin fragmentation and calcification.
- In Western and developed countries, systolic blood pressure increases with lower rate of increase in diastolic pressure.

Respiratory

- Lung elastic recoil decreases as a result of collagen and elastic changes.
- Chest wall compliance decreases due to stiffening of the chest wall.
- Respiratory muscle strength decreases.
- Lung volumes change as a consequence of the above changes.
  - Increase in residual volume and functional residual capacity.
  - Decrease in vital capacity and expiratory flow rates.
- Gas exchange.
  - Decrease in arterial pO2, due to ventilation-perfusion mismatch.

Gastrointestinal

- Esophageal motility decreases due to lower amplitude contractions after swallowing (presbyesophages).
- Gastric mucosa thins, acid-producing parietal cells atrophy, and gastric acid secretion decreases.
- Small and large intestinal mucosa atrophies, reducing absorptive surface area and decreasing the ability to absorb sugars, calcium, vitamin B12, and iron.
- Liver decreases in size but maintains function; however, the microsomal enzyme function declines.

Renal

- Renal mass decreases with primarily cortical losses of nephrons, glomeruli, and capillaries.
- Renal plasma flow decreases.
- Glomerula filtration rate (GFR) falls.
- Creatinine clearance progressively declines 1% per year after age 40 with no change in serum creatinine levels, because creatinine generation also decreases.
- Ability to retain sodium (Na) declines.
- Ability to concentrate urine declines.

Musculoskeletal

- Decrease in muscle weight compared to total body weight.
- Decreased muscular strength and endurance associated with decrease in number of muscle fibers.
- Hyaline cartilage water content declines.
- Bone loss is universal, but rate is highly variable; loss is more rapid in women after menopause than in men.

Hematopoietic

- Overall red cells, hemoglobin, hematocrit, white cells, and platelets maintain normal values and functions.
- Active bone marrow decreases and marrow fat increases but remains adequate for hematopoiesis.

Immune System

- Thymic involution begins about age of puberty.
- Number of T- and B-lymphocytes does not change.
- T-lymphocyte function declines.
  - Decreased response to skin tests.
  - Production of interleukin-2 is reduced.
- B-lymphocyte function is not as clear.
  - Immunoglobulins IgM and perhaps IgG levels decline.
  - Immunoglobulin production to a challenge (vaccine or antigen) is lowered response and shortened duration.

Endocrine

- Progressive decline in carbohydrate tolerance.
  - Primary defect in insulin resistance as post-receptor defect.
- Metabolic clearance rate of thyroid hormone decreases but thyroxine (T4) levels are normal.

Genital/Sexual Function

Women

- With menopause, rapid decline of estrogen and progesterone.
- Hormonal changes cause atrophic changes of uterus, vagina, external genitalia, and breasts.
- Sexual activity decreases, but exact role of biologic changes and sociocultural factors are unknown.

Men

- Testosterone levels remain level.
- Prostate gland increases in size due to hyperplasia.
- Erectile and ejaculatory function declines; postejaculatory refractory period increases.
- Sexual response is delayed due to reduced penile sensitivity and increased threshold for tactile stimulation.

Note: From Stanford, E.P., & Schmidt, M.G. (1991). *Guidelines for education: Geriatric health care professionals* (pp. 18-20). Used with permission. Diane L. Schneider, MD, UCSD School of Medicine, prepared this for the San Diego Geriatric Education Center publication.

as well as the appropriate interventions of care from a nursing perspective, including patient education and treatment, will assist nurses in caring for these individuals. Strategies suggested include: control of blood pressure, preventative measures accompanied with those of treatment for hyperparathyroidism, appropriate dialytic prescriptions (i.e., dialyzer and dialysate), corrective action for anemia (i.e., epoetin alfa), and aluminum overload control (Ismail et al., 1993).

Respiratory system. Several changes occur within the respiratory system that affect an older person, and can be of more concern if that person is on dialysis. The chest wall and musculoskeletal changes include the calcification of the costal cartilage, weakening of the respiratory muscles, and osteoporosis of the ribs and vertebrae. Because of these changes, there is a reduction in the efficiency of the respiratory system and the maximal inspiratory and expiratory force. This affects the supply of oxygen and removal of carbon dioxide, impacting vital organs and tissue functioning (Miller, 1995).

The lungs become smaller with decreases in muscle tone, and the vasculature is affected. Gas exchange is compromised so that there is a decrease in arterial pO2 (Miller, 1995). This age-related change accompanied by the technology of hemodialysis can cause some difficulties for the elderly patient. The renal patient is usually anemic, resulting in decreased oxygen transfer within the body due to the smaller amount of red blood cells. Epoetin alpha has lessened anemia in many patients. However, anemia persists in some who require supplemental oxygen and even transfusions at intervals. Renal patients are vulnerable to pulmonary edema and must therefore be monitored closely when infusions of any kind of fluids are necessary.

The elastic recoil of the lungs is also changed with aging. It is reduced somewhat and has an effect on the expansion and retraction of the lungs. This results in an increase of the residual volume, while the forced expiratory volume is decreased. This change in recoil also affects airflow rates, with an overall decrease in the efficiency of the lungs (Miller, 1995).

It is very important for the nephrology nurse to become familiar with normal breath sounds and the process of auscultation. Variations that affect the physical and mental well-being of the elderly dialysis patient may be identified through proper assessment and then may be treated effectively prior to any debilitating consequences.

Renal system. Although renal anatomy and physiology have been addressed in Chapter 7, it is necessary at this point to reemphasize specific aspects related to the aging process. It is generally accepted that there is a progressive decline in the overall renal functioning once a person reaches early adulthood, and this is the result of changes in renal structure and vasculature. However, this is a controversial issue because of longitudinal studies which suggest that this is more pathological rather than due to the inevitable decline of functioning cells related to the aging process (Rowe & Kahn, 1987). Anatomical changes specific to the normal aging of one's kidneys include a decrease in the weight of the kidney (Roessle & Roulet, 1932) and total renal mass, resulting primarily from the vascular changes in the cortex (Goyal, 1982). There is a decrease in the cells within the glomeruli due in part to sclerosis, and a decrease in the tubules that experience some hypertrophy (Oliver, 1939). The basement membranes of these two areas thicken, and the size of individual cells increase (Goyal, 1982).

Accompanying the physiological changes noted above, there are impairments in various areas of functioning. Some of these include: (a) decreases in the renal plasma flow (RPF) and glomerular filtration rate (GFR), which affects the filtration fraction ("calculated by dividing GFR by effective RPF") (Radke, 1994, p. 184); (b) decreased concentrating ability (Lindeman & Goldman, 1986); (c) reduced sodium retention, thought to be related to changes in the renin-aldosterone system (Radke, 1994); (d) decrease in urinary excretion of calcium, thought to be partially related to the reduction in renal mass and serum calcium levels (Radke, 1994); and (e) impaired potassium excretion due to a lowered aldosterone level (Kee, 1992).

Normally, the kidneys adapt and function adequately as physiological changes occur within the human body. However, stress induced by acute and chronic illnesses may cause an upset in the homeostatic state of the kidneys, possibly resulting in renal failure for that individual.

Psychosocial Challenges and Realities

Theoretical foundation/base. Throughout one's life span, learning accompanied by many changes in behavior take place due to adaptation to environmental factors. As with every stage of life, old age can be met and experienced with upheaval or serenity. Following are the views of two theorists who have expressed their ideas of developmental levels and the accompanying behaviors that the demands of these levels bring about as individuals grow older.

Havinghurst (1952) addresses the last segment of the developmental tasks of adulthood as that of later maturity. He states that a developmental task is one that "arises at or about a certain period in the life of the individual, successful achievement of which leads to his happiness and to success with later tasks, while failure leads to unhappiness in the individual, disapproval by the society, and difficulty with later tasks" (p. 2). During this period of old age, the individual adjusts to physical changes, retirement, living with the spouse who has retired, changes in income, establishment of living arrangements that are physically satisfactory, and affiliation with one's peers while also assimilating social roles and obligations.

Erikson (1963) looks at life as a continuum with four major phases subdivided into eight stages. A review of the last phase, that of old age, addresses individuals of 60 or more years. It is further subdivided into ego integrity versus despair. The first of these, ego integrity, refers to individuals' sense of peace, as well as their view of past life and self with satisfaction. They are able to let go and look toward the future with contentment. Despair, on the other hand, is used by individuals, who wish they could go back to earlier days and change the past.

Stressors of aging. As an individual ages, changes and transitions take place that are considered stressors. These can be viewed as good or bad depending on the effect they have on individual persons. Specific stressors for the elderly have been identified that affect them psychologically, but are often overlooked because of the portrayal of old age as a time of tranquility and contentment. According to Gonchar and Itschaki (1986), the older population actually experiences more stressors than younger generations. Common emotional reactions for this age group include that of grief, guilt, loneliness, rage, depression, helplessness, and anxiety (Butler, Lewis, & Sunderland, 1991). Accompanying these are those situational crises that may occur with some older persons, but not all, and possibly at the same time causing an added stress on the elderly person. These include: widowhood; marital problems; sexuality; financial difficulties; physical changes and discomfort (to include sensory loss and chronic pain); disability; hospitalization; the process of death and dying (which encompasses concern for one's self as well as loved ones) (Butler et al., 1991); ageist attitudes; retirement; and relocation (Miller, 1995). Geriatric nephrology patients may reveal a variety of emotional reactions to the need for dialysis treatments, including depression, anger, despair, shock, and grief over the loss of a body function (Gonchar & Itschaki, 1986).

The impact of life events are important to consider because they can have an effect on the overall well-being of individuals. Miller (1995) has differentiated the meaning of life events as they occur within older individuals' lives from those of younger adults. She believes that:

1. Events for an older person are frequently associated with loss;
2. Several events are more likely to occur within a short time span;
3. They last for a longer period of time; and,
4. Powerlessness is often felt by the individual (Miller, 1995, p. 58).

Sexuality. Sexuality, as identified in the previous section, is one of the stressors for an elderly person. It is an often overlooked aspect of care, and because of this, it will be addressed here as a means of stressing its importance within the holistic framework for elderly individuals. Whether it be a hug, holding of hands, flirting, a sexual fantasy, or sexual intercourse, elderly individuals have as much a right to express their sexual feelings as any other human being. Dysfunction in this area of behavioral responses for this population can be attributed not only to the aging process and physiological changes, but also societal attitudes and myths regarding sexual expressions/nonexpressions; chronic illnesses; lack of a friend or spouse; the fact that many elderly individuals of today were not educated regarding methods of sexual expression (Comfort, 1974); and medications/drugs and alcohol (Ferrini & Ferrini, 1992). Keep in mind also that elderly nephrology patients are affected by their chronic renal failure as noted in Chapter 10.

Aging physiology and sexual responses. As with other body systems, the reproductive system changes as one grows older, causing a need for adaptations in sexual activity. For females, sexual response changes include: a slower vaginal lubrication with a decreased amount produced, a thinning of the vaginal lining, less flexibility of the vagina, and a decrease in the intensity organisms. Males experience: a decrease in the urgency of the sex drive; a longer time to have an erection, with the penis also not as firm as in previous years; disappearance of the erection prior to orgasm; more stimulation needed for ejaculation, which is then less forceful(if one does ejaculate) and with a smaller amount of semen; and a longer refractory period (Byer & Shainberg, 1991).

Societal attitudes and myths. There is an array of societal myths that tend to override the actual feelings and practices of the elderly. Two common misconceptions are mentioned here:

1. Sex is not practiced by the elderly. Contrary to popular beliefs, sexual activity occurs well into the ninth decades by some individuals. It has been found that those who were most active in their younger years tend to be the most active in later years (Dressel & Avant, 1983).
2. Elders do not enjoy sex. Unless severely compromised by physical difficulty and inhibition, older individuals can enjoy sex as much as a younger adult. Of course, it must be kept in mind that the sexual drive can differ for an individual from one time to another (as in younger life), and that each person has individual sexual desires and needs (Dressel & Avant, 1983).

Chronic illnesses. Individuals are more susceptible to chronic illnesses as they grow older. The elderly nephrology patient may therefore be dealing with not only renal failure, but also other illnesses that may already be causing sexual dysfunction. Some of the chronic illnesses identified as having an effect on sexual expression include: diabetes, arthritis, cancer

Table 17-3
Sexual counseling of the geriatric nephrology patient - The PLISSIT model.

Levels of Counseling	Purpose	Patient Outcomes
Permission	Allows patients to discuss sexual concerns openly and without hesitation, with reassurance from health care professionals.	Understanding that the sexual problems encountered are normal and that sexual activity is still permitted.
Limited **I**nformation	Provides patients with reading materials in layman's terms concerning sexual changes related to renal disease and the aging process. These are then discussed with health care professionals.	Patients are reassured through written information and have a more thorough understanding of the effects of renal disease accompanied by aging as it relates to sexual activity.
Specific **S**uggestions	Suggestions are presented by health care professionals for improving the sexual problems of patients.	The strategies provided allow patients alternatives from which to choose for expressing sexuality.
Intensive **T**herapy	Assistance is provided by certified sex therapists.	Patients benefit from therapists educated in the field of sex therapy when the previous three levels are unsuccessful.

Note: Adapted from Garden (1994) for nephrology patients.

(Foundation for Medical Education and Research, 1983), cardiovascular disease, hypertension, primary hypothyroidism, and mental illness (Garden, 1994).

Lack of partner or spouse. Lack of a sexual partner tends to be a problem more with women than men. This has been found to be due to two specific reasons: women outlive men, so there is a decreased number of males from which to choose (Ferrini & Ferrini, 1992; Yurick, 1989).

Educational background. It is important that information regarding physiological changes in the normal aging process and any usual occurring changes brought about by a disease be shared with the patient and partner. Knowing what is normal will help relieve some of the guilt often experienced by elderly individuals when sexual activity and relationships are hindered. Education also involves dissipating any myths to which they are susceptible, and introducing alternative methods for expressing sexuality such as a change in coital positions and suggesting ways to express compassion and warmth. Information on the availability of medical and surgical interventions, if necessary, should also be provided.

Medications/drugs and alcohol. Many pharmacological agents and alcohol consumed by the elderly can have an effect on sexual activity, both physically and psychologically. Some of the medications that can have an adverse effect are included in the following classifications: hypertensives, benzodiazepines, antihistamines, antispasmodics, antidepressants, and antiparkinson agents (just to name a few) (Garden, 1994). Blood levels indicative of large amounts of alcohol intake, also correlate with diminished sexual performance, including temporary impotence for men with a potential for loss of erections if the intake is chronic (Ferrini & Ferrini, 1992). Women often experience decreased libido and orgasms (Ferrini & Ferrini, 1992; Miller, 1995).

Sexual counseling. Viewed from a rehabilitative standpoint, sexual counseling is best addressed by individuals who have received specific training and are personally skilled with sexual counseling. This may be any member of the multidisciplinary team, particularly nurses, social workers, and nephrologists. Because talk about sexual activity was usually taboo for the older person during the early developmental years, it is often the health care provider who will first mention sexual activity and potential problems to an individual. Physical assessment and a sexual history may reveal some problems that could be reversed through some minor interventions, or even through surgery, if it is of a more-serious nature. A method suggested by Garden (1994) that is often used in sexual counseling is *PLISSIT*. This four-step method could be used with elderly nephrology patients as well, and is summarized in Table 17-3.

Depression. Depression, with respect to the patient with chronic renal failure, has been addressed in Chapter 10, and certainly relates to all patients with this chronic condition. However, it must not be overlooked that the elderly patient may be experiencing depression related to other life events.

Although depression has been shown to be less frequent among older adults than those who are younger, it has been identified as the most common functional psychiatric disorder for the elderly (Meyers & Alexopoulas, 1988). Burnside (1988) noted that older adults are concerned mainly with poor health, which can lead to depression. Other causes of depression include: loss, medication, drug and substance abuse, failure to thrive, loneliness, and isolation (Hogstel, 1995). It has also been noted that increasing dependence and inability to perform activities of daily living may cause depression, or make an already diagnosed condition of depression worse (Parmelee, Katz, & Lawton, 1992).

Assessing the elderly depressed patient can be difficult, because the cause is not always readily recognized. Using the strategies suggested in the next section on assessment will facilitate this part of the nursing process. Interventions will then depend on those areas of concern for the elderly person, and may include counseling, education, and referrals to outreach programs.

Coping with life. Growing old can be a challenge to any individual. How one accepts these challenges will help to determine the state of mind and body, which in turn can cause a fluctuation in the individual's self-esteem. A self-esteem disturbance may be identified in such life circumstances as retirement, loss of spouse, physical disability, the impact of ageism associated with negative stereotypes, decreased social interaction, and loss of control over environmental issues (Taft, 1985).

The mental capacity of individuals will depend on how well coping can be employed with the changes in their lives. Defense mechanisms used in old age are methods of coping with the frustrations, anxieties and uncertainties presented in everyday living as well as those situational crises that occur. Individuals will experience life events from different perspectives, thereby adding, maintaining and discarding defense mechanisms as the situations dictate, and depending on the personal perception that they have of each event. Denial, projection, fixation, regression, displacement, counterphobia, and idealization have been identified as the main ones used by older people (Butler et al., 1991).

Problems that may surface if a crisis situation ensues, that is, ones that coping mechanisms cannot assist, include depression, loneliness, isolation, and a lowered self-esteem. Also, chronic illness, as in the case of elderly persons with renal disease, has been noted to increase the incidence of psychiatric disorders (Rodin & Voshart, 1986; Wells, Golding, & Burnam, 1988). However, several researchers have shown that psychiatric morbidity does not increase with those on hemodialysis in comparison to continuous ambulatory peritoneal dialysis (CAPD) patients (Iordanidis et al., 1993; Morris & Jones, 1989; Wolcott & Nissenson, 1988).

Through research, factors have been identified as having an effect on the coping strategies used by hemodialysis patients, primarily of a younger generation. These include physical condition, predialysis personality, dialysis treatment, family reactions, reactions of the multidisciplinary team members (Kaplan De-Nour & Czaczkes, 1972) as well as age, sex, nutritional status, immunological competence, personality, family, and social and demographic parameters (Kimmel, Weihs, & Peterson, 1993). The coping strategies identified were both emotion-focused (Blake & Courts, 1996) and problem-focused (Gurklis & Menke, 1988; Murdaugh, 1987). Little research, however, has been conducted in the area of coping strategies specific to geriatric nephrology patients, who are often incorporated within the adult sampling of a study. This leaves a significant gap regarding the care of this population.

Spirituality. That dimension of care, often overlooked in nursing, is the spiritual development which contributes to the mental health of older adults. This may be due to the fact that often objective data in the form of signs and symptoms, accompanied by pathological changes, tend to be foremost in our thoughts of what consists of comprehensive nursing assessment. When considering the spirituality of a geriatric patient, background assessment includes all other aspects of life as discussed in this chapter (physical, pathological, and social), but also the individual's culture, religious, and ethnic background. It must be kept in mind that spirituality is often what gives meaning to life's experiences for the elderly, and assists with their coping strategies necessary to deal with problems associated with illnesses, losses, and longevity in general (Brooke, 1987). Reed (1991) summarizes healthy spirituality as that which "fosters a concern for others and self, a sense of meaning and enjoyment in life, commitment to purposes greater than the self, a sense of relatedness, and a means for moving through a debilitating sense of guilt, anger, and anxiety" (p. 17).

Comprehensive Nursing Assessment and Interventions

Performance of a patient-specific, accurate and comprehensive assessment of the elderly person provides information necessary to analyze individual strengths and weaknesses. The alterations of geriatric functioning may be pinpointed through an integration of biological, psychological, and social data. The assessment should encompass genetics, culture, and nutrition as well as a person's adaptation to changes in health and functioning, outside support, living arrangements, economic status, recent life situations, and disease/illness (Campbell, 1995). The assessment may be conducted by means of observations, interviews, and physical assessment and include both subjective and objective data. Knowing the expected changes that occur with normal aging, as noted in Table 17-2 can help to identify what is abnormal. The individuality of the aging process has a diversity of presentations.

Nursing Strategies/Adaptations

Assessment of the elderly person may be conducted in much the same manner as with other age groups. There are, however, several considerations needing adaptations that should be taken into account. These include time, environmental conditions, and communication techniques. Other factors that need to be included within these are sensory deficits and cognitive changes.

Time. Time of day is a consideration that may mean the difference between obtaining accurate and specific information from that which is given too quickly. Elderly people may not do well at certain times of day, and it is important to establish times suitable for them. It has been suggested that morning is the most reliable time for assessing an elderly individual (Enloe, 1993). This may be partially attributed to the fact that one's sleep pattern is different than when younger, with the elderly often taking a nap during the afternoon. It also helps individuals to know not only the reason for the interview/questioning, and how the feedback will be used, but also the length of time needed to obtain this valuable information. Because elderly individuals tend to tire easily, have slower functioning, a longer history to share, and more problems to discuss, multiple interviews for shorter periods of time will assist in eliciting the needed data (Eliopoulos, 1990). Thirty minutes has been identified as a sufficient amount of time for an assessment period (Campbell, 1995).

Environmental conditions. It is important to consider the environmental setting during an interview. The room should be well lit, but without the brightness of direct sunlight and florescent lights which can cause an irritating glare for elderly individuals (Eliopoulos, 1990). Chairs should be padded slightly and have a straight back for comfort. Have available pillows and blankets, especially when patients are lying on an examination table or are having a dialysis treatment, and minimize the length of time they need to be in this position. Room temperature should be at a comfortable level, keeping in mind that these individuals chill easily due to the decrease in the amount of body fat. Extraneous noises should be kept to a minimum, especially if there is a hearing problem. And, finally, allowing for as much privacy as feasible will produce an atmosphere conducive for an effective exchange of information and assessment (Campbell, 1995; Eliopoulos, 1990; Enloe, 1993).

Communication techniques. Unless one's specialty is psychiatric nursing, the tendency is to be so focused on the task at hand (i.e., dialysis procedure) that the basic skill of listening is often forgotten. The nurse should be positioned so as to allow the elderly individual to lip read as a supplement to hearing loss if this should be the case. Give the elderly individual enough time to express herself/himself, allowing for a deficit for reaction time. Use open-ended questions to extract the individual's perceptions and viewpoints (Eliopoulos, 1990). This cohort, however, likes to reminisce, and although it is good to allow this to gain insight into the background of the individual's problems (Campbell, 1995), it may be necessary to also redirect the questioning. Use lay terms, refraining from medical jargon and terms that may not be understood. At times, it will also be necessary to use family members to assist with signs and symptoms, because the elderly tend to underreport information, which may be due to problems with mental clarity or fear that they may be seen as senile. However, initial interviewing of individuals alone should be conducted so as to obtain information directly from them to prevent interference from family members who often try to answer for patients. If it is agreed upon by the patient to have another family member present, then this is done. If not, the family may still be approached separately for their input (Enloe, 1993). Where language is a barrier, interpreters may be needed to facilitate the interaction. The nurse must also be aware of and respect the ethnic and cultural diversity related to viewpoints of health functioning (Campbell, 1995).

Observing for nonverbal communication and outward physical appearance of the individual by the nurse cannot be overemphasized. This in itself may answer many questions or lead to effective assessment that otherwise may be overlooked. Even simple observations of physical mobility when requested to move from one position to another may indicate some problems not identified by the patient (Eliopoulos, 1990).

Assessment Tools and Interventions

Organization of the data collection material and selectivity of information solicited are important aspects to consider during the assessment process. An array of geriatric assessment tools are available, and it has been suggested by Santo-Novak (1988) that seven key points need to be addressed in the assessment of the elderly person: chief concerns, health history, medication history, recent life changes, daily activities, cognitive patterns, and support systems. It is up to the nurse to decide what tools would be valuable to assess each of these areas, and which would best facilitate the care planning of the patient within the nephrology facility. To obtain a holistic overview of the patient, the nephrology nurse must not only review that information obtained by the nephrologist, but also use this information to obtain further data. Collaborative assessment facilitates the care of these patients for optimal outcomes and includes specifics concerning the biological, psychological, and social functioning of the individual.

Biological data. A health history, physical assessment, and laboratory data are components of the biological information needed to obtain an overview of the physical aspect of an individual. Though these are specifically objective data, it is also necessary to obtain subjective input from the patient and from the other health team members. Both medical and nursing diagnoses can be a challenging process for health care professionals. The older person often presents with signs and symptoms, as well as objective data that can be attributed to a multitude of reasons, making it difficult to pinpoint a specific problem. Assessment of biological data is ongoing and is often interrelated with both psychological and social behavioral manifestations. Campbell (1995) has suggested points to consider when identifying physiological and psychological problems:

- there is a proven decline in the biological makeup of an older individual of tissues and organ systems;
- depression has an impact on psychological functioning; and
- psychological changes can be the result of changing pathophysiology (Foreman & Gradowski, 1992).

As noted by Campbell (1995), the cognitive functioning of an individual can be affected physiologically by: "cardiovascular problems, metabolic disorders, hematological disorders, neurological disorders and deficits, and iatrogenic disorders" (p. 91).

Interventions are dependent on the diagnoses and the specific problems identified. Education and then follow-up assessment may encompass such things as ways to enhance dietary compliance, medication change to include reinforcement of reasons for changes and the potential side effects, significance of laboratory values, support groups and counseling, disease process education, and self-care information.

Psychological/emotional data. The nephrology nurse must keep in mind that geriatric CRF patients will or have already experienced some of the changes that come about with old age. The most recent changes that have occurred within individuals' lives, accompanied with the psychosocial problems that face them as patients with renal disease, can prove to be a very overwhelming situation. Finding the appropriate time for assessing individuals is not always an easy task. However, as a general rule, allowing patients some time to stabilize on treatment instead of obtaining psychosocial information at the initiation of the treatment regimen may help to obtain data easier and be more accurate (Schumacher, Olschewski, & Schulgen, 1991). Analyzing the results should then assist in developing patient-specific interventions, leading to optimal outcomes.

Nephrology nurses should explore the patients' problems and their perceptions of their problems. Through the use of the therapeutic communication suggested at the beginning of this section, with emphasis on open-ended questions and utilization of listening skills, the nurse can act as a sounding board and facilitate verbalization of the patient's thoughts and feelings. Then, in collaboration with the patient, attempts to explore alternatives, problem-solve, and find solutions can be conducted. As an advocate, the nurse should also collaborate with the interdisciplinary team and elicit appropriate assistance, thereby helping patients to acquire and use the various resources available to solve or gain control of their problems.

Several interventions are suggested here to assist an elderly individual toward psychological stability. These include:

1. Education - Evaluating first the emotional readiness, or motivation to learn as well as the experiential readiness, or the background knowledge, values and attitudes will assist in developing the instructional content and methods needed for a particular individual. Also, keeping in mind the needs and goals of the elderly person will help.
2. Enabling and empowerment - Through this process, assistance is provided to individuals to gain control of issues and factors affecting their lives (Gibson, 1991). Nephrology nurses can facilitate this gain of control and self-care for patients through the provision of knowledge, skills, and resources (Thomas, 1992). Positive as well as negative feedback is important in this process to encourage continuance of personal growth and development.
3. Enhancement of self-esteem - Through a review of research findings and study of the chronically ill, Miller (1992) has suggested five strategies that an individual can use to increase his/her self esteem: cognitive control, interpersonal relationships, self-affirmation, role performance review and modifications, and self-care competence (p. 406). These are noted in Figure 17-1 with accompanying outcomes that can be used for evaluation purposes. Although not specific to the geriatric patient, these ideas could easily assist the elderly patient toward a more positive view of self. The nurse, as part of the therapeutic environment to assist in the care of the elderly individual, needs to identify the strengths and abilities of older persons, and emphasize these qualities to them. By doing so, self-esteem is positively enhanced.

Figure 17-1
Strategies to enhance self-esteem.

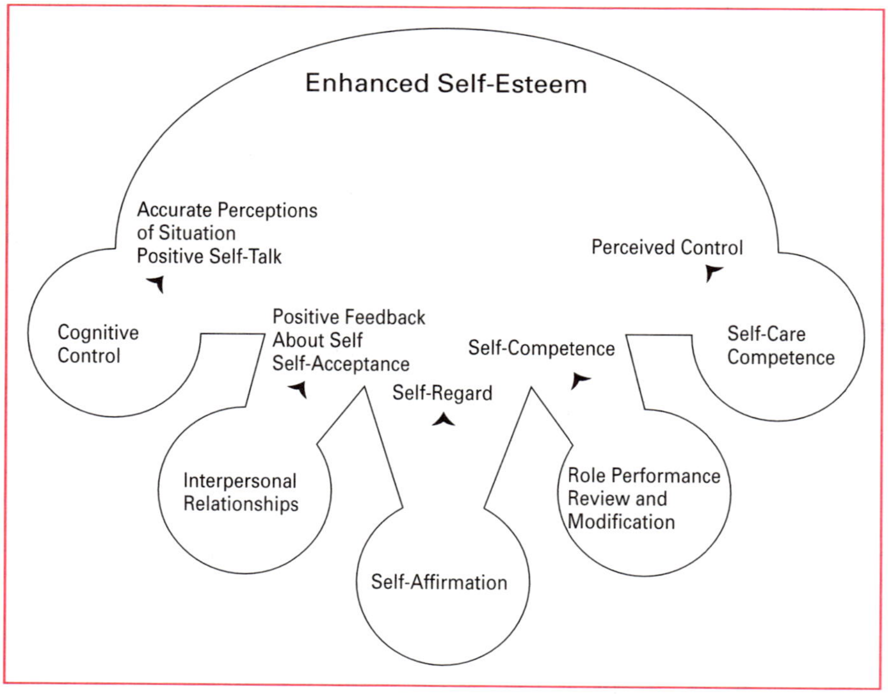

Note: From Miller, J. (1992). Enhancing self-esteem. In J. Miller (Ed.), *Coping with chronic illness: Overcoming powerlessness* (2nd ed.) (pp. 397-412). Philadelphia: F.A. Davis Company. Reprinted with permission.

4. Support groups - Participation in support groups may help to express feelings and anxieties, eliciting feedback and problem solving solutions from others who have experienced similar situations. They may be in the form of groups specific to certain conditions and circumstances such as chronic renal disease, widowhood, or depression. Educational groups about a certain interest of the patient, or groups formed based on age of the participants such as senior citizen activity groups may be useful. Other ideas for groups may include reminiscing, remotivation, music and dance, guided autobiography, and travel clubs. Groups are often not used by the elderly patient due to financial concerns, transportation, time restraints of the dialysis treatments, and even lack of knowledge about the availability of resources and what they provide. Interventions in this respect should be directed toward the limiting conditions as a means of assistance toward participation.
5. Social support networks - Encouragement to utilize social support systems can provide a sense of well-being and give meaning to the elderly person's life. Family, group, peer, or counseling can provide a means of support during troubled times of anger, confusion, depression, and anxiety. All of these support systems, of course, depend on availability at the time of need. Family support may be marginal, especially if members are not situated within the same geographic area. Yet there are those that actually hinder the patient's progress and independence through their constant bedside attendance. Whatever the situation, this source of support needs to be utilized to the patient's best advantage.

Much of the information addressed above is dependent on the cognitive functioning of the individual. When the nurse assesses cognitive functioning, she does so to determine whether there is a progressive change in the mental status of the individual, and to help determine what interventions may be useful to the individual at the time. Such tools as the Short Portable Mental Status Questionnaire (SPMSQ) by Pfeiffer (1974) and the Mini-mental Status Exam (Folstein, Folstein, & McHugh, 1975) are valuable memory and cognitive resources.

Social/functional data. Assessing the social functioning of an individual reflects the degree of competence, independence and autonomy. If problems exist, these can tend to reduce socialization in general, leading to isolation and emotional problems of loneliness and even depression (Eliopoulos, 1990). Consideration in the social assessment of these individuals should include the social support network, family support, financial status, independency with regards to activities of daily living and functional ability, image, cognitive functioning, and environmental adequacy (Kaiser, 1990).

A social assessment consists of basic identifying data about the person such as full name, address, telephone number, next of kin, insurance information, and use of other outside agencies. The nurse should identify the environmental adequacy of living conditions, such as the compatibility of the physical condition of the residence to the needs of the patient, security of the home and neighborhood, and the availability of a support network (i.e. neighbors, family and friends) and means of transportation for other commodities besides those of dialysis treatment appointments. Financial status is also of great importance, because without monetary support, many social activities, whether it be recreational in nature or one of necessity such as doctors' appointments, cannot be accomplished. Often, this information is obtained by the social worker in a dialysis facility, but is of great importance for the nurse to be aware of in the holistic frame of care.

Functional status can have a great impact on the socialization of the individual. According to Nelson and Mayfield (1994), "functional assessment is a systematic attempt to objectively measure performance in the areas of daily living, activities of daily living (ADL), instrumental activities of daily living (IADL), mental status, social status, and economic resources" (p. 120). Functional deficits may not always be something that older individuals are aware of because they tend to diminish slowly and adaptations are made accordingly. Requesting an explanation of a typical day from the individual may lead to some very evident problems and situations that simple interventions may make a little more easier and more comfortable. Identify the routine of such ADLs as eating, grooming and dressing, transferring self from one area to another, and toileting. Know what they can do with regards to IADLs such as shopping, housekeeping chores, and transportation, among others (Reban & Millsap, 1992). Along with these verbal and written accounts, however, the nurse must observe how well the patient is accomplishing tasks, for an older person may answer according to what they think the interviewer wants to hear or for fear of consequences if questions are answered inappropriately. Observations of transfer from a wheelchair to the dialysis chair, walking with or without mechanical assistance, and even noting the method of transportation and timeliness with appointments are important assessments.

Interventions are dependent upon the specific areas of need as identified by the assessment above. Several suggestions include:

1. Identification of resources - Nurses can provide the elderly patient, with the assistance of the interdisciplinary team, a list of community resources based on the interests of the patient, to facilitate socialization. Talking with the patient and helping that individual to understand why particular groups and activities have been suggested, and providing informational literature about them, will encourage their participation. It may encompass developing new skills or hobbies, or personal sharing with others about a skill already mastered. Budget restraints may be somewhat relieved if provided information about a community class on financial management, talking with appropriate financial advisors, or referred for financial assistance. Maintaining or increasing functional status and independence could be facilitated through established physical therapy programs with a goal of maximizing optimal level of functioning, thereby increasing self-worth.
2. Provision of necessary assistance - Whether it be assistance from the help of a home aide who can assist with the shopping or housecleaning, or mechanical assistance in the form of a wheelchair or walker, these measures can facilitate the ease with which things can be accomplished and make everyday living more bearable.

Renal Replacement Therapies

An influx of those elderly patients within the United States being treated for CRF has been noted particularly since the initiation of Medicare funding in 1972 and the Federal Age Discrimination Act of 1975. Although these exist, there is still much concern in the areas of ethical, economic and social considerations when placing an individual on some form of renal replacement therapy (RRT). As with younger patients, the quality of an elderly individual's life along with supplying adequate dialysis is of utmost importance. These viewpoints are incorporated within the following discussion of each of the three modalities of hemodialysis (incenter and home), peritoneal dialysis, and transplantation.

Hemodialysis

In-center hemodialysis tends to be the primary form of RRT chosen for the elderly patient (Ross & Rutsky, 1990; USRDS, 1996), mainly because the individual cannot perform self-care dialysis (Ross & Rutsky, 1990). Both internal and external physical changes due to the aging process, other chronic conditions, and mental impairments can make it difficult for the individual to function without assistance. These areas need to be assessed initially and throughout any dialytic therapy so that adequate treatment for the elderly patient may be provided.

There are several factors that support the use of

incenter hemodialysis as compared to home hemodialysis and peritoneal dialysis. During home hemodialysis, which is used least of all the dialytic therapies, the support of another individual during the time of treatment is necessary. Often, the spouse is the other person available. It must be kept in mind that this individual may also be elderly and may not be capable or willing to assume the responsibilities of caring for the sick partner. Also, for peritoneal dialysis, it is important for another individual, whether family or friend, to understand the functioning and treatment of this modality as well as the patient. Again, the support of another may be a requirement, depending on the abilities of the elderly patient to perform the procedure safely and effectively. In comparison also to peritoneal dialysis, there may be more control of anorexia and malnutrition (Young et al., 1991) and less stress on pulmonary function (Winchester, 1984) with the use of hemodialysis, whether it be in-center or home.

Hemodialysis necessitates the creation of a vascular access. However, controversy exists regarding the kind of access that needs to be developed. Geriatric patients with complications of diabetes and hypertensive vascular disease tend to have difficulty with high-efficiency dialysis and may not do well with an arterio-venous (AV) fistula (Windus, Jendrisak, & Delmez, 1992). These particular individuals may do better with other methods of vascular access available. Also, problems of graft erosion may occur due to the skin changes of the elderly (Didlake, Raju, Rhodes, & Bower, 1991). Nephrology nursing care should include the consistent monitoring of not only the surgical sites, but also of the integrity of the skin to prevent undo bruising and tearing.

The hemodialysis procedure is not without its complications for the geriatric patient. Ismail et al. (1993) addresses several considerations as potentials for morbid events for this cohort, including hypotension, hypoxemia, gastrointestinal bleeding, subdural hematomas, infection, and reduced adequacy of dialysis.

Blood pressure control can be a challenging effort for the health care provider caring for any individual during the hemodialysis procedure. When dialyzing the geriatric patient, a lower cardiac reserve and autonomic dysfunction may make this a difficult process when attempting to ultrafiltrate (Henrich, 1990). Compromised because of these problems, the body does not always respond effectively to the volume shifts, resulting in hypotension whose "sequelae may include seizures, cerebral infarction, myocardial ischemia, aspiration pneumonia, and vascular access thromboses" (Ismail et al., 1993, p. 762). Careful monitoring of the dry weight and ultrafiltration no more than 1 L/hr has been recommended for the geriatric patient (Ismail et al., 1993).

Elderly CRF patients with a decreased cardiac or pulmonary reserve may be at risk for hypoxemia that occurs for most patients at the beginning of the hemodialysis treatment. Another area of concern is the fact that older patients are at risk for gastritis induced by the uremia and specific drugs, and angiodysplasia. Subdural hematomas due to elderly falls can be complicated by the systemic heparinization needed for the hemodialysis treatment. The elderly are also more prone to infections due to a compromised immune system (Ismail et al., 1993).

The last concern to be mentioned in this section is that of adequacy of dialysis. Because of the complications of the elderly person during the hemodialysis treatment (i.e., nausea and vomiting, hypotension, cramping) the treatment may be discontinued prematurely, so that the individual has not obtained the adequate amount of treatment. Physical changes of the elderly patient can also affect the dialysis prescription adversely. This includes a lowered blood urea nitrogen from a decreased intake of protein, and a lowered creatinine from a reduced muscle mass. Without consideration of these changes, the nephrologist may prescribe an inadequate treatment based on the standard of treatment of Kt/V or urea reduction ratio (Ismail et al., 1993).

Peritoneal Dialysis

The second most common dialytic therapy utilized by the elderly population is that of peritoneal dialysis (USRDS, 1996). Reasons for selecting or not choosing this method tends to be based on physical as well as psychosocial considerations, which all have a bearing on the individual's functional capacity as well as the quality of life.

Because of the steady state of peritoneal dialysis, this method is particularly helpful for those that have a diminished cardiovascular reserve which can be critical in the treatment of hemodialysis when attempting to remove fluid and maintain blood pressure control (Wizemann, Timio, Martin, & Kramer, 1993). There is also a homeostasis exhibited with the blood chemistries, including the maintenance of a higher hematocrit.

As with other CRF populations, maintaining independence and self-care can be viewed as an advantage of this method of dialytic therapy. A decrease in either of these areas can threaten the self-esteem of the elderly person. Psychological adaptation has been shown to be better with dialysis done in the home setting, particularly that of chronic ambulatory peritoneal dialysis (Levey, 1988). At the same time, however, peritoneal dialysis can also be an advantage for the dependent person who has some form of support with administration of this method. Assistance for the elderly can be in the form of paid helpers in the home, utilization in nursing homes, and adult day care centers specific to peritoneal dialysis patients

(Nissenson, Diaz-Buxo, Adcock, & Nelms, 1990).

Although vascular access for this treatment is avoided, insertion of a peritoneal catheter is indicated, which can be a potential risk for fluid leaks, hernia formation and infection (Nissenson, et al., 1990). The sensory losses of eyesight and touch, and the increased difficulty with manual dexterity could be classified as problems for this cohort, although technological advances have made it easier for individuals to administer peritoneal dialysis, overcoming these complications. There is also a potential for respiratory distress with the pressure of the fluid in the peritoneal cavity.

Transplantation

Renal transplantation, the third option for RRT, is not often selected by the elderly CRF population and their treating nephrologists. The 1996 Annual Data Report showed that at the end of 1993, approximately 5.1% of patients transplanted for that year were 65 years and above (USRDS, 1996). Although it may be considered, reluctance to use this modality stems from the fact that there continues to be a shortage of cadaver kidneys, nephrologists still feel that transplantation is a high risk for elderly patients, and results of transplantation and the use of the immunosuppressant drugs available during the 1970s were poor (Ismail, Hakim, & Helderman, 1994).

It is felt that the success rate of elderly transplant patients is based on several factors, one of these being the preoperative selection and evaluation of the patient. Although the criteria is basically the same as that for any other CRF patient, as discussed in Chapter 23, special evaluation procedures may be employed if indicated due to patient symptoms or incidence of specific problems in the elderly population. For example, there may be a need for additional invasive cardiac testing, gall bladder evaluation, barium enemas, and mammograms (females) or rectal exams (males with enlarged prostate).

Another factor of importance that influences the success rate of elderly transplantation is the increased awareness of the elderly changes in pharmacokinetics, demonstrating a need for lower dosages of immunosuppressants. With this change, the graft survival rates have increased. Allograft loss can now be attributed mainly to patient death, with leading causes of cardiovascular problems and infections (Ismail et al., 1994).

Who Makes the Choice?

The geriatric patient should be well informed of the advantages and disadvantages of the three modalities available for his/her renal failure. If capable of making decisions, the patient, along with the family and health care professionals, should choose that method which would maximize the quality of life for him/her. Consideration should be given to physical, social and psychological issues when making the choice.

Nutritional Issues of Adequacy

As in the treatment of other nephrology patients, older individuals must also have dietary restrictions. Adequate caloric intake with a decrease of protein, potassium, phosphorus, sodium, and fluid will assist in the maintenance of weight, while curbing complications (Stall, 1986). Dietary restrictions and listings of foods recommended/contraindicated in each of these areas have already been addressed in Chapter 11.

The dietary management and nutritional status specific to that of an elderly CRF patient can be a complex issue. It is important to keep in mind that these individuals have developed a lifelong history of eating habits, which extend from such sources as tradition, ethnic background and religious preferences (Ebersole & Hess, 1994). But no matter what has preceded their current dietary intake, the nephrology nurse needs to be aware that a common problem among the elderly in general is that of malnutrition. This is seen as a deficiency of essential nutrients and calories with deviations in dietary patterns , which can result in risk factors for the elderly (Ebersole & Hess, 1994). Factors needing to be considered which have an effect on nutritional status include physiological and psychosocial issues, as well as environmental, and pathological conditions (Stiles, 1993). Proper assessment, education and monitoring of the individual is necessary in each of these areas for the prevention of malnutrition and assurance of proper nutritional intake.

Physiological Considerations

As an individual ages, sensory changes occur. There are conflicting results from research conducted in the area of taste receptors and changes that occur in the elderly population (Miller, 1995). When comparing these studies, however, one can conclude that there is a *potential* decrease in the number of taste buds (which are located on the tongue, palate and tonsils), and *possibly a change* in taste sensitivity of sweet, sour, salty, and bitter which don't necessarily affect the taste sensation for the elderly but may have an effect (Bartoshuk & Weiffenbach, 1990; Weiffenbach & Bartoshuk, 1992). Stimulation of the appetite is dependent also on the ability of an individual to smell. Olfactory changes that occur include a decrease in the sensory cells of the mucosa and those at the olfactory bulb located at the brain (Ebersole & Hess, 1994). Accompanied with the problems of renal disease, these losses can make it difficult for an individual to obtain proper intake if the food is not palatable, or does not smell good.

Other physiological disturbances that affect nutritional intake include environmental factors such as smoking and medications. Saliva production, diminished from such causes as medications and disease, can have an effect on the digestion process occurring in the mouth, which in turn can have an effect on the amounts and kinds of food ingested. Other problems include that of constipation (possibly due to medications and a lowered activity level) and dental changes (gum disease, no dentures, or ill-fitting dentures) that make it difficult to chew food. Dentures will also cover the secondary taste areas of the palate, making it difficult to taste the food. Other physical concerns that may occur with the elderly include lactose intolerance, impaired vitamin D metabolism, and atrophic gastritis (Stiles, 1993).

Psychosocial Considerations

Assessment of psychosocial considerations can shed an interesting light on the potential for malnutrition. As an individual grows older, changes occur in the area of financial status. This can cause a strain on the individual when the lower income needs to cover medications, medical bills, housing repairs, and other necessities of life, as well as food. This can lead to a decrease in purchasing food, as well as an increase in consuming inappropriate foods and drinks. The consumption of alcohol, for example, makes it difficult to maintain adequate nutrition within a renal diet. Isolation and loneliness, depression, and bereavement are other concerns, not exclusive to the elderly, but of such a nature so as to cause serious consequences within this population if not identified. Also, those individuals that are confused, forgetful, and/or disoriented tend to receive improper nutrition.

Environmental Considerations

Transportation may be a physical impediment to the purchase of food because the elderly individual is unable to get to the grocery store. Preparation of the food once it is purchased can also be a difficult task for the individual. It may be that he/she is wheelchair bound and finds it difficult to get around in the kitchen to prepare a meal, or if physically incapable of preparing a meal, is dependent on the availability of someone to do the cooking. The elderly person, with strict financial constraints, may live in substandard housing without a refrigerator to store certain items or not own a stove on which to prepare a meal (Ebersole & Hess, 1994).

Pathological Considerations

Often the elderly have more than one chronic condition, and this in itself may present difficulties with eating. Stiles (1993) lists the following complications which all have an effect on nutritional status. Some of the perplexing issues of each have been added for clarity: Parkinson's disease (shaking), alcoholism (depressant), swallowing disorders (inability to swallow foods without difficulty necessitating other means of feeding), cancer (nausea and vomiting), cardiopulmonary disease (restricted diet), diabetes (restricted diet), drug-nutrient interactions (medications cause anorexia, or the drug interferes with nutrient absorption [Kaiser, 1990]), malabsorption syndromes (inability to absorb adequate calories and nutrients), surgery or trauma (difficulty eating depending on cause and/or increased need for caloric intake to potentiate healing process), recurrent infections (increases need for caloric intake for healing, which is already a difficult process to maintain) and renal disease (restricted diet and uremia which can have a negative effect on appetite).

Addressing Nutritional Issues

Although dietitians are a requirement for the interdisciplinary team, it is essential that the nephrology nurse is aware of the issues that surround the nutritional status of the geriatric CRF patient. Accurate assessment of those areas identified in the previous sections can assist the elderly individual toward adequate nutritional intake. It may simply be a means of knowledge deficit and an unclear understanding of the restrictions of the renal diet that may be the cause for dietary noncompliance. Educating the elderly without cognitive impairment is possible, although repetition and reinforcement of factual information may be necessary, as well as the provision of adequate time for comprehension. Adjusting the instructional design for presentation of information to accommodate any hearing loss may be indicated. (Refer to section on educating the elderly in this chapter). Guidelines proposed by Henrich (1990) to assess the nutritional status of the elderly dialysis patient includes the monitoring of weight loss, indicated as the "best predictor of insidious malnutrition" (p. 340), attention to a low serum albumin level, the protein catabolic rate, protein intake, and energy stores measured by triceps skin fold.

Consistency in monitoring laboratory values, as well as physical, psychosocial, environmental, and pathological conditions is a step toward nutritional stabilization. This in turn can have an effect on the quality of life of the elderly individual.

Drug Therapy

Special considerations must be taken into account when medicating the elderly patient. One of these is polypharmacy, which often accompanies chronic illnesses, and is a common occurrence especially among the elderly population. LeSage (1991) describes polypharmacy as the "concurrent use of several different drugs" which may be of the same therapeutic class, used to treat "coexisting disease or a single illness" (p. 274). In fact, 3 to 12 medications may be indicated for the geriatric patient and prescribed at the same time (Lamy, 1980), with an average of 10.7 prescriptions used within a year (Yee, Williams, & O'Hara, 1990). This often leads to a complex drug regimen, which can result in devastating consequences for the older individual. LeSage (1991) has identified other causes for potential complications with drug use which include:

1. Misdiagnosis of an ailment,
2. More than one prescriber who does not know what others have already given the patient, leading to duplicate medications and drug-drug interactions,
3. Self-medication with over the counter drugs and drugs of other individuals without consultation with health care professionals,
4. Hoarding of medications that have been discontinued, for "later use if necessary", and
5. Failure to accurately assess the individual for underlying causes of a problem sometimes leading to the treatment of one drug's side effects with another drug .

As the body ages, changes occur in pharmacodynamics (drug effects at site of action) and pharmacokinetics (absorption, distribution, metabolism and excretion of a drug) that can lead to morbid adverse effects (Schwertz & Buschmann, 1989). Because of these changes, along with the practices of drug usage of the geriatric patient, there is always the danger of health risks and complications.

Pharmacodynamics

Two types of pharmacodynamic alterations have been identified in the elderly. The first of these are changes at the cellular level (Schwertz & Buschmann, 1989). There may be an increase or decrease sensitivity to a drug due to the number of receptors as well as the attraction of the drug to the receptors (Kane et al., 1994).

The second pharmacodynamic alteration is that of "homeostatic vitality" (Schwertz & Buschmann, 1989, p. 31). That is, the body responds with adverse drug reactions, and may inhibit the primary intention of the drug. Serious adverse reactions have been demonstrated with cardiovascular and psychotropic drugs (Kane et al., 1994). Reactions from these and other drugs have also been noted in the areas of the respiratory, thermo-regulatory, and renal systems (Roberts & Tumer, 1988).

Research continues in the area of pharmacodynamic alterations with the elderly. And, although some drugs have shown these effects and dosages have been adjusted, research is still needed for further dosage requirements on specific drugs (Kane et al., 1994).

Pharmacokinetics

As an individual ages, both physiological and anatomical changes occur in the gastrointestinal tract, the site of most *absorption* of oral drugs. Changes include decreased motility and secretion of gastric acid as well as a decline in blood flow and decrease surface area of the intestine (Ebersole & Hess, 1994; Gerber & Brass, 1990; Vitting, 1986.) Although these changes occur, research has not shown that absorption of oral drugs is significantly affected as one ages (Plein & Plein, 1981).

Absorption of those drugs administered by intramuscular injection or topical administration may also be affected due to physiological changes and affect the permeability and concentration of a medication. Consideration needs to be given to tissue perfusion and skin hydration which may be decreased in the elderly individual (Duchin, 1985).

Plasma protein binding and body composition are the determining factors of drug *distribution* within the body. Throughout the aging process, serum albumin, total body water, and lean body mass tend to decline. On the other hand, body fat increases, with a greater amount in men than women. These changes cause alterations in both the half-life of a drug as well as volume distribution (Kane et al., 1994).

The *metabolism* of drugs in the liver and enzyme activity based on environmental factors has made it difficult to predict changes specific to the elderly in this area. Studies are needed that take into account specific factors such as gender, smoking, combinations with other drugs, and even atmospheric pollutants and their effect on the metabolism of specific drugs consumed by a geriatric patient. It is suggested, however, that unless a person has severely impaired liver function, one still cannot make assumptions that an older individual has the same metabolism as a younger one (Kane et al., 1994).

The elderly are at high risk for toxic effects and enhanced actions of a drug when *excretion* is affected, specifically drugs that are dependent on the kidney for this process. These drugs have been found to have a longer half-life, be eliminated from the body more slowly, and reach a higher concentration (Kane et al., 1994). As the glomerular filtration rate (GFR) declines, the clearance of a drug is decreased. The loading dose of a drug usually remains the same, but the drug regimen will be altered in one of three ways: reduced dosages at the same intervals; same dosages but administered less frequently; or, alterations in both the dosages and intervals (Duchin, 1985).

Compliance Issues

Noncompliance due to overuse, underuse, or misuse may occur because of uncomfortable side effects experienced by the drugs, inability to read the labels correctly or open the bottles with ease, thoughts that more than the prescribed dosage may have a better effect, financial constraints to purchase the prescribed medications, memory lapses as to whether a particular medication has been taken, transportation problems obtaining the medications, and misunderstanding of the use of a particular medication, appropriate times and dosages

Table 17-4
Considerations for teaching elderly patients with CRF.

Patients
- Assess their immediate concerns and priorities.
- Assess their personal values and lifestyle.
- Determine their reading level.
- Determine their mental status.
- Assess any physical disabilities (i.e., visual, auditory, or musculoskeletal impairments).
- Determine the appropriate time for reviewing information.
- Assess for medications that influence alertness and comprehension.

Environment
- Provide an area with adequate lighting.
- Provide an area that is comfortable.
- Provide an area conducive to concentration.

Instructional Design
- Use multimedia methods such as pamphlets, audiotapes, and videotapes.
- Use written materials with large type and bold print.
- Use posters.
- Allow patients to control the pace of the presentation.
- Keep educational sessions short (30 minutes or less).
- Reinforce information using different approaches.

Note: From Mathers, T. (1995). Epoetin alfa - Focus on the geriatric patient (Educational supplement sponsored by Amgen, Inc.). *ANNA Journal, 22*(5), 494-497. Adapted from Stewart & Walton (1992) and Matheson (1994). Reprinted with permission.

prescribed. Knowledge deficit with regards to the foods that can alter a drug's reactions as well as malnutrition are also important considerations. All of these reasons can have a significant influence on the therapeutic medication levels of the individual and must be monitored closely.

Nursing Interventions

The geriatric patient with CRF is particularly vulnerable to medication problems due not only to the aging process, but the fact that his/her kidneys are not able to excrete many of the medications and must rely on dialytic therapy to do this. A holistic approach for care of the geriatric nephrology patient is suggested to enhance the safe practice of pharmacotherapy as well as the quality of life. Knowledge of the specifics of each drug taken by these patients, including dosages, therapeutic levels and actions, potential side effects, and adverse reactions as well as a general understanding of the effects of renal failure on drug excretion and pharmacogeriatrics is necessary for effective patient care. A change in the geriatric patient should not be attributed to old age, but should automatically alert the nurse to careful evaluation of the pharmacological condition of the individual.

Assessment, monitoring, and evaluation of the geriatric CRF patient cannot be viewed lightly. This should include the following assessments and considerations:

1. A complete medical history and list of personal physicians.
2. A drug history which includes a listing of the medications, dosages, and times of administration for each medication they are now taking, versus what they are suppose to be taking. Identify all prescription and non-prescription drugs, those they take belonging to other individuals, and those prescribed by each of their other physicians.
3. Appropriate serum levels of specific medications to assure that the therapeutic levels are maintained, as well as those serum values affected by medications.
4. Mental status examination.
5. Effects and reactions to each medication with documentation of findings to provide for effective follow-up.
6. The patient's overall understanding of the individualized drug regimen, and educating them (repeatedly if necessary) on the important aspects of each drug including their responsibility to help monitor the effects and report any unusual problems.
7. Compliance with regard to underuse, misuse, and nonuse of drugs, taking into account any changes with physical, psychological, social, and economic status.
8. Use of one pharmacy to assist in the control of the drug regimen.

9. Use of alternative methods (such as stress reduction methods, diet therapy, and psychotherapy) to decrease the amount of drugs administered (Schwertz & Buschmann, 1989).
10. Assurance that the patient understands the reasoning for change of dosage and discontinuation of medications, discouraging hoarding while encouraging compliance.

It is the responsibility of all health care professionals caring for the geriatric nephrology patient, as well as the patient, to promote effective pharmacotherapy. Communication and thorough patient care planning will also assist in the advancement of the quality of that individual's life.

Education - Adaptation For Life's Changes

Providing education to the geriatric CRF population can be a challenging, yet rewarding experience if approached in the right manner. The educator, whether it be the nephrology nurse, dietitian, social worker, or other health care professional, must make individualized modifications based on the needs of that elderly person. Not only do the effects of renal disease on these persons need to be considered, but also the aging process with respect to biopsychosocial changes.

When planning for an educational session, three areas are important to consider: the person to be instructed, the teaching environment, and the instructional design of the presentation. Elements of these three areas are highlighted in Table 17-4. A thorough assessment accompanied by appropriate interventions based on these findings will lead to successful accomplishment of the goals established for the educational session as well as those of the patient.

Elderly CRF Patients

The principles of adult learning, as addressed in Chapter 27, are important to keep in mind when the educator tries to accomplish in providing information to the elderly person. Because of the uniqueness of each adult with regards to the learning process, a specific definition of an adult learner can not be identified (Polson, 1993). However, there are some general characteristics that affect the individual as s/he grows older, and these must be kept in mind by the educator: multiple and significant individual roles, lifestyle based on values, beliefs and attitudes of past experiences, developmental level, recent and remote educational experiences, financial commitment, and definitive educational goals (Polson, 1993). Other factors which may influence learning also include the individual's reading ability, knowledge about the topic to be presented to include personal perceptions and misconceptions, ethnic and cultural backgrounds, religious practices (Collett, 1988), meaningfulness of the material to be presented, a need for concrete ideas and tasks, and timing of the instruction (Dall & Gresham, 1982).

The three behavioral objectives, which are often viewed as domains, are important components of the learning process. These include: cognitive, affective, and psychomotor. When assessing cognition, the intellectual perspective of individuals is checked, including orientation to time, place and person. Affectively, one's attitude and feelings with regard to physical health and status, the medical regime and/or proposed topic of discussion is assessed by observation and direct questioning. An assessment of the psychomotor skills gives nurses feedback regarding functional status of the neurological and musculoskeletal systems combined (Alywahby, 1989).

Aging with respect to physical and pathophysiological changes can have a significant impact on the teaching methods utilized and the individual's readiness for learning. The physiological changes can have an effect on the comprehension as well as the ability to participate in the learning process. One must keep in mind that the older individual is capable of processing information, unless cognitively impaired. The effects of aging on the central nervous system, however, can slow the individual down with this processing, requiring a little more time for comprehension and resulting in an increase in response time (Weinrich, Boyd, & Nussbaum, 1989).

Environmental Conditions

It is important that the teaching environment is conducive to learning, one that actually promotes the process. To accomplish this, those areas to be assessed include the physical location and setting and the physical comfort of the patient within this setting.

The ideal location for receiving instruction is that which is familiar to the patient, i.e. home setting, work setting (Ager, 1986; Dellasega, 1990). In the case of the patient that has renal failure requiring some form of dialysis, the dialysis facility itself is one that is or will soon become familiar surroundings to the patient, and can be considered a good location for instruction, provided that other accommodations are also met. These include appropriate lighting without glare, distractions and background noises minimized, padded straightback chairs and adjustable table heights, a comfortable and relaxing temperature, adequate ventilation, assurance of privacy, and an organized and neat work area (Ager, 1986; Dellasega, Clark, McCreary, Helmuth, & Schan, 1994; Matheson, 1994). These will not only accommodate the physical changes that have occurred with the elderly person, but also enhance the psychological aspect.

Instructional Systems Design

The goals for teaching an older person include the maintenance or improvement of functioning for

Figure 17-2
Comparison of the nursing process (NP) and instructional systems design (ISD).

NP	Common Descriptors	ISD
Assess	Determination of patient's needs	Analyze
Plan	Development of appropriate interventions	Design and Develop
Intervene	Implementation of meaningful measures	Use
Evaluate	Analysis of outcomes	Evaluate

that individual and the provision of skills for their survival (Redman, 1984). Variables relevant to the enhancement of learning and improved performance make up an instructional systems design (ISD) model. According to Rossett (1991), the ISD is composed of the steps of analysis, design, development, use, and evaluation, with the analysis or needs assessment as a part of every phase of the process. This is comparable to that of the nursing process. Figure 17-2 reflects this comparison.

Analysis. The first approach to designing a presentation is the conduction of a needs assessment of the elderly patient. Identification of any mental, physical, or psychological conditions, and the patient's attitudes, values, or beliefs about the disease process or topic of presentation may alert the instructor to factors that will facilitate or even impede the learning process. Once accomplished, the teacher can then proceed to design an individualized format with teaching methods and techniques to communicate pertinent information that is needed by the patient based on mutual and realistic goals established at this time.

Design and development. Although basic concepts and information to be presented will be of a generic nature, individualization based on the needs assessment, taking into account the physical and psychosocial factors, will assist the instructor to design the program and develop appropriate and meaningful material. Utilization of multimedia methods such as pamphlets, audiotapes, and videotapes (for some patients), written materials with large type and bold print, and poster presentations, all well organized, relevant, simple, and concrete, will facilitate learning (Ager, 1986; Matheson, 1994; Stewart & Walton, 1992). It has been also suggested that the use of previous knowledge to teach elderly patients will improve their learning (Knowles, 1980; Theis, 1991).

Use. Throughout the implementation of the plan, educational sessions should be well organized and kept to a minimum of 30 minutes in length for the older patient (Matheson, 1994). Material should be presented at a comfortable pace controlled by the patient so that s/he may absorb the information without feeling rushed, and reinforced through the use of the various methods identified above (Ager, 1986; Matheson, 1994). According to Okun (1977), also allowing the patient the choice of task will assist in the fulfillment of one's personal needs and pre-established goals (p. 148).

Evaluation. Although identified as the last step in the instructional design model, evaluation is a step that should also be continuous throughout the implementation process. The patient can be evaluated for understanding of the information being presented and for any previously unidentified problems. Evaluation at the end of a session can then provide feedback of knowledge gained and that yet to be achieved. Further plans can then be made for future presentations.

Educational Outcomes

Assessing and making accommodations in the three areas of concern, that is the patient, environment, and instructional design, will facilitate nursing care for the elderly patient. If also accompanied by support and respect, rapport can be established and a working relationship fostered leading toward achievement of patient and educational goals.

Ethical Aspects of Care

Technological advances in nephrology and in medical care in general, accompanied by the increase in the well being and health status of an aging society, have caused an increase in ethical dilemmas. It has been noted that, because of this, physiologic age, rather than chronologic age must be kept in mind when caring for the elderly individual (Cummings, 1990).

Among the issues of concern for the elderly nephrology patient are those of allocation of resources, particularly that of equitable access to care and transplantation (Brodeur, 1990; Cummings, 1990), quality of life (Cummings, 1990), autonomy and decision making, and death and dying concerns (Brodeur, 1990; Husebye & Kjellstrand, 1987). These issues encompass those principles of respect, beneficence, and justice, as addressed in Chapter 5 and exemplified by a case study of an elderly patient in the same chapter. These must be a central focus of concern for the nephrology nurse to facilitate quality care in collaboration with the other interdisciplinary team members so that patient preferences are considered and addressed.

Allocation of Resources

Health care reform has been an issue of great debate among politicians, health care professionals, and those individuals who feel strongly about equitable access to care. Elderly individuals, no matter what their age or place of residence, have resources available to them in the form of nephrology care. This includes access to dialysis facilities, home care in the form of hemodialysis and peritoneal dialysis, and nephrology treatment provided either in nursing homes or through transportation from nursing homes to dialysis facilities. However, one issue of concern with nephrology care is the availability of donor kidneys for transplantation for this population. Although the formation of UNOS with their nondiscriminatory policy facilitated the transplant of those individuals over the age of 65, there is still considerable ethical concerns among nephrology professionals as to the appropriateness of this procedure for someone whose life span has just about reached its conclusion. This is especially evident when it concerns young living related donor kidneys to elderly persons (Cummings, 1990).

Situations may arise that call for other advanced technologies due to multiple comorbid conditions that are so frequent among the elderly. These are the ones that may not be as easily accessed, thereby limiting the resources available to this population.

Quality of Life

Ethical issues revolving around the quality of life is of particular interest when it pertains to a geriatric patient. A question that often arises is, "Who should determine the quality of life of an elderly person?" If geriatric individuals are mentally competent, should they not be the ones to decide how much quality there is to their own lives? A study conducted by Meers et al. (1995) compared the perceptions of a group of hemodialysis patients (ages 19-85) with that of their health care providers with regards to their quality of life. In this small but mixed age sample, the results showed that the majority of discrepancies were in the psychosocial dimensions, with the patients showing greater adaptation and coping with their renal disease than perceived by the health care providers. Another perspective is the comparison of younger patients to older ones. Older persons tend to report a greater satisfaction with life (United States Congress, 1989). However, viewpoints vary in studies specific to that of the elderly nephrology population. This cohort has been shown to do well physically and psychologically with chronic dialysis (Schultz & Powers, 1987), while others show a lower level of psychological well-being when compared with their peers not on dialysis (Kutner, Brogan, Fielding, & Hall, 1991). Some have also demonstrated a higher degree of dependence and depression when compared with other age groups of dialysis patients (McKevitt, Jones, & Marion, 1986).

Another area of concern for nephrology patients in particular are the reimbursement rates for dialysis treatments that do not cover the comorbid conditions mentioned earlier and do not take into account the severity of illnesses. This could jeopardize the overall quality of care given to these patients.

Several things need to be taken into consideration when research is conducted with the elderly nephrology patient regarding quality of life issues: (a) the time of day; (b) the time allowed to answer the questions; (c) the amount of time it takes to ask the questions; and (d) allowance for stabilization with dialytic treatment, which was suggested by Schumacher et al. (1991). The problems that exist with measuring and analyzing the quality of life, in conjunction with inadequate tools that have not been proven as valid and reliable for use with the geriatric population, have brought about non-conclusive evidence regarding the status of elderly persons.

Autonomy and Decision Making

The principle of autonomy allows an individual the freedom to choose a plan from alternatives, and then act upon that plan. This involves respect for the elderly person and their values and beliefs. The elderly nephrology patient, unless cognitively impaired to the point of incomprehension, has the ability to consider the available alternatives of treatment modalities and to choose among them, utilizing the principle of autonomy. Difficulty expressing this autonomy may arise when patients are affected by a chronic illness that tends to lend itself to dependence. Physical dysfunctions, psychologic factors, and social factors may encourage dependency on the health care providers, as well as those persons caring for the individual at home.

Informed consent and advance directives play a significant role in the demonstration of autonomy and decision making by the patient. According to McCullough, Rhymes, Teasdale, and Wilson (1995), "a meaningful informed consent process creates a common ground between beneficence-based and autonomy-based clinical ethical judgment" (p. 577). To achieve this, a nine-step process has been proposed by these same authors from a physician perspective, and is one that can be easily adapted for use with the geriatric nephrology patient (p. 577). These steps and their adaptations include the following:

1. Patient understanding of renal disease, the alternative treatments available and prognosis of each.
2. Enhancement of patient knowledge through correction of statements made concerning renal disease and the alternative treatments.
3. Explanation of the nephrologist's best clinical judgment regarding the patient's condition and

the treatments.
4. Enhancement of cognitive understanding by the physician and supportive efforts of the nurse to the patient.
5. Identification of the patient's values and beliefs.
6. Evaluation of alternatives by the patient, with clarification by the nephrologist and nurse.
7. Preferences are identified by the patient, based on their values and beliefs.
8. Recommendation made by the nephrologist, keeping patient preferences and own clinical judgment in mind.
9. Plan is mutually agreed upon.

Encompassed throughout this process, are the three components identified by Cassel (1990) which are important for informed consent and include communication and respect for the geriatric patient: all information is provided, the patient makes an uncoercive and free decision, and the patient making the decision is competent (p. 41). This informed consent process would be conducted by the nephrologist and reinforced by the nephrology nurse, fostering choice and control by the patient. Should patients be unable to make their own decisions and participate in the process above, another may speak on the patient's behalf. This is often the next of kin or even someone that has been designated in writing as the *Durable Power of Attorney for Health Care* by the patient, the latter known as an advance directive. These representatives indicate how they feel the patient would respond if s/he was able to do so, and makes known any wishes of the patient, participating in the decision-making process. Another form of advance directive is that of the *Living Will*, written by the patient prior to incompetency, of his wishes regarding any form of aggressive treatment. Many older patients prefer that family members be the surrogate decision makers (Shawler, High, Moore, & Velotta, 1992). It is important, however, that nurses still provide guidance in these matters, encouraging the elderly patient to discuss their concerns and wishes with their family members so that their preferred method of treatment will be carried out. Staff members need to also be aware of the wishes of the patient, so that appropriate patient care is provided (Miller, 1995).

Death and Dying

The main cause of death in the elderly can be attributed to chronic illnesses (Ebersole & Hess, 1994). It has been found that this cohort tends to accept death more easily because of their position on life's continuum (McCormick, 1993a). In the case of the nephrology patient, this may be one of the reasons for the discontinuation of dialysis occurring more frequently in the elderly, especially when accompanied by the issue of quality of life (Husebye & Kjellstrand 1987). Another concern of the elderly is the fear of placing a burden on others (Maddocks, 1995). This may stem from the fact that they realize their increased dependency and needs. It must be kept in mind that one's perception plays a significant role in this particular viewpoint.

Discontinuation of any medical regime usually occurs when the physician and/or patient see the continuation of treatment as a burden rather than a benefit. A decrease in neurological and functional status is often the main reason that the decision is made to withhold or withdraw from dialysis (Holley, Faulks, & Moss, 1991). Other issues that come into the decision making process include factors affecting the quality of life, such as major events in life (other than a diagnosis of renal disease), having an effect on one's coping abilities (McCormick, 1993b). Husebye and Kjellstrand (1987) found that the only thing which increases the risk of discontinuation of dialysis treatments is life in a nursing home.

Whatever the reasons may be, the nephrology nurse has the responsibility to have respect for one's self-determination, provide information, support, and comfort to an individual who decides to discontinue dialysis treatment. Consideration should be given to the competency of the patient, the fact that the patient is voluntarily making the decision without coercion, and that the patient is well informed of the consequences accompanying the discontinuation of treatment (McCormick, 1993b). Although goals and treatment may be adjusted for a dying individual, Brodeur (1990) believes that "... one does not cease to need compassionate, caring and technological medical interventions". Otherwise, provision of care is given as long as accepted by the patient.

Rehabilitation and Elderly Patients

Individuals change physiologically and psychologically throughout life in response to unique personal lifestyles and their values and beliefs. These may be associated with such things as eating, drinking and smoking, as well as inherited risks due to familial diseases, pathological changes, and accidental occurrences. As these situations occur, some individuals may be able to make adaptations to accommodate for these changes, assisting themselves toward maintenance of an optimal level of functioning. Others need outside assistance, depending on the circumstances, to achieve this functioning. Often referred to as rehabilitation, this process has as its goal that of improvement in the physical capabilities of the individual and an improved quality of life (Blagg, & Fitts, 1994). Kutner (1994) refers to patients with a chronic disease (i.e. renal disease), when she states that "maximizing functioning and well-being should be primary objectives of care" (p. 321).

Rehabilitation of the elderly patient can be a challenge to both the health care professional as well as the elderly person. Biopsychosocial issues can play a significant role in the accomplishment of an improvement in the quality of life for the individual, and often one problem can lead to another. For example, a decrease in stamina due to physiological changes may lead to an inability to perform activities of daily living, which in turn can lead to dependency and even depression and isolation. It has been shown that a higher level of functioning of an older individual can have a positive impact on independence and be a predictor of life satisfaction (Branch, 1987; Osberg, McGinnis, DeJong, & Seward, 1987).

According to Stineman and Granger (1994), geriatric rehabilitation programs are comprised of some key elements to facilitate the care of this population. These include (pp. 514-551):

1. A reduction in disabling effects if rehabilitation is initiated early (p. 514);
2. Identification of needs of the elderly;
3. Physical and verbal exchange between patients and staff;
4. Establishment of rapport, to include the patient, family and team members;
5. A balance of the various treatment modalities;
6. Environmental and equipment adaptations with personal prescriptions and appropriate patient training;
7. Educational programs;
8. An interdisciplinary team approach with communication between and among the rehabilitation team and with others in all phases of the process, including the referral phase and post rehabilitation follow-up; and,
9. A program based on realistic individual goals and expectations, reemphasized in each stage of the rehabilitation process.

Many of the statements above are basic elements for rehabilitation, regardless of age. However, like all other aspects of geriatric care, one must approach the individual from a holistic perspective, so as to make the rehabilitation process patient specific to assist in achieving maximal functioning for that individual. One must keep in mind that the elderly patient on dialysis may have problems other than that of renal disease, generated by the aging process. These will often make the return to a predialysis level a complicated and difficult task.

Components of Elderly Rehabilitation

As a first step toward rehabilitation, assessment of this population must include their sense of control and health outlook (Kutner, Cardenas, & Bower, 1992). Personal strengths and weaknesses need to be identified. One's physical ability, social functioning, sense of well-being, and perspective on what constitutes a quality life must also be taken into account (James-Rogers, 1994). All of this can be accomplished if age appropriate tools are used. Then, keeping in mind the five core objectives of encouragement, education, exercise, employment, and evaluation as established by the Life Options Advisory Council (Medical Education Institute, 1995), and the fact that individuals become less homogenous as they grow older, the rehabilitation program can be individualized according to identified needs and goals.

Active participation is required for any rehabilitation program to be successful (Bower, 1989). Many times this involves *encouragement* from the physician, staff, family, and peers who form a support for the individual. Psychological status of the elderly patient can also be improved by encouraging the individual to engage in activities that promote a healthy outlook on life.

Education, keeping in mind the specific needs of the geriatric patient (as addressed in the educational section of this chapter), is very important to include in this aspect of care. Helping the elderly person to understand the need for knowing about oneself and what is happening with regards to their care facilitates an improvement in their self-worth. The health care professional should not assume that the patient knows all there is to know because of age and past experiences, or that the patient will not listen. Each person is an individual and must be approached as such.

Physical *exercise* as one aspect of rehabilitation is an important component of all patient health care plans, including those of the elderly. Considering the CRF patient, the capacity for exercise is reduced as chronic renal failure progresses. For this reason, it has been suggested that rehabilitation be started as early as possible in the course of chronic renal failure with continuing management (Blagg & Fitts, 1994). Decrease in exercise and activity specific to the dialysis patient have been attributed to fatigue, time restraints, and hospitalizations, to include access surgeries (Blagg & Fitts, 1994). For the elderly, time restraints may not be as much a problem (depending on one's social calendar and activity level), as are the other factors mentioned. Hospitalizations, in particular, are even more frequent for the elderly dialysis patient. As exercise programs with the older adult are initiated, physiological changes plus endurance and functional capacity need to be monitored. Suggested exercises to slow the rate of physical degeneration include walking, swimming, and bicycling. The individual who engages in self care, in addition to finding a means to decrease the fatigue that accompanies the dialysis treatments, assisted by the health care team, will facilitate their own rehabilitation.

Employment does not necessarily mean a job requiring a paycheck. Although the number of older workers is increasing (Shrey & Hursh, 1994), there are still those who view themselves as retired. These are the ones that need to consider vocational and recreational activities. Work may include the responsibilities of being a homemaker, a volunteer worker, a gardener, or activities such as painting, swimming, or golfing. Recognition and praise for one's achievements will enhance self-worth and well-being.

Evaluation is continuous throughout the rehabilitation process and needs to be accompanied by outcome analysis. This will assist the team in determining whether the program established for a particular geriatric patient is appropriate. Other factors/issues of a physical or psychological nature may surface throughout the process, and it is at this point that reassessment and further planning need to be addressed.

Considerations for Implementation

As with any new program, the elderly person must be thoroughly assessed so as to ascertain wants and needs, and then the instructional design made specific to that patient. Utilization of principles of adult learning make the material or activities relevant to daily activities are ones that will interest the geriatric person. Include the family caregivers whenever possible to reinforce and encourage the rehabilitation process, promoting independence and self-care. Keep in mind, however, that a dialysis facility cannot always provide the necessary rehabilitation for the geriatric patient. Therefore, community-based services may need to be utilized. Several factors that must be kept in mind when making arrangements for these individuals include: accessibility to services, acceptability by the patient who is concerned not only with staff and services but sensitivity to cultural diversity, appropriateness of the services provided based on outcome analyses, and reimbursement for services rendered (Frank & Miller, 1994). This can cause a shift in scheduling of a patient's dialysis treatments, which is not always an easy task in today's world of dialytic technological advances and fast pace environments. Patience, understanding and positive feedback on the part of the nephrology nurse and other interdisciplinary members will encourage participation and enhance compliance and self-esteem, personal development, and an overall enhanced well-being for the elderly patient.

Caregivers

Emotional and material support is given through a family as developmental changes occur within its familial system. Although we often view elderly individuals as recipients of care, they are frequently the source of giving to the rest of the family. In this sense they may provide support in the form of being good listeners; giving advice; providing financial support and child care; providing a home for divorced children; serving as family historians; and providing religious stability and cultural identification (Ebersole & Hess, 1994).

Reversal of roles within the family may be due to the increased dependency of elderly persons, where children provide the care for parents. The stress of caring for individuals with a chronic illness such as renal disease, particularly elderly individuals who are dependent on others to accomplish such tasks as remembering medication, needing transportation to treatment centers and physicians' appointments, and needing assistance in ADLs cannot be overemphasized when it involves family members. When all that has been presented in this chapter is compounded with the fact that the elderly need extensive assistance to accomplish these things, the experience for anyone can be overwhelming and even devastating to the relationships of family members.

A literature review, conducted by Beach (1993), pointed out various themes that tend to emerge in the literature with respect to caregivers. These appear to be related to balancing the elderly person's needs with their other daily activities, hindrance in the social activities of caregivers, limited assistance by other family members (i.e., siblings and children) to assist in the caregiving, and use of institutions when exhausted physically and/or emotionally (p. 35). Subjective experiences in the study conducted by Beach (1993) were categorized into three specific areas that the health care providers need to be mindful of when considering the caregivers: role strain, sense of self, and problem solving/coping.

It is important for the nurse to aid the patient in identifying those who can be of assistance and then mobilize these resources. As one grows older, the loss of key members in the family, as well as the accessibility of others may place some difficulty in this process. Children may be living in other areas of the country, and spousal support may be available, but more often than not, these individuals are also elderly. They may have health problems which interfere with giving care to the partner. In addition, their own health may be neglected in their efforts to care for their spouse. It is also important to keep in mind the physical and emotional status of the caregivers. These individuals may need information on sources of support for themselves including counseling and knowledge about respite care, so that quality time and care can be given to the dependent elderly person.

Gerontological Research

A review of the literature reveals that, until recently, nephrology nursing research has often integrated the elderly subjects (ages 65 and older) as part of the overall adult population, instead of viewing them as a separate entity. This could be attributed to several reasons: awareness of the increasing nephrology geriatric population has spawned new research; the elderly were not identified previously by researchers as having separate needs with regards to research so the same methodology was followed as with other patient populations; and, research may be considered to be difficult to conduct with the geriatric population alone due to the unpredictability of the physical and mental status of these individuals to participate, and the attrition rate from a study.

Research is not without its problems when considering the changes that occur with the aging process. This calls for some adaptations in the tools and in the conduction of the research to facilitate the reliability and validity of the research procedure and a concern for the ethical issues that revolve around the use of geriatric subjects and research in general.

Methodological Considerations

When conducting research with the elderly population, there are several problems that confound the process. One of these is the sampling process. It is difficult to locate a representative sample of this population (Gueldner & Hanner, 1989). The research topic can have a bearing on this aspect, for often this will lead to specific areas such as nursing homes, senior citizens centers, hospitals, and so forth, depending on the research question. Heterogeneity is another concern, for this population is a very diverse group (Gueldner & Hanner, 1989; Zimmer et al., 1985). Although chronologically the age may be the same, they are very unique in their ways of living, their background and experiences, and ideas and beliefs, which need to be considered when conducting a study. Another concern is that of the psychometric properties of the instruments available. These are often obtained for other populations, but not always for the elderly, and can actually be inappropriate for use with this population. Shaw (1992) has highlighted some of the main problems with regards to the physical changes that occur with aging having an affect on reliability, and has also identified some threats to validity. These are demonstrated in Tables 17-5 and 17-6. It has been suggested by several authors (Gueldner & Hanner, 1989; Uman & Urman, 1990) that tools considered for a study of geriatric patients be reevaluated with regards to these properties, and that pilot testing be conducted with the specific population being considered for study.

Ethical Issues

Federal regulations regarding the research on human subjects reflect respect for persons with regards to their autonomy, informed consent, protection, and the need for the studies conducted (McCullough et al., 1995). However, difficulty ensues when dealing with elderly patients who do not understand what is being done due to their cognitive and physical impairments, and those that are institutionalized. Even though research needs to be done in these areas of concern, it presents ethical and legal dilemmas.

Currently, the guidelines for the protection of human subjects are the same, no matter what the age of the population being studied (Kapp, 1990). It is believed that separate guidelines need to be developed to protect the elderly persons being considered for research, and those compiled by Kapp (1990) as suggested by others (Dubler, 1987; Melnick, Dubler, & Weisbard, 1984) include: having the elderly person grant permission to be utilized as a research subject while still competent (should they be later incapacitated), permission granted by consent auditors, and placing increased responsibility on institutional review boards to monitor research (p. 628).

Future Implications

Research in the field of geriatric nephrology nursing is growing and as long as appropriate measurements are utilized and the research conducted in a scientific manner, it will continue to provide guidelines for the future. Future nephrology research that provides consistent comparisons among a homogenous sample (to include such variables as medical and functional status, as well as age) and then study the effectiveness of interventions, will facilitate innovative approaches toward a higher quality of life to be experienced by the elderly population.

Summary

It is the responsibility of every nephrology nurse caring for elderly dialysis patients to know about their special needs. This includes being knowledgeable about the changes that occur with the aging process that deal with the biopsychosocial aspects of life, and also those changes that occur with renal disease and its potential effects and changes of care that must be considered for the older patient. Knowledge is also needed concerning the nursing process and the importance of instructional design. Then, utilization of appropriate interventions that change the patient and/or the environment for the benefit of the patient, will facilitate health changes conducive to maintaining an optimal level of functioning.

Nephrology nursing roles have changed and evolved over the years, and must continue to do so as technological advances change care, and as diversity persists between and within the populations being served. As the number of geriatric patients increase, care must be directed toward efficient and effective health care services. And as an increasing number of these patients become consumers of nephrology care, a holistic perspective must be integrated into the framework and maintained for the enhancement of quality care. If specific services needed by an individual can not be provided by the dialysis facility and nephrology health care providers, then resources in the form of outside community services must be considered.

Table 17-5
Physical changes in aging with research implications.

Physical Changes	Implications	Suggestions
Perceptual		
Diminished lens accommodation; retinal atrophy, cataracts, glaucoma.	Presbyopia, decreases visual acuity; able to discriminate yellow, orange, and red better than blue, green, or purple.	Use large print for questionnaires; use light yellow or buff paper.
Smaller pupil size.	Increased sensitivity to light.	Use nonglare paper.
Decreased tear production.	Conjunctival dryness, eye fatigue.	
Inner ear atrophy.	Presbycusis (decreased hearing acuity); difficulty hearing high tones.	Provide clear verbal and written instructions about the research; sit at the side on which the subject's hearing is better; maintain eye contact with the subject; speak clearly, use low tones; give adequate time for responses.
Skeletal		
Muscle atrophy; calcification of joints.	Decreased strength; postural changes; fatigue and joint pain.	Provide a comfortable environment and seating when interviewing or administering questionnaires.
Genitourinary		
Muscle weakness; prostatic enlargement.	Prone to frequency and urgency.	Be sure accessible bathroom facilities are available; check for bladder discomfort before beginning interviews.
Cardiovascular System		
Decreased force of heart contraction; decreased circulation to coronary arteries.	Decreased stroke volume.	Consider the individual's energy level.
Respiratory System		
Stiffening of alveolar surfaces; decreased respiratory muscle tone.	Decreased respiratory vital capacity.	Consider the individual's oxygenation and energy level.
Skin		
Becomes dry, thin, with less subcutaneous fat; slower epidermal and dermal cell production; fewer sweat glands.	Decreased perspiration and ability to regulate body temperature; prone to decubitus ulcers.	Provide a comfortable environment and seating when interviewing or administering questionnaire; check comfort of room temperature.
Metabolism		
Decrease in size and number of cells in all glands.	Lower metabolic rate, hypothyroidism, less capacity for tissue adaptation to stress.	Keep questionnaire short and simple; ensure environmental comfort; do not hurry elderly subjects.
Nervous System		
Atrophy of the brain and brain cells; accumulation of lipofuscin in central nervous system cells; atherosclerosis.	Slower responses; fatigue; decreased adaptability.	Explain the importance of the research; provide both written and verbal instructions about the research; keep the instructions simple; decrease extraneous environmental distractions; avoid time pressure; consider the individual's physical comfort and energy level.

Note: From Shaw, R. (1992). Nursing research: Threats to reliability and validity in gerontology. *Journal of Gerontological Nursing 18*(8), 31-37. Reprinted with permission.

Table 17-6
Threats to internal and external validity with suggestions for research design.

Threat	Suggestions
Internal Validity	
Statistical conclusion validity: use of shortened tools designed for ease of administration with the elderly.	Collect observational data; use chart data.
Ambiguity about the direction of causal influence.	Randomization; longitudinal design.
History	Randomization.
Attrition	Obtain large number of subjects, several different samples; include mortality and morbidity statistics in analysis; evaluate reasons why subjects drop out of the study.
External Validity	
Interaction of selection and treatment.	Evaluate possible competing variables; delineate between young-old and old-old; discuss exclusion of disoriented subjects or those who refuse to participate; obtain a large number of subjects; compare sample demographic data with census demographic data available for the target population.
Measurement effect	Pilot-test tools that have not been evaluated on older subjects.

Note: From Shaw, R. (1992). Nursing research: Threats to reliability and validity in gerontology. *Journal of Gerontological Nursing 18*(8), 31-37. Reprinted with permission.

References

Ager, C. (1986). Teaching strategies for the elderly. *Physical & Occupational Therapy in Geriatrics, 4*(4), 3-14.

Alpert, M. (1995). Cardiovascular risks for hemodialysis and peritoneal dialysis patients. *Nephrology News & Issues, 9*(5), 12,14,16,18.

Alywahby, N. (1989). Principles of teaching for individual learning of older adults. *Rehabilitation Nursing, 14*(6), 330-333.

American Association of Retired Persons [AARP]. (1996). *A profile of older Americans.* Washington, DC: Program Resources Department, American Association of Retired Persons (AARP) and Administration on Aging (AoA), U.S. Department of Health and Human Services.

American Association of Retired Persons [AARP], Health Advocacy Services Program Department. (1986). *The eyes have it!* Washington, DC: Author.

American Association of Retired Persons [AARP], Health Advocacy Services Program Department. (1984). *Have you heard? Hearing loss and aging.* Washington, DC: Author.

Anderson, J., Kraus, J., & Sturgeon, D. (1993). Incidence, prevalence, and outcomes of end-stage renal disease patients placed in nursing homes. *American Journal of Kidney Diseases, 21*(6), 619-627.

Bartoshuk, L. & Weiffenbach, J. (1990). Chemical senses and aging. In E.L. Schneider & J.W. Rose (Eds.), *Handbook of the biology of aging* (pp. 429-433). New York: Academic Press.

Beach, D. (1993). Gerontological caregiving: Analysis of family experience. *Journal of Gerontological Nursing, 19*(12), 35-41.

Blagg, C., & Fitts, S. (1994). Dialysis, old age, and rehabilitation. *Journal of the American Medical Association, 271*(1), 67-68.

Blake, C., & Courts, N. (1996). Coping strategies and styles of hemodialysis patients by gender. *ANNA Journal, 23*(5), 477-482, 507.

Bower, J. (1989). The Yangtze syndrome: Pull man from Yangtze, responsible for man's life. *Contemporary Dialysis and Nephrology, 10*, 30-37.

Branch, L.G. (1987). Assessing physical function in the elderly. *Clinical Geriatric Medicine*, 3, 29-31.

Brodeur, D. (1990). Ethical principles in geriatric nephrology. *American Journal of Kidney Diseases, 16*(4), 372-374.

Brooke, V. (1987). The spiritual well-being of the elderly. *Geriatric Nursing, 8*(4), 194-195.

Burnside, I. (1988). *Nursing and the aged* (3rd ed.). New York: McGraw-Hill.

Butler, R., Lewis, M., & Sunderland, T. (1991). *Aging and mental health: Positive psychosocial and biomedical approaches* (4th ed.). (L. Sharp & C. Geldis, Eds.). New York: Macmillan Publishers.

Byer, C., & Shainberg, L. (1991). *Dimensions of human sexuality* (3rd ed.). Dubuque, IA: William C. Brown.

Campbell, J. (1995). Assessment. In M. Hogstel (Ed.). *Geropsychiatric nursing* (2nd ed.) (pp. 73-95). St. Louis: Mosby Year Book.

Cassel, C. (1990). Ethical problems in geriatric medicine. In C. Cassel, D. Riesenberg, L. Sorensen, & J. Walsh (Eds.), *Geriatric medicine* (2nd ed., pp. 38-47). New York: Springer- Verlag.

Chen, H. (1994). Hearing in the elderly: Relation of hearing loss, loneliness, and self-esteem. *Journal of Gerontological Nursing, 20*(6), 22-28.

Collett, C. (1988). Assessing the patient education needs of the elderly. *Medical Times, 116*(11), 95-99.

Comfort, A. (1974). Sexuality in old age. *Journal of the American Geriatric Society, 22*, 440- 442.

Coyne, M., & Hojlo, C. (1985). Physiologic aspects of aging. *Occupational Health Nursing, 33*(3), 117-122.

Cummings, N. (1990). Ethical issues in geriatric nephrology: Overview. *American Journal of Kidney Diseases, 16*(4), 367-371.

Dall, C., & Gresham, L. (1982). Promoting effective drug-taking behavior in the elderly. *Nursing Clinics of North America, 17*(2), 283-290.

Dellasega, C. (1990). Self-care for the elderly diabetic. *Journal of Gerontological Nursing, 16*(1), 16-20.

Dellasega, C., Clark, D., McCreary, D., Helmuth, A., & Schan, P. (1994). Nursing process: Teaching elderly clients. *Journal of Gerontological Nursing, 20*(1), 31-38.

Didlake, R., Raju, S., Rhodes, R., & Bower, J. (1991). Dialysis access in patients older than 65 years. In B. Sommer & M. Henry (Eds.), *Vascular access for hemodialysis-II* (pp. 166-172). Boston: W.L. Gore and Associates, Precept Press.

Dimond, M., & Jones, S. (1983). *Chronic illness across the life span.* Norwalk, CT: Appleton- Century Crofts.

Dressel, P. & Avant, W. (1983). Range of alternatives. In R. Weg (Ed.). *Sexuality in later years: Roles and behavior* (pp. 185-207). New York: Academic Press.

Dubler, N.(1987). Legal judgments and informed consent in geriatric research. *Journal of the American Geriatric Society, 35*, 545-549.

Duchin, K. (1985). Pharmacodynamics and pharmacokinetics of drugs in the elderly. In E. Zawada, Jr., & D. Sica, *Geriatric nephrology and urology* (pp. 215-228). Littleton, MA: PSG.

Ebersole, P., & Hess, P. (1994). *Toward healthy aging: Human needs and nursing response* (4th ed.). St. Louis: Mosby YearBook.

Eliopoulos, C. (1990). *Health assessment of the older adult* (2nd ed.). Redwood City, CA: Addison-Wesley.

Enloe, C. (1993). Assessment in the elderly. In D. Carnevali & M. Patrick (Eds.), *Nursing management for the elderly* (3rd ed., pp. 21-49). Philadelphia: J.B. Lippincott Company.

Erikson, E. (1963). *Childhood and society.* New York: W. W. Norton.

Ferrini, A., & Ferrini, R. (1992). Sexuality. In A. Ferrini, & R. Ferrini (Eds.), *Health in later years.* Madison, WI: Brown & Benchmark.

Folstein, M., Folstein, S., & McHugh, P. (1975). Mini-mental state: A practical method for grading the cognitive state of patients for the clinician. *Journal of Psychiatric Research, 12*, 189-198.

Foreman, M., & Gradowski, R. (1992). Diagnostic dilemma: Cognitive impairment in the elderly. *Journal of Gerontological Nursing, 18*(9), 5-12.

Foundation for Medical Education and Research. (1993). Sexuality and aging. In H. Cox (Ed.). *Aging* (10th ed.) (pp. 45-49). Guilford, CT: The Dushkin Publishing Group.

Frank, J., & Miller, L. (1994). Community-based rehabilitation for the elderly. In G. Felsenthal, S. Garrison, & F. Steinberg (Eds.). *Rehabilitation of the aging and elderly patient* (pp. 477-485). Baltimore: Williams & Wilkins.

Garden, F. (1994). Sexual function in the elderly. In G. Felsenthal, S. Garison, & F. Steinberg (Eds.), *Rehabilitation of the aging and elderly patient* (pp. 319- 325). Baltimore: Williams & Wilkins.

Gerber, J., & Brass, E. (1990). Drug use. In R. Schrier (Ed.), *Geriatric medicine* (pp. 91-103). Philadelphia: W.B. Saunders Company.

Gibson, C. (1991). A concept analysis of empowerment. *Journal of Advanced Nursing, 16*, 354-361.

Gonchar, J., & Itschaki, N. (1986). Psychosocial factors in the geriatric nephrology patient. In M. Michelis, B. Davis, & H. Preuss (Eds.), *Geriatric nephrology* (pp. 153-159). New York: Field, Rich and Associates.

Goyal, V. (1982). Changes with age in the human kidney. *Experimental Gerontology, 17*, 321- 331.

Gueldner, S., & Hanner, M. (1989). Methodological issues related to gerontological nursing research. *Nursing Research, 38*(3), 183-185.

Gurklis, J., & Menke, E. (1988). Identification of stressors and use of coping methods in chronic hemodialysis patients. *Nursing Research, 37*(4), 236-248.

Havinghurst, R.J. (1952). *Developmental tasks and education.* New York: David McKay.

Henrich, W. (1990). Dialysis considerations in the elderly patient. *American Journal of Kidney Diseases, 16*(4), 339-341.

Hogstel, M. (1995). *Geropsychiatric nursing* (2nd ed.). St. Louis, MO: Mosby YearBook.

Holley, J., Faulks, C., & Moss, A. (1991). Nephrologists' reported attitudes about factors influencing recommendations to initiate or withdraw dialysis. *Journal of the American Society of Nephrology, 1*, 1284-1288.

Husebye, D. & Kjellstrand, C. (1987). Old patients and uremia: Rates of acceptance to and withdrawal from dialysis. *International Journal of Artificial Organs, 10*, 166-172.

Iordanidis, P., Alivanis, P., Iakovidis, A., Dombros, N., Tsagalidis, I., Balaskas, E., Derveniotis, V., Ierodiakonous, C., & Tourkantonis, A. (1993). Psychiatric and psychosocial status of elderly patients undergoing dialysis. *Peritoneal Dialysis International, 13* (Suppl. 2), S192-S195.

Ismail, N., Hakim, R., Oreopoulos, D., & Patrikarea, A. (1993). Renal replacement therapies in the elderly: Part 1, hemodialysis and chronic peritoneal dialysis. *American Journal of Kidney Diseases, 22*(6), 759-782.

Ismail, N., Hakim, R., & Helderman, H. (1994). Renal replacement therapies in the elderly: Part II. Renal transplantation. *American Journal of Kidney Diseases, 23*(1), 1-15.

James-Rogers, A. (1994). Rehabilitation and the elderly dialysis patient. *Dialysis & Transplantation, 23*(9), 517-518.

Kaiser, F. (1990). Principles of geriatric care. *American Journal of Kidney Diseases, 16*(4), 354-359.

Kane, R., Ouslander, J., & Abrass, I. (1994). *Essentials of clinical geriatrics* (3rd ed.) New York: McGraw-Hill Book Company.

Kapp, M. (1990). Medical treatment and the physician's legal duties. In C. Cassel, D., Riesenberg, L., Sorensen, & J. Walsh (Eds.), *Geriatric medicine* (2nd ed.) (pp. 623-639). New York Springer-Verlag Publishers.

Kaplan De-Nour, A., & Czaczkes, J. (1972). Personality factors in chronic hemodialysis patients causing non-compliance with medical regimen. *Psychosomatic Medicine, 34*, 333-344.

Kee, C. (1992). Age-related changes in the renal system: Causes, consequences, and nursing implications. *Geriatric Nursing, 13*(2), 80-83, 89, 93.

Kimmel, P., Weihs, K., & Peterson, R. (1993). Survival in hemodialysis patients: The role of depression. *Journal of the American Society of Nephrology, 4*(1), 12-25.

Knowles, M. (1980). *The modern practice of adult education.* Chicago: Follet.

Kutner, N. (1994). Assessing end-state renal disease patients' functioning and well-being: Measurement approaches and implications for clinical practice. *American Journal of Kidney Diseases, 24*(2), 321-333.

Kutner, N., Cardenas, D., & Bower, J. (1992). Rehabilitation, aging and chronic renal disease. *American Journal of Physical Medicine and Rehabilitation, 71(2), 97-101.*

Kutner, N., Brogan, D., Fielding, M., & Hall, D. (1991). Older renal dialysis patients and quality of life. *Dialysis & Transplantation, 20(4), 171-175.*

Lamy, P. (1980). *Prescribing for the elderly.* Littleton, MA: PSG.

LeSage, J. (1991). Polypharmacy in geriatric patients. *Nursing Clinics of North America, 26*(2), 273-289.

Levey, N. (1988). Effects of medical advances and political climate upon psychonephrology. *General Hospital Psychiatry, 10*, 278-279.

Lindeman, R., & Goldman, R. (1986). Anatomic and physiologic age changes in the kidney. *Experimental Gerontology, 21*, 379-406.

Lubkin, I.M. (1990). *Chronic illness: Impact and interventions.* Boston: Jones and Bartlett.

Maddocks, I. (1995). Management of the dying patient. In W. Reichel (Ed.), *Care of the elderly: Clinical aspects of aging* (4th ed.) (pp. 561-569). Baltimore: Williams & Wilkins.

Mathers, T. (1995). Epoetin alfa - Focus on the geriatric patient: Case study of the anemic patient. *ANNA Journal, 22*(5), 494-497.

Matheson, L. (1994). Improving patient outcomes: Educating the elderly. *Dialysis & Transplantation, 23*(9), 514-516.

McCormick, T. (1993a). Ethical issues. In D. Carnevali & M. Patrick (Eds.), *Nursing management for the elderly* (3rd. ed.) (pp. 53-72). Philadelphia: J.B. Lippincott Company.

McCormick, T. (1993b). Ethical issues in caring for patients with renal failure. *ANNA Journal, 20*(5), 549-555.

McCullough, L., Rhymes, J., Teasdale, T., & Wilson, N. (1995). Preventive ethics in geriatric practice. In W. Reichel (Ed.), *Care of the elderly: Clinical aspects of aging* (4th ed.) (pp. 573- 586). Baltimore: Williams & Wilkins.

McKevitt, P., Jones, J., & Marion, R. (1986). The elderly on dialysis: Physical and psychosocial functioning. *Dialysis & Transplantation, 15*, 130, 134-137.

Medical Education Institute. (1995, September/October). Bridges to renal rehabilitation: Focus on the 5 E's. *Renal Rehabilitation Report, 3*(5), 5-10.

Meers, C., Hopman, W., Singer, M., MacKenzie, T., Morton, A., & McMurray, M. (1995). A comparison of patient, nurse, and physician assessment of health-related quality of life in end-stage renal disease. *Dialysis & Transplantation, 24*(3), 120-124, 139.

Melnick, V., Dubler, N., & Weisbard, A. (1984). Clinical research in senile dementia of the Alzheimer's type: Suggested guidelines addressing the ethical and legal issues. *Journal of the American Geriatric Society, 32*, 531-536.

Meyers, B., & Alexopoulas, G. (1988). Geriatric depression. *Medical Clinics of North America, 72*(4), 847-863.

Mignon, F., Michel, C., Mentre, F., & Viron, B. (1993). Worldwide demographics and future trends of the management of renal failure in the elderly. *Kidney International, 43*(Suppl. 41), S-18-S-26.

Miller, C. (1995). *Nursing care of older adults: Theory and practice* (2nd ed.). Philadelphia: J.B. Lippincott Company.

Miller, J. (1992). Enhancing self-esteem. In J. Miller (Ed.), *Coping with chronic illness: Overcoming powerlessness* (2nd ed.) (pp. 397-412). Philadelphia: F.A. Davis Company.

Morris, P., & Jones, B. (1989). Life satisfaction across treatment methods for patients with end-stage renal failure. *Medical Journal of Australia, 17*, 428-432.

Murdaugh, C. (1987). Coping responses of spouses of MI patients and hemodialysis patients. *Journal of Cardiovascular Nursing, 2*(1), 67-74.

Nelson, M., & Mayfield, P. (1994). Health assessment. In M. Hogstel (Ed.), *Nursing care of the older adult* (3rd ed.). Fort Worth, TX: Delmar Publishers.

Nissenson, A., Diaz-Buxo, J., Adcock, A., & Nelms, M. (1990). Peritoneal dialysis in the geriatric patient. *American Journal of Kidney Diseases, 16*(4), 335-338.

Okun, M. (1977). Implications of geropsychological research for the instruction of older adults. *Adult Education, 27*, 139-155.

Oliver, J. (1939). Urinary system. In E. Cowdry (Ed.), *Problems of aging: Biological and medical aspects* (pp. 257-277). Baltimore: Williams & Wilkins.

Osberg, J., McGinnis, G., DeJong, G., & Seward, M. (1987). Life satisfaction and quality of life among disabled elderly adults. *Journal of Gerontology, 42*, 228-230.

Parmelee, P., Katz, I., & Lawton, M. (1992). Incidence of depression in long-term care settings. *Journal of Gerontology, 47*(6), m189-m196.

Pfeiffer, E. (1974). A short portable mental status questionnaire for assessment of organic brain deficit in elderly patients. *Journal of the American Geriatrics Society, 23*(10), 422-441.

Plein, J., & Plein, E. (1981). Aging and drug therapy. *Annual Review of Gerontological Geriatrics, 2,* 211.

Polson, C. (1993, September). *Teaching adult students. Idea Paper No. 29*, Center for Faculty Evaluation and Development, Division of Continuing Education, Kansas State University.

Radke, K. (1994). The aging kidney: Structure, function, and nursing practice implications. *ANNA Journal, 21*(4), 181-190.

Reban, A., & Millsap, P. (1992). Assessment of older adults. In M. Hogstel (Ed.). *Clinical manual of gerontological nursing.* St. Louis, MO: Mosby YearBook.

Redman, B. (1984). *The process of patient education* (5th ed.). St. Louis, MO: C.V. Mosby.

Reed, P. (1991). Spirituality and mental health in older adults: Extant knowledge for nursing. *Family and Community Health, 14*(2), 14-25.

Roberts, J., & Tumer, N. (1988). Pharmacodynamic basis for altered drug action in the elderly. *Clinical Geriatric Medicine*, 4, 127-149.

Rodin, G., & Voshart, K. (1986). Depression in the medically ill: An overview. *American Journal of Psychiatry, 143(6)*, 696-705.

Roessle, R., & Roulet, F. (1932). *Nieren, in mass und zahl in der pathologie.* Berlin and Wien, Germany: Julius Springer.

Ross, C., & Rutsky, E. (1990). Dialysis modality selection in the elderly patient with ESRD: Advantages and disadvantages of peritoneal dialysis. *Advances in Peritoneal Dialysis 6*(Suppl.), 11-18.

Rossett, A. (1991). Needs assessment. In G. Anglin (Ed.), *Instructional technology: Past, present, and future.* Englewood, CO: Libraries Unlimited.

Rowe, J., & Kahn, R. (1987). Human aging: Usual and successful. *Science*, 237, 143-149.

Santo-Novak, D. (1988). Seven keys to assessing the elderly. *Nursing88, 18*(8), 60-63.

Schleifer, C. (1990). Peritoneal dialysis in nursing homes. *Advances in Peritoneal Dialysis, 6*(Suppl.), 86-91.

Schreiner, G. (1990). Prevention of renal disease and conservation of renal function. *American Journal of Kidney Diseases, 16*(4), 360-366.

Schultz, K., & Powers, M. (1987). Adjustment of older patients to hemodialysis. *Dialysis & Transplantation, 16*, 234-242.

Schumacher, M., Olschewski, M., & Schulgen, G. (1991). Assessment of quality of life in clinical trials. *Statistics in Medicine*, 10, 1915-1930.

Schwertz, D., & Buschmann, M. (1989). Pharmacogeriatrics. *Critical Care Nursing Quarterly, 12*(1), 26-37.

Shaw, R. (1992). Nursing research: Threats to reliability and validity in gerontology. *Journal of Gerontological Nursing 18*(8), 31-37.

Shawler, C., High, D., Moore, K., & Velotta, C. (1992). Clinical considerations: Surrogate decision making for hospitalized elders. *Journal of Gerontological Nursing, 18*(6), 5-11.

Shrey, D., & Hursh, N. (1994). Protecting the employability of the working elderly. In G. Felsenthan, S. Garrison, & F. Steinberg (Eds.). *Rehabilitation of the aging and elderly patient* (pp. 487-496). Baltimore: Williams & Wilkins.

Stall, S. (1986). Dietary considerations for the geriatric nephrology patient. In M. Michelis, B. Davis, & H. Preuss (Eds.), *Geriatric nephrology* (pp. 117-122). New York: Field, Rich and Associates.

Stewart, K., & Walton, R. (1992). Teaching the elderly. *Nursing 92, 22*(10), 66, 68.

Stiles, N. (1993, July 13). *Sanders Brown Summer Series Workshop: Geriatric nutrition*, Lexington, KY.

Stineman, M., & Granger, C. (1994). Outcome studies and analysis: Principles of rehabilitation that influence outcome analysis. In G. Felsenthan, S. Garrison, & F. Steinberg (Eds.). *Rehabilitation of the aging and elderly patient* (pp. 511-522). Baltimore: Williams & Wilkins.

Svanborg, A., Bergstrom, G., & Mellstrom, D. (1982). *Epidemiological studies on social and medical conditions of the elderly.* Copenhagen: World Health Organization.

Taft, L. (1985). Self-esteem in later life: A nursing perspective. *Advances in Nursing Science, 8(1)*, 77-84.

Theis, S. (1991). Using previous knowledge to teach elderly clients. *Journal of Gerontological Nursing, 17*(8), 34-38.

Thomas, N. (1992). Measurement of quality of life for elderly people on dialysis. *British Journal of Nursing, 1*(6), 281-284.

Uman, G., & Urman, H. (1990). The challenges of conducting clinical nursing research with elderly populations. *AORN Journal, 52*(2), 400-406.

United States Congress, Office of Technology Assessment (1989). Life-sustaining technologies and the elderly: Excerpts of Congressional OTA study. *Nephrology News & Issues, 3*(10), 21-24.

United States Renal Data System [USRDS]. (1996). *USRDS 1996 Annual Data Report.* Bethesda, MD: National Institutes of Health.

U.S. Senate Special Committee on Aging. (1991). *Aging America: Trends and projections.* Washington, DC: U.S. Department of Health and Human Services.

Vitting, K. (1986). Drug metabolism in the elderly nephrology patient. In M. Michelis, B. Davis, & H. Preuss (Eds.), *Geriatric nephrology* (pp. 54-57). New York: Field, Rich and Associates.

Weiffenbach, J. & Bartoshuk, L. (1992). Taste and smell. *Clinics in Geriatric Medicine, 8,* 543- 555.

Weinrich, S., Boyd, M., & Nussbaum, J. (1989). Teaching the elderly: Adaptations for aging changes. *Journal of Gerontological Nursing, 15(11)*, 17-21.

Wells, K.B., Golding, J.M., & Burnam, M.A. (1988). Psychiatric disorder in a sample of the general population with and without chronic medical conditions. *American Journal of Psychiatry, 145*, 976-981.

Winchester, J. (1984).Peritoneal dialysis and pulmonary function. *Chest, 86*, 806-806.

Windus, D., Jendrisak, M., & Delmez, J. (1992). Prosthetic fistula survival and complications in hemodialysis patients: Effects of diabetes and age. *American Journal of Kidney Diseases, 19*, 448-452.

Wizemann, V., Timio, M., Martin, A., & Kramer, W. (1993). Options in dialysis therapy: Significance of cardiovascular findings. *Kidney International, 43*(Suppl.), S85-S91.

Wolcott, D., & Nissenson, A. (1988). Quality of life in chronic dialysis patients: A critical comparison of continuous ambulatory peritoneal dialysis and hemodialysis. *American Journal of Kidney Diseases, 11*, 402-412.

Yee, B., Williams, B., & O'Hara, N. (1990). Medication management and appropriate substance use for elderly persons. In C.B. Lewis (Ed.), *Aging: The health care challenge* (2nd ed.)(pp. 298-329). Philadelphia: F.A. Davis Company.

Young, G., Kopple, J., Lindholm, B., Vonesh, E., De-Vecchi, A., Scalamagna, A., Castelnova, C., Oreopoulos, D., Anderson, G., & Bersgtrom, J. (1991). Nutritional assessment of CAPD patients: An international study. *American Journal of Kidney Diseases, 17,* 462-471.

Yurick, A., Spier, B., Robb, S., & Ebert, N. (1989). *The aged person and the nursing process* (3rd. ed.). Norwalk, CT: Appleton & Lange.

Zimmer, A., Calkins, E., Hadley, E., Ostfeld, A., Kaye, J., & Kaye, D. (1985). Conducting clinical research in geriatric populations. *Annals of Internal Medicine, 103*, 276-283.

Chapter Highlights

- Care for the elderly differs from that of a younger population due to changes which occur as a result of the aging process. The number of these individuals is increasing when compared to the total population, and will continue to do so on into the 21st century. Most elderly persons over the age of 65 have at least one chronic illness.
- The fact that individuals are living longer can be attributed to several reasons: (a) emphasis on health promotion, (b) prevention of and technological advances providing treatment for cardiovascular conditions, (c) control of infectious diseases, and (d) improvements in maternal care during pregnancy and child care immediately after and during early childhood.
- The median age of a new patient initiating RRT is 63 (USRDS, 1996), with vascular diseases identified as the leading cause (Mignon, Michel, Mentre, & Viron, 1993).
- The small number of dialysis patients in nursing homes is believed to be attributed to transportation problems, finances, and nursing home reluctance to accept dialysis patients (Schleifer, 1990).
- Issues of concern for the elderly include those related to physiology and psychosocial perspectives. Points addressed that are of a physiological nature includes changes in the five senses, cardiovascular system, respiratory system, and the renal system. Psychosocially, the geriatric population experiences more stress than the younger generation (Gonchar & Itschaki, 1986) including grief, guilt, loneliness, rage, depression, helplessness, and anxiety (Butler, Lewis, & Sunderland, 1991).
- A comprehensive nursing assessment of the geriatric patient should include adaptations in time, environmental conditions, and communication techniques. The tools used to obtain the assessment depends on which would best facilitate the care planning of the patient.
- The primary form of RRT chosen for the elderly patient is in-center hemodialysis, with the second most common dialytic therapy being peritoneal dialysis.
- Malnutrition is a common nutritional problem among the elderly. Proper assessment of nutrition involves consideration of physiological, psychosocial, environmental, and pathological conditions.
- It is important to consider three specific areas when preparing to educate the geriatric nephrology person: the patient, the environmental conditions, and the instructional design. Comparable to the nursing process, the Instructional Systems Design model, according to Rossett (1991), consists of an analysis, design and development, use, and evaluation.
- Ethical dilemmas for the elderly nephrology patient have increased due to technological advances and medical care, and the well being and healthy status of this growing population. Several issues involve: allocation of resources, quality of life, autonomy and decision making, and death and dying. A nine-step process for informed consent has been formulated by McCullough, Rhymes, Teasdale and Wilson (1995) and adapted in this chapter for use with the elderly nephrology patient.
- Rehabilitation can play a role in the quality of life of an elderly individual. Incorporating the core objectives of encouragement, education, exercise, employment, and evaluation, as identified by the Life Options Advisory Council, will promote this perspective of geriatric nephrology care.
- Emotional and material support is given through a family system, and it is important to identify those who can be of assistance to the dependent elderly person, and then mobilize these resources. Concern for the caregiver's welfare and its effect on the care of the geriatric patient is also important.
- Methodological changes are important to consider in the conduction of research for the geriatric population, so that their participation is not hindered or influenced by inadequate preparation.
- It has been suggested by Santo-Novak (1988) that seven key points need to be addressed in the assessment of the elderly person, among them: chief concerns, health history, medication history, recent life changes, daily activities, cognitive patterns, and support system.

UNIT 6

Treatment of Renal Disease: Therapies and Approaches

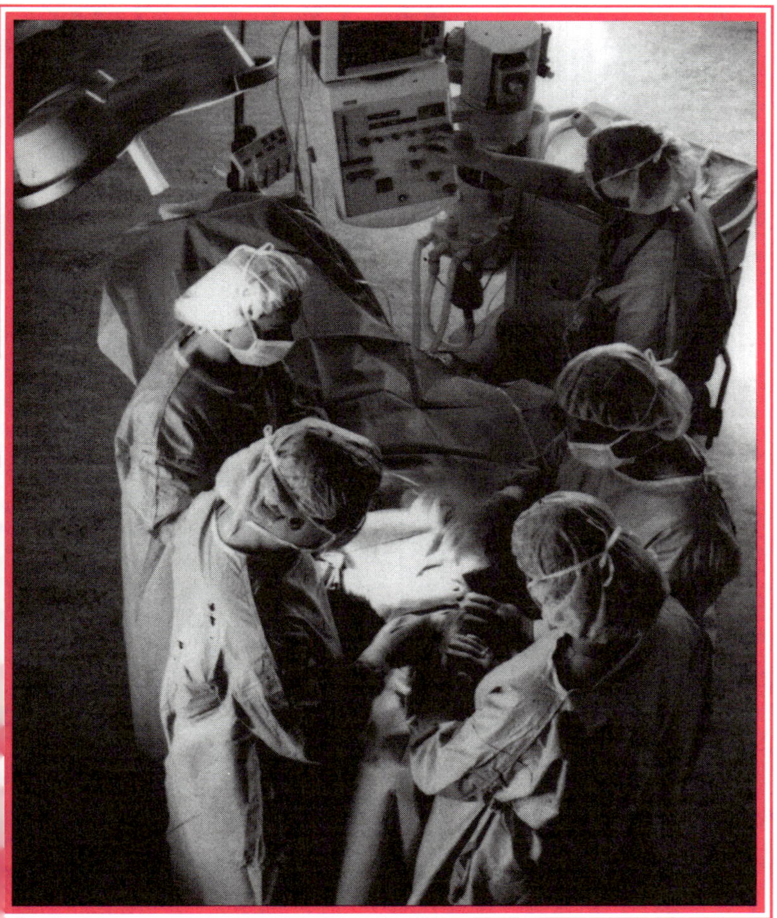

Unit Contents

Chapter 18
Conservative Management 517
Sally S. Russell, MN, RNC

Chapter 19
Hemodialysis 525
Patricia Baltz Salai, MSN, RN, CRNP, CNN

Chapter 20
Continuous Renal Replacement Therapy 577
Christy A. Price, RN, MSN, CNN

Chapter 21
Therapeutic Plasma Exchange . . 589
Christy A. Price, RN, MSN, CNN

Chapter 22
Peritoneal Dialysis. 603
LaVonne Burrows, MS, RN, CNN, and Barbara F. Prowant, BSN, RN, CNN

Chapter 23
Transplantation 661
Christine Mudge, MS, RN, PNPc/CNS, CNN; Laurie Carlson, MSN, RN; and Patricia Brennan, MSN, RN

CHAPTER 18

Conservative Management of Renal Failure

Sally S. Russell, MN, RNC

Chapter Contents

Identification of High-Risk Patients . . . 519
Discovery of Renal Function . . . 519
Blood Pressure Control . . . 519
Diabetes Mellitus Control . . . 520
Dietary Control . . . 520
Necessity for Restrictions, Types of Restrictions . . . 520
Control of Anemia . . . 520
Control of Renal Osteodystrophy . . . 521
Prevention of Infection . . . 522
Causes and Concerns . . . 522
Drug Therapy Complications: Nephrotoxicity, Half-Life Implications 522
Integumentary Care . . . 522
Pruritus, Infection, and Treatment . . . 522
Sexual Dysfunction Concerns . . . 522
Summary . . . 522
References . . . 523
Chapter Highlights . . . 524

Conservative Management of Renal Failure

Sally S. Russell, MN, RNC

Progressive renal failure is the result of ongoing and irreversible destruction of kidney structures. The progression of renal failure usually occurs in three stages: (a) diminished renal reserve when the glomerular filtration rate (GFR) is about 50% of normal; (b) renal insufficiency, which represents a GFR reduction of about 20%-30% of normal; and (c) end-stage renal disease, where the GFR is 10% of normal (Price & Wilson, 1997, pp. 691-692). The use of dialysis is necessary for survival in end stage renal disease. Therapeutic measures used to retard deterioration of renal function are a priority in renal insufficiency and are used to treat renal failure for as long as they are successful in maintaining optimal physical well-being.

Therapeutic measures used to manage chronic renal failure (CRF) usually begin with the use of conservative management techniques. Conservative management techniques such as maintenance of fluid and electrolyte imbalance, healthy diet, and relief from uremic symptoms assist patients to maintain an optimal quality of life. Andreoli, Carpenter, Plum, and Smith (1991) report that people with a GFR lower than 10 ml/min have been managed conservatively for short periods of time quite successfully while other forms of treatment are discussed and evaluated.

Primary nursing interventions can protect remaining renal function and prevent further damage, especially the renal complications from hypertension (HTN) and diabetes. The nursing plan includes (a) dietary control; (b) medication administration, with attention to evaluation of the drug's side effects; (c) assessment of fluid and electrolyte control; (d) patient comfort; and (e) patient education. The purpose of this chapter is to describe those measures and nursing interventions used to preserve renal function for as long as possible without dialysis or transplantation. Those measures used to conservatively manage CRF and the nursing interventions that will aid in the attainment of this goal, will be emphasized.

Identification of High-Risk Patients

Discovery of Renal Dysfunction

Given the complexity of many individuals' health status, it is not uncommon for reduced renal function to occur during a stay in health care facilities for reasons other than renal-related symptoms. Nurses may identify those at risk for loss of renal function in all patient care settings by reviewing laboratory values, especially serum creatinine, and assessing for side effects of diagnostic and treatment procedures. Patients with renal insufficiency having procedures with a high risk for fluid loss, such as surgery or X-rays requiring patients to have fluids withheld for a protracted period of time, may need administration of IV fluids prior to the procedure to prevent an increased loss of glomerular function. Upon completion of these procedures, observing for volume depletion is mandatory while recognizing that medications may be even more nephrotoxic than usual if patients are indeed hypovolemic. Proteinuria is also an independent risk factor for progression of renal function loss.

Encouraging and educating patients about the importance of following through with dietary and medication regimens for the treatment of HTN and diabetes is paramount to preventing further glomerular loss.

Blood Pressure Control

Nephrosclerosis, the renal disease that occurs as a result of hypertension, develops over a long period of time and is treated by controlling hypertension (Richard, 1995). Blood pressure control slows the progression of renal disease (Richard, 1995) while HTN causes several changes in the kidneys, including atherosclerosis of the glomerular membrane. As the vessels thicken perfusion diminishes, leading to decreased blood supply to the kidney. Hypoxia leads to diminished kidney function, causing diminished concentrating ability that gives rise to an increase in blood urea nitrogen (BUN) – especially if fluid deprivation has occurred – and development of proteinuria (Andreoli et al., 1991). HTN is also an early indicator of renal failure. It may occur after an increased renin production by the kidneys secondary to decreased intravascular volume.

The initial treatment of HTN consists of sodium and fluid restrictions plus diuretics followed by antihypertensive agents when restriction of sodium and fluid alone is not sufficient (Baer, 1995). One primary classification of drugs used to control HTN in renal failure patients is beta adrenergic blocking agents. These may be used to decrease heart rate and cardiac output, prolong decreased velocity of mechanical systole, and inhibit renin secretion. Physicians often prescribe Propanolol (Inderal®), which requires close monitoring of the patient's apical pulse and blood pressure because either may drop below a tolerable level. Inderal® also causes fluid retention and potentiates the hypoglycemic action of insulin, triggering nurse observation of weights and blood sugars. Antihypertensive agents contraindicated for use in patients with compromised renal function are potassium-sparing diuretics such as triamterone, spironolactone, or amiloride.

Some patients respond better to angiotensin-converting enzyme (ACE) inhibitors. These drugs block the conversion of angiotensin I to angiotensin II, decreasing sodium and water retention and inhibiting peripheral resistance throughout the body. Proteinuria, especially in patients with renal disease, may occur with the use of ACE inhibitors with an increase in potassium levels (Baer, 1995). Captopril (Capoten®) and enalapril (Vasotec®) often control HTN in patients with renal insufficiencies. Because ACE inhibitors control HTN, they slow the progression of renal disease, especially in diabetic nephropathy (Anderson, Fedje, & Pulliam, 1993). To prevent the progression of renal failure, nurses should observe serum creatinine, potassium, and blood pressure in the plan of care because of the risk of hyperkalemia and blood pressure changes. The drugs may decrease GFR too. When GFR decreases, drugs accumulate and cause an increase in side effects and toxicities that must be a concern to nurses caring for these patients.

Calcium channel blockers prevent entry of calcium into the cell, thereby decreasing the mechanical activity of vascular smooth muscle and decreasing peripheral vascular resistance. Nifedipine (Procardia®) and nicardipine (Cardene®) are calcium channel blockers that also inhibit renin activity. Both calcium channel blockers and ACE inhibitors have demonstrated ability to decrease amounts of protein in the urine, an important effect since proteinuria is an independent risk factor for progression of renal function loss.

Nurses can monitor the effectiveness of ACE inhibitors and calcium channel blockers by taking blood pressure with patients in supine, sitting, and standing positions. Patients may experience lightheadedness, nausea, and orthostatic hypotension from volume depletion if treatment too rapidly lowers blood pressure in a body that has adapted to HTN over a long period of time.

Diabetes Mellitus Control

Diabetic nephropathy is the most frequent cause of chronic renal failure (Andreoli et al., 1991) . Twenty five percent (25%) 25% of CRF patients have diabetes mellitus with 50% of juvenile onset diabetics developing CRF with 20 years of the onset of their diabetes (Richard, 1995). Diffuse glomerulosclerosis presents along with arteriosclerosis in the arterioles of the kidneys (Andreoli et al., 1991, p. 234). Since these changes occur over a long period of time, extreme care and monitoring of blood sugar is required.

Tight control of blood sugar has been found to dramatically slow the progression of diabetic complications, especially during the early stages of renal impairment. As the decrease in renal function diminishes, (Anderson, Fedje, & Pulliam, 1993), hyperglycemia becomes less important; even patients with a significant amount of renal function loss have been found to benefit from the control of diabetes. Information from the Diabetes Control and Complications Trial (DCCT) report improved renal function glucose control in diabetic renal failure patients whose glucose remains stable (Anderson et al., 1993). Thus, nurses may contribute to preventing renal function by educating patients about glucose control. Nursing interventions that focus on long-term control of blood sugar from the outset, especially in patients with insulin dependency, will be the highest priority in the early stages of diabetic nephropathy to prevent kidney damage.

Glucose intolerance is common in renal failure, and diabetic patients may have difficulty with insulin and carbohydrate requirements as their renal function decreases because of tissue insensitivity to insulin, a delay in the production of insulin by the pancreas, and an increase in the half-life of insulin related to the kidneys inability to breakdown insulin (Lancaster, 1995). For patients with anorexia, adjustment of insulin dose will prevent hypoglycemia (Andreoli et al., 1991). Gluconeogenesis does not always occur normally in some uremic patients who may experience hypoglycemia. Other diabetic patients in renal failure experience hyperglycemia because uremia may cause defects in the uptake and/or metabolism of glucose by body tissue (Andreoli et al., 1991). Blood sugar also increases when urinary excretion decreases. Nurses therefore must closely monitor blood sugar, frequently adjust insulin dosage, and modify the diet to maintain stable blood sugar levels.

Dietary Control

Necessity for Restrictions, Types of Restrictions

The conservative management of renal failure includes dietary modification to decrease the kidneys' workload (Hoffart, 1995) and preserve renal function. Protein restriction reduces demand on the kidney to excrete waste products of protein metabolism. Phosphorus restriction often accompanies protein restriction. Phosphorous accumulates in renal insufficiency because long-term severe protein restriction needs careful monitoring to avoid malnutrition (Cooper & Chapman, 1995). Cooper and Chapman recommend no more than 0.8–1 gm protein/Kg/day. Eggs, milk, poultry, and lean meat provide high biologic value and can be supplemented with essential amino acids (Cooper & Chapman, 1995). Caloric intake from fats and carbohydrates must be high to prevent use of protein for energy and heat production. Nurses can collaborate with dieticians to provide nutritional counseling and education to ensure adequate nutrition for growth, healing, and health.

In early renal insufficiency polyuria may be present and sodium wasting may occur because of the increased workload of the remaining functioning nephrons (Price & Wilson, 1997). Many authorities determine sodium replacement to be most accurate if based on the measurement of urinary sodium excretion. Once fluid retention occurs, restriction of sodium to 1-3 gm and water to 1500-2000 ml/day is recommended (Hoffart, 1995). Nursing assessment must include monitoring blood pressure and daily body weight.

In general, potassium need not be restricted until the urinary output drops to less than 1000 ml/day (Hoffart, 1995). Because fecal excretion of potassium increases (Hoffart, 1995) as renal secretion decreases, it takes longer for potassium to become a problem compared to sodium. Many patients with renal insufficiency have potassium levels that are consistently above normal. These levels are tolerated well since the elevation occurred over a long enough period of time to allow the body to adapt. These levels are tolerated well since the elevation occurred over a long enough period of time to allow the body to adapt (Cooper & Chapman, 1995). Sodium polystyrene exonate (Kayexalate®) 30-50 gm with 20% sorbitol may be used for treatment of hyperkalemia (Cooper & Chapman, 1995), and is given orally or as a retention enema. This is an effective chronic treatment, but not fast enough for acute hyperkalemia. Nursing care of persons receiving Kayexalate includes (a) observing for the desired effect of lowered potassium levels; and (b) assessing the effect this treatment has on the plasma fluid volume level.

As renal function decreases the kidney excretes less H+, causing acidemia. Acidemia may interfere with protein metabolism and may lead to muscle wasting and cardiac dysfunction (Cooper & Chapman, 1995). Conservative treatment consists of dietary restrictions of alkali products such as sodium bicarbonate until the serum bicarbonate level reaches 15 mg/dl, at which time more aggressive therapy such as dialysis may be required (Cooper & Chapman, 1995). Patients often take sodium bicarbonate or sodium citrate to buffer the additional acid. Because these substances contain sodium, they may raise blood pressure. Sodium citrates also increase aluminum absorption leading to aluminum toxicity, which may be associated with dementia in patients with renal failure (Cooper & Chapman, 1995). While calcium carbonate may provide an agent for acidemia, its effectiveness has not been as easily maintained with these subjects as with other drugs (Cooper & Chapman, 1995).

Control of Anemia

Anemia occurs because of the decrease in erythropoietin production in the failing kidneys. Anemia often causes activity intolerance and severe fatigue. Anabolic steroids stimulate erythropoietin production in nonrenal tissue but increase sodium and water retention, diminishing their success. Recombinant erythropoietin stimulates red blood cell production like natural epoetin alfa (EPO) by acting on bone marrow. The therapeutic goal for patients receiving EPO is a hematocrit level ranging from 32%-38% (Baer, 1995). Those patients with iron deficiency receive folic acid, vitamin B12, and iron. As the patient's appetite increases, the dietary intake may also change, requiring a reassessment of the nutritional plan. By elevating the hemoglobin and hematocrit, often patients have increased activity tolerance, improved sexual function, and an overall perception of an increased quality of life.

A second cause of anemia in patients with renal failure may be upper gastrointestinal (GI) bleeding. Bleeding may be seen in the form of epistaxis, vomiting of coffee ground materials as well as bright red emesis, or blood in the stools (Gallagher-Lepak, 1994). Nurses caring for these patients may need to institute safety measures such as protection of the nasal mucosa by ensuring air humidity is adequate especially if patients are receiving oxygen. Other measures to prevent GI bleeding may include the use of antacids. Duodenitis and gastritis are reported in 10%-60% of patients with moderate to severe renal failure (Cooper & Chapman, 1995). Cimetidine (Tagamet®), ranitidine, and famotiden relieve symptoms of gastritis by preventing acid uptake. Because antacids such as Maalox®, Mylanta®, or Tums® should be avoided (McKentry, p. 825) due to interference with the absorption of H2 receptor antagonists, they should be given at different times.

Control of Renal Osteodystrophy

Osteodystrophy occurs in all renal patients to some degree, necessitating nursing care aimed at both increasing calcium levels and at prevention of fractures. Concern must be given to the integrity of the skeletal system in all renal patients since recovery from a fractured bone is difficult.

When phosphate excretion diminishes in the failing kidney, serum levels rise. Dietary restriction of phosphate intake is usually restricted to 4-10 mg/kg/day (Hoffart, 1995) and phosphate binders reduce serum levels. Aluminum hydroxide antacids (Amphogel®, Alternagel®) bind the phosphate in the GI tract, increasing phosphate excretion in the stool. These binders are now rarely used because dementia and osteomalacia are complications of aluminum absorption. Instead, calcium carbonate (Tums®) and calcium acetate (PhosLo®) are being used to raise Ca and decrease absorption from the bone. The increased Ca and P may combine and precipitate to form deposits in the soft tissues of the body (Gallagher-Lepak, 1994). These soft-tissue calcifications may occur anywhere throughout the body but seem to occur most frequently in the fingers and toes (Andreoli et al., 1991). Patients may need stool softeners to decrease discomfort and increase compliance with the antacid regimen because both aluminum-based and calcium-based antacids cause constipation.

Synthetic vitamin D, available in oral preparations such as calcitriol (Rocaltrol®) and in IV form such as calcitriol (Calcijex®), promotes the absorption of calcium from the GI tract. Normal serum calcium levels in hypocalcemic CRF patients can usually be maintained with an oral dose of 0.5-1.0 mcg/day after reaching desired serum levels (Deglin & Vallerand, 1995) if medicinal therapy is not effective.

Removal of a portion of the parathyroid glands to decrease the production and secretion of PTH may be necessary to preserve the skeletal system. In a few situations a total parathyroidectomy is performed in order to stop the erosion of calcium from the bones, although it also requires control of serum calcium and frequent monitoring of the calcium level.

Prevention of Infection

Causes and Concerns

Studies have suggested that renal patients are vulnerable to infection because of a compromised immune system and a diminished inflammatory response (Gallagher-Lepak, 1994; Andreoli et al., 1991). Nurses may protect patients from drug nephrotoxicity, which may occur with the use of antimicrobials since these are known to be harmful to the kidneys (Baer, 1995). If nephrotoxicity occurs sodium and potassium may rise, and these may mask symptoms of a supra infection.

Drug Therapy Complications: Nephrotoxicity, Half-Life Implications

Because many drugs are bound to protein for transport, renal patients may experience increased drug availability due to diminished plasma proteins (Baer, 1995). Drug toxicity and half-life may increase. Patient teaching must emphasize the need for follow-up care and monitoring medication regimens. The pathways of some drugs, such as insulin may decrease and patients may require less insulin.

Integumentary Care

Pruritis, Infection, and Treatment

Sixty to eighty percent (60%-80%) of chronic renal failure patients experience pruritus (Shoop, 1994). When the severity of the problem is assessed by nurses, plans of care should include comfort measures. Tepid baths have been effective for some patients while bath oils and lotions have helped others. However, no one measure works independently. Uncontrollable itching may have an impact on the integument system. Because open skin increases infection, nurses should encourage patients to wear gloves.

Sexual Dysfunction Concerns

Depression occurs frequently in renal failure patients due to restricted diet, pharmacologic regimen, and the chronicity of the disease itself. In those patients with depression, physiological causes of impotence occur as a result of vascular changes, neuropathy causing bladder dysfunction, sensory deficits leading to inability to sustain erection and delayed ejaculation, and hormonal changes that may lower testosterone levels. Treatment of this phenomenon is mostly a medical plan, but nurses may be the initial health care professionals to hear these concerns from patients. Follow-up must be done sensitively and professionally in order to maintain open communication with patients.

Summary

The length of time that patients can be maintained on conservative management varies considerably and depends on the progression of renal failure. This is difficult for patients who desire to remain in control of a disease that may not be controllable. While patients are being conservatively managed is the best time for decisions regarding future therapies to be made. Making these decisions while there is time to consider all ramifications, and for patients and significant others to discuss the positive and negative aspects of these therapies, is the most desirable aspect of this plan. Developing a plan before complications occur is also desirable as mental status may change, and neuropathies and changing emotional well-being could make decision-making more difficult. Helping patients to take a primary part in the plan of care will be one of the most important accomplishments that can be achieved. Education about treatment and its options, and encouraging an active part in the decision-making process will give patients information that could be used to assume control over their lives, renal failure, and future health care.

References

Anderson, S., Fedje, L., & Pulliam, J. (1993). Slowing the progress of renal failure. *Patient Care*, pp. 102-121.

Andreoli, T.E., Carpenter, C.J., Plum, F., & Smith, L.H. (Ed.). (1991). *Cecil essentials of medicine* (2nd edition) (pp. 167-191). Philadelphia: W.B. Saunders Company.

Baer, C.L. (1995). The pharmacologic aspects of renal failure. In L. Lancaster (Ed.), *Core curriculum for nephrology nursing* (third edition) (pp. 173-206). Pitman, NJ: American Nephrology Nurses' Association.

Cooper, A.B., & Chapman, A.B. (1995). Renal failure. In J. Mladenovic (Ed.), *Primary care secrets* (pp. 241-246). Philadelphia: Hanley & Belfus.

Deglin, J.H., & Vallerand, A.H. (1995). *Davis' drug guide for nurses* (4th edition). Philadelphia: F.A. Davis Company.

Gallagher-Lepak, S. (1994). Renal failure. In C. Mattson Porth (Ed.), *Pathophysiology: Concepts of altered health States*.(pp. 684-696.) Philadelphia: J.B. Lippincott Company.

Hoffart, N. (1995). Nutrition in renal failure, dialysis, and transplantation. In L. Lancaster, (Ed.), *Core curriculum for nephrology nursing* (third edition) (pp. 153-172). Pitman, NJ: American Nephrology Nurses' Association.

Lancaster, L. (1995). Systemic manifestations of renal failure. In L. Lancaster (Ed.), *Core curriculum for nephrology nursing* (pp. 73-108). Pitman, NJ: American Nephrology Nurses' Association.

Price, S., & Wilson, L. (1997). *Pathophysiology*. St. Louis, MO: Mosby Year-Book.

Richard, C.L. (1995). Causes of renal disease. In L. Lancaster (Ed.), *Core curriculum for nephrology nursing* (pp. 51-72). Pitman, NJ: American Nephrology Nurses' Association.

Shoop, N. (1994). Pruritus in end stage renal disease. *ANNA Journal, 21*(2), 147-153.

Readings

Chambers, J.K. (1993). Renal insufficiency: Implications for care of the medical-surgical patient. *MEDSURG Nursing, 2*(1), 33-40.

Mladenovic, J. (1995). Bleeding and thrombocytopenia. In J. Mladenovic (Ed.), *Primary care secrets*.(pp. 256-258.). Philadelphia: Hanley & Belfus.

Chapter Highlights

- Primary nursing interventions can protect remaining renal function and prevent further damage, especially the renal complications from hypertension (HTN) and diabetes.

- Given the complexity of many individuals' health status, it is not uncommon for reduced renal function to occur during a stay in health care facilities for reasons other than renal-related symptoms.

- Nephrosclerosis, the renal disease that occurs as a result of hypertension, develops over a long period of time and is treated by controlling hypertension (Richard, 1995). Blood pressure control slows the progression of renal disease (Richard, 1995) while HTN causes several changes in the kidneys, including atherosclerosis of the glomerular membrane.

- Calcium channel blockers prevent entry of calcium into the cell, thereby decreasing the mechanical activity of vascular smooth muscle and decreasing peripheral vascular resistance.

- The conservative management of renal failure includes dietary modification to decrease the kidneys' workload (Hoffart, 1995) and preserve renal function.

- Anemia occurs because of the decrease in erythropoietin production in the failing kidneys. Anemia often causes activity intolerance and severe fatigue. Anabolic steroids stimulate erythropoietin production in nonrenal tissue but increase sodium and water retention, diminishing their success.

- Osteodystrophy occurs in all renal patients to some degree, necessitating nursing care aimed at both increasing calcium levels and at prevention of fractures. Concern must be given to the integrity of the skeletal system in all renal patients since recovery from a fractured bone is difficult.

- Studies have suggested that renal patients are vulnerable to infection because of a compromised immune system and a diminished inflammatory response . . . . Nurses may protect patients from drug nephrotoxicity, which may occur with the use of antimicrobials since these are known to be harmful to the kidneys (Baer, 1995).

- Depression occurs frequently in renal failure patients due to restricted diet, pharmacologic regimen, and the chronicity of the disease itself . . . Treatment of this phenomenon is mostly a medical plan, but nurses may be the initial health care professionals to hear concerns from patients. Follow-up must be done sensitively and professionally.

CHAPTER 19

Hemodialysis

Patricia Baltz Salai, MSN, RN, CNN, CRNP

Chapter Contents

Basic Principles 527
Semipermeable Membrane 527
Diffusion 527
Ultrafiltration 528
Clearance 530
The Hemodialysis System 530
The Dialyzer 530
The Blood Circuit 532
Dialysis Solution (Dialysate) 533
The Dialysate Circuit 534
Optional System Components 535
Water Treatment for Dialysis 536
Methods of Water Purification 536
Vascular Access for Hemodialysis 537
Temporary/Acute Vascular Access 538
Permanent Vascular Access 542
The Hemodialysis Prescription 549
Amount of Dialysis 549
Dialysis Solution 550
Delivery of Adequate Treatment 552
Anticoagulation During Hemodialysis 552
Heparin Prescription 552
Assessing Anticoagulation During Hemodialysis 554
The Hemodialysis Procedure 555
Predialysis Equipment Preparation 555
Predialysis Patient Assessment and Preparation 555
Vascular Access Assessment and Preparation 556

Chapter Contents

- Beginning the Treatment 556
- Intradialytic Monitoring 556
- Termination of the Hemodialysis Treatment 557
- Postdialysis Patient Assessment. 557
- Postdialysis Blood Work 561
- Postdialysis Equipment Care 562

Complications of Hemodialysis 562
- Hypotension 562
- Muscle Cramps 564
- Chest Pain 564
- Fever and Chills 565
- Dialysis Disequilibrium Syndrome 565
- Acute Hemolysis 566
- Air Embolism 566
- Dialyzer Reactions 567
- Dysrhythmias 568
- Cardiac Arrest 568
- Seizures 568
- Exsanguination 569
- Dialysis Encephalopathy 569
- Neutropenia/Complement Activation 569
- Hypoxemia 570
- Hemodialysis-related Amyloidosis 570
- Hemodialysis-related Interleukin-1 Stimulation 570

Special Procedures Related to Hemodialysis 571
- Sorbent Hemodialysis 571
- Isolated Ultrafiltration 571
- Treatment of Drug Overdose or Poisoning 572
- Dialyzer Reuse 572

Summary 573

References 573

Chapter Highlights 575

Hemodialysis

Patricia Baltz Salai, MSN, RN, CNN, CRNP

Hemodialysis, first used clinically in the treatment of renal failure in 1947, remains the most commonly prescribed renal replacement therapy in this country. It is used successfully in the treatment of persons with acute and chronic renal failure (Gutch & Stoner, 1993; Keen et al., 1995).

The purpose of this chapter is to describe the hemodialysis process, discuss patient outcomes and response to therapy, identify potential complications related to this mode of renal replacement therapy, and discuss the nursing care of the patient receiving hemodialysis.

Basic Principles

Dialysis is a process through which the composition of two solutions are changed when they are exposed to each other through a semipermeable membrane (Van Stone & Daugirdas, 1994). During hemodialysis, the solute composition as well as the water content of a person's blood is altered through exposure of the blood, in that manner, to a physiologically ideal electrolyte solution. Removal of excess plasma water and uremic toxins as well as correction of electrolyte and acid-base imbalances can be accomplished in patients with chronic renal failure (CRF) or acute renal failure (ARF). The hemodialysis process reestablishes body fluid solute concentrations that can no longer be maintained by the patient's natural kidneys (Sargent & Gotch, 1989).

Semipermeable Membrane

The semipermeable membrane used for hemodialysis is located inside the artificial kidney or dialyzer (see Figure 19-1 for dialyzer design). The semipermeable membrane separates the dialyzer into two compartments, the blood compartment and the dialysate or dialysis solution compartment. Perforated by small pores, the membrane separates the patient's blood from the dialysis solution and allows water and small molecular weight molecules from both solutions to pass through the pores. Large solutes such as blood cells and proteins cannot pass through the small openings and thus are retained in their respective compartments (Van Stone & Daugirdas, 1994).

Solute removal during hemodialysis occurs primarily through the process of diffusion. Solutes are also dissolved in water molecules that are transported across the membrane and from the patient's blood during the process of ultrafiltration. The thickness and surface area of the semipermeable membrane, as well as the number of pores, determine in part the amount of water and solute movement between the solutions (Ismail & Hakim, 1991).

Diffusion

Ismail and Hakim describe diffusion as the movement of solutes through a semipermeable membrane from an area of greater concentration to an area of lesser concentration (see Figure 19-2). During hemodialysis, solutes move from the blood into the dialysis solution and from the dialysis solution into the blood. Solutes highly concentrated in the blood of a uremic patient, such as urea, creatinine, and potassium, move into the dialysis solution where these substances are absent or pre-

Figure 19-1
General scheme for dialyzer design.

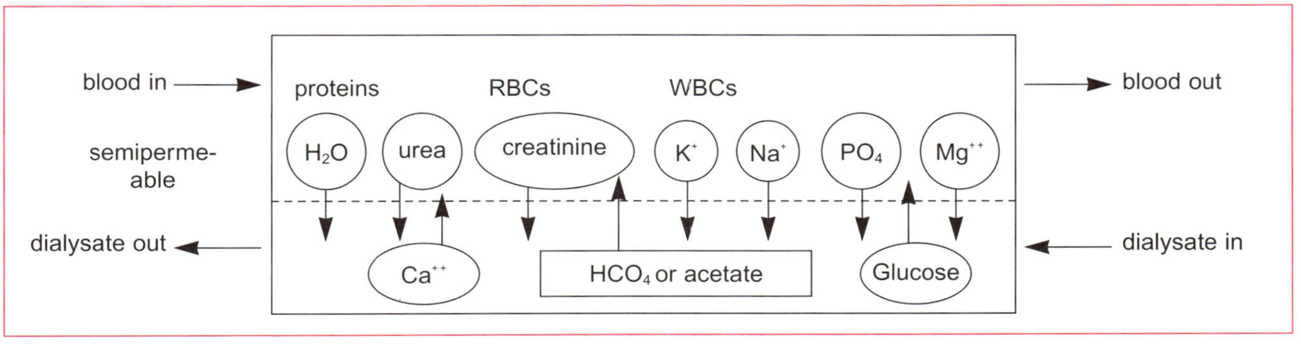

sent in low concentrations (Ismail & Hakim, 1991). At the same time, solutes that are present in a higher concentration in the dialysis solution than in the patient's blood, move through the membrane from the dialysis solution into the blood. Buffers such as acetate and bicarbonate are examples of solutes that diffuse from the dialysis solution to the blood (Rockel et al., 1988).

There are several factors identified to affect diffusion, particularly the rate at which it occurs, during hemodialysis. These factors include membrane surface area and thickness, the number of pores in the membrane, the concentration gradient between the blood and the dialysis solution, blood and dialysate flow rates, solution temperatures, membrane resistance, and the molecular size, weight, and charge of the solutes (Ismail & Hakim, 1991).

As the surface area of the semipermeable membrane increases, the space available for contact between the blood and the dialysis solution increases. As the amount of contact increases, diffusion increases. The numerous conventional dialyzers available for hemodialysis vary greatly in surface area, allowing for selection of dialyzer according to patient need. Most of the membrane surface inside the dialyzer is effective surface area for dialysis. Portions of the membrane are obstructed by internal structures and potting compounds within the dialyzer (Gutch & Stoner, 1993; Ismail & Hakim, 1991).

Some membranes contain a greater number of pores per square meter, thus are more porous than others. Increased porosity also enhances the rate of diffusion. A larger number of openings in the membrane creates the potential for greater movement of solutes through the membrane (Ismail & Hakim, 1991).

The difference between the amounts of solutes contained in the solutions on either side of the semipermeable membrane is the concentration gradient. The larger the difference, or the higher the concentration gradient, the faster diffusion of solutes occurs from the area of greater concentration to the area of lesser concentration. One explanation for this phenomenon is that with higher concentrations of solutes in a solution, there are more collisions of moving molecules with the porous membrane, thus more transfer of solutes out of the more concentrated solution (Ismail & Hakim, 1991; Van Stone & Daugirdas, 1994).

Diffusion of molecules in hemodialysis, particularly small molecules, is also flow-dependent. The rate of blood flow and dialysis solution flow through the dialyzer is an important factor that influences the rate of diffusion that occurs during hemodialysis. If blood and dialysate were to be left in constant static contact with each other inside the dialyzer, diffusion of solutes across the membrane would occur rapidly at the beginning, when the concentration gradient was highest. Diffusion, however, would slow down as the contents of the two solutions became similar and equilibrium was achieved. At that point, diffusion would continue to occur back and forth across the membrane; however, solute concentrations of the solutions would remain the same. This concentration equilibrium is prevented during hemodialysis by continuously replacing the dialysis solution with fresh unused solution and by circulating undialyzed blood through the blood compartment (Van Stone & Daugirdas, 1994).

Blood flow rates and dialysis solution flow rates through the dialyzer can be adjusted to either increase or decrease diffusion or clearance of small molecules such as creatinine. Since large molecules are much less dependent on flow rates, clearance of these molecules cannot as readily be enhanced by an increase in either rate (Ismail & Hakim, 1991).

The rate of diffusion of any given solute is also determined, in part, by the molecular size and weight of the molecule. The larger the molecular weight, the slower the solute diffuses across the membrane. Because large molecules move more slowly, they have fewer collisions with the membrane. Passage of large molecules through the membrane may also be hindered because the pores are smaller than the molecules. The charge of the molecule may also affect the rate of diffusion. Molecules may be repelled by like-charged molecules on the other side of the membrane (Daugirdas & Ing, 1994; Levine, 1991).

Solution temperature affects the rate of diffusion because of its effect on the movement of molecules in the solution. Molecules in a warmed solution move faster and thus collide with the membrane more often and move through the membrane more frequently if other factors are conducive to diffusion. During the hemodialysis procedure, the dialysate is warmed to maintain warmth of the blood circuit. This warming may also enhance the diffusion of solutes.

The final factor that affects diffusion is described as membrane resistance. The resistance to the diffusion of molecules occurs primarily because of a layer of unstirred fluid that remains adjacent to the membrane inside the dialyzer blood compartment. Because the solutes have diffused out of the fluid and the fluid has equilibrated with the dialysis solution, it acts to decrease effective concentration gradient and thus decrease the rate of diffusion. This phenomenon is thought to occur despite adequate blood and dialysis solution flow rates and occurs to a greater degree in thicker, less porous membranes. Thinner, more porous membranes have lower membrane resistance (Ismail & Hakim, 1991).

Ultrafiltration

Ultrafiltration is the process through which water removal is accomplished during hemodialy-

Figure 19-2
Diffusion and ultrafiltration.

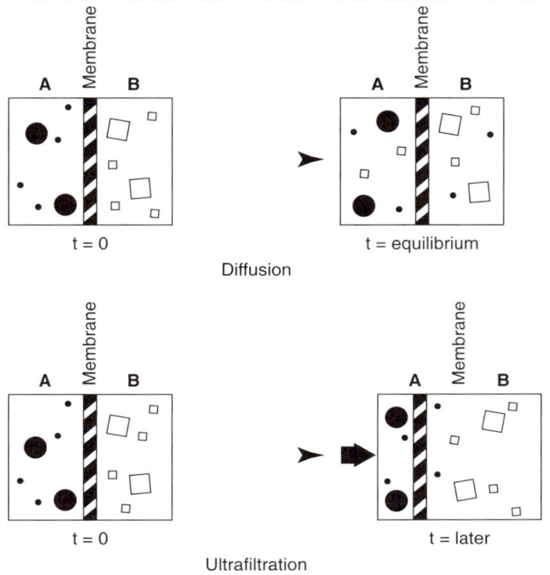

The processes of diffusion (top) and ultrafiltration (bottom). As shown, in both processes, small molecular weight solutes can cross the semipermeable membrane, whereas larger solutes are held back.

Note: From Van Stone, J.C., & Daugirdas, J.T. (1994). Physiologic principles. In J.T. Daugirdas & T.S. Ing (Eds.), *Handbook of dialysis* (2nd ed., pp. 13-29). Boston: Little, Brown. Reprinted with permission.

sis. It is defined by Ismail and Hakim (1991) as the bulk movement of a solvent across a semipermeable membrane. A solvent is fluid in which electrolytes and nonelectrolytes are dissolved to form a solution. Water is the solvent in all body fluids.

The driving force in ultrafiltration is the hydrostatic pressure gradient across the dialyzer membrane (Ismail & Hakim, 1991) (see Figure 19-2). The transport of water across the membrane, however, is affected not just by hydrostatic pressure, but by osmotic pressure, as well as pressure within the dialysate compartment of the dialyzer. Hydrostatic pressure within the blood compartment is positive pressure generated by the force of the moving bloodflow against the membrane. When this positive pressure is greater than the osmotic pressure within the blood and the hydrostatic pressure within the dialysis solution compartment, it forces water molecules through the membrane pores and into the dialysis compartment.

Dialysis solution pressure is usually a negative pressure. However, with most hemodialysis systems, positive pressure can also be generated if necessary (Lazarus, 1982; Van Stone & Daugirdas, 1994). Both the blood compartment pressure and the dialysis solution pressure are measured in mmHg. The combined transmembrane pressure (TMP) exerted on the dialysis membrane can be determined by subtracting the dialysis solution pressure, usually a negative number, from the blood compartment pressure (Ismail & Hakim, 1991).

The capability of the hemodialyzer membrane to remove water varies widely throughout dialyzer types and membrane compositions. Just as the amount of chemical clearance that occurs during hemodialysis is, among other factors, a function of the dialyzer membrane capability for diffusion, water removal is dependent, in part, upon the ultrafiltration capability of the membrane being used. This capability is expressed as the ultrafiltration coefficient, which is a measurement of the permeability of the dialyzer membrane to water and is expressed as the number of milliliters (ml) of water that will cross the membrane per millimeters of mercury (mmHg) of transmembrane pressure during 1 hour (Ismail & Hakim, 1991; Van Stone & Daugirdas, 1994).

All dialyzers have specified ultrafiltration coefficients so that the appropriate one can be matched to the clinical situation. For example, a dialyzer with a higher ultrafiltration coefficient may be chosen for a hypervolemic patient with a normal to elevated blood pressure to facilitate rapid fluid removal during hemodialysis. Conversely, a patient who appears to be euvolemic or minimally volume overloaded and will require little fluid removal during hemodialysis may be more appropriately treated using a dialyzer with a lower ultrafiltration coefficient.

As with diffusion, there are factors that affect ultrafiltration during hemodialysis. The manufacturer reported ultrafiltration coefficients of dialyzers are determined in in-vitro measurements. The true in-vivo coefficients have been found to range 5-30% lower than those reported by the manufacturers. This difference is thought to be due to blood protein and hematocrit variances among patients as well as to such factors as partial dialyzer clotting, which reduces effective membrane surface area during hemodialysis in the clinical setting (Ismail & Hakim, 1991; Van Stone & Daugirdas, 1994).

Hemodialysis systems that require the operator to calculate and set the TMP does not provide for as accurate fluid removal as the systems that control the amount of ultrafiltration volumetrically. The latter measures the volume of ultrafiltrate as it is removed, then continuously calculates and adjusts the TMP to ensure that the desired fluid removal is occurring. In systems without volumetric control, the operator must observe the blood compartment and dialysate pressures and adjust the TMP as necessary. These adjustments are made only periodically when the nurse assesses the patient. Without the continuous adjustment of the volumetric ultra-

Figure 19-3
Hollow fiber hemodialyzer.

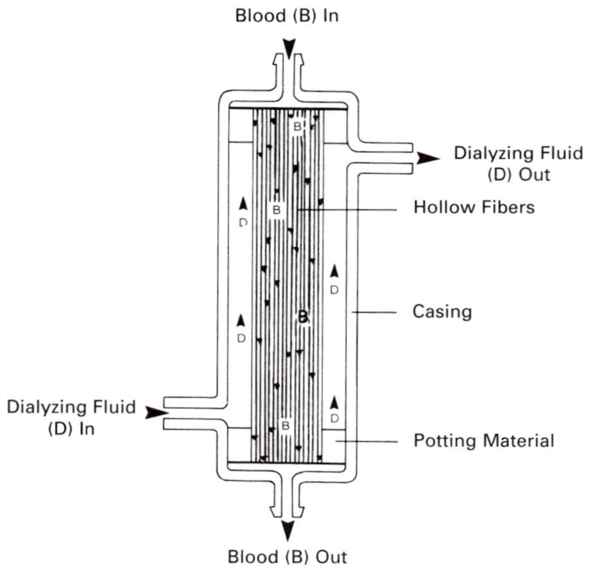

Note: From Wick, G.S., & Parker, J. (1984). *Protecting the future of quality care through an understanding of hemodialysis principles.* Pitman, NJ: The American Nephrology Nurses' Association. Reprinted with permission.

filtration controller, fluid removal varies throughout the treatment and may not be accurate (Van Stone & Daugirdas, 1994). Fluid removal using a highly fluid permeable dialyzer with a high ultrafiltration coefficient is best controlled volumetrically (Ray et al., 1982).

Clearance

The concept of clearance is used by nephrologists when assessing the ability of the natural kidneys to remove metabolic waste products from the blood stream. It is also used in hemodialysis to refer to removal of a substance from the bloodstream during a specific unit of time. It is an empirical measurement of the volume of blood that is totally cleared of a particular substance per unit of time (1 minute) (Ismail & Hakim, 1991).

In hemodialysis, clearance is used to indicate the performance of a dialyzer. It is affected by the blood flow rate through the dialyzer and the solute concentration (Gutch & Stoner, 1993). The percent reduction in the blood concentration of a given waste product is multiplied by the blood flow rate to obtain a hypothetical volume of blood that is being totally cleared of the substance (Van Stone & Daugirdas, 1994).

Clearance of solutes in hemodialysis occurs as a function of both diffusion and ultrafiltration. Ultrafiltrate contains waste products as dissolved solutes. Thus, when large volumes of water are removed, more solutes are removed in the water in addition to those removed by diffusion (Lazarus, 1982). Since clearance is dependent upon both diffusion and ultrafiltration, the same factors that have been previously described to affect those processes will have an impact on clearance during hemodialysis. Clearance increases as the blood flow rate through the dialyzer increases. Clearance also increases as the dialysis solution flow rate is increased. However, the effect is not as great as with changes in the blood flow rate.

Dialyzer efficiency is another factor. Membranes that are thin with large pores and a large surface area allow maximum contact between the dialysis solution and the blood, thus enhancing clearance. The molecular weight of a substance affects the clearance of that substance as previously described in the discussion of diffusion. Vascular access recirculation can also affect the clearance obtained during a hemodialysis treatment. Recirculation will be addressed in greater detail in the discussion of vascular access (Van Stone & Daugirdas, 1994).

The Hemodialysis System

There are two important components of the hemodialysis system, the dialysate or dialysis solution circuit and the blood circuit. The blood circuit contains the dialyzer, the structure in which diffusion and ultrafiltration occur.

The Dialyzer

Structure. The hemodialyzer is designed with two internal compartments, one to contain blood and the other for dialysis solution. The two compartments are separated by a semipermeable membrane. The membrane surface area between the two compartments is maximized by using a membrane that is divided into either multiple hollow fibers or multiple parallel plates.

There are four ports on the dialyzer, two end ports for blood and two side ports for dialysis solution. Blood enters the dialyzer through the port on one end, flows through the blood compartment, and leaves the dialyzer via the port on the opposite end. Dialysis solution enters one side port on the dialyzer, flows through the dialysate compartment, and exits the dialyzer through the remaining side port. Dialysis solution, in most cases, runs countercurrent to the blood, and thus it enters the side port on the same end of the dialyzer from which the blood exits (Ismail & Hakim, 1991; Van Stone, 1994).

The hollow fiber dialyzer, sometimes called a capillary dialyzer, is the most commonly used at the present time (see Figure 19-3). It consists of

Figure 19-4
Parallel plate hemodialyzer.

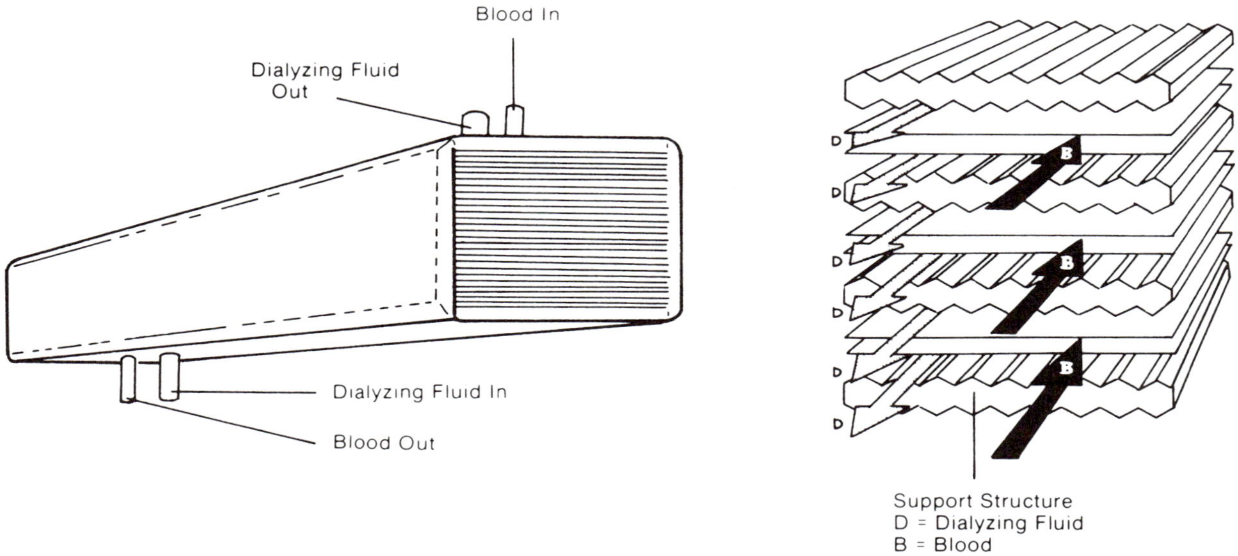

Note: From Wick, G.S., & Parker, J. (1984). *Protecting the future of quality care through an understanding of hemodialysis principles.* Pitman, NJ: The American Nephrology Nurses' Association. Reprinted with permission.

10,000 or more capillary-like tubes of membrane tightly bound in a bundle that provides a high ratio of membrane surface area to blood volume. Blood enters the end of the dialyzer and flows through the center of the tubes while dialysis solution circulates around the outside of the fibers. Parallel plate dialyzers consist of sheets of membrane laying on top of one another over supporting structures (see Figure 19-4). Blood and dialysis solution pass through alternate spaces between the membrane sheets (Ismail & Hakim, 1991; Van Stone, 1994).

Advantages of hollow fiber dialyzers include the small amount of blood required to fill the blood compartment (low priming volume) as well as a low resistance to blood flow through the dialyzer because of the large number of blood passages. The volume of blood required to fill the dialyzer does not increase with the application of TMP, making precise control of ultrafiltration much easier. One disadvantage is the potential for a higher residual blood volume due to clotting in the fibers. Blood channels within a hollow fiber dialyzer are extremely small, making clotting a common problem. The need for the use of potting compound to anchor the fibers to the ends of the dialyzer can be a disadvantage. Depending on the chemical composition of this material, removal of disinfectant solutions such as ethylene oxide may be difficult, thus placing the patient at risk for exposure to a toxic substance (Gutch & Stoner, 1993; Van Stone, 1994).

In the past, the primary disadvantage of the parallel plate dialyzer was the increase in the dialyzer blood volume when TMP was applied. During application of a high TMP, the membranes in a parallel plate dialyzer will bulge somewhat, resulting in larger blood spaces. Newer, better designed parallel plate dialyzers do not react in this fashion (Van Stone, 1994).

Membrane composition. The semipermeable membranes used in hemodialysis are composed either of cellulose, substituted cellulose, or synthetic materials. Cellulose dialyzers such as Cuprophane® are processed from cotton fibers. This is the most commonly used dialyzer membrane material. Substituted cellulose such as cellulose acetate is composed of polymer groups chemically bonded to acetate. Synthetic materials used for dialyzer membranes, include polyacrylonitrile and polymethyl methacrylate. These are not cellulose-based. There are also cellulosynthetic membranes, which are made by adding synthetic material to liquified cellulose during formation (Ismail & Hakim, 1991; Van Stone, 1994).

Each of the membrane types exhibits specific characteristics, which are delineated in Table 19-1 as advantages and disadvantages. Cellulose and substituted cellulose membranes offer similar small and middle molecule clearances. Synthetic mem-

Table 19-1
Dialyzer membrane types.

Dialyzer Membrane Type	Advantages	Disadvantages
Cellulose	Good small and middle molecule clearances	High degree of complement activation Not highly biocompatible
Substituted cellulose	Low degree of complement activation Good small and middle molecule clearances	Some complement activation
Synthetic	Biocompatible Low degree of complement activation High permeability, particularly in mid-molecule range High ultrafiltration rates	Evidence of activation of the coagulation cascade

Figure 19-5
Diagram of components of a typical hemodialysis system.

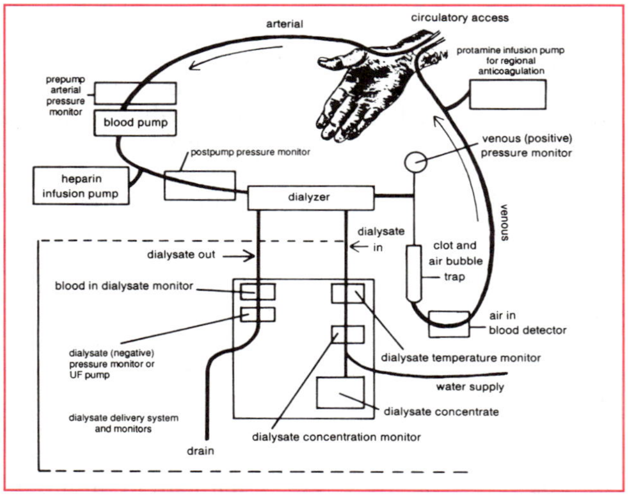

Note: From Keen, ML., Lancaster, L.E., & Binkley, L.S. (1995). Hemodialysis. In L.E. Lancaster (Ed.). (1995). *ANNA Core Curriculum for Nephrology Nursing* (3rd ed., p. 214). Pitman, NJ: American Nephrology Nurses' Association. Reprinted with permission.

branes exhibit enhanced clearances, including clearance of larger molecules and high ultrafiltration coefficients (Hoenick, 1988).

Synthetic dialyzers are associated with less dialysis-related leukopenia as well as a low degree of complement activation (Gutch & Stoner, 1993; Hoenick, 1988). Hydroxyl groups on the surface of cellulose membranes are believed to activate the complement system in the blood flowing through the dialyzer. This effect is reduced if the dialyzer is reused and occurs to a much lesser extent with substituted cellulose membranes. Synthetic membranes are associated with a very low degree of complement activation. Leukopenia and complement activation will be addressed in greater detail in the discussion of hemodialysis complications (Cheung, 1990; Van Stone, 1994).

Noncellulosic membranes have two unique characteristics: high permeability to solutes, particularly in the mid-molecule range, and high ultrafiltration rates. The chemistry of these membranes yields a larger pore size (Gutch & Stoner, 1993).

The Blood Circuit

Blood lines. Blood lines carry the blood from the patient's vascular access site to the dialyzer (arterial line) and from the dialyzer back to the patient's access (venous line). Along the lines, there are various ports for infusion, blood drawing, and pressure monitoring. The blood lines are shown in Figure 19-5, which diagrams the components of a typical hemodialysis system.

Blood pump. A roller-style blood pump moves blood from the patient's vascular access, through the

Table 19-2
Components of standard acetate-containing and bicarbonate-containing dialysis solutions.

Component	Acetate-containing (mEq/liter)	Bicarbonate-containing (mEq/liter)
Sodium	135-145	135-145
Potassium	0-4.0	0-4.0
Calcium	2.5-3.5	2.5-3.5
Magnesium	0.5-1.0	0.5-1.0
Chloride	100-119	100-124
Acetate	35-38	2-4*
Bicarbonate	0	30-38
Dextrose	11	11
PCO_2(mm Hg)	0.5	40-100
pH	Variable	7.1-7.3

* The acetate is in the form of acetic acid in the "acid" component concentrate. On mixing with the bicarbonate component, the hydrogen reacts with an equimolar amount of bicarbonate to form CO_2.

dialyzer, and back to the patient. This device is necessary to overcome the resistance in the dialyzer and the vascular access and does so by creating positive pressure within the extracorporeal system. The pump compresses segments of the blood tubing and forces the blood forward through the blood line (Gutch & Stoner, 1993; Keen et al., 1995; Van Stone, 1994).

Monitoring devices. Pressure monitors are present along the blood lines. One is located proximal to the dialyzer and, usually, to the pump as well. The other is located just distal to the dialyzer. The monitor prior to the dialyzer monitors is what is referred to as arterial pressure. If it is located before the blood pump, it guards against excessive suction by the pump, on the vascular access. If the arterial pressure monitor is located between the blood pump and the dialyzer, it monitors the resistance within the dialyzer. If elevated, this resistance to the blood being pushed into the dialyzer by the pump may be an indicator of dialyzer clotting. It also helps estimate pressure within the blood compartment of the dialyzer (Ismail & Hakim, 1991; Van Stone, 1994).

The venous pressure monitor is located on the blood line distal to the dialyzer. It monitors resistance to blood return in the vascular access. This pressure is used when calculating TMP for ultrafiltration (Ismail & Hakim, 1991).

The monitoring devices measure the pressures in millimeters of mercury (mmHg) and continuously ensure that each remain within specific acceptable limits, usually within a range of 50 mmHg. If either pressure rises above the acceptable high limit or drops below the acceptable low limit, an audible alarm sounds, the blood pump halts, and the venous blood line is clamped distal to the venous monitor (Ismail & Hakim, 1991).

Both the arterial and venous monitors can help protect the patient in the event of an accidental disconnection. In that scenario, pressures within the blood lines usually approach zero rapidly, dropping below the acceptable low pressure limits and activating the pressure alarms.

Also present on the venous blood line is an air detector. The air detector is located adjacent (distal) to a chamber or trap on the venous blood line that serves to catch small amounts of air that may come through the line. The purpose of the detector is to prevent air that may have inadvertently entered the blood circuit from being returned to the patient (Van Stone, 1994). If air is detected in the line, an audible alarm is initiated, the blood pump stops, and a clamp closes over the line, completely halting movement of blood back to the patient. The venous blood line must pass through both the air detector and the line clamp to be functional.

Dialysis Solution (Dialysate)

The dialysis solution, or dialysate, is composed of water, a buffer such as acetate or bicarbonate, and specific concentrations of electrolytes such as sodium, chloride, potassium, and magnesium. These substances are in the solution in concentrations that mimic an ideal plasma water. Most dialysate also contains glucose or dextrose (Lazarus, 1982). Table 19-2 lists the components of acetate-containing and bicarbonate-containing dialysis solutions.

The buffer is added to the dialysis solution for acid neutralization during hemodialysis. Most individuals generate 50-100 mEq of nonvolatile acid each day as a result of the metabolism of food. In persons with normal renal function, this acid is excreted by the kidneys or neutralized. In the absence of renal function, however, this acid cannot be excreted, so it must be buffered or neutralized during dialysis. This buffering occurs due to the diffusion of either acetate or bicarbonate from the dialysis solution into the blood (Van Stone, 1994).

When an acetate-based dialysis solution is used, acetate diffuses across the membrane into the bloodstream and is eventually metabolized by the liver. An end product of this metabolism is bicarbonate, which is used to buffer acids. At the same time that acetate is diffusing into the patient, the absence of bicarbonate molecules in the dialysis solution allows diffusion of bicarbonate from the blood, out of the patient. Therefore, during the first hour of hemodialysis, the plasma bicarbonate level may not increase but actually fall. By the end of a

Figure 19-6
Single proportioning system.

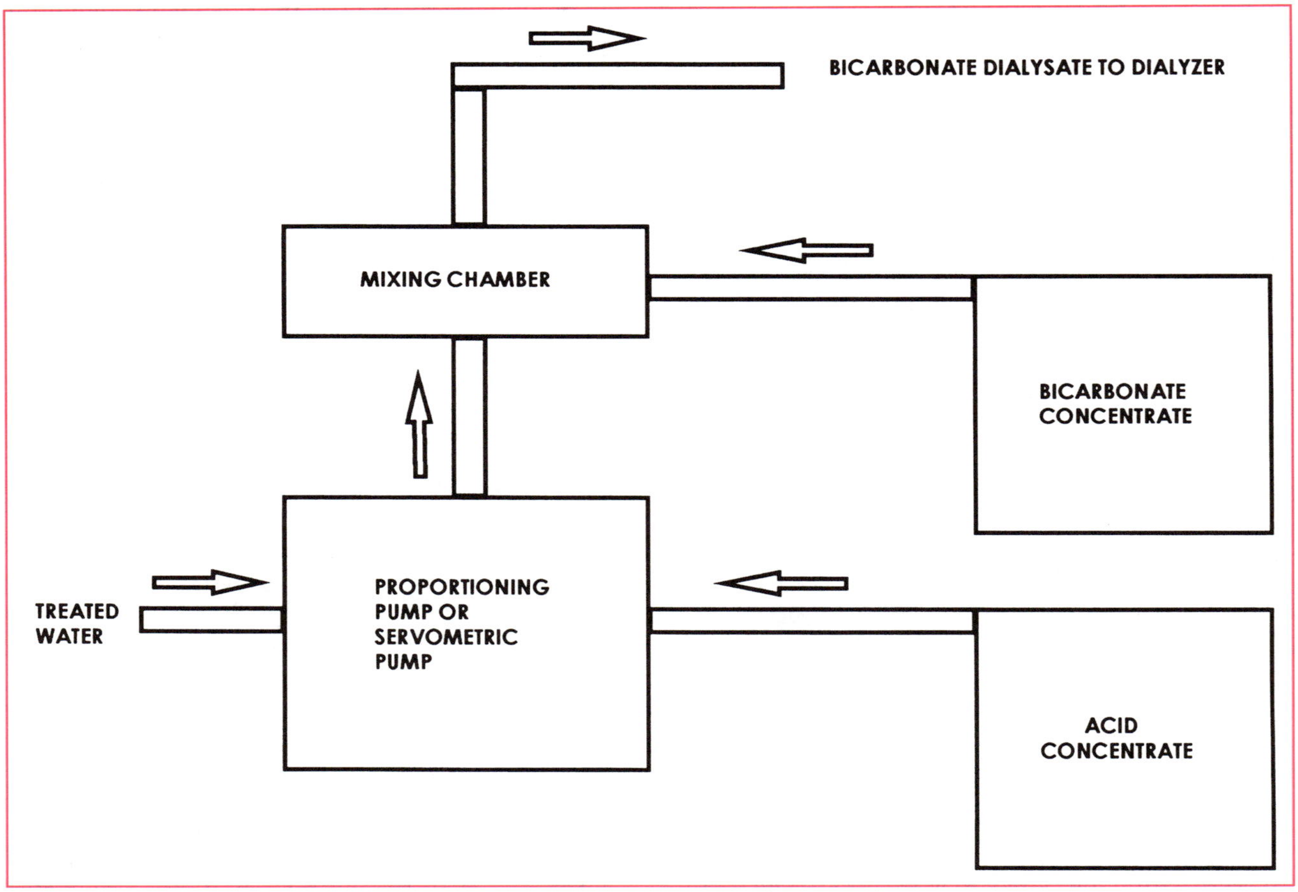

Note: From Keen, ML., Lancaster, L.E., & Binkley, L.S. (1995). Hemodialysis. In L.E. Lancaster (Ed.). (1995). *ANNA Core Curriculum for Nephrology Nursing* (3rd ed., p. 214). Pitman, NJ: American Nephrology Nurses' Association. Reprinted with permission.

4-hour treatment, however, plasma bicarbonate will rise as much as 2-4 mEq/liter (Van Stone, 1994). Plasma bicarbonate levels may, however, continue to rise for a period of time after the dialysis treatment is terminated because of the delay in conversion of acetate to bicarbonate in the liver.

The use of bicarbonate-based dialysis solution prevents the loss of bicarbonate molecules from the blood because bicarbonate is present on the other side of the membrane. Bicarbonate diffuses across the semipermeable membrane from the dialysis solution and into the blood. There is no delay in the increase of serum bicarbonate such as that which occurs with an acetate-based solution. By the end of a 4-hour hemodialysis treatment, the rise in plasma bicarbonate will be similar to that with acetate dialysate (Van Stone, 1994).

The Dialysate Circuit

There are various types of dialysate delivery systems. They include the batch system, central and individual proportioning systems, and regenerative (sorbent) dialysate systems. Regenerative dialysate systems will be discussed in a later section of this chapter.

The batch system uses a machine with a large reservoir, approximately 200 liters, in which purified water is mixed with appropriate amounts of electrolytes and a buffer to form a dialysis solution. The dialysis solution from the reservoir is circulated through the dialyzer in a single pass fashion and then discarded. The remaining solution is continuously stirred to prevent precipitation of the solutes. This system allows for individualization of hemodialysis treatments and can be used for remote treatments in areas where treated water is not available. The equipment, however, tends to be large and cumbersome, and the 200 liters of dialysis solution renders the machine heavy and difficult to move at times.

Proportioning systems are the most commonly used dialysate delivery systems for hemodialysis. With a central proportioning delivery system, all dialysis solution for the entire unit is produced by a single machine that mixes a liquid concentrate, in specific proportion, with purified water. The final product solution is then pumped to each individual hemodialysis machine. Although there may be a lower initial equipment cost with this type of system, there are limitations. Dialysis solution contents cannot be modified or individualized according to specific patient needs because every patient dialyzes with the same solution (Van Stone, 1994).

Individual proportioning systems allow for individualization and modification of dialysis treatments. Each hemodialysis machine proportions and mixes a liquid dialysate concentrate with water. Thus, dialysis prescriptions can be varied throughout the patient population (Van Stone, 1994).

Dialysate lines. These lines carry dialysis solution from the machine's proportioning unit, or the reservoir in a batch system, to the dialyzer and then from the dialyzer to the drain. Several devices located along this circuit monitor the composition and temperature of the final dialysis solution product as well as for the presence of blood in the dialysate leaving the dialyzer. The proportioning system can be examined in Figure 19-6.

Monitoring devices. The concentration of the final dialysis solution is measured as reflected by its electrical conductivity or capacity to conduct an electrical charge. This type of measurement is possible because the primary solutes in the dialysis solution are electrolytes, which carry electrical charges. Proper proportioning by the machine of purified water and dialysate concentrate is monitored by a meter that continuously measures the electrical conductivity of the product before it enters the dialyzer. This monitor notifies the nurse of a malfunction in the proportioning unit or other problems, such as an empty concentrate container, before an excessively dilute or concentrated dialysis solution is delivered to the dialyzer. Exposure of the patient's blood to a severely hyposmolar solution can result in rapid hemolysis or significant hyponatremia (Van Stone, 1994).

When the conductivity monitor senses an increase or a decrease in conductivity outside of the acceptable range, an audible alarm sounds, and the machine converts to a dialyzer bypass mode. During that time, the dialysis solution is shunted around the dialyzer, directly into the drain, allowing for determination and correction of the problem without harm to the patient (Van Stone, 1994).

The hemodialysis system contains a heater that maintains the temperature of the dialysis solution near body temperature. This prevents the patient's blood from cooling during the treatment. It is very important that proper solution temperature be maintained. Exposure to a cool solution can cause a cold feeling and shivering in the patient. More seriously, it can lead to hypothermia in an unconscious patient. A dialysis solution temperature of 42 degrees centigrade or more can lead to hemolysis. A temperature sensor continuously monitors the solution temperature. If an increased or decreased temperature outside of acceptable limits is sensed, the machine converts to dialyzer bypass, and an audible alarm sounds (Van Stone, 1994).

A blood detector monitor is located on the dialysate outflow line, which carries used dialysis solution from the dialyzer to the drain. It monitors for the presence of blood, which indicates a rupture or break in the dialyzer membrane. The presence of blood in the dialysate causes an audible alarm, stops the blood pump, and closes the venous blood line clamp, protecting the patient from further blood loss and preventing entrance of dialysis solution into the patient's bloodstream (Van Stone, 1994).

Dialysate outflow pressure is monitored on hemodialysis machines by the ultrafiltrate controllers. This number is used in conjunction with blood outflow pressure to calculate transmembrane pressure (Van Stone, 1994).

Optional System Components

Heparin pump. Virtually all hemodialysis machines have a pump that will continuously infuse heparin for anticoagulation during the treatment. Heparin is infused from a syringe into the arterial blood line, just proximal to the dialyzer (Van Stone, 1994). Some heparin pumps can be set to automatically stop infusing at some time during or near the end of the treatment. However, others must be controlled manually, requiring the nurse to discontinue the infusion when desired.

Ultrafiltration (UF) controller. Because manual calculation of transmembrane pressure (TMP) leaves room for potential human error, precise UF control is a good feature for a hemodialysis machine. Volumetric controllers, the most advanced type, measure the volume of dialysis solution to and from the dialyzer, then make appropriate adjustments in TMP to ensure prescribed fluid removal.

In most cases, ultrafiltrate is removed at a constant rate throughout the treatment. However, programmable UF controllers allow for rate adjustment, such as removal of most of the fluid during the initial part of the treatment. With programmable controllers, the operator can design any fluid removal pattern desired for the patient (Van Stone, 1994).

Variable sodium. This option permits rapid alteration of dialysis solution sodium concentration as well as individualization of the dialysis treatment. The sodium concentration is usually altered by changing the proportion of the mixture of concentrate and water. This, however, also changes the concentration of all other electrolytes in the solution as well (Van Stone, 1994).

In a typical hemodialysis treatment using variable sodium, the patient initially dialyzes with a dialysate sodium concentration of 145 mEq/liter. Throughout the treatment, the dialysate sodium is decreased in steps to 140 mEq/liter for the final hour. This feature allows the patient to have the benefits of a high sodium dialysate such as fewer intradialytic symptoms and hypotension. It also has been shown to decrease the need for nursing interventions throughout the treatment because the patient is more stable. Decreasing the dialysate sodium to 140 mEq/liter for the final hour reduces the risk of high interdialytic weight gains and blood pressure that have often been associated with high dialysate sodium levels of 145 mEq/liter or higher (Jenson et al., 1994).

Single needle devices. These devices allow dialysis with only a single blood pathway. A solitary line from the vascular access attaches to a Y tube connector which, in turn, attaches to the blood lines. Intermittently, the venous blood line is clamped while blood is drawn into the system through the arterial blood line. When the pressure within the system increases, the blood pump stops and the venous line clamp is released. Blood is returned to the patient either by the pressure in the system or through the use of a second pump (Van Stone, 1994).

Although single needle devices allow for the convenience of use of a single lumen catheter or a solitary needle, there are limitations. Access recirculation is higher. Also, TMP estimation is less accurate because dialyzer compartment pressure varies so widely with movement of the blood. Dialyzer blood compartment pressure must be estimated by adding the minimum pressure plus half of the pulse pressure (maximum minus minimum pressure) (Van Stone, 1994).

Water Treatment for Dialysis

During hemodialysis, the patient's blood is often exposed to more than 120 liters of water. This is greater than 20 times the amount the average person would normally drink during a 24-hour period. Thus, substances that are not harmful in drinking water may be harmful in water used for hemodialysis. Small molecular weight substances in the water have direct access to the patient's bloodstream, so it is very important that the purity of the water used for hemodialysis be known and controlled (Gutch & Stoner, 1993; Van Stone, 1994).

Despite the exposure of the patient's blood to water during hemodialysis, this water need not be completely sterile. The dialyzer membrane normally acts as a barrier to both bacteria and endotoxin. Bacteria levels, however, should be maintained at less than 200 colonies per ml in the water and below 2000 colonies per ml in the final dialysis solution. These levels are maintained through periodic disinfection of the water system and, in some cases, use of bacteriological water filters (Van Stone, 1994).

The pyrogen outbreaks that have been reported in hemodialysis centers have most commonly been reported to be associated with the use of bicarbonate-containing dialysis solution as well as with the use of high-flux membranes. There are multiple factors that appear to contribute to this phenomenon. Some bicarbonate powders and concentrates are contaminated with bacteria or endotoxin that can accumulate if the machine is not cleaned well between treatments. Additionally, the large pores in high-flux membranes may allow for more exposure of the blood to bacteria and endotoxin. Some bacterial products in the dialysate appear to stimulate blood monocytes to produce interleukin 1 (IL-1). High levels of IL-1 can result in pyrexia and possibly other side effects during hemodialysis (Van Stone, 1994).

Calcium carbonate is the most common impurity in water. Other substances are also commonly found such as sodium, chloride, iron, magnesium, chloramine, nitrates, manganese, aluminum, copper, zinc, iodide, and fluoride. These substances in excess, exposed to the patient's blood, can lead to serious complications. For example, nitrates can lead to myoglobinemia, a condition in which red cell hemoglobin cannot carry or transport oxygen. Copper and chloramine can lead to hemolysis (hemolytic anemia) and both fluoride and aluminum can aggravate uremic bone disease (Gutch & Stoner, 1993; Van Stone, 1994).

Trace elements found in water include arsenic, silver, strontium, and tin. The types of elements found in the water are dependent upon the minerals common to the geographic area that are picked up as rain water travels through the air to the ground. The air contains carbon dioxide and sulfur dioxide which combine with water to form weak carbonic and sulfuric acid solutions (Gutch & Stoner, 1983).

Methods of Water Purification

Several methods of water purification are available for use in hemodialysis.

Filtration. A filtration system mechanically filters water through a membrane. Suspended particles such as mud, sand, rust, and algae are left behind and removed. Dissolved particles, such as ions, remain in the water that moves through the membrane (Gutch & Stoner, 1993).

Absorption (activated charcoal filter). An activated charcoal filter removes chloramines, organic matter, and lower molecular weight materials from the water. These substances are nonionic contami-

Figure 19-7
Deionization.

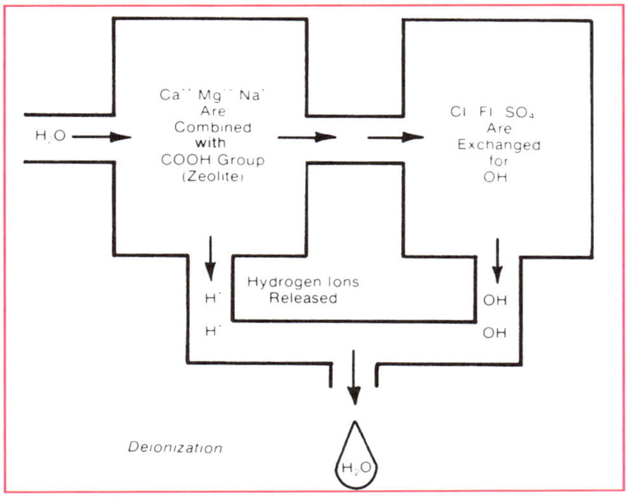

Note: From Wick, G.S., & Parker, J. (1984). *Protecting the future of quality care through an understanding of hemodialysis principles.* Pitman, NJ: The American Nephrology Nurses' Association. Reprinted with permission.

Figure 19-8
Reverse osmosis.

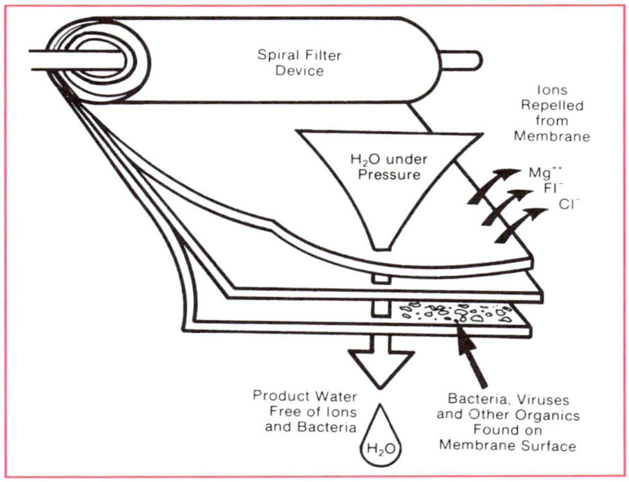

Note: From Wick, G.S., & Parker, J. (1984). *Protecting the future of quality care through an understanding of hemodialysis principles.* Pitman, NJ: The American Nephrology Nurses' Association. Reprinted with permission.

nants (Gutch & Stoner, 1993; Van Stone, 1994).

Water softening. Hardness of water is produced primarily by calcium and magnesium. The water softening process replaces calcium and magnesium ions with sodium ions while the water passes through an exchange resin bed. This exchange occurs on a milliequivalent per milliequivalent basis. Thus, for example, for each calcium ion (++) removed, two sodium ions (+) are exchanged. This process results in a higher quality water that extends the life of the reverse osmosis membrane (Gutch & Stoner, 1993).

Deionization. The deionization process uses an ion-exchange resin similar to that in a water softener (see Figure 19-7). The resin used for deionization, however, is more sophisticated, and its use results in the removal of all charged particles in the water (Van Stone, 1994).

The deionizer consists of two resin beds, one anion bed, and one cation bed. Each is composed of grains of ion exchange resins. In the anion bed, chloride, fluoride, sulfates, nitrates, bicarbonate, and other negatively charged ions are exchanged for hydroxide ions (OH-). In the cation bed, positively charged ions such as calcium, magnesium, and sodium combine with larger molecules and release hydrogen ions (H+). The released hydrogen and hydroxide ions combine to form water molecules (Gutch & Stoner, 1993).

The ion exchange beds tend to exhaust suddenly. Therefore, standby beds are necessary so a conversion can be made. The life of the beds depends upon water composition and/or the volume of water moving through the system.

Reverse osmosis. This method uses a semipermeable membrane to remove both organic matter and electrolytes from the water (see Figure 19-8). As water is pushed through the membrane, the passage of smaller molecular weight substances such as urea, sodium, and chloride is restricted due to the extremely small size of the membrane's pores. In this manner, more than 90% of impurities are removed. Bacteria and viruses are also rejected by the membrane, so the product water approaches distilled quality (Gutch & Stoner, 1993; Van Stone, 1994).

Reverse osmosis frequently produces water sufficient for dialysis, depending on the degree of contamination of the initial water supply. The product water is continuously monitored for conductivity to detect membrane leaks (Gutch & Stoner, 1993).

For maximum water quality, this system should be used in conjunction with a charcoal filter. Chloramines and oxidant compounds such as chlorine and ammonias, which are used as bacterial agents in some city water supplies, cross the reverse osmosis membrane. A carbon filter will remove those substances (Gutch & Stoner, 1993).

Vascular Access for Hemodialysis

Circulatory access is the lifeline for patients depending on hemodialysis for survival. Since the first permanent access for hemodialysis was created in 1960 by Scribner and Quinton, there have been innumerable advances in this technology. This section will discuss the various types of vascular access used not only for hemodialysis but for continuous renal replacement therapies and therapeutic plasma exchange.

Temporary/Acute Vascular Access

Vascular access is frequently needed to emergently provide renal replacement therapy for patients with acute renal failure (ARF). Temporary access is also used to treat patients during the maturation period of a permanent access, or during revision of a permanent hemodialysis or peritoneal dialysis access. It is also required for patients needing hemoperfusion or therapeutic apheresis (Gutch & Stoner, 1993; Raja, 1994).

Central venous catheterization has become a well-accepted method used for temporary access for hemodialysis. This is accomplished through percutaneous cannulation of the femoral, subclavian, or internal jugular veins with single or double lumen catheters. Single lumen catheters are used to both pull blood from and return blood to the patient. A Y connection is attached to the end of the catheter, and blood is alternately pulled from the patient, passed through the dialyzer, and pushed back to the patient with the help of a single needle device (Bander & Schwab, 1992; Ismail & Hakim, 1991; Raja, 1994).

Double lumen catheters are used most commonly. They contain a partition or septum inside the catheter lumen, separating it into two blood pathways. One lumen opens at the tip of the catheter, and one opens at another site along the side of the catheter. This allows blood to be pulled from the patient via one lumen and returned to the patient through the other lumen with less recirculation. Long-term patency and complication rates of the two catheters are comparable (Ismail & Hakim, 1991; Raja, 1994).

Subclavian vein catheters. The subclavian vein is a common insertion site for acute dialysis catheters (see Figure 19-9). A catheter at this site can be left in place for several weeks and, once inserted, allows the patient to be comfortable, be ambulatory, remain at home, and receive hemodialysis as an outpatient. In addition to those advantages, the catheter can be used for hemodialysis almost immediately after insertion (Hartigan & Thomas-Hawkins, 1995; Raja, 1994).

The catheter can be inserted by a physician at the bedside, with the nurse assisting as needed. The right side is preferred for insertion for a number of reasons. The dome of the right lung is lower than the left, which decreases the chance of pneumothorax during insertion. Also, there is a relatively straight line to the atrium, and the thoracic duct is not endangered during the process of insertion. The side where a new arteriovenous fistula or graft has been or will be placed as well as the side previously used for a transvenous pacemaker insertion should not be for subclavian catheter insertion because of an increased risk of subclavian vein thrombosis (Ismail & Hakim, 1991; Raja, 1994).

Figure 19-9
Technique of subclavian vein cannulation.

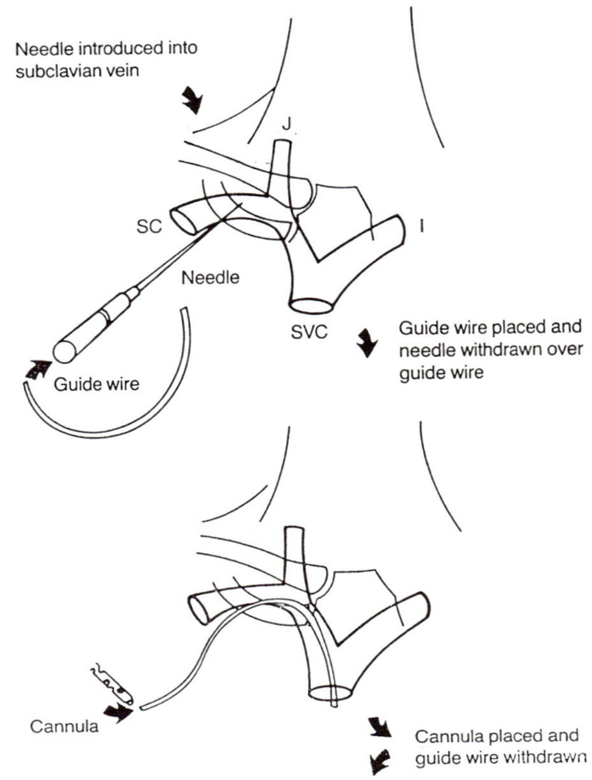

Note: From Bell, PR.F., & Veitch, P.S. (1990). Vascular access for hemodialysis. In A.R. Nissenson, R.N. Fine, & D.E. Gentile (Eds.). *Clinical dialysis* (2nd ed., pp. 26-44). Norwalk, CT: Appleton & Lange. Reprinted with permission.

Strict aseptic technique should be adhered to during catheter insertion with the physician wearing a sterile surgical gown and gloves as well as a mask. Proper positioning is essential to distend the subclavian vein. The patient should be placed in Trendelenburg position with a rolled towel placed longitudinally under the back between the scapulae. The patient's head should then be turned 45 degrees away from the side of insertion (Ismail & Hakim, 1991; Raja, 1994).

To prepare for catheter insertion, the skin is prepped with a disinfectant solution, and the physician anesthetizes the area. The subclavian vein is cannulated with a small (18-gauge) needle, then with an introducer. A guidewire is inserted into the vein through the introducer. The catheter is fed over the guidewire and is advanced into the superior vena cava (SVC) until the tip of the catheter is just above the junction of the superior vena cava and the right atrium. The guidewire is then removed, and each catheter lumen is heparinized.

After the catheter is sutured securely at the hub, its position must be confirmed by radiography. The nurse should ensure the catheter is never used for dialysis until a physician examines the x-ray and confirms the catheter placement in the SVC. The catheter insertion site is covered with a sterile dressing, which is changed at each dialysis session, or more frequently as needed (Bander & Schwab,1992; Ismail & Hakim, 1991; Raja, 1994).

There are several disadvantages to the use of a subclavian vein catheter for hemodialysis. Although it is considered a safe method of temporary access, complications can occur. Thrombosis or stenosis of the subclavian vein are possible complications that can affect venous outflow of the extremity or of subsequent accesses in the extremity. The catheter should not be inserted into a bacteremic patient until the patient's infection is being treated. In addition, the catheter must be removed if the patient develops positive blood cultures and has no other obvious source of infection. Removal is also recommended if purulent drainage is noted at the catheter exit site. Insertion may be difficult or impossible in a patient in pulmonary edema who is unable to tolerate placement in the Trendelenburg position. Finally, major life-threatening, insertion-related complications can occur. These include pneumothorax, puncture of the subclavian artery or the SVC, pericardial tamponade resulting from vessel erosion, arrhythmias secondary to endocardial irritation if the guidewire is passed too far, brachial plexus injury, superficial infections, and bacteremia (Ismail & Hakim, 1991; Raja, 1994).

Postinsertion complications include pneumothorax, hemothorax, arterial perforation, tissue perforation, and dysrhythmias (Hartigan & Thomas-Hawkins, 1995). Later complications include catheter infection and catheter-related septicemia. Local catheter infections include exit site or tract infections and catheter infections. Tract infections are often found when pus or inflammation is noted at the catheter exit site. Cultures of the purulent material will confirm the involved organism. Tract infection as well as catheter-related septicemia has been found to occur in up to 20% of catheters. These infections are usually secondary to staphylococcus epidermidis or staphylococcus aureus. Management of infection is to administer antibiotics based on the culture results for at least 7-10 days. Removal of the catheter is also an appropriate measure if there is purulent exudate at the catheter exit site, if the patient develops a temperature greater than 38 degrees centigrade, or if the patient has positive blood cultures. A new catheter can be inserted on the opposite side or at another site after 24-48 hours of treatment if the patient's blood cultures are negative (Bander & Schwab, 1992; Raja, 1994).

The catheter itself may become infected. The catheter material or a fibrin sheath may become colonized with bacteria if the patient is bacteremic from another source, or the catheter may become infected because of contamination when opened and connected to dialysis equipment. Again, treatment of this infection includes antibiotic therapy and, usually, catheter removal (Bander & Schwab, 1992).

Sepsis is a common complication of any central venous catheter. Prompt initiation of antibiotic therapy based on clinical symptoms, even prior to blood culture results, is important in the management of sepsis. Antibiotics can be modified according to culture results. Treatment should continue for 7-10 days, or 4-5 days after clinical signs and symptoms have resolved. Except in the extremely rare situation where the patient would be placed at significant risk during reinsertion of another catheter and is not clinically septic, catheter-related sepsis should also be treated by removal of the catheter. If the decision is made, however, to leave the catheter in place, the patient should be observed for a clear clinical response to the antibiotic therapy in less than 24 hours. The catheter must be removed if this response does not occur. If the patient responds to the antibiotic therapy, and the catheter is left in place, antibiotics should continue to be administered for 2-3 weeks (Bander & Schwab, 1992; Raja, 1994).

Most catheter-related infections can be prevented through an aseptic insertion and handling of the catheter and by minimizing the number of caregivers through restriction of the performance of dressing changes and catheter use to dialysis staff only. Interdialytic use of the catheter for infusions or blood draws should be avoided. A catheter that has become dislodged should never be pushed back into the patient. This can lead to infection, if not puncture of a vein. Dislodged catheters must be removed. A new catheter can be reinserted using the process of insertion of a new guidewire through the old catheter prior to removal and threading of a new catheter over this wire. The practice of replacing problem-free catheters every 2-3 weeks is still popular in some hemodialysis centers. The rationale for this practice is that the incidence of catheter-related sepsis is very low, approximately 5%, in catheters left in place less than 2 weeks. Other physicians feel that the risks associated with catheter insertion are greater than the risk of infection from a catheter left in place. In these centers, well-functioning, noninfected catheters are not routinely removed and replaced at specific time intervals (Bander & Schwab, 1992; Ismail & Hakim, 1991; Raja, 1994).

Thrombosis of the subclavian catheter is a common problem that can result in poor blood flow through the catheter. Whenever a foreign material such as a catheter is introduced into a vein, the immediate response of the vascular system is to initiate the formation of a clot. Endothelial injury may result in the release of thromboblastic substances that cause platelet aggregation at the insertion site. A clot may form on the interior surface of the catheter, or a fibrin sleeve may develop on the exterior surface and extend to the catheter tip over time. This is prevented by heparinization of the catheter lumen(s) between dialysis treatments. If clotting occurs, a thrombolytic agent such as urokinase or streptokinase may be placed in the catheter lumen(s) and allowed to dwell for 20-30 minutes, then aspirated. The use of urokinase has been shown in several studies (Brown et al., 1989; Schwab & Butler, 1988; Wachs, 1990) to safely restore patency by dissolving the clot. There is also evidence that it extends catheter life and reduces the number of catheter replacements, thus reducing patient risk as well as nursing and physician time. A mural thrombus may also develop along the vein wall secondary to endothelial injury. This type of thrombus usually resolves spontaneously with catheter removal; however, anticoagulation or thrombolytic therapy may be necessary (Bander & Schwab, 1992; Northsea, 1994; Raja, 1994).

Subclavian vein stricture or narrowing occurs following 20-50% of subclavian catheter insertions. Clinically significant subclavian vein thrombosis occurs in less than 20% of cases. Signs and symptoms of stricture and thrombosis are similar and include swelling of the involved arm, the development of collateral venous circulation in the affected shoulder, increased venous resistance during hemodialysis, and compromised flow through any subsequent AV fistulas or grafts placed in the extremity. Strictures are treated with balloon angioplasty with varying degrees of success. Thrombosis may be treated by systemic anticoagulation. Heparin is usually administered, followed by warfarin. This type of therapy is successful, most of the time, in decreasing edema in the extremity. Thrombolytic therapy is not usually effective and may be dangerous. Balloon angioplasty is used, with varying degrees of success, to treat subclavian vein strictures (Bander & Schwab, 1992; Raja, 1994).

Nursing management of central venous catheters include the use of aseptic technique when initiating or terminating dialysis, catheter exit site care and sterile dressing change at each hemodialysis treatment, and assessment of the patient for signs and symptoms of local or systemic infection (Hartigan & Thomas-Hawkins, 1995).

Femoral vein catheters. Femoral vein catheters are a relatively easy access to place for acute dialysis. A single or double lumen catheter is placed by the physician into the femoral vein and advanced into the inferior vena cava. Often, a femoral vein catheter is used for one dialysis treatment, then is removed. Therefore, it is safe for use in bacteremic patients (Ismail & Hakim, 1991; Raja, 1994).

The catheter can be inserted in either femoral vein as long as there is no history of surgery or thrombosis of the femoral vein or a history of aortofemoral or femoral-popliteal bypass surgeries. For insertion, the patient is placed supine, with the leg rotated outward. The groin should be shaved and skin prepped with an antibacterial agent such as povidone-iodine. The physician first locates the femoral pulse, which assists in location of the femoral vein that is 2 centimeters below the inguinal ligament and approximately 1 centimeter medial to the femoral pulse. Once the vein is located, the site is anesthetized. A small-gauge needle, an introducer, and then a guidewire are inserted into the vein. The catheter is inserted over the guidewire, and the wire is removed. Complications associated with insertion are puncture of the femoral artery, retroperitoneal bleeding, femoral vein thrombosis, and phlebitis (Ismail & Hakim, 1991; Raja, 1994).

Infection and thrombosis are not major complications of the femoral catheter since the catheter is usually removed after each treatment or after 1-2 days. If a second hemodialysis treatment is expected to be performed within 48 hours of insertion, the catheter can be left in. The patient must remain in the hospital on bed rest while the catheter is in place. This is the main disadvantage of the femoral catheter reported by patients (Raja, 1994).

A primary advantage of this access is the easy insertion. Insertion is possible in a semi-recumbent position; therefore, it is a good option for patients unable to tolerate the Trendelenburg position. Other advantages include the low infection rate, the catheter's safety for use in bacteremic patients, and the extremely low incidence of major complications associated with the catheter (Ismail & Hakim, 1991; Raja, 1994).

The nurse caring for the patient with a femoral catheter should observe for hematoma at the insertion site and assess distal pulses in the extremity before, during, and after insertion. The nurse should also be aware of signs of retroperitoneal bleeding, which include restlessness, hypotension, pain, decreased pulses, decreased outflow of blood, and increased venous pressure during dialysis. Care should be taken to ensure venous stasis after catheter removal by applying pressure to the insertion site for 20 minutes before applying a pressure dressing. Patients should be instructed to remain in bed with leg flat if the catheter is to be left in place for several dialysis treatments (Hartigan & Thomas-Hawkins, 1995).

Figure 19-10
Scribner shunts.

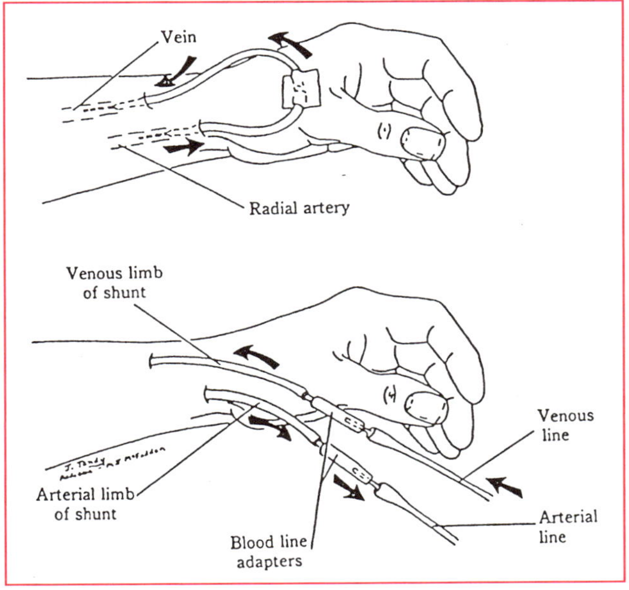

Note: From Raja, R.M. (1994). Vascular access for hemodialysis. In J.T. Daugirdas & T.S. Ing (Eds.). *Handbook of dialysis* (2nd ed., pp. 53-77). Boston: Little, Brown. Reprinted with permission.

Jugular vein catheters. Jugular vein catheters are also used for acute or temporary hemodialysis access. It is a popular access in the critical care setting in patients on ventilators, as the risk of pneumothorax is virtually eliminated. Many clinicians now view the jugular vein site as preferable to the subclavian vein in any patient. The high frequency of occurrence of vein thrombosis and stenosis with subclavian vein catheters make that site less preferable (Bander & Schwab, 1992; Raja, 1994).

As with the subclavian access, the right side is preferred for insertion of a jugular vein catheter. The right internal jugular has a straight path to the atrium. For insertion, the patient is supine and placed in Trendelenburg position (15 degrees). The head is extended and turned away from the side of the venipuncture. Insertion in patients who cannot lie in Trendelenburg is more difficult, but not impossible (Raja, 1994).

A jugular vein catheter can be left in place for up to several weeks, and ambulation is possible. The main disadvantage is that the catheter is often in an awkward position that impairs neck mobility. It is also, because of its position, often difficult to affix to the skin. The advantages include low risk of pneumothorax or hydrothorax, and a much lower incidence of delayed vessel stricture. Infection rates are similar to the subclavian catheter. Complications such as catheter infection, sepsis, and catheter thrombosis are treated in the same manner as those occurring in a subclavian vein catheter (Bander & Schwab, 1992; Ismail & Hakim, 1991; Raja, 1994).

External arteriovenous shunt. This access was first developed in 1960 by Scribner and Quinton for use as a semipermanent vascular access for both acute and chronic hemodialysis (see Figure 19-10). It consists of two hard Teflon cylinders or vessel tips, one implanted in an artery and one in a vein, connected to pieces of Silastic tubing. The tubing is connected in an end-to-end fashion to establish an external arteriovenous shunt. The continuous flow of blood through the tube usually prevents clotting without anticoagulation (Hartigan & Thomas-Hawkins, 1995; Ismail & Hakim, 1991; Raja, 1994).

The forearm (radial artery to cephalic vein) and the leg (posterior tibial artery to long saphenous vein at ankle) are the common sites for shunt placement. The upper arm is also sometimes used. The ankle site has the advantage of sparing upper extremities for subsequent permanent access (Ismail & Hakim, 1991; Raja, 1994).

Insertion of an external shunt is usually performed in the operating room, but can be performed at the bedside in a critical care setting. A local or regional anesthetic is used. The extremity may need to be elevated to prevent or reduce edema after insertion. The shunt should never be used for blood draws or infusions (Raja, 1994).

Currently, the shunt is rarely used for hemodialysis. The main advantage of a shunt is that it is available for immediate use for dialysis. Shunts are, however, prone to a fairly high incidence of infection and a higher incidence of thrombosis than other types of vascular access. Shunts are difficult (and sometimes impossible) to declot and often result in loss of peripheral vessels for permanent access placement. Accidental or intentional dislodgement or disconnection can be life-threatening. The advent of percutaneous access devices, which do not require the skill of a vascular surgeon for placement, has rendered it virtually obsolete. It may, however, still be used for continuous renal replacement therapies and, occasionally, as a temporary access (Bander & Schwab, 1992; Hartigan & Thomas-Hawkins, 1995; Raja, 1994).

Nursing care of the external arteriovenous shunt includes daily cleansing and dressing of the cannulae insertion sites as well as monitoring of the patient for signs and symptoms of localized and systemic infection. Patency of the shunt must be checked every 12 hours by evaluation of proximal pulsation at the venous limb and by listening for a bruit at that site. The external loop should also be observed. Cool temperature of the loop and separation of blood and plasma in the tubing indicate clotting. Thrombosis of the shunt is common, particularly in individuals with frequent hypotension, dehydration, or a hypercoagulable state. The use of anticoagulants or antiplatelet agents may prevent or decrease the incidence of clotting. Although a gauze dressing should be maintained over the shunt and exit sites at all times, circumferential tape around the extremity should be avoided. This can compromise venous return, which may result in thrombosis of the shunt. The patient should have bulldog clamps available, perhaps attached to the dressing, in case of disconnection (Raja, 1994).

Patient education should center on daily care of the shunt as well as observations to be made daily. The patient should be aware of signs and symptoms that require notification of the nurse or physician. Management of emergency situations such as dislodgement or disconnection is a crucial aspect of patient education. As dislodgement or disconnection could lead to exsanguination and loss of life, patients should be continuously monitored for signs of depression or feelings of hopelessness (Hartigan & Thomas-Hawkins, 1995).

Although declotting of a thrombosed shunt is seldom successful, it may be attempted if there are no signs of infection or phlebitis. The physician can use a #3 Fogarty catheter for declotting. The procedure is performed by insertion of the catheter into the clotted shunt, inflation of the catheter balloon, and withdrawal of the catheter along with the clot. After a successful declot procedure, the physician may consider administration of a heparin infusion. This is accomplished by insertion of a "T" tube connector in place of the usual straight connector between the limbs of the shunt. Heparin solution can then be infused continuously into the connector for 1-2 days. Since the most common cause of shunt thrombosis is poor venous return, a shunt angiogram may be ordered after a declot procedure (Ismail & Hakim, 1991; Raja, 1994).

Infection is a major complication of the external shunt. If the patient develops a fever, cultures should be obtained from the exit sites, and blood cultures should be drawn from the opposite arm. Usual treatment includes immediate antibiotic therapy and, in septicemia, shunt removal (Raja, 1994).

Permanent Vascular Access

One of the most important aspects in the total management of a patient with CRF is the establishment and maintenance of permanent vascular access. Dialysis access problems, however, remain responsible for much of the morbidity and cost associated with ESRD treatment as they account for up to 25% of hospitalizations in dialysis patients. Careful planning and preservation of the extremity prior to placement of the access, proper maturation, and prevention of complications after placement should be the focus of nursing care (Berkoben & Schwab, 1995).

Primary arteriovenous fistula (AVF). The primary AVF is the preferred long-term access for patients with CRF. It should be created 2-6 months

Figure 19-11
Typical sites for AV fistulae are indicated in this drawing.

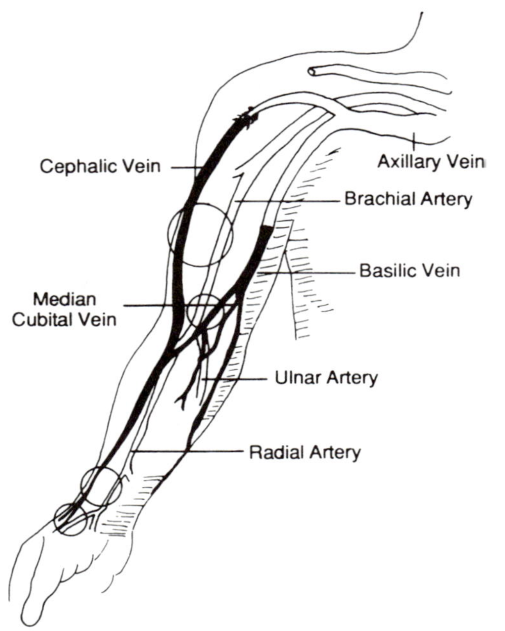

Note: From Hartigan, M.F., & Thomas-Hawkins, C. (1995). Circulatory access for hemodialysis. In L.E. Lancaster (Ed.). (1995). *ANNA Core Curriculum for Nephrology Nursing* (3rd ed., p. 265). Pitman, NJ: American Nephrology Nurses' Association. Reprinted with permission.

prior to anticipated initiation of dialysis therapy. An AVF is the safest and longest-lasting permanent vascular access, with a reported 3-year survival rate of 65-75%. It is preferable to the synthetic graft because of long-term patency and lower infection rates (Berkoben & Schwab, 1995; Ismail & Hakim, 1991; Raja, 1994).

The AVF is created in the operating room with a regional anesthesia. A subcutaneous anastomosis is created between an artery and a vein, allowing arterial blood to flow through the vein, causing venous engorgement and enlargement while preserving distal blood flow. There are several types of anastomoses used in the creation of an AVF. A side of artery to side of vein, end of artery to end of vein, end of artery to side of vein, or end of vein to side of artery connection can be created. During the next several months following creation, the fistula goes through a maturation process in which the venous limb dilates and the vessel wall thickens. This allows repeated insertion of large bore needles for hemodialysis (Hartigan & Thomas-Hawkins, 1995;

Ismail & Hakim, 1991). Typical sites for AVF are shown in Figure 19-11.

After the AVF matures, the veins proximal to the anastomosis are used for placement of both needles required for hemodialysis. The arterial needle is placed most distally, but at least 3-5 centimeters from the anastomosis. The venous needle is placed proximal to the arterial needle and at least 5 centimeters away. This lessens the possibility of recirculation of dialyzed blood during hemodialysis. The arterial needle can be inserted, pointing away from or toward the heart, and the venous needle is inserted pointing toward the heart. The manner in which the needles are inserted can affect the longevity of the AVF. Grouping of venipunctures in one or two areas can result in weakening of the vessel wall and subsequent aneurysm formation. Rotation of needle sites and use of the entire length of the AVF increases the life of the access (Ismail & Hakim, 1991; Raja, 1994).

Postoperative nursing care of the patient with an AVF includes observation for signs and symptoms of infection, frequent assessment of patency (i.e., palpation for thrill or auscultation for bruit over anastomosis site), elevation of the extremity after surgery to reduce edema, and avoidance of tight circumferential dressings around the extremity. Patient education should include these things as well as instruction in exercises aimed at increasing blood flow to the extremity, speeding dilatation of the arterialized blood vessels (Raja, 1994).

Advantages of the AVF include lower incidence of thrombosis and infection compared to other forms of vascular access, increased safety compared to external devices, low level of daily care, and lack of implanted synthetic materials that could lead to an allergic response. Well-developed AVFs have been reported to have the greatest longevity (3-year patency rate of approximately 70%) and lowest incidence of complications of all vascular accesses used for hemodialysis. The main disadvantage of the primary AVF is the length of time required for maturation before it is ready for use for hemodialysis (Hartigan & Thomas-Hawkins, 1995).

Complications of the AVF include primary nondevelopment, poor blood flow, recirculation, thrombosis, steal syndrome, venous hypertension, aneurysm/pseudoaneurysm formation, infection, and high-output congestive heart failure (Stackiewicz, 1994; Raja, 1994).

Primary nondevelopment of AVFs can occur for a number of reasons, including insufficient vasculature such as poor arterial flow or small vein size or can be due to a less than optimal anastomosis or venous hypertension. Diagnosis is made through assessment of degree of fistula maturation and Doppler ultrasound to determine blood flow and assess for proximal vessel stenosis. Ligation of distal veins is the treatment of choice (Hartigan & Thomas-Hawkins, 1995).

The most common cause of poor flow from an AVF is partial obstruction secondary to clotting or fibrosis. Fibrosis often occurs as a result of multiple venipunctures. Poor flow can lead to thrombosis, so early detection and treatment is important. High venous pressures and excess negative pressures at the arterial site are common signs of partial obstruction and should be indications for further workup (Raja, 1994).

Fistulograms can be used to assess patency in patients who have demonstrated signs of possible obstruction. Injection of angiography dye can often locate the area of obstruction. Although this test can identify an abnormality, it cannot give information about function of the access. Screenings such as venous pressure readings and recirculation studies should be used as predictors to select cases for fistulograms. Duplex Doppler Color Flow studies and intravascular ultrasound may accurately measure AVF blood flow and access patency. Intravascular ultrasound also provides information on composition and precise intraluminal dimensions of stenotic lesions (Stackiewicz, 1994).

Patency of the AVF can be assessed by palpating for a thrill or auscultating for a bruit over the anastomosis site. Measurement of venous pressure on the venous blood line is important in the assessment of access patency. Consistently increasing venous pressure can, in most cases, reliably identify patients at risk for significant venous stenosis and allow for early intervention, which may reduce the incidence of thrombosis and prolong access viability (Stackiewicz, 1994).

Percutaneous transluminal angioplasty (PCTA) is a method of correction of venous stenosis. More than 50% of stenotic and occlusive lesions are improved following PCTA. Although the recurrence rate is 25%, most lesions can be successfully treated with repeat angioplasty. Successful correction of venous stenosis will result in prolongation of access life (Berkoben & Schwab, 1995; Stackiewicz, 1994).

In the absence of sufficient forward blood flow through the AVF during hemodialysis, dialyzed blood returning to the access through the venous needle will reenter the extracorporeal circuit via the arterial needle. This direct recirculation of dialyzed blood through the extracorporeal circuit is usually a result of venous stenosis proximal to the venous needle and reduces effective urea clearance. It can also be caused by incorrect needle placement, inappropriately high blood flow setting, hypotension, low cardiac output, volume depletion, or arterial stenosis (Berkoben & Schwab, 1995; Raja, 1994; Stackiewicz, 1994).

Urea recirculation tests can identify patients

with significant venous stenoses. Although there are several methods for performing a recirculation study, consistency in technique and timing is important in each method in order to obtain accurate, reproducible, and interpretable results. Blood samples should be obtained during the first hour of dialysis before cardiac output and blood pressure have been greatly affected by ultrafiltration. They also should be obtained at a standard extracorporeal blood flow rate (Berkoben & Schwab, 1995; Stackiewicz, 1994).

The most widely used method of obtaining blood samples for recirculation is a three-needle method in which blood is obtained simultaneously from the arterial blood line, the venous blood line, and a peripheral vein in the contralateral arm. Other techniques are used in which the arterial and venous line samples are obtained at the standard blood flow rate. Then the peripheral blood sample is obtained from the arterial line either at a reduced blood flow rate of 50 ml per minute or with the blood flow halted (see the two-needle procedure in Table 19-3) (Berkoben & Schwab, 1995).

Recirculation values of 15-20% have been found to be highly predictive of venous stenosis or occlusion. Fistulography should be considered in patients in which urea recirculation exceeds these levels (Berkoben & Schwab, 1995).

Thrombosis of the AVF can occur soon after surgery or as a late event. Early thrombosis usually occurs because of technical factors during the surgery or the premature use of the AVF for dialysis. Late thrombosis is commonly preceded by poor flow through the AVF, but may be precipitated by periods of dehydration, hypotension, or hypercoagulability. AVF thrombosis can also occur as a result of fistula compression during sleep or possibly because of excessive compression of the access to achieve hemostasis after hemodialysis. Although there is no conclusive evidence implicating repetitive occlusion as a risk factor for thrombosis, nurses should never totally occlude an access to achieve hemostasis (Hartigan, 1994). It had been thought that higher hematocrit levels secondary to the treatment of anemia with erythropoietin would lead to increased rates of access thrombosis. However, this has not been found to be the case when hematocrits are maintained within the recommended range (Berkoben & Schwab, 1995).

Declotting of the AVF can be performed either by surgically opening and cleaning the vessel with a Fogarty catheter, or medically, with a thrombolytic agent such urokinase. Once thrombosis has occurred, long-term salvage of the access may be difficult. However there may be an obstruction that is correctable (Raja, 1994).

Ischemia of the distal extremity, commonly called *steal syndrome*, occurs most commonly in patients with previously compromised circulation, such as older patients, or patients with diabetes mellitus or atherosclerosis. For example, with the side-to-side radiocephalic anastomosis, approximately one-third of the blood through the anastomosis normally comes from the ulnar artery via the palmar arch. Because of this, the AVF regularly steals blood from the ulnar artery system. Symptoms include pain in the hand upon exercise, a cold, clammy feeling, and, in extreme circumstances, rest pain and appearance of nonhealing ulcers. Venous hypertension resulting in edema and pain of the distal extremity may also occur as the result of a side-to-side anastomosis and transmission of arterial pressure to veins of the hand. Both problems may be relieved by conversion of the anastomosis from side of vein to end of vein (Raja, 1994).

Aneurysm and pseudoaneurysm of the venous limb of the anastomosis are common complica-

Table 19-3
Procedure for drawing noninvasive, two needles, stop flow percent recirculation.

1. Measure within the first 30 minutes after prescribed blood flow is established.
2. Samples are drawn simultaneously from the arterial and venous lines into syringes labeled "arterial" and "venous," then placed in tubes labeled "arterial sample" and "venous sample."
3. Ultrafiltration is reduced to minimum.
4. The blood pump is stopped.
5. Clamp arterial needle and blood lines.
6. Separate the arterial needle and blood lines.
7. Withdraw 10 ml from the arterial needle line, keep sterile, and set aside.
8. Within 30 seconds of stopping blood flow, withdraw 5 ml from arterial needle line and place in tube. Label "Systemic Sample."
9. Return the 10 ml of sterile blood that was set aside.
10. Reconnect arterial needle and blood lines.
11. Reestablish blood flow.

Formula for percent recirculation of vascular access:

$$\frac{S-A}{S-V} \times 100 = \%\ \text{recirculation}$$

Note: From Hartigan, M.F., & Thomas-Hawkins, C. (1995). Circulatory access for hemodialysis. In L.E. Lancaster (Ed.). (1995). *ANNA Core Curriculum for Nephrology Nursing* (3rd ed., p. 267). Pitman, NJ: American Nephrology Nurses' Association. Reprinted with permission.

tions. Aneurysms occur most commonly at the anastomosis site but can occur in other areas of the vessel as the result of repeated cannulation of the same site. Dilatation of the vessel wall and a bounding pulse over the area are commons signs. Pseudoaneurysm is the most common of the two lesions and occurs secondary to extravasation of blood after removal of the dialysis needles. Most are treated conservatively by observation and by avoidance of the area for venipunctures. However, if there is marked thinning of the overlying skin, surgical repair becomes necessary to avoid rupture. Nurses can aid in preventing aneurysms and pseudoaneurysms by rotating cannulation sites and by ensuring venous stasis when needles are removed. Patients with aneurysms or pseudoaneurysms should be taught to avoid trauma at the site and to report signs and symptoms of infection immediately (Hartigan & Thomas-Hawkins, 1995; Raja, 1994).

Infection of the AVF is rare, but is usually secondary to staphylococcus aureus when it occurs. Often it is due to a break in aseptic technique during cannulation, poor hygiene of the access extremity, or bacterial seeding from another infected site. Prophylactic antibiotic treatment may help avoid resultant access infection in patients undergoing invasive procedures. Diagnosis is based on local signs of infection or inflammation, and confirmation is made with local and blood cultures. Treatment of an infected AVF with systemic antibiotics is often curative when accompanied by local care. The need for surgical revision or access loss, however, may result (Hartigan & Thomas-Hawkins, 1995; Ismail & Hakim, 1991; Raja, 1994).

Nurses should use strict aseptic technique during cannulation of an AVF and avoid cannulation through an obviously inflamed area. The AVF and the patient should always be assessed for signs and symptoms of infection prior to cannulation. The patient should be instructed to report any signs or symptoms of local or systemic infection and to inform staff of any scheduled invasive procedures (Hartigan & Thomas-Hawkins, 1995).

High cardiac output congestive heart failure can result due to the high blood flow rate through the AVF, particularly in patients with severe anemia or preexisting cardiovascular disease. Blood flow rates through the AVF can range from 200 to 600 ml per minute. High output CHF is unusual with a radiocephalic AVF, but can occur more frequently in upper arm or femoral AVFs (Hartigan & Thomas-Hawkins, 1995; Raja, 1994). Signs include tachycardia, pulmonary rales, shortness of breath, and/or jugular vein distension despite the patient being at or near estimated dry weight. Diagnosis is confirmed when cardiac studies show marked changes in cardiac output with transient occlusion of the fistula. The usual treatment is then surgical narrowing or banding of the fistula. Until the problem is corrected surgically, measures such as wrapping the fistula with an elastic bandage when not being used may help to decrease cardiac output. The patient should also be instructed to minimize his or her activity and interdialytic weight gains in the interim (Hartigan & Thomas-Hawkins, 1995; Raja, 1994).

Although the AVF is certainly the preferred vascular access for many reasons, it is not the most commonly found access in most dialysis centers. As the percentage of elderly diabetic patients increases in the dialysis population, the number of patients requiring the use of synthetic grafts has also increased. Many elderly and diabetic patients do not have suitable vascular anatomy for construction and maturation of endogenous AVFs. Approximately 25% of AVFs fail to mature after construction. Fewer than one-third of current dialysis patients have functional primary AVFs. Most of these patients are dialyzed using synthetic arteriovenous grafts.

Arteriovenous grafts. The arteriovenous (AV) graft is a type of access created when an arteriovenous connection is made using a tube graft from a biologic source or one made of synthetic material. Common sources of biologic grafts include the autogenous saphenous vein, human umbilical vein, and the bovine carotid artery. Biologic grafts, although once used in many patients, have been virtually replaced by synthetic arteriovenous grafts. Synthetic grafts are created with tubes of materials such as polytetrafluoroethylene (PTFE). Although the AV graft can be used sooner than the AVF and cannulation is often easier, this access is not as desirable as a direct connection of an artery to a vein because of lower patency rates and higher complication rates. The AV graft, however, has the advantage of being a useful alternative in patients, such as the elderly or diabetics, in which an AVF cannot be successfully created (Berkoben & Schwab, 1995; Hartigan & Thomas-Hawkins, 1995; Ismail & Hakim, 1991; Raja, 1994).

AV grafts are placed in the operating room, usually using regional anesthesia. The grafts are either placed as a straight graft or as a loop graft with the ends of the graft attached to the sides of the artery and the vein (see Figure 19-12). Straight grafts may be placed in the forearm (radial artery to basilic vein) or in the upper arm. Loop grafts are placed in the forearm (brachial artery to basilic vein) or in the upper arm or the thigh. Grafts in upper arms and thighs are associated with higher complication rates (Ismail & Hakim, 1991; Raja, 1994).

Prophylactic antibiotics are commonly administered preoperatively or intraoperatively when a graft is inserted. Postoperative care and nursing management is the same as for the AVF. Grafts can theoretically be used immediately for hemodialysis, but this practice is not recommended. It is preferable to wait for a 3-4 week (minimum 2-week) maturation period. This delay allows healing of the subcutaneous tunnel. The tunnel fills in with granulated tissue that will stabilize and reseal the graft after cannulation. Earlier use, prior to healing of the tunnel, could result in extravasation and spread of blood though the tunnel with subsequent hematoma and graft compression (Berkoben & Schwab, 1995; Hartigan & Thomas-Hawkins, 1995; Raja, 1994).

To perform hemodialysis, both needles are placed directly into the graft. The arterial needle is inserted in the section of the graft closest to the artery-graft anastomosis and should be placed at least 3 centimeters away from the anastomosis. The venous needle is inserted into the section of the graft closest to the venous anastomosis, at least 5 centimeters from the arterial needle site. Special care should be taken when placing needles in loop grafts to ensure that they are oriented to the flow of blood through the graft. The majority of forearm loop grafts will have the arterial limb on the medial (ulnar) side. In about 20% of cases, however, the arterial limb may lie on the radial aspect of the forearm. Care should also be taken when needles are removed from the graft. The needles should be removed at the same angle at which they were inserted to avoid further tearing of the graft wall. Pressure should be applied to the insertion site, only after the needle is totally removed, both over the site of skin insertion as well as over the site of graft entry (Hartigan & Thomas-Hawkins, 1995; Raja, 199).

PTFE grafts are durable and will withstand multiple venipunctures, thrombectomies, and revision. They do not, however, last forever, and will eventually fail as a result of multiple needle punctures. The 3-year patency rate associated with arteriovenous grafts is approximately 30%, much lower than the 70% long-term patency rate described with AVFs (Raja, 1994).

Patient education related to grafts should focus on assessment of the graft for patency and measures to maintain patency. As with the AVF, the patient should be taught to palpate for a thrill at the venous anastomosis daily and to notify the physician if it is absent. The patient should be instructed to avoid circumferential pressure around the access extremity, such as wearing a watch or a tight sleeve, and to avoid sleeping on the arm with the graft. The patient should also be aware that no blood pressures or venipunctures should be taken in the extremity with the graft.

Recognition of the signs and symptoms of a graft infection or sepsis is another skill that should be taught to the patient and family. Ideally, the patient needs to be able to detect these symptoms early and report appropriately to the physician or nurse.

Figure 19-12
Graft AV fistulae.

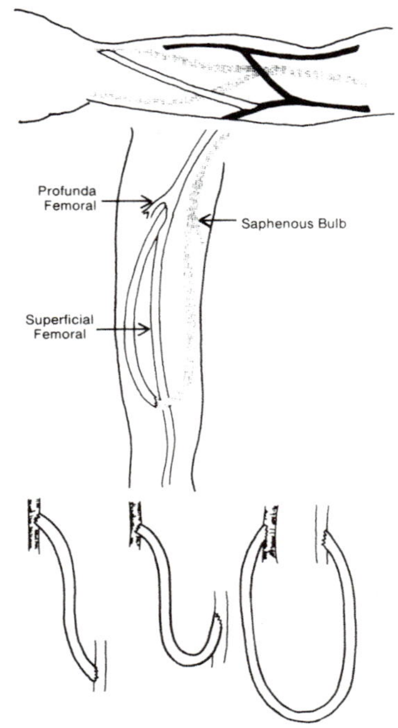

Top: graft interposed between radial artery and basilic vein. Middle: graft interposed between superficial femoral artery and saphenous vein. Bottom: various arrangements for AV grafts (straight, curved, loop).

Note: From Hartigan, M.F., & Thomas-Hawkins, C. (1995). Circulatory access for hemodialysis. In L.E. Lancaster (Ed.). (1995). *ANNA Core Curriculum for Nephrology Nursing* (3rd ed., p. 271). Pitman, NJ: American Nephrology Nurses' Association. Reprinted with permission.

Complications of the AV graft include stenosis, thrombosis, infection, poor flow, aneurysm/pseudoaneurysm, steal syndrome, venous hypertension, and high cardiac output CHF. Stenosis at the venous anastomosis or in the vein immediately proximal to it is a common complication and the most common cause of poor flow through grafts. It often leads to graft thrombosis. Intimal fibromuscular hyperplasia is the cause of stenosis and is most common at the venous end (Ismail & Hakim, 1991; Raja, 1994).

Clinical indicators suggestive of stenosis include frequent clotting, difficult needle placement, and persistent arm edema. A venous pressure greater than 50 mmHg before starting the blood flow as well as a venous pressure greater than 100 mmHg at a 200 ml per minute blood flow rate also indicates stenosis at the venous end. This is demonstrated by a high pressure in the dialyzer and blood outlet line during hemodialysis. Access recirculation of more than 15% is another indicator. Physical findings at the access site indicating stenosis include a discontinuous, harsh, high-pitched systolic bruit. Attention to these indicators as predictors of imminent graft failure is important. Early detection of stenoses enhances the possibility of correction of the lesion and extension of useful graft life (Berkoben & Schwab, 1995; Raja, 1994).

Further evaluation of the stenosis can be achieved by use of the Color Doppler Ultrasound, which allows imaging of blood flow through the AV graft. It is a noninvasive procedure that appears to be promising as a useful tool for detecting stenoses and microaneurysms. Low blood flow rates may be predictive of venous outflow obstruction. Digital subtraction angiography can also be used to evaluate stenoses. This test provides a well-defined view of the proximal anastomosis. It is not a good screening tool since it is an invasive study, but is useful in follow-up of stenotic lesions (Berkoben & Schwab, 1995; Raja, 1994).

Angioplasty of the stenotic lesion has an initial success rate of 90-95% with a 30-40% reduction venous pressure. Restenosis is common after 1 year. Only 40% of accesses will be functional at that time. Restenosis rates in subclavian veins is higher (70% at 6 months). As with the AVF, restenoses can often again be corrected with angioplasty. If the stenosis is large, a jump graft around the lesion may be used (Berkoben & Schwab, 1995; Ismail & Hakim, 1991).

Thrombosis is the most common complication and, as in the AVF, may occur early or late. Early is usually attributable to surgical problems, hypotension, premature graft use with hematoma formation in the tunnel, or anatomic causes. Late thrombosis is usually secondary to venous outflow tract stenosis, in fact, up to 80% have been linked to anatomic lesions. The majority of venous stenoses are found within 2-3 centimeters of the vein-graft anastomosis. Most are secondary to progressive intimal hyperplasia and fibrosis (Berkoben & Schwab, 1995; Ismail & Hakim, 1991).

Treatment of thrombus with balloon declotting or thrombolytic therapy should be followed by angiographic assessment of the graft. Injection of streptokinase directly into the clotted graft under high pressure (pulsed-spray therapy) and manual massage of the clot is successful in 60-70% of cases. Recurrent thromboses occurring despite good flow or other apparent cause may be treated with oral anticoagulation or antiplatelet therapy. Venous stenosis related to AV grafts can be treated with balloon angioplasty as described with the AVF. Surgical bypass of the venous stenosis has proven successful in the treatment of venous stenoses. The bypass method, however, extends the graft, thus possibly eliminating future access sites (Berkoben & Schwab, 1995; Ismail & Hakim, 1991).

Infection is more common with AV grafts than with AVFs and is also more serious. Including both local and systemic infections, the incidence is 5-20% of grafts. Septicemia may occur without local signs of infection. Infection is the second most common cause of graft loss. Signs and symptoms include erythema, edema, pain, fluid collection around the graft, fever, and chills during hemodialysis (Berkoben & Schwab, 1995; Hartigan & Thomas-Hawkins, 1995; Ismail & Hakim, 1991; Raja, 1994).

Common causes of AV graft infection are break in aseptic technique during cannulation or surgical procedure, poor hygiene of access extremity, and bacterial seeding from another infected site. Most common causal organisms include *Staphylococcus aureus, Staphylococcus epidermidis*, and, rarely, E. coli or other gram negative organisms. Staphlococcus aureus infection is particularly worrisome because this organism tends to lead to other infections such as endocarditis, osteomyelitis, meningitis, and others. Longer antibiotic courses, up to 4-6 weeks, are often prescribed for patients with staphylococcus aureus infection, in an attempt to prevent such metastasis. Blood cultures should be obtained at the conclusion of the antibiotic therapy to ensure adequate treatment of the infection (Berkoben & Schwab, 1995; Hartigan & Thomas-Hawkins, 1995; Ismail & Hakim, 1991; Raja, 1994).

In addition to antibiotic therapy, treatment may include local revision of the infected segment. The extent of the surgery required depends upon the extent of the infection. Incision and drainage or a partial graft removal and bypass grafting may eradicate the problem. This may salvage the graft; however, removal of the graft is often necessary. Hemorrhage can occur due to rupture of an infected graft, particularly if the initial sign of the infection has been bleeding through eroded skin over the graft. This clinical sign mandates graft removal (Berkoben & Schwab, 1995; Ismail & Hakim, 1991; Raja, 1994).

Measures to prevent graft infection include prophylactic antibiotics when patients undergo procedures capable of inducing bacteremia such as dental extraction or cleaning or gastrointestinal manipulation. Also, avoiding graft utilization for at least 2 weeks after insertion, when edema and inflammation have abated, as well as avoiding high risk locations such as the groin can minimize the risk of infection. Nurses should ensure that adequate skin preparation with an antimicrobial solution is accomplished prior to needle insertion for dialysis. Patient-related risk factors such as poor personal hygiene or practices such as intravenous drug use should be included in patient education (Berkoben & Schwab, 1995; Raja, 1994).

Aneurysms and pseudoaneurysms are common problems with grafts, more so than with AVFs. They usually can be corrected with local resection and interposition of a new graft segment. As with AVFs, rotation of cannulation sites and appropriate pressure to achieve venous stasis after needle removal are measures found to be successful in prevention of this problem (Hartigan & Thomas-Hawkins, 1995).

Steal syndrome, or ischemia of the distal extremity, can occur with grafts and necessitate surgical revision. It is caused when normal arterial blood supply to the distal extremity is shunted through the access, thus depriving the distal extremity of oxygenated blood (Raja, 1994).

Nursing management of steal syndrome centers on symptom control. Placing the graft extremity in a dependent position gives the distal extremity more circulation due to gravity and may reduce pain. Keeping the distal extremity warm may also help. The patient should be instructed in meticulous skin care for the extremity to avoid breakdown (Hartigan & Thomas-Hawkins, 1995).

Venous hypertension and high cardiac output congestive heart failure can be seen with AV grafts just as with AVFs. Management of these complications is addressed in the discussion of the primary AVF.

Cuffed double-lumen silastic catheters. Double-lumen silastic catheters with felt cuffs are used, in some instances, for vascular access in chronic hemodialysis patients. The catheter is subcutaneously tunneled and surgically implanted into a large vein via the internal jugular or subclavian vein (see Figure 19-13). After insertion, there is ingrowth of connective tissue at the cuff, which greatly reduces the rate of infection and holds the catheter in place. Disadvantages include thrombosis and infection, although infection appears to occur less frequently in cuffed catheters than in those without cuffs (Berkoben & Schwab, 1995; Hartigan & Thomas-Hawkins, 1995).

Some centers report catheter survival rates of 75% at 1 year and 50% at 2 years. Thus, it is becoming an alternative form of long-term vascular access for certain types of patients. The most common of these catheters is the PermCath (Quinton Instrument Co., Seattle, WA), but there are other catheters that are also used (Berkoben & Schwab, 1995; Raja, 1994).

Use of the PermCath is indicated in patients in whom it is difficult to readily insert an AVF or graft. It can provide a long-term access in children, diabetics, and morbidly obese patients. It is also useful in patients who have exhausted all other access sites and in patients who experience high output congestive failure with a primary AVF or an AV graft. The PermCath is also indicated for use as a temporary access in patients awaiting maturation of a permanent access (Berkoben & Schwab, 1995; Hartigan & Thomas-Hawkins, 1995; Raja, 1994).

The preferred insertion site is the internal jugular vein. The subclavian vein can be used, but the incidence of thrombosis and stenosis is higher there. Important on insertion is the alignment of the arterial port on the catheter tip away from the caval wall to avoid adherence to the wall during HD. The catheter is inserted through a subcutaneous tunnel and into the vein (Berkoben & Schwab, 1995; Raja, 1994).

Figure 19-13
Cuffed double-lumen hemodialysis catheter inserted through a subcutaneous tunnel into the right internal jugular vein.

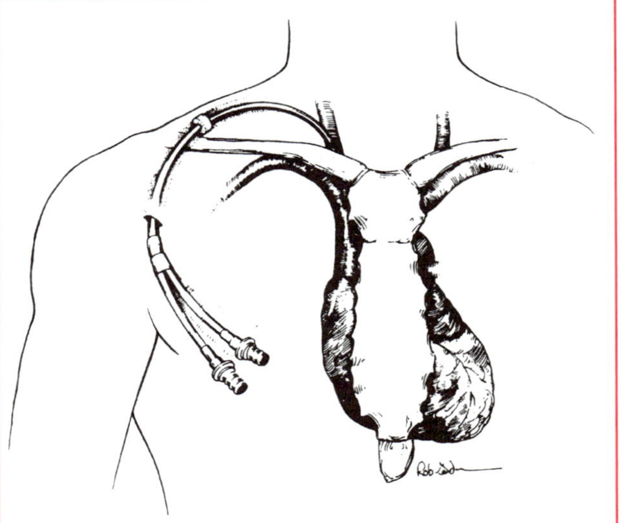

Note: From Berkoben, M., & Schwab, S.J. (1995). Maintenance of hemodialysis vascular access patency. *ANNA Journal, 22*(1), 17-24. Reprinted with permission.

A major disadvantage of the PermCath is that lower blood flow rates are usually achieved. Although the life of the catheter can be nearly as long as that for a synthetic graft, blood flow rates through the catheter have been found to average only 250 ml per minute. Since many patients require higher blood flow rates to achieve adequate hemodialysis, the long-term use of these catheters should be restricted only to those patients who have no other access option (Berkoben & Schwab, 1995; Moss et al., 1990).

Complications are similar to those of acute catheters, with thrombosis and infection being the most common. As with temporary catheters, occlusion secondary to thrombus has been safely and successfully relieved with thrombolytic agents such as urokinase. This practice has almost eliminated the need for catheter replacement due to thrombosis (Northsea, 1994).

Catheter exit site infection, with or without bacteremia, is treated similarly to acute catheters. Bacteremia with most central lines is usually an indication for catheter removal. However in patients with a PermCath in place, the catheter may represent the last readily-available form of access. Some centers report good results with antibiotics and changing the catheter over a guidewire. Infection and insufficient blood flow continue to be the most frequent reasons cited for catheter failure. Nursing care, as with temporary catheters, should focus on prevention and recognition of infection. Frequent assessment of the patient for clinical signs of inadequate dialysis should also be performed (Berkoben & Schwab, 1995; Moss, et al., 1990; Raja, 1994).

Without well-functioning vascular access, other hemodialysis technology is rendered virtually useless. Nursing has an important role in maintaining adequate vascular access. The most crucial of nursing interventions related to vascular access are those aimed at prevention of complications. Those measures include use of strict aseptic technique, rotation of cannulation sites, and minimizing trauma with cannulation, as well as prevention of blood flow interruption to the access such as hypotensive episodes or occlusion during hemostasis. Patient education should focus on proper hygiene and optimal nutrition (Hartigan, 1994).

The Hemodialysis Prescription

In 1976, as a result of the need to develop an assessment tool for dialysis adequacy, the National Institutes of Health commissioned a multicenter study to examine and compare various hemodialysis regimens regarding patient outcomes. Thus, the National Cooperative Dialysis Study (NCDS) was conducted between 1978 and 1983. A group of 151 hemodialysis patients were randomized into high and low treatment groups and monitored for a minimum of 6 months. The amount of dialysis delivered to each patient was measured using the kinetic model of Kt/V. This formula computes the amount of dialysis using the parameters of dialyzer clearance (K), time on dialysis (t), and the volume of urea distribution in the patient (V). It also takes into account the patient's normalized protein catabolic rate (NCPR) (Depner, 1991; Levin et al., 1991; Threlkeld, 1991).

The NCDS revealed that dialysis prescription had an effect on the occurrence of medical complications and hospitalization rates in hemodialysis patients. Patients who received less dialysis, those with Kt/V levels of 0.8 or less, developed worsening uremic manifestations such as gastrointestinal, cardiac, and hematologic problems. Those patients with Kt/V levels between 0.9 and 1.5 had much lower morbidity rates. The results of this study provided the nephrology community with two important tools. A measurable definition of adequate dialysis resulted: a Kt/V of 1.0 or higher (Depner, 1991; Threlkeld, 1991).

Although there continues to be argument about the appropriate target Kt/V for hemodialysis (1.0-1.4), kinetic modeling provides nephrologists and nephrology nurses with a tool for determining individualized dialysis prescription and for monitoring the effectiveness of treatment delivery (Burrows-Hudson, 1995; Depner, 1991; Threlkeld, 1991). Kinetic modeling and target Kt/V is used in the nephrology field to determine adequacy of treatment.

Since the 1980s, there has been a continuous evolution of the concept of adequacy. The term *adequacy*, when used by nephrology professionals, indicates the effect of renal replacement therapy to overcome most uremic symptoms and allow for maximum patient rehabilitation. It refers to a clinical endpoint and a predictor of morbidity and mortality (Burrows-Hudson, 1995; Ronco et al., 1994). Burrows-Hudson (1995) suggests that the nephrology community has settled, after much discussion, on the term *adequate* when the goal of dialytic therapy is actually to optimize. How to best measure adequate or optimal therapy is still under discussion.

Currently, the nephrology health care team looks at several indicators in addition to Kt/V to determine adequacy of and patient response to therapy. Measurements such as hematocrit and albumin as well as assessment of patient symptoms, fluid volume status, bone disease, and functional status and well-being are examined in conjunction with Kt/V to determine patient response to therapy and to individualize the patient's hemodialysis prescription.

Amount of Dialysis

Length of time on dialysis, dialyzer clearance, and adequate blood flow rate are the most important determinants of the amount of dialysis. These factors are taken into account when prescribing a dialysis treatment and can be adjusted to achieve the desired results. Results are based on the removal of uremic toxins, represented by urea.

Nephrologists usually prescribe dialysis treatment time as well as the dialyzer and blood flow rate to achieve greater than a 65% reduction in the blood urea nitrogen (BUN) during the treatment. This measurement is called the urea reduction ratio (URR). The URR indicates the amount of urea removed during a specific dialysis session. It does not account for urea removed with UF nor does it take residual renal function into account as does the Kt/V measurement. Although URR does not give a complete picture of dialysis adequacy, it is used to trend adequacy because one can predict what URR needs to be accomplished to achieve a specific Kt/V. In general, a URR of 65% will translate into an approximate Kt/V of 1.2 in an average sized adult.

Predialysis BUN is not a good parameter for use in determination of the dialysis prescription as it is greatly affected by the patient's protein intake. Time on dialysis is frequently the first parameter to be adjusted to changes in the predialysis BUN or to the urea reduction rate. An exception to the desired

65% reduction in BUN is a treatment such as the first in a patient with severe azotemia or hyponatremia, or in which disequilibrium syndrome is a risk. For this patient, only a 30% reduction in BUN is desired. This lower urea reduction is often accomplished with a shortened treatment length, a slower concurrent blood flow rate, and a lower efficiency dialyzer. After the first treatment, blood flow rate is increased over several treatments, to the desired level (300-450 ml/minute) as is the treatment length increased to 3-4 hours. The dialyzer may also be changed to a higher efficiency one (Daugirdas, 1994; Levin, 1991; Threlkeld, 1991).

When prescribing a dialyzer, consideration should be given to possible differences between the in-vitro calculations of clearance and the actual in-vivo clearances in the clinical setting. In-vivo clearances are often lower (Threlkeld, 1991).

Dialysis Solution

All dialysis solution (dialysate) is based in either acetate or bicarbonate. Bicarbonate is the base of choice when choosing a solution unless the patient is at risk for metabolic or respiratory alkalosis. Bicarbonate dialysate is best particularly for treatments in which a high BFR is used. The usual level of bicarbonate is 35 mEq/liter. The hemodynamically stable patient can be dialyzed with an acetate-based solution of 35-38 mEq/liter (Daugirdas, 1994).

Dialysate sodium is usually 135-145 mEq/liter; however, most dialysis treatments are performed with a dialysate sodium of 140 mEq/liter. If the patient has marked predialysis hypernatremia or hyponatremia, it can be adjusted accordingly. Solution with a sodium level of 3-4 mEq/liter lower than serum sodium should not be used unless absolutely necessary as it will cause the blood returning to the patient to be hyponatremic compared to the interstitial fluid. This will result in water leaving the hypernatremic blood and moving into the interstitial and intracellular spaces, causing a rapid decrease in circulating blood volume even with low UF rates. This could lead to hypotension or cramps and could contribute to or exacerbate disequilibrium. Thus, it is best to keep dialysate sodium at or slightly above plasma level (Daugirdas, 1994; Ismail & Hakim, 1991).

Dialysate sodium levels greater than 140 mEq/liter have, at times, been associated with increased thirst, increased interdialytic weight gains, and hypertension. Recent studies have shown that high and variable sodium dialysate can be used successfully in preventing and treating dialysis disequilibrium (Jenson et al., 1994). This concept will be discussed further in the section on hemodialysis complications.

Potassium in dialysate can range from 0 to 4.5 mEq/liter, with most treatments using a range from 2 to 4 mEq/liter. Zero potassium dialysate is rarely used due to risk of too rapid lowering of serum potassium, resulting in arrhythmias. Also, correction of severe acidosis during HD will cause a shift of potassium, into the cells, further lowering the serum potassium and possibly leading to arrhythmias as well. For patients with a prehemodialysis potassium of 5.5, a dialysate containing 2 mEq/liter of potassium should be adequate. However, for patients on digitalis, the level should be higher, such as 2.5-3 mEq/liter. If the patient's serum potassium is greater than 7, a 2 mEq/liter dialysate can be used; however it may rapidly decease the serum potassium. Lab values should be monitored and dialysate potassium adjusted during the treatment as necessary (Daugirdas, 1994).

There is evidence that a dialysate calcium of less than 3.0 mEq/liter can predispose patients to hypotension. If the patient has predialysis hypocalcemia, a higher dialysate calcium should be used, or ionized calcium will be lowered further, predisposing the patient to seizures (Daugirdas, 1994; Ismail & Hakim, 1991).

For acute hemodialysis, the dialysate should always contain 200 mg/dl of dextrose. Septic patients, diabetics, and patients on beta blockers are also at risk for low blood glucose levels during hemodialysis and should be dialyzed with a solution that contains dextrose. Dextrose in the dialysate may also decrease hemodialysis side effects (Daugirdas, 1994). Many centers now routinely use dextrose-containing dialysis solutions for all chronic and acute hemodialysis patients.

Normally, fluid removal needs will vary with each dialysis session. More than 4 liters removal rarely needs to occur with the first acute or chronic hemodialysis treatment, even if the patient is in pulmonary edema. Fluid removal calculations should always take prime and rinse volumes into account. Isolated ultrafiltration is a safe method of fluid removal in acute dialysis if large amounts of water need to be removed. This will be discussed in greater detail in the Special Procedures section of the chapter.

Slower fluid removal at a constant rate is usually a successful method. The dialysis treatment can be extended to 4-5 hours with a slow blood flow rate and a slow ultrafiltration rate to accomplish this. To ensure a constant fluid removal rate, it is best to use an ultrafiltration controller whenever possible. If dialysate sodium is set lower than the plasma sodium level, the UF rate should be initially lower to compensate for osmotic contraction of blood volume, which occurs as sodium is rapidly decreased (Daugirdas, 1994).

During acute dialysis, hypotension should be avoided at all times. It can cause further renal damage and delay of recovery. Since it is often difficult to estimate a dry weight for an acutely ill patient, careful fluid removal is the key to prevention of hypotension during acute hemodialysis.

Table 19-4
Heparinization methods for hemodialysis.

ROUTINE HEPARINIZATION	MINIMAL (TIGHT) HEPARINIZATION
Target Clotting Times: 180% of baseline during dialysis 140% of baseline at end of dialysis	**Target Clotting Times:** 140% of baseline during and at the end of dialysis if using constant infusion method 125% of baseline during and at the end of dialysis if using repeated bolus method
Constant Infusion Method: - Obtain baseline clotting time - Administer initial bolus dose of heparin (Example: 2000 units) - Wait 3-5 minutes, then initiate dialysis - Monitor clotting times every hour - Begin heparin infusion (Example: 1000 units/hour) - Adjust the infusion rate to maintain clotting time at 180% of baseline - Stop heparin infusion 1 hour prior to the end of dialysis - Measure clotting time at end of dialysis	**Constant Infusion Method:** - Obtain baseline clotting time - Administer initial bolus dose of heparin (Example: 750 units) - Initiate dialysis - Begin heparin infusion (Example: 600 units/hour) - Monitor clotting times every 30 minutes - Adjust heparin infusion rate to maintain clotting time at 140% of baseline - Continue heparin infusion until the end of the dialysis treatment
Repeated Bolus Method: - Obtain initial clotting time - Administer initial bolus dose of heparin- higher dose than with constant infusion method (Example: 4000 units) - Monitor clotting times every hour and if less than 150% of baseline, give an additional bolus of heparin (Example: 1000-2000 units) and recheck clotting time in 30 minutes.	**Repeated Bolus Method:** - Obtain initial clotting time - Administer initial bolus dose of heparin (Example: 1000-1200 units) and if less than 125% of baseline, give an additional small bolus of heparin (Example: 500 units) and recheck clotting time in 15 minutes

***NOTE:** For routine heparinization, clotting times are performed on a regular basis only until the patient's optimal heparin prescription is determined. Clotting times can be restarted if a change is noted in the patient's coagulation pattern.

Delivery of Adequate Treatment

An adequate hemodialysis prescription is only the beginning of an adequate treatment. Ongoing evaluation of treatment parameters and successful delivery of the prescribed treatment are as important as, or more important than, the determination of treatment parameters. Nephrology nurses have the most crucial role in ensuring that hemodialysis patients receive the treatment that has been prescribed (Threlkeld, 1991).

Levin (1991) described the requirements for ensuring adequate therapy: an appropriate prescription, a high level of nursing expertise, an efficiently operating hemodialysis machine, satisfactory access to the circulation, an informed patient, and ongoing data collection and review. Based on these stated requirements, it is clear that there are many reasons why adequate therapy is often not achieved despite an adequate prescription.

Inadequate blood flow rates during hemodialysis are a common problem, often secondary to a less than satisfactory vascular access. Thrombosis and stenosis of AVFs and grafts often result in inadequate blood flow for the prescribed treatment. Access recirculation, discussed earlier in the chapter, is a problem often underrecognized, especially with the use of higher blood flow rates in high flux dialysis. Often the blood pump is set to deliver a blood flow rate of up to 400 ml/minute but is actually delivering a substantially reduced volume because of recirculation. This is not always readily apparent to the operator. Frequent monitoring of recirculation studies can help reduce the impact of this problem (Levin et al., 1991).

Nephrology nurses must remain aware of the need for adequate blood flow and achieve the prescribed rate as quickly as possible when initiating hemodialysis. The nurse should also avoid transient reductions in the blood flow rate, as in hypotensive events. The value of blood flow rate reduction has never been proven. Delays in achieving prescribed blood flow rate and transient reductions lead to inadequate delivery of the prescribed dialysis. (Keen et al., 1995; Levin et al., 1991; Threlkeld, 1991)

Failure to adhere to prescribed dialysis time can also result in inadequate treatment. Interruptions in dialysis due to complications and alarms must be taken into account when looking at actual dialysis time. Hemodialysis machines that measure actual dialysis time or liters of blood processed help to reduce this error. Merely timing treatments according to the clock on the wall will almost always lead to underdialysis. Patients need to be informed of the importance of dialysis time and the reasons that clock time may not be an accurate measurement of dialysis time (Levin et al., 1991; Threlkeld, 1991).

In addition, the nurse must remain aware of practices related to dialysis time such as early termination of treatments. Some patients will regularly fail to comply with the prescribed dialysis treatment time by missing treatments or by demanding shortened treatments. Patient education related to time and the consequences of underdialysis may influence the patient to adhere to the prescribed treatment (Levin et al., 1991; Threlkeld, 1991).

Continuous monitoring of Kt/V, NPCR, and, in some cases, residual renal function, is vital to ensuring an appropriate dialysis prescription and in assessing patient response to therapy. Although increased nursing and physician time is required for this review, it is essential that the hemodialysis prescription be reassessed on a routine basis, such as monthly (Levin et al., 1991; Threlkeld, 1991).

Nephrology nurses play a vital role in ensuring positive patient outcomes through adequate delivery of the hemodialysis prescription. In addition, the nursing assessment is crucial in determining the patient's response to therapy. The nurse should monitor the patient for uremic signs and symptoms, fluid volume status, anemia, nutritional status, and signs and symptoms of bone disease. This comprehensive assessment along with measurement of the Kt/V and determination of the patient's functional status, quality of life, and well-being provide a total picture of the patient and his or her response to therapy.

Anticoagulation During Hemodialysis

During a hemodialysis treatment, the patient's blood comes into contact with tubing, membrane, and other parts of the extracorporeal circuit. Any of these surfaces may initiate clotting of the blood in the circuit, which may lead to occlusion of the circuit.

Anticoagulation with heparin is the usual method of preventing clotting in the extracorporeal system. Heparin, extracted from beef lung or pork intestine, works by bonding to circulating antithrombin III, resulting in a rapid inactivation of clotting factors II, IX, XI, and XII. The half-life of heparin is 30-120 minutes (Caruana & Keep, 1994).

Heparin Prescription

Routine heparin (see Table 19-4). Heparin can be administered systemically, without fear of initiation of a bleeding episode, in stable patients with no abnormal bleeding risk. The usual target range for activated clotting times (ACTs) is 150-180% of the baseline value drawn prior to dialysis. The ACT at the end of the HD treatment should be less than 140% of baseline. In azotemic patients, such as many with acute renal failure or at the initiation of chronic dialysis, when the baseline ACT is prolonged out of the normal range, further prolongation of the ACT to 180% of baseline during HD may be associated with bleeding and may not be necessary (Caruana & Keep, 1994; Ismail & Hakim, 1991).

One technique for administration of routine systemic heparin is by giving a bolus initial loading dose followed by a constant heparin infusion. Another method is administration of a bolus followed by repeated bolus injections as necessary. With the constant infusion method, the initial bolus dose is lower (approximately 2000 units) than with the repeated bolus method (approximately 4000 units). This difference exists because, with the constant heparin infusion, the initial dose is required to prolong the ACT only to the baseline plus 80%. With the bolus method, the initial dose must prolong the ACT to much higher than 180% to allow for the decrease in ACT that occurs between bolus doses. If using the Lee White Clotting Time (LWCT) to monitor anticoagulation, the goal is considerably higher than with ACT, and it is much higher than 140% of the baseline at the end of the treatment (Caruana & Keep, 1994).

The initial bolus dose of heparin required to elevate the ACT to 180% of baseline will vary from patient to patient, depending on the patient's sensitivity to heparin and the potency of the heparin being used. A dose such as 2000 units is chosen for the initial bolus. An ACT or whole blood partial thromboplastin time (WBPTT) can be checked 3 minutes after giving the initial 2000 units. If prolongation of the clotting time is insufficient, a second bolus can be administered immediately. Prolongation of the ACT will be directly proportional to the amount of heparin given. For example, if the initial bolus increased the clotting time by 50 seconds, then a second bolus of half the initial dose will prolong the ACT an additional 25 seconds (Caruana & Keep, 1994).

If the patient is extremely uremic, such as an acute renal failure patient with platelet dysfunction, the initial bolus dose should be reduced to avoid bleeding. Consideration should also be given to reduction of the initial dose of heparin in a shortened session of hemodialysis, especially if using the repeated bolus method of administration. If the initial dose anticoagulates the patient excessively, the clotting time may still be markedly prolonged after the treatment ends.

The infusion rate necessary to maintain the WBTT or ACT at 180% of baseline can vary from 500 to 3000 units/hour. The required infusion rate is dependent upon patient sensitivity to heparin as well as the heparin half-life. Once a steady state is achieved, the infusion rates will be directly proportional to the prolongation of the clotting time. For example, if an infusion rate of 1000 units/hour is causing an ACT prolongation of 40 seconds, then an infusion rate of 1500 units/hour will prolong the ACT an additional 20 seconds (Caruana & Keep, 1994).

Once the nurse knows the current prolongation of the clotting time, he or she can predict, based on that and the half-life of the heparin, the prolongation at the end of the treatment, assuming no further heparin is administered. This is important for deciding when to terminate the heparin infusion during dialysis. For example, if the prolongation of the ACT is 50 seconds and the half-life of the heparin is 1 hour, then in 1 hour the heparin will have reduced by 50%, at which time the prolongation of the ACT will be only 25 seconds. Heparin half-life ranges from 30 minutes to 2 hours; however, the average is 50 minutes in dialysis patients (Caruana & Keep, 1994).

Tight or minimal heparin (see Table 19-4). The target range of ACT or WBPTT for patients with mild to moderate risk of active bleeding is much lower, usually 140% of baseline. Again, some patients will have prolonged baseline ACTs due to uremia or other factors. The prolongation of the ACT for these patients can be based on the average baseline ACT for the patients in the unit (Caruana & Keep, 1994).

The best method for administration of a tight or minimal heparin prescription is the initial bolus followed by a constant infusion. The constant infusion technique avoids the rise and fall in clotting times that occurs with the repeated bolus method. A repeated bolus method can be used, if necessary; however the target ACT should be only 125% of baseline to avoid prolongation of the clotting time out of the desired range immediately after administration of the boluses (Caruana & Keep, 1994).

The initial bolus dose of heparin to achieve a 40% prolongation of the baseline ACT or WBPTT can range from 300 to 2000 units. Most centers start with an initial dose of 750 units and then recheck the ACT at 3 minutes. If the clotting time is not sufficiently prolonged, a supplemental bolus dose is given at that time. The amount of heparin given in the supplemental dose depends upon the prolongation achieved with the 750 units. Again, the amount of prolongation of the clotting will be directly proportional to the amount of heparin given. For example, if 750 units prolonged the ACT by 30 seconds, then an additional 375 units will prolong it an additional 15 seconds (Caruana & Keep, 1994).

For tight or minimal heparin, the average hourly infusion rate will be 600 units/hour, but it can vary depending on patient sensitivity to heparin and heparin potency. If the initial dose of 750 units prolonged the ACT much more or less than expected, then the hourly infusion rate should be adjusted as necessary. Close monitoring of the patient's clotting time is crucial to a successful tight heparin regimen. Studies have shown that patients between 50 and 90 kg do not appear to have differences in heparin sensitivity based on weight, so heparin doses do not have to be adjusted for this factor (Caruana & Keep, 1994).

Heparin-free dialysis. Heparin-free dialysis is the method of choice for patients who are actively bleeding or are at high risk for bleeding. There are also patients in whom heparin is contraindicated, such as those with thrombocytopenia or other coagulopathies, who will benefit from heparin-free dialysis (Caruana & Keep, 1994).

A variety of techniques are used for performing heparin-free dialysis. However most regimens include the following: a heparin rinse, a high blood flow rate, and a periodic saline rinse. The heparin rinse is a rinse of the extracorporeal circuit with heparinized saline, then with plain saline prior to starting dialysis to avoid giving heparin to the patient. The blood flow rate is set as high as tolerated during dialysis. A periodic rapid saline rinse of the dialyzer is done every 15-30 minutes. Approximately 100-250 ml is administered with each rinse, so the ultrafiltration calculations must be adjusted accordingly. The rinsing allows inspection of a hollow-fiber dialyzer while reducing the dialyzer propensity for clotting (Caruana & Keep, 1994; Ludlow, 1989).

There is no evidence that suggests that hollow fiber dialyzers are better than parallel plate dialyzers for use in heparin-free dialysis. With the use of heparin-free dialysis, the literature shows that complete dialyzer clotting will occur in only 5% of treatments. Blood or lipid emulsion administration during dialysis may increase the risk of this clotting (Ludlow, 1991; Caruana & Keep, 1994).

Regional citrate anticoagulation. This is an alternative to heparin-free dialysis. Since calcium is required in the coagulation process, lowering of the ionized calcium level of the blood in the extracorporeal circuit anticoagulates the blood. The extracorporeal ionized calcium level is lowered by infusion of trisodium citrate into the arterial blood line and by using a dialysate containing zero calcium. The trisodium citrate complexes calcium; thus to avoid returning blood with a dangerously low calcium level to the patient, the process is reversed by an infusion of calcium chloride into the venous blood line, distal to the dialyzer. Approximately one-third of the remaining citrate is dialyzed out, and the remainder is metabolized safely by the patient (Caruana & Keep, 1994).

Any dialyzer can be used for regional citrate anticoagulation. However, UF capability must be sufficient to remove the extra fluid administered hourly to the patient in the two infusions, approximately 300 ml/minute. The dialysate will usually be bicarbonate based, but this is primarily because this method is used in acute renal failure patients, who are often unstable and in the critical care setting. A zero calcium dialysate must be used. The trisodium citrate solution is administered into the arterial blood line prior to the dialyzer, and the calcium carbonate solution is administered just distal to the dialyzer in the venous blood line.

Baseline blood is obtained for clotting studies (ACT or WBPTT) and for serum calcium level. The citrate infusion is initiated at 270 ml/hour, and the calcium carbonate infusion is started at 30 ml/hour. The patient's calcium level is checked at 30 minutes and as necessary, thereafter. The calcium infusion is adjusted to maintain a normal serum calcium level in the patient. Samples for clotting times are obtained from the arterial line, downstream from the citrate infusion, to determine the effect of the infusion. Clotting times should be prolonged by 100%. The rate of infusion of the citrate can be increased to achieve this prolongation up to a rate of 420 ml/hour, or reduced as necessary to maintain the 100%.

If the dialyzer goes into bypass mode, the effect of the zero calcium dialysate will be eliminated, so the citrate infusion should be decreased by 50% and the calcium infusion discontinued until dialysate flow to the dialyzer has been restored. At the end of the treatment, both solutions are stopped simultaneously, and the patient's blood is rinsed back as usual (Ludlow, 1989; Caruana & Keep, 1994).

This method of anticoagulation has several advantages over heparin-free dialysis. The blood flow rate does not need to be high. Clotting almost never occurs, and the patient is not at risk for bleeding due to heparin. Saline flushes are not required. There are also disadvantages. Blood calcium level must be monitored throughout the treatment. Two infusions are required, one of citrate and one of calcium carbonate. Citrate metabolism generates bicarbonate, so use of this technique will result in a greater than usual increase in serum bicarbonate during the treatment. Therefore, it should be used only if absolutely necessary and with caution in patients at risk for alkalemia. If this method is used chronically, the dialysate bicarbonate level must be reduced to avoid metabolic alkalosis (Caruana & Keep, 1994; Ludlow, 1989). The technique is time-intensive for the nurse performing the hemodialysis treatment.

Assessing Anticoagulation During Hemodialysis

Optimally, anticoagulation should be individualized based on baseline clotting times, according to the procedures described above. Many dialysis facilities, however, are unable to use ACTs due to regulations resulting from the Clinical Laboratory Improvement Amendments (CLIA) of 1988. Therefore, it is essential that nephrology nurses use the observation skills they depended upon to determine heparin dose prior to ACTs (Breiterman-White, 1995).

Visual inspection of the dialyzer during a hemodialysis treatment is important in assessing the effects of anticoagulation. The extracorporeal circuit can be better visualized if rinsed with saline. Visual signs of clotting in the system include extremely dark blood, shadows, or black streaks in the dialyzer, and clot formation in the drip chambers and the arterial header of the dialyzer. Other signs of clotting are the rapid filling of the transducer filters with blood, indicating increased pressure within the system, and a venous chamber that fills repeatedly with blood or foam (Breiterman-White, 1995).

Changes will be seen in the arterial and venous pressures, depending upon where the clotting is occurring in the extracorporeal circuit. If a post-pump arterial pressure monitor is used, the difference between the arterial and venous pressures can indicate the location of the clotting. An increased arterial pressure and lower venous pressure, in this case, indicates that clotting is occurring in the dialyzer or the arterial chamber. If the clotting is occurring distal to the venous chamber, venous pressure and arterial pressures are both increased. A clotted venous needle can also cause both pressures to be elevated (Breiterman-White, 1995; Caruana & Keep, 1994).

It is useful to note the amount of clotting in the dialyzer after dialysis. A few clotted fibers or some clots in the header are not unusual; however, large amounts of clotting are indicative of a need for increased anticoagulation. In programs doing reuse, fiber bundle volume test can provide information related to dialyzer clotting during dialysis (Caruana & Keep, 1994).

If the nurse notes evidence of clotting in the system and adjusts the heparin dose during the treatment, the heparin regimen for the next treatment should be modified in the same manner and the outcome evaluated. When determining an appropriate heparin prescription, the nurse should also be aware that concomitant use of some other medications may alter the effects of heparin. The use of oral anticoagulants, salicylates, cephalosporins, and nonsteroidal antiinflammatory drugs may enhance the effects of heparin and place the patient at risk for bleeding if the HD heparin dose is not adjusted. The reverse is true of digitalis, tetracyclines, nicotine, and antihistamines, which counteract the heparin effect. Patients using those medications may need more heparin during HD. The nurse would also be aware that the patient's heparin requirements may increase with the use of recombinant erythropoietin and the resultant increase in hematocrit (Breiterman-White, 1995).

All techniques for tight or minimal heparinization, regional citrate anticoagulation, and regular systemic heparinization use blood tests for clotting times to determine dosage and effects of anticoagulation. Blood for clotting studies should be drawn from the arterial line, prior to any heparin insertion site, to reflect the clotting status of the patient, not that of the extracorporeal circuit. The exception to this is with regional citrate anticoagulation where the blood is drawn from the arterial line at a point after the citrate infusion. The goal with this method is to determine the clotting status of the blood in the dialyzer (Caruana & Keep, 1994; Ludlow, 1989).

There are several methods for testing clotting times. Whole blood partial thromboplastin time (WBPTT) is a test that accelerates the blood clotting time by the addition of a reagent called Thrombofax to the blood. The mixture is then heated and tilted every 5 seconds until a clot forms. The prolongation of the WBPTT is linearly related to the heparin dose given during dialysis (Caruana & Keep, 1994).

The activated clotting time (ACT) test is similar to the WBPTT but uses an activator to accelerate the clotting process. The ACT is less reproduceable than the WBPTT, especially at low heparin levels. However, devices that continuously turn or tilt the tube and detect clot formation standardize the test and increase reproduceability of the results (Caruana & Keep, 1994).

The Lee-White clotting time (LWCT) is performed by adding 0.4 ml of blood to a glass tube and inverting the tube every 30 seconds until the blood clots. There is no accelerant in the tube; therefore a long period of time is required before clotting occurs and there is poor standardization and reproduceability. This is the least desirable method of monitoring clotting during hemodialysis (Caruana & Keep, 1994).

Several new techniques for anticoagulation are being studied in an effort to improve this important aspect of the dialysis treatment. The use of more specific low molecular weight heparins, natural and synthetic prostaglandins and other antiplatelet agents, protease inhibitors, the thrombin inhibitor hirudin, and extracorporeal device modifications such as the use of Heparinase cartridges to remove heparin from the circuit are being tested (Caruana & Keep, 1994).

The Hemodialysis Procedure

Predialysis Equipment Preparation

Dialysis systems should be prepared according to manufacturer recommendations. Thorough rinsing of the dialyzer is important during setup. This aids in removing allergens such as the commonly used dialyzer disinfectant, ethylene oxide, which can lead to a dialyzer reaction. While priming the dialyzer with dialysate, the blood compartment should be rinsed with at least 2 liters of normal saline. After the rinse, the dialysis should be initiated within 5-10 minutes. If the system sits longer, it will leach ethylene oxide into the rinsing fluid. If more than 10 minutes elapse, the dialyzer should be rinsed briefly a second time just prior to use (Daugirdas, 1994).

Predialysis Patient Assessment and Preparation

Vital signs and weight are important components of the predialysis assessment. The predialysis weight should be compared with the postweight from the previous treatment and with the patient's estimated dry weight (EDW). Other parameters such as blood pressure, pulse, findings upon auscultation of the heart and lungs, the presence or absence of edema, and an interdialytic history should be considered along with the weight to determine the true volume status of the patient. Any large weight gain accompanied by dyspnea and orthopnea should prompt a complete cardiorespiratory examination including auscultation of the lungs, assessment of the patient for edema, and auscultation of the heart. Cardiac or respiratory signs of volume overload without an accompanying large weight gain should prompt a reassessment of the patient's EDW.

Hypertension predialysis is often volume-related. However, it may be renin mediated. If renin is a factor, the blood pressure may increase during hemodialysis despite fluid removal. The meaning of predialysis hypertension should be evaluated with the weight and other parameters mentioned above (Daugirdas, 1994).

Patients with hypertension routinely prior to hemodialysis may be counseled to hold antihypertensive medications the morning of hemodialysis. This may help to limit hypotension during the treatment, particularly in patients requiring a large fluid removal. Whether or not to administer antihypertensive medication prior to hemodialysis may be a factor for a patient receiving early morning dialysis, but may not be as important if the dialysis treatment is scheduled later in the day.

Measurement of the patient's temperature before dialysis is important. The temperature is often less than normal prior to HD, and a rise of 0.5 degrees centigrade during HD is normal. This phenomenon will be addressed in greater detail in the discussion of interleukin-1 later in the chapter. Predialysis fever is a serious finding suggestive of infection or bacteremia and should be investigated (Daugirdas, 1994).

The interdialytic history is a very important part of the nursing assessment. It can provide valuable information that is helpful in interpretation of physical findings. For example, a brief interdialytic dietary history can be helpful in the interpretation of interdialytic weight gain in the reassessment of the patient's estimated dry weight.

Vascular Access Assessment and Preparation

The patient's access site should be examined for patency and signs of infection prior to each dialysis. Cannulation of the access should occur only after the skin is cleansed with povidone iodine solution. For an AVF, the tourniquet is placed proximal to the access. Needle insertion is done with the needle at a 45-degree angle and with the bevel up. With the AV graft, the skin is prepared in the same fashion, but a tourniquet is never used. Local anesthesia, whether topical or administered intradermally, may or may not be used to decrease the pain of the needle insertion (Rockel et al., 1988). Appropriate sites for venipuncture are discussed in the vascular access portion of the chapter.

If a percutaneous venous catheter is being used for dialysis, the heparin instilled at the end of the previous treatment as well as any clots are aspirated from each limb. Patency is checked by irrigation of each lumen with normal saline in a syringe (Rockel et al., 1988).

Blood sample acquisition is done via the needle prior to heparinization as heparin interferes with some tests. Blood acquisition through the catheter should be done only after adequate flushing of the catheter lumen with blood and normal saline.

Beginning the Treatment

Once the vascular access has been prepared and, if appropriate, cannulated, the initial dose of heparin is administered into the venous limb of the catheter or the venous needle. Two or three minutes should be allowed for systemic absorption prior to starting the blood circulation through the extracorporeal circuit (Rockel, 1988).

The blood lines are then connected to the access, and the blood flow is started slowly, allowing the circuit to fill gradually with the patient's blood. The priming solution in the system can be either given to the patient or discarded. If the patient is to receive the prime, both the arterial and venous blood lines should be connected to the access prior to starting the blood pump. If the patient is volume overloaded or is not receiving the solution for another reason, the procedure is different. The arterial blood line is connected to the access, and the priming fluid is allowed to drain from the circuit while it is being displaced by blood until the blood reaches the venous air trap (chamber). At that time, the venous line is connected to the access.

Once both blood lines are attached to the access, the blood flow rate is slowly increased to the desirable level. Arterial and venous pressures are noted and limits set. The air detector is set manually, if it is not automatic, prior to the nurse's leaving the patient.

Intradialytic Monitoring

Blood circuit. Arterial pressure, also referred to as inlet pressure or prepump pressure, is monitored during hemodialysis. It is usually negative 20 to negative 50 mmHg in conventional dialysis and is as low as negative 200 mmHg in high efficiency hemodialysis. If the access is not providing sufficient blood to the pump, the suction proximal to the pump will increase, causing a lower arterial pressure. The alarm will sound, shutting off the blood pump. The suction must be relieved to deactivate the alarm and resume the blood flow (Van Stone, 1994).

Causes of excessive inflow suction include improper positioning of the arterial needle with the bevel up against the vessel wall or not entirely in the vessel. Hypotension causing decreased blood flow through the access, spasm of the access vessel (AVF only), stenosis of the arterial anastomosis of an AV graft, clotting in the access or in the arterial needle, kinking of the arterial line, or collapse of or decreased blood flow into the access secondary to position of the patient's arm (i.e., arm bent at elbow or arm elevated above heart level) are other causes (Van Stone, 1994).

Nursing management related to arterial pressure monitoring or alarm situations includes assessment of the problem to determine the cause of pressure changes or alarms as well as troubleshooting the problem. If an arterial pressure alarm occurs, the nurse should reduce the blood flow rate to the point that inflow suction decreases enough to allow the alarm to stay off. This will allow the nurse time to ascertain the problem and correct it.

The nurse should first ensure that the patient's blood pressure is not unusually low. If it is, it should be corrected by fluid replacement or reduction in the UF rate. If the problem is not hypotension, needle position should be suspected. The arterial needle should be repositioned by moving it up or down slightly or by rotating it to change the position of the bevel. An attempt to restore the blood flow to the previous rate is appropriate after adjustment of the needle. Needle adjustment can be attempted again if the low arterial pressure is still present (Van Stone, 1994).

The nurse may consider placement of another arterial needle and dialyze through it in an attempt to achieve a greater blood flow rate. The original needle can be left in place with a syringe attached to the end until the treatment is completed. If the suction cannot be corrected, dialysis can be continued at a slower blood flow rate. The dialysis time, however, should be lengthened to compensate for this.

Stenosis at the inflow to the vascular access should be suspected if excessive inflow suction persists despite the above measures. This can be further confirmed by occlusion of the access between the arterial and venous needles. If the arterial pressure moves farther to the negative when the access is occluded, this suggests that some of the blood flowing into the arterial needle was coming from the venous portion of the access (Van Stone, 1994). Further evaluation of this problem should be done and is discussed in the vascular access section of the chapter.

Venous pressure or outflow pressure is also monitored on the blood circuit. Ideally, the pressure should remain between +50 mmHg and +100 mmHg. Venous pressure may be as high as +200 when dialyzing with an AV graft because high arterial pressure in the graft is often transmitted to the venous line. High blood flow rates when using a smaller gauge needle can result in higher venous pressures as can clotting in the venous blood line, in the filter of the venous air trap, in the venous needle, or in the venous limb of the vascular access. Stenosis or spasm in the venous limb of the access or at the graft vein anastomosis of an AV graft can cause an increased pressure. Improperly positioned venous needle and kinked venous blood line should always be ruled out (Van Stone, 1994).

If clotting of the venous line or filter is the reason for the increased pressure, it can be confirmed by rinsing of the line with saline. If necessary, a new venous line can be primed and substituted for the clotted one. The presence of obstruction, such as clotting in the venous needle or venous limb of the access, can be confirmed by irrigating the venous needle or limb with a syringe of normal saline and noting the resistance. To evaluate for stenosis, the same type of test can be performed as with arterial pressure, occluding the access between the arterial and venous needles. In this case, if the venous pressure rises when the access is occluded, it suggests that stenosis downstream is causing the outflow obstruction (Van Stone, 1994).

An elevated venous pressure reflects a high blood compartment pressure which can cause excessive UF during hemodialysis because of increase in the TMP. The use of a UF controller will correct this problem.

As previously mentioned, the extracorporeal blood circuit is armed with an air detector that constantly monitors the blood returning to the patient for the presence of air. The danger of air accidentally entering the blood circuit is greatest between the arterial access site and the blood pump, where the pressure within the system is negative. Common sites of air entry include around the arterial needle if inflow suction is very high, tubing connections that may be slightly loose or leaky, a broken pump segment on the tubing, and the infusion set connected to a normal saline infusion. The administration of albumin or medications in vented bottles can lead to air entering the system if the bottle is not observed continuously during the infusion. The patient is also at risk of an air embolus if an air rinse is used to return the patient's blood at the end of a treatment. Therefore, this practice should be avoided (Van Stone, 1994).

Dialysate circuit. Conductivity and temperature are continuously monitored on the dialysate circuit. A properly functioning bypass valve, which diverts dialysate away from the dialyzer, will protect the patient from dialysate with an abnormal conductivity or temperature. The dialysate is also monitored for the presence of hemoglobin, which would indicate a blood leak inside the dialyzer. Small blood leaks cannot always be discerned by observing the dialysate line. False alarms do occur and may be due to air bubbles within the dialysate lines. A blood leak should always be confirmed with a test of the effluent using a test strip such as those used to test for hemoglobin in the urine. If a blood leak is confirmed, the dialysate compartment pressure should be set to –50 mmHg or lower to minimize entry of bacteria or endotoxin from the dialysate into the bloodstream. Small leaks in hollow fiber dialyzers may seal themselves off. However, with most leaks, the blood should be returned and dialysis discontinued or restarted with a new circuit (Van Stone, 1994).

Patient monitoring. The patient's vital signs, including blood pressure and pulse, should be monitored at least every 15 minutes during acute hemodialysis and at least hourly during chronic hemodialysis. The patient should also be monitored for hemodialysis complications. These will be discussed in detail in a later section of the chapter.

Termination of the Hemodialysis Treatment

The blood in the extracorporeal circuit is returned to the patient by displacing it in the circuit with normal saline. The patient usually receives 100-300 ml of normal saline during the rinseback procedure. When the venous blood line is light pink, the normal saline infusion is stopped. If the patient's blood pressure is low at the end of the treatment, more normal saline can be infused as necessary to raise the BP. Use of air to return blood to the patient is not recommended because of the high incidence of air embolism with this procedure.

Once the blood is returned to the patient, the needles are removed from the AVF or graft, and venous stasis is achieved with the application of pressure to the venipuncture sites. If a catheter was used for dialysis, the catheter lumens are rinsed with normal saline and heparinized before the caps are replaced and the limbs clamped.

Postdialysis Patient Assessment

The postdialysis weight should be compared with the preweight and the EDW. If weight loss is

Table 19-5
Hemodialysis complications.

Complication	Etiology	Signs/Symptoms	Prevention	Treatment
Hypotension	Reduction in cardiac output Decrease in systemic vascular resistance Splanchnic vasodilatation due to food ingestion Anemia Low dialysate sodium Antihypertensive medications Hypoalbuminemia Aggressive UF Acetate dialysate Unstable cardiovascular status	Low BP (may be associated with nausea, vomiting, diaphoresis, or cold clammy skin) Warm feeling (early sign) Dizziness Tachycardia Loss of consciousness and seizures	Ensure accurate predialysis weights Frequent assessment of EDW Withhold antihypertensive medications prior to dialysis Monitor hematocrit Teach patient to restrict interdialytic fluid intake Teach patient early signs and symptoms of hypotension	Place patient in Trendelenburg position Reduce UF rate If necessary to reverse low BP, administer normal saline and/or osmotic agents
Muscle Cramps	Excess fluid removal Hypoosmolality Hypotension	Pain Tightness in muscle group	Frequent assessment of EDW Use of dialysate with appropriate sodium and potassium concentrations Sodium modeling Use of osmotic agents Stretching of affected muscles	Application of heat to muscle group Volume expansion, if indicated
Chest Pain	Anemia Coronary artery spasm Arteriosclerotic heart disease Severe volume depletion	Pain or tightness in chest Pain may be accompanied by diaphoresis, nausea, dyspnea	Monitor hematocrit Utilize appropriate UF target Assess and treat volume depletion Frequent assessment of EDW	Administer nitroglycerin and related drugs as ordered Administer oxygen as indicated Temporarily decrease UF rate Discontinue dialysis, if severe
Fever/Chills	Infection Pyrogens/Endotoxins	Temperature elevation during or shortly after dialysis (infection) Temperature elevation within first 45-75 minutes of dialysis (pyrogen/endotoxin exposure) Cold feeling Involuntary shaking Rarely, hypotension	Proper water treatment, disinfection of equipment, reuse procedures, and preparation of dialysate Clean technique in preparation of dialysate and system Preparation of extracorporeal circuit limited to 2 hours prior to initiation of dialysis treatment	Assess for signs and sources of infection Obtain blood cultures, inlet and outlet dialysate and water cultures Administer antipyretics and antibiotics as ordered

Table 19-5
Hemodialysis complications (continued).

Complication	Etiology	Signs/Symptoms	Prevention	Treatment
Dialysis Disequilibrium	Rapid decrease in BUN Rapid pH changes Electrolyte shifts	Occur during or soon after dialysis Headache Nausea, vomiting Hypertension Restlessness Increased pulse pressure Decreased sensorium Convulsions Coma Death	Slower urea removal during dialysis (short treatments, less efficient dialyzer, slow BFR) High sodium dialysate/sodium modeling Administration of an osmotic agent Assessment for signs and symptoms	Early recognition of signs and symptoms Termination of the dialysis treatment, if necessary Treat symptoms supportively
Acute Hemolysis	Hypotonic or hypertonic dialysate solutions High dialysate temperature Blood exposure to toxins such as copper, chloramines, nitrates, formaldehyde, or bleach Rarely, RBC trauma from roller pump or high negative pressure in circuit	Chest and/or back pain Dyspnea Clear or translucent blood in venous blood line Localized burning and pain in access return site Dysrhythmias Hyperkalemia Acute decrease in hematocrit Pink plasma in centrifuged blood	Alarms in working order Appropriate check of dialysate temperature and conductivity prior to dialysis Regular preventive maintenance of monitors and alarms Monitor pre-pump arterial pressure Proper water preparation for dialysis If appropriate, test for bleach and formaldehyde in system	Discontinue dialysis without reinfusing blood Monitor vital signs Assess for dysrhythmias, dyspnea, hypotension Administer oxygen, as indicated Check hematocrit, electrolytes If appropriate, replace volume or transfuse
Air Embolism	Defective or disarmed air detector Loose connection or leak in the extracorporeal circuit prior to blood pump Empty air-vented IV containers attached to circuit prior to blood pump	Dependent on position of patient when air infused Feeling and sight of air rushing into circulation Chest pain Dyspnea Coughing Cyanosis Visual problems Confusion Hemiparesis Death	Correct use of air detector Secure all connections Return patient's blood with saline rinse, not air rinse During dialysis, administer normal saline as a bolus rather than a continuous infusion Observe infusion sites carefully	Stop infusion of air immediately Place patient in Trendelenburg position on left side Assess vital signs Administer oxygen Notify physician
Dialyzer Reaction	Type A: Hypersensitivity to dialyzer sterilant Uncertain Type B: Complement activation by dialyzer membrane Reduced with reuse	Type A: Acute bronchoconstriction Initially, feeling of uneasiness, agitation, chest tightness, dyspnea, nausea Coughing, wheezing Urticaria, facial edema Respiratory stridor Type B: Back pain Chest pain Hypotension	Type A: Use of a different dialyzer Type B: Use of synthetic membranes Reuse of cellulosic membranes	Type A: Symptom management If severe, terminate dialysis without reinfusing blood

Table 19-5
Hemodialysis complications (continued).

Complication	Etiology	Signs/Symptoms	Prevention	Treatment
Dysrhythmias	Electrolyte and pH changes Removal of antiarrhythmic medications with dialysis	Irregular pulse Possible hypotension	Dialysate potassium at least 2 mEq/liters for patients on digitalis Monitor heart rate and rhythm Monitor EKG in high risk patients	Administer antiarrhythmic agents as ordered Discontinue dialysis for severe symptomatic dysrhythmias Treat symptoms supportively
Cardiac Arrest	Electrolyte imbalance Dysrhythmias Myocardial infarction Cardiac tamponade Large air embolism Hemolysis Exsanguination Hyperthermia	Absence of pulse Lack of spontaneous respiratory effort Unresponsiveness	Prevent conditions that can lead to cardiac arrest Careful assessment of patient during dialysis EKG monitoring for high risk patients	Begin CPR as appropriate Discontinue dialysis and return blood to patient, if appropriate
Seizures	Dialysis disequilibrium Electrolyte imbalances Hypotension Dialysate composition errors	Convulsions May be unresponsive	Avoid/counteract large drop in BUN Frequent monitoring of BP Support BP throughout treatment	Support airway, as necessary Replace volume, if indicated Administer anticonvulsant medications as ordered
Exsanguination	Accidental or traumatic separation of blood lines, needles dislodged from access site, or caps loosened from dialysis catheter Dialysis membrane rupture with failure of blood leak detector Rupture of AVF anastomosis or aneurysm	Obvious source of bleeding Shock Seizures Cardiac arrest	Secure all bloodline and access connections/caps Carefully secure needles with tape Ensure conditions that allow visualization of extracorporeal circuit at all times Ensure properly functioning blood detector and pressure alarms Place blood lines in pump properly	Stop bleeding at any site Return all appropriate blood to patient If blood loss significant, administer volume expander, oxygen, and possibly transuse Notify physician
Dialysis Encephalopathy	Accumulation of aluminum in body from water used to prepare dialysate or large quantities of aluminum-based phosphate binders	Speech disturbances Myoclonus Seizures Gait changes Intellectual deterioration EEG changes Osteodystrophy Anemia	Use appropriately treated water for dialysis Use non-aluminum phosphate binders Assess for early signs and symptoms	Early recognition of signs and symptoms Serum aluminum chelation to decrease body aluminum stores

Table 19-5
Hemodialysis complications (continued).

Complication	Etiology	Signs/Symptoms	Prevention	Treatment
Neutropenia	Use of cellulosic dialyzer membranes Activation of complement cascade and neutrophil accumulation in pulmonary vasculature	Hypotension Nausea/vomiting Chest pain	Use of synthetic dialyzer	Draw all CBC's prior to dialysis
Hypoxemia	Hypoventilation secondary to acetate dialysate Intrapulmonary diffusion block due to neutrophil aggregation in lungs	Possible dyspnea, cyanosis in already compromised patients	Use of substituted cellulose or synthetic dialyzer Use of bicarbonate dialysate	Administer oxygen
Amyloidosis	Repeated immune stimulation with long-term dialysis on cellulosic membranes	Carpal synovial amyloid deposits Cystic bone deposits Carpal Tunnel Syndrome	Use of substituted cellulose or synthetic dialyzers	Treat symptomatically
Interleukin-1 Stimulation	Interaction between dialyzer membrane and monocytes during dialysis	Long-term catabolic changes over the years of muscle, fat, the liver, connective tissue resulting, in part, in wasting and negative nitrogen balance Transient elevation of body temperature during dialysis Headache	Possibly reduced with substituted cellulose or synthetic membranes Possibly reduced with reuse	Treat symptomatically

greater or less than anticipated, nursing measures should be taken. The calculations related to ultrafiltration such as TMP should be reviewed for errors such as failure to include the priming solution or rinse solution. With high permeability (high efficiency) dialyzers, small errors in TMP can result in large errors in fluid removal (Daugirdas, 1994).

Whether or not there has been difficulty in maintaining desired TMP throughout, the entire treatment should be assessed. Changes in venous pressure and hypotensive episodes are examples of events that result in changes in the TMP. The dialyzer should be observed for signs of clotting that could reduce dialyzer permeability. Coating of the membrane with clots or protein can result in decreased ultrafiltration capability of the dialyzer (Daugirdas, 1994).

The nurse should also remember that TMP based on the in vitro value reported for the membrane may result in less or more fluid removal than expected. The in vitro ultrafiltration values tend to differ from the actual in vivo values in the clinical setting. In vitro values are usually found to be higher than in vivo values, therefore if weight loss is other than expected and no obvious cause can be found, differences in these values may be the reason for the discrepancy.

Postdialysis Blood Work

Serum samples obtained immediately postdialysis can give information regarding urea removal, correction of acidosis, and normalization of electrolytes. However, movement of these substances between body fluid compartments will continue after dialysis is completed. If acetate dialysate was used, correction of acidosis will continue, and a sample 1-2 hours after completion of dialysis will be more representative of the postdialysis status (Daugirdas, 1994).

Postdialysis Equipment Care

After the treatment, the dialysis machine is stripped of the disposable blood circuit equipment such as blood lines, intravenous bags, and syringes. If the center performs dialyzer reuse, the dialyzer is prepared for this procedure, which will be discussed later in the chapter. If reuse is not employed, the dialyzer is discarded with the other equipment. The machine is rinsed with treated water to remove all dialysate from the circuit. After the rinse is completed, disinfection of the machine is performed.

Complications of Hemodialysis

The most common complications of hemodialysis are, in descending order of frequency: hypotension (20-30% of hemodialysis treatments), muscle cramps (5-20%), nausea and vomiting (5-15%), headache (5%), itching (5%), chest pain (2-5%), back pain (2-5%), and fever and chills (<1%) (Bregman et al., 1994). These and other complications of the therapy are discussed in detail in this section as well as listed in Table 19-5.

Hypotension

Hypotension is the most frequent complication of hemodialysis. Symptomatic hypotension is the most frequently observed side effect during acetate hemodialysis. Studies show that hypotension is related to both the patient's situation and to the type of dialysis employed (Zuchelli, 1987). Twenty percent of all hemodialysis patients experience hypotension during a routine treatment. Sequelae include nausea and vomiting, decreased mental status, posttreatment malaise and fatigue, and self-limited seizures (Ismail & Hakim, 1991). Hypotension becomes a clinical problem when it occurs too often to permit the performance of dialysis and to achieve the goals of keeping the patient free of uremic symptoms and excess fluid (Zuchelli, 1987).

The most common cause for intradialytic hypotension is a rapid decrease in blood volume and a decrease in cardiac output. The mean arterial pressure (MAP) is determined by the peripheral vascular resistance (PVR) and the cardiac output (CO). The CO is a function of stroke volume and heart rate. Stroke volume depends upon the plasma volume and myocardial contractility. During hemodialysis, a decrease in plasma volume will lead to decreased blood pressure if compensatory changes in heart rate, PVR, or myocardial contractility do not occur. When the UF rate is high because of a large weight gain, fluid is removed from the vascular space at a faster rate than the rate at which plasma refilling occurs (fluid moves in from intracellular and interstitial fluid compartments). Maintenance of blood volume during hemodialysis depends upon rapid refilling of the blood compartment from surrounding compartments. If the plasma refilling rate is low and the patient is unable to maintain adequate or increased PVR, hypotension will result (Bregman et al., 1994; Ismail & Hakim, 1991).

Decreased blood pressure during dialysis is largely a reflection of the large amount of fluid relative to plasma volume that is removed during an average hemodialysis treatment. These rapid decreases in blood volume can be due to large interdialytic weight gains of greater than 3% of the body weight, resulting in the need for a high UF rate to accomplish a large fluid removal during a short dialysis treatment. As the patient approaches his or her EDW, the rate at which the blood compartment fills from surrounding spaces is diminished. A decrease in blood volume will result in a decrease in cardiac filling, in turn a decrease in cardiac output, and ultimately a decrease in blood pressure (Ismail & Hakim, 1991).

Excessive UF rates bringing the patient below his or her EDW or to a target weight set too low can lead to hypotension during and after the hemodialysis treatment. Inaccurate weights, either the EDW or the predialysis weight, result in inappropriate UF calculations, thus removal of inappropriate amounts of fluid. Failure to use UF controllers can put the patient at risk for errors in fluid removal and postdialysis weights below the EDW. If a UF controller is not available, less permeable dialyzers should be used so that changes in TMP will cause smaller changes in actual fluid removal. Ideally, the UF rate should be constant throughout the HD treatment. Without a UF controller, fluid removal can fluctuate considerably, causing transient rapid UF rates and resultant hypotension (Bregman et al., 1994; Ismail & Hakim, 1991).

Dialysate sodium levels can also affect the patient's intradialytic blood pressure. When dialysate sodium is less than plasma sodium, the blood returning to the patient from the dialyzer will be hypotonic in relation to fluid in surrounding spaces. To maintain equilibrium, water will leave the blood compartment, causing an acute decrease in blood volume. This effect is most pronounced early in the treatment. Excessive sodium removal secondary to inappropriately low dialysate sodium levels, such as less than 36 mEq/liter, reduces plasma sodium level and further exacerbates plasma volume reduction during UF (Bregman et al., 1995; Ismail & Hakim, 1991).

Lack of vasoconstriction can also cause hypotension during hemodialysis. Blood volume depletion causes a state in which CO is limited by cardiac filling. Any minor decrease in PVR can precipitate a drop in blood pressure because the CO cannot increase enough to compensate. Use of acetate-containing dialysate solution can lead to vasodilatation (Bregman et al., 1994).

Core body heating is a powerful stimulus for vasodilatation, resulting in both arterial and venous vasodilatation. Dialysate at body temperature or warmer can facilitate this dilatation. The use of colder dialysate solution can reduce the incidence of hypotension during HD, presumably by preventing temperature-induced vasodilatation. For some patients, it seems beneficial to use cooler dialysate for treatments in which large interdialytic fluid gains must be removed (Bregman et al., 1994; Ismail & Hakim, 1991).

Splanchnic vasodilatation is common secondary to food ingestion during HD. Dilatation causes an increase in capacity of those blood vessels, resulting in a decrease in systemic blood pressure. This food effect lasts at least 2 hours. Patients prone to hypotension may need to avoid food intake immediately predialysis or during dialysis to avoid a hypotensive episode (Bregman et al., 1994).

Tissue ischemia that occurs during hypotension causes the release of adenosine. Adenosine blocks the release of norepinephrine from sympathetic nerve terminals and also has intrinsic vasodilator properties. Thus, hypotension can perpetuate itself through this release of adenosine and its effects. This tissue ischemia effect may also be the reason that anemic patients are prone to hypotension (Bregman et al., 1994). Hypotension during hemodialysis is a common problem in diabetic patients due to autonomic neuropathy. In these patients, arteriolar constriction in response to volume depletion is impaired. Thus, they have a decreased ability to maintain a normal blood pressure during hemodialysis.

Many antihypertensive medications, such as hydralazine, impair vasoconstriction. Beta blockers decrease cardiac contractility and limit the increase in heart rate that should occur. Patients may be told to hold medications until completion of the hemodialysis treatment. Most antihypertensive medications, narcotics, and angiolytics should be withheld up to 4 hours before hemodialysis (Ismail & Hakim, 1991).

PVR may be acutely decreased during hemodialysis because of many vasoactive substances that can be administered with dialysis or released by the cells. Aggregation of neutrophils in the extracorporeal system and sequestration of neutrophils in lungs may produce pulmonary hypertension and a fall in CO and blood pressure. Release of cationic proteins and release of chemical inflammatory mediators from cells may induce acute allergic and potent vasodilatory effects. Interleukin-1 is released in response to exposure of whole blood to cellulose membranes. This release of interleukin-1 and its effects will be discussed in greater detail later in the chapter (Zuchelli, 1987).

Cardiac factors are also a common cause of decreased blood pressure during hemodialysis. The heart's ability to maintain or increase CO in response to volume depletion plays a major role in prevention of hypotension. Hypertrophy and dilatation of the left ventricle, increased age, atherosclerosis, and coronary artery disease can all limit this response. Diastolic dysfunction secondary to a stiff hypertrophied heart results in the inability to maintain CO in response to a minor decrease in filling pressures. Decreased cardiac reserve can also be due to the chronic high output state secondary to the anemia of chronic renal failure and the presence of an AVF or AV graft (Zuchelli, 1987). Uremic autonomic neuropathy or use of beta blockers can also inhibit responses necessary to increase the blood pressure, such as an increase in the pulse rate (Ismail & Hakim, 1991).

Uncommon causes of intradialytic hypotension include pericardial tamponade, myocardial infarction, occult hemorrhage, septicemia, arrhythmias, dialyzer reaction, hemolysis, and air embolism (Bregman et al., 1994).

Nursing management of intradialytic hypotension should focus on early detection, measures to support or restore blood pressure, and prevention. Early detection is the key to prevention of serious consequences resulting from hypotension. Making patients aware of the signs and symptoms of hypotension that they should report to the nurse will help in early detection of the problem. Other important measures are close observation of the patient and monitoring vital signs more frequently in patients prone to hypotension.

When hypotension is discovered, the patient should be placed in Trendelenburg position if respiratory status allows. The UF rate should be decreased to as near zero as possible. It can be resumed at a later time, possibly at a slower rate, once vital signs have stabilized. Slowing of the blood flow rate may help in certain instances. With parallel plate dialyzers, a decrease in blood flow rate as well as a decrease in dialysate negative pressure results in a decrease in pressure in the blood compartment of the dialyzer. This shrinks the total volume of the extracorporeal circuit. If acetate dialysate is being used, then a decrease in blood flow rate will reduce transfer of acetate to the patient. When a UF controller is not available, slowing of the blood flow rate makes it easier to limit the amount of UF. If a hollow fiber dialyzer, bicarbonate dialysate, and a UF controller are being used, then a decrease in the blood flow rate should not be done initially unless the hypotension is severe or unresponsive to other measures (Bregman et al., 1994).

Reversal of hypotension can often be accomplished with a bolus of normal saline solution, 100 ml or more, as necessary, rapidly administered via the venous blood line. As an alternative, hypertonic sodium chloride, hypertonic glucose, mannitol, or albumin solutions can be used to treat the low blood pressure. Unless cramps are present, hypertonic sodium chloride seems to be no more effective than normal saline solution. Nasal oxygen administration may be of benefit by helping to prevent tissue ischemia and improve myocardial function (Bregman et al., 1994).

Most of the time, intradialytic hypotension can be prevented by accurate assessment of the patient, frequent evaluation of the patient's EDW, and use of an ultrafiltration controller whenever possible. The nurse should ensure that the predialysis weight is accurate, especially when the patient has weighed himself or herself. The weight should be compared to the postdialysis weight from the previous treatment and to the EDW. A predialysis weight near to or less than the EDW may suggest that the patient has had some actual weight loss and call for reevaluation of the EDW. The predialysis blood pressures and pulse as well as a complete nursing assessment of the patient's volume status should also be done to determine the need for a change in the EDW. If the patient is below his or her EDW, further weight removal with dialysis should be avoided until the EDW is adjusted. The use of variable sodium dialysate has been found to be successful in preventing intradialytic hypotension in many patients (Jenson et al., 1994).

Patients who are prone to hypotension during hemodialysis should be instructed to withhold their antihypertensive medications prior to their treatment. A daily or BID dose can be given after the treatment. Patient education regarding the signs and symptoms of hypotension as well as dietary counseling regarding fluid restriction is also important.

A dialysis machine with an ultrafiltration controller should be used whenever possible, especially in patients who are prone to hypotension. Dialysate sodium level should be at or above the patient's plasma sodium level, and bicarbonate dialysate should be used anytime the patient dialyzes with a high blood flow rate or with a high-efficiency dialyzer. In selected patients prone to hypotension, the dialysate solution temperature may be decreased to 35-36% degrees centigrade during hemodialysis. This may need to be done only when the patient has had a large interdialytic weight gain (Bregman et al., 1994).

Muscle Cramps

Muscle cramps occur in about 10% of hemodialysis treatments. They are most common after a large fluid gain when a patient requires rapid UF during hemodialysis. Commonly, the cramps accompany a hypotensive episode; however, they can occur alone. The pathophysiology of dialysis-associated muscle cramps is not well understood, but a popular theory is that extracellular volume contraction associated with a rapidly changing osmolality causes the cramping. Hypokalemia has also been cited as a likely cause (Keen et al., 1995).

Severe and prolonged cramps, beginning during the latter part of dialysis and persisting after the treatment ends, can occur when the patient has been dehydrated below his or her EDW. Use of a low sodium dialysate that acutely lowers the plasma sodium concentration can result in constriction of blood vessels in an isolated muscle group (Bregman et al., 1994; Ismail & Hakim, 1991).

When hypotension and muscle cramps occur at the same time, the hypotension may respond to volume expansion, but cramps may or may not persist. The UF rate can be temporarily decreased, and muscle bed blood vessels can be dilated by the administration of normal saline, hypertonic sodium chloride, or hypertonic glucose solutions. The disadvantage of using normal saline is that weight reduction during hemodialysis will be less. A disadvantage of hypertonic sodium chloride (10 ml of 23%) is hyperosmolality, resulting in postdialysis thirst. The use of hypertonic glucose (50 ml of 50%) is better in nondiabetics (Bregman et al., 1994; Ismail & Hakim, 1991).

Stretching of the muscles through dorsiflexion of the foot, either manually or by standing, may help relieve the cramps. Application of heat to the muscle group can also help. Prevention of hypotensive episodes will eliminate the majority of cramping episodes. Frequent assessment of EDW to ensure accuracy is also important.

Use of dialysate with appropriate sodium and potassium levels will help in the prevention of muscle cramps. Sodium modeling, starting with a high dialysate sodium (150-155), then a programmed linear decrease to 135-140 at the end of the treatment, can accomplish this without causing the postdialysis thirst and large interdialytic weight gain that usually accompany the use of high sodium dialysate. High weight gains are also associated with a more pronounced hyponatremia predialysis; thus osmolality changes during dialysis can also be accentuated (Ismail & Hakim, 1991).

Chest Pain

Chest pain can occur during hemodialysis as a result of coronary artery disease, anemia, and severe decrease in intravascular volume. Nursing management includes reduction of the UF rate to zero until the blood pressure increases and discontinuation of dialysis if chest pain is severe. If present, volume depletion is treated with normal saline or other volume expanders. Nitroglycerine should be given only if the patient's blood pressure is stable (Ismail & Hakim, 1991).

Assessment of the patient to determine the appropriate EDW and UF goal are preventive measures for prevention of chest pain. Measures to maintain adequate hematocrit, such as Epogen and transfusions as necessary, will help prevent chest pain secondary to anemia. Nitroglycerine and related maintenance drugs should be prescribed as needed for the patient with coronary artery disease (Levine, 1991).

Fever and Chills

Fever and chills during dialysis can occur for a number of reasons. Fever can be related to infection, pyrogens, or endotoxins (Ismail & Hakim, 1991). Chills are a cold feeling with involuntary shaking, sometimes accompanied by hypotension.

Fever secondary to infection usually occurs at the start of dialysis or shortly after the end of the treatment. Fever at the start of hemodialysis suggests that the patient has been infected by contaminated equipment or dialysate. Fever developing within the first 1-2 hours after completion of hemodialysis implies that the infection has occurred during the termination procedure (Ismail & Hakim, 1991).

Fever and chills occurring during the course of dialysis are most likely secondary to a pyrogenic reaction. Leaching of endotoxin from the membrane causes a pyrogenic reaction (Ismail & Hakim, 1991).

Nursing management of this problem includes assessment of the patient for signs and sources of infection, such as access, respiratory, urinary tract, and so forth. Obtaining cultures of blood, dialysate, and water is important. Antipyretics should be administered for patient comfort. In an undiagnosed febrile reaction, empiric treatment with antibiotics such as vancomycin and aminoglycosides should be considered until culture results are available (Ismail & Hakim, 1991).

Careful sterilization of equipment, especially in high flux dialysis, can help prevent febrile reactions. Bicarbonate-based solution from concentrate should be prepared immediately before hemodialysis and should not be stored long because it supports bacterial growth. Other equipment preparation such as proper reuse procedures are also important. Proper disinfection of the water system, dialysis equipment, and concentrate containers is essential (Ismail & Hakim, 1991).

Dialysis Disequilibrium Syndrome

Dialysis disequilibrium syndrome is a set of systemic and neurologic symptoms, often associated with characteristic EEG findings, occurring during or soon after a hemodialysis treatment. It often occurs when a severely uremic patient is dialyzed aggressively (Bregman et al., 1994; Ismail & Hakim, 1991).

The etiology of dialysis disequilibrium is controversial. The most popular theory is that cerebral edema, or an acute increase in brain water content, occurs when the plasma solute level is rapidly lowered during dialysis, leaving the urea concentration and osmolality of the brain cells and cerebral spinal fluid much higher than that of the plasma. Water then shifts from the plasma into the brain tissue. Another theory is that acute changes in pH of the cerebral spinal fluid during hemodialysis is the cause of the syndrome. This pH change is caused by a more rapid diffusion of carbon dioxide than bicarbonate across the blood-brain barrier (Bregman et al., 1994; Ismail & Hakim, 1991).

Dialysis disequilibrium syndrome was more problematic several years ago when patients with a high BUN were commonly subjected to prolonged dialysis. Milder forms may still be seen in acute and chronic dialysis patients today (Ismail & Hakim, 1991).

Signs and symptoms of mild disequilibrium syndrome include headache, hypertension, restlessness, nausea, and vomiting. Headache is a common symptom associated with hemodialysis, and nausea and vomiting also occur in up to 10% of routine hemodialysis treatments. Therefore, some episodes of disequilibrium go unrecognized. Although most nausea and vomiting in stable patients are associated with hypotension, they can also be an early manifestation of disequilibrium syndrome. As the syndrome progresses or becomes more severe, seizures, decreased sensorium, and coma can occur. Death may even result (Bregman et al., 1994).

Nursing management of mild disequilibrium syndrome includes recognition of early signs and symptoms. Since nausea, vomiting, restlessness, and headache are nonspecific symptoms, it is difficult to be certain that they are secondary to disequilibrium. If these mild symptoms occur in an extremely uremic patient, however, measures should be taken to decrease the efficiency of the dialysis treatment, such as decreasing the blood or dialysate flow rates. This action would also decrease the pH change. Hyperosmolar agents such as hypertonic sodium chloride or glucose solutions or mannitol can be administered to decrease movement of water out of the plasma. A dialysate sodium concentration of greater than 140 mEq/liter has been found in some studies to be useful in maintaining a higher serum osmolality during hemodialysis, thus preventing or alleviating some of the symptoms and discomforts associated with disequilibrium. However, adverse effects secondary to a high dialysate sodium, such as high interdialytic weight gains and elevated blood pressure, have limited its use for this complication. Jenson et al. (1994) demonstrated the successful use of both high and variable sodium dialysate in reducing dialysis disequilibrium symptoms without significant adverse effect. If none of these measures are effective, the treatment may need to be terminated earlier than planned if symptoms persist (Bregman et al., 1994; Jenson et al., 1994).

The occurrence of signs and symptoms of severe disequilibrium such as seizures, obtundation, or coma necessitates the immediate termination of the dialysis treatment. Seizures are treated with maintenance of the airway and ventilation. Mannitol administered intravenously may be of benefit. Coma is treated supportively and usually subsides within 24 hours if due to disequilibrium (Bergman et al., 1994; Ismail & Hakim, 1991).

Acute Hemolysis

Acute hemolysis during hemodialysis is a medical emergency and is almost always due to a problem with the dialysis solution. Overheated dialysis solution can cause hemolysis. Hypotonic dialysis solution from insufficient concentrate to water ratio or the opposite hypertonic dialysate can also lead to hemolysis.

Dialysis solution contamination with metals, organic substances, and inorganic substances in the water used to prepare the dialysate can lead to hemolysis. These contaminants include zinc, copper from pipes, nitrates, and chloramines from the water supply, as well as bleach and formaldehyde used to disinfect the water system and HD machines (Ismail & Hakim, 1991) In rare instances, hemolysis can occur because of erythrocyte trauma in an improperly functioning roller blood pump or high negative pressure in the extracorporeal circuit (Bregman et al., 1994; Keen et al., 1995).

Signs and symptoms of hemolysis include chest pain or tightness, back pain, and dyspnea. The patient may also complain of burning in the access return site and experience hypotension. A port wine or cherry pop appearance of the blood in the venous line postdialyzer indicates hemolysis. Centrifuged samples of hemolyzed blood will show a pink discoloration of the plasma (Bregman et al., 1994; Ismail & Hakim, 1991).

If massive hemolysis is not detected early, hyperkalemia may occur due to the release of potassium from the hemolyzed red blood cells. This can lead to EKG abnormalities, muscle weakness, and possibly to cardiac arrest. Lab results may also reveal a marked decrease in hematocrit and hyponatremia (Bregman et al., 1994).

Nursing management of hemolysis includes immediate halting of the blood pump and clamping of the arterial and venous blood lines. The hemodialysis treatment should be terminated without returning postdialyzer blood to the patient. Monitoring of the patient's vital signs, being alert for signs of arrhythmias, and administration of oxygen is indicated. Volume replacement should also be given if necessary (Bregman et al., 1994).

Blood samples for hematocrit and electrolytes should be obtained, and the nurse should prepare to treat hyperkalemia or low hematocrit. Samples of dialysate should be analyzed to determine the cause if the hemolysis is not related to a faulty blood pump (Ismail & Hakim, 1991).

Once stabilized, the patient should be assessed for the need for continued hemodialysis or isolated UF. He or she also should be assessed for the need for continued observation for delayed hemolysis, which may occur for some time after the treatment ends (Bregman et al., 1994).

Prevention of hemolysis is accomplished with appropriate dialyzer bypass mechanisms on the hemodialysis machine to protect the patient from temperature or conductivity deviation in the dialysis solution. The conductivity and temperature monitors must be working properly to alert the nurse and trigger the bypass mechanism. Proper preventive maintenance will ensure that these devices are functioning adequately to safeguard the patient. Proper water preparation and monitoring of prepump arterial pressures are also measures that may prevent hemolysis.

Air Embolism

Air embolism is a potential catastrophic complication of hemodialysis that can lead to death. Therefore, it must be quickly detected and treated.

An air embolism can be caused during hemodialysis if air enters the extracorporeal circuit via faulty connections, intravenous containers, or from the dialysate compartment. The air detector on the blood circuit should protect the patient, as discussed earlier. However if the air detector is not armed or is malfunctioning, air may be allowed to move through the venous blood line, past the air detector and into the patient (Ismail & Hakim, 1991).

Signs and symptoms of an air embolus depend somewhat upon the position of the patient at the time the air enters the blood stream. In patients who are seated or in bed with head elevated, air will tend to pass up the jugular vein into the cerebral venous system without entering the heart. This causes obstruction of cerebral venous return with loss of consciousness, seizures, and possibly death. If the patient is recumbent, air tends to enter the heart and form foam in the right ventricle, which then passes on into the lungs. At this point the patient will exhibit dyspnea, cough, and chest pain. In a patient lying on the right side, the air may go to the pulmonary arteries, resulting in acute pulmonary hypertension. Some air may also pass into the left ventricle with resulting arterial embolism to the brain and the heart. This can cause arrhythmias and acute neurologic dysfunction. The patient may exhibit sudden dyspnea, cyanosis, respiratory arrest, and loss of consciousness. If the patient is in Trendelenburg position at the time the air enters, air will pass to the lower extremities, causing patchy cyanosis. Air remaining in the legs may prevent the grave consequences outlined above (Bregman et al., 1994; Ismail & Hakim, 1991).

Regardless of patient position, classic signs will

be foam or air pockets in the venous blood line, as well as the patient calling out in alarm at the feeling of air rushing into the venous system. If air has entered the heart, a churning sound may be heard on auscultation of the heart (Ismail & Hakim, 1991).

Nursing management of an air embolus includes immediate clamping of venous blood line and halting of the blood pump to discontinue infusion of air into the patient. The patient should immediately be placed into Trendelenburg position and on his or her left side with chest and head tilted downward. This traps air in the right ventricle, away from the pulmonary valve. Cardiorespiratory support by administration of 100% oxygen by mask, or via endotracheal tube if patient is unconscious, may be indicated. Aspiration of air from the ventricle with a percutaneously inserted needle can be attempted by the physician. Monitoring of vital signs is crucial (Bregman et al., 1994; Ismail & Hakim, 1991).

The nephrology nurse has a vital role in prevention of air embolism during hemodialysis. Preventive measures include use of air detector at all times, taping of connections, and administration of normal saline in bolus form instead of as a continuous infusion. Vented intravenous bottles should not be used in the extracorporeal circuit if at all possible. The heparin infusion should always be administered into the blood line at a point after the blood pump (Bregman et al., 1994; Ismail & Hakim, 1991).

Dialyzer Reactions

This is a broad group of events that includes anaphylactic reaction as well as many less adverse reactions of uncertain origin. These events were often called "first use syndrome" in the past because they presented more often with a new dialyzer, as opposed to a reused dialyzer. However, similar reactions occur with reused dialyzers. Dialyzer reactions are described in two categories, Type A and Type B.

Type A: A Type A dialyzer reaction is more severe than a Type B reaction. Although milder symptoms such as dyspnea, feeling of warmth at the exit site or throughout the body, and a sense of impending doom are common initial symptoms, anaphylaxis, cardiac arrest, and death may ensue. Somewhat milder cases may present with itching urticaria, cough, sneezing, watery eyes, or gastrointestinal symptoms such as abdominal cramping or diarrhea (Bregman et al., 1994).

Symptoms usually occur in the first few minutes of hemodialysis, but may sometimes be delayed for up to 30 minutes or more. Severe reactions are infrequent but represent a major cause for concern. The most severe cases have some features in common. The symptoms start within a few minutes of the initiation of hemodialysis. The patient complains of feeling hot and flushed and may become anxious and agitated. Dyspnea, itching, wheezing, chest pain, back pain, abdominal pain, nausea and diarrhea, and, in some cases, the feeling of impending death are common signs and symptoms. The patient's blood pressure may be low or high. Cardiorespiratory arrest is rare. These severe reactions have occurred in patients with every type of dialyzer and membrane. The reaction may be immunologic or toxic in nature (Bregman et al., 1994; Rault & Silver, 1985).

The etiology of Type A reactions varies. Ethylene oxide was implicated initially in about two-thirds of patients because they were found to have elevated serum titers of antibodies to ethylene oxide-altered proteins. Ethylene oxide was used by manufacturers to sterilize almost all hollow fiber dialyzers in the 1980s, and it tended to accumulate in the potting compound inside the dialyzer. The reaction was observed most often during the first use of a dialyzer and less in dialyzers after reuse. Today, ethylene oxide reactions are uncommon because manufacturers are taking care to remove it, while some have changed potting compound materials to reduce absorption of ethylene oxide (Bregman et al., 1994).

Reactions mediated by the bradykinin system were initially reported in patients both dialyzed with the AN69 membrane and treated with angiotensin-converting enzyme (ACE) inhibitors. The negatively charged AN69 membrane activates the bradykinin system, and effects are magnified because of the ACE inhibitors, since the angiotensin-converting enzyme inactivates bradykinin. It is unclear to what extent ACE inhibitors and other PAN-based membranes or non-PAN membranes cause the same type of reaction. ACE inhibitors may be just amplifying a dialyzer reaction occurring by some other mechanism (Bregman et al., 1994).

Type A reactions have occurred with high-flux dialyzers used with bicarbonate dialysate, which may implicate contamination of the dialysate. Sometimes anaphylactic-type dialyzer reactions have been linked to reuse settings, the problem seeming to be associated with bacteria or endotoxin contamination of the water used for the reuse procedures. However, often the cause is unknown (Bregman et al., 1994).

Occasionally, allergic reactions have been associated with heparin. These reactions have usually been mild, but some reactions to heparin have reportedly led to anaphylaxis. When a patient seems to be allergic to all dialyzers, and dialysate contamination has been ruled out, a heparin allergy should be considered and a trial of heparin-free dialysis or citrate anticoagulation initiated (Bregman et al., 1994).

Complement activation may be a cause of anaphylactic Type A reactions, but this is controversial. Complement activation during hemodialysis with cuprammonium cellulose dialyzers has been reported to be increased in patients prone to hypersensitivity reactions. Complement has been associated with various symptoms, including respiratory distress and poor tolerance to dialysis (Bregman et al., 1994; Rockel, 1988).

Eosinophilia is common in hemodialysis patients, and some reports show that prevalence increases with time on hemodialysis therapy. It has been suggested that eosinophilia could be a part of the dialyzer first use syndrome and thus related to the membrane. In some patients, adverse effects could be related to the Cuprophane® membrane. In this study, in patients with persistent eosinophilia, counts were significantly decreased after a change from cellulose membranes to PAN membranes. The study concluded that eosinophilia was at least partly related to cellulose membranes (Venherwegen et al., 1988).

Nursing management of a Type A reaction is based on symptom management. Hemodialysis should be stopped immediately and blood lines clamped. The blood in the lines and dialyzer should be discarded without returning the blood to the patient. Immediate cardiorespiratory support may be required in an anaphylactic reaction, so the nurse should be prepared for this. Intravenous antihistamines, steroids, or epinephrine may be given according to the severity of the reaction. Patient education regarding signs and symptoms is important in early recognition and intervention (Bregman et al., 1994).

Prevention of Type A reactions can be accomplished by proper rinsing of the dialyzers prior to use to rid them of residual ethylene oxide and other allergens. One may consider switching to gamma-radiated dialyzers as opposed to ethylene oxide sterilized dialyzers. Administration of antihistamines before dialysis may help. Placing the patient on a reuse program and putting new dialyzers through the reprocessing procedure prior to the first use have been found to be valuable preventive measures. Avoidance of the use of AN69 dialyzers in patients taking ACE inhibitors may be beneficial (Bregman et al., 1994).

Type B: Type B reactions are more common than Type A but are nonspecific and less severe. The etiology is unknown. Complement activation has been implicated, but its role has never been proven. If reuse is beneficial in preventing this reaction, it is not known if this effect is due to to the protein coating of the membrane from previous uses resulting in increased biocompatibility, or due to washout of potentially toxic substances from the dialyzer during previous uses and reprocessing (Bregman et al., 1994).

The principal sign of a Type B reaction is chest pain, which may or may not be associated with back pain. Symptoms may occur within the first few minutes of hemodialysis or may be delayed up to 1 hour.

Nursing management of a Type B dialyzer reaction is supportive in nature. Oxygen per nasal cannula should be administered. Myocardial ischemia is common, so any angina should be treated promptly. Dialysis can usually be continued because symptoms usually abate after the first hour (Bregman et al., 1994).

Prevention of Type B reactions can be accomplished by placing the patient on a reuse program, although benefits of reuse are controversial. Changing to a different dialyzer membrane that will cause less complement activation such as substituted cellulose (cellulose acetate) or a synthetic membrane may help (Bregman et al., 1994).

Dysrhythmias

Arrhythmias are common in hemodialysis, especially in patients with underlying heart disease receiving digitalis. They are caused by electrolyte and pH shifts during hemodialysis as well as by removal of antiarrhythmic drugs during the course of the treatment (Bregman et al., 1994).

Nursing management includes the use of appropriate dialysate potassium levels (never less than 2 in a patient on digitalis). The patient's pulse and blood pressure should be monitored for changes and cardiac monitoring or EKGs as necessary. Antiarrhythmic drugs should be administered as ordered. Prevention is the most important focus of nursing care.

Cardiac Arrest

Cardiac arrest during hemodialysis can occur for a number of reasons, including electrolyte imbalances, myocardial infarction, arrhythmias, cardiac tamponade, or a result of technical complications. Signs and symptoms include absence of pulse, respiration, and asystole or ventricular fibrillation on the monitor (Bregman et al., 1994).

Nursing management is supportive, with initiation of CPR, discontinuation of hemodialysis, and return of the blood to the patient. Prevention of causes as well as careful patient assessment before dialysis and during dialysis are important nursing measures. Cardiac monitoring should be considered for high-risk patients on HD (Ismail & Hakim, 1991).

Seizures

Seizures occurring during hemodialysis can be from various etiologies. Seizures associated with uremia or dialysis tend to be generalized in nature and can occur during or after the treatment. The etiology of seizures include hypotension, dialysis disequilibrium, electrolyte imbalances, and known seizure disorders. Children as well as patients with high predialysis BUN or severe hypertension are most prone to seizures during hemodialysis (Ismail & Hakim, 1991).

Nursing management includes measures to minimize osmotic changes during hemodialysis as described in the discussion of dialysis equilibrium. The use of a higher dialysate sodium level (140) and infusion of an osmotic agent, such as mannitol, in the first 2 hours of treatment, can be effective, especially if the BUN is greater than 150. Seizures can also be prevented with avoidance of a rapid decrease in BUN. Measures to prevent this rapid reduction in BUN were also discussed earlier. They include the use of small surface area dialyzers, a low blood flow rate, short treatment time, and concurrent dialysate flow as in the prevention of disequilibrium. Bicarbonate dialysate may also be of value (Bregman et al., 1994; Ismail & Hakim, 1991).

If a patient is at high risk for seizures, administration of an anticonvulsant medication should be considered. If the patient's routine anticonvulsant medication is dialyzable, then an additional dose during hemodialysis may be necessary (Ismail & Hakim, 1991).

Exsanguination

Exsanguination during HD can occur due to breaks in the extracorporeal system or due to access problems. Separation of the blood lines, needle dislodgement, or dialyzer rupture are all potential causes. As previously mentioned, arterial and venous pressure alarms on the hemodialysis blood circuit should alert the nurse to these problems because of the resultant rapid decline in system pressures when a break occurs in the system (Bregman et al., 1994).

Access problems can include rupture of the AVF aneurysm or anastomosis, separation of external shunt at the connector, or separation of a catheter from the catheter cap (Bregman et al., 1994).

Signs and symptoms include obvious bleeding, leading to shock and seizures. Nursing management is to minimize the blood loss by clamping both sides of the separated blood line, catheter, or ruptured dialyzer and by stopping the blood pump. Pressure should be applied to any bleeding site. Symptoms should be treated with oxygen and volume expanders as indicated (Bregman et al., 1994).

Prevention includes securing all connections, catheter caps, and needles with tape. Visualization of the entire extracorporeal circuit is important throughout the dialysis treatment. Use of appropriate pressure monitors and blood leak detectors can cause early detection of problems and prevention of exsanguination.

Dialysis Encephalopathy

Dialysis encephalopathy is a neurologic disorder occurring primarily in patients receiving chronic hemodialysis for many years. Aluminum toxicity is largely accepted as the common cause of this progressive disorder (Ismail & Hakim, 1991).

Early neurologic signs and symptoms include stuttering or stammering, but can progress to personality changes, myoclonus, seizures, and progressive dementia. EEG changes include multiple bursts of delta or theta activity, occasionally accompanied by spikes. These changes can be found 4-6 months before symptoms develop and may persist throughout the course of the disorder (Ismail & Hakim, 1991).

Other evidence of aluminum toxicity may be found, such as microcytic hypochromic anemia in the absence of iron deficiency. Aluminum-associated bone disease (osteomalacia) may be present. Plasma aluminum levels of greater than 200 ug/ml is strongly suspicious, and toxicity cannot be ruled out at a level as low as or less than 100 ug/ml. Rises in plasma aluminum of more than 200 ug/ml after a deferoxamine (DFO) stimulation test is very suggestive of an increased tissue burden of aluminum. A rise of more than 400 ug/ml is highly predictive. A bone biopsy from the iliac crest with stain for aluminum is diagnostic. Aluminum toxicity does not necessarily need to be debilitating or fatal if there is early diagnosis and treatment (Ismail & Hakim, 1991).

Nursing management includes chelation of aluminum with DFO. This is continued until basal levels of aluminum are only slightly increased and there is only a small rise of 20-30 ug/ml after DFO administration. One gram of DFO is given intravenously two times per week during the last 30 minutes of the hemodialysis treatment. The best management, however, is prevention (Ismail & Hakim, 1991).

Use of appropriately-treated water for hemodialysis is an important factor in prevention. Substitution of calcium preparations for aluminum-based gels for phosphate binding is also important (Ismail & Hakim, 1991).

Neutropenia/Complement Activation

Dialyzer membranes made of unsubstituted cellulose will have on their surfaces many exposed hydroxyl groups that can activate the complement cascade in the blood flowing through the dialyzer. The complement fragments will then cause circulating neutrophils to migrate to the lungs where they will localize next to the blood vessel walls, resulting in neutropenia. After 30-60 minutes of hemodialysis, the circulating neutrophil count will again rise to normal levels or even above normal. Substituted cellulose membranes have the hydroxyl groups chemically covered, so they cause much less activation of complement resulting in less neutropenia. This neutrophil accumulation in the pulmonary vasculature is a recognized phenomenon during hemodialysis and has been implicated in the hypoxemia that occurs in some patients early in hemodialysis (Bregman et al., 1994; Lazarus, 1982).

Signs and symptoms such as nausea and vomiting, hypotension, chest pain, and back pain may be due to neutropenia and complement activation, but this is controversial. The majority of patients on cellulose acetate membranes are dialyzed without these symptoms (Bregman et al., 1994).

Complement activation may delay recovery of renal function in acute renal failure because it causes sequestration of neutrophils in the glomeruli. The white blood cell count may also be transiently reduced by 50-80% during dialysis with a cellulose membrane. Thus, all CBCs should be drawn before treatment (Bregman et al., 1994).

Hypoxemia

During hemodialysis, the pO_2 drops anywhere from 5 to 30mmHg. This fall is not clinically significant in a normal patient but may be dangerous for the HD patient with preexisting pulmonary or cardiac disease. There are several possible reasons for this drop in pO_2 (Bregman et al., 1994).

Hypoventilation can be implicated. Acetate dialysate can result in loss of CO_2 from the blood passing through the dialyzer. This leads to hypocapnia, which causes the patient to hypoventilate slightly. Contributing to this is CO_2 consumption during acetate metabolism. Bicarbonate dialysate has an elevated CO_2 due to the way the solution is made, so it does not cause hypocapnia. Bicarbonate, however, can cause alkalosis, particularly if the dialysate bicarbonate level is greater than 35 mEq/liter. Transfer of bicarbonate from the dialysate to the blood can result in metabolic alkalosis, which is a well-known cause of hypoventilation and hypoxemia (Bregman et al., 1994; Hoenick, 1988).

Intrapulmonary diffusion block secondary to leukocyte (neutrophil) aggregation in the pulmonary vasculature can also result in hypoxemia. Some studies have suggested that the alveolar to arterial oxygen gradient is increased very early during HD as a result of neutrophils in the capillaries (Hoenick, 1988).

Supplemental oxygen should be administered during dialysis to acutely-ill patients or those whose clinical course might be compromised by even mild hypoxemia. Nasal oxygen is usually sufficient to prevent hypoxemia (Bregman et al., 1994; Lazarus, 1982).

In high-risk patients, consider the use of a dialyzer made of substituted cellulose or synthetic materials to reduce complement activation and neutrophil aggregation in the pulmonary vasculature. Bicarbonate dialysate should be used with a bicarbonate level low enough to not result in alkalemia (Bregman et al., 1994).

Hemodialysis-related Amyloidosis

Hemodialysis-related amyloidosis is a concern in patients receiving long-term hemodialysis. Carpal tunnel syndrome due to amyloid infiltration of the B2 microglobulin protein is a frequent complication of long-term therapy. Perineural amyloid deposits are formed in B2 microglobulin fibrils and are responsible for the carpal tunnel syndrome. The prevalence appears to be higher in patients on hemodialysis longer than 7 years. In addition to the carpal synovial deposits, cystic bone deposits, particularly in the hips and shoulders, have been reported. However, the extent of systemic amyloid deposition has not been determined (Laurent et al., 1988; Vanderbraucke et al., 1988; Varga, 1987).

Many studies have examined this phenomenon and have found that carpal tunnel syndrome occurs in up to 37% of long-term HD patients. The prevalence correlated with length of time on dialysis. In an 18-year study involving 468 HD patients (Laurent et al., 1988), 68 patients required surgery for nerve entrapment, with 40 of those patients requiring surgery on both sides. Three patients experienced a relapse of the problem and repeat surgery. The mean time between the first hemodialysis treatment and surgery for carpal tunnel syndrome was 12 years. Bone cysts were seen in 28 patients (Laurent et al., 1988; Varga, 1987).

Studies have found bone amyloidosis only in patients dialyzed on Cuprophane® membranes, which are considered to be poorly biocompatible. This could mean that deposition of amyloid may be due to repeated immune stimulation during hemodialysis. B2 microglobulin plasma levels are known to be higher in patients dialyzed with Cuprophane® membranes than in those using PAN membranes.

Hemodialysis-related Interleukin-1 Stimulation

Hemodialysis causes an interaction between the dialyzer membrane and monocytes in the patient's blood, which may result in a local inflammatory response. This response leads to increased monocyte production and induction of interleukin-1 (IL-1). Microbial content of the dialysis solution may also contribute to this IL-1 production. An increased level of IL-1 can cause long-term systemic effects as well as acute changes during and shortly after the HD procedure (Dinorella et al., 1988).

Most patients undergoing an uncomplicated hemodialysis procedure exhibit a slight but consistent rise in body temperature throughout the course of the treatment and for awhile after the procedure. This phenomenon is poorly understood but is consistent with IL-1's ability to induce fever. Headache during HD may also be a result of the induction of prostaglandin E2 (PGE2) by IL-1 in the cerebral tissue. The vasodilatory effect of PGE2 is thought to be responsible for the headache. IL-1 can produce slow-wave sleep, and many HD patients are known to sleep during the procedure (Dinorella et al.,1988).

Long-term changes from accumulation of IL-1 over the years include catabolic changes in muscle, fat, the liver, and connective tissue, which may

Figure 19-14
Flow path for the REDY system.

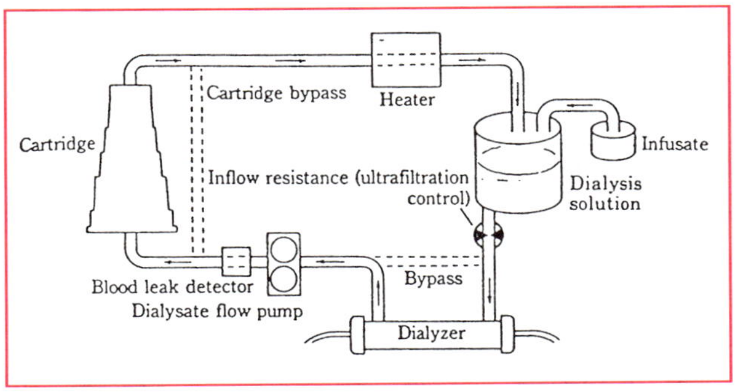

Note: From Roberts, M., & Daugirdas, J.T. (1994). REDY sorbent dialysis. In J.T. Daugirdas & T.S. Ing (Eds.), *Handbook of dialysis* (2nd ed., pp. 198-217). Boston: Little, Brown. Reprinted with permission.

account in part for some of the wasting and negative nitrogen balance found in hemodialysis patients. It causes abnormal lipid metabolism by inhibiting lipoprotein lipase activity in the liver and adipocytes. IL-1 may also contribute to the bone disease suffered by renal failure patients (Dinorella, 1988).

Amyloid deposition may also be related to IL-1. IL-1 may stimulate or activate monocytes, and there appears to be a possible relationship between B2 production and monocyte production when blood is exposed to dialysis membranes (Dinorella, 1988).

Special Procedures Related to Hemodialysis

Sorbent Hemodialysis

Sorbent hemodialysis is a type of portable HD treatment that allows for custom HD without the need for water treatment or even a water supply (see Figure 19-14). Electricity is all that is required to perform HD with this system, which makes it popular in some centers for acute dialysis (Gutch & Stoner, 1993).

Sorbent HD uses a small volume of dialysate which, after passing through the dialyzer, is recirculated through a cartridge of adsorbent materials. The dialysate is chemically regenerated within the cartridge. During regeneration, metabolic waste products, which have been transferred from the blood to the fluid during HD, are removed, and electrolyte content and pH of the solution are restored. During regeneration, conversion of urea to ammonium carbonate, adsorption of creatinine and other nonionized solutes, and ion exchanges in resins occur. The result is a dialysis solution that can be reused for dialysis (Gutch & Stoner, 1993).

As used dialysate enters the sorbent cartridge, it first passes through a carbon layer, which removes heavy metals and oxidants. The dialysate then comes in contact with a bed containing urease, an enzyme that converts urea to ammonium ions and releases sodium and hydrogen ions. Carbonate ions equilibrate with hydrogen ions to form bicarbonate and carbon dioxide. Calcium, magnesium, and potassium ions are exchanged for sodium ions. The third layer in the cartridge contains hydrated zirconium oxide, which removes phosphate and fluoride. The final layer contains activated carbon, which binds creatinine, uric acid, and guanidine by adsorption (Gutch & Stoner, 1993).

An electrolyte infusion called infusate is added to the regenerated dialysate just before it is returned to the dialyzer. It adds calcium and magnesium to keep the desired concentration of these ions in the dialysate. Potassium can be added or omitted at this point, depending on the patient's need (Gutch & Stoner, 1993).

Over the course of the treatment, the composition of the dialysate tends to change. Sodium rises over time because of the release of sodium ions in exchange for ammonium, calcium, magnesium, and potassium ions. Bicarbonate, chloride, and pH also increase over time. Ammonia levels tend to increase because of urease breakdown into ammonium and carbonate (Gutch & Stoner, 1993).

Disadvantages of sorbent hemodialysis include expense. The cartridges are moderately expensive and not always is one cartridge adequate for a dialysis treatment. A second cartridge may need to be used if ammonia accumulates in the fluid of the patient, or if the patient is very large or catabolic. The separate infusate system also adds to the cost of the treatment (Gutch & Stoner, 1993).

The main disadvantage is that there is a quantitative limit to the amount of urea that can be digested by urease and to the amount of ammonium that can be bound to the zirconium phosphate. There is also a lower than normal dialysate flow rate secondary to resistance in the cartridge (Gutch & Stoner, 1993).

Isolated Ultrafiltration

This is a procedure that allows for fluid removal in isolation from diffusion during HD. Studies have shown that it is easier to remove fluid with fewer symptoms during sequential or isolated UF. During conventional acetate HD, there can be significant reduction in plasma volume and cardiac output while total peripheral resistance remains unchanged. During isolated UF, similar reductions in plasma volume and cardiac output are accomplished by a significant increase in total PVR. Thus the result is an unchanged MAP during fluid removal (Zuchelli, 1987).

During isolated UF, ultrafiltration across a high-flux membrane is used to remove large quantities of fluid in the first hour or so of treatment. In the second part of dialysis, dialysate is passed through the dialyzer and clearance occurs, but no fluid is removed. Isolated UF can be performed also at the end of a hemodialysis treatment (Lazarus, 1982).

Treatment of Drug Overdose or Poisoning

Hemoperfusion is the process of using an absorptive cartridge in a hemodialysis circuit to treat overdose or poisoning. Absorptive cartridges are effective in removing many drugs or intoxicants. They are also more efficient than hemodialysis in removing barbiturates, other sedatives, tranquilizers, antidepressants, cardiovascular agents, and various herbicides and insecticides (Gutch & Stoner, 1993).

Decreased platelets are a consequence of the hemoperfusion procedure, but this phenomenon usually reverses within 24 hours. Decreased leukocytes may occur in some patients. Cartridges have limited capacity (Gutch & Stoner, 1993).

Dialyzer Reuse

Dialyzers, after use, can be rinsed free of blood, chemically cleaned, disinfected, and reused. This is a safe and effective practice that is applied to the treatment of about 70% of HD patients in the United States. Most reuse is done with hollow fiber dialyzers. The average number of times a dialyzer is reused varies between centers but may average greater than 10 uses (Kaufman et al., 1994).

The reprocessing process involves rinsing and cleaning, performance measurements, disinfection, and inspection. Removal of residual blood and dialysate from the dialyzer is done with a pressurized rinse of both blood and dialysate compartments shortly after HD. The dialyzer is then cleansed with a 1% bleach solution to dissolve proteinaceous deposits that may occlude fibers. Use of bleach in too high concentrations can cause membrane damage. Hydrogen peroxide and peracetic acid are commonly used agents to clean. Hydrogen peroxide, however, does not remove proteins deposited on the dialyzer membranes so the UF coefficient may decrease over time in dialyzers cleansed with that agent. Reuse is performed on either automated or manual systems (Kaufman et al., 1994).

Tests of dialyzer performance are done to check the integrity of the membrane and its clearance and UF capabilities. The dialyzer is first pressure-tested for leaks through a process that generates a TMP gradient across the membrane and observes for a fall in pressure in either compartment. The fiber bundle volume indirectly measures changes in membrane clearance. It is measured by purging the filled blood compartment with air and measuring the volume of the fluid that is displaced. A reduction in fiber bundle volume of 20% corresponds to a 10% reduction in urea clearance, which is the maximum decrease acceptable for continued use. In any patient, repeated failure to reach a target number of reuses because of fiber bundle volume test failure suggests clotting in the fibers during dialysis. A review of the heparinization prescription should follow. In-vitro UF can also be measured as a direct measurement of mass transfer properties. In-vitro UF is measured by determining the volume of water passing through the membrane at a given pressure and temperature (Kaufman et al., 1994).

Once tested, the dialyzer must undergo disinfection, a physical or chemical process that renders all living organisms inactive. Disinfection can be accomplished through the use of germicide or heat. Common germicides are formaldehyde and a peracetic acid-hydrogen peroxide solution. Heat sterilization obviates concerns related to germicide use, such as ensuring adequate removal of the substance from the dialyzer, but its efficacy is still under investigation. The dialyzer is heated in a 105-degree convection oven for 20 hours. Polysulfone is the only material that has been proven to be heat resistant (Kaufman et al., 1994).

Before use for the next dialysis treatment, a final inspection of the dialyzer is performed. The dialyzer should not be used if it has an abnormal or unaesthetic appearance such as overall brownish or black discoloration, if there are clots visible in the header, or if bands of clotted fibers are present (Kaufman et al., 1994).

In preparation for dialysis with a reused dialyzer, visual inspection should again be done to note any discoloration. The dialyzer should be checked to make certain that it is the proper dialyzer belonging to the patient. Patients should also be taught to check the dialyzer to ensure it has their name on it (Kaufman et al., 1994).

The dialyzer should be tested for the presence of disinfectant to ascertain if that part of the procedure has been done. It is then rinsed, primed, and prepared for hemodialysis. Monitoring of the patient includes observation for symptoms such as fever and chills, which may indicate contamination of the dialyzer. The nurse should also observe for dialyzer failure such as leaks, deviation in UF rates, progressive increase in the patient's serum creatinine, or deterioration in the patient condition such as development of uremic symptoms (Kaufman et al., 1994).

Although there are concerns cited to be associated with dialyzer reuse, there are many clinical benefits. Reuse allows for wider use of costlier, high-efficiency dialyzers. This allows us to increase the amount and efficiency of dialyzers for our patients. High efficiency membranes tend to be expensive; therefore, given the uncertainties regarding reimbursement, reuse affords the opportunity for centers to use these dialyzers (Kaufman et al., 1994).

Some dialyzer reactions associated with cellulosic membranes may be decreased with reuse. It has been advocated that new dialyzers be reprocessed even prior to initial use. In cellulose membranes, reuse lessens the degree of membrane-induced complement activation and the resultant transient neutropenia, which may be due to the protein coating during its initial use. Bleach can remove this protein, however, so the use of bleach will reverse this effect. Nonreused cellulose dialyzers have been found to cause a chronic suppression of several aspects of the immune system. These effects occur less in patients enrolled in a reuse program (Kaufman et al., 1994).

Concerns include those related to reuse center on the substance used for disinfection, the possibility of contamination and transmission of infection, the potential for decreased dialyzer performance over time, and others (Kaufman et al., 1994).

Summary

The patient receiving hemodialysis presents many challenges for the nephrology nurse. The cornerstone of practice for nephrology nurses caring for the hemodialysis patient is a strong knowledge base in the effects of this treatment, the management of treatment complications, maintenance of vascular access, and assessment of patient response to therapy. This sound knowledge base is vital for positive patient outcomes.

References

Bander, S., & Schwab, S. (1992). Central venous angio access for hemodialysis and its complications. *Seminars in Dialysis, 5*(2), 121-128.

Berkoben, M., & Schwab, S. (1995). Maintenance of permanent hemodialysis vascular access patency. *ANNA Journal, 22*(1), 17-24.

Brown, L.H., Wantroba, I., & Simonson, G. (1989). Reestablishing patency in an occluded central venous access device. *Critical Care Nurse, 9*(5), 114-118, 120-121.

Bregman, H., Daugirdas, J.T., & Ing, T.S. (1994). Complications during hemodialysis. In J.T. Daugirdas & T.S. Ing (Eds.), *Handbook of dialysis* (2nd ed., pp. 149-168). Boston: Little, Brown & Company.

Breiterman-White, R. (1995). A review of heparin use in hemodialysis and peritoneal dialysis. *ANNA Journal, 22*(5), 491-493.

Burrows-Hudson, S. (1995). Nephrology clinical outcomes. Part 1: Mortality, morbidity, adequacy of treatment, and quality of life. *ANNA Journal, 22*(2), 113-121.

Caruana, R.J., & Keep, D.M. (1994). Anticoagulation. In J.T. Daugirdas & T.S. Ing (Eds.), *Handbook of dialysis* (2nd ed., pp.13-29). Boston: Little, Brown.

Cheung, A.K. (1990). Membrane biocompatibility. In A.R. Nissenson, R.N.Fine, & D.E. Gentile (Eds.), *Clinical dialysis* (2nd ed., pp. 69-96). Norwalk, CT: Appleton & Lange.

Daugirdas, J.T. (1994). Acute hemodialysis prescription. In J.T. Daugirdas & T.S. Ing (Eds.)., *Handbook of dialysis* (2nd ed., pp.178-191). Boston: Little, Brown.

Daugirdas, J.T. (1994). Chronic hemodialysis prescription: A urea kinetic approach. In J.T. Daugirdas & T. S. Ing (Eds.), *Handbook of dialysis* (2nd ed., pp. 192-220). Boston: Little, Brown.

Depner, T. (1991). Standards for dialysis adequacy. *Seminars in dialysis, 4*(4), 245-252.

Dinorella, C., Koch, K., & Shaldon, S. (1988). Interleukin-1 and its relevance in patients treated with hemodialysis. *Kidney International, 33*(24), S-21–S-26.

Gutch, C., & Stoner, M. (1993). *Review of hemodialysis for nurses and dialysis personnel* (5th ed.). St. Louis, MO: C.V. Mosby Company.

Hartigan, M.F. (1994). Vascular access and nephrology nursing practice. Existing views and rationale for change. *Advances in Renal Replacement Therapy, 1*(2), 155-162.

Hartigan, M.F., & Thomas-Hawkins, C. (1995). Circulatory access for hemodialysis. In L.E. Lancaster (Ed.), *ANNA Core Curriculum for Nephrology Nursing* (3rd ed., pp.259-289). Pitman, NJ: American Nephrology Nurses' Association.

Hoenick, N. (1988). Comparison of membranes used in treatment of end-stage renal failure. *Kidney International, 33*(24), S-44–S-48.

Ismail, N., & Hakim, R. (1991). Hemodialysis. In D.Z. Levine (Ed.), *Care of the renal patient* (2nd ed., pp 220-246). Philadelphia: Saunders.

Jenson, B.M., Dobbe, S.A., Squillace, D.P., & McCarthy, J.T. (1994). Clinical benefits of high and variable sodium concentration dialysate in hemodialysis patients. *ANNA Journal, 21*(2), 115-120.

Kaufman, A.M., Godmere, R.O., & Levin, N.W. (1994). Dialyzer reuse. In J.T. Daugirdas & T. S. Ing (Eds.), *Handbook of dialysis* (2nd ed., pp.137-148). Boston: Little, Brown.

Keen, M.L., Lancaster, L.E., & Binkley, L.S. (1995). Hemodialysis. In L.E. Lancaster (Ed.), *ANNA Core Curriculum for Nephrology Nursing* (3rd ed., pp. 207-258). Pitman, NJ: American Nephrology Nurses' Association.

Laurent, G., Calemard, E., & Charra, B. (1988). Dialysis related amyloidosis. *Kidney International, 33*(24), S-32–S-34.

Lazarus, J. (1982, October). Dialytic therapy: Principles and clinical guidelines. *Hospital Practice,* 111-133.

Levin, N., Gotch, F., Bednar, B., Gallagher, N., & Peterson, G. (1991). Kinetics and quality assurance: Prescription therapy through kinetic modeling. *ANNA Journal, 18*(3), 269-290.

Ludlow, M. (1989). Heparin-free dialysis. *ANNA Journal, 16*(4), 295-297.

Moss, A., Vasilakis, C., Holley, J., Foulks, C., Pillai, K., & McDowell, D. (1990). Use of a silicone dual-lumen catheter with a Dacron cuff as a long-term vascular access for hemodialysis patients. *American Journal of Kidney Diseases, 16,* 211-215.

Northsea, C. (1994). Using urokinase to restore patency in double lumen catheters. *ANNA Journal, 21*(5), 261-264, 273.

Pollak, V., et al. (1988). Dialyzer membranes: Syndromes associated with first use and effects of multiple use. *Kidney International, 33*(24), S-49–S-52.

Raja, R.M. (1994). Vascular access for hemodialysis. In J.T. Daugirdas & T.S. Ing (Eds.), *Handbook of dialysis* (2nd ed., pp. 53-77). Boston: Little, Brown.

Rault, R., & Silver, M. (1985). Severe reactions during hemodialysis. *American Journal of Kidney Diseases,* 5(2), 128-131.

Rockel, A., et al. (1988). Ethylene oxide and hypersensitivity reactions in patients on hemodialysis. *Kidney International, 33*(24), S-62–S-67.

Ronco, C., Conz, P., Bosch, J.P., Lew, S.Q., & LaGreca, G. (1994). Assessment of adequacy in peritoneal dialysis. *Advances in Renal Replacement Therapy, 1*(1), 15-23.

Roy, T., Ahrenholz, P., Falkenhagen, D., & Klinkmann, H. (1982). *The International Journal of Artificial Organs, 5*(3), 131-135.

Sargent, J.A., & Gotch, F.A. (1989). Principles & biophysics of dialysis. In J.F. Maher (Ed.), *Replacement of renal function by dialysis* (3rd ed., pp.4-143). Boston: Kluwer Academic Publishers.

Schulman, G., & Hakim, R. (1994). Hemodialysis membrane biocompatibility in acute renal failure. *Advances in Renal Replacement Therapy, 1*(1), 75-82.

Schwab, S., & Butler, G. (1988). Prospective evaluation of a dacron cuffed hemodialysis catheter for prolonged use. *American Journal of Kidney Diseases, 6*(2), 166-169.

Stackiewicz, L. (1994). Nursing assessment: Preservation of

angio-access. *Dialysis & Transplantation* (6), 331-334.

Threlkeld, J. (1991). Nursing implications in kinetic modeling. *ANNA Journal, 19*(2), 178-181.

Van Stone, J.C. (1994). Hemodialysis apparatus. In J.T. Daugirdas & T. S. Ing (Eds.)., *Handbook of dialysis* (2nd ed., pp.30-52). Boston: Little, Brown.

Van Stone, J. C., & Daugirdas, J.T. (1994). Physiological principles. In J.T. Daugirdas & T. S. Ing (Eds.), *Handbook of dialysis* (2nd ed., pp.13-29). Boston: Little, Brown.

Vandenbraucke, J., et al. (1988). Capsulo synovial and bone amyloidosis: Biocompatibility phenomenon of hemodialysis? *Kidney International, 33*(24), S-35–S-36.

Vanherweghen, J., et al. (1988). Membrane-related eosinophilia in hemodialysis. *Kidney International, 33*(24), S-73–S-74.

Varga, J., et al. (1987). Lack of amyloid in fat aspirates from patients undergoing long-term hemodialysis. *Archives of Internal Medicine, 147*(8), 1455-1457.

Zuchelli, P. (1987). Hemodialysis-induced symptomatic hypotension. A review of pathophysiological mechanisms. *The International Journal of Artificial Organs*, 139-144.

Chapter Highlights

- Hemodialysis, first used clinically in the treatment of renal failure in 1947, remains the most commonly prescribed renal replacement therapy in this country.
- Dialysis is a process through which the composition of two solutions is changed when they are exposed to each other through a semipermeable membrane.
- Diffusion is the movement of solutes, through a semipermeable membrane, from an era of greater concentration to an area of lesser concentration.
- Ultrafiltration is the process through which removal is accomplished during hemodialysis. It is defined by Levine (1991) as the bulk movement of a solvent across a semipermeable membrane.
- Hemodialysis refer to removal of a substance from the bloodstream during a specific unit of time. It is an empirical measurement of the volume of blood that is totally cleared of a particular substance per unit of time (1 minute).
- The hemodialyzer is designed with two internal compartments, one to contain blood and the other for dialysis solution. The two compartments are separated by semipermeable membrane. The membrane surface area between the two compartments is maximized by using a membrane that is divided into either multiple hollow fibers or multiple parallel plates.
- The dialysis solution, or dialysate, is composed of water, specific concentrations of electrolytes such as sodium, chloride, potassium, and magnesium, and a buffer such as acetate or bicarbonate. These substances are in the solution in concentrations that mimic an ideal plasma water. Most dialysate also contains glucose or dextrose (Lazarus, 1982).
- During hemodialysis, the patient's blood is exposed to more than 120 liters of water. This is greater than 20 times the amount the average person would normally take in orally in a 24-hour period. Thus, substances that are not harmful in drinking water may be harmful in dialysis water. Small molecular weight substances in the water have direct access to the patient's bloodstream, so it is very important that the purity of the water used for hemodialysis be known and controlled.
- Vascular access is frequently needed to emergently provide renal replacement therapy for patients with acute renal failure (ARF). Temporary access is also utilized to treat patients during the maturation period of a permanent access, or during revision of a permanent hemodialysis or peritoneal dialysis access.
- The primary AVF is the preferred long-term access for patients with CRF. An AVF is the safest and longest-lasting permanent vascular access, with a reported 3-year survival rate of 65-75%. It is preferable to the synthetic graft because of long-term patency and lower infection rates.
- Ischemia of the distal extremity, commonly called steal syndrome, occurs most commonly in patients with previously compromised circulation, such as older patients, or patients with diabetes mellitus or atherosclerosis.
- Nurses should ensure that adequate skin preparation with an SP antimicrobial solution is accomplished prior to needle insertion for dialysis. Patient-related risk factors such as poor personal hygiene or practices such as intravenous drug use should be included in patient education.
- Use of the PermCath is indicated in patients in whom it is difficult to readily insert an AVF or graft. It can provide a long-term access in children, diabetics, and morbidly obese patients. It is also useful in patients who have exhausted all other access sites and in patients who experience high output congestive failure with a primary AVF or an AV graft.
- In 1976, as a result of the need to develop an assessment tool for dialysis adequacy, the National Institutes of Health commissioned a multicenter study to examine and compare various hemodialysis regimens in regard to patient outcomes. Thus, the National Cooperative Dialysis Study (NCDS) was conducted between 1978 and 1983.

Chapter Highlights (continued)

- The NCDS revealed that dialysis prescription had an effect on the occurrence of medical complications and hospitalization rates in hemodialysis patients. The results of this study provided the nephrology community with two important tools. A clear, measurable definition of adequate dialysis resulted (a Kt/V of 1.0 or higher). It also provided nephrologists with a tool for determining dialysis prescription and monitoring of the effectiveness of treatment delivery.

- An adequate hemodialysis prescription is only the beginning of an adequate treatment. Ongoing evaluation of treatment parameters as well as successful delivery of the prescribed treatment are as important as the determination of treatment parameters. Nephrology nurses have the most crucial role in ensuring that hemodialysis patients receive the treatment that has been prescribed.

- Levin described the requirements for ensuring adequate therapy: an appropriate prescription, a high level of nursing expertise, an efficiently operating hemodialysis machine, satisfactory access to the circulation, an informed patient, and ongoing data collection and review.

- Heparin-free dialysis is the method of choice for patients who are actively bleeding or are at high risk for bleeding. There are also patients in whom heparin is contraindicated, such as those with thrombocytopenia or other coagulopathies, who will benefit from heparin-free dialysis.

- The predialysis weight should be compared with the postweight from the previous treatment and with the patient's estimated dry weight (EDW). Other parameters such as blood pressure, pulse, findings upon auscultation of the heart and lungs, the presence or absence of edema, and an interdialytic history should be considered along with the weight to determine the true volume status of the patient.

- Serum samples obtained immediately postdialysis can give information regarding urea removal, correction of acidosis, and normalization of electrolytes. However, movement of these substances between body fluid compartments will continue after dialysis is completed.

- The most common complications of hemodialysis are, in descending order of frequency: hypotension (20-30% of hemodialysis treatments), muscle cramps (5-20%), nausea and vomiting (5-15%), headache (5%), chest pain (2-5%), back pain (2-5%), itching (5%), and fever and chills (<1%).

- When the UF rate is high because of a large weight gain, fluid is removed from the vascular space at a faster rate than the rate at which plasma refilling occurs (fluid moves in from intracellular and interstitial fluid compartments). Maintenance of blood volume depends upon rapid refilling of the blood compartment from surrounding compartments. If the plasma refilling rate is low and the patient is unable to maintain adequate or increased P/VR, hypotension will result.

- Nursing management of intradialytic hypotension should focus on early detection, measures to support or restore blood pressure, and prevention.

- Arrythmias are common in hemodialysis, especially in patients with underlying heart disease receiving digitalis. They are caused by electrolyte and pH shifts during hemodialysis as well as by removal of antiarrhythmic drugs during the course of the treatment.

- Sorbent hemodialysis is a type of portable HD treatment which allows for custom HD without the need for water treatment or even a water supply.

- During isolated UF, ultrafiltration across a high-flux membrane is used to remove large quantities of fluid in the first hour or so of treatment.

- Dialyzers, after use, can be rinsed free of blood, cleaned, disinfected, and reused. This is a safe and effective practice that is applied to the treatment of approximately 70% of HD patients in the United States.

CHAPTER 20

Continuous Renal Replacement Therapy

Christy A. Price, RN, MSN, CNN

Chapter Contents

Historical Review of Treatment of Acute Renal Failure 579
CRRT Technologies, Hemofilters, and Equipment 579
Responsibilities of Health Care Professionals 583
Nursing Care Before CRRT 583
Nursing Care During CRRT 584
Nursing Care After CRRT 585
Nursing Literature and Research Related to CRRT 585
Summary 586
References 586
Chapter Highlights 588

Continuous Renal Replacement Therapy

Christy A. Price, RN, MSN, CNN

The treatment of acute renal failure in the United States has military roots coinciding with the treatment of war casualties during World War II, Korean police action, and the Vietnam conflict. The clinical experience gained from these difficult periods in history has led to changes, which in current practice allow nephrology and critical care professionals to effectively manage the fluid, electrolyte and acid/base abnormalities that occur secondary to acute kidney dysfunction. Although hemodialysis remains a treatment option in an intensive care unit, the purpose of this chapter is to address continuous renal replacement therapy as the treatment of choice. The technical aspects related to the different approaches of employing continuous therapy will be covered. The roles of the nephrology and critical care nurses as they relate to the preprocedure, intraprocedure, and postprocedure assessment and intervention will be addressed. Finally, the nursing literature and current research will complete the chapter.

Historical Review of Treatment of Acute Renal Failure

The mortality and morbidity associated with acute renal failure (ARF) was extremely high during the two world wars. The multisystem sequelae and sepsis that often accompany ARF secondary to traumatic injuries and/or gunshot wounds led to the triage of many soldiers to the "expectant" category. Primarily in Europe during the 1940s, researchers were slowly making progress in dialysis-related delivery systems and hemodialyzers. In 1948, the first successful use of hemodialysis in the United States was reported as a treatment for ARF related to self-administration of vaginal mercury to induce a spontaneous abortion (McBride, 1987). During the Korean police action, military nephrologists were able to use hemodialysis successfully, which led to saving many young lives. Upon returning to civilian practice, these military physicians provided valuable experience for the training of future nephrologists. Shortly thereafter, nurses became involved in the delivery of hemodialysis and care of the patients with ARF.

After the passage in 1972 of PL 92-603, which assured Medicare coverage for patients with chronic renal failure (CRF), more physicians and nurses were needed to provide dialytic therapy to the growing patient population. It is this expanded coverage and availability for the treatment of CRF that led to an increase in the number of professionals with the knowledge and experience to safely and effectively treat ARF during the Vietnam conflict and more recently the Persian Gulf conflict.

Whether on a battle ground or in a hospital intensive care unit (ICU), since 1982 nephrology professionals have not had to rely on hemodialysis (HD) or peritoneal dialysis (PD) for the treatment of ARF. Continuous renal replacement therapy (CRRT) has received popular acceptance in Europe and the United States, particularly for hemodynamically unstable patients who are unresponsive to conservative management with pharmacologic and dietary interventions. In the simplest form, CRRT is an arterial to venous extracorporeal whole blood circuit that uses the patient's mean arterial pressure (MAP) as a driving force to propel blood through the circuit and create an ultrafiltration of plasma water. In military situations and/or civilian settings, many nephrologists and nephrology nurses have embraced CRRT because it is recognized as meeting the total 24-hour needs of the patient for hourly fluid and electrolyte balance, adjustment of acid/base status, and continuous removal of uremic toxins. Furthermore, correction of the patient's clinical profile can be accomplished while maintaining hemodynamic stability and providing essential nutritional and pharmacokinetic support.

CRRT Technologies, Hemofilters, and Equipment

The early literature describing CRRT highlighted the benefits of continuous fluid removal for patients with renal dysfunction (Kramer et al., 1980). The extracorporeal circuit required arterial and venous vascular access and a hemofilter as a highly porous device for removal fluid and small molecular weight plasma contents. A continuous heparin infusion was used to maintain anticoagulation of the system. Replacement fluids were administered continuously or intermittently to balance the hourly fluid removal. Figure 20-1 provides a pictorial view of basic CRRT components.

The first acronyms for these treatments were CAVH (continuous arteriovenous hemofiltration), CAVU (continuous arteriovenous ultrafiltration), and SCUF (slow continuous ultrafiltration) respectively (Paganini & Nakamoto, 1980; Lauer et al.,

Figure 20-1
Arterial, ultrafiltrate line, and venous blood lines, hemofilter, and CAVHD port.

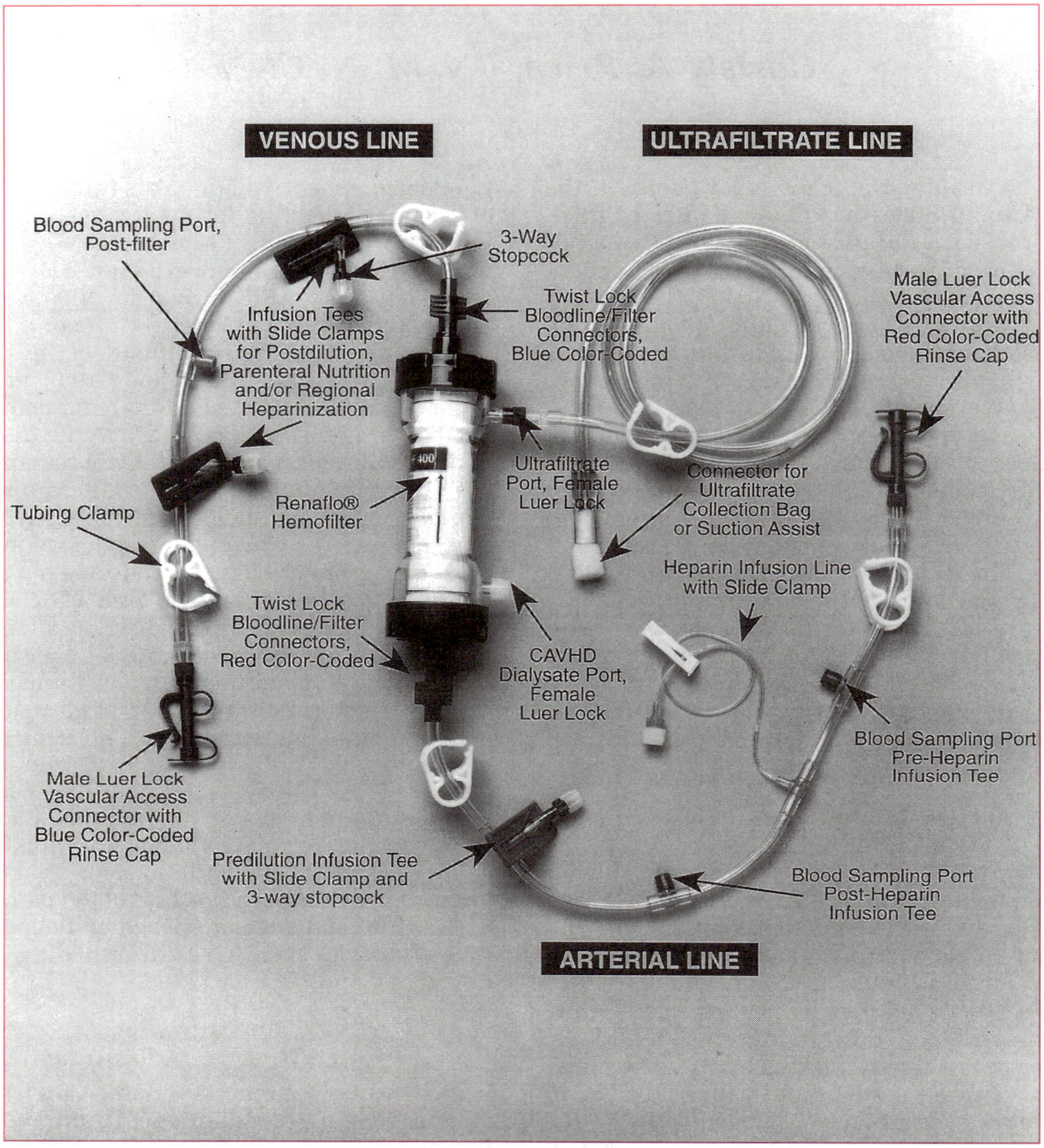

Note: Printed with permission from Renal Systems.

1983; Kaplan, Longnecker, & Folkert, 1984; Kiely, 1984; Golper, 1985; Bosch, 1986; Paganini, 1988; Price, 1989a). A basic definition of these procedures is: an arteriovenous extracorporeal circuit with the patient's whole blood flowing through a hemofilter to create an ultrafiltrate of plasma. A hemofilter is a medical device of either hollow fiber or parallel plate membrane geometric design that allows plasma water and dissolved contents to freely move across the membrane and out of the patient's blood. Ultrafiltrate is plasma water free of formed cells and protein, and it is isotonic with plasma for small molecules, for example, electrolytes, creatinine, and urea. The system is blood pressure-dependent as the driving force for the blood flow rate (BFR), and it uses a gravity drain for ultrafiltration into a fluid collection container. Ideally the patient's systolic blood pressure (SBP) is constantly > 90 mmHg and the MAP is > 70 mmHg. This is required to assure a positive pressure on the

Table 20-1
Formulae and calculations for monitoring CRRT.

A. Blood flow rate
- Qbi = (Qf x Hct outlet) / (Hct outlet - Hct inlet)
- QBi = blood flow rate in ml/min
- Qf = ultrafiltation rate in ml/min
- Hct inlet = hematocrit prehemofilter in percent
- Hct outlet - hematocrit posthemofilter in percent

B. Ultrafiltration rate
- UFR = TV / 60 min
- UFR = ultrafiltration rate in ml/min
- TV = total volume of ultrafiltrate in 1 hour

C. Sieving coefficient for solute removal
- Sieving coefficient = ultrafiltrate level/ plasma level
- Sieving coefficient = ratio of the ultrafiltrate concentration of a solute to the plasma concentration of the solute

D. Fluid replacement using net loss concept
- Total fluid output - total fluid intake = volume of fluid loss
- Volume of fluid loss - prescribed net loss = fluid replacement
  - Total fluid output = urine, gastric tubes, chest tubes, stool, UF, insensible loss, etc.
  - Total fluid intake = IVs, blood products, oral, nutritional support, etc.
  - Net loss must be in physician's orders
  - Replacement fluid will be infused over following hour

blood side of the hemofilter membrane and an uninterrupted BFR through the circuit, which can be calculated using the formula from Table 20-1. For most patients, the BFR will range from 50 - 200 ml/min.

The plasma ultrafiltrate is collected and measured hourly to calculate the ultrafiltration rate (UFR). The formula is included in Table 20-1. The tubing to the gravity drain ultrafiltrate collection device characteristically is straight and 40 cm long, which generates a negative, or pulling, pressure. The combination to the positive pressure reflective of the MAP and negative pressures generated by the gravity drain set up creates the hourly UFR. Consideration of the total amount of fluid removed must also calculate the influence of the patient's oncotic, or plasma proteins, pressure, which acts to retain fluid in the intravascular space. As in the human kidney, oncotic pressure opposes ultrafiltration. Without appropriate oncotic pressure, the patient would not have the ability to maintain a proper intravascular volume and considerable third spacing of fluid would occur into the tissues. With appropriate oncotic pressure (albumin level approximately 4.0 gm/ml), the intravascular space remains fully expanded, and the excessive fluid can be removed as the whole blood passes through the hemofilter. If the patient has a low serum albumin or low oncotic pressure, the amount of hourly fluid removal could be very high, particularly if the patient is hypertensive, which causes a higher positive pressure in the CRRT circuit.

The use of CRRT is limited to an ICU setting where close hourly monitoring and fluid adjustments are possible. The original intent of CAVH and SCUF was to augment existing renal function and decreased urine output. The most conservative of the CRRT therapies for fluid removal is SCUF. Generally, the patient is not anuric, but requires ultrafiltration of an extra 100 - 300 ml of fluid/hour for a short period of time, possibly 12 - 48 hours. Replacement fluid for the ultrafiltrate is usually not necessary. A typical patient profile might be an individual with renal insufficiency who is status-post myocardial infarction, or a patient with moderate oliguria who is resistant to diuretics.

When the patient's clinical status is more critical, or involves multisystem failure, CAVH provides a therapeutic advantage. With CAVH the hourly UFR can range from 200 - 800 ml of fluid, which is poorly tolerated by most hemodynamically unstable patients. The patient may be oliguric or anuric. If replacement fluid is not delivered intravenously (IV) every hour, the patient may experience significant hypotension and other cardiac abnormalities. Physicians will prescribe a hourly net loss of fluid as their goal for the patient, for example 100 - 300 ml/hr. The physician's orders will also prescribe the type of replacement fluid to be infused, for example, normal saline with potassium, 5% dextrose and .45% normal saline, or 5% albumin solution. The replacement is customized to meet the patient's unique needs. Critical care nurses will monitor the patient's hemodynamic parameters, document the intake and output fluid volumes, and then calculate the amount of fluid to be replaced. In a patient scenario, the total fluids intake might be 500 ml and the total fluids output might be 800 ml. If the planned net loss of fluid per hour is 200 ml, the nurse would administer 100 ml of the replacement fluid over the next hour (800 - 500 = 300 actual fluid loss; then 300 - 100 = 200 net fluid loss) (see Table 20-1).

The replacement fluid is infused either predilution in the arterial blood tubing, before the hemofilter, or postdilution in the venous blood tubing, after the hemofilter, as labeled in Figure 20-1.

The preference for the replacement fluid administration is physician dependent. Predilution will dictate the use of more solution, but it may decrease the anticoagulation requirements and increase clearance of plasma contents because of the hemodilution effect of expanding the blood volume. Postdilution is simpler to comprehend because none of the fluid is lost in the ultrafiltrate, easier to calculate for intake and output, and less expensive because generally less replacement fluid is needed.

In addition to maintaining and calculating the BFR, UFR and fluid requirements, the CRRT circuit requires an ongoing method of anticoagulation to maintain the long-term patency. A patient clinical presentation may require the application of CRRT for a short period, that is 24 - 48 hours, or a prolonged period of > 2 weeks. Heparin therapy is the standard means of assuring patency of the extracorporeal circuit. Heparin administration is prescribed usually as a bolus dose to be given prehemofilter at the initiation of CRRT. Depending on the patient's injuries or wounds, postsurgical status, and risk for hemorrhage, the heparin dose may range from 0 - 2000 units IV bolus. During the course of therapy, an hourly heparin infusion may be prescribed that may range from 0 to 5 - 10 u/kg. The heparin administration may be regulated by the platelet count, partial prothrombin time (PTT), prothrombin time (PT), or activated clotting time (ACT). The experience of health care professionals, available hospital equipment, and established ICU protocols will dictate the use of heparin therapy. There is no standard or universally accepted approach.

For several years, CAVH and SCUF served the nephrology and critical care community well for the treatment of ARF. However, in the late 1980s, a new dimension was added to the CRRT system. Fluid and moderate solute removal could be achieved with CAVH or SCUF, but for patients who had no kidney function, the removal of uremic toxins and electrolytes was inadequate. Continuous arteriovenous hemodiafiltration or hemodialysis (CAVHD) was introduced for the treatment of patients who required considerable adjustment for serum electrolyte abnormalities, intervention for severe acid/base disturbance, and correction of moderate to severe uremia (Geronemus, 1988).

In the ARF setting, therapy for correction of fluid overload is of paramount importance. Equally important is the removal of toxins that under normal conditions would be excreted through the kidneys. Clearance of metabolic waste products is a goal of renal replacement therapy. Clearance of plasma substances is achieved by convection during CAVH. Adequate clearance can be achieved if the patient is not extremely catabolic and/or nephrology service is consulted early in the ARF setting. There is only minimal clearance achieved using SCUF because of the low hourly UFR. Convective clearance is the removal of a substance along with fluid, that is, the ultrafiltrate. The plasma contents are essentially carried across the hemofilter membrane. In this situation, clearance is reflective of the sieving coefficient (see Table 20-1). The more ultrafiltrate generated, the higher will be the clearance of molecules. The measurement is based on every 100 ml of fluid ultrafiltrated.

With CAVHD, the CRRT system is not dependent on convective clearance alone. Adding a dialysate solution to run countercurrent to the patient's blood flow in the extracorporeal circuit permits diffusion of substances across the hemofilter membrane. Plasma contents will move in the direction of higher concentration to lower concentration. The dialysate solution will customarily be prescribed for concentration of sodium, potassium, calcium, bicarbonate, and possibly glucose. Solutions similar to PD solutions may be used, that is, Na: 134 mEq/L; K: 0 - 4 mEq/L; Ca: 2.5 - 3.5 mEq/L; HCO3: 25 - 35 mEq/L; Mg: 0.5 - 1.5 mEq/L; and glucose: 0 - 1500 mg dextrose/L. If the patient's serum level is higher than the dialysate level, then that particular substance will diffuse across the membrane with the ultrafiltrate. During CAVHD, the dialysate flow rate (DFR) may range from 1 - 3 L/hr, or 16.7 - 50 ml/min. CAVHD rapidly replaced CAVH for critically ill patients whose health care needs necessitated more intense management. The clearance of plasma water contents is improved by having convection and diffusion principles operational. However, this complicates a rather simple procedure and added to the expense of providing the therapy (Henrich, 1993). Patients who might benefit from CAVHD are patients who have sustained severe traumatic injuries or burns, patients with extremely compromised cardiac function, and/or patients who are statuspost extensive vascular repair surgery.

Although CAVH and CAVHD satisfied the needs of patients with ARF, physicians and nurses were frustrated with the inconsistency inherent in the arteriovenous circuit and related BFR. When a patient's MAP dropped, the driving force for the CRRT was impaired, which led to a decrease in ultrafiltration and clearances. Additionally, the interruptive nature of the arteriovenous blood flow led to earlier clotting of the system secondary to periods of stasis. The arteriovenous system necessitated sometimes very prolonged cannulation of usually a femoral artery with a large catheter. Occasionally, patients who would benefit from CRRT do not have the arterial vascular integrity to support the large indwelling catheter.

With these considerations at hand, nephrologists relied on their experience with the blood pump-assisted system of HD. Continuous venovenous hemofiltration (CVVH) and continuous venovenous hemodialysis (CVVHD) were introduced as alternatives for CAVH and CAVHD, respectively. These techniques further complicated the simple CRRT system, but they have allowed for a greater number of patients to be treated (Mehta, 1993;

Paganini, 1993). The patient's MAP does not influence the BFR with CVVH or CVVHD, but in lieu of the MAP, a blood pump is set from 50 - 200 ml/min. Problems can arise during periods of hypotension because the BFR is not altered, nor is the UFR lowered to compensate for the decreased MAP. The patient may continue to lose intravascular fluid volume and quickly develop a fluid deficit. However, during the venovenous approach to CRRT the infusion of heparin is more consistent, therefore, clotting of the hemofilter may be less problematic. The venovenous system equipment requirements add to the expense of providing CRRT and to the nurse's time and attention for monitoring patient care. Continuous venovenous therapy mandates a blood pump, air alert detector, and venous pressure alarm. CVVHD requires the use of one or more dialysate delivery pumps to maximize the therapy for achieving diffusive clearance (Bonnardeaux et al., 1992). Some ICU protocols allow for another pump on the ultrafiltrate tubing to control the UFR, which adds equipment and cost to CRRT. A pump-controlled UFR or continuous suction-controlled UFR set-up negates the original gravity drain approach to CRRT for collecting the ultrafiltrate. Patients who would be candidates for these therapies are diabetics, patients with advanced cardiovascular disease, elderly patients with significant arteriolosclerosis or atherosclerosis, and/or neonatal or pediatric patients.

The treatment of ARF has changed considerably over the years. Likewise, the practice of CRRT has changed. The advantage of CRRT over standard acute HD is that there are five approaches in the health care professionals' armamentarium of therapies. Treatment can be provided on a continuous basis, rather than attempting to fit the patient's needs into a time-prescribed therapy, like 3 or 4-hour treatment with HD. The approach to CRRT most often is based on the knowledge and skill of the nephrology and critical care professionals, the availability of necessary equipment, and the patient's clinical status. Treatment with planned patient outcomes and expected goals guides the use of CRRT.

Responsibilities of Health Care Professionals

In a collaborative effort, the American Nephrology Nurses' Association (ANNA) developed *Standards of Clinical Practice for Continuous Renal Replacement Therapy,* and these standards were reviewed and subsequently endorsed by the American Association of Critical Care Nurses (AACN) (Price, 1993). Nursing professionals recognize collaboration and communication must exist for successful management of patients receiving CRRT. Unlike the nursing care for patients receiving HD, where the lines of responsibility are fairly well defined, there is a blending of nursing roles and care, when CRRT is the treatment of choice. The continuous nature of CRRT over hours or days requires a delineation of who will provide the care and when the necessary nursing interventions will occur. Of equal importance is the delineation of physicians' responsibilities for the nephrologists and intensivists. However, this chapter will only address the nursing care from the perspective of pre-CRRT assessment, intra-CRRT monitoring and interventions, and post-CRRT evaluation.

Nursing Care Before CRRT

When critically ill patients present to the hospital emergency room or develop ARF while hospitalized, intensive monitoring and intervention are often required. Critical care nurses are always responsible for the total nursing management of ICU patients. This includes following the nursing process of systematic data collection, setting expected patient outcomes, planning nursing interventions accordingly, and evaluating the patient's response to the nursing care provided. A total body systems physical assessment is completed upon admission to the ICU, and then at the beginning of each nursing shift. Using the cephalocaudal approach, the nurse incorporates any findings that are caused by ARF, or may be exacerbated by the ARF, for example, fluid imbalance and cardiac dysrhythmias. Additionally, the critical care nurse assesses findings of available pertinent laboratory analyses and diagnostic tests. This might include serum chemistries, arterial blood gases, urine analysis, and blood and/or urine cultures. Diagnostic procedures might include renal biopsy, radiography, ultrasound, flow scans, computed tomography (CT), and/or magnetic resonance imaging (MRI) studies.

After the nephrologist has been consulted regarding the patient's medical problems, nephrology nurses are alerted to the possibility of providing dialysis. Often the nephrologist and a nephrology clinical nurse specialist (CNS) will collaborate on the type of dialysis that would best meet the patient's needs. If CRRT is the selected renal replacement modality, the physician and the CNS, or another nephrology nurse, review the patient's clinical presentation, the need for fluid and/or solute removal (urea and creatinine), and the availability of arterial and venous vascular access. Ideally, a critical care CNS and a nephrology CNS jointly plan the nursing care of the patient. Based on each of these considerations, SCUF, CAVH, CAVHD, CVVH, or CVVHD will be prescribed. Figure 20-2 provides a pictorial view of each of the CRRT therapies.

A nephrology nurse will prepare the CRRT system to assure removal of all air, sterilant, and packing agents. This is necessary to avoid an adverse reaction upon initiation of the therapy. After priming the system with heparinized normal saline (5000 u/L), the nephrology nurse usually takes the CRRT system to the patient's ICU bedside. Before proceeding with the initiation of CRRT, the nephrology nurse completes an assessment of the patient's condition. Additionally she/he completes, or consults with the critical care nurse regarding the total patient physical assessment. The nephrology nurse reviews the nursing documentation and the physician's orders and progress notes. Collaboratively the nurses perform an assessment of the vascular access(es) that has been placed either by the nephrologist, the intensivist, or the surgeon. The nephrology nurse and the responsible critical care nurse discuss the intended interventions and assure that all appropriate supplies are readily available, that is, replacement fluids, dialysate, heparin infusion, and pump-assisted equipment.

Ideally, the nurses work together to initiate the treatment. The arteriovenous or venovenous vascular access(es) are flushed per protocol, the blood tubing is connected using strict sterile technique, and the extracorporeal blood circuit is established. If prescribed, the nephrology nurse will administer a heparin bolus into the arterial blood line. The heparin infusion will be started and gradually increased based on the ICU protocol, which generally requires monitoring the patient's activated clotting time (ACT), partial prothrombin time (PTT), or prothrombin time (PT), and titrating the heparin infusion for delivery of the correct dose. There is no universal or standard approach for anticoagulation therapy related to CRRT, but rather hospital-specific guidelines.

The nurses monitor the patient's response to the initiation of the treatment. Particularly the patient's blood pressure and pulse are observed to avoid sudden changes that indicate cardiac distress. During the first 30 minutes of treatment, the nurses observe the ultrafiltrate for color and amount. The BFR and UFR can be calculated (see Table 20-1). If a venovenous approach is used, the BFR is slowly increased as ordered, usually from 50 to 150 ml/min. If the UFR is high, that is greater than 200 ml of collected ultrafiltrate in less than 30 minutes, the replacement fluid is started to avoid significant vascular collapse and hypotension. The replacement prescription is based on an assumed net loss of fluid every hour. The nurses must collect the information to calculate the total intake and output each hour (see Table 20-1). Finally, if prescribed, a dialysate solution is prepared on a fluid administration pump to be delivered countercurrent to the BFR. This dialysate solution is delivered to the space on the outside of the hollow fiber or parallel plate membrane to promote clearance of small molecular weight solutes across the membrane by diffusion. The nurses share the responsibility for assuring correct solution and delivery rate as prescribed in the physician's orders.

Figure 20-2
Diagrams of continuous renal replacement therapies.

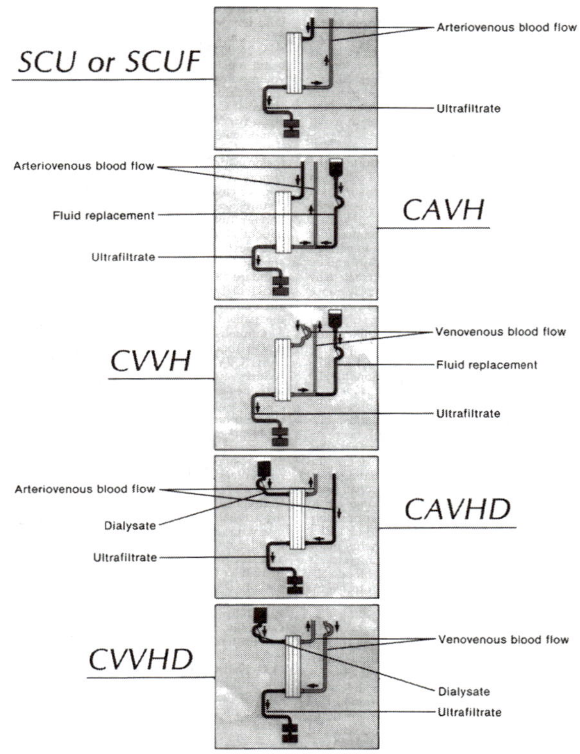

Note: Printed with permission from Cobe Gambro-Hospital Medical, Inc.

Nursing Care During CRRT

Once the therapy is ongoing and the patient remains stable, critical care nurses assume primary responsibility for the CRRT treatment (Bosworth, 1992). However, a nephrology nurse or CNS is expected to visit the patient daily or more often if necessary, and complete a physical assessment of the patient and an equipment assessment of the CRRT system. After consulting with the nephrologist, if patency of the system is suspect, a nephrology nurse arranges for discontinuation of the present CRRT circuit and reinitiation of CRRT with a new hemofilter and tubing. A nephrology nurse checks daily laboratory analyses to assess adequacy of clearances and ultrafiltration, which might also necessitate a new hemofilter and tubing, if the therapy is not meeting expected goals. The nephrologist and nephrology CNS usually collaborate on making adjustments in the CRRT system, and the CNS assists the critical care nurse with the necessary interventions. A nephrology nurse must always be available by telephone or pager to assist critical care nurses with nursing care related to CRRT.

In performing routine intensive care, the critical care nurse consults with the intensivist or nephrologist and relates the nursing assessment and any changes in the patient's clinical course. A nephrology CNS and a critical care CNS, working together for the patient and involved nursing professionals, is the best means of assuring successful clinical application of CRRT. Relying on their individual expertise, these nurses will enhance the probability of successful management of patients with ARF. Appropriate nursing policies, procedures, and standards of practice are developed and communicated to all professional nurses. Particularly important during the intratherapy period, all nurses must comprehend and follow protocols for intervening to resolve problems related to CRRT, or make adjustments based on evaluation of the patient's response to therapy. Some of the most frequent patient complications that may occur are hypotension, cardiac dysrhythmias, excessive fluid loss, electrolyte imbalance, acid/base abnormalities, neuromuscular changes, local and/or systemic infection, and blood loss. Some of the most frequent CRRT circuit problems that may occur are disconnection of blood lines at the vascular access site, clotting of the hemofilter, blood leak in the hemofilter, physical damage to the hemofilter plastic case, and malfunctioning pump-assisted equipment. The patient-related problems often are related to the patient's underlying diagnosis, comorbid factors, and/or need to make changes in the CRRT circuit, for example, advancing CAVH to CAVHD or changing the replacement fluid prescription. The supply or equipment-related problems mandate changing the sterile set-up, increasing attention to all tubing connections, having the hemofilter clearly visible at all times (that is, not covered with bed linens), increasing anticoagulation delivery, monitoring for positional or kinked catheters, and securing biomedical assistance for equipment support. If the system should clot, the critical care nurse must disconnect the tubing from the vascular access(es) and focus on maintaining patency of the access until a new system is available.

Nursing Care After CRRT

With resolution of the patient's ARF or with a decision to withdraw therapy, the CRRT circuit is discontinued. Often this task is a joint responsibility shared by nurses. If the ARF has resolved, the critical care nurse assumes total responsibility for managing the patient's nursing care. After a day or two, if the vascular access(es) is no longer needed, either the nephrology or critical care nurse will remove the catheter(s). Often shortly afterwards, the patient is transferred out of the ICU. If the patient's condition has deteriorated and the prognosis is poor, the nurses, physicians, and family discuss the decision to withdraw care and prepare for comfort measures only. At this time written advance directives, living will, and/or durable power of attorney become extremely important to assure that the patient's wishes are followed.

Nursing Literature and Research Related to CRRT

The medical professional literature covering CRRT dates back to the 1970s, and is vast. The introduction of CRRT into clinical practice involved nephrology and critical care nurses from the very beginning, but often the nurses' contributions were only acknowledged as a note of appreciation from manuscript authors. The earliest nursing publication appeared in the *AANNT Journal* in 1981 (Rainone & Littman). Nursing involvement with CRRT during the early 1980s was primarily the work of two critical care nurses, Gayle Whitman and Susan Dirkes, and this author, Christy Price. The Cleveland Clinic in Ohio, under the physician direction of Emil Paganini, MD, has been heavily involved in research related to CRRT, and nursing assistance has been recognized in joint physician and nurse publications. Paganini, Fisque, Whitman, and Nakamoto (1982) published the first studies using SCUF in the treatment of ARF. Several years later Cindy Bosworth, RN, was the primary author of a paper published from data collected on using pump-assisted ultrafiltration and dialysate delivery during CAVHD (Bosworth, Swann, & Paganini, 1990). An early reference guide for CRRT was coauthored by physicians and a nurse from the University of Michigan in 1984, but the 1989 edition specifically listed the contributing professionals (Mault, Dirkes, Swartz, & Bartlett, 1989). Rabetoy, Mosley, Duke, and Price (1989) collaboratively presented a review of the literature and summarized their early experience with CRRT being practiced in a military teaching hospital.

After the above initial nurse-coauthored publications, nurses independently published in nursing journals. The nursing literature addressed the principles and procedures related to CRRT, but several articles appeared that outlined nursing interventions, continuous critical care monitoring, potential patient and system complications, and expected patient outcomes (Williams & Perkins, 1984; Kiely, 1984; Cant, 1984; Locke, Groth, & Lees, 1985; Winkelman, 1985; Whittaker, Brown, Grabenbauer, & Cauble, 1986; Palmer, Koorejian, London, Dechert, & Bartlett; 1986; Lawyer, 1987; Bell, 1988, Wedel, 1988; Dirkes, 1989; Kaplow & Bendo, 1989; Paradiso, 1989; Price, 1989a, 1989b). These authors represent a mix of nephrology and critical care nurses in professional positions as inservice coordinator, clinical nurse specialist, clinical staff nurse, and/or nursing director of a particular ICU or renal unit.

The nursing literature after the 1980s became less descriptive of the principles and supplies and began to focus on specific areas of concern and on patient presentations. The first comprehensive nursing care plan using nursing diagnoses was published in 1990 by four critical care nurses (Coloski, Mastrianni, Dube, & Brown, 1990). An experienced nephrology nurse investigated the cost comparisons between HD, PD, and CRRT (Lees, 1991). Although it is not universally practiced, the treatment of ARF using CRRT was recommended as the treatment of choice and as collaborative practice between intensive care physicians and nurses, and nephrology physicians and nurses (Price, 1991 b). Nephrology nurses reported an alternative to standard heparin anticoagulation using trisodium citrate (Ashton, Mehta, Ward, McDonald, & Aguilar, 1991). Butler (1991) presented nutritional considerations for patients with ARF requiring renal replacement therapy. Successful medical and nursing management of a patient with hepatorenal syndrome using CAVH has been reported (Chmielewski, Zellers, & Eyer, 1990). The experience of Canadian nurses with CAVH and CAVHD has appeared in the literature (Graham & Urquhart, 1990). The clinical application of CAVH for treating neonates and pediatric patients has demonstrated the increasing popularity of CRRT over conventional HD and PD (Stapleton & Wright, 1991; Hendrix, 1992). Several nurse authors focused on preventing complications, nursing management, and the advantages of CRRT (Bosworth, Paganini, Consentino, & Heyka, 1991; Lievaart & Voerman, 1991; Pinson, 1992; Stark, 1992; Price, 1992).

Researchers continue to investigate the most optimal means of managing patients with continuous therapies. Adequate nutrition remains a primary concern, and it is being addressed by nurses (Chima et al., 1993; Hagland, 1993). A case presentation involving a severely injured trauma patient using CVVHD has been reported (Strohshein, Caruso, & Greene, 1994). The application of dialysis therapies for treatment of ARF as a sequelae of sepsis highlighted nursing challenges (Price, 1994).

ANNA added content related to CRRT in the 2nd edition of the *Core Curriculum for Nephrology Nursing* (Price, 1991 b). AACN included discussion of CRRT in the Fourth edition of the *Core Curriculum for Critical Care Nursing* (Stark, 1991). Nursing professionals have worked closely in providing the necessary knowledge and clinical skills to the practice environment.

Summary

The treatment of ARF continues to evolve as pharmacologic agents and medical devices improve. All technological advances present new opportunities and challenges for professionals. Possibly nowhere else in health care has a diagnosis and treatment had more of an impact on collaborative practice than with ARF and CRRT. Nurses and the physicians have benefitted, but the true beneficiaries have been critically ill patients.

References

Ashton, D., Mehta, R., Ward, D., McDonald, B., & Aguilar, M. (1991). Recent advances in continuous renal replacement therapy: Citrate anticoagulated continuous arteriovenous hemodialysis. *ANNA Journal, 18*(3), 269-267, 329.

Bell, S. (1988). CAVH in pediatrics: Meeting the challenge...continuous arteriovenous hemofiltration. *ANNA Journal, 15*(1), 25-26.

Bonnardeaux, A., Pichette, V., Quimet, D., Geadah, D., Habel, F., & Cardinal, J. (1992). Solute clearances with high dialysate flow rates and glucose absorption from the dialysate in continuous arteriovenous hemodialysis. *American Journal of Kidney Diseases, 19*(1), 31-38.

Bosch, J. (1986). Continuous arteriovenous hemofiltration (CAVH): Operational characteristics and clinical use. *AKF Nephrology Letter, 3*(3), 15-26.

Bosworth, C. (1992). SCUF/CAVH/CAVHD: Critical differences. *Critical Care Nursing Quarterly, 14(*4), 45-55.

Bosworth, C., Swann, S. & Paganini, E. (1990). Evaluation of the IMED infusion pumps in extracorporeal continuous therapy circuits. *Dialysis & Transplantation, 19*(1), 26-28.

Bosworth, C., Paganini, E., Consentino, F., & Heyka, R. (1991). Long-term experience with continuous renal replacement therapy in intensive care unit acute renal failure. *Contributions in Nephrology, 93*, 13-16.

Butler, B. (1991). Nutritional management of catabolic acute renal failure requiring renal replacement therapy. *ANNA Journal, 18*(3), 247-259.

Cant, J. (1984, January). Haemofiltration. *Nursing Mirror*, pp. 3-6.

Chima, C., Meyer, L., Hummell, A., Bosworth, C., Heyka, R., Paganini, E., & Werynski, A. (1993). Protein catabolic rate in patients with acute renal failure on continuous arteriovenous hemofiltraton and total parenteral nutrition. *Journal of American Society of Nephrology, 3*(8), 1516-1521.

Chmielewski, C., Zellers, L., & Eyer, J. (1990). Continuous arteriovenous hemofiltration in the patient with hepatorenal syndrome: A case study. *Critical Care Nursing Clinics of North American, 2*(1), 115-122.

Coloski, D., Mastrianni, J., Dube, R., & Brown, L. (1990). Continuous arteriovenous hemofiltration patient: Nursing care plan. *Dimensions of Critical Care Nursing, 9*(3), 130-142.

Dirkes, S. (1989). Making a critical difference with CAVH...continuous arteriovenous hemofiltration. *Nursing 1989, 19*(11), 57-60.

Geronemus, R. (1988). Slow continuous hemodialysis. *Transactions of ASAIO, 34*, 59-60.

Golper, T. (1985). Continuous arteriovenous hemofiltration in acute renal failure. *American Journal of Kidney Diseases, 6*(6), 373-386.

Graham, K., & Urquhart, G. (1990). Continuous arteriovenous hemofiltration/dialysis. *Canadian Critical Care Nursing Journal, 7*(1), 18-24.

Hagland, M. (1993). The management of acute renal failure in the intensive therapy unit. *Intensive & Critical Care Nursing, 9*(4), 237-241.

Hendrix, W. (1992). Dialysis therapies in critically ill children.

AACN Clinical Issues in Critical Care Nursing, 3(3), 605-613.

Henrich, W. (1993). Arteriovenous of venovenous continuous therapies are not superior to standard hemodialysis in all patients with acute renal failure. *Seminars in Dialysis, 6*(3), 174-176.

Kaplan, A., Longnecker, R., & Folkert, V. (1984). Continuous arteriovenous hemofiltration. *Annals of Internal Medicine, 100*, 358-367.

Kaplow, R., & Bendo, K. (1989). QA in continuous arteriovenous hemofiltration. *Dimensions of Critical Care Nursing, 8*(3), 170-174.

Kiely, M. (1984). Continuous arteriovenous hemofiltration. *Critical Care Nurse, 4*(4), 39-43.

Kramer, P., Kaufhold, G., Grone, H., Wigger, J., Rieger, D., Matthaei, D., Stokke, T., Burchardi, H., & Scheler, F. (1980). Management of anuric intensive care patients with arteriovenous hemofiltration. *International Journal of Artificial Organs, 3*(4), 225-230.

Lauer, A., Saccaggi, A., Ronco, C., Belledonne, M., Glabman, S., & Bosch, J. (1983). Continuous arteriovenous hemofiltration in the critically ill patient. *Annals of Internal Medicine, 99*(4), 455-460.

Lawyer, L. (1987). *Clinical experience and application of continuous arteriovenous hemodialysis in the intensive care unit.* Reprint from the Third International Symposium on Acute Continuous Renal Replacement Therapy.

Lees, P. (1990, April). Acute renal replacement treatment alternatives. *Contemporary Dialysis & Nephrology*, pp. 22-27.

Lievaart, A., & Voerman, H. (1991). Nursing management of continuous arteriovenous hemodialysis. *Heart & Lung, 29*(2), 152-160.

Locke, S., Groth, N., & Lees, P. (1985). Continuous arteriovenous hemofiltration: An alternative to standard hemodialysis in unstable patients. *ANNA Journal, 12*(2), 127-131.

Mault, J., Dirkes, S., Swartz, R., & Bartlett, R. (1989). Continuous hemofiltration: A reference guide for SCUF, CAVH, and CAVHD. Ann Arbor, MI: University of Michigan Medical Center.

McBride, P. (1987). *Genesis of the arterial kidney.* Deerfield, IL: Baxter Healthcare Corporation.

Mehta, R. (1993). Renal replacement therapy for acute renal failure: Matching the method to the patient. *Seminars in Dialysis, 6*(4), 253-259.

Paganini, E., & Nakamoto, S. (1980). Slow continuous ultrafiltration in oliguric renal failure. *Transaction of ASAIO, 26*, 201-204.

Paganini, E., Fisque, J., Whitman, G., & Nakamoto, S. (1982). Amino acid balance in patients with oliguric acute renal failure undergoing slow continuous ultrafiltration (SCUF). *Transactions of ASAIO, 28*, 615-620.

Paganini, E. (1988). Slow continuous hemofiltration and slow continuous ultrafiltration. *Transactions of ASAIO, 34*, 63-66.

Paganini, E. (1993). Continuous renal replacement is the preferred treatment for all acute renal failure patients receiving intensive care. *Seminars in Dialysis, 6*(3), 176-179.

Palmer, J., Koorejian, K., London, J., Dechert, R., & Bartlett, R. (1986). Nursing management of continuous arteriovenous hemofiltration for acute renal failure. *Focus on Critical Care, 13*(5), 21-30.

Paradiso, C. (1989). Hemofiltration: An alternative to dialysis. *Heart & Lung, 18*(3), 282-290.

Pinson, J. (1992). Preventing complications in the CAVH patient. *Dimensions of Critical Care Nursing, 11*(5), 242-248.

Price, C. (1989a). Continuous arteriovenous ultrafiltration: A monitoring guide for ICU nurses. *Critical Care Nurse, 9*(1), 12-19.

Price, C. (1989b). Continuous renal replacement therapy from a professional nursing perspective. *Nephrology News & Issues, 3*(7), 31-34.

Price, C. (1991a). Continuous renal replacement therapy. In L. Lancaster (Ed.). *Core curriculum for nephrology nursing* (2nd ed.) (pp. 323-340). Pitman, NJ: American Nephrology Nurses' Association.

Price, C. (1991b). Continuous renal replacement therapy: The treatment of choice for acute renal failure. *ANNA Journal, 18*(3), 239-244.

Price, C. (1992). An update on continuous renal replacement therapies. *AACN Clinical Issues in Critical Care Nursing, 3*(3), 597-604.

Price, C. (1993). Standards of clinical practice for continuous renal replacement therapy. In S. Burrows-Hudson (Ed.). *Standards of clinical practice for nephrology nursing.* Pitman, NJ: American Nephrology Nurses' Association.

Price, C. (1994). Acute renal failure - A sequelae of sepsis. *Critical Care Nursing Clinics of North America, 6*(2), 359-372.

Rabetoy, G., Mosley, C., Duke, M., & Price, C. (1989). Continuous arteriovenous hemofiltration (CAVH). *Dialysis & Transplantation, 18*(3), 120-125, 128.

Rainone, A., & Littman, E. (1981). The use of the Amicon filter in dialysis related complications. *AANNT Journal, 8*(3), 32-33.

Stapleton, S., & Wright, J. (1992). Continuous arteriovenous hemofiltration: An alternative dialysis therapy in neonates. *Journal of Neonatal Nursing, 11*(4), 17-29.

Stark, J. (1992). Dialysis options in the critically ill patient: Hemodialysis, peritoneal dialysis, and continuous renal replacement therapy. *Critical Care Nursing Quarterly, 14*(4), 40-44.

Stark, J. (1991). The renal system. In J. Alspach (Ed.), Core curriculum of critical care nursing (4th edition) (pp. 472-608). Philadelphia: W.B. Saunders Company.

Strohshein, B., Caruso, D., & Greene, K. (1994). Continuous venovenous hemodialysis. *American Journal of Critical Care, 3*(2), 92-100.

Wedel, S. (1988). Continuous arteriovenous hemofiltration. *Current Reviews in Respiratory and Critical Care, 11*(5), 34-40.

Whittaker, A., Brown, C. Grabenbauer, K., & Cauble, L. (1986). Preventing complications in continuous arteriovenous hemofiltration. *Dimensions of Critical Care Nursing, 5*(2), 72-79.

Williams, V., & Perkins, L. (1984). Continuous ultrafiltration. *Critical Care Nurse, 4*, 44-49.

Winkelman, C. (1985). Hemofiltration: A new technique in critical care nursing. *Heart & Lung, 14*(3), 265-271.

Chapter Highlights

- Continuous renal replacement therapy (CRRT) has received popular acceptance in Europe and the United States, particularly for the hemodynamically unstable patient who is unresponsive to conservative management with pharmacological and dietary interventions.

- The use of CRRT is limited to an ICU setting, where close hourly monitoring and fluid adjustments are possible. The original intent of CAVH and SCUF was to augment existing renal function and decreased urine output.

- For several years, CAVH and SCUF served the nephrology and critical care communities well for the treatment of ARF. However, in the late 1980s, a new dimension was added to the CRRT system. Fluid and moderate solute removal could be achieved with CAVH or SCUF, but for patients who had no kidney function, the removal of uremic toxins and electrolytes was inadequate. Continuous arteriovenous hemodiafiltration or hemodialysis (CAVHD) was introduced for the treatment of patients who required considerable adjustment for serum electrolyte abnormalities, intervention for severe acid/base disturbance, and correction of moderate-to-severe uremia (Geronemus, 1988).

- Continuous venovenous hemofiltration (CVVH) and continuous venovenous hemodialysis (CVVHD) were introduced as alternatives for CAVH and CAVHD, respectively. These techniques further complicated the simple CRRT system, but they have allowed for a greater number of patients to be treated (Paganini, 1993; Mehta, 1993).

- Treatment can be provided on a continuous basis, rather than attempting to fit the patient's needs into a time prescribed therapy, like 3 or 4-hour treatments with HD.

- Nursing professionals recognize collaboration and communication must exist for successful management of patients receiving CRRT.

- Particularly important during the intratherapy period, all nurses must comprehend and follow protocols for intervening to resolve problems related to CRRT, or make adjustments based on evaluation of the patient's response to therapy.

CHAPTER 21

Therapeutic Plasma Exchange

Christy A. Price, RN, MSN, CNN

Chapter Contents

Historical Review of Therapeutic Apheresis 591
Therapeutic Plasma Exchange (TPE) 591
Development of Specific Therapies 592
Intermittent Flow Centrifugation 592
Continuous Flow Centrifugation 593
Membrane Plasma Separators 593
Cascade or Secondary Plasma Filtration 594
Similarities and Differences Between TPE and HD 595
Indications 595
Pretreatment Nursing Assessment 595
Vascular Accesses 595
Equipment and Supplies 595
Intraprocedural Monitoring for TPE 596
Postprocedural Nursing Care 597
Nursing Literature and Research Related to TPE 598
Summary 599
References 599
Chapter Highlights 601

Therapeutic Plasma Exchange

Christy A. Price, RN, MSN, CNN

Nephrology nurses are recognized for their unique knowledge and skill in performing extracorporeal therapies safely and effectively. This technical proficiency coupled with their holistic approach to patient care has lead to vast expansion and contribution of nephrology nurses' role within the health care arena. The purpose of this chapter is to address the historical progression of nephrology nursing's clinical involvement with therapeutic plasma exchange (TPE). Centrifuge and membrane technology equipment and systems will be described. Hemodialysis and plasma exchange will be compared and contrasted from technical and patient care perspectives. The clinical indications will be addressed by presenting the literature from nephrology and other specialty nursing groups.

Historical Review of Therapeutic Apheresis

Apheresis simply means to separate a part from its whole. It is the umbrella term used to describe all blood separation techniques. TPE and cytapheresis are the two primary categories of apheresis.

Therapeutic Plasma Exchange (TPE)

TPE was introduced for medicinal purposes in the early 1900s. It was described as a process for removing blood factors and relief of toxaemia (Abel, Rowntree, & Turner, 1914). As with other beginning approaches for improving an individual's health status, physicians were not always certain if a benefit would be realized from their prescriptions. A bloodletting procedure, or technique of cannulating a vein for the removal of whole blood, was a rather aggressive approach for removal of plasma. If the patient did receive a beneficial response from this intervention, there was an uncertainty as to why it occurred. The simple explanation provided the patient may have been a description of a process for removing toxins, poisons, or "bad" substances that were the cause of their illness. The short and long-term adverse effects were unknown. Possible complications were anemia, electrolyte imbalance, vascular collapse, immune suppression, and infection.

After this crude beginning, plasmapheresis, plasma exchange or TPE, as it is currently identified, became a therapy of more widespread application. With refinement of the technology and procedures, it became a frequent practice of blood banking facilities for plasma donations and for therapeutic applications. Each plasma removal technique will be fully explained in the next section of this chapter. However to summarize, as the medical indications for prescribing plasma exchange increased, intermittent therapies advanced to continuous flow techniques and eventually plasma membrane separators. Plasma exchange therapy gained acceptance when the patient's disease or syndrome was characterized as antibody or immune complex mediated, monoclonopathy or for replacement of certain plasma factors (Dau, 1983; Ward, 1984; Kaplan, 1995).

Cytapheresis is the collection of one particular formed cell by means of centrifuge apheresis equipment. The procedure could be performed for the removal of white cells, red cells or platelets. Cytapheresis is clinically indicated for the reduction of a particular cell in an individual patient, or for donation of a particular cell to another individual or self in the future. An example for these procedures would include routine red cell reduction, which is a treatment for a patient who has hemochromatosis, a disease characterized by an inborn error in iron metabolism leading to very elevated iron levels that result in excessive pathological iron deposits throughout the body. The treatment plan may include cytapheresis for the removal of stored iron through red cell reduction. Plateletapheresis is an example of a procedure performed with the intention of collecting platelets from a healthy individual. The purpose of platelet collection is for transfusion of platelets to achieve hemostasis, such as for a severely injured trauma patient, intraoperatively to control blood loss or to treat severe thrombocytopenia. Presently, peripheral stem cell collection with preservation of these cells until the patient completes a course of chemotherapy is becoming a widespread practice. Stem cells are immature cells that can become normal blood cells. The healthy stem cells are retransfused back to the patient where they can differentiate into white cells.

With the introduction of hemodialysis (HD) in the early 1950s, researchers, engineers, and physicians recognized that whole blood could be processed extracorporeally using membrane technology for the correction of metabolic, electrolyte,

Figure 21-1
Advances in therapeutic apheresis time line.

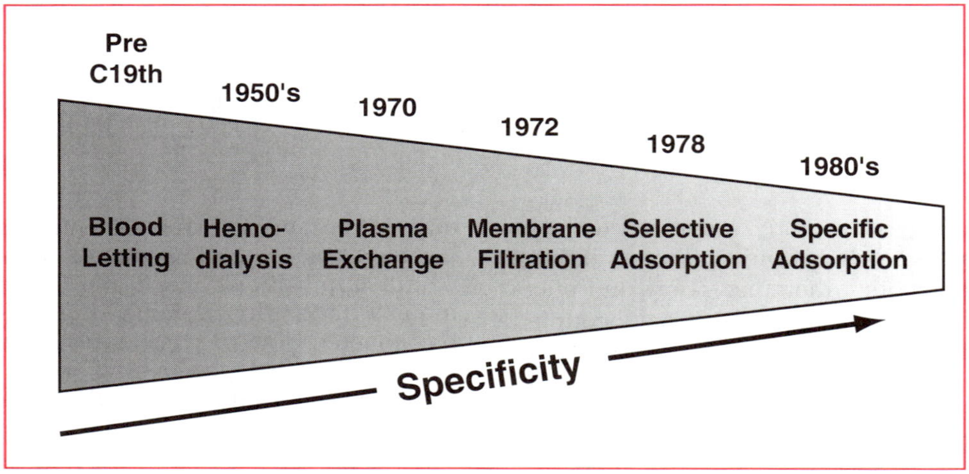

and fluid imbalances. The dialyzer membrane has a particular molecular weight (MW) above which substances cannot be removed. Uremic toxins, specifically urea (MW 69 daltons) and creatinine (MW 113 daltons) could be removed along with other small molecular weight substances typically less than 10,000 daltons. High-flux, or synthetic dialyzer membranes have the ability to remove molecules up to 50,000 daltons. An example is beta 2 microglobulin, which has a MW of 11,800 daltons. The clearance capacity of the human kidney is controlled by several factors, one of which is that substances over 69,000 daltons are poorly removed. Proteins, immunoglobulins and antibodies have molecular weights of 69,000 to over 1 million daltons. Therefore, they require a much more porous membrane to effectively use TPE to treat immune complex or antibody mediated diseases or syndromes, or to remove large plasma factors.

It is this development of a membrane technology approach to TPE that has lead to nephrology nurses' roles in the care of patients for whom TPE is prescribed. The similarity in the equipment and procedural considerations between HD and TPE is the primary reason for establishing a TPE program in a dialysis unit. (Price, 1987; Gerhardt, Ntoso, Koethe, Lodge & Wolf, 1992). However, the expertise of nephrology nurses in patient assessment and treatment monitoring is essential to providing safe and effective therapy. Nephrologists and nephrology nurses are becoming more interested and involved in research related to the numerous applications of TPE in treating acute and chronic illnesses. Additionally, the newer therapies of secondary cascade filtration and immunoadsorption therapy are gaining widespread acceptance for certain identified patient populations. Figure 21-1 provides a pictorial view of the advancement of extracorporeal therapies.

Development of Specific Therapies

Intermittent Flow Centrifugation

The early equipment for TPE used centrifugal forces to separate whole blood into its formed elements and plasma. The original machines relied on anticoagulating and pumping blood into a bowl that rotates, and thereby separates the blood components by their density (Gardner & Gilcher, 1990; Hakim & Siami, 1994). The red cells, having the highest density, move toward the center and the plasma, being the lightest component, moves out to the periphery of the bowl. The white cells and platelets align themselves between the red cells and the plasma according to their respective density. Any of the components can be discarded, collected, or reinfused depending on the indication and goals of performing the procedure. The intermittent nature of the blood flow and removal of a blood component or plasma generally results in a longer procedure time and some intravascular fluid imbalance being experienced by patients. For intermittent flow centrifuge TPE procedures, the standard anticoagulant is acid-citrate dextrose (ACD). Vascular access is achieved by cannulating usually only one antecubital vein with a 17-gauge needle.

Although these machines continue to be used in clinical practice, they are being replaced by continuous flow centrifuge machines. A centrifugal process for separating blood components is necessary for removing or collecting one particular component, for example, platelets, but centrifugation is not necessary for simple separation of plasma.

Figure 21-2
Continuous centrifuge apheresis.
A. Extracorporeal blood and plasma circuit.
B. Therapeutic plasma exchange channel.

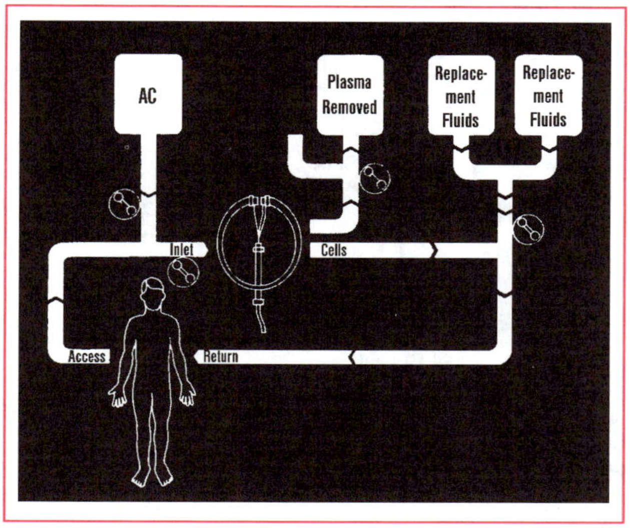

A. Extracorporeal blood and plasma circuit.

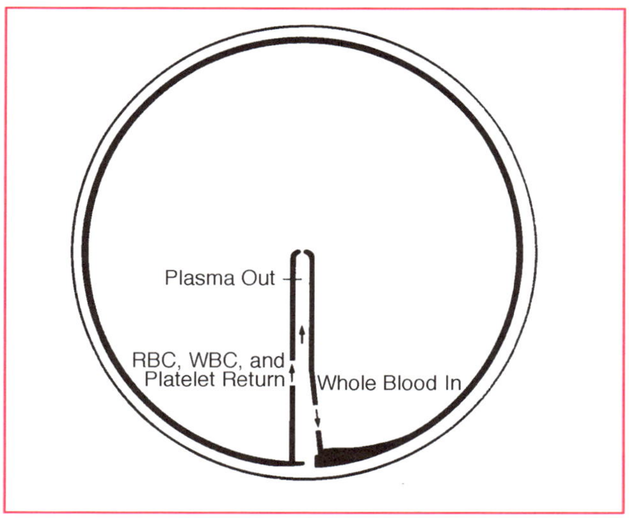

B. Therapeutic plasma exchange channel.

Note: Printed with permission from Cobe BCT, Lakewood, CO.

Continuous Flow Centrifugation

As the name implies, continuous flow machines use an uninterrupted blood flow path. The whole blood enters into a rotating channel, or space, that generates a centrifugal force. The spinning blood into the channel separates into cellular elements and plasma (Senack, 1990; Hakim & Siami, 1994). The red cells move to the outside of the channel and the plasma moves toward the inside, and similar to an intermittent system the white cells and platelets divide the remaining space. Any blood component can be collected, discarded or reinfused. The continuous nature of these procedures helps to avoid intravascular fluid shifts once the treatment is ongoing, but this also requires two sites for vascular access — blood flow out to the machine and blood return to the patient. The anticoagulation method is called acid-citrate dextrose (ACD) (see Figure 21-2).

Continuous flow centrifugal therapies are preferred because of increased patient comfort and usually decreased treatment time. Cytapheresis procedures are performed in blood banks or donor collection centers. Relative few nephrology nurses are involved with cytapheresis and therefore, continuous flow centrifuge equipment.

Membrane Plasma Separators

In 1983, the first medical devices for membrane TPE were introduced in the United States. A plasma membrane separator device is similar to a hemodialyzer in appearances, that is, either hollow fiber or parallel device, but the membrane properties are significantly different. Whereas, conventional dialyzers remove blood components up to 10,000 daltons, and high-flux, high permeable dialyzers remove elements up to 50,000 daltons, plasma separators are capable of removing plasma and all dissolved components up to 3 million daltons in size (Asaba, Rekola, Bergstrand, Wasserman, & Bergstrom, 1980). Although this extracorporeal circuit for TPE looks quite similar to an HD circuit (see Figure 21-3), there are major differences in the ways of priming, monitoring, and performing TPE (Price, & McCarley, 1993). Membrane plasma separation has been proven to be as effective as the centrifuge techniques for the removal of plasma, plasma proteins, and other plasma components (Samtleben et al., 1984; Wood, Bond & Jacobs, 1984). The continuous flow extracorporeal circuit requires use of a central line dual lumen catheter or permanent vascular access, that is an arteriovenous fistula or synthetic graft. The anticoagulation of choice is heparin.

TPE has been recognized as part of the core curriculum content for clinical nephrology nurses (Price, 1995). Clinical practice standards have been written to guide patient care (McCarley, Wingard & White, 1993). Nephrology nurses are recognized for their expertise with extracorporeal therapies, sys-

Figure 21-3
Membrane plasma exchange circuit.

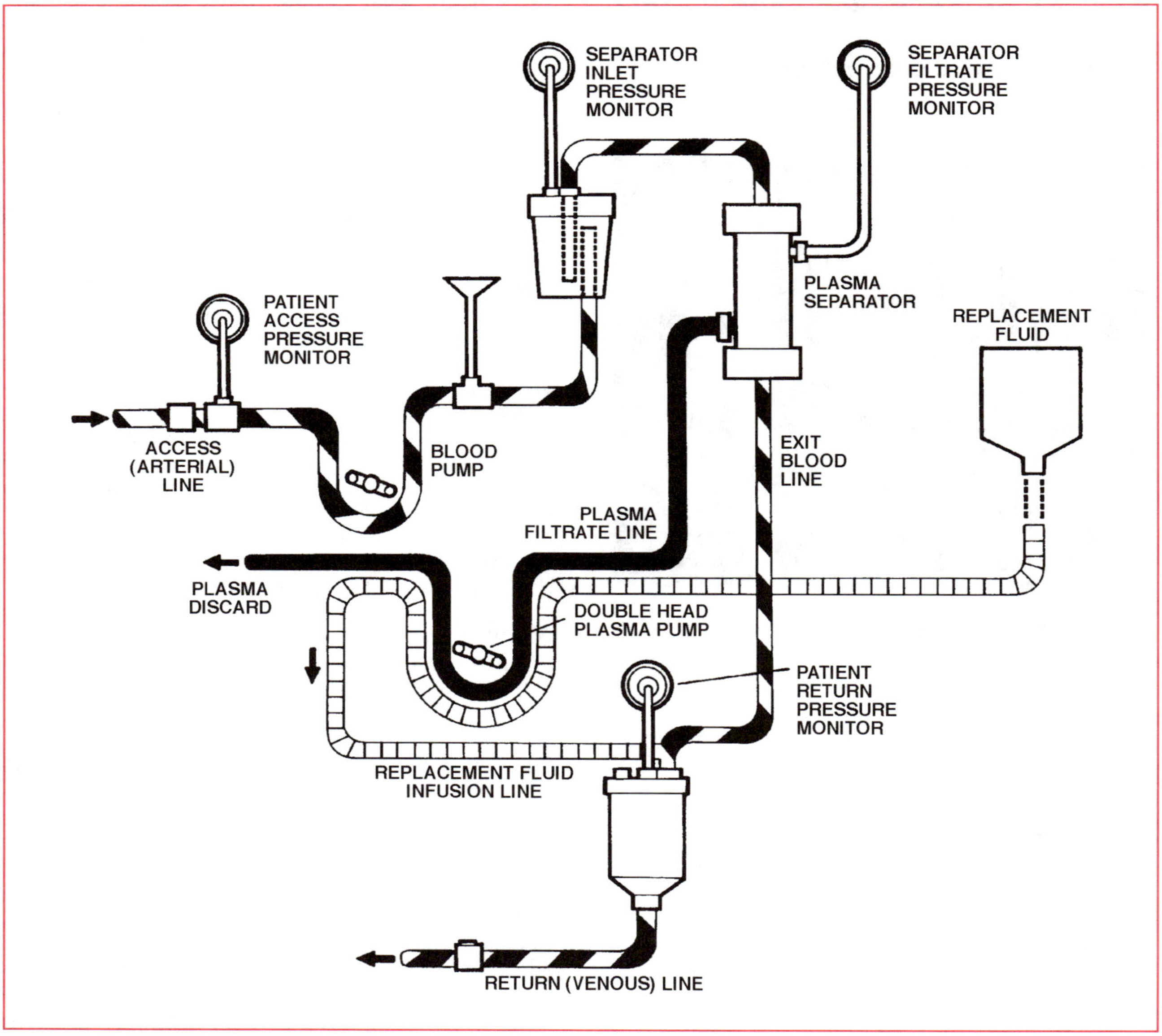

Note: Printed with permission from Apheresis Technologies Inc., Palm Harbor, FL.

tematic anticoagulation, and sophisticated technology and equipment. The total body systems nursing assessment required for a patient receiving TPE and/or HD is the identical first step of the nursing process (Price & McCarley, 1994). TPE has been a natural transition and incorporation of membrane technology into nephrology nursing's scope of practice. However, cytapheresis and related procedures have not become a major component in nephrology clinical practice.

Cascade or Secondary Plasma Filtration

As illustrated in Figure 21-1, the wave of the future is incorporating plasma filtration therapies under the parent heading of apheresis. Selective adsorption of a particular plasma component by perfusing the separated plasma through a secondary column may become the therapy of choice as these techniques are further researched (see Figure 21-4). Currently in the United States, there is only one secondary column available, and it is limited to the treatment of idiopathic thrombocytopenia purpura (ITP) (Guthrie & Oral, 1989). Cascade plasma filtration requires a dual lumen catheter or a permanent arteriovenous vascular access. Anticoagulation therapy is prescribed cautiously

Figure 21-4
Cascade, or secondary, plasma filtration circuit.

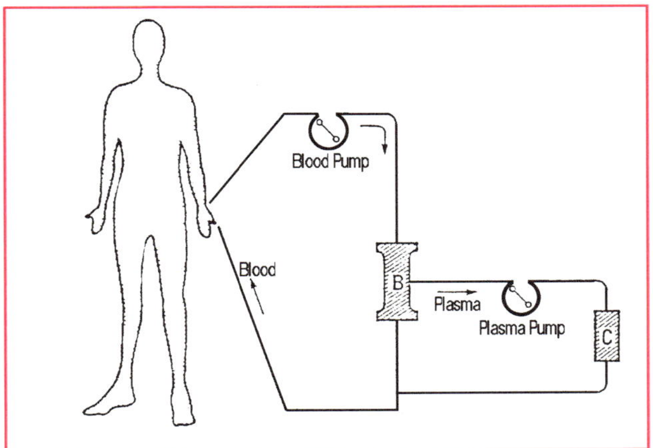

Note: Printed with permission from Apheresis Technologies Inc., Palm Harbor, FL.

because of the patient's underlying thrombocytopenia. The significant increase in TPE being performed by nephrology nurses has lead to their involvement with secondary filtration therapy. It is again a natural extension of procedural skills and nursing assessment required.

Similarities and Differences Between TPE and HD

HD and TPE share many of the same equipment and supplies, although the indications are quite different. The performance of TPE by membrane technology involves an extension of preexisting HD skills, principles, protocols and nursing assessment. Table 21-1 provides a comparison between the two procedures.

Indications

HD is prescribed when a patient has acute renal failure, chronic renal insufficiency in the setting of fluid or electrolyte imbalance or chronic renal failure. TPE is prescribed when a patient is diagnosed with a disease or syndrome involving autoantibodies, alloantibodies, monoclonal proteins, immune complexes, unidentified plasma factors, or for the replacement of certain plasma factors (Dau, 1983; Ward, 1984; Hakim & Siami, 1994). TPE may be recommended for certain drug overdoses or ingestion of poisonous substances (Rabetoy, Price, Findlay, & Sailstad, 1990; Kale, Thomson, Provenzano & Higgins, 1993; Chu, Mantin, Shen, Baskett & Sussman, 1993). The goal for HD may be to reduce the patient's intravascular blood volume, but the expectation for TPE is that the patient will remain euvolemic. TPE involves replacing the discarded plasma with an equal volume of a replacement fluid.

Pretreatment Nursing Assessment

A total body systems assessment is identical for HD and TPE. As the initial step in the nursing process, a complete patient assessment is an expectation before proceeding with any nursing intervention. The physical assessment for a patient receiving TPE may focus on a certain body system, depending on the medical diagnosis (Price & McCarley, 1994). Unlike a patient being treated with HD for renal failure, a patient receiving TPE may not have renal dysfunction. The etiology for the primary condition may involve hematology/oncology, neurology, cardiology, dermatology, nephrology, gastroenterology, obstetrics/gynecology and/or transplantation. Although serial monitoring of serum electrolytes and complete blood count (CBC) is standard operating procedure, laboratory analyses may also include following titers for antibodies, identified markers of disease activity, drug levels, circulating immune complexes, and immunoglobulins. Pulmonary function tests, nerve conduction tests, and cardiac stress tests are a few of the invasive and noninvasive diagnostic examinations that may be required depending on the patient's diagnosis. It is important that the nephrology nurse is aware of the need for such testing and the findings to appropriately plan the nursing component for total patient care. Finally, prior to initiating TPE, it may be the responsibility of the nephrology nurse to calculate the patient's plasma volume. This may be estimated at 40 ml/min, using a formula for estimated plasma volume (EPV) (Kaplan, 1992) or by using a nomogram for plasma volume (Buffaloe & Heineken, 1983; Price, 1995).

Vascular Accesses

HD may be performed using two single lumen catheters, a Scribner shunt, a dual lumen catheter, or a permanent arteriovenous fistula or graft. For TPE any of these vascular accesses are acceptable. The placement, monitoring, use, and nursing care of the vascular access are the same for both procedures (refer to Chapter 19 in this book). The primary difference is that unlike HD where the standard blood rate is 200 to 450 ml/min, the usual blood flow rate for membrane plasma exchange is 100 to 150 ml/min. TPE performed by intermittent or continuous flow centrifuge technique may range from 30 to 90 ml/min.

Equipment and Supplies

Standard HD requires the use of a hemodialysis machine with the appropriate blood pump, dialysate delivery system, ultrafiltration controls, pressure monitors, and an air alert detector. The disposable supplies include a dialyzer, arterial and venous blood tubing and dialysate concentrate

Table 21-1
Comparison of HD and TPE.

	HD	TPE
.9% NaCl priming	1000 ml	1000 to 3000 ml
vascular access	dual lumen catheter dialysis needles	dual lumen catheter dialysis needles
equipment	dialysis machine	dialysis machine & plasma pump TPE machine
tubing	arterial & venous	arterial & venous plasma discard fluid replacement
initial heparin	zero to > 8000 u	zero to 100 u/kg
heparin infusion	zero to >2000 u/hr	1000 to 2000 u/hr
systemic ACTs	125 to 250 sec	200 to > 400 sec
ACTs obtained	postdialyzer	preplasma filter
heparin administered	predialyzer	postplasma filter
treatment time	3 to 4 hours	1.5 to 3 hours
fluid replacement	normal saline	normal saline 2.5% - 5% albumin FFP
staffing (acute care)	one nurse	one nurse
patient diagnosis	ARF or CRF drug overdose	every organ system drug overdose

Key
ARF = acute renal failure
CRF = chronic renal failure
FFP = fresh frozen plasma
HD = hemodialysis
TPE = therapeutic plasma exchange

solutions. Heparin (1000 u/ml) is available to be given by the nurse as prescribed. Normal saline (.9% NaCl) is used as necessary for priming the system, fluid replacement during the treatment ,and returning the patient's blood at termination of the treatment.

Centrifuge TPE will require the use of a dedicated machine, as previously described. Membrane TPE may involve a dedicated machine or the use of a standard dialysis machine, but the essential equipment needs include a blood pump, pressure monitoring devices, an air alert detector and a plasma pump that is ideally a dual track pump. Dialysate is never used when performing TPE. The disposable supplies include a plasma membrane separator, TPE arterial and venous blood tubing, a plasma discard line, and a fluid replacement line. Heparin is the standard anticoagulant, but a physician may elect to use citrate anticoagulation from a protocol adapted for performing hemodialysis. Heparinized .9% NaCl is used as the priming solution for preparing the extracorporeal circuit. However, the replacement fluids will vary depending on the patient's diagnosis and anticoagulation parameters; that is, platelet count, prothrombin time, partial prothrombin time or fibrinogen level. Plasma replacement fluids may involve a combination of crystalloids, colloids, and/or fresh frozen plasma (FFP).

Intraprocedural Monitoring for TPE

Like HD, TPE requires continuous monitoring of the patient's hemodynamic status. Vital signs, that is, blood pressure and pulse, are recorded every 15 to 20 minutes. If blood products are being administered, the patient's temperature must also be checked before and after each unit. It is imperative when monitoring the patient's vital signs that the underlying diagnosis is taken into consideration, as often patients with neurologic disorders will be hypotensive. During TPE the patient should remain euvolemic, therefore, hypotension generally is not related to a fluid imbalance. However, as with HD, normal saline must be available for immediate bolus infusion, and the patient is placed in Trendelenburg to treat hypotension.

During TPE, the nurse is continuously monitoring the plasma discard volume and plasma replacement fluid. It is the nurse's responsibility to make certain the output and intake are balanced. The plasma replacement fluid may be .9% NaCl, Lactate Ringers, a 2.5% to 5% albumin solution, or FFP. It is a nursing responsibility to assure that the correct solution and amount is administered by following the physician's prescription. A typical prescription may instruct the nurse to remove 3 liters of plasma and replace the plasma with 1 liter of .9% NaCl and 2 liters of 5.0% albumin solution.

Standard initial heparin prescriptions for HD range from 0 to 8000 units IV, followed by hourly doses of 0 to 2000 units. Patients who are being treated for acute renal failure tend to receive less heparin than chronic renal failure patients. Similarly, patients receiving TPE may have a range of heparin doses depending on the patient's diagnosis. A heparin bolus of 0, or 50 to 100 units/kg of body weight is administered at the initiation of the treatment. If the patient has significant thrombocytopenia, heparin may be contraindicated. The nurse will monitor activated clotting times (ACTs) every 20 to 30 minutes and administer a heparin bolus of 1000 to 2000 units, if indicated. Anticoagulation therapy during TPE is prescribed in consideration of the patient's diagnosis, platelet count, hematocrit, prothrombin time (PT), and fibrinogen level. It may vary from no heparin to systemic range anticoagulation, generally with ACTs maintained higher than during an HD treatment, that is, greater than 300 seconds. Depending on the patient's pretreatment PT or fibrinogen level, FFP may be used as part of the plasma replacement fluid (Refer to Chapter 19 for further discussion of ACTs).

Potential complications that require continuous monitoring during TPE are hypotension, fluid imbalance, electrolyte imbalance, air embolism, blood leak, and hemolysis. Hypotension and fluid imbalance have been addressed. The first intervention would be fluid recessitation with follow-up assessment for possible etiologies.

All small molecules, including electrolytes, are removed along with the plasma. The nurse checks the pretreatment sodium, potassium, calcium and magnesium serum levels, and if they are not within normal to possibly high normal ranges, the physician is consulted for appropriate intervention. Often patients are prescribed routine oral calcium supplementation to avoid hypocalcemia. Generally, if other electrolyte replacement is necessary it can be provided through dietary or nutritional changes. Intravenous replacement may be indicated if the patient is not eating well, or the levels are critically low and need a faster replacement route for correction. If during TPE, the patient complains of tingling over fingers or face, numbness around the mouth, nausea or feeling "washed out," or develops muscle flaccidity or tetany, the physician is consulted and along with serum labs for calcium, potassium and magnesium, an electrocardiogram is obtained.

If the air alert detector is not armed, or if the equipment is faulty the patient is at risk for receiving an air embolism. Monitoring of the situation is an expected nephrology nurse responsibility. Should an air embolism be suspected, the treatment is immediately stopped, the patient is placed in Trendelenburg on her/his left side and oxygen is administered. The rationale for these actions is to trap any air in the right atrium of the heart, and prevent it from escaping into the carotid arteries causing a cerebral embolism. The patient is likely to become hypotensive and, possibly hypoxic. Preparations for possible cardiac resuscitation are made.

Occasionally, a product fault may occur, and it may result in a broken hollow fiber or parallel plate that allows a small amount of blood to leak into the plasma discard. This is not a medical emergency, but the treatment should be discontinued. Unlike HD, the patient can safely have the blood returned because there is no possibility of contamination with nonsterile dialysate. A new TPE system is prepared if the treatment is to be continued.

During HD, hemolysis may occur secondary to a contaminant in the dialysate, like chloramine, or secondary to the dialysate being too warm, that is, greater than 40.5º C. During TPE, hemolysis may also occur. However, the causes are different, and the situation is not a medical emergency, as with HD. Unlike HD, the patient's blood may be returned during TPE. Hemolysis may occur because the transmembrane pressure for TPE has been exceeded, or because the plasma filter is significantly clotted. There is no nonsterile dialysate as a possible etiology for the hemolysis as in HD. Monitoring for hemolysis is an ongoing procedural concern, and it is usually avoided. Under normal circumstances, plasma is light to moderately dark yellow. When hemolysis occurs the discarded plasma changes to an orange color. If hemolysis should occur, the intervention is to simply stop the plasma exchange and flush the filter with normal saline to reestablish pressure equilibrium within the system. Generally only a very small amount of whole blood is actually hemolyzed, and the red cell fragments and free hemoglobulin are discarded with the plasma.

Postprocedural Nursing Care

After the appropriate plasma volume has been exchanged, the plasma pump is turned off, and the patient's whole blood is returned via the venous line. The TPE circuit is disposed of as contaminated waste, as the plasma filters are not reused as in HD. The vascular access is given appropriate attention that will vary depending on the access used.

The nephrology nurse completes a posttreatment assessment and evaluation. Vital signs, subjective responses and laboratory analyses are obtained. The patient is allowed 15 to 30 minutes to adjust and stabilize her/his blood pressure and pulse back to baseline parameters. Most patients will be transferred back to their hospital room, although other patients will return home. Patients and/or other hospital personnel are instructed on the two most frequent postprocedural complications, that is bleeding and infection.

During TPE heparin therapy may be provided, but also unlike HD, clotting proteins, particularly fibrinogen, are removed. This increases the patient's risk for postprocedural bleeding. Precautions must include allowing no invasive procedures for the next 24 hours. This includes surgery, and/or intraarterial and spinal punctures. Likewise, intravenous catheters should not be attempted unless absolutely necessary for several hours. Patients are cautioned about protecting themselves against blunt trauma, falling against a hard surface, shaving cuts, or vigorous teeth brushing. Protocols should be in place that prohibit discontinuing central line catheters until possibly 24 hours after TPE, and a fibrinogen or PT level has been recorded. Hospital staff should be prepared to hold direct pressure against the site for 15 to 20 minutes.

Patients receiving TPE are at high risk for secondary or opportunistic infections. Many will be receiving steroids or cytotoxic agents as part of their treatment regimen. Any patient with an indwelling central line catheter and undergoing intermittent invasive procedures is considered at high-risk for infection. Patients are to be instructed to report to the nurses any ill feeling, sweating, chills, or fever. Hospital staff monitor for signs and symptoms of systemic infection, including hemodynamic instability, hyperthermia, and elevated white cell count with an abnormal differential. Signs of local infection include observing for induration, erythema, drainage, and warmth. Appropriate interventions are taken immediately because a patient receiving TPE can become septic quickly.

The long term care, monitoring, and clinical outcomes of patients receiving TPE will vary greatly and will be directly related to the patient's primary diagnosis. Depending on the patient's presentation and disease course, the patient's illness may be resolved or cured, placed in a state of remission, or require long term chronic treatments. The healthcare professional must tailor their therapeutic interventions, patient education, and psychosocial support in consideration of the immediate circumstances and clinical situation.

Nursing Literature and Research Related to TPE

Over the past decade, there have been more published reports of the nursing care provided for patients treated with TPE. TPE has become recognized as a safe and effective therapy. The involvement of various nursing specialties demonstrates some of the clinical applications.

Neuroscience nurses have recognized the therapeutic value of TPE and the related nursing concerns for patients diagnosed with Guillain-Barre Syndrome, myasthenia gravis, and neuromuscular respiratory failure (George, 1988; Hood, 1990; Weeks, 1991; Parobeck, Burnham, & Laukhuf, 1992; Hinkle, Albanese, & McGinty, 1993). The primary nursing concern with these neurologic disorders is respiratory depression or arrest. Function of the cranial nerves, gag reflex, and ability to swallow are monitored closely to assure the patient has a protected airway. These patients may have a self-limited condition that will resolve over a period of weeks to months, or they may have a chronic condition that could require repeated courses of TPE over their lifetime.

Professional nurses who specialize in perinatology neonatal nursing have been confronted with pregnant women needing TPE for the treatment of myasthenia gravis and Guillain-Barre Syndrome (Burke, 1993; Graves & Oates, 1994). This may be a frightening situation for all because the goal of therapy is to sustain normal fetal growth and development without complications, while treating the mother's disorder.

A patient who developed Stevens-Johnson Syndrome secondary to medication reaction has been reported in the nursing literature. (Sherry, 1993) The florid and painful rash that occurs may resolve with conventional prescription of steroids and antihistamines, skin lotions, and hygiene care.

Critical care nurses have experienced an increased use of TPE for critically ill patients with a variety of clinical presentations, including those already mentioned plus thrombotic thrombocytopenic purpura (TTP), idiopathic thrombocytopenic purpura (ITP), cardiac transplantation, cardiac surgery, and familial hypercholesterolemia (Bell, 1989; Cohen, 1989; Ellis, 1994; Folkes, 1990; Pfister & Bullas, 1990; White-Williams, 1993; Ellenberger, Haas & Cundiff, 1993; Eggenberger, Coker & Menezes, 1993; Krnsak, 1994). ITP is a hematological syndrome resulting from the presence of antiplatelet antibodies. Patients may present with neurologic deficits, renal failure, and/or gastrointestinal or cerebral hemorrhage. TTP is believed to be a nonimmunological syndrome that mimics ITP with either a fulminant or subacute presentation. All transplant patients develop antibodies against the donor organ, and occasionally TPE is prescribed in conjunction with pharmacologic management. Familial hypercholesterolemia is a genetic disorder characterized by elevated levels of serum cholesterol that are not amenable to the standard therapy of diet, exercise, and cholesterol lowering agents.

With the changes in technology, nephrology nursing literature has increased content related to their scope of practice for the treatment of rapidly progressive glomerulonephritis (RPGN), Goodpasture's Syndrome, hemolytic uremia syndrome (HUS), hyperviscosity syndrome, cryoglobulinemia, as well as all diseases previously listed (Price, 1987; Duff & Dugas, 1991; Wiseman, 1993; Wingard, 1993; Klee, McAfee, & Greenleaf, 1993; Neumann & Urizar, 1994; Price & McCarley, 1994; Isaacs, 1994; Graves & Oates, 1994). Antibody mediated renal diseases are often treated with TPE. Paraproteinemias are disorders of the blood in which a particular protein becomes elevated, resulting in changes of the pressures in the vascular space and disruption of normal clotting processes.

Along with the professional health care community becoming increasingly aware of the value of TPE, the general public has been informed of this wonder of modern medicine through lay public journals, like *Woman's Day* and *Saturday Evening Post* (Coudert, 1993; Martin, 1993).

Summary

As the science and technology related to TPE and cascade, or immunoadsorption therapy are advanced, the role of nephrology nurses will parallel these developments. As evidenced by the several specialty nurses involved, collaborative practice will continue to be of great importance for the sharing of education and support for patients and professionals. Reinforced by their expertise with HD, nephrology nurses will be called upon to develop specific TPE protocols and practices related to vascular accesses, anticoagulation prescriptions, treatment regimens, and expected patient outcomes. Experience with the Medicare ESRD program will assist nephrology nurses in designing appropriate checks and balances as society debates the long-term treatment of chronic disease. Similarly, the evolution of the treatment of acute renal failure as a component of multisystem failure should serve nephrology nurses as a guide for end-of-life patient care considerations.

Nephrology nurses have been at the forefront of aggressive, invasive health care practices for the treatment of acute illness and chronic disease. This past experience is an asset as their scope of practice expands to encompass caring for patients and families when TPE is the treatment of choice.

References

Abel, S., Rowntree, L., & Turner, B. (1914). Plasma removal with return of corpuscles (plasmapheresis). *Journal of Pharmacol. Exp. Ther., 5*, 625-641

Asaba, H., Rekola, S., Bergstrand, A., Wasserman, H., & Bergstrom, J. (1980). Clinical trial of plasma exchange with a membrane filter in the treatment of crescentic glomerulonephritis. *Clinical Nephrology, 14*(2), 60-65.

Bell, J. (1989). Understanding and managing myasthenia gravis. *Focus on Critical Care, 16*(1), 57-65.

Buffaloe, G., & Heineken, F. (1983). Plasma volume nomograms for use in therapeutic plasma exchange. *Transfusion, 23*(4), 355-358.

Burke, M. (1993). Myasthenia gravis and pregnancy. *Journal of Perinatology Neonatal Nursing, 7*(1), 11-21.

Chu, G., Mantin, R., Shen, Y., Baskett, G., & Sussman, H. (1993). Massive cisplatin overdose by accidental substitution of carboplatin. *Cancer, 72*(12), 3707-3714.

Cohen, J. (1989). Reducing cholesterol: Strategies for increasing patient awareness. *Critical Care Nurse, 9*(3), 25-28.

Coudert, J. (1993). I was trapped in a useless body (pregnant woman suffers from Guillian-Barre syndrome). *Woman's Day, 57*, 56-60.

Dau, P. (1983). *Therapeutic plasma exchange disease compendium.* Lakewood, CO: Cobe Laboratories, Inc.

Duff, B., & Dugas, A. (1991). A clinical picture of a patient with thrombotic thrombocytopenia purpura. *CANNT Journal, 1*(4), 23-24.

Eggenberger, E., Coker, S., & Menezes, M. (1993). Pediatric Miller Fisher syndrome requiring intubation: A case report. *Clinical Pediatrics, 32*(6), 373-376.

Ellenberger, B., Haas, L., & Cundiff, L. (1993). Thrombotic thrombocytopenia purpura: Nursing during the acute phase. *Dimensions of Critical Care Nursing, 12*(2), 58-65.

Folkes, M. (1990). Transfusion therapy in critical care nursing. *Critical Care Nursing Quarterly, 13*(2), 15-28.

Gardner, J. & Gilcher, R. (1990) Haemonetics V-50 and plasma collection system: Common concerns and troubleshooting. *Journal of Clinical Apheresis, 5*, 106-109.

George, M. (1988) Neuromuscular respiratory failure: What the nurse knows may make the difference. *Journal of Neuroscience Nursing, 20*(2), 110-117.

Gerhardt, R., Ntoso, A., Koethe, J., Lodge, S., & Wolf, C. (1992). Acute plasma separation with hemodialysis equipment. *Journal of American Society of Nephrology, 2*, 1455-1458.

Graves, G., & Oates, M. (1994). Therapeutic plasma exchange for Guillian-Barre syndrome during pregnancy. *ANNA Journal, 21*(4), 277-278.

Guthrie, T., & Oral, A. (1989). Immune thrombocytopenia purpura: A pilot study of staphylococcal protein A immunomodulation in refractory patients. *Seminars in Hematology, 26*(2), 3-9.

Hakim, R., & Siami, G. (1994). Plasmapheresis. In Daugirdas & Ing (Eds.), *Handbook of dialysis* (2nd ed.) (pp. 218-241). Boston: Little, Brown & Company.

Hinkle, J., Albanese, M., & McGinty. (1993). Development of printed teaching materials for neuroscience patients. *Journal of Neuroscience Nursing, 25*(2), 125-129.

Hood, L. (1990). Myasthenia gravis: Regimens and regimen-associated problems in adults. *Journal of Neuroscience Nursing, 22*(6), 358-364.

Isaacs, P. (1994). Combined therapy management for patients with thrombolytic thrombocytopenic purpura. *ANNA Journal, 21*(4), 196-197, 199.

Kale, P., Thomson, P. Provenzano, R., & Higgins, M. (1993). Evaluation of plasmapheresis in the treatment of an acute overdose of carbamazepine. *Annals of Pharmacotherapy, 27*(7-8), 866-870.

Kaplan, A. (1995). General principles of therapeutic plasma exchange. *Seminars in Dialysis, 8*(5), 294-298.

Kaplan, A. (1992). Toward the rational prescription of therapeutic plasma exchange: The kinetics of immunoglobulin removal. *Seminars in Dialysis, 5*(3), 227-229.

Klee, K., McAfee, N., & Greenleaf, K. (1993). Pediatric case study: Hemolytic uremic syndrome. *ANNA Journal, 20*(4), 505-506.

Krsnak, J. (1994). Immunoadsorption column treatment for refractory ITP. *ANNA Journal, 21*(4), 198-199.

Martin, L. (1993, July-August). Mommy, why don't you hug me? (women suffers from Guillian-Barre syndrome). *Saturday Evening Post, 265*, 60-67.

McCarley, P., Wingard, R., & White, R. (1993). Therapeutic plasma exchange. In S. Burrows-Hudson (Ed.), *ANNA standards of clinical practice for nephrology nursing* (2nd ed.) (115-135), Pitman, NJ: American Nephrology Nurses' Association.

Neumann, M., & Urizar, R. (1994). Hemolytic uremic syndrome: Current pathophysiology and management. *ANNA Journal, 21*(2), 137-143.

Parobeck, V., Burnham, S., & Laukhuf, G. (1992). An unusual nursing challenge: Guillian-Barre syndrome following cra-

nial surgery. *Journal of Neuroscience Nursing, 24*(5), 251-255.
Pfister, S., & Bullas, J. (1990). Acute Guillian-Barre syndrome. *Critical Care Nurse, 10*(10), 68-73.
Price, C. (1987). Therapeutic plasma exchange in a dialysis unit. *ANNA Journal, 14*(2), 103- 108.
Price, C., & McCarley, P. (1993). Technical considerations of therapeutic plasma exchange as a nephrology nursing procedure. *ANNA Journal, 20*(1), 41-46.
Price, C., & McCarley, P. (1994). Physical assessment for patients receiving therapeutic plasma exchange. *ANNA Journal, 21*(4), 149-154, 201.
Price, C. (1995). Therapeutic plasma exchange. In L. Lancaster (Ed.), *Core curriculum for nephrology nursing* (3rd ed.) (pp. 347-365). Pitman, NJ: American Nephrology Nurses' Association.
Rabetoy, G., Price, C., Findlay, J., & Sailstad, J. (1990). Treatment of digoxin intoxication in a renal failure patient with digoxin-specific antibody fragments and plasmapheresis. *American Journal of Nephrology, 10*, 510-521.
Samtleben, W., Randerson, D., Blumenstein, M., Habersetzer, R., Schmidt, B., & Gurland, H. (1984). Membrane plasma exchange: Principles and application techniques. *Journal of Clinical Apheresis, 2*(2), 163-169.
Senack, E. (1990). Cobe: 2997 TPE Spectra, troubleshooting and common concerns. *Journal of Clinical Apheresis, 5*, 110-114.
Sherry, M. (1993). Wound care. A rash cure. Stevens-Johnson syndrome. *Nursing Times, 89*(25), 68, 71.
Ward, D. (1984). Therapeutic plasmapheresis and related apheresis techniques. In *Update to Harrison's principles of internal medicine,* (volume 5, pp. 67-95). New York: McGraw-Hill.
Weeks, D. (1991). Washing the blood, *RN, 54*(5), 60-64.
White-Williams, C. (1993). Immunosuppressive therapy following cardiac transplantation. *Critical Care Nursing Quarterly, 16*(2), 1-10.
Wingard, R. (1993). Familial hypercholesterolemia treated by plasma exchange and immunoadsorption. *ANNA Journal, 20*(1), 84-85.
Wiseman, K. (1993). New insights on Goodpasture's syndrome. *ANNA Journal, 20*(1), 17-26.
Wood, L., Bond, R., & Jacobs, P. (1984). Comparison of filtration to continuous-flow centrifugation for plasma exchange. *Journal of Clinical Apheresis, 2*(2), 155-162.

Chapter Highlights

- Therapeutic plasma exchange (TPE) and cytapheresis are the two primary categories of apheresis.
- The similarity in the equipment and procedural considerations between HD and TPE is the primary reason for establishing a TPE program in a dialysis unit.
- The expertise of nephrology nurses in patient assessment and treatment monitoring are essential to providing safe and effective therapy.
- The goal for HD may be to reduce the patient's intravascular blood volume, but the expectation for TPE is that the patient will remain euvolemic. TPE involves replacing the discarded plasma with an equal volume of a replacement fluid.
- The physical assessment for a patient receiving TPE may focus on a certain body system, depending on the medical diagnosis (Price & McCarley, 1994). Unlike a patient being treated with HD for renal failure, a patient receiving TPE may not have renal dysfunction.
- Potential complications that require continuous monitoring during TPE are hypotension, fluid imbalance, electrolyte imbalance, air embolism, blood leak, and hemolysis.
- If other electrolyte replacement is necessary, it can be provided through dietary or nutritional changes.
- The two most frequent postprocedural complications are bleeding and infection.
- Neuroscience nurses have recognized the therapeutic value of TPE and the related nursing concerns for patients diagnosed with Guillian-Barre Syndrome, myasthenia gravis, and neuromuscular respiratory failure.
- Professional nurses who specialize in perinatology neonatal nursing have been confronted with pregnant women needing TPE for the treatment of myasthenia gravis and Guillian-Barre Syndrome.
- Critical care nurses have experienced an increased use of TPE for critically ill patients with a variety of clinical presentations, including those already mentioned plus thrombotic thrombocytopenic purpura (TTP), idiopathic thrombocytopenic purpura (ITP), cardiac transplantation, cardiac surgery, and familial hypercholesterolemia.
- As the science and technology related to TPE and cascade or immunoadsorption therapy are advanced, the role of nephrology nurses will parallel these developments.
- Reinforced by their expertise with HD, nephrology nurses will be called upon to develop specific TPE protocols and practices related to vascular accesses, anticoagulation prescriptions, treatment regimens, and expected patient outcomes.

CHAPTER 22

Peritoneal Dialysis

LaVonne Burrows, MS, RN, CNN
Barbara F. Prowant, BSN, RN, CNN

Chapter Contents

Historical Perspectives of Peritoneal Dialysis 605
Utilization of Peritoneal Dialysis 605
Principles of Peritoneal Dialysis 606
Peritoneal Anatomy and Physiology 607
Solute Removal/Transport 608
Description of the Peritoneal Dialysis Process 613
Patient Selection for Peritoneal Dialysis 618
Peritoneal Dialysis as the Preferred Option 618
Peritoneal Dialysis Absolute Contraindications 618
Peritoneal Dialysis Relative Contraindications 619
Access 620
Acute Catheters 620
Chronic Catheters 620
Peritoneal Dialysis Prescription 625
Evaluation of Peritoneal Membrane Characteristics 625
Application of Membrane Classification to the Dialysis Prescription 626
Elements of the Dialysis Prescription 628
Dialysis Solution 629
Nursing Interventions/Procedures 631
Nursing Management of the Home PD Patient 632
Adequacy of Peritoneal Dialysis 636
Definition of Kt/V 636

Chapter Contents

Individualization of PD Therapy 638
- Modifications of Initial Prescription 638
- Changes in Clearance Over Time 638
- Tools to Individualize the PD Prescription 639

Infectious Complications 639
- Peritonitis 639
- Exit Site Infections 644
- Tunnel Infections 645

Noninfectious Complications 646
- Catheter Insertion 646
- Catheter Malfunction/Malposition 647
- Increased Intra-abdominal Pressure 648
- Miscellaneous Complications 649
- Metabolic Complications: PD Specific Considerations 651
- Endocrine and Reproductive Complications 651
- Nutritional Status 652

Patient Outcomes 653
- Metabolic Control 653
- Modality Survival 653
- Morbidity and Mortality 654

Summary 654

References 655

Chapter Highlights 658

Peritoneal Dialysis

LaVonne Burrows, MS, RN, CNN
Barbara F. Prowant, BSN, RN, CNN

Peritoneal dialysis (PD) is a treatment modality available for use in individuals with chronic renal failure. A relatively simple form of renal replacement therapy, PD generally is performed by the patient at home often without the need for complex machines and equipment. PD has a shorter history than hemodialysis (HD) as a treatment for ESRD patients, and there is still much to learn about the capabilities of PD and its optimal application. This chapter reviews the principles of PD, discusses the application of the therapy, reviews nursing care appropriate for this patient population, and indicates possible areas for nursing research.

Historical Perspectives of Peritoneal Dialysis

As early as 1923, the German physician and professor G. Ganter reported using the peritoneal membrane as a dialyzing surface in animals and was the first known to use peritoneal dialysis to filter wastes from uremic humans (Ganter, 1950). In contrast, the first working hemodialysis machine and artificial kidney was used by Dr. Willem Kolff in the early 1940s, with the first hemodialysis treatment in the United States performed in January, 1948 (Fishman, Kroop, Leijer, & Hyman, 1949). Technical complications, principally the lack of a suitable, long-term access to the peritoneal cavity and infectious complications, hampered further development of peritoneal dialysis as a treatment option. Although these complications prevented widespread use, interest in PD persisted. Problems associated with the anticoagulation required for hemodialysis and limited availability of hemodialysis spurred interest in PD, which was viewed as having potential for home dialysis. In 1967, Henry Tenckhoff developed a silicone, double cuffed catheter, allowing long-term access to the peritoneal cavity (Tenckhoff & Schechter, 1968). This facilitated the application of PD as a viable, long-term treatment modality for ESRD patients. Until 1976, intermittent PD (IPD) was used; patients were treated at a dialysis center three or more times per week for a 10 to 14 hour IPD treatment, or, in some cases, patients performed IPD at home. Drs. Jack Moncrief and Robert Popovich developed the concept of continuous ambulatory peritoneal dialysis (CAPD) in 1976. This allowed patients to perform PD at home, exchanging dialysis solution four to five times daily without being attached to IPD but remaining free to move around, resulting in more widespread use of the treatment modality.

Infections and protein loss remained the major problems associated with PD. The use of collapsible fluid containers helped diminish peritonitis rates by obliviating the need for a vent, resulting in a closed system for infusion of dialysis solution. Discontinuing the practice of using water baths to warm the PD solution also decreased the peritonitis rate, presumably by minimizing introduction of bacteria from unsterile water. More recently, introduction of "Y set" disconnect PD delivery systems has significantly decreased peritonitis rates. Several variations of peritoneal dialysis are currently in use, including (a) manual and automated systems, (b) straight line and disconnect apparatus, and (c) intermittent and continuous techniques. Key events in the history of PD are summarized in Table 22-1.

Utilization of Peritoneal Dialysis

PD is used as the treatment modality for end-stage renal disease by nearly 70,000 patients worldwide (Nissenson, 1994). Utilization rates for PD vary significantly by country. For example, in Japan, only 6% of ESRD patients are treated with PD, in Mexico the figure is 89%, and in the United States approximately 16% of patients use some form of peritoneal dialysis for their maintenance renal replacement therapy (Baxter Renal Care, 1996). Alexander and Honda (1993) report that more than 70% of children (15 years of age and younger) in the United States use some form of PD as their dialysis therapy. They attribute this high rate of use to the psychosocial, educational, and emotional advantages of treating children at home, as well as to the continuous biochemical and fluid control, patient mobility, easing of dietary restrictions, and simplicity of operation previously noted by Popovich et al. (1981). Many factors influence modality selection, including medical considerations, number and severity of co-morbid conditions, age, cultural and lifestyle issues, self-care ability, financial reimbursement issues and health care delivery systems, and personal preference. The

Table 22-1
Development of peritoneal dialysis.

1877	Wegner studied peritoneal lavage in animals.
1894	Starling and Tubby described absorption from the peritoneal cavity.
1923	Ganter described peritoneal dialysis in uremic animals and reported the first use of peritoneal dialysis for uremia in a human.
1959	Sterile peritoneal dialysis solution becomes available commercially.
1964	Boen developed the first closed automated delivery system.
1964	Palmer designed a silicone catheter for chronic use.
1965	Weston and Roberts designed an acute stylet catheter.
1966	Lasker developed an automated cycler.
1967	Tenckhoff designed the silicone double-cuff catheter.
1972	Fully automated, reverse osmosis system developed.
1976	Popovich and Moncrief described continuous ambulatory peritoneal dialysis technique.
1978	FDA approved peritoneal dialysis solution in polyvinyl bags for use in the United States.
1981	Diaz-Buxo et al. described continuous cycling peritoneal dialysis.
1980s	New CAPD systems, cycling machines, and catheter design developed, as well as variations in dialysis prescription and regimens.
1994	Sixteen percent of the U.S. dialysis population on PD.

Figure 22-1
Baxter Worldwide Survey on Peritoneal Dialysis, 1995.

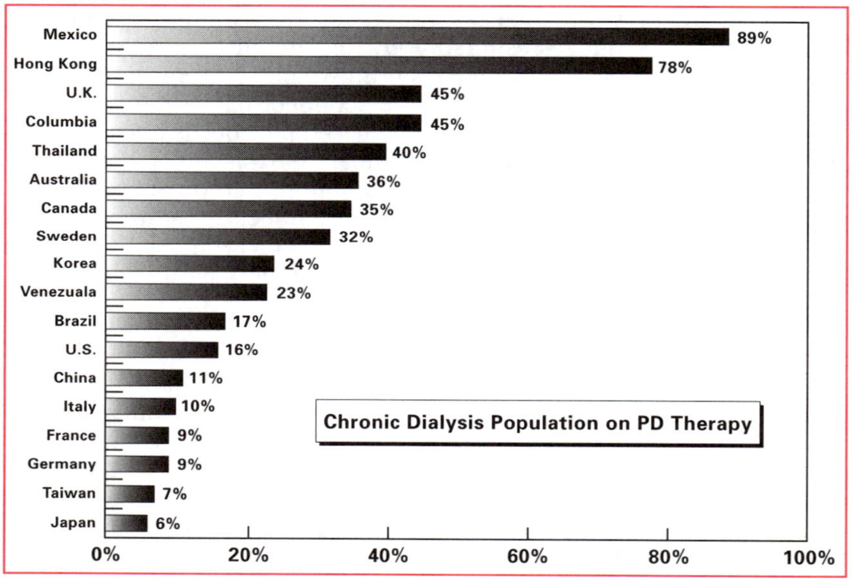

Note: From Baxter Renal Care. (1996). A look at worldwide use of peritoneal dialysis. *Nephrology News & Issues, 10*(4), 17–18. Reprinted with permission.

use of PD as a treatment modality worldwide is illustrated in Figure 22-1.

Principles of Peritoneal Dialysis

Dialysis is defined as the removal of certain crystalloids and fluids from the blood and lymph by the difference in their rate of diffusion through a semi-permeable membrane (Anderson & Anderson, 1994). For dialysis to occur, whether HD or PD, three components are required: blood, dialysis solution, and a semi-permeable (dialyzing) membrane. PD uses the blood present in the microcirculation of the abdominal cavity adjacent to the peritoneal membrane. The heart serves as the blood pump, with much slower blood flow rates than HD. Generally, dialysis solution used in PD is commercially prepared and pre-packaged; it *must* be sterile. The peritoneal membrane serves as the dialyzing membrane with each individual patient having unique membrane characteristics.

A comparison of several basic characteristics of PD and HD is presented in Table 22-2. In general, PD is less efficient than HD primarily due to the slower blood flow rates. To compensate for the less

Table 22–2
Comparison of peritoneal dialysis (PD) to hemodialysis (HD).

	PD	HD
Access	PD catheter	Vascular catheter, fistula, or graft
Blood flow rates	Capillary blood flow	300–500 ml/minute
Blood propulsion	Heart	Mechanical blood pump
Dialysis solution	Sterile	Non-sterile
Dialysis solution delivery system	2–3 liters per exchange	Continuous flow
Dialysis solution volume	8–15 liters per day duration (3–5 hours)	500–700 ml/minute for treatment
Dialyzing membrane	Peritoneal membrane; biocompatible	Synthetic fiber; not totally biocompatible
Membrane characteristics	Predetermined for each individual	Many choices available
Efficiency	Low	Moderate to high
Time Required	24 hours/continuous or >10 hours overnight 7 days/week	3–5 hours/treatment 3 treatments/week

efficient nature of PD, required dialysis time is much longer for PD compared to hemodialysis. The continuous or near continuous removal of toxins and fluid is more physiologic, mimicking native kidney function, and better tolerated than HD by individuals susceptible to problems associated with rapid fluid or electrolyte shifts. The dialyzing membrane cannot be manipulated in PD, whereas in HD many choices of dialyzers with a variety of membrane characteristics can be prescribed. Comparing PD to HD is difficult; although these two renal replacement therapies have similarities, they work quite differently. Nolph (1992) notes that weekly dialysis clearances of urea for PD are only 60% of the thrice weekly clearances of HD, yet both PD and HD yield comparable patient outcomes.

Peritoneal Anatomy and Physiology

The peritoneal membrane is a serous membrane consisting of two layers: the visceral peritoneum covering the abdominal organs and the parietal peritoneum lining the outer walls of the abdominal cavity (Guyton, 1976) (see Figure 22-2). The peritoneal membrane is continuous and forms a closed sac in males; in females, the Fallopian tubes and ovaries open into the peritoneal cavity. The average surface area of the membrane in adults is 1–2 meters squared, and approximates body surface area (Twardowski, 1995).

The primary purpose of the peritoneum is to provide a smooth contact surface between the abdominal wall and the intra-abdominal organs, with approximately 100 milliliters (ml) of transudate present under normal circumstances to facilitate movement of the peritoneal layers. In average sized adults, this space can be enlarged by instillation of fluid to a capacity of 2 liters or more without undue distress. The peritoneal membrane consists of the vascular wall, the interstitium, the mesothelium, and adjacent fluid films that contribute to impedance of the diffusion of substances, or peritoneal membrane resistance. Nolph, Miller, Rubin, and Popovich (1980) identified at least six sites of resistance: (a) R1-fluid films within peritoneal capillaries; (b) R2-the capillary endothelium; (c) R3-the capillary basement membrane; (d) R4-the interstitium; (e) R5-the mesolthelium; and (f) R6-stagnant fluid films within the peritoneal cavity. The permeability of the tissue between the peritoneal capillary lumen and the peritoneal cavity filled with dialysis solution varies among individuals; these characteristics can and should be determined to select an appropriate PD prescription. Studies to determine peritoneal membrane permeability characteristics include the peritoneal equilibration test (PET) and peritoneal function test (PFT), which are discussed later in this chapter.

The arteries of the abdominal wall supply the blood for the parietal peritoneum; venous return enters the systemic circulation. The visceral peritoneum receives its blood supply from the mesenteric and celiac arteries, with this blood re-entering the circulation through the liver via the portal vein.

Lymphatic drainage of the peritoneal cavity is

Figure 22-2
The peritoneal membrane.

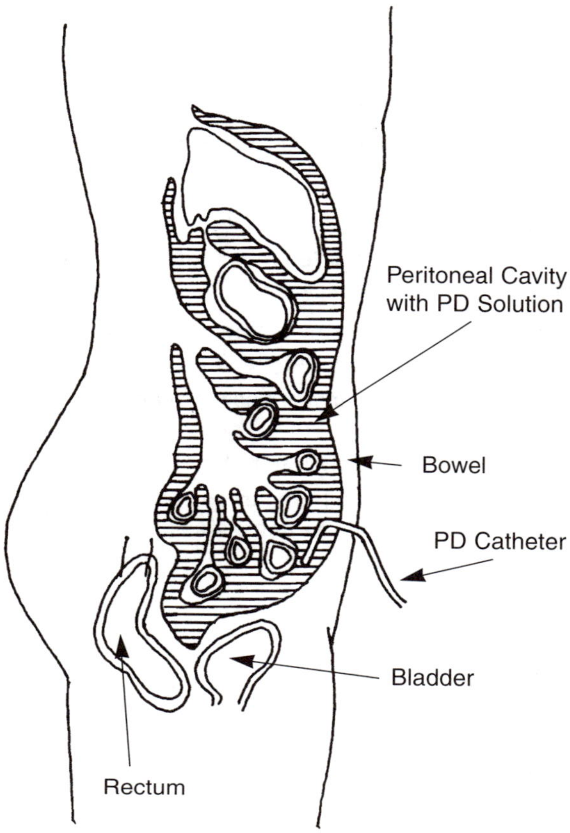

very active, but the role of this lymphatic absorption in PD has been largely ignored until recently. "Diaphragmatic contractions actively pump fluid from the peritoneal cavity into and through the diaphragmatic lymphatics and lymph drains" (Twardowski, 1995, p. 336). The lymphatics thought to have the most impact in PD are those immediately beneath the diaphragm (Twardowski). The rate of lymphatic absorption can be approximated by determining the rate of disappearance of albumin. Because albumin is such a large molecule (molecular weight 68,000 daltons), it is absorbed almost exclusively by lymphatic convection, and can be used as a marker to determine the rate of lymphatic absorption. Lymphatic absorption of fluid when the peritoneal cavity is filled with 1–2 liters of fluid occurs at a rate of 0.5 to 1.5 milliliters per minute (Sorkin & Diaz-Buxo, 1994), with higher rates of absorption in children compared to adults. Increased lymphatic absorption is thought to play a role in some patients who experience difficulty with fluid removal or loss of ultrafiltration (Sorkin & Diaz-Buxo), but this remains a diagnosis of exclusion. Until methods of easily determining lymphatic absorption are available to the clinician, measurement of lymphatic absorption rates is limited to a research setting.

Host defenses for the peritoneal cavity are somewhat limited, since normally no anatomical access exists for bacterial invasion. Host defenses include circulating immunocompetent cells (i.e., macrophages), humoral substances (i.e., cytokines, platelet activating factor), and chemotaxis, or the attraction of cells towards infected areas (Vanholder, Van Loo, De Smet, & Ringoir, 1995). Institution of PD includes placement of a catheter into the peritoneal cavity to allow introduction of dialysis solution; however, this same catheter may serve as a portal of entry for pathogens. Additionally, the introduction of large volumes of dialysis solution serves to dilute the normal host defenses, leaving the individual more vulnerable to infection. Recent studies have indicated that the dialysis solution itself is somewhat bioincompatible; its acidic pH results in some degree of direct toxicity to macrophages (Coles, 1995). This combination of factors contributes to a predisposition to infection, the most common complication of PD.

The greater omentum, which descends from the stomach in front of the small intestines and sometimes extends to the pelvis (Gray, 1977), plays a role in localizing and combating infection. The omentum is capable of absorbing or walling off various foreign bodies (Wilkie, 1911). However, because the PD catheter is a foreign body, omental wrapping of the catheter can occur.

Solute Removal/Transport

Dialysis is used to remove toxic substances from the blood of uremic individuals. A review of key terms is useful in understanding the principles of dialysis. For example, any liquid capable of dissolving substances is called a *solvent.* Any substance that dissolves in a solvent (liquid) to form a solution is called a *solute.* In dialysis, blood and dialysis solution are the solvents, and the various toxins (urea, creatinine, sodium, potassium, and others) are the solutes.

Diffusion. Transport or clearance is achieved principally via the process of diffusion. *Diffusion* can be defined as the movement of solutes through a semi-permeable membrane, with net movement occurring from an area of greater concentration to an area of lesser concentration. Urea, creatinine, potassium, sodium, and various other substances move from the blood to the dialysis solution, provided the concentration of the solute is greater in the blood than in the dialysis solution and the solute is small enough to pass through the membrane. A number of factors affect the rate of diffusion of a solute, including (a) concentration gradient, (b) membrane permeability, (c) size (weight) of the solute, (d) membrane surface area, (e) volume of dialysis solution, and (f) length of time dialysis solution is allowed to dwell in the peritoneal cavity.

The degree of difference between the concentration of the substance on either side of the membrane is called the *concentration gradient*, and this influences the rate of diffusion. The steeper the concentration gradient, the faster the solute diffuses. Over time, the concentration of the solute begins to equalize or equilibrate across the membrane, resulting in a diminishing of the concentration gradient and therefore a slowing in the rate of diffusion.

Membrane permeability is the term generally used to refer to the number and size of the openings in the membrane; permeability reflects the ease with which solutes can pass through the membrane. A highly permeable membrane allows solutes to pass freely unless the solute is larger than the membrane openings. A membrane with low permeability characteristics impedes the diffusion of solutes.

The size and weight of the solute also affects the rate of diffusion, with smaller, lighter solutes (for example, urea) diffusing much more quickly than large solutes (for example, Vitamin B12). Extremely large molecules may not diffuse across the membrane. In contrast to HD, where synthetic membranes have pores small enough to completely restrict movement of large molecules such as proteins, the peritoneal membrane does allow some transport of large molecules, including proteins (Sorkin & Diaz-Buxo, 1994). However, large molecules cross the peritoneal membrane primarily by convective transport, not diffusion (see Convective transport), while small molecules cross the peritoneal membrane primarily by diffusion. To facilitate comparison of relative size, Table 22-3 lists the molecular weight of a few solutes in PD.

Surface area of the peritoneal membrane influences rate of diffusion. Because peritoneal membrane surface area approximates body surface area, a large adult has more surface area available for diffusion than a small adult, with an increase in the total diffusive capacity. Infants and children have a peritoneal membrane surface area that is proportionately greater than adults (Fine & Tejani, 1994), resulting in more efficient solute diffusion. The degree of solute removal relative to the quantity of solute generated determines whether or not the removal is adequate for an individual patient (see Adequacy of Peritoneal Dialysis).

The volume of dialysis solution in the peritoneal cavity also influences the transport and removal of solutes, in part due to the interaction of dialysate volume and effective peritoneal membrane surface area. A larger volume increases the surface area of the membrane in contact with dialysis solution, thus increasing effective functional surface area. The increase is limited by the absolute surface area of the membrane; if all membrane surfaces are in contact with solution, additional volume will not increase functional diffusive surface area. Additional volume *will* result in the net removal of more solute, since more solute is needed in the dialysis solution to reach equilibrium with the serum concentration. Simply stated, more urea will be required to raise 3 liters of dialysis solution to a concentration equal to blood urea levels than would be required to raise 2 liters of dialysis solution to the same level.

The length of time dialysis solution is left in the peritoneal cavity affects total diffusive clearance. Urea can serve as an example to illustrate this point. There is no urea in dialysis solution, thus the blood level of urea will be significantly higher than zero, creating a steep concentration gradient. The urea from the bloodstream crosses the peritoneal membrane by diffusion and enters the dialysis solution, rapidly at first, then more slowly as the urea concentration between the two compartments (dialysate and blood) becomes more nearly equal. Eventually, if the dialysis solution is allowed to remain in the peritoneal cavity, the concentration of urea in the blood and the concentration of urea in the dialysis solution will be the same. This is referred to as *equilibration*. Urea molecules will still cross the peritoneal membrane, but without a concentration difference or gradient, there will be no *net* change in the concentration of urea in the blood or dialysis solution. For additional net solute transfer to occur, the dialysis solution must be drained from the peritoneal cavity and fresh dialysis solution infused, re-establishing the concentration gradient. It is important to note that equilibration for different substances will occur at different times. A small molecule such as urea moves readily across the membrane and equilibrates more rapidly than larger molecules. When prescribing the timing of PD exchanges, the rates of diffusion of key solutes must be considered. Table 22-4 summa-

Table 22–3
Comparison of molecular weights of selected solutes.

Substance	Molecular Weight(daltons)
Urea	60
Creatinine	113
Glucose	180
Albumin	68,000

Table 22–4
Factors affecting diffusion.

Factors	Effects
Molecular size	Large molecules diffuse more slowly. Small molecules diffuse more readily.
Concentration gradient	A large difference in the concentration of the solute between the two compartments increases the rate of diffusion.
Membrane permeability characteristics	A highly permeable membrane has a high rate of diffusion. A membrane with low permeability has a lower rate of diffusion.
Effective membrane surface area	Large surface area increases the rate of diffusion.
Volume of dialysis solution	An increase in the volume of dialysis solution may increase net diffusive capacity.

rizes the factors that affect diffusion and thus net removal to toxins in PD.

Osmosis/ultrafiltration. The movement of a *solvent* (liquid) through a semi-permeable membrane from an area of lower concentration to an area of higher concentration *of the solute* is called *osmosis. Ultrafiltration* is defined as the removal of a solvent (fluid). Ultrafiltration can be the result of a pressure gradient or an osmotic gradient. Pressure gradients are used in HD to achieve ultrafiltration. In PD, dextrose in the dialysis solution provides an osmotic gradient responsible for ultrafiltration achieved. Water is the fluid removed (Sorkin & Diaz-Buxo, 1994).

To induce the movement of water across the membrane, a solute must create a concentration gradient. A solute that diffuses readily through the semipermeable membrane will not create an osmotic gradient; an osmotically active solute must either not diffuse through the membrane, or must diffuse slowly, thus creating a disequilibrium between the two compartments on either side of the membrane (see Figure 22-3). To illustrate, two solutions (A and B) are separated by a semi-permeable membrane. Solution A has a large number of small solute particles in solution capable of diffusing through the membrane; Solution B has large solute particles in solution, too large to diffuse through the membrane. Over time, the small particles from Solution A diffuse across the membrane, reaching equilibrium. Since the large solutes in Solution B cannot cross the membrane, an osmotic gradient is created, which results in the movement of water through the membrane to equalize the concentration between the two compartments.

The *volume* of fluid in each of the two compartments may be unequal, as in this illustration, but the solution *concentration* will equalize. As is true with diffusion, the greater the difference in concentrations across the membrane, the faster the rate of ultrafiltration. The initial movement of water in the example cited will be faster than when the two solutions are nearly equilibrated.

Osmotic ultrafiltration, the fluid removal process active in PD, occurs as a result of the addition of dextrose to the dialysis solution. Dextrose is a large molecule that does not cross the peritoneal membrane rapidly, and thus is capable of creating an osmotic gradient, attracting water from the patient's blood across the membrane to dilute to dialysis solution. Factors that affect the rate of ultrafiltration include (a) colloid osmotic and oncotic pressure in the capillary beds, (b) individual peritoneal membrane characteristics, (c) degree of osmotic pressure gradient (the concentration of dextrose in the solution), and (d) length of time the dialysis solution is left in the peritoneal cavity.

Colloid osmotic or *oncotic pressure* in the capillary beds refers to the "pull" or osmotic pressure created within the capillary by the plasma proteins. Capillary oncotic pressure serves to hold water in the capillary, not allowing water to move into the peritoneal cavity. The degree to which this is a factor varies and can be affected by certain disease states.

Individual membrane permeability characteristics important to diffusion also influence ultrafiltration, but with a near opposite effect. A highly permeable membrane, although allowing rapid diffusion, also permits more rapid absorption of dextrose with a resulting decrease in ultrafiltration. At the other extreme, a peritoneal membrane with low permeability characteristics impedes the absorption of dextrose, resulting in marked ultrafiltration, but

Figure 22-3
Two solutions separated by a semi-permeable membrane.

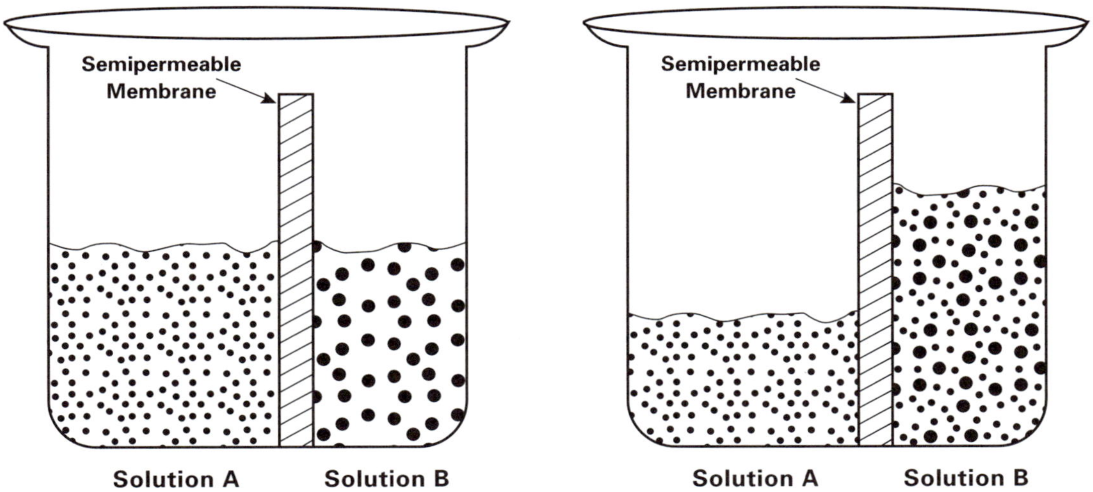

Solution A contains small particles that diffuse through the membrane. Solution B contains large particles that cannot cross the membrane. These particles create an osmotic pressure gradient that causes water to cross the membrane.

limited diffusion of solutes.

The degree of osmotic pressure within the peritoneal cavity is determined by the osmolality of the dialysis solution. Dextrose used in dialysis solution is the D-glucose monohydrate, which has a molecular weight 10% higher than anhydrous glucose; therefore, although dextrose concentration of dialysis solution closely parallels glucose, the terms are not interchangeable. "For this reason, the dextrose concentrations listed on the dialysis solution bottle are 10% greater than the true glucose concentrations" (Sorkin & Diaz-Buxo, 1994, p. 249). Various concentrations of dextrose solutions are available for use in peritoneal dialysis: 1.5%, 2.5%, 3.5% and 4.25% dextrose (1.36, 2.27, 3.17, or 3.86% glucose, respectively). The higher the concentration of dextrose in the solution, the higher the osmotic gradient created. This results in an increased volume of fluid that ultrafiltrates from the blood and surrounding tissues of the individual.

The length of time the dialysis solution is left in the peritoneal cavity is significant in determining the net ultrafiltration. As with diffusion, the movement of water continues until the concentration is equal on both sides of the semi-permeable membrane. In a closed system with an osmotic substance incapable of crossing the membrane, once equilibrium is reached it becomes a steady state. This is not the case in PD for two reasons: (a) the osmotic substance used (dextrose) *does* cross the peritoneal membrane, and (b) the system is *not closed*, since dialysate is also absorbed via the lymphatics.

Upon initial instillation of the dialysis solution into the peritoneal cavity, fluid moves relatively rapidly from the blood and interstitial spaces of the individual into the peritoneal cavity. With time, the rate of fluid movement from the blood into the peritoneal cavity decreases, due to both the dilution of the hypertonic solution by the water that has already crossed the membrane and the gradual absorption of dextrose across the membrane. Equilibrium is achieved within a period of hours, the exact time depending on individual membrane characteristics, the dextrose concentration of the fluid infused, and the volume of fluid infused. If the dialysis solution is allowed to remain in the peritoneal cavity, dextrose absorption continues. As dextrose is absorbed into the blood, water moves *back* across the membrane, *re-entering* the tissue and blood. Thus, the volume of fluid in the peritoneal cavity peaks, then declines as the dextrose and water move into the patient's bloodstream. Some fluid is also re-absorbed from the peritoneal cavity back into the patient through the lymphatic system. *Net ultrafiltration* is the volume of water drawn into the peritoneal cavity less the volume reabsorbed (into the peritoneal vasculature or by the lymphatic system). The factors influencing osmosis/ultrafiltration and their effects are summarized in Table 22-5.

Table 22–5
Factors affecting osmosis/ultrafiltration.

Factors	Effects
Peritoneal membrane permeability characteristics	A highly permeable membrane increases the rate of dextrose absorption, resulting in more rapid loss of the osmotic pressure gradient and decreased ultrafiltration. Low membrane permeability maintains the osmotic gradient longer, sustaining ultrafiltration.
Dwell time	Extremes in dwell time tend to produce less ultrafiltration. Very short dwells may not allow time for water movement. Very long dwells allow fluid to be reabsorbed.
Dialysis solution dextrose concentration	Higher dextrose concentration (2.5%, 4.25%) increases ultrafiltration. Lower dextrose concentration (1.5%) decreases ultrafiltration.

Dextrose absorption has some disadvantages including elevation of blood glucose levels, weight gain, and elevated serum triglyceride levels. Therefore, alternatives to dextrose as the osmotically active component in peritoneal dialysis solutions have been explored. Amino acids have been considered for use as an osmotic agent, due to their large molecular weight and the potential that any absorption of amino acids might benefit the PD patient. Williams et al. (1982) conducted an early trial of a dialysis solution containing 2 grams/deciliter of amino acids on 6 patients. Ultrafiltration volumes were similar to 4.25% dextrose solution, and the amino acids that were absorbed were considered beneficial for the patient, since protein loss is one of the potential drawbacks to PD. This prompted the authors to conclude "that intraperitoneal administration of amino acids is effective and well-tolerated in patients on CAPD" (Williams et al., p. 124). A later study by Bruno et al. (1989) evaluated the use of a 1% amino acid dialysis solution. Six CAPD patients used the amino acid solution for one exchange per day. Nitrogen balance, plasma cholesterol and triglyceride levels improved, but were accompanied by an increase in weight in already overweight patients and an increase in acidosis. No toxic effects to the peritoneal membrane were apparent, but long-term biocompatibility of these solutions has not yet been established. The principal barriers to use of amino acid solutions are cost and metabolic acidosis. Thus, alternatives to dextrose as the osmotic agent in PD solution are not in widespread use. This is an area where research may be of significance in the future, to help determine if there is a group of patients for whom the additional cost of amino acid dialysis solution would be beneficial overall, if risk of malnutrition, hospitalizations, or death could be decreased. Nurses should participate with other members of the health care team in designing and implementing such research.

Convective transport. Unlike diffusion, convective transport does not require a solute concentration gradient (Keshaviah, 1995), but does increase significantly as molecular size of the solute increases. Convective transport occurs as a result of the frictional forces between the solvent (water) and the solute. As osmotic forces cause water to move across the membrane, some solutes in solution are carried across the membrane with the water, a phenomenon also known as "solute drag." Convection may account for little small molecule clearance, but is much more effective than diffusive transport for removing large molecular weight solutes (Twardowski, 1995).

Clearance. Clearance is a measure commonly used to quantify renal function and dialysis efficiency. "Plasma clearance is defined as a hypothetical volume of plasma that is completely cleared of a given solute per unit of time" (Sorkin & Diaz-Buxo, 1994, p. 254). Creatinine or urea clearances for the purpose of evaluation of renal function generally are expressed in ml/minute; dialysis effectiveness can also be expressed as a clearance, generally expressed in liters per week (L/wk). Urea and creatinine are the solutes most frequently measured in the clinical setting and represent small to middle molecule clearances. The concentration of a substance in the drained, or "spent" dialysate can be measured in a laboratory. Measurement of the concentration of specific solutes in dialysate and plasma has resulted in the establishment of "standard" dialysate to plasma ratios for these solutes for a given dwell time (see Figure 22-4).

To estimate a clearance, the dialysate to plasma ratio for the solute at the given dwell time is determined from the standard curves. This number is multiplied by the volume of spent dialysate drained from the patient, and an approximate clearance is determined. For example, a patient who infuses 2 liters (L) of dialysis solution 4 times daily drains 9.5 L of spent dialysate: 8 L + 1.5 L of ultrafiltrate (ultrafiltrate contains an equal amount of solute, and therefore adds to the total clearance achieved). Each 2 L exchange remains in the peritoneal cavity for approximately 6 hours, with a standard dialysate to plasma ratio for creatinine of 0.8 (the creatinine level in the dialysis solution is 80% of the plasma level after 6 hours). To calculate the estimated creatinine clearance, simply multiply the volume of drained dialysate by 0.8 to get the liters of plasma cleared per day, then multiply by 7 to estimate weekly clearance. In this example, 9.5 L x 0.8 (D/P) x 7 = 53.2 L/week. Creatinine clearance formulas are summarized in Table 22-6.

Calculation of an actual clearance requires collection of the spent dialysate, and use of a formula for clearance. Many centers calculate the clearance of the dialysis and the residual renal clearance, and combine these to evaluate the total effective clearance achieved for the patient. Other centers only consider the dialysis clearance since residual renal clearance declines over time. Current recommendations for creatinine clearance are controversial, but there is a general consensus that no less than 50 L/wk creatinine clearance is required, with some experts recommending as much as 70 L/wk creatinine clearance (see Adequacy of Peritoneal Dialysis).

Description of the Peritoneal Dialysis Process

PD consists of delivering dialysis solution into the peritoneal cavity, allowing time for diffusion and ultrafiltration, then draining the spent dialysate

Figure 22-4

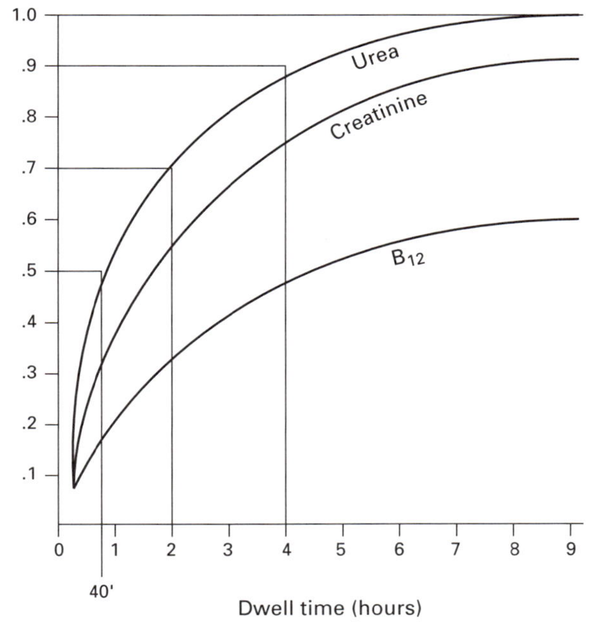

Rate of entry of urea creatinine, and vitamin B12 into peritoneal dialysis solution that has been left in the abdomen. Results are expressed as the ratio of the level in dialysate (D) to the level in plasma (p). Typical D/P ratios for urea at time points of 40 minutes, 2 hours, and 4 hours are indicated.

Note: From Sorkin, M.I., & Diaz-Buxo, J.A. (1994). Physiology of peritoneal dialysis. In J.T. Daugirdas & T.S. Ing (Eds.), *Handbook of dialysis* (2nd ed., p. 246), Copyright, 1994, Little, Brown, & Company. Reprinted with permission.

Table 22–6
Creatinine clearance formulas.

Definition — volume of blood cleared of creatinine in 1 minute

Formula for calculation of urinary creatinine clearance:

$$\frac{\text{Volume of urine in ml/min x Urinary concentration of creatinine in mg/dl}}{\text{Plasma concentration of creatinine}}$$

Cockroft - Gault formula for estimation of urinary creatinine clearance*:

$$\frac{\text{(140 - age) x (body weight in kgs)}}{\text{72 x serum creatinine in mg/dl}}$$

Formula for estimation of dialysate creatinine clearance in L/week:

Dialysate creatinine/Plasma creatinine **
x 24 hour dialysate volume in L x 7 days

* times 0.85 for females
** from Peritoneal Equilibration Test

Table 22–7
Variations of peritoneal dialysis.

Form of Peritoneal Dialysis	Abbreviation	Description
Continuous ambulatory peritoneal dialysis	CAPD	Dialysis solution dwelling 24 hours/day; manual exchange
Continuous cyclic peritoneal dialysis	CCPD	Dialysis solution dwelling 24 hours/day; cycler used for at least some exchanges
Intermittent peritoneal dialysis	IPD	Dialysis solution dwelling less than 24 hours/day; cycler usually used
Nightly intermittent peritoneal dialysis	NIPD	Dialysis daily done overnight; cycler used
Tidal peritoneal dialysis	TPD	Cycler dialysis with initial fill, subsequent cycle volumes maintain dialysis solution in the peritoneal cavity until completion of treatment
Automated peritoneal dialysis	APD	Describes any form of PD where a cycler is used (CCPD, IPD, NIPD, TPD)

from the cavity. This process is then repeated to achieve adequate dialysis. A variety of PD delivery systems are currently in use.

Exchange or cycle. A peritoneal dialysis exchange consists of three phases: (a) *infusion* of dialysis solution into the peritoneal cavity, (b) allowing the solution to remain in the cavity or *dwell*, and (c) allowing the dialysate to *drain* out of the peritoneum. In manual forms of PD, infusion is accomplished by placing the dialysis fluid container higher than the patient's abdomen and allowing fluid to flow into the peritoneal space by gravity. A 2 L container takes approximately 10–12 minutes to infuse, with the limiting factor for rate of infusion being patient comfort. Dwell time is prescribed, and should be tailored to meet the individual patient's dialytic needs (see Individualization of PD Therapy). The drain phase of the cycle simply reverses the process of infusion, with the container for spent dialysate positioned lower that the patient's abdomen, and drainage achieved by gravity flow. Drainage takes somewhat longer than infusion, approximately 20–30 minutes for a 2 L inflow volume. As mentioned previously, osmosis and ultrafiltration generally result in the drained volume of dialysate being more than the volume originally infused.

In automated forms of PD, an exchange is sometimes referred to as a cycle. However, the process still consists of an infusion or inflow, dwell, and drain phase. Depending on the specific cycler used, the fill and drain phases may be accomplished by gravity flow (as with the manual forms of PD), or may use low pressure pumps. To minimize risk of trauma to the peritoneal membrane, care should be taken to avoid any high pressure pumps for infusion or drainage of PD solution into or out of the peritoneal cavity.

Types of peritoneal dialysis. Peritoneal dialysis in clinical practice has evolved into several variations (see Table 22-7). PD may be performed as a continuous or an intermittent therapy. Continuous forms of PD include continuous ambulatory PD (CAPD) or continuous cyclic PD (CCPD). In both CAPD and CCPD, dialysis solution is constantly in the peritoneal cavity, 24 hours a day, 7 days a week; the only time there is not fluid dwelling is during the actual infusion and drain phases of each exchange. CAPD is a manual technique, consisting of usually 3-5 exchanges per day. Daytime exchanges are spaced throughout the waking hours, with a longer exchange overnight. CCPD uses a machine, called a cycler, that automates the infusion and drain phases of the exchange. Most often, cycler exchanges are done at night while the patient sleeps, a reverse of the CAPD pattern. The cycler is prepared with tubing and enough dialysis solution for all exchanges to be delivered for the night, typically 4-6 cycles of $\geq$ 2 L for a total of 8–12 L or more of dialysis solution required each treatment. The patient connects to the cycler, which drains the fluid already in the peritoneal space, and infuses the next exchange. At the end of the session, the cycler fills the patient with dialysis solution for a long daytime dwell, and the patient disconnects from the cycler. A recent variation combines CCPD and CAPD, with the patient using a cycler at night and doing a daytime manual exchange as well.

Intermittent forms of PD may be either manual or automated with a cycler. Nightly intermittent PD

Figure 22-5
Y-Disconnect system.

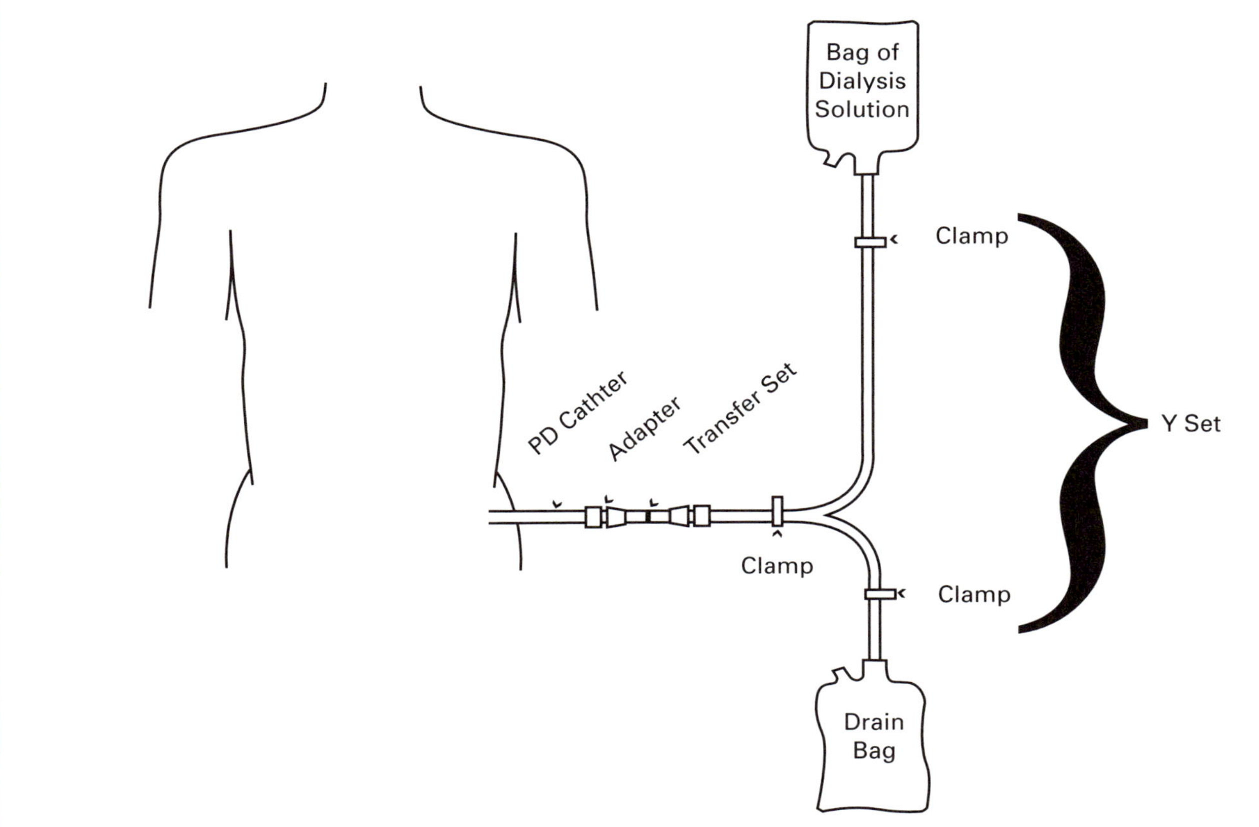

(NIPD) refers to the same pattern of exchanges as CCPD, except the spent dialysate is drained prior to disconnecting from the cycler for the day. The absence of dialysis solution during the day results in no dialysis taking place during the day; therefore, NIPD is an intermittent therapy. Intermittent PD (IPD) can also be done in a dialysis unit or clinic; however, this form of PD is rarely used since treatments may require 10-12 hours each, 5-6 days per week. Despite the time invested, it is difficult to achieve adequate dialysis with this method.

Tidal peritoneal dialysis (TPD) is a form of cycler dialysis occasionally used, primarily in pediatric patients. A volume of dialysis solution is infused and allowed to dwell, as with other forms of automated peritoneal dialysis (APD), but when the drain begins, only a portion of the fill volume is drained. Fresh dialysis solution is infused, replacing some of the drained fluid and maintaining a prescribed volume of PD solution in the peritoneum during the entire treatment. The concept is to avoid the time during the drain and infusion when little or no dialysis solution is dwelling, and thus, no dialysis can take place. Also, by adding a volume of fresh dialysis solution, a steeper concentration gradient is re-established. At the end of the cycling session, all dialysate is drained. If continuous therapy is prescribed, fresh dialysis solution is infused for the long dwell. The advantages of TPD include maximizing clearances and avoidance of down time during the dialysis treatment. Disadvantages are the need for more dialysis solution (since dialysate is drained well before equilibrium is achieved) with its associated costs, and the need for a much more sophisticated cycler.

All forms of PD using a cycler are correctly referred to as automated PD (APD). No distinction is made between the continuous and intermittent forms when using the term APD.

Systems for PD delivery. A number of delivery systems are available for use in PD. Systems commonly used for CAPD are (a) disconnect systems, (b) a straight manual system with a spike connector, (c) a straight manual system with a luer connector and recessed spike, and (d) systems using an assist device to transfer the spike, with or without an

Figure 22-6
Straight manual PD system.

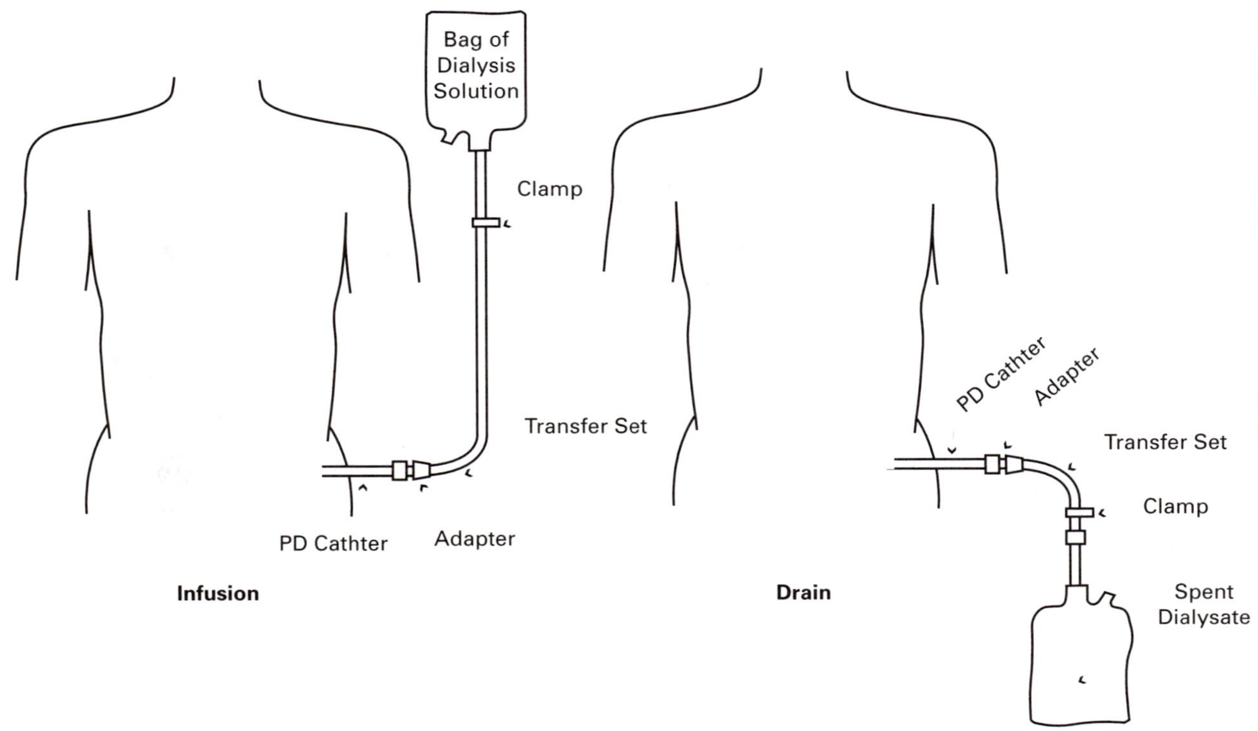

ultraviolet light for disinfection.

Disconnect systems allow the patient to have only the PD catheter and a short transfer tubing, with a protective sterile cap attached to the end. Unlike the standard manual system, the empty bag is disconnected from the patient once the dialysis solution is infused, instead of being worn, until the next exchange. This minimizes the alteration in body image, making PD more attractive to some patients. Additionally, the disconnect system employs the principle of flush before fill. The system (sometimes called a Y-set or Y-disconnect system) consists of a Y-shaped tubing. The base of the Y connects to the transfer set. One arm of the Y connects to the bag of fresh dialysis solution, the other arm to a drain bag. The patient first "flushes" a small volume of dialysis solution from the new bag into the drain bag, removing air and also flushing the tubing *after* connection to the transfer set, presumably washing any bacteria that may have been introduced via touch contamination away from the patient and into the drain bag. The spent dialysate in the peritoneal cavity is then drained, and the next exchange infused (see Figure 22-5). Finally, the Y-set tubing is disconnected and a protective disconnect cap is placed on the end of the transfer set to prevent contamination until the next exchange.

The two examples of "straight" systems include (a) a transfer tubing attached directly to the catheter adapter on one end and the bag of dialysis solution at the other, using either a spike (similar to those used on intravenous [IV] tubing) or (b) the recessed spike with a luer adapter to connect to the bag. Dialysis solution is infused into the peritoneum, and the empty bag is folded and worn under the clothing. After the prescribed dwell time, the empty bag is unfolded and placed below the level of the patient's abdomen, the fluid is drained into the bag, and the process is repeated with fresh solution (see Figure 22-6). Extreme care must be taken to avoid the introduction of bacteria into the system, since straight systems infuse dialysis solution directly into the peritoneum after the system has been opened; any touch contaminant at the end of the

Table 22–8
Key elements of standard versus disconnect CAPD exchange procedures.

Standard*	Disconnect*
Empty bag from previous inflow attached, worn under clothing with long transfer set.	Short transfer set with protective cap at end worn under clothing between exchanges.
- Begin draining spent dialysate into bag.	- Prepare new Y-disconnect system (dialysis solution and empty bag).
- Clamp at end of drain and place spent dialysate bag on work surface.	- Connect transfer set to Y-disconnect system.
- Prepare new bag of dialysis solution.	- Flush fresh dialysis solution from new bag into drain bag (away from patient).
- Transfer spike (or other connecting device) from spent dialysate bag to new solution bag.	- Drain spent dialysate into empty bag of Y-disconnect system.
- Infuse fresh dialysis solution.	- Infuse fresh dialysis solution.
- Fold empty container and replace under clothing until next exchange.	- Disconnect Y-disconnect system & replace protective cap.
Note: After system is opened, dialysis solution flows directly into peritoneal cavity	**Note:** After system is opened, fluid is flushed into the drain bag prior to infusing into peritoneal cavity flush before fill.

*Both procedures require handwashing and aseptic technique. Masks must be worn any time the system is opened.

transfer set will be infused directly into the peritoneal cavity and can cause an infection. Most of these systems include the use of a disinfectant at the connection between the bag and the transfer tubing, such as some form of povidone-iodine solution. To minimize the risk of infection, the exchange procedure should be done in a clean room with minimal drafts, using good handwashing and aseptic technique. Use of masks by all persons in the room is recommended to minimize airborne bacteria or other contaminants.

Use of an assist device is an alternative to the standard manual system. These devices were designed to decrease the rate of peritonitis by avoiding the manual transfer of the spike prior to insertion into the new bag and by adding a disinfection system. Although also infusing fresh dialysis solution directly into the peritoneal cavity after the spike is transferred, these devices physically move the spike from the bag of spent dialysate to the bag of fresh dialysis solution, and may expose the spike to an ultraviolet light to kill bacteria prior to inserting the spike into the new bag.

Key elements of standard versus disconnect CAPD exchange procedures are listed in Table 22-8. To date, Y-disconnect systems have provided lower infection rates than other CAPD delivery systems. Piraino, Bernardini, and Sorkin (1988) paired 37 patients using a standard spike system with 37 patients using a disconnect system, matching the groups for sex, age, insulin dependent diabetes, and time of PD. They found a significantly lower infection rate with the bagless disconnect system, reporting not only fewer episodes of peritonitis but fewer catheter exit site infections. The decrease in peritonitis was attributed to the flush before fill technique, while the decreased exit site and catheter infection rates were considered related to the decrease in trauma to the catheter exit site by the bagless system. In 1992, Port, Held, Nolph, Turenne, and Wolfe analyzed data collected by the United States Renal Data System (USRDS), which validated these findings. USRDS data were analyzed for time to first peritonitis episode by connection technique on virtually all patients started on CAPD between January 1 and June 30, 1989. Regarding time to first episode of peritonitis, 1,133 using a standard connection manual system (spike) averaged 9 months until the first episode of peritonitis, 916 UV system patients averaged 13.4 months, and 1,067 patients using the Y-disconnect system averaged 15 months.

Benefits of a bagless CAPD system include clinically significant reductions in infection rates and quality of life improvements associated with eliminating the need to wear a bag between exchanges. These systems also involve an increase cost, since the tubing and empty dialysis bag are discarded after each exchange, not reused for dialysate outflow as with manual systems where the bag remains attached until the drain phase.

Cyclers, like disconnect systems, allow the patient to be free from a bag. Advantages to NIPD include a daytime free from the need to perform dialysis exchanges, which may facilitate the individual's employment or activities outside the home. Since dialysis solution is infused with the patient supine, intra-abdominal pressure is minimized; this may benefit patients with existing hernias or a high risk for hernias or leaks. Disadvantages include the need to have dialysis machinery in the home and the additional equipment when traveling, although newer models of cyclers are increasingly portable. (It may be prudent to teach patients who use cyclers to perform CAPD for use during travel or in the event of a power loss.) Often, the patient is required to have 10 hours or more of dialysis, and being connected to the cycler for this length of time may interfere with other activities. Some cycler systems allow the patient to connect to the machine, infuse the initial exchange, disconnect for a period of a few hours, then reconnect to the cycler for the remainder of the exchanges prescribed, thereby enhancing patient freedom and satisfaction. Cyclers have built in alarms to safeguard the patient from incomplete filling, which would result in underdialysis, or overfilling, which would result in increased abdominal pressure and patient discomfort. These alarms may interfere with the patient's sleep patterns, especially until he or she learns to avoid practices that may contribute to alarm conditions. The patient needs to know how to correct these alarm conditions, when to report problems, and to whom to report problems or turn to for assistance.

Patient Selection for Peritoneal Dialysis

When a patient reaches chronic renal failure and a renal replacement therapy is required to sustain life, a number of factors may influence the choice of treatment modality. These include clinical and functional factors, cost considerations, and lifestyle or patient preference. As managed care systems continue to grow, all of these factors must be considered as well as the relationship between the choice of alternative dialysis prescriptions and outcomes. Although little research data has been published on this topic, a study called CHOICE (Choices for Health Outcomes in Caring for ESRD) is currently underway to (a) explore factors influencing the choice of particular dialysis prescription, (b) assess patient outcomes and costs of alternative dialysis prescriptions in the United States, and (c) formulate optimal dialysis strategies that consider the perspectives of patients, providers, and payers (Powe et al., 1996). Not surprisingly, physician and other health care providers' bias has been postulated as influencing current practice patterns. Results from the CHOICE study, projected to conclude June 30, 1999, should provide helpful information to guide practice in the future.

Peritoneal Dialysis as the Preferred Option

PD is a treatment option for most ESRD patients, and is the preferred treatment for certain patients. Individuals with poor vasculature, in whom hemodialysis access may be difficult or impossible to place and maintain, may be managed on peritoneal dialysis. Patients with severe heart disease, such as congestive heart failure or cardiomyopathy, may benefit from the continuous nature of peritoneal dialysis. Alpert, Huting, Twardowski, Khanna, and Nolph (1995) reviewed 46 studies relating to CAPD and the heart, and concluded that CAPD can decrease left ventricular volume, improve left ventricular function in some patients, and produce symptomatic improvement in patients with refractory congestive heart failure. The intermittent hemodialysis schedule results in the accumulation of fluid and toxins for 2–3 days between treatments and more rapid shifts of fluids and solutes during the dialysis treatment itself. This may make it difficult for many patients with severe heart disease to tolerate HD. PD allows for continuous removal of fluid and toxins, and may be better tolerated. "Failure to thrive" on HD is another potential indication for PD; if a kidney transplant is not suitable or not available, PD offers another possibility for a positive outcome.

Peritoneal Dialysis Absolute Contraindications

PD may not be a treatment option for certain individuals due to medical contraindications. Individuals with a history of multiple abdominal surgeries may have adhesions and scarring resulting in inadequate functional peritoneal membrane surface area. This can result in inadequate solute removal with limited clearance capacity, and may preclude the provision of adequate dialysis via PD. Even patients who have been maintained on PD for a period of time may have changes in the peritoneal membrane, resulting in a peritoneal space that becomes loculated into small pockets instead of being continuous and allowing dialysis solution to infuse and drain freely. These anatomical changes interfere with the movement of dialysis solution into and out of the cavity, making PD therapy incapable of providing adequate clearances, or, in some cases, interfering with the mechanical function of the peritoneal catheter because multiple adhesions or scar tissue prevent the flow of dialysis solution into and out of the peritoneal cavity (Zawada, 1994).

Hypercatabolic or extremely large patients may require more clearance than can be achieved with PD. Since the membrane characteristics are predetermined for each individual, some patients with large clearance requirements may be unable to achieve adequate dialysis despite manipulation of other elements of the PD prescription (volume of dialysis solution, number of exchanges, timing of exchanges). In this case, transplant or HD are the treatments of choice. Occasionally, a combination of peritoneal and HD is attempted, but reimbursement and lifestyle considerations make this an uncommon choice.

Rarely, an individual may have a patent opening between pleural and peritoneal cavities that allows dialysis solution to flow from the peritoneal space into the pleural space; this rules out PD as a treatment option as long as the passage remains patent. It may be desirable to intervene and correct this anatomical defect, allowing PD therapy following closure of the peritoneal-pleural opening.

Peritoneal Dialysis Relative Contraindications

Several conditions may be considered relative contraindications for PD; in these cases, the risks and benefits of peritoneal dialysis must be carefully considered. A decision is made on an individual basis, weighing clinical outcomes, quality of life issues, patient preference, and cost considerations. Morbid obesity raises questions of whether PD is the optimal renal replacement therapy, since dextrose absorption and associated caloric intake from the dialysis solution may worsen the obesity and may begin a vicious cycle of weight gain, increased mass, and increased requirement for dialysis solution, resulting in yet greater glucose absorption.

The volume of dialysis solution in the abdomen adds weight, changes body alignment, and increases intra-abdominal pressure. Chronic back pain can be exacerbated by carrying 2 L or more of dialysis solution in the peritoneal space, especially with continuous therapies when the dialysis solution is in the peritoneal cavity while the patient is active. In some situations, an intermittent form of PD may allow the patient to have dialysis solution dwelling only at night while supine, thus avoiding additional back strain. Patients with abdominal hernias that have not been surgically repaired may be poor candidates for PD; the dialysis solution creates increased intra-abdominal pressure, increasing the risk that an unrepaired hernia could protrude or even strangulate. In most cases, surgical repair of the hernia allows PD to be a viable treatment option. However, because hernias may recur, these patients must be closely monitored for signs or symptoms of recurrent hernia.

Table 22–9
Factors affecting modality selection.

Clinical
- Body surface area/obesity
- Co-morbid conditions (vascular, cardiac, pulmonary)
- Residual renal function
- Membrane characteristics and functional surface area

Functional
- Tolerance to increased intra-abdominal pressure
- Family and social support

Cost

Patient Preference
- Lifestyle considerations
- History of compliance

Diverticular disease may create problems with infectious complications. Thin-walled intestinal diverticula may allow fecal matter to penetrate into the surrounding tissue. This fecal material is rich with bacteria; if this fecal material should leak into the peritoneal cavity in the presence of the glucose containing dialysis solution, peritonitis is a near certainty. Peritonitis of this etiology is characterized by high cell counts and multiple organisms, generally gram negative bacteria that are intestinal flora (see Peritonitis). Nursing considerations include close monitoring of these patients, follow-up of hazy effluent, tracking for repeated episodes of peritonitis, close attention to the causative organisms, and monitoring closely for enteric organisms. Repeated peritonitis in patients with a history of diverticular disease may be cause to recommend a change in dialysis modality to HD. Recent abdominal surgery with drains remaining in the abdomen or with recent bowel anastamosis is another relative contraindication to PD, for similar reasons.

Some dialysis centers consider the presence of an intra-abdominal vascular graft a contraindication for PD. The increased risk of an abdominal infection associated with PD is thought to predispose these patients to infection of the intra-abdominal vascular graft (Zawada, 1994).

Chronic obstructive pulmonary disease is

another relative contraindication for PD since the increased intra-abdominal pressure created by the dialysis solution exerts pressure on the diaphragm. In cases of severe pulmonary disease, the limitations of diaphragmatic excursion caused by the pressure from the dialysis solution may exacerbate the disease. Table 22-9 summarizes the factors affecting modality selection.

Access

Access to the peritoneal cavity is required for any type of PD. "A successful peritoneal access device must transfer large volumes of dialysate into and out of the peritoneal cavity in a minimal amount of time, while maintaining normal anatomy, histology, bacteriology, and physiology of the surrounding tissues" (Ash, Carr, & Diaz-Buxo, 1995, p. 295). Peritoneal catheters provide a route for dialysis solution to pass from outside the body into the peritoneal cavity, enabling acute or chronic PD. Catheter types and insertion methods may vary depending on the urgency associated with initiation of PD therapy and the anticipated duration of that therapy.

Acute Catheters

Acute peritoneal catheters are generally straight and relatively rigid. They are inserted using either a metal stylet or over a guidewire. These semirigid catheters may be made of nylon or polyethylene; many have catheter wings sutured to the skin surface to secure the catheter in position (Ash, 1993). Acute peritoneal catheters can be inserted at the bedside, used immediately, and removed at the bedside. Although this is an advantage for patients needing PD urgently, a number of potential complications are associated with the use of acute catheters. Placement complications include preperitoneal placement, bowel or bladder perforation, and rupture of a major vessel. Preperitoneal placement, where the catheter fails to enter the peritoneal space, results in slow dialysis solution inflow, pain with inflow, and sometimes localized swelling. Preperitoneal placement is treated by removal of the catheter and re-insertion elsewhere in the abdomen. Perforation of abdominal organs or major vessels is extremely rare, but may require surgical intervention. Bowel perforation presents with feces or gas in the effluent or watery diarrhea; bladder perforation presents with polyuria and glycosuria. Treatment may require surgical repair, but in some cases it is possible to remove the catheter and observe the patient while administering antibiotics (Ash & Daugirdas, 1994). Perforation of a major abdominal vessel results in grossly bloody effluent, fall in hematocrit, and signs of shock. This requires emergency surgical intervention.

Since acute catheters have no barriers to prevent bacteria from migrating into the peritoneal cavity, the risk of infection is great. Fluid may leak along the catheter tract, further increasing the infection risk, as the dextrose rich dialysis solution provides an excellent growth medium for bacteria. Limiting the time the catheter is left in place helps lessen the infection risk; acute catheters should be left in no longer than three days (Ash, 1993). Since acute renal failure usually requires dialytic therapy for longer than 3 days, catheters designed for chronic use are often used even for treatment of acute renal failure.

Prior to placement of an acute PD catheter, nursing management includes assessment of the patient for a history of abdominal operations or trauma, and noting abdominal scars, ostomy stomas, or any other physical findings significant to catheter placement. Findings should be discussed with the healthcare professional who will be placing the acute PD catheter. Patient education should include an explanation of the need for PD, the rational for catheter placement, and what to expect during the catheter placement procedure. Additionally, nursing care includes placing an absorbent, sterile, non-occlusive dressing over the catheter exit site, immobilizing the PD catheter, and vigilant monitoring for early signs or symptoms of infection. In general, dressings should be left intact and reinforced to minimize contamination and manipulation of the catheter.

Chronic Catheters

Catheters designed for chronic use are made of soft, flexible materials such as silicone rubber or polyurethane, and consist of three segments: the intraperitoneal, subcutaneous, and external segments. The intraperitoneal segment contains numerous side holes and an open tip for fluid flow. It generally is 11-15 cm in length, although various lengths of catheters are available for use for patients from neonates to large adults. Outside the peritoneal cavity, the subcutaneous segment of the catheter tunnels through the muscle and subcutaneous fatty tissue to a stab wound opening called the exit site. This subcutaneous segment is usually 5–7 cm in length, and may be either straight or arcuate (curved in the shape of an arch). The external segment extends from the opening in the skin or exit site, with the external end of the catheter attached to a connector or adapter made of titanium metal or plastic polymers. The adapter allows the catheter to be attached to a tubing called a transfer set, which connects to one of several available PD delivery systems.

Chronic PD catheters may have one or two extraperitoneal cuffs made of Dacron® polyester or velour. When present, these cuffs serve to secure the catheter in position, present a barrier to movement of micro-organisms into the peritoneal cavity, and help prevent the leaking of fluid out of the peritoneal space. A double cuff catheter has the deep or inner cuff positioned near the peritoneal membrane in the abdominal musculature to facilitate rapid tis-

Figure 22-7
Chronic peritoneal dialysis catheters.

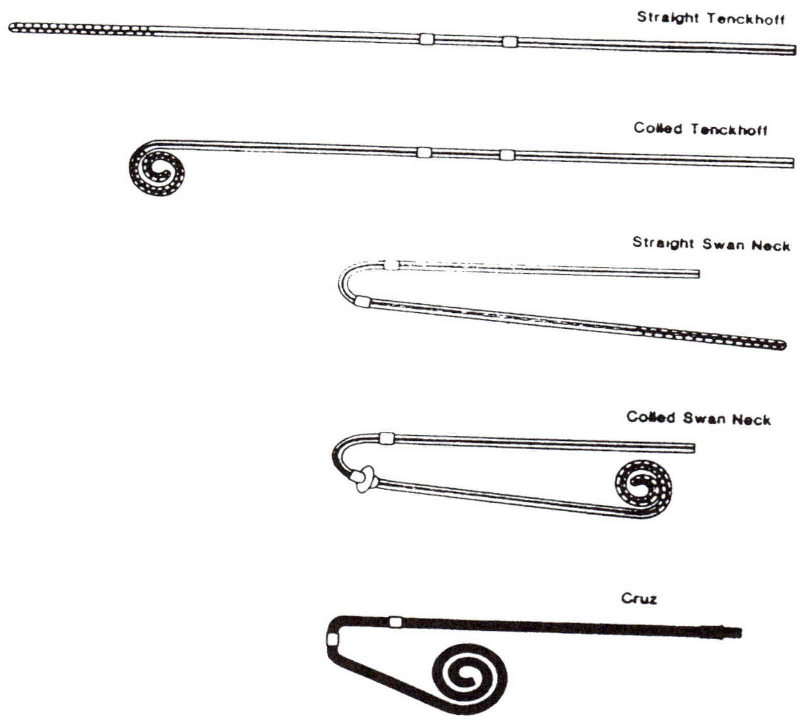

From top: double-cuff Tenckhoff with straight intraperitoneal segment; double-cuff Tenckhoff with coiled intraperitoneal segment; double-cuff Swan Neck with straight intraperitoneal segment; Swan Neck Missouri catheter with flange and bead at preperitoneal cuff, and coiled intraperitoneal segment; Cruz catheter with coiled intraperitoneal segment.

Note: From Prowant, B.F., & Gallagher, N.M. (1995). Peritoneal dialysis. In L. Lancaster (Ed.), *Core curriculum for nephrology nursing* (3rd edition) (p. 291). Pitman, NJ: American Nephrology Nurses' Association. Reprinted with permission.

sue ingrowth, and the outer cuff buried in the subcutaneous tissue approximately 2 cm below the skin exit site (Ash, 1993). Upon placement of the PD catheter, a local inflammatory response to the cuff material results in a fibrous plug being formed; this serves to hold the catheter in position, helps prevent fluid from leaking out along the sinus tract beside the catheter, and provides a barrier to bacterial migration along the catheter tract or tunnel (Ash). Single cuff catheters may have either the deep or the subcutaneous cuff. A retrospective analysis of catheter type and survival demonstrated that catheters with a single deep cuff had a shorter survival than catheters with a single subcutaneous cuff or double cuff catheters (Linblad, Hamilton, Nolph, & Novak, 1988).

The tip of the intraperitoneal segment of the catheter should be in the lower quadrant of the abdomen between the visceral and parietal layers of the peritoneum. There is less omentum in the lower abdominal quadrants, and outflow is generally improved with this placement. Presumably, the effects of gravity on the fluid in the peritoneal space draw the fluid toward the pelvis, where the catheter tip is located. Catheters are made with a radiopaque stripe to allow visualization of the intraperitoneal segment via abdominal x-ray. Catheter migration out of the lower abdomen may occur and is associated with an increased incidence of fluid outflow problems. To minimize this risk, catheters such as the Toronto-Western have discs in the intraperitoneal segment to help secure them in position. The Toronto-Western catheter also has a disc-ball shape at the pre-peritoneal cuff to allow fixing the catheter relative to the parietal peritoneum. Placement with the catheter tip toward the left lower quadrant is preferred; a right lower quadrant position may predispose to upward migration of the catheter, thought to be associated with the upward peristalsis of the ascending segment of the large bowel. The intraperitoneal segment of the catheter may be straight, coiled, or a column-disc design (see Figure 22-7).

The shape of the catheter within the tunnel can be either straight or arcuate (an inverted V). The Missouri catheter developed by Twardowski has an arcuate or swan neck-shaped catheter tunnel segment to enable the intraperitoneal segment of the catheter to be directed downward, while also maintaining a downward external tunnel direction. This is thought to decrease the risk of exit site infection (ESI) (Twardowski, Prowant, Nichols, Nolph, & Khanna, 1992).

In a meta-analysis of studies of chronic PD catheter complications by Ash et al. (1995), conclusions drawn indicate little difference in the infection rates (peritonitis and catheter) between single and double cuff catheters, although double cuff catheter infections were *slightly* lower. Over 50% of double cuff Tenckhoff catheters develop complications within 12 months (unchanged over the past 10 years), and catheters with a shape that fixes the cuff relative to the parietal peritoneum (column-disc, Toronto-Western disc-ball, and Missouri catheters) have fewer exit site infections presumably related to preventing extrusion of the external catheter cuff.

Insertion methods. Peritoneal catheters can be inserted by a surgical procedure, via peritoneoscope, or via a blind percutaneous insertion technique. Surgical placement of chronic peritoneal catheters remains the most common method used. This method allows visualization of the tissues through which the catheter will pass, and is the only insertion method that can be used with the column-disc catheter. The catheter is inserted through the subcutaneous tissue, the rectus sheath, and the anterior fascia and parietal peritoneum, with bleeding controlled with electrocautery. Care is taken to avoid injury to the bowel or other visceral organs. An air space (pneumoperitoneum) may be created between the parietal and visceral peritoneum, and the catheter carefully advanced toward the pelvis. A purse-string suture is used to secure the catheter at the level of the posterior rectus fascia. This procedure is usually done under local anesthesia in combination with some sedation, allowing the patient to confirm the position of the catheter tip by telling the surgeon where pressure is felt as the catheter tip is advanced. If pressure is felt near the bladder, the catheter may be too far anterior, and may be repositioned at that time by the surgeon. Inflow and outflow of fluid through the PD catheter should be checked while in the operating room, allowing quick correction of problems with flow that are immediately apparent (J. Gibson, personal communication, May 30, 1996).

In traditional surgical procedures, the external segment of the PD catheter is brought through the skin as part of the surgical placement procedure. Moncrief et al. (1993) advocate an alternate approach, the Moncrief-Popovich catheter access technique, where the external segment is buried in the subcutaneous tissue for approximately 6 weeks, and is then exteriorized in a separate procedure. This minimizes the risk of transfer of bacteria from external areas into the peritoneal cavity by allowing adequate time for healing and tissue ingrowth in the cuffs prior to having the catheter exteriorized, thus eliminating a potential passageway for bacterial invasion and decreasing the incidence of peritonitis. In a 2-year prospective randomized trial involving 59 patients, Park et al. (1995) found this technique resulted in a decreased incidence of peritonitis irrespective of the PD fluid delivery system used. The average peritonitis free interval was 14.8 months versus 8.8 months between the two groups.

Placement of the peritoneal catheter via trocar is still used in some centers. A 2–3 cm skin incision is made over the deep cuff site, a needle is inserted, and fluid is instilled. During this procedure, the patient is asked to contract the abdominal wall. The trocar, with an internal stylet in place, is inserted; passage through the abdominal wall and peritoneal membrane are determined by a pop that is felt as the trocar is advanced. When the stylet is removed, dialysate should drain indicating proper positioning of the trocar in the peritoneal space. The peritoneal catheter is then advanced through the trocar, and a suture may be placed around the deep cuff. The subcutaneous tunnel is created by using the trocar, inserting it into the skin (after making a small incision) at the location of the exit site and tunneling toward the primary incision. The catheter is then pulled back through this newly created subcutaneous tunnel to the exit site.

In a similar procedure, the peritoneal catheter may be inserted by use of a needle followed by a guidewire, much like insertion of central venous catheters. The exit site and tunnel are created as in surgical implantation (Ash et al., 1995).

An alternative to blind percutaneous techniques or surgical placement is peritoneoscopic placement. The peritoneoscope provides visualization of the anatomical landmarks to facilitate proper catheter positioning and minimizes the risks associated with blind placement.

Catheter care. Infection is one of the potential complications of peritoneal catheters, regardless of insertion method. Infection can occur within the peritoneal cavity (peritonitis), along the subcutaneous tract (tunnel infection), or at the skin exit site (exit site infection). To minimize this risk, prophylactic pre-operative broad spectrum antibiotics are recommended. Because antibiotic penetration into the coagulum is poor, it is important to administer antibiotics prior to a catheter insertion procedure to ensure adequate antibiotic concentrations in the blood and tissue fluids before the coagulum forms (Prowant & Twardowski, 1996).

Nursing management prior to catheter insertion includes assessment of the patient history and abdomen (as discussed for acute catheter placement), administration of pre-operative antibiotics, skin preparation, and patient education. The essential elements of the catheter insertion procedure should be explained to the patient to encourage participation and cooperation and to facilitate proper catheter insertion. Prior to the procedure, the patient's bladder should be emptied to minimize the risk of bladder perforation, and constipation should be resolved to decrease the risk of bowel perforation. The skin exit site should be marked prior to the catheter placement procedure whenever possible. The exit site should be positioned in a place where it can be readily visualized for routine care, avoiding the belt line, skin folds, and the diaper area for ostomy appliances, if applicable. Clear visualization facilitates early recognition of any signs or symptoms of inflammation or infection. Avoiding skin folds helps ensure that the exit site remains clean and dry without harboring moisture that might predispose to bacterial colonization or infection. Avoiding the beltline minimizes traumas, one of the key contributors to exit site infection, and avoiding the diaper area for stoma appliances helps diminish the risk of cross-contamination. Proper placement of the catheter exit site decreases the risk of exit site infection.

Nursing considerations during the immediate post-placement period depend, in part, on the insertion method used. Surgical placement minimizes the risk of bleeding or perforation of abdominal organs, although there have been reported instances of bladder or bowel perforation even with open surgical procedures. Catheter inflow and outflow should be brisk. The patient will be recovering from whatever anesthesia was required for the surgery; therefore, routine post-anesthesia monitoring is indicated. The relatively large incision through the peritoneal membrane, compared to other techniques, predisposes to fluid leaks if the catheter is used for dialysis in the early post-operative period. To avoid leaks, it is preferable to wait 7–14 days before using the catheter for CAPD; however, if peritoneal dialysis *must* be initiated sooner, the patient should be supine whenever there is dialysis solution dwelling, and small volume exchanges should be used to minimize intra-abdominal pressure that could contribute to leaks. Post-operative turning and deep breathing are acceptable, but coughing should be avoided due to the associated increase in intra-abdominal pressure and increased risk of leaks (Twardowski et al., 1986).

Blind percutaneous techniques minimize the size of the opening in the peritoneal membrane, thus decreasing the risk of fluid leaks. Because the technique can be performed at the bedside (often by the nephrologist) using local anesthesia, little or no anesthesia recovery is required. Since bedside percutaneous procedures are done "blindly," there is an increased risk of intra-abdominal organ perforation, bleeding, or malpositioning of the catheter. Problems with catheter placement can often be identified by the patient's signs and symptoms. For example, pain during inflow of dialysis solution may indicate preperitoneal placement; poor outflow may indicate catheter kinks, malposition, or other forms of obstruction, such as omental wrap; cloudy or foul-smelling drainage may indicate bowel perforation; sudden or significant increase in volume of voidings may indicate bladder perforation; and persistently bloody outflow may indicate hemorrhage. Any of these signs or symptoms require intervention, and may require catheter removal or surgical exploration to correct the problem. (See Noninfectious Complications). Vigilant nursing monitoring of the patient following catheter placement is essential in identifying potential problems early, thus facilitating early intervention to correct problems and proceed with dialysis therapy.

Peritoneoscopic placement combines many advantages of surgical and "blind" placement techniques. It allows visualization as with surgical placement and creates a small peritoneal opening, minimizing leaks. The chief disadvantages are the initial cost of the equipment and the need for training in peritoneoscopy for the operator (nephrologist or surgeon). This type of catheter placement is increasingly popular (Ash & Daugirdas, 1994) and has the lowest incidence of complications of all insertion methods (Ash et al., 1995). Nursing care includes assessment for complications as previously mentioned, noting avoidance of coughing, monitoring for leaks, and assessing for signs or symptoms of infection.

A variety of catheter break-in protocols are used, with the key elements establishing and maintaining catheter patency, minimizing intra-abdominal pressure, and maintaining the sterility of the system. Catheter patency is established by infusion of sterile normal saline or dialysis solution, generally with added heparin. Patency is maintained by either the initiation of regular dialysis exchanges or by intermittent "flushing" of the catheter with sterile normal saline or dialysis solution, again with added heparin. Low intra-abdominal pressure is maintained by using low inflow volumes, minimizing coughing, and keeping the patient supine while fluid is dwelling. Nursing care must ensure sterility of the system during all required procedures. Careful monitoring of the spent dialysate and the

Table 22–10
Principles of exit-site care post–catheter implantation.

- Restrict care to experienced PD staff or trained patients.
- Use aseptic technique: both mask and gloves.
- Avoid irritating or toxic solutions for cleansing.
- If povidone iodine and hydrogen peroxide are used, limit to the skin surrounding the exit and keep out of the sinus or wound.
- Use absorbent dressings.
- Immobilize the catheter.
- Keep exit as dry as possible.
- Do not submerge exit until completely healed.
- Culture exit and monitor frequently if healing does not progress.
- Continue sterile dressings until exit is healed.

Note: From Prowant, B.F., & Twardowski, Z.J. (1996). Recommendations for exit care. *Peritoneal Dialysis International, 16* (suppl. 3), S94-S99. Reprinted with permission.

catheter exit site for signs or symptoms of infection is an ongoing nursing assessment.

Immediately following catheter placement, or following catheter exteriorization in the case of a catheter left buried for several weeks, a sterile dressing is applied over the catheter exit site. Tissue reaction to the catheter is characterized by scab formation, granulation tissue, and then epithelialization of the sinus tract. Current recommendations for nursing management to promote healing include securing the catheter, applying a sterile dressing, and leaving this dressing in place for approximately 1 week (Prowant & Twardowski, 1996).

The dressing must be changed if it becomes wet, but it is preferable to leave the catheter immobile and undisturbed during the initial healing. Care should be taken to instruct the patient to keep the dressing clean and dry. Initial dressing changes should be done by professional nurses familiar with PD.

Twardowski and Prowant (1996b) analyzed the characteristics and outcomes of 43 PD catheter exit sites to determine the length of time until the catheter healing is complete, including firm tissue ingrowth into the cuff(s) and epidermal growth into the sinus tract. Scabs are visible in nearly all cases during the first week after catheter implantation, diminish by week 3, and are gone by week 4. Exit color is described as pink or pale pink throughout the 6-week period. Epithelialization of the sinus tract begins in week 2 or 3, but covers only half the visible sinus tract by week 5 even in the optimally or fast healing exits. As a result, some dialysis units continue sterile dressing changes by PD nursing staff once or twice weekly during this healing process, or at least until the sutures are removed at the incision. If this is impossible, a prudent recommendation for routine care during the healing period would be to maintain the integrity of the sterile dressing as long as possible (up to 1 week), avoid showering or other exposure to water at the catheter exit site, cleanse the catheter exit site gently and carefully, and minimize manipulation of the catheter until the initial 6-week period has passed. Sutures at the exit site are not recommended; they serve no purpose, tend to promote infection, and have the added risk of a nick in the peritoneal catheter during the suture removal process (Albee, 1995). Factors that promote healing include proper positioning of the external cuff, approximately 1 cm - 2 cm from the skin (2 cm - 3 cm in obese individuals); securing the external segment of the catheter to avoid tension on the cuff; directing the tunnel segment either laterally or downward; and peri-procedural administrating systemic antibiotics (Albee). Generally accepted principles for nursing care of the exit site immediately postinsertion are listed in Table 22-10 (Prowant & Twardowski, 1996).

Once healed, frequent catheter exit site care is recommended, usually in conjunction with showering or bathing, daily or three to four times weekly. For patients who prefer a tub bath, it is preferable not to submerge the catheter exit site in the bath water; this water is filled with many skin bacteria that might adversely affect the exit site. The site should be examined closely on a regular basis, preferably daily. A well-healed exit site is clean, free of debris and signs of inflammation, with skin color either normal or slightly darker than that of the surrounding skin. Redness, tenderness, bleeding, drainage, or breaks in the skin should be treated promptly (see Exit Site Infections). After a thorough inspection, the exit site should be cleansed. Prowant et al. (1988) found use of antibacterial soap and water more effective for routine cleansing of the site than either a sterile dressing or a povidone-iodine paint; Luzar et al. (1990) found povidine-iodine more effective in preventing infection. Differences in study design of note included the type of soap used for the soap and water methods (Prowant et al. used antibacterial soap, although Luzar et al. by design excluded disinfectant soaps), and while Luzar et al. discouraged "prolonged tub bathing," submerging the catheter exit site in water was not forbidden as was the case in the Prowant et al. study. Doyle (1996) conducted a 6-year retrospective study to determine the incidence of exit site infection and found a higher exit site infection rate with the use of hydrogen peroxide and povidone-iodine. She advocates the use of soap and water for well-healed exit sites and a non-ionic wound cleanser for new sites. Additional nursing research to validate or repudiate these findings would provide clearer direction for PD patients and professionals. Swimming, using hot tubs, and other activities involving submerging the exit site are generally discouraged. If individuals engage in such activities, it should be recommended that the exit site be protected with an occlusive film dressing or ostomy device, and the site cleansed as soon as possible after the activity. The external segment of the catheter should be secured in such a way as to avoid tension or trauma to the exit site that might result in a break in the skin; tape or catheter securing devices may be used for this purpose.

Goals of routine care are to keep the catheter exit site clean, to maintain intact tissue at the site to minimize risk of bacterial invasion, and to closely observe the site to facilitate early detection and treatment of any problems. Principles of care for the healed catheter exit site are summarized in Table 22-11 (Prowant & Twardowski, 1996).

Some protocols include the use of an antistaphylococcal ointment on the skin surrounding the exit site. More nursing research is needed to evaluate exit site care procedures for efficacy and patient compliance considerations as well as the impact of such protocols on exit site infection rates and causative organisms.

Peritoneal Dialysis Prescription

The PD prescription consists of several elements, and is tailored to meet the needs of each individual patient for both clearance and fluid removal (see Table 22-12). Elements include the composition of the dialysis solution, the number and volume of exchanges, the system used to deliver the exchanges (manual or automated), and the timing of the exchanges. Peritoneal membrane characteristics must also be considered, but cannot be prescribed (see Description of the Peritoneal Dialysis Process). Because the other elements of the PD prescription must be adjusted based on the membrane characteristics, it is logical to determine these characteristics as soon as possible and tailor the PD prescription around them.

Evaluation of Peritoneal Membrane Characteristics

The peritoneal membrane for each individual has unique permeability characteristics. As Ronco, Conz, Bosch, Lew, and La Greca (1994) note, one of the most critical factors in overall efficiency of the dialysis system in PD is membrane permeability. Because there are fewer variables of the dialysis prescription that can be manipulated in PD compared to HD, determining these permeability characteristics is essential.

Peritoneal Equilibration Test (PET).

Table 22-11
Principles of care for the healed catheter exit site.

- Cleanse daily, every other day, or at least 2–3 times/week.
- Cleanse any time the exit is wet or dirty.
- Wash hands well prior to exit care.
- Inspect the exit and tunnel.
- Use a cleansing agent with antibacterial properties; liquid soap is preferred.
- Do not forcibly remove crust, scab, or cuticle.
- Gently dry the exit.
- Anchor the catheter.

Note: From Prowant, B.F., & Twardowski, Z.J. (1996). Recommendations for exit care. *Peritoneal Dialysis International, 16* (suppl. 3), S94-S99. Reprinted with permission.

Table 22-12
Elements of the PD prescription.

- Composition of PD solution
- Number of exchanges
- Volume of exchanges
- Timing of exchanges
- Delivery system
- Peritoneal membrane permeability*

* Must be considered, but cannot be prescribed

Table 22-13
D/P and D/Do ratios.

Dialysate to Plasma (D/P) Ratios — Dialysate concentration of solute divided by plasma concentration

Dialysate to Initial Dextrose (D/Do) Ratios — Dialysate dextrose concentration divided by initial dextrose concentration of dialysis solution

Standard Peritoneal Equilibration Test Sample Times	
0 Dwell	Dialysate
2 Hour Dwell	Dialysate and Serum
4 Hour Dwell	Dialysate

Table 22–14
Implications of peritoneal membrane characteristics.

Permeability	Solute Clearance	Ultrafiltration
Low	Poor	Excellent
Low average	Fair	Good
High average	Good	Fair
High	Excellent	Poor

Twardowski et al. (1987) developed the peritoneal equilibration test (PET), a standardized test to determine these membrane characteristics. In brief, a standard PET consists of draining the peritoneal cavity after an overnight dwell, infusing 2 L of 2.5% dextrose dialysis solution, and allowing this to dwell for 4 hours. Samples of dialysate are obtained at 0 hours (immediately after infusing the fresh solution), 2 hours, and 4 hours; a blood sample is obtained at 2 hours; and the volume of spent dialysate drained after the 4 hour dwell is measured (Schmidt & Prowant, 1991). Dialysate to plasma (D/P) ratios are determined for urea and creatinine for each of the sample times. Likewise, dextrose concentration at the time of each sample collection is divided by the initial dialysate dextrose concentration to determine a D/Do ratio (see Table 22-13). D/P ratios indicate the rate of diffusion for the solute measured, typically urea and creatinine, while D/Do ratios indicate the rate of dextrose absorption. Together, these data are compared to standard curves of membrane permeability, determined by averaging results from over 100 patients (Twardowski et al., 1987). The peritoneal membrane is then classified in one of four categories of permeability: low, low average, high average, or high. The degree of permeability correlates with the ability of the patient's membrane to transport solutes; highly permeable membranes allow solutes to diffuse readily, while low permeability characteristics are associated with slow diffusion. Dextrose absorption reflects the ability of the membrane to maintain an osmotic pressure gradient, thus enabling ultrafiltration of water. Low membrane permeability maintains the osmotic gradient for a relatively long time, resulting in the achievement of large ultrafiltration volumes; high membrane permeability implies rapid dextrose absorption and smaller drain volumes (Prowant & Schmidt, 1991). General implications of the membrane permeability characteristics are summarized in Table 22-14.

A disadvantage of a standard PET is the time required to collect samples. Patients must come to the clinic prior to doing their first exchange in the morning, and must remain at or near the clinic for the entire test, over 4 hours. To address these concerns, an alternative to the standard PET, the "Fast" PET, was developed (Twardowski, 1990). For this test, the patient is instructed to drain the peritoneal cavity at home, infuse 2 L of 2.5% dextrose dialysis solution, and then come to the health care facility. There, the dialysate is drained at the end of the 4-hour dwell, blood is drawn, and the same D/P and D/Do ratios are calculated for the 4-hour sample. The advantages of the "Fast" PET are patient convenience, minimal staff time, and ease of performance for both the patient and the dialysis staff. A disadvantage is limited data, which increases the risk of inaccurate assessment of the peritoneal membrane permeability. Because there is only one value, collection and laboratory errors cannot be readily determined. In a standard PET, several values should trend similarly to the standard PET curves. (see Figure 22-8).

Peritoneal function test (PFT). Yet another method for determining membrane permeability characteristics is the peritoneal function test (PFT) developed by Gotch and Keen (1995). In this test, samples from each exchange done during the test day are collected (usually by the patient at home), noting the time, total drain volume, and dextrose concentration of each exchange. If the patient produces 100 ml or more of urine output, a 20 - 30-hour urine collection is also required. A serum sample is collected from the patient when the samples are brought to the dialysis facility, and the exchange infused that morning is drained for a sample. From this data, a number of indices can be calculated, including peritoneal and renal clearances of urea and creatinine, protein losses and requirements, and estimated glucose absorption. Peritoneal membrane permeability characteristics are determined. Advantages of the PFT include ease of completion for dialysis staff and patients; because the test is done primarily by the patient at home, an extended (several hour) stay at the dialysis facility is unnecessary. Disadvantages are the potential for error due to inaccurate specimen collection or measurement and recording of drain volumes by patients.

Application of Membrane Classification to the Dialysis Prescription

Specific forms of PD should be matched to peritoneal membrane characteristics to optimize the dialysis prescription. For example, patients with high permeability are excellent candidates for NIPD: the short nighttime cycles match the rapid diffusion expected with this membrane to provide good clearances, plus eliminating the long daytime exchange minimizes the chance of fluid absorption with little decrease in clearance. Conversely, a patient with low transport characteristics requires a longer dwell time to allow time for diffusion of

Figure 22-8
Peritoneal equilibration test curves.

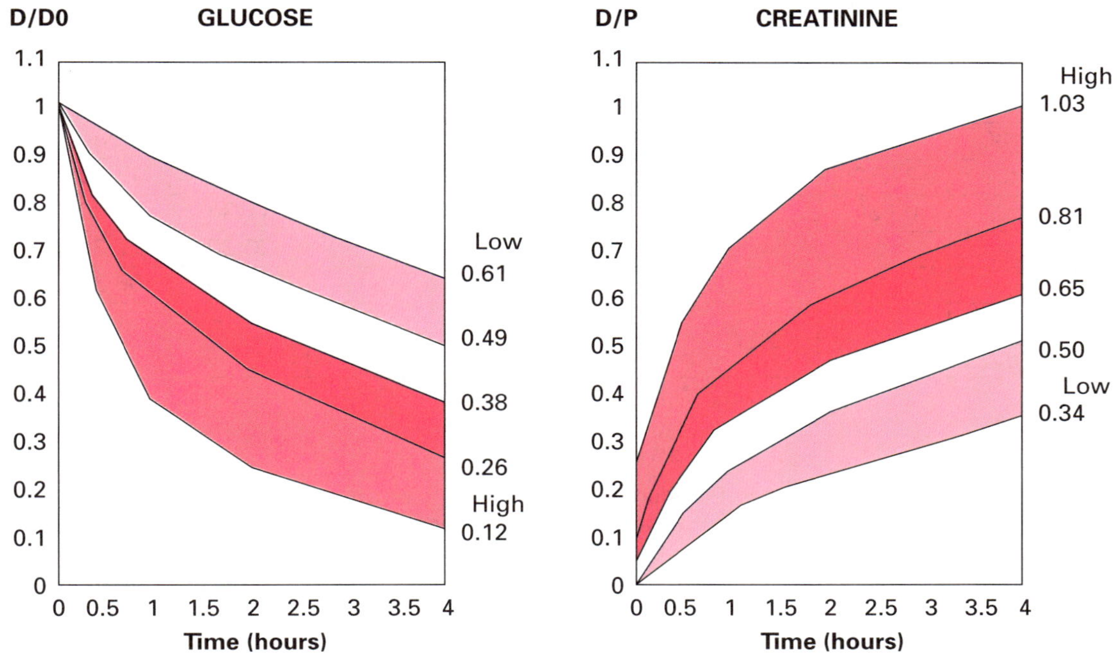

Peritoneal equilibration test curves for corrected creatinine dialysate to plasma (D/P) ratios (right figure) and dialysate glucose to dialysis solution glucose ratios at time 0 (D/DO) (left figure); determined from 103 equilibration studies in 86 patients.

Note: From Prowant, B.F., & Schmidt, L.M. (1991). The peritoneal equilibration test: A nursing discussion. *ANNA Journal, 18,* 361-366. Used with permission.

solutes, but fluid ultrafiltration occurs readily. Thus, patients with low average transport characteristics are generally good candidates for CAPD, provided the total clearance achieved is adequate. Patients with very low transport characteristics may be unable to achieve adequate dialysis and may not be suitable candidates for PD; it may be impossible to provide enough volume of dialysis solution to compensate for the slow diffusive transport of solutes (see Adequacy of Peritoneal Dialysis). Individuals in the high average and low average categories generally can be managed on either CAPD or APD. The dialysis prescription is adjusted to meet both clinical and lifestyle needs of the individual (see Individualization of Peritoneal Dialysis Therapy). One of the biggest challenges for the PD nurse and other members of the multidisciplinary team is to develop a PD prescription that optimizes the patient's peritoneal membrane permeability characteristics, provides adequate dialysis via a delivery system that minimizes risk of complications, and meets the patient's lifestyle needs.

Peritoneal membrane permeability characteristics are remarkably stable, demonstrated by highly reproducible PET results (Burkart, 1995). Nevertheless, a PET should be repeated if there is an unexplained change in peritoneal clearance, because it can change over time in some individuals. Disease states such as peritonitis may alter permeability temporarily, with *acute* inflammation *temporarily increasing* permeability, but these changes are usually transient, with membrane function returning to near baseline after the acute infection is resolved. Long-term changes in the peritoneal membrane have been noted, generally thought to be related to scarring or adhesions with concomitant loss of peritoneal membrane surface area. Selgas, Bajo, Peso, and Jimenez (1995) reviewed 25 studies of peritoneal membrane transport reported in the literature from 1979-1992. Study results indicated either no change in solute transport in long-term PD patients, or an increase in the transport of low to middle molecular weight solutes. Further, patients with a large number of days with peritoneal inflammation (frequent or pro-

Table 22–15
Sample exchange schedules of CAPD.

Exch	4 Exchanges			5 Exchanges			6 Exchanges		
#	Inflow	Drain	Dwell	Inflow	Drain	Dwell	Inflow	Drain	Dwell
1	07:00	11:30	4.5	07:00	10:30	3.5	07:00	10:00	3.0
2	12:00	16:30	4.5	11:00	14:30	3.5	10:30	13:30	3.0
3	17:00	21:30	4.5	15:00	18:30	3.5	14:00	17:00	3.0
4	22:00	06:30	8.5	19:00	22:30	3.5	17:30	20:00	2.5
5				23:00	06:30	7.5	20:30	22:30	2.0
6							23:00	06:30	7.5
Total			22.0			21.5			21.0

longed episodes of peritonitis) showed a decreased ultrafiltration capacity, prompting the authors to observe "the greatest threat to peritoneal durability appears to be the effects of severe peritonitis which fails to resolve quickly and completely" (p. 329). Sclerosing peritonitis appears to be the most severe form of peritoneal membrane damage; it is sometimes referred to as end-stage peritoneal disease, with membrane damage thought to be due to a fibroblastic reaction and considered irreversible (Rodby & Korbet, 1994). Nursing implications of these findings include close on-going monitoring of the patient. If a patient who has been doing well on a given prescription of PD shows evidence of changes such as a decrease in outflow volume or return of uremic symptoms, repeating the PET or PFT should be considered, particularly if there have been repeated infections or a fungal peritonitis. This will determine if changes have occurred in the peritoneal membrane characteristics and will guide the health care team in adjusting the dialysis prescription accordingly.

Elements of the Dialysis Prescription

The elements of the PD prescription include number of dialysis exchanges per day, volume of each exchange, timing of the exchanges (dwell time), dextrose concentrations of PD solution used, and the integration of the dialysis regimen into the patient's lifestyle. Each element of the PD prescription listed can be manipulated to facilitate optimal dialysis. It is critical to include the patient in determining the specific individual dialysis prescription, because the most carefully planned and precisely honed PD prescription will be ineffective if the patient does not carry it out. Dialysis literature has an abundance of information regarding the noncompliant patient, but prescribing a dialysis regimen that the patient finds intolerable is a certain way to assure noncompliant behavior and a less than optimal outcome.

The number of exchanges required per day is an essential element of the PD prescription. For most CAPD patients, 4 to 6 exchanges daily are prescribed, with 4 the most common. A typical schedule for 4, 5, and 6 exchanges daily is included as Table 22-15. Note the daytime dwells are 4 or more hours in duration with 4 exchanges, while the single long-dwell exchange overnight is typically 8 hours in duration. As the frequency of exchanges increases, the total dwell time for the day decreases, due to the increased time required for draining and filling the peritoneum. As mentioned earlier, this is down time; with little or no dialysis solution in the peritoneal cavity, no dialysis can take place. With CAPD exchanges, there is a point of diminishing return; that is, the benefit gained from increased dialysate flow is offset by the loss of effective dwell time. Add to this the logistic difficulties associated with frequent exchanges, and the time commitment of requiring 6 exchanges daily would leave little time available for the patient to pursue other activities.

CCPD patients generally have 5 to 8 exchanges, with the night-time exchanges delivered by the cycler having a dwell time of 1–2 hours, and the single long-dwell exchange during the day typically 8–12 hours in duration. IPD is done either during the day with no fluid left in at night, or with a cycler at night with no fluid dwelling during the day. The former may be done at a dialysis center by dialysis personnel, but is no longer a common form of therapy. The latter, NIPD, is usually done at home with 4 to 8 exchanges or cycles done overnight; the exact number of exchanges prescribed should be based on peritoneal membrane permeability characteristics.

The volume of each exchange can be varied to

benefit the patient, with exchange volumes in adults generally 2 L, 2.5 L, or 3L. Patient size, blood levels of uremic toxins, and degree of residual renal function combine to determine the clearance required from PD. As illustrated above, increasing the number of exchanges has limits in terms of overall effectiveness in increasing clearance. Increasing the volume of each exchange can be an alternate strategy for increasing total dialysate flow and clearance, either alone or as an adjunct to increased number of exchanges. Potential problems associated with an increase in exchange volume include dyspnea, leak, discomfort, and change in body image (Twardowski, Burrows, & Prowant, 1984). These factors should be considered before determining exchange volume. Problems related to increased intra-abdominal pressure may be addressed in part using the larger volumes selectively, perhaps at night when the patient is supine. A CAPD patient may be able to tolerate a larger volume for the overnight exchange than for the daytime exchanges, or a CCPD patient might use larger volumes for overnight cycles than for the daytime dwell. Exchange volumes in infants and children are based on weight and body size (see Chapter 15 on the Pediatric Patient).

Management of the number of exchanges and the volume of each exchange is aimed at enhancing the dialysate flow, defined as the number of exchanges per day times the volume of each exchange. Inflow of dialysis solution influences clearance, because the volume of solution infused affects the volume of drained dialysate, which can be used to estimate clearance (in conjunction with the D/P ratio-see Clearance). Thus, a 2 L exchange done 5 times daily will result in 10 L of dialysis solution inflow as will a 2.5L exchange done 4 times daily. Differences in these two prescriptions include the dwell time for each exchange, the time involved for the actual exchange procedures, and the issues of patient tolerance to larger volumes just discussed. Cost may also differ for the two prescriptions, depending on the supplier. It is important to note that although the volume of dialysis solution infused is the same for each of the two prescriptions, the estimated clearance may be different because of differences in individual peritoneal membrane characteristics, differences in dextrose concentrations used, and resulting differences in drain volumes. These issues will be discussed in more detail in determining adequacy of PD.

The dextrose concentration of the dialysis solution is varied to achieve fluid balance and to maximize clearance. Lower dextrose concentrations create less osmotic pressure, and less fluid is removed by ultrafiltration; higher dextrose concentrations result in more ultrafiltration, with larger drain volumes anticipated. Fluid status should be assessed daily, fluid removal needs determined, and dextrose concentrations selected based on these factors. Since clearance of solutes is influenced by the volume of dialysate drained, and dextrose concentration influences drain volumes, the dextrose concentration has an impact on the total clearance achieved. Although more hyperosmolar solutions increase drain volumes and thereby enhance clearances, evidence indicates that these solutions suppress phagocytosis (Coles, 1995) and should be used sparingly if possible.

Table 22–16
Composition of peritoneal dialysis solution.

	Standard	Low Magnesium	Low Calcium
Sodium (mEq/L)	132	132	132
Calcium(mEq/L)	3.5	3.5	2.5
Magnesium (mEq/L)	1.5	0.5	0.5
Chloride (mEq/L)	102	96	95
Lactate (buffer)	35	40	40

Dialysis Solution

Solution used for peritoneal dialysis is sterile with electrolyte composition and pH designed to correct the imbalances caused by lack of adequate renal function. The concentration of electrolytes in commercially available solutions is represented by Table 22-16. Dextrose is used as the osmotic agent; however, recent evidence suggests the dextrose in dialysis solution may be associated with an increase in lipids and may contribute to the formation of advanced glycosylation end products. This has resulted in exploration of alternatives (Coles, 1995).

Buffers in PD solution may be either lactate or acetate, with a pH ranging from 5.2 - 5.5. Bicarbonate would be an "ideal" buffer because it would correct the metabolic acidosis without requiring metabolism and would be more physiologic hence more biocompatible. However, its use to date has been precluded by two problems: (a) the dialysis solution must be formulated at an acid pH to prevent the dextrose from caramelizing during sterilization, and (b) calcium precipitates in the presence of bicarbonate and an alkaline pH (Diaz-Buxo, 1995). Concern about the long-term effects of bioincompatible dialysis solution and the clinical implications for PD patients have prompted ongoing research for a more biocompatible solution. Coles (1995) reports initial clinical trials of a bicarbonate based dialysis solution with a neutral pH. This solution requires a two-bag system, one containing sodium bicarbonate, the other containing

Table 22-17
Preparation of PD solution.

Check solution bag for each of the following prior to use:
• Correct solution type (standard, low calcium, etc.) • Correct dextrose concentration • Correct volume of solution • Expiration date • Solution clarity • Integrity of solution container

the remaining constituents; the two bags are mixed immediately prior to infusion. Maintaining the two solutions in separate container avoids carameliza-tion during the sterilization process and formation of precipitates, but creates a more complex system for patients to manage. Should trials of this solution prove successful, nursing will be faced with the challenge of training patients to use this system successfully at home. Another promising alterna-tive is a low pH pyruvate fluid that is reportedly less toxic than lactate (Coles, 1995). This would be cheaper and less complicated than the two bag bicarbonate solution and may be available for use in the future.

Low calcium solutions may be indicated for patients using calcium salts as phosphate binders or for those using vitamin D supplements for sup-pression of parathyroid hormone, based on their serum calcium concentrations. Low magnesium solutions may be indicated for patients using mag-nesium containing antacids as phosphate binders; however, more research into the effectiveness of magnesium as a phosphate binder is needed before widespread use of these compounds is likely (Diaz-Buxo, 1995). Standard dialysis solution contains no potassium, because hyperkalemia is common in CRF patients; however, in some PD patients, hypokalemia may develop requiring potassium supplements. Digitalized patients should be moni-tored closely to ensure serum potassium concentra-tions are maintained within the desired range to minimize risk of cardiac dysrhythmias.

Most dialysis solutions currently available are packaged in polyvinyl, collapsible bags, often enclosed in a nonsterile outer wrapping. However, rigid plastic containers may be used with either PD or with disconnect systems for CAPD.

Nursing considerations. Summarized in Table 22-17, nursing considerations specific to the dialy-sis solution include noting the expiration date, appropriate dextrose concentration and volume; checking the solution container integrity; observing solution clarity; and ensuring the dialysis solution is at an appropriate temperature. The expiration date is marked on each bag of fluid, with the month and year noted. Fluid may be used until the end of the month printed on the container, but fluid past its expiration date must be discarded since sterility and stability of the electrolyte composition cannot be assured.

The dextrose concentration is printed on the container, but may be difficult to read through the outer wrap, particularly for patients with visual impairment. Most manufacturers of PD solution have adopted a color code to designate the dextrose concentration, making it easier for patients to dif-ferentiate between dextrose concentrations without opening the protective outer wrapping. The tip pro-tector that covers the portion of the system that the patient connects to is colored coded, with yellow often used for 1.5% dextrose, green for 2.5% dex-trose, and red for 4.25% dextrose. The volume of the solution is also printed on the container, as well as the container's volume capacity. Because more hypertonic solutions create more of an osmotic gra-dient, these solutions may come in a larger sized container to allow for the anticipated additional drainage volume from ultrafiltration. For example, a 2 L 4.25% dextrose solution may come in a 3 L sized container to accommodate both the original fill volume and the anticipated ultrafiltration vol-ume.

A small amount of moisture on the outside of the container may be the result of condensation, and is generally found inside the outer wrap. Any moisture present should be wiped away, and the container checked carefully for possible leaks, which are most likely to occur at the seams along the sides of the solution container. Containers with leaks should be discarded, because they are no longer sterile. Dialysis solution should be clear; any turbidity or appearance of cloudiness may indicate contamination, and the fluid should be discarded.

Most patients do not tolerate infusion of room temperature dialysis solution, experiencing abdom-inal discomfort and cramping. Warming PD solu-tion to approximately body temperature is recom-mended. This not only increases comfort for the patient, but enhances blood flow (cold solution causes vasoconstriction) and may enhance or facil-itate diffusion. Dry heat is the preferred method for warming the solution. A heating pad placed in an insulated container with the bags of PD solution is frequently used; solution is warm enough to infuse within a few hours. Warm water baths are *not* rec-ommended, since the water is not sterile and may inadvertently contaminate the system during the exchange procedure. Heating dialysis solution in the microwave is safe and effective (Wadhwa, Kenward, Kenney, & Rowe, 1983; Armstrong &

Zalatan, 1992), but care must be taken to avoid overheating. Infusing solution that is hotter than body temperature can cause pain, increase in body temperature, sweating, flushing, and possibly cardiac dysrhythmias. Should this occur, the hot dialysis solution should be drained immediately, hyperthermia or cardiac irregularities treated as indicated, and the method used to warm the solution carefully evaluated to prevent future problems, because burns of the peritoneal membrane with subsequent inflammation and scarring are possible (Prowant & Gallagher, 1995).

Any form of PD results in production of spent dialysate. This fluid should be handled much as urine with recommended disposal via a sanitary sewer. HIV has been isolated from spent dialysate of HIV infected patients, thus appropriate Universal Precautions should be taken when handling all spent dialysate. The reader is referred to current Centers for Disease Control and Prevention recommendations for disposal of blood or body fluids known to be contaminated by the HIV virus.

Nursing Interventions/Procedures

When providing direct, hands-on care for the PD patient, the nurse should be familiar with several procedures to adequately meet the needs of this patient. Although it is beyond the scope of this chapter to provide specific procedural information, the types of procedures commonly associated with patients receiving PD are reviewed briefly. This is followed by a section addressing the home management of the PD patient, which addresses non-procedural elements of nursing care for the home PD patient.

Transfer set change. The tubing that is attached to the catheter itself, called a transfer set, requires periodic changing to avoid breaks in integrity from normal wear. This procedure is generally done at the dialysis unit by the PD nurse at intervals recommended by the manufacturer of the transfer set, generally every few months, or following a known contamination of the transfer set. Specific procedures vary, but all require strict attention to aseptic technique using masks and sterile gloves. Care must be taken to minimize the risk of introducing bacteria while the PD system is open. Any clamps used on the PD catheter must not have "teeth" or rough edges that might damage the catheter.

Addition of medications. Certain conditions may require the addition of medications to the dialysis solution, the intraperitoneal (IP) route of administration. This procedure may be done by the PD nurse or by the patient or trained helper for home patients. PD solution containers have a medication port for use in adding medications, but it is essential to use aseptic technique when entering the PD system. Specific procedures preparing the medication port vary, but if the outer port is not sterile, should include use of a disinfecting solution with an appropriate procedure documented to decrease bacteria. A 5-minute povidone iodine soak of the medication port and medication vial has been used with good results, but is time consuming. Exploration of the efficacy of other disinfecting agents, shorter preparation time, or alternate disinfection procedures (e.g., a friction scrub instead of a soak) may prove useful and could potentially simplify the process of adding medications and enhance patient compliance. Additional nursing research in this area would be beneficial to guide future nursing practice. In addition to proper preparation of the medication port, it is important to use a needle of sufficient length to penetrate through the medication port and into the PD solution. To verify that the needle has penetrated into the solution, the syringe can be "flushed" with dialysis solution by withdrawing dialysis solution into the syringe and reinjecting this solution prior to removing the needle from the port. Mixing the medication with the dialysis solution by gently tilting the bag is recommended. Should sterile specimens of dialysate be required, usually for culture in a suspected case of peritonitis, the same procedure can be used with the bag of spent dialysate. (Specimens for laboratory analysis such as cell counts or dialysate solute levels are not required to be sterile).

Common additives to PD solution include heparin, insulin, potassium chloride, and antibiotics. Heparin 1000 units per 2 L is used to help prevent aggregation of substances in the dialysate that might obstruct flow, such as visible fibrin or a large number of cells. Drug transport is influenced by body distribution, protein-binding tendency, lipid or water solubility, molecular weight, and peritoneal permeability. The molecular size of heparin is too large to cross the peritoneal membrane. Therefore, heparin is not systemic when given intra-peritoneally. Since a slow drain may indicate accumulation of fibrin in quantities too small to be visible, heparin may be added for sluggish outflow. In cases of peritonitis, large numbers of white blood cells make the spent dialysate appear cloudy, and heparin is added to PD solution until the effluent is no longer cloudy. Bloody effluent is another indication for IP heparin to prevent formation of clots that could occlude the catheter or tubing. (Frank bleeding is addressed in Noninfectious Complications).

Insulin can be added to the PD solution for control of blood sugar in diabetic patients. Only regular insulin is used: beef, pork, or recombinant human. Required insulin doses may be larger than the doses given subcutaneously previously because a portion of the insulin binds with the bag and tubing itself, and not all of the insulin added to the dialysis solution is absorbed into the bloodstream by the end of the dwell. The amount of insulin lost in the drained solution will vary based on individual membrane permeability characteristics and dwell time of the

Table 22–18
Common intraperitoneal medications.

Medication	Indications for use
Heparin	Slow dialysate drainage Fibrin in dialysate Cloudy effluent associated with peritonitis Bloody dialysate (unless frank bleeding)
Regular insulin	Blood sugar control (May be used alone or in combination with oral agents or subcutaneous insulin)
Antibiotics Cephalosporins Aminoglycosides Vancomycin	Peritonitis Exit or tunnel infections Miscellaneous infections

exchange in which IP insulin is administered. Advantages of IP insulin include ability to dose more frequently than with subcutaneous insulin (4 or more times daily depending on the number of exchanges), avoidance of a subcutaneous stick for the patient, and a more physiologic absorption pattern. Insulin administered via the IP route may be absorbed more quickly into the portal circulation with resulting improvements in blood glucose control (Grefberg, Danielson, Nilsson, & Berne, 1987). Disadvantages of IP insulin include the potential increased dose requirement with associated increased cost, the increase in infection risk associated with entering the PD system to add the medication, and the difficulty in managing glucose control for patients with NIPD or CCPD, with exchanges done primarily at night while glucose loads from meals occur primarily during the day.

Potassium chloride may be indicated for patients prone to hypokalemia. As mentioned, PD solution contains no potassium chloride. Individual requirements should be determined based on biochemical analysis of serum potassium levels, with from 1 to 4 milli Equivalents potassium chloride per L being prescribed. It is important to note that potassium chloride is dispensed in single dose vials with no preservative. Even if the contents are not completely used, they must be discarded once punctured to minimize risk of infection.

Antibiotics for treatment of peritonitis or exit site infection are frequently given IP. Specific doses and frequency vary based on culture results identifying the causative organism and its antibiotic sensitivities. Some antibiotics, such as vancomycin, require a minimum dwell time of 6 or more hours for adequate absorption. Antibiotics for non-dialysis related infections can also be given IP, because the antibiotic is absorbed into the bloodstream. This may be a convenient form of antibiotic administration for home patients who require parenteral antibiotic therapy. Amphotericin B and generic vancomycin have been associated with a "chemical peritonitis," which features cloudy effluent with or without abdominal pain (Piraino, Bernardini, Johnston, & Sorkin, 1987). Appropriate resources should be consulted before administering any medication via the IP route for specific dosage or any required precautions. If patients are to administer these medications at home, they need education to facilitate safe and effective outcomes, including instructions for reconstitution of medications supplied as a powder. Common intraperitoneal medication are listed in Table 22-18.

Nursing Management of the Home PD Patient

Nursing management of the PD dialysis patient primarily occurs in an outpatient setting, and consists of three phases: (a) initial education and training, (b) ongoing monitoring and support, and (c) problem solving interventions if complications arise.

The initial education of the patient beginning PD is a critical nursing intervention. Ideally, the PD nurse should be involved in predialysis patient education, enabling the nurse to discuss with the patient the advantages and disadvantages of PD to facilitate an informed decision regarding preferred renal replacement modality. Diaz-Buxo (1996) indicates that appropriate patient selection along with responsible training and close monitoring enhance the probability of successful PD. An initial nursing assessment of the patient includes determining pertinent nursing and medical history, current physical findings, educational level, and readiness for learning. Special attention should be paid to visual acuity and manual dexterity, since the choice of PD system can be tailored to maximize chances of individual patient success. After this assessment is complete, a teaching plan for the patient is developed. It is important to involve the patient when developing the teaching plan, setting goals, and establishing desired outcomes. Severe uremia may impair the patient's ability to learn, and frequent rest periods may be required during patient education sessions. Patients need to have a basic understanding of the processes involved in peritoneal dialysis, since this will assist them in trouble shooting and decision making at home. The goal of PD training is to provide the patient with the knowledge and skills necessary to successfully perform the dialysis prescription, to identify problems early, and to recognize when to seek professional assistance. In addition, the patient should have adequate

Table 22-19
Sample home training patient education outline.

I. Review of Renal Function
  A. Normal function
  B. Alterations associated with renal disease
    1. Physiologic manifestations
    2. Emotional manifestations
II. Principals of Peritoneal Dialysis
  A. Definitions
  B. Processes
  C. Access
  D. Benefits / complications and risks
  E. Lifestyle adaptation
    1. Nutrition
    2. Mobility
  F. Financial considerations
III. Home Treatment
  A. Principals of asepsis
  B. Treatment procedures
  C. Troubleshooting
  D. Management of emergencies
  E. Home treatment records
  F. Supply ordering and inventory
  G. Medical waste disposal / infection control
  H. Equipment maintenance and disinfection
  I. Follow-up care
IV. Laboratory and Radiologic Tests
  A. Routine tests
    1. Purpose
    2. Frequency
    3. Procedure
V. Nutrition *
  A. Requirements
    1. Energy
    2. Protein
    3. Sodium and fluid
    4. Potassium
    5. Calcium / phosphorus balance
    6. Vitamins and minerals
  B. Incorporation into lifestyle
    1. Shopping
    2. Preparation
    3. Dining out
VI. Medication Therapy
  A. For each medication - name, purpose, dose, route, timing (relationship to diet), side effects, interactions
VII. Psychosocial Issues **
  A. Rehabilitation / adjustment
  B. Sexuality
  C. Counseling services
  D. Resources
    1. Patient organizations
    2. Financial resources
VIII. Patient Rights and Responsibilities
  A. Involvement in plan of care and modality selection
  B. Right to informed consent
  C. Confidentiality
  D. Grievances mechanism
IX. Facility Orientation
  A. Support services
    1. Telephone numbers for routine and emergency access (nurses, physicians)
    2. Introduction to all members of multi-disciplinary team / roles clarification
    3. Facility schedule/hours
X. Emergency Procedures
  A. During treatment
  B. Disaster planning
    1. Earthquake
    2. Hurricane
    3. Blizzard
    4. Power failure

*In collaboration with dietitian
**In collaboration with social worker

Note: Adapted from American Nephrology Nurses' Association. (1993). *Standards of clinical practice for nephrology nursing.* Pitman, NJ: Author. Reprinted with permission.

resources available to deal with simple problems.

The essential elements to be taught to CAPD patients, summarized in Table 22-19, were adapted from *ANNA Standards of Clinical Practice for Nephrology Nursing* (1993). Emphasis should be placed on preventing complications and recognizing early signs and symptoms of complications, chiefly peritonitis, exit site infection, dehydration, and fluid overload. Additional information may be indicated for specific patients, such as the addition of IP medication or administration of subcutaneous medications such as recombinant human erythropoeitin. CCPD patients need the same information, plus details about cycler set-up and management of cycler alarm conditions. Use of a training checklist can facilitate comprehensive patient education as well as simplify documentation of this education.

Once implementation of the teaching plan is completed, evaluation of patient education is required. Return demonstration is an effective method to determine if procedures or other motor skills have been mastered. To safely dialyze at home, patients must also be able to identify problems and state appropriate actions to take should such problems arise. Evaluation of initial PD training may include a written quiz, a question and answer session, or both. Some centers advocate having a nurse other than the nurse primarily responsible for the training do the comprehensive review.

Once the patient has completed training, home dialysis begins. The role of the PD nurse shifts to ongoing monitoring and support of the home patient, using a variety of strategies. The patient returns to the facility periodically for follow-up care. At this time, the nurse and other members of the multidisciplinary team can review the patient's progress, current status, and address problems. Clinic visits allow physical assessment and should include an evaluation of fluid balance, the condition of the exit site, and, if an exchange is done, exchange technique and the clarity of the spent dialysate. Patients should keep a home dialysis record that includes daily weights, vital signs, number of exchanges done each day, dextrose concentration, and medications added. A sample of a home record form is included as Table 22-20. An area for comments assists in identifying problems, since sometimes patients do not recall all of their questions at the clinic visit. Review of this information can help the nurse identify trends and may indicate areas where review with the patient could be beneficial. Routine monthly bloodwork typically consists of a chemistry profile and hematology assessment. Additional tests done less frequently include assessment of parathyroid hormone, aluminum levels, hepatitis screening, and adequacy testing such as Kt/V urea or creatinine clearance.

Between clinic visits, telephone calls provide another method for follow-up. Some centers call the patients routinely, while others rely on patients to contact the facility should a problem requiring assistance arise. Routine telephone calls are a cost effective way to avoid complications. Nursing research is needed to validate the effectiveness of routine follow-up, but Devins and Binik (1996) cite medical research indicating patients receiving so-called telephone house calls had significant health benefits, a survival advantage, and lower overall health care costs compared to a usual-care control group. Visits by nurses to the PD patient's home are another way to evaluate patient status and identify potential problems. In an 18-month study including 36 home visits, Ponferrada et al. (1993) concluded that although home visits are time intensive, an initial home visit provided beneficial insights that cannot be replaced by other types of evaluations.

Since PD is a home therapy, the issue of patient compliance is important. Unlike an inpatient or even in-center treatment, patients are responsible for the daily dialysis treatments. When outcomes do not meet expectations, careful evaluation of all potential causes must be explored, including the possibility that the prescribed dialysis treatment is not the delivered dialysis treatment. A trusting relationship between the patient and the dialysis staff is important to encourage candor. Patients who fear remonstration will not likely confess to skipping some exchanges. It is extremely important to involve the patient in the development of the PD prescription. The patient must "buy in" to the need to carry out the prescription; therefore, the health care team must work with the patient to assure the prescribed treatment is possible for the patient to carry out on a day-to-day basis. Holley (1995) notes that psychologic and non-compliance related dropout from CAPD, reported in up to 25% of patients (Holden & Gaumer, 1987), has not been studied extensively. Further study and design of interventions to prospectively address these issues is needed. Computer generated estimates of clearances can help determine expected clearances, using peritoneal membrane characteristics coupled with the number, timing, volume, and dextrose concentrations of exchanges. Actual clearance measurements can be compared to projected clearances to evaluate whether exchanges are being carried out on a regular basis. If a patient has been missing exchanges prior to the collection of dialysate for testing, creatinine accumulates. During the collection of dialysate for testing, the patient likely will do all prescribed exchanges, with a resultant wash out effect producing higher than expected clearance. This information must be interpreted carefully, however, since errors in either the measurement of exchange volumes, solute concentration, or the time of the collection (more than 24 hours) can also result in overestimation of clearance. Furthermore, errors in estimating creatinine generation may result in some patients consistently exceeding predicted clearances. Use of all available sources of information to evaluate compliance with the dialysis prescription helps determine if a change in prescription is required. Invoices from supply companies reveal if adequate dialysis solution has been ordered and delivered to carry out the prescription. Non-compliance may require additional teaching, and ultimately the suitability of a home dialysis modality may need re-evaluation.

Patients with CRF have a variety of needs that are best addressed by a multidisciplinary team consisting of the nephrologist, nephrology nurse, social worker, dietitian, and the patient. The contribution of each team member is important to maximize patient outcomes.

Emergency management may be required for PD patients, and PD patients must be taught whom to contact for both dialysis and non-dialysis related emergencies, both during regular clinic hours and after hours. Should a PD patient require treatment through an emergency room, health care professionals providing such care should be advised the

Table 22-20: Peritoneal dialysis home record sheet.

Date	Wt.	Sitting B/P	Standing B/P	Pulse	1.50%	2.50%	4.25%	Medications	Comments
1									
2									
3									
4									
5									
6									
7									
8									
9									
10									
11									
12									
13									
14									
15									
16									
17									
18									
19									
20									
21									
22									
23									
24									
25									
26									
27									
28									
29									
30									
31									

Month____________, 19____ Name ________________________

Table 22-21
Kt/V.

Definition — a way to quantify dose of dialysis treatment, where K is clearance (both dialysis and residual renal), t is time, and V is volume in which the solute is distributed (body water).
Formula
$\frac{\text{K [total clearance in ml/min] x t [time in minutes]}}{\text{V [in ml]}}$

patient is on PD. Care of the PD catheter and performance of PD procedures should be carried out by only professionals trained and experienced in PD. Specific interventions required for management of PD related emergencies and complications are addressed below.

Adequacy of Peritoneal Dialysis

Much emphasis has been placed on the importance of delivering an adequate dose of dialysis to CRF patients. It is important to note the distinction between adequate and optimal dialysis. *Adequate* refers to the amount of dialysis required to avoid untoward outcomes, while *optimal* dialysis indicates additional dialytic therapy would offer no benefit. Inadequate dialysis has been associated with an increase in morbidity (hospitalizations) and mortality (death). Most of the research on adequacy of dialysis has been in a hemodialysis setting, but a recent multi-center study involving 10 Canadian and 4 US dialysis centers (CANUSA Peritoneal Dialysis Study Group, 1992) was designed to help evaluate adequacy of PD as defined by clinical outcomes. The CANUSA study uses a prospective, analytical design, enrolling consecutive new PD patients from each of the 14 participating centers. Since patient membrane characteristics and personal preference for a particular form of PD must be considered, random assignment to different PD techniques is not possible. However, baseline factors that might predict clinical outcomes are recorded for each patient enrolled. Findings recently published (CANUSA Peritoneal Dialysis Study Group, 1996) indicate 680 patients were enrolled; a weekly Kt/V of 2.1 and a weekly creatinine clearance of 70 L per 1.73 meters squared were associated with an expected 2-year survival rate of 78%. A decrease of 0.1 unit Kt/V per week was associated with a 5% increase in the relative risk of death; likewise, a decrease of 5L/1.73 meters squared creatinine clearance was associated with a 7% increase in relative risk of death.

In the early days of CAPD, 4 exchanges of 2 liters per day was prescribed to virtually all patients. Dextrose concentrations were varied to control fluid status, but were not universally recognized as important in determining the amount of clearance achieved. As more is learned about the variables involved in peritoneal dialysis, the need to consider a number of individual factors is increasingly apparent. Zabetakis, Krapf, DeVita, Gleim, and Michelis (1993) completed a prospective study of 26 patients beginning PD to determine the required dialysate volume to achieve a predetermined daily creatinine clearance considered to provide adequate dialysis. They found only 6 of these 26 patients, or 23%, could be adequately dialyzed by the standard prescription of 4 exchanges of 2 liters daily. The determination that the patient is receiving "adequate" dialysis based exclusively on serum biochemical indices or clinical assessment (including the subjective sense of well-being of the patient) is no longer advised. Burkart (1994) suggests clinical assessment of adequacy of dialysis consists not only of the absence of signs or symptoms of uremia, but also control of blood pressure, anemia and other biochemical parameters, and the patient's subjective sense of well being. Actual determination of the clearance is recommended as an adjunct to the aforementioned indicators, since Keshaviah (1995), Burkart, and others have demonstrated that inadequate dialysis may occur for a period of time prior to patients becoming symptomatic. Increasing the dialysis dose after symptoms of inadequate dialysis occur may not "correct" for the period of inadequate dialysis, demonstrated by higher morbidity and mortality rates in underdialyzed patients, even if dialysis dose is later increased.

Definition of Kt/V

Dialysis adequacy is a relatively recent concept: prior to the current decade, many units never measured the amount of dialysis delivered. Gotch and Sargent (1985) developed the concept of Kt/V, where K is the urea clearance, t the treatment time, and V the volume of urea distribution in the hemodialysis setting. Keshaviah et al. (1990) applied these indices to peritoneal dialysis patients. Urea, the bulk waste product of protein catabolism, accumulates in body water. The concept of Kt/V is to determine the removal or clearance (K) of this waste (urea) from the patient's total body water (V) over a period of time (t).

Hemodialysis calculations are complex, given the intermittent nature of the therapy and the various compartments of body water where urea is distributed. Determination of Kt/V in peritoneal dialysis patients is more straightforward than in hemodialysis, due to the continuous nature of the therapy and the near steady state of urea concentration in various compartments of body water. For continuous therapies (CAPD and CCPD), a 24-hour collection of spent dialysate and urine are required, as well as a single blood sample. The total drained volume of dialysate is measured; the concentration of urea in the dialysate is measured then multiplied by the drained dialysate volume to determine the dialysate urea output. This value divided by the serum urea concentration yields a dialysis urea clearance for 24 hours. Urine clearance is calculated similarly, using urine volume and urea concentrations divided by serum urea. Kt/V per 24 hours is calculated by summing dialysis and urine clearance of urea and dividing this by the patient's total body water (Ponferrada & Van Stone, 1995). Kt/V is generally expressed as a weekly clearance. A sample formula is included as Table 22-21. It is important to note that the value for Kt/V is "unit-less," because all the units cancel out in the calculation.

Nursing considerations to facilitate determination of an accurate Kt/V value include adequate patient instructions and attention to detail in specimen handling. The measurement of dialysate volume must be accurate; the dialysate specimen analyzed for urea must be a representative sample for the total volume of spent dialysate. Ideally, the PD patient brings to the laboratory or dialysis unit all the individual bags of spent dialysate for the 24-hour collection period. If this is the collection method used, all spent dialysate should be thoroughly mixed together prior to collecting the sample for analysis, enabling collection of a truly representative sample. Alternately, a representative sample of spent dialysate can be collected from each bag of spent dialysate and the samples mixed or values averaged during the specimen processing. It is important to be as accurate as possible; the Kt/V determined is a daily value that is then multiplied by 7 to determine the weekly value. Therefore, any error in the sampling or chemical analysis becomes magnified sevenfold.

Nutritional status of the PD patient is closely related to adequacy of dialysis, with nutritional indicators such as serum albumin levels correlating closely with patient outcomes (See Morbidity and Mortality). The protein catabolic rate (PCR) can be estimated by measuring the presence of urea and protein in the dialysate and urine. The PCR estimates dietary protein intake, and may be more accurately referred to as urea nitrogen appearance (UNA). By determining the level of urea nitrogen, a waste product of protein metabolism, the protein equivalent of urea nitrogen appearance can be derived. In other words, the amount of protein intake required to generate the given level or urea can be estimated. For patients in a steady state, this estimate is fairly accurate, but in very catabolic patients who are breaking down protein stores, the PCR may overestimate protein intake. Since protein and urea are so closely inter-related and urea is used as one of the key markers for determining adequacy of dialysis, it is important to determine nutritional status and protein intake to interpret dialysis adequacy measurements. Underdialysis of peritoneal patients could be masked by a concomitant reduction in protein intake. If less protein is consumed, less urea is generated, resulting in a lower BUN; this lower BUN level could be interpreted as improved dialysis with higher clearances responsible for the lower BUN unless the nutritional status and protein intake are taken into consideration (Schleifer, Teehan, Brown, & Raimondo, 1993). A weekly Kt/V urea of 1.7 is currently accepted in most facilities as adequate dialysis for continuous therapies (CAPD or CCPD) and 2.2 for intermittent therapies (NIPD or IPD) (Nolph, 1991). Additional research is underway that may bring into question whether this is adequate dialysis, or if additional dialysis must be delivered to minimize the risk of poor outcomes. Preliminary data from the CANUSA study (CANUSA Peritoneal Dialysis Study Group, 1996) suggest that even a Kt/V of 1.7 may be inadequate.

Additional study is needed to validate appropriate levels of PD as well as to pinpoint the specific risks of underdialysis. A subjective global assessment focusing on nutritional status of PD patients (McCann, 1996) has been demonstrated to correlate reasonably well with Kt/V, and may be a useful clinical tool to evaluate adequate dialysis between actual laboratory assessments of PD adequacy. Results from the clinical assessment tool have correlated well with laboratory assessment of dialysis adequacy with two exceptions. Patients with many co-morbid conditions tend to be evaluated by the nursing assessment as underdialyzed when by laboratory data they may be receiving adequate dialysis. This is presumably because their multiple illnesses result in symptoms that mimic symptoms associated with uremia and underdialysis, thus subjectively appearing underdialyzed. Likewise, patients who are relatively healthy with the exception of their renal disease may display few symptoms of underdialysis based on the subjective nursing assessment, while laboratory findings indicate the need for additional dialysis (Ponferrada & Prowant, 1996). It is important to use the subjective and objective data together to most accurately evaluate patient status and develop the most effective plan of care.

Creatinine clearance has been previously discussed in terms of measurement of residual renal function. The creatinine clearance achieved by dialysis is often evaluated in conjunction with the Kt/V to determine adequacy of dialysis. Since Kt/V is based on urea, a small molecule (molecular weight 60) and creatinine is a somewhat larger molecule (molecular weight 113), clearances vary. It seems prudent to evaluate adequacy based on both Kt/V and creatinine clearance as well as patient's subjective feelings of well being, control of co-morbid conditions, blood pressure and anemia control, and physical assessment findings.

Individualization of PD Therapy

The dose of dialysis delivered has a significant impact on patient outcomes. It is important to ensure each patient is receiving the dialysis schedule that best meets his or her biochemical clearance requirements while balancing the demands of PD with lifestyle considerations to enhance modality survival as well as patient survival and quality of life. Individualization of PD therapy has two major goals: (a) to determine what prescription achieved adequate dialysis for the individual patient based on physical factors such as size, dietary intake, residual renal function, and peritoneal membrane characteristics; and (b) to develop a dialysis prescription that the patient is willing and able to carry out on a daily basis. From a nursing perspective, the key term in the phrase dialysis dose delivered is *delivered*. If a prescribed PD regimen does not fit the patient's lifestyle, he or she is unlikely to carry out the prescription on a daily basis. Therefore, although the prescription may be adequate, the delivered dialysis dose may not be sufficient to avoid untoward outcomes.

Modifications of Initial Prescription

Initially, a patient is started on a dialysis schedule based on estimated needs. Residual renal function may be known. If not, it can be estimated by serum creatinine, and the initial dialysis prescription determined on the basis of this limited information, assuming "average" peritoneal membrane characteristics. As soon as is possible, however, a peritoneal equilibration test or some other form of assessment of peritoneal membrane permeability and function should be performed to identify membrane characteristics for the individual patient. This information allows the physician and nurse to modify the initial dialysis prescription to best meet the needs of the patient. The number, volume, and timing of exchanges are reviewed.

When dealing with a patient who appears to be underdialyzed, Burkart (1994) recommends (a) evaluating whether the dwell times are most appropriate for the individual patient based on membrane characteristics; (b) monitoring for the loss of residual renal function, which could require additional dialysis clearance; (c) reviewing with the patient timing of exchanges; and (d) encouraging the use of more hypertonic dialysis solution for the longer dwells to achieve adequate ultrafiltration to maintain clearances. In general, patients with highly permeable peritoneal membranes benefit from shorter dwell times and either more frequent exchanges or IPD to maximize clearance while still achieving adequate ultrafiltration for fluid control. A long dwell time for patients with high permeability of the membrane results in small outflow volumes, little clearance (due to the low outflow volume), with no net ultrafiltration or even fluid absorption. Patients with low peritoneal membrane permeability need longer dwell times to allow time for solutes to cross the peritoneal membrane and enter the dialysis solution; short dwell times for these patients results in large drain volumes but little solute clearance and potentially inadequate dialysis.

Frequent assessment of patient's fluid status, dialysate drain volumes, and blood chemistry results validate the appropriateness of the dialysis prescription. Once the patient has been on peritoneal dialysis for a period of a few weeks, a Kt/V should be determined. It is useful to wait for several weeks after beginning dialysis prior to determining the Kt/V, to ensure the patient has reached a steady state, and is not clearing urea that has accumulated during the pre-dialysis period of renal insufficiency, a so called wash out effect.

Changes in Clearance Over Time

Even after the dialysis prescription has been individualized for the patient, a number of factors may still influence the required dialysis dose. Over time, residual renal function has been documented to continue to decline. Although this occurs more slowly in patients on PD than those on HD (Schmidt, 1995), it does occur. Burkhart (1995) contends that PD patients who have been on dialysis for a period of 2-3 years tend to develop uremic symptoms and are more likely to be transferred to HD primarily because of the loss of solute clearance from residual renal function of their native kidneys. Should the contribution of the residual renal function be unrecognized, the dialysis prescription will not be adjusted to compensate for the loss of residual function with inadequate dialysis as the logical result. The decline of residual renal function is not linear, but may occur suddenly perhaps as the result of an acute insult to the kidneys. Even though patients in CRF have little renal function, care should be taken to preserve this function for as long as possible. Avoidance of nephrotoxic medications, such as antibiotics, as well as avoidance of contrast media that is nephrotoxic are interventions that may assist in preserving function. Nurses should instruct PD patients to note the volume of urine output, and to let the nurse or physician know if there is a sudden change in urinary output. Sudden changes in volume of urine output may herald the loss of residual function, and a urinary clearance or Kt/V determination may be warranted to ensure the appropriate dialysis dose is being delivered. When nephrology professionals recognize the contribution to total clearance provided by this residual function, appropriate adjustments in the prescribed dose of PD can be made proactively, avoiding the adverse effects of inadequate dialysis.

There is evidence that in some individuals the peritoneal membrane itself undergoes changes in permeability. Selgas et al. (1995) note that many patients do not remain on PD due to functional instability of the peritoneal membrane, with loss of ultrafiltration and severe anatomical changes as the principal reasons. Their study of 67 adult patients indicate that the PET is an acceptable measure of peritoneal diffusive transport, noting it is the most widely used due to its simplicity. If changes in peritoneal membrane permeability are suspected, the PET can be repeated to evaluate current membrane functioning. Some facilities routinely repeat the PET or a similar measure of membrane characteristics at pre-determined intervals, while others repeat these tests only if there are clinical indications of a change in the membrane. Loss of ultrafiltration is one of the most frequent changes reported, and should be suspected if the patient reports increased use of hypertonic exchanges, decreasing drain volumes for the same dextrose concentration and dwell time, or difficulty maintaining fluid balance (increased incidence of fluid overload).

Bio-incompatibility of dialysis solution is thought to contribute to membrane changes over time, as are repeated episodes of peritonitis. Certain organisms may predispose to sclerosing of the peritoneal membrane, limiting the functional membrane surface area and decreasing clearance or causing loss of ultrafiltration. This problem might manifest as increased BUN and/or creatinine or as clinically evident symptoms. Again, tests of adequacy or membrane permeability assist in diagnosing the changes and making appropriate changes in the PD prescription. In severe cases, the patient may require a change in dialysis modality to HD for adequate therapy.

Tools to Individualize the PD Prescription

A number of variables affect dialysis efficiency in peritoneal dialysis as previously discussed: the number of exchanges, the volume of each exchange, the dwell time, individual membrane permeability, and dextrose concentration used (by affecting spent dialysate volume). The inter-relationship between these variables is complex, and manipulating one element of the prescription influences others. In an effort to project what effect prescription changes will have on overall clearances, computer programs have been developed to assist the nephrology team to evaluate the anticipated effect of changes in each of these variables. Several computer programs are available to simulate the effects of changes. Data entered includes PET information and pertinent laboratory values, the volume of exchanges, usual dextrose concentration, and dwell times. The computer uses this data to project the approximate clearance. Various combinations can be entered, using the computer projections to select the schedule most likely to produce the desired result. Schedules for CAPD, CCPD, and IPD can be simulated. These simulations are helpful, but only predict clearances. This does not eliminate the need to measure actual Kt/V. A very good correlation exists between computer projections and actual data.

Another use for the computer simulation is to evaluate suspected problems with compliance. If an actual Kt/V is significantly greater than projected, one explanation could be that the patient has been altering the dialysis prescription, perhaps skipping exchanges prior to the collection. The resultant build-up of urea can lead to higher than expected clearances during the collection period. Caution in interpretation is advised, however, since other sources of error could account for the variance.

Infectious Complications

Infection is the primary complication associated with PD. The most common infections include peritonitis, soft tissue infections of the catheter exit site, and subcutaneous tunnel infections. Predisposition to infection results from a combination of factors: a foreign body, a newly created portal of entry for bacteria, and dilution of host defenses by large volumes of dialysis solution (Coles, 1995). Although infections usually respond to antibiotic therapy, they cause increased costs for the diagnosis and treatment, and may result in hospitalizations, deterioration in nutritional status, and even a change in renal replacement therapy in a small sub-set of patients.

Peritonitis

Many advances have significantly lowered the incidence of peritonitis, but it remains the leading cause of catheter loss, transfer to HD (temporarily or permanently), and a major cause of hospitalization for PD patients. Peritonitis can result in death to PD patients, either directly from sepsis or indirectly from associated complications. The incidence of peritonitis for CAPD patients is approximately one episode every 12-18 patient months. Cycler patients have a slightly lower peritonitis rate – approximately one episode every 18-24 patient months – generally attributed to fewer connections required with cycler dialysis (Leehey, Gandhi, & Daugirdas, 1994).

Definitions. Peritonitis is defined as inflammation of the peritoneal cavity with *infectious peritonitis* caused by micro-organisms, *viral peritonitis* by viruses, and *fungal peritonitis* by fungi. Peritonitis is suspected when the dialysis effluent is cloudy. A culture of the dialysis effluent is positive in most cases of peritonitis, but a positive culture is not required for the diagnosis. There is a large volume of drained dialysate, which may explain the relatively high number of dialysate cultures with no growth; the small volume of spent dialysate used in the culture may not contain the offending organism. Use of blood culture bottles or concentrating the effluent prior to inoculating the culture media may enhance the probability of growth, with subsequent identification of the causative organism and its antibiotic sensitivities. With appropriate culture technique, growth of causative organisms and a positive identification occur in approximately 90% of cases (Leehey, Gandhi, & Daugirdas, 1994). A white blood cell (WBC) count of >100 cells per cubic millimeter with a predominance of neutrophils (> 50%) supports the diagnosis of peritonitis. (WBC counts > 50 cells per cubic millimeter are used to define peritonitis for patients already on antibiotics.) Gram stain of the effluent is recommended since this may identify micro-organisms rapidly and can assist in early implementation of the appropriate antibiotic therapy.

Culture negative, cloudy dialysate that meets the cell count criteria is usually caused by bacteria that have not grown on culture, but other potential causes of cloudy dialysate should be considered. Blood or fibrin can make the dialysate appear cloudy or hazy, requiring a differential diagnosis to rule out peritonitis. Blood in the spent dialysate will result in cell counts with higher than usual numbers of red blood cells, not WBC's, and the experienced observer can usually identify fibrin. Another cause for cloudy dialysate can be an eosinophilic response, an "allergic" type reaction. This is generally evidenced by cloudy dialysate within the first three months of initiating PD; the elevated WBC count shows an increased number of eosinophils on differential analysis. This is frequently asymptomatic and resolves spontaneously in most cases. Certain antibiotics, specifically generic vancomycin and amphotericin administered IP, have been associated with a *"chemical" peritonitis* (Piraino et al., 1987). This chemical peritonitis is dose related, and resolves with discontinuation of the drug therapy; certain brands of vancomycin are less likely to result in cloudy effluent, providing an option for treatment if vancomycin is the drug of choice. Pancreatitis can cause cloudy sterile dialysate; when this is the case, amylase values in the effluent will be elevated (Piraino, 1995). Table 22-22 presents diagnostic criteria for peritonitis.

Relapsing peritonitis refers to an episode of peritonitis where initial improvement is followed by a reappearance of symptoms, positive cultures, or elevated neutrophils. *Recurrent peritonitis* is reappearance of symptoms within 2 weeks of the completion of antibiotic therapy with the same organism (and same antibiotic sensitivities) on culture. An *episode of peritonitis* is a reinfection or new infection when it occurs more than 4 weeks after completion of therapy, and may or may not be the same organism as the previous episode (Prowant & Gallagher, 1995).

Signs and symptoms. The hallmark sign of peritonitis is cloudy peritoneal fluid, present in 99% of cases; abdominal tenderness occurs in 80% of cases, with rebound tenderness in up to half of cases, depending on severity and time from onset of infection to patient evaluation (Leehey, Gandhi, & Daugirdas, 1994). Patient symptoms include abdominal pain, which varies in intensity from severe pain to mild discomfort, nausea, vomiting, fever, and, rarely, chills. Fibrin strands are often present in the dialysis effluent during peritonitis.

Portals of entry. Transluminal, periluminal, hematogenous, and transmural can all serve as portals of entry for bacteria. Transluminal (through the catheter lumen) is the most common route, usually resulting from contamination during the exchange procedure, with bacteria entering the system via touch or airborne contamination, and being carried into the peritoneal cavity along with the dialysis solution. Transluminal contamination is also possible when the peritoneal dialysis system is opened for procedures. Episodes of peritonitis that occur following catheter transfer tubing set changes, accidental disconnections, or known holes in the catheter itself indicate an external contamination and subsequent bacterial introduction into the peritoneal cavity. Recurrent or relapsing peritonitis may be associated with *biofilm*. Certain bacteria are thought to coat the internal lumen of the catheter with a substance, or biofilm. These bacteria may harbor in this film, then re-infect the peritoneal cavity once antibiotic therapy is completed or stopped.

Periluminal entry refers to bacterial invasion along the outer surface of the catheter. The preperitoneal and subcutaneous cuffs are designed to help minimize this route of entry. Since acute catheters do not have these cuffs, patients with acute catheters are more prone to infection via this portal of entry. Likewise, patients with catheter exit site or tunnel infections are at high risk for peritonitis, since the bacteria have penetrated through the outer barriers of skin and the subcutaneous catheter cuff (if present).

Bacteria in the bloodstream can cause an infection of the peritoneal cavity, but this hematogenous route of entry is relatively uncommon. In this case, peritonitis is a secondary infection; an example is *Mycobacterium tuberculosis*. This route of infection may result from transient bacteremia, and may follow dental procedures or sigmoidoscopy with biopsy (Prowant & Gallagher, 1995).

Transmural infections refer to the passage of bacteria through the bowel wall. Often this is a result of a leak of normal bowel flora through a weakened area of bowel, such as is common with diverticular disease, but can also occur from a bowel perforation. For this reason, patients with diverticular disease are at higher risk for peritonitis. Nursing measures to minimize this risk include advising these patients to avoid constipation and to follow appropriate dietary guidelines.

Causative organisms. Gram positive organisms are responsible for the majority (55%-80%) of peritonitis episodes (Walshe & Morse, 1990). Coagulase-negative staphylococci, predominately *Staphylococcus epidermidis,* are the most common of the gram positive organisms for peritonitis (Piriano, 1995). These cases are thought to be related to touch contamination, and generally result in mild cases that respond well to the antibiotic therapy. The increased use of disconnect systems, with the "flush before fill" technique, has decreased the incidence of peritonitis from this group of organisms. *Staphylococcus aureus* is the next most common causative organism, causing a more severe form of peritonitis with abdominal pain, nausea, vomiting, and even fever in approximately one third of cases (Piraino). Use of disconnect systems has not decreased the incidence of *S. aureus* peritonitis, which is frequently associated with concomitant catheter infections, thus implicating a perilumenal portal of entry. Evaluation for *S. aureus* colonization in the nares or on the skin, particularly at the catheter exit site, with subsequent treatment of the carrier state, holds promise for decreasing the infections caused by this organism (see Exit Site Infections). Gram negative organisms are the cause of 17%-30% of peritonitis episodes (Walshe & Morse), with the decrease in some gram positive peritonitis resulting in an increase in relative probability of a gram negative peritonitis. *Escherichia coli, Klebsiella,* and *Enterobacter* species are normal bowel flora, and peritonitis caused by these organisms implies transmural contamination, although touch contamination with dirty hands could also be a possibility. Multiple gram negative organisms and/or anaerobic organisms are most likely from a bowel perforation. These peritonitis episodes may be especially severe, with increased morbidity and mortality (Brunier, 1995) and require aggressive therapy and close monitoring. *Pseudomonas* species have been considered environmental contaminants, frequently found in soil and water (Brunier). These organisms typically cause infections in the presence of a foreign body (catheter) or in an immunodeficient state, including renal failure (Piraino). Not surprisingly, *Pseudomonas* infections are frequently associated with catheter infections, and have a significantly higher incidence in PD patients who are HIV positive (Piraino). These infections are difficult to eradicate, frequently resulting in catheter loss and even patient death.

Fungal peritonitis is infrequent. Risk factors for developing a fungal peritonitis include prior antibiotic therapy, immunosuppression, or bowel perforation (Prowant & Gallagher, 1995). Yeasts such as *Candida albicans* are the predominant cause. Symptoms range from mild to severe. Prognosis with fungal peritonitis is grave. Catheter removal nearly always is required; delay in catheter removal is associated with an increased risk of death (Piraino, 1995).

Mycobacterium tuberculosis rarely causes peritonitis. A hydrophobic organism (Wiseman, 1995), its portal of entry is hematogenous contamination (Vas, 1993). The slow rate of growth of this organism makes it difficult to obtain positive culture and identification of the organism. It also helps protect the organism from some antibiotics, and requires a prolonged course of treatment (Protic & Hardy, 1993).

Table 22-22
Diagnostic criteria for peritonitis.

At least 2 of the following conditions:

- Symptoms of peritoneal inflammation
- Cloudy effluent with a white blood cell count > 100 cells/mm3 and differential with > 50% neutrophils
- Positive gram stain or culture demonstrating micro-organisms

Clinical course. Normal host defenses including neutrophils and macrophages attempt to destroy invading bacteria introduced into the peritoneal cavity. The acidity of dialysis solution, hypertonicity, and large volume of solution combine to impair the normal defenses (Holmes, 1993). The incubation for a touch contamination is 24-48 hours, while incubation for endogenous infections may be shorter (Prowant & Gallagher, 1995). Home patients should be instructed to notify appropriate health care personnel for any break in the PD delivery system so the need for prophylactic antibiotics can be evaluated. Keane et al. (1993) note there are no data to support *or* refute whether use of prophylactic antibiotics after a break in sterile technique effectively prevents peritonitis. Some centers use this strategy to minimize risk, but additional research is needed to demonstrate the effectiveness as well as to determine the optimal treatment regimen. Even though no known contamination has occurred, when cloudy fluid is noted, treatment should be initiated immediately for best results. Home patients must be instructed to report the *first* cloudy drain bag, especially if associated with abdominal discomfort. Using sterile technique, a specimen of the cloudy fluid is drawn for culture and sensitivities, white blood cell count with differential, and Gram's stain. The Gram stain allows treatment to be tailored to either gram positive or gram negative organisms; if no organisms are seen, antibiotic coverage for both gram positive and gram negative organisms is recommended until the causative organism is known (Piraino, 1995). Although the Gram stain may show a single organism, this does not preclude the presence of multiple organisms; therefore, Gram's stain results as a guide for initiation of therapy should be considered preliminary data (Keane et al.). Some centers advocate one or two rapid exchanges to flush contaminants from the peritoneal cavity, but this practice is controversial because recent evidence indicates this may actually impair host defenses for the previously mentioned reasons (acidic pH, dilutional effects).

Antibiotic therapy is begun, most often using the IP route. Antibiotic transport across the peritoneal membrane is bi-directional; therefore, oral, IP, or IV route of antibiotic administration may be effective. IP is the preferred route because generally it is more convenient for the patient. Broad spectrum drugs such as cephalosporins are most commonly used, either alone or in combination with aminoglycosides. With the increase in resistant strains of *Staphylococci*, the use of vancomycin has expanded. Current concerns about development of vancomycin resistant organisms may lead to still other recommendations for antibiotic therapy (Hospital Infection Control Practices Committee [HICPAC], 1995). Some antibiotics (i.e., cephalosporins) are usually given IP with each exchange; others (i.e., vancomycin) are given intermittently (weekly) and may require a prolonged dwell time (at least 6 hours) for best IP absorption (Vas, 1993). It is beyond the scope of this chapter to review specific antibiotic regimens and dosages, but the reader is referred to information published by the Ad Hoc Advisory Committee on Peritonitis Management (Keane et al., 1993) or to more recent publications for specific information of this type. Symptoms should begin to abate within 24–48 hours after initiation of treatment. Addition of heparin 1000 units/L of dialysis solution is recommended until the fluid is clear to prevent fibrin formation, minimizing the risk of peritoneal adhesions and avoiding catheter obstruction (Brunier, 1995).

Refractory peritonitis refers to cases where symptoms do not diminish after 48–96 hours of appropriate treatment. In such cases, a repeat culture, Gram stain, and cell count should be obtained, and therapy adjusted appropriately. If a 3 to 5 day course of intensified therapy does not result in improvement, the PD catheter should be removed and antibiotic therapy continued for an additional period of approximately 1 week (Leehey et al., 1994). Other indications for catheter removal include fungal peritonitis, infections also involving the catheter tunnel and exit site, and infections from intestinal leaks with fecal peritonitis. Peritonitis from fecal contamination is associated with a high mortality rate, and surgical intervention may be required (Vas, 1993).

Signs and symptoms of sclerosing peritonitis include abdominal pain, diminishing ultrafiltration, and hemoperitoneum (blood in the peritoneum). A definitive diagnosis requires either a peritoneal biopsy or CT imaging of bowel wall thickening and adhesions. The patient with sclerosing peritonitis must transfer to HD for maintenance renal replacement therapy. Mortality rates are extremely high with sclerosing peritonitis. Other, reversible forms of peritoneal damage may respond to resting the peritoneum using HD as a temporary treatment modality, then returning the patient to PD; Selgas et al. (1995) reported success in such cases with a one month rest of the peritoneum.

Nursing management. The best nursing strategy for managing peritonitis is to prevent episodes by teaching patients to use strict aseptic technique to prevent introduction of bacteria. Attention to detail during exchange procedures cannot be overemphasized. Additionally, patients should be encouraged to report touch contamination and breaks in the closed system so prophylactic antibiotics can be administered. The seriousness of repeated episodes of peritonitis must be conveyed to the patient, since repeated episodes may result in scarring of the peritoneal membrane and ultimately can result in PD no longer being an effective form of renal replacement therapy for this patient.

Once the patient presents with an episode of peritonitis, assessment of his or her clinical condition is essential. Symptomatic treatment of nausea, vomiting, or fever may be indicated, based on the severity of symptoms and established practices of the center. In addition to assessing the patient, the nurse should carefully inspect the catheter and tubing for possible small holes or tears that might have resulted in bacterial entry and subsequent peritonitis. In the absence of an obvious source for contamination, a history is taken to attempt to identify the portal of entry. The nurse should ask if the patient recalls any recent break in aseptic technique. A review of the exchange procedure is indicated. If the patient is too sick during the acute episode, a time should be planned for this review in the near future, when symptoms improve. It is important to interact positively with the patient during the review, with the stated goal of preventing future episodes of infection, not to be reproachful or punitive. A patient who feels reprimanded during an episode of peritonitis may delay reporting similar symptoms in the future, which can postpone treatment and perhaps result in more serious consequences from the infection.

The specimens of spent dialysate for the WBC count and differential and Gram stain should be processed quickly to ensure accurate results and to facilitate initiation of appropriate treatment. Depending on the antibiotic therapy chosen, the patient may need to add medications to subsequent bags of solution, or the PD nurse may be able to mix antibiotics in solution for the patient to use. If the patient will be required to add antibiotics, it is important to review dosage, frequency, reconstitution, and administration procedures as appropriate. Addition of IP heparin is recommended until fluid clears, and for patients who do not routinely add IP medications, a review of this procedure is indicat-

Table 22–23
Calculation of peritonitis rates.

Expressed as 1 episode per number of patient months
Actual patient days divided by average days per month (365 divided by 12 or 30.42) = total patient months
Total patient months divided by # episodes of peritonitis = peritonitis rate

Example — Your dialysis unit follows 30 patients. In the past three months (June, July, and August), 3 patients experienced an episode of peritonitis.
First, determine the number of actual patient days:
92 days (# days in June, July, and August) x 30 patients = 2760
Next, divide actual patient days by average days per month:
2760 divided by 30.42 = 90.73 patient months
Finally, divide patient months by the number of episodes of peritonitis
90.73 divided by 3 = 30.24.
Rate — The peritonitis rate is 1 episode per 30.24 patient months.

Expressed as 1 episode per number of patient years
patient days divided by 365 for total patient years
Patient years divided by # episodes of peritonitis yields rate

Example — Using the data above:
First, determine the number of actual patient days, or 2760
Next, divide by 365
2760/365 = 7.56 patient years
Finally, divide patient years by the number of episodes of peritonitis
7.56/3 = 2.52.
Rate —The same peritonitis rate expressed this way is 1 episode per 2.52 patient years.

Expressed as episodes per patient year
actual patient days divided by 365 = total patient years
episodes of peritonitis divided by total patient years = rate

Example — Using the data above:
2760 patient days divided by 365 = 7.56 total patient years
3 episodes divided by 7.56 patient years = 0.40 episodes per patient year.

Note: Exit site infection rates can be calculated in the same way.

ed as well. Patients who are treating peritonitis on an outpatient basis should know when to expect to see improvement in symptoms and in the appearance of the spent dialysate. Many centers follow these patients, usually by telephone, on a frequent (daily) basis at least until fluid clears and there is evidence the treatment is effective.

During an episode of peritonitis, the peritoneal membrane becomes more permeable. Although this may facilitate solute clearance, it also results in a decrease in ultrafiltration. Initially, if the patient is experiencing nausea and vomiting, this can be helpful since the nausea and vomiting can predispose to dehydration. However, more hypertonic exchanges and even shorter dwell times may be required to achieve ultrafiltration and avoid volume overload if the patient continues his or her usual fluid intake. The increased permeability along with use of more hypertonic dialysis solution also combine to increase glucose absorption. Diabetic patients will be prone to hyperglycemia, so blood glucose levels should be monitored closely, with appropriate adjustments in therapy to maintain glucose control (Leehey et al., 1994). Protein loss across the peritoneal membrane also increases secondary to the higher permeability. Patients should be advised to eat more protein during episodes of peritonitis.

Peritonitis rates can be calculated as one episode per given interval (expressed as patient months or years), or as a number of episodes per patient year. Table 22-23 illustrates these methods of calculating peritonitis rates.

Exit Site Infections

Infection of the catheter exit site has a significant impact on morbidity of peritoneal dialysis patients, longevity of catheters, and PD modality survival. Exit site infections are reported at a rate of approximately 1 episode every 24–48 patient months (Leehey et al., 1994), and may occur alone or in association with a tunnel infection and/or peritonitis episode (in approximately 20% of cases). Infection of the exit site may be either acute or chronic.

Signs and symptoms. Unlike peritonitis, defining characteristics of exit site infections are not yet accepted universally. After a thorough evaluation of the exit site, presence of two or more of the following signs and symptoms are generally classified as an exit site infection: (a) erythema, (b) induration, (c) tenderness, (d) purulent drainage with or without crust, or (e) positive culture of exudate. To better understand the need for the presence of at least two of the above mentioned signs and symptoms to diagnose an exit site infection, a review of each may be helpful. Erythema, alone, may indicate inflammation or irritation, but not necessarily an infection. Induration can be the result of scar tissue from trauma or previous infections, but not always an indication of a current infectious process. Tenderness can result from recent surgery for catheter placement or a part of the normal healing process. It also may be associated with recent exit site trauma, which, while predisposing to a subsequent exit site infection, does not indicate infection when present in isolation. Regarding purulent drainage with or without crust, serum and white blood cells exuded by granulation tissue in the catheter sinus tract suppress bacterial proliferation, but this exudate often forms a crust around the catheter (Twardowski & Prowant, 1996b). Purulent drainage in the absence of any localized signs or symptoms at the catheter exit site may indicate a tunnel infection, while clear drainage at the exit site may indicate a dialysate leak, or serous fluid. The presence of a positive culture in the absence of other symptoms does not constitute an exit site infection because well-healed, uninfected exits sites are usually colonized with bacteria. Exit site infection occurs when there is *bacterial invasion* of the soft tissue surrounding the catheter exit site, not just colonization.

Scabs are formed by dried blood, either post operatively after the creation of the exit site or following trauma that causes bleeding. Although any break in intact skin at the exit site may increase the risk of infection, the presence of a scab alone does not indicate infection. Excessive granulation tissue is thought to be a response to inflammation, and usually is accompanied by infection (Twardowski & Prowant, 1996a).

Acute exit site infection refers to a new onset infection, with a duration of less than 4 weeks. Acute infections may occur either in the immediate post-implantation period or much later. *Chronic exit site infection* refers to an ongoing infection, where symptoms have persisted for more than 4 weeks, or where symptoms wax and wane without eradication of the infection.

Causative organisms. Bernardini, Holley, Johnston, Perlmutter, and Piraino (1991) conducted a retrospective analysis of over 300 CAPD related infections over a 10-year period to determine trends in infections. These results indicate *Staphylococcus aureus* as the most common infecting organism for catheter exit site infections (averaging 49% of all infections), followed by other gram positive organisms (primarily *Staphylococcus epidermidis*), with *Pseudomonas aeruginosa* the most common gram negative organism. This report of 10-year trends emphasized the significance of exit site infections when noting "catheter removal tended to parallel catheter infection rather than peritonitis" (p. 33). Thus, exit site infection may affect technique survival even more than the number of peritonitis episodes.

Treatment. Treatment of exit site infections usually includes systemic antibiotic therapy (via oral, IP, or IV routes) and intensified local care, sometimes including topical antibiotic preparations. As previously noted, there is less agreement on the definition of exit site infection than peritonitis; likewise, there is less uniformity of treatment regimens.

Recent research by Piraino (1990) linked *S. aureus* infections with colonization of patients with the organism, a so-called carrier state. Treatment to eradicate *S. aureus* carriage through use of oral Rifampin and/or 2% mupirocin ointment in the anterior nares resulted in a significant reduction in *S. aureus* infection rates in their reviews. Cyclic or ongoing treatment may be required to prevent recurrence of the carrier state, but additional research is needed to determine the optimal frequency and any associated problems. Nolph (1992) noted prophylactic use of antibiotics following catheter exit site trauma may reduce the chances of subsequent infections.

Nursing management. As with peritonitis, the most effective nursing management of exit site infections begins with prevention strategies. Care of the PD catheter immediately post implantation was previously discussed.

Nursing research by Prowant et al. (1988) demonstrated fewer exit site infections with a routine exit site care procedure that includes cleansing the site with antibacterial soap and securing the catheter, compared with either a sterile dressing change or exit site care that includes the use of a povidone-iodine paint.

Moore (1989) evaluated a gauze dressing changed daily compared with a dressing of

Blisterfilm® changed every five days, and found that the latter resulted in fewer infections. In general, there is agreement that routine care for the well-healed exit site should be done regularly, either daily or at least every few days. Routine care begins with good handwashing, followed by any dressings removal. The exit site is then inspected carefully, looking for any signs or symptoms of infection. Any problems noted should be reported to the nephrology nurse immediately. Purulent drainage, if present, should *not* be cleansed away by the patient, but rather left until a culture can be obtained. If no abnormalities are noted, the patient can proceed with gentle cleansing using an antibacterial liquid soap or other prescribed solution. The skin is carefully dried with a clean towel, and the catheter secured to the skin to minimize risk of trauma. Dressings are optional, but should be worn if soiling is likely or to minimize rubbing from tight clothing.

Prowant and Twardowski (1996) noted that improved nutrition, control of glycemia in diabetics, and use of prophylactic antibiotics for *S. aureus* nasal carriers may reduce the incidence of exit site infection. They list the following two additional keys to prevention: (a) avoidance of trauma (defined as any break the integrity of the skin at the exit site), and (b) avoidance of gross contamination of the exit site. The principles of catheter exit site care for a well-healed site are included as Table 22-11; for an infected exit site as Table 22-24.

Submersion of the exit site increases risk of infection from water-borne organisms. The use of ostomy appliances or other waterproof dressing over the exit and catheter may be used to minimize this exposure for patients who swim in clean ocean water or chlorinated private pools. Patients should be instructed to avoid lakes, public pools, whirlpools, and hot tubs because of the increased risk associated with these sources of water.

Some centers use sterile dressing changes as part of localized care of an infected exit site. Evaluation of the current care regimen in use at the time the catheter exit site became infected seems prudent. Because there is often an increase in the drainage at the site during an episode of infection, more frequent cleansing of the exit site is generally advised. Excessive or exuberant granulation tissue (proud flesh) is associated with exit infection or inflammation. This tissue can be cauterized using silver nitrate sticks. Care must be taken to avoid damaging healthy tissue and possibly disrupting the sinus tract; therefore, it is advisable for the physician or nurse to apply the silver nitrate to the granulation tissue, not the patient or partner. Use of magnification to visualize the granulation tissue facilitates its removal while avoiding damage to intact skin.

The subcutaneous cuff of the peritoneal catheter may extrude from that tissue and become visible at the exit site. If this occurs, the cuff may irritate the skin and predispose the area to inflammation and infection. Treatment options include (a) careful observation with intervention only if symptoms occur, or (b) removal of the external cuff through a cuff shaving procedure. Care must be taken to avoid damage to the skin or the peritoneal catheter itself. Catheter replacement is required if the catheter integrity is breached during the cuff shaving procedure, or for chronic infection unresponsive to treatment. One potential cause of cuff extrusion is the tendency for a straight catheter placed in an arcuate shaped tunnel to resume its straight shape, thus forcing the subcutaneous cuff towards the skin surface and even causing this cuff to extrude. Twardowski et al. (1986) advocate the use of catheters with a pre-formed arc to achieve a downward tunnel direction toward the exit site without the increased risk of cuff extrusion.

Table 22–24
Principles of nursing care for the infected exit site.

- Culture all exudate.
- Cauterize exuberant granulation tissue.
- Use sterile dressings.
- Immobilize the catheter.
- Increase frequency of exit care to at least once daily.
- Do not use cytotoxic agents in the sinus.
- Do not forcibly remove crusts or scabs.
- Reassess exit every 7-10 days.

Note: From Prowant, B.F., & Twardowski, Z.J. (1996). Recommendations for exit care. *Peritoneal Dialysis International, 16 (Suppl. 3), S94-S99. Used with permission.*

Tunnel Infections

Infection of the soft tissue tunnel of the PD catheter is often classified with exit site infections, because it can be difficult to differentiate between the two in many cases. Exit site infections have the potential to invade into the subcutaneous tunnel, and may even involve the peritoneal cavity, resulting in an exit/tunnel/peritonitis (translumenal portal of entry). It is possible to have a tunnel infection not associated with an exit site infection. These cases can be difficult to diagnose because the only symptom may be repeated episodes of peritonitis (Fox & Tzamaloukas, 1994). Luzar et al. (1990) defined a tunnel infection as erythema, edema, and/or tenderness of the subcutaneous tunnel with or without discharge and positive culture.

Signs and symptoms of a tunnel infection include the presence of (a) a palpable thickening over the tunnel, (b) edema and erythema over the tunnel segment, (c) pain and tenderness along the tunnel, (d) an abscess over the catheter tunnel, or (e) purulent drainage from the catheter exit site (Prowant & Gallagher, 1995). Ultrasound may be used to evaluate for fluid in the tunnel and indium scans can evaluate for pus; however, the sensitivity of these diagnostic tests has not been established (Fox & Tzamaloukas, 1994). Catheters at high risk for development of tunnel infection include those with one or more of the following: (a) an extruded subcutaneous cuff, (b) delayed healing, (c) a concurrent exit site infection, (d) post trauma, and (e) dialysate leak.

Treatment options for tunnel infection are somewhat limited. Antibiotic therapy similar to that used with exit site infections may be prescribed. Opening the tunnel through a procedure called deroofing is occasionally attempted. Tunnel infection treatments have had limited success; most tunnel infections lead to catheter loss (Prowant & Gallagher, 1995).

Modification of the catheter itself is being explored as a possible means to decrease the number of infections in peritoneal dialysis. The material used to make catheters and their cuffs is one avenue that is being explored for possible modification to reduce infection rates. Silver is known to have antibacterial properties, with good biocompatibility when incorporated in bioprosthetic materials. Using silver to coat peritoneal catheters may help decrease infectious complications (Dasgupta, 1995). Tradition Dacron® cuffs on peritoneal catheters decrease vascularization and result in a fibrous plug. A new tissue implant, the Seare's spatially specific porous biomaterial (SSPM) implant creates open cell porosity and development of new vasculature (Lefton, 1995). Recent changes in catheter shape have been discussed. Nurses should participate in research designed to explore and validate benefits of such catheter design modifications.

Noninfectious Complications

A number of noninfectious complications may be associated with PD. These include problems associated with catheter insertion, catheter position or function, increased intra-abdominal pressure, discomfort or pain, and fluid volume status.

Catheter Insertion

Insertion of a PD catheter is a relatively low-risk procedure, but there can be some associated complications. Complications of placement of rigid catheters intended for acute PD were discussed in the section on peritoneal access. Complications associated with the use of long-term PD catheters may not be apparent at the time of insertion, but may present hours, days, or even weeks following insertion.

Bleeding into the peritoneal cavity, with resulting pink-tinged dialysate, is usually a benign event. Blood does not cause abdominal pain, and small amounts may make the effluent hazy with only a slight pink appearance. Therefore, it is easily confused with peritonitis. Cell counts are useful for differential diagnosis because the white cell count will not be elevated with blood tinged dialysate. Blood may appear with menstruation, ovulation, or following colonoscopy (Steiner, 1993). Pink-tinged dialysate is relatively common, and can be treated by administering IP heparin to prevent clot formation that could obstruct the catheter, or by flushing the peritoneum with dialysis solution to facilitate clearing. Hemoperitoneum associated with abdominal pain or the presence of clots indicate a more serious problem that requires further evaluation. If the effluent is not pink but red, a hematocrit and cell count should be done. Hematocrits of 2% or red blood cell counts of 60,000 cells per cubic centimeter indicate significant bleeding, and surgical exploration to ligate the bleeding source may be required (Ash et al., 1995). At a rate of 0.4%, the incidence of serious hemorrhage requiring transfusion is rare (Zappacosta, 1993).

Pericatheter leaks may occur, and are more likely when the catheter is used immediately after placement. Leaks present as moisture or fluid around the skin exit site, and must be differentiated from serous fluid associated with the newly created exit site. Because dialysis solution contains high concentrations of dextrose (relative to serum), the use of a dextrose stick or other tests to determine glucose content may be helpful in the differential diagnosis. To avoid this problem, it is recommended to postpone catheter use for the immediate postoperative period, usually 1–2 weeks. If the catheter must be used, small volumes should be instilled with the patient supine to minimize pressure and lessen the risk of leak. Pericatheter leaks not only delay healing and ingrowth of the cuff(s), the dextrose rich dialysis solution predisposes to infection. The Moncrief-Popovich method of catheter insertion lessens this complication, by allowing 6 weeks for tissue healing prior to exteriorization of the catheter.

Fluid can also leak into the subcutaneous tissue, evidenced by rapid inflow, poor outflow, and diminished return volumes along with tissue edema. Edema may be present within the abdominal wall or may be in the dependent areas, such as the scrotum or labia. Diagnosis may be empiric via clinical assessment findings, or radiographic studies involving the use of contrast may be used. As with external leaks, stopping PD may allow for tissue to ingrow and seal the area where the leak is occurring. In rare instances, the catheter may require replacement.

Perforation of the bowel by the peritoneal catheter most often occurs during insertion, with the highest risk associated with percutaneous insertion methods. Rare cases of erosion of the bowel wall by the indwelling catheter have also been reported (della Volpe, Iberti, Ortensia, & Veronesi, 1984). Patients with adhesions are at higher risk for bowel perforation. Signs and symptoms of bowel perforation include a foul smell, cloudy dialysate with particulate matter, and profuse watery diarrhea (Zappacosta, 1993). Treatment of bowel perforation includes removal of the catheter, temporarily maintaining the patient on hemodialysis, and use of antibiotics to clear infection. The bowel puncture is usually managed nonsurgically. PD catheter replacement can be attempted once infection has cleared and the bowel has healed.

Bladder perforation can usually be avoided by emptying the bladder prior to the insertion procedure. If perforation of the bladder occurs, it manifests as an increase in voiding volume that tests positive for glucose along with lower than expected PD drain volumes. Bladder perforation requires removal of the PD catheter and possible insertion of a urinary catheter. Zappacosta (1993) reports replacing the PD catheter and resuming PD immediately, with the urinary catheter left in place for a week before its removal.

Incisional pain following catheter insertion is generally mild and responsive to analgesics. Deep breathing to maintain pulmonary hygiene is recommended, but coughing should be discouraged to avoid increased intra-abdominal pressure. Use of narcotic analgesics may predispose to constipation, so nursing measures to avoid this complication should be employed as indicated. The use of stool softeners and bulk laxatives may be required. Fluid intake should be individualized to the patient, but care must be taken to avoid fluid overload in the CRF patient.

Catheter Malfunction/Malposition

Adequate inflow of dialysis solution with poor outflow can indicate catheter malfunction, catheter tip migration, catheter malposition, omental wrapping of the catheter, or trapping of the catheter between loops of bowel. Nursing management is aimed at determining the cause of the outflow problems and intervening to correct the underlying cause(s). Logic dictates addressing the most likely and most readily correctable potential cause first, and progressing to more remote possibilities. The process begins by looking for kinks in the tubing, presence of fibrin, or unopened clamps. Kinks must be straightened and clamps opened appropriately to allow flow; fibrin is treated with IP heparin (see below). Next, a nursing history evaluates bowel function, and constipation is corrected if indicated. Patients should be taught to avoid constipation, using a combination of diet, exercise, and medications as needed.

In the absence of these problems as the cause of poor outflow, malposition of the catheter should be suspected. Simple catheter tip migration generally presents as adequate inflow, poor outflow when the patient is upright, but good outflow when the patient assumes a supine or side-lying position. By having the patient attempt to drain dialysate in a variety of positions, including supine positions, the position of the catheter tip can be estimated empirically depending on the success of drain attempts. Catheter position can be demonstrated by radiographic studies; an abdominal x-ray will show the catheter's position within the abdomen. If the catheter must be repositioned for adequate function, use of a J-wire or laporoscopic techniques may be employed. Rarely, catheter revision or replacement is required.

Omental wrapping of the catheter may displace the catheter upward, and results in a one-way obstruction to flow. Use of radiopaque contrast infused through the catheter (using sterile technique) may demonstrate omental wrapping, characterized by occlusion of some or all of the openings in the catheter. Contrast media infused through the catheter remains near the catheter, trapped by the omentum, not free-flowing into the cavity. If the impedance to flow is significant, partial omentectomy may be indicated, either surgically or laporoscopically with catheter replacement required in severe cases.

A fibrin plug in the catheter can occur, resulting in partial or complete obstruction of dialysate flow. Early symptoms include slow drains, often followed by slow inflow of dialysis solution, then total obstruction. Fibrin may be visible in effluent, but may not be seen until the dialysate cools, allowing the fibrin to congeal and become more apparent. Addition of heparin to dialysis solution to avoid obstruction is usually effective if symptoms are recognized early. The use of IP heparin is desirable, since this intervention can be safely accomplished by the patient or caregiver at home. If total obstruction to flow has occurred, intervention by a health care professional may be required. Urokinase can be infused using an accepted protocol and/or a J-wire used to attempt to clear the obstruction. Determining whether or not a kink is present in the internal portion of the catheter causing the obstruction is essential prior to using these interventions. Abdominal x-ray will demonstrate kinks in the intra-peritoneal segment of the catheter; both a flat plate (frontal) view and side view may be required. An important point to remember is that a catheter can become kinked even after having been in place for some time as a result of catheter migration within the peritoneal cavity.

Loss of catheter integrity can occur over time. This may result from accidental trauma, inappropriate sampling through the catheter, use of clamps with teeth that damage the catheter, or from use of inappropriate cleansing agents that damage the catheter material itself. Emerging trends in exit site care aimed at preventing infection from *S. aureus* include use of mupirocin at the exit site; however, mupirocin applied directly to polyurethane catheters can lead to damage to the catheter itself (Pirano & Faller, 1995). If this technique for exit site care is advocated, careful patient education is required to ensure the mupirocin is applied only to the skin surrounding the catheter, not the catheter itself. At each clinic visit or hospitalization, the nurse should inspect the catheter for signs of wear or trauma. Should these signs be noted, the nurse should review with the patient or caregiver the routine practices; the history may indicate the source of the problem. Patients or caregivers should be instructed to avoid practices that increase risk of damage to the catheter. Should a break in catheter integrity occur that results in an opening in the system, usually evidenced by a leak, dialysis should be stopped immediately and the catheter clamped (using a clamp with a smooth surface). The clamp should be placed between the break in the catheter and the patient. This serves to decrease the risk of bacterial contamination of the peritoneal cavity. If the external catheter segment is of adequate length, the catheter can be trimmed with the segment including the hole in the catheter removed. A tubing change procedure is done, trimming the catheter with sterile scissors, then replacing the adapter and connecting the sterile transfer tubing. For a short external segment, a splicing procedure can be attempted using a commercially available kit that includes a splicing device, an additional segment of catheter material, and a glue or cement. In rare instances, the catheter may require replacement.

Increased Intra-abdominal Pressure

Instillation of dialysis solution into the peritoneal cavity results in an increase in intra-abdominal pressure. A number of potential complications are associated with this increased pressure and include hernias, dialysis solution leaks, and hemorrhoids. Additionally, pre-existing conditions such as pulmonary disease may be aggravated by the pressure of dialysis solution on the diaphragm. A feeling of fullness in the abdomen can occasionally contribute to gastrointestinal complaints, such as early satiety or even nausea. PD patients should be evaluated for predisposition to these concerns, and steps taken to minimize the risk of these complications.

The key determinants of intra-abdominal pressure are volume of dialysis solution instilled, patient position, and patient activity. Larger volumes produce higher pressures, increasing almost linearly; for any given volume of dialysis solution, the supine position results in the lowest intra-abdominal pressure, with standing next lowest, and sitting creating the highest pressure. Activities such as coughing or straining create extremely high pressure, although for a short duration (Twardowski et al., 1986). Patients at risk for development of hernias should be instructed to avoid activities that create high pressures, such as heavy lifting. Should such activity be unavoidable, it would be preferable for the patient to engage in these activities with an empty peritoneal cavity. Exercise to strengthen abdominal muscles may be effective, if a suitable program can be developed and the patient is willing to comply. Since increased intra-abdominal pressure is one of the key factors predisposing to recurrent hernia, nursing interventions should focus on minimizing this pressure. Patients generally tolerate larger exchange volumes at night while supine with fewer symptoms of discomfort than the same volume while upright.

Hemorrhoids may occur or be aggravated by the increase in intra-abdominal pressure. Nursing measures to prevent constipation are indicated to minimize straining and the emergence of hemorrhoids. Local treatment of hemorrhoids to reduce swelling and relieve symptoms may also be required, and severe cases can be surgically treated.

Likewise, PD patients may experience gastrointestinal symptoms, such as dyspepsia, reflux, anorexia, and early satiety. Increased intra-abdominal pressure can predispose to reflux; the accompanying feeling of fullness may contribute to anorexia, and glucose absorption may promote early satiety. Diabetic PD patients may already suffer from decreased gastric motility (diabetic gastroparesis), with PD contributing to or exacerbating these symptoms. Patients can be advised to eat several smaller meals a day, or to plan meal times to allow eating while the peritoneum is empty or near empty, such as between exchanges or during the drain phase. Limiting fluid intake to allow use of lower dextrose concentration minimizes the glucose absorption and its negative effects on appetite.

Cardiopulmonary compromise in PD patients may occur. A decrease in cardiac output and stroke volume is thought to be related to changes in venous return from the increased intra-abdominal pressure. Pulmonary excursion can be impaired by the intra-abdominal pressure, and in cases where cardiopulmonary function is marginal to begin with, patients may become symptomatic. Decreased exchange volumes may diminish symptoms; however, it is important to maintain adequate dialysis. Despite these issues, continuous removal of fluid and wastes may be better tolerated by patients with decreased cardiac function than the rapid shifts associated with hemodialysis. Nursing interventions include frequent assessment of the patient's pulmonary status, including evaluation of skin color, pulmonary effort, use of accessory muscles for respirations, and any symptoms such as shortness of breath or a change in exercise tolerance. If symptoms of pulmonary disease worsen, an alternate dialysis modality such as HD may be better tolerated by the patient.

Miscellaneous Complications

Although infrequent, abdominal pain not related to a catheter placement procedure may occur. Sensations of rectal or suprapubic pain or discomfort may be related to the catheter itself; these sensations usually subside after some time for most patients. Rapid inflow of dialysis solution can contribute to abdominal discomfort, as can solution that is too hot or cold. Some patients are particularly sensitive, and may experience discomfort from the acidic pH of the dialysis solution or hypertonic solution. Nursing intervention is determined by the etiology of the discomfort. For patients experiencing discomfort from the catheter itself, instilling dialysis solution generally lessens symptoms. Slowing inflow rates, especially during initial exchanges, is effective in managing discomfort from rapid infusion. Alternating hypertonic exchanges with less concentrated dialysis solution diminishes symptoms; sodium bicarbonate can be added to dialysis solution if acidic pH is the cause of discomfort. Ensuring dialysis solution temperature within an acceptable range prior to infusion prevents pain as well as other sequelae from inappropriate temperature (Prowant & Gallagher, 1995).

Shoulder pain represents referred pain from the diaphragm, most commonly caused by the presence of air in the peritoneal cavity. In most cases, introduction of air occurs during the exchange procedure. Disconnect systems in widespread use require priming the tubing with dialysis solution prior to infusing each exchange to eliminate air from the system. Incomplete priming or omitting this step can result in air being introduced to the peritoneal cavity. Nursing procedures such as transfer tubing changes also require priming tubings to avoid introduction of air. Delivery systems with vents allow air to enter the system, and should be avoided. Another source of air in the peritoneal cavity is a bowel perforation. Assessment of a patient with shoulder pain includes evaluating for a history of known air infusion and reviewing exchange technique to determine if tubings are completely primed. An abdominal X-ray will demonstrate any free air present in the peritoneum. Catheter position can be determined to evaluate for mechanical irritation of the diaphragm, another potential cause of shoulder pain. Bowel perforation typically results in peritonitis, and is readily identified. To remove air, at the end of the dwell phase, the patient assumes a knee-chest position with the head down or a Trendelenburg position; the initiation of the drain (using standard procedure) follows. This maneuver encourages passive movement of the air toward the lower pelvis, near the position of the tip of the peritoneal catheter, and the fluid outflow facilitates removal of the air through the catheter. Follow-up teaching to prevent reaccumulation of the air is indicated and generally well received once relief of shoulder pain is accomplished.

Back pain can result from the alteration in body mechanics associated in the increased abdominal volume and its associated weight. Individuals with weak musculature, poor posture, or neuromuscular disease are at high risk for back pain. Renal osteodystrophy or other types of bone disease can also contribute to symptoms of back pain. Interventions include encouraging proper body mechanics and body alignment and promoting good posture. Strengthening exercises may be helpful in some cases. Minimizing exchange volume decreases strain, but it may not be possible to achieve adequate dialysis. Use of IPD, with fluid dwelling while the patient is supine, reduces back strain, and may be an acceptable alternative.

Acute hydrothorax can result from structural defects in the diaphragm (Boeschoten et al., 1987). A pre-existing structural defect or weakness in the diaphragm, coupled with the normally negative intra-thoracic pressure and the increased intra-abdominal pressure created by PD can result in movement of dialysis solution from the peritoneal to the thoracic cavity. Signs and symptoms imitate those of a pleural effusion, with rapid shallow respirations, diminished breath sounds on the affected side, and X-ray evidence of the presence of fluid around the lung. A diagnostic thoracentesis would produce fluid high in glucose, and of similar chemical composition of dialysis effluent. Treatment of severe pleural effusions requires discontinuation of PD. Resolution of symptoms is generally rapid, but severe cases may require therapeutic thoracentesis to relieve pressure on the lung and restore adequate gas exchange. Repair of the structural defect may be necessary before resumption of PD, either through surgical intervention or via pleurodesis (Posen & Sachs, 1979). Nursing care includes careful monitoring of respiratory status.

Alterations in fluid volume are common complications with peritoneal dialysis. Hypovolemia occurs when too much fluid volume is removed by the PD or when intake is inadequate. Volume overload is the result of excessive intake or inadequate volume removal. Volume status of a PD patient is assessed in much the same manner as for any other patient, but special considerations should be considered. Intake and output records for an acute setting must reflect dialysis inflow and outflow volumes, in addition to oral and IV fluid intake and urinary and other drainage (nasogastric, wound drains, etc.) as output volumes. Daily weights are a useful tool for monitoring fluid balance, particularly in a chronic setting. PD fluid adds to the weight,

Table 22-25
Signs and symptoms of fluid volume status.

	Fluid Overload	Dehydration
Blood pressure	Generally increased No change or increases on standing	Generally decreased Orthostatic drop upon standing
Heart rate	Rate changes non-specific	Generally increased
Jugular vein	Full, distended	Flat
Tissue turgor	Full, may have pitting edema	Poor, skin lax and wrinkled
Weight	Increased	Decreased
Pulmonary	Diminished breath sounds, may have rales May have nonproductive cough	Clear breath sounds

and must be taken into account as part of the baseline weight for CAPD patients. Since the ultrafiltration volume varies with dextrose concentration and dwell time, it is recommended to weigh CAPD patients immediately following infusion of dialysis solution at the same time each day to minimize variables that contribute to fluctuations in weight. Many centers have CAPD patients weigh after infusing the first exchange each day. CCPD or IPD patients may weigh either with PD fluid dwelling or with an empty peritoneum; consistency is key for weight to be an accurate indicator of fluid balance trends.

Blood pressure (BP) is also useful to evaluate fluid balance. Sitting and standing BPs taken in succession can reveal an orthostatic drop in BP, potentially an early sign of hypovolemia. An important fact to remember is that many diabetic patients may have orthostatic BP drops unrelated to fluid volume. Both daily weights and BP readings are useful tools to evaluate fluid status of home patients.

Presence of fluid in the interstitial spaces, or edema, can also be an indication of volume status. Protein malnutrition can result in low serum albumin levels, which predispose to movement of fluid from the vascular space into the interstitial spaces, and may result in edema not directly related to volume overload. Again, individual patient trends are important. Patients can be taught to check for dependent edema, and to report changes to the appropriate health care professional. Table 22-25 summarizes signs and symptoms of fluid volume status.

Nursing interventions for volume overload require evaluation of the patient's current PD schedule, fluid intake, and dietary patterns. Adjustments may be needed in the dextrose concentration of dialysis solution used, with more hypertonic solutions to increase ultrafiltration and fluid removal. A decrease in oral fluid intake may help minimize the required fluid removal. Salt intake often drives thirst, making fluid restriction compliance difficult. Consult with the dietitian to assist the patient in identifying sources of sodium in the diet that may be driving fluid ingestion.

Loss of ultrafiltration can lead to volume overload. The exchange dextrose concentrations used and the drain volumes achieved need to be evaluated to determine if this is likely. Most home PD patients do not measure spent dialysate, but can tell the nurse if the bags are as full as usual. As mentioned previously, peritonitis causes increased membrane permeability, with associated rapid glucose absorption and decreased ultrafiltration. Determine if the PD effluent is clear when dealing with a home patient.

Nursing interventions for hypovolemia include an evaluation of the patient's oral intake, evaluation of all sources of fluid loss (diarrhea, sweat, emesis), and a review of PD dextrose concentrations used recently. Patients new to PD simply may be using inappropriate dextrose concentrations, resulting in fluid imbalances. Changes in dietary intake often require changes in the dextrose concentration of dialysis solution used; if no adjustment in PD solution is made, fluid imbalances can result. Advising the patient to alter the dextrose concentration being used is often all that is needed to correct fluid imbalances. During episodes of nausea or gastrointestinal distress, dehydration is more likely. Even in the absence of significant loss of fluid in the form of emesis, intake may be decreased with the potential for volume depletion. If hypovolemia is mild, use of salty food or broth to increase serum sodium and encourage thirst and fluid intake can address the fluid deficit. Broth is especially helpful, since it may be tolerated even with some mild nausea. More severe dehydration, particularly if associated with severe nausea or vomiting, may require use of antiemetic medications, IV fluids, or even hospitalization in rare cases. Nurses must collaborate with other members of the health care team to determine the underlying causes of volume status changes if these are not readily apparent. Some examples include (a) an underlying medical condition that is the source of symptoms; (b) depression, which can contribute to changes in dietary intake; and (c) a lack of understanding of the required dietary restrictions. Thus, the physician, nurse, dietitian, and social worker as a team are best equipped to identify the cause and develop a plan with the patient to avoid fluid imbalances in the future.

Documentation of patient teaching to minimize or avoid complications is an important nursing intervention. Graham-Macaluso (1991) published a concise review of information to teach patients to facilitate dealing with complications of PD, as well as sample care plans.

Metabolic Complications: PD Specific Considerations

Anemia is a common complication of CRF, although patients on PD typically have less severe anemia than those on HD. A number of factors are thought to contribute to the higher hemoglobin levels in PD patients. There is no blood loss associated with the treatment modality, as with intermittent HD treatment. Residual renal function has been shown to be preserved for a longer period of time in PD patients than in patients undergoing HD (Nolph, 1990; Schmidt, 1995), and perhaps this preservation of residual renal function includes the ability of the native kidneys to continue production of some endogenous erythropoietin. Fox et al. (1995) demonstrated a decrease in requirement for exogenous erythropoietin in PD patients with higher residual function and with enhanced peritoneal creatinine clearance. Due to the continuous or near continuous (daily) nature of PD, the level of uremic toxins remains lower than in HD during the interdialytic period (days between hemodialysis treatments). One hypothesis, called the "peak concentration hypothesis" (Keshaviah & Nolph, 1989) contends that the highest level of urea during an intermittent dialysis cycle is critical for determining toxicity, not the average level. Thus, continuous dialysis results in a lower peak of urea, and could contribute to higher hemoglobins by extending the life of the red blood cells. For PD patients who require medical management of their anemia, recombinant human erythropoietin (rHuEPO) and iron replacement therapy may be given, and rHuEPO can be given IV, IP, or subcutaneously (SC). IV administration, common in HD since blood access is already established, is rarely used in PD because IV access is not readily available. With IP administration of rHuEPO, not all of the drug may be absorbed by the end of the dwell time, resulting in loss in the effluent and resulting higher dosing requirements; therefore cost considerations make this route of administration impractical. As a result, SC is the most common route of rHuEPO administration in PD patients.

Endocrine and Reproductive Complications

A variety of endocrine disorders are associated with CRF. Three of primary concern are gonadotrophins and sexual function, reproduction, and growth hormone.

Nursing care for patients experiencing chronic illness such as renal failure should include addressing sexual functioning. Physiologic complications of the disease process influence the individual's sexual functioning, with abnormalities resulting from derangements of pituitary or gonadal hormones, psychologic problems, medications that affect sexual functioning, or from anemia or malnutrition commonly associated with CRF (Akmal, Bughi, & Kaptein, 1995). Circulating testosterone levels are generally decreased (Akmal et al.). Specific problems in sexual functioning include erectile dysfunction in men, and decreased libido in men and women. Using a multidisciplinary team approach, physicians, social workers, counselors, and clergy may assist nurses and patients in dealing with these issues.

Infertility is common in both men and women with chronic renal failure (CRF). Menstrual dysfunction is observed in over 90% of women with CRF, and over half of these are amenorrheic (Akmal et al., 1995). Most uremic women, including those with normal menstruation, have an anovular hormonal pattern. Despite this, Hou (1994) reports finding at least 68 case reports of pregnant women receiving dialysis for renal failure. She notes that although fertility is decreased in dialysis patients, it is common enough that contraceptive education should be provided to CRF patients of child-bearing age. Diagnosis of pregnancy in CRF patients can be difficult, since the more common symptoms of pregnancy (amenorrhea, nausea, fatigue) are often attributed to CRF. Complications such as hypertension and bleeding contribute to the 52% successful pregnancy rate reported by Hou. Intensive dialysis to keep blood chemistries as near normal as possible is recommended. Theoretically, the continuous nature of PD should enhance chances for a successful pregnancy, but this is yet to be substantiated by research.

Growth retardation in infants and children with renal insufficiency generally results in failure to reach optimal adult stature. Interference with normal growth patterns has been attributed to malnutrition, metabolic acidosis, anemia, and renal osteodystrophy. Correction of nutritional abnormalities has disappointingly little effect on growth (Tonshoff & Fine, 1995). Continuous forms of PD demonstrate an initial improvement in growth rates, but over time these growth patterns show a relative decline (Tonshoff & Fine). The impact of renal disease on growth depends largely on the age of the child at the onset of the disease. Infants have the most rapid growth rate normally, and are significantly affected by CRF. Onset of puberty is generally delayed in children with CRF, generally by about 2 years (Tonshoff & Fine). Recent work has also implicated alterations in the growth hormone/insulin-like growth factor axis. Introduction of recombinant human growth hormone (rhGH) therapy in 1988 has had promising initial results. Specifics related to optimal dosing at various stages of growth and development have yet to be established.

Diabetics maintained on PD may have blood glucose control by oral agents, SC insulin administration, or IP insulin administration. In determining the insulin requirements for a diabetic initiating dialytic therapy, several factors should be considered, such as (a) Will the correction of uremia and control of uremic symptoms have an impact on the individual's dietary intake? (b) Does dialysis remove some kind of "anti-insulin factor" rendering insulin more effective? and (c) What effect will the glucose load associated with PD have on blood glucose control? In a retrospective study of insulin requirements of dialysis patients, Grefberg et al. (1987) compared HD patients maintained on SC insulin, PD patients maintained on SC insulin, and PD patients maintained on IP insulin. They found no significant change in the insulin dose required with either the HD or PD patients using SC insulin, but did find a significant decrease in insulin dose requirements for PD patients on IP insulin. Additionally, the group using IP insulin demonstrated better metabolic control of blood glucose levels. One possible explanation is the likelihood that IP insulin is administered more frequently, usually 4 times daily and usually at or near mealtimes. Furthermore, IP insulin may enter the portal circulation either directly or more rapidly than when given SC, with a more efficient inhibitory action on hepatic glucose production.

Nutritional Status

Nutritional management in the CRF patient is addressed in detail in Chapter 10. PD patients present some specific nutritional issues that must be included when planning care for this population. Protein losses and glucose absorption must be considered when planning dietary interventions aimed at maintaining optimal nutrition for PD patients. Compared to HD, the dietary restrictions of fluid and electrolytes for PD may be more liberal, due largely to PD being a continuous or nearly continuous form of therapy.

Protein losses through the drained dialysate vary, but average between 5 and 15 grams per day (Shuler & Wolfson, 1994). Losses vary from one individual to another but tend to remain relatively constant in a given patient based on the peritoneal membrane permeability characteristics. Protein intake for peritoneal dialysis patients should be at least 1.2 grams per kilogram per day. It is important to recall that membrane permeability increases during an episode of peritonitis, with a resulting increased protein losses (from 50% to 100% of baseline), which may persist as long as several weeks following successful treatment of the peritonitis (Shuler & Wolfson, 1994). Appropriate increases in dietary protein intake should be advised during infectious episodes. Collaboration with the renal dietitian to address specific cases is invaluable.

Glucose absorption is directly proportional to the quantity infused; use of hypertonic exchanges increases the glucose load. On average, 70% of the glucose infused in the dialysis solution is absorbed. This caloric intake may be up to 30% of the daily total (Grodstein, Blumenkrantz, Kopple, Moran, & Coburn, 1981). Oral intake of carbohydrates may be decreased to compensate for this glucose absorption, and total non-protein caloric intake (including those calories from the dialysis solution) should range between 35 to 45 kilocalories per kilogram of ideal body weight (Shuler & Wolfson, 1994). Potential nutritional consequences of the glucose "load" associated with PD include weight gain and hyperlipidemia. A variety of approaches may be employed to manage weight gain, including fluid management to minimize use of hypertonic exchanges, dietary restrictions on caloric intake, and an exercise program based on the patient's overall clinical condition and exercise tolerance. Treatment of hyperlipidemia may require use of pharmacologic agents if use of hypertonic exchanges cannot be avoided and dietary interventions prove unsuccessful.

In general, potassium restrictions for PD patients are more liberal than for HD patients. In some instances, potassium may need to be supplemented for PD patients. Although potassium can be added to the dialysis solution, generally oral supplements are used to avoid hypokalemia; there is less risk of contamination and oral potassium supplements are less expensive than injectable potassium. Sodium and fluid restrictions typically are also more liberal than for HD. Phosphorus is poorly removed by PD, and requires continued dietary restriction as well as the use of phosphate binders, frequently calcium carbonate or calcium acetate. Patients must be instructed to take calcium with meals if it is intended as a phosphate binder because calcium preparations taken between meals increase serum calcium levels and have little effect on phosphorus absorption. A low calcium PD solution is available for use for patients prone to hypercalcemia, allowing better control of serum calcium levels.

Malnutrition in PD patients is of concern (Young et al., 1991). Marckmann (1988) estimates that 30-40% of all dialysis patients have some degree of malnutrition. The causes of malnutrition in PD patients are multifactorial. Inadequate dialysis may result in symptoms including nausea and vomiting. Underlying disease processes such as diabetes mellitus may predispose to delayed gastric emptying. Early satiety from glucose absorption and the full feeling from dialysis fluid in the abdomen may contribute to inadequate dietary intake. In an effort to avoid weight gain, some patients voluntarily decrease oral intake, resulting in inadequate intake of needed nutrients leading to malnutrition; other patients decrease oral intake without conscious effort, presumably related to early satiety. Depression secondary to the chronic disease state may result in decreased food intake in some patients. Malnutrition may be addressed through use of nutritional counseling, use of supplements, and, in severe cases, tube feedings. Intraperitoneal nutrition (IPN) refers to the use of amino acid dialysis solutions as a nutritional intervention strategy for PD patients suffering from malnutrition. Early studies have focused on tolerance and effect on biochemical parameters and ultrafiltration, as well as efficacy of therapy. Oren et al. (1983) studied 6 PD patients, alternating infusion of 1% amino acid containing dialysis solution with dialysis solution containing glucose. At the end of the 4-week trial, there was no significant change in fasting serum albumin levels. However, there was an increase in serum transferrin and total body nitrogen, prompting the conclusion that the nutritional status of these patients was improved. More recently, Bruno et al. (1989) conducted a similar study on 6 PD patients over a 6-month period, using one daily exchange of 1% amino acid dialysis solution. Measurements were taken prior to beginning the amino acid dialysis solution, during the trial period, and then 3 months after discontinuing use of amino acid solution in this long-term, cross-over study. Data indicated an improvement in nutritional status, evidenced by a positive nitrogen balance during the trial period that trended back towards baseline values after termination of the amino acid dialysis solution. Weight gain and slight worsening of systemic acidosis were the problems noted by these investigators. To date, widespread use of IPN has been limited by economic considerations; the amino acid solution is expensive with variable reimbursement, and not all nephrology professionals are convinced the use of IPN has enough of a positive effect to be considered cost-effective. Recent data on morbidity and mortality that demonstrate the significance of albumin levels and other nutritional indicators as predictors of hospitalization and death may have an impact on the future of IPN. Additional study is needed to determine if the use of IPN might avoid other, perhaps more costly events, such as hospitalization.

Patient Outcomes

Three major areas are considered when evaluating patient outcomes of PD. These include metabolic control, modality survival, and morbidity/mortality.

Metabolic Control

Peritoneal dialysis is capable of maintaining biochemical parameters within acceptable limits for most patients, as reviewed in the section of adequacy of PD. Despite the fact that PD as a modality delivers lower clearances than HD, overall control of biochemical parameters in many patients is essentially equivalent to that achieved by HD. As Blake (1996) notes, HD may initially appear "to be superior in that the total weekly small solute clearance delivered is typically 50–100% greater than PD" (p. 75), but the continuous clearance may be more efficient in removing different solutes. Although the intermittent nature of HD treatments lead to peaks and troughs in urea, creatinine, acid-base balance, and hydration, PD more closely resembles native renal function. The long-term clinical significance of this is unclear, but may prove important. Ronco et al. (1994) address the differences in intermittent and continuous dialysis, suggesting that in intermittent therapies, some body compartments are not cleared of wastes at all, resulting in a rebound of toxins. This explains the need for higher Kt/V values to reflect the same amount of solute removal and level of patient well being in intermittent therapies.

Modality Survival

The continuous nature of PD, although perhaps a clinical benefit, requires the patient or care giver to perform tasks several times daily. Over time, this can lead to fatigue or burn out. Historically, PD has experienced poor technique survival, particularly after 3 to 5 years. Maiorca, Cancarini, Brunori, Camerini, and Manili (1992) reviewed and reappraised studies on morbidity and mortality in CAPD, comparing it with HD. Method survival is better for HD. However, they concluded that the difference is completely accounted for by peritonitis; that is, once the patients who were switched from PD to HD as a result of peritonitis were removed from the analysis, technique survival for both HD and PD were the same. This echoes findings of Jindal and Hirsch (1994) whose 3-year study of 155 patients demonstrated an 86% technique survival rate. The primary cause for drop-out from CAPD was peritonitis, with only 1 patient transferring to HD as a result of inadequate dialysis on PD. In contrast, a report in *Nephrology News & Issues* ("Growth in PD," 1995) listed inadequate dialysis as the number one reason for discontinuing PD and switching to HD, followed by infectious complications. Interpretation of findings from studies on PD technique failure is compounded by inconsistent definitions. One study considered switching from a home form of PD to IPD as technique failure, even though the patient was still being dialyzed via the peritoneal membrane in-center (Jindal & Hirsch, 1994); other studies included as PD "drop-outs" only patients who no longer used any form of PD.

Psychologic factors may also contribute to technique failure and change in modality. Nissenson (1994) laments that quality of life in chronic PD patients has not been adequately assessed, citing lack of standardization of instruments used for measurement, no control groups, and short-term studies with small populations. Holley (1995) also notes that psychologic reasons for patient dropout from PD are not uniformly defined, but generally include patient choice, patient inability to cope, reduced mental ability, and noncompliance. PD patients using partners to perform their treatment were more likely to transfer from PD (33% compared to 25% 18 months after beginning treatment) (Holley). Nurses can assist patients in coping with stresses associated with daily self care by individualizing the therapy to integrate with the patient's lifestyle. Additional nursing research is needed to identify or develop a comprehensive instrument for measurement of factors contributing to quality of life, patient "burn-out," and noncompliance. Once this is occurs, nurses can explore interventions that might enhance modality survival and improve compliance.

Morbidity and Mortality

Morbidity (defined as rate of hospitalization) and mortality (death) of patients on PD is frequently compared to HD. To date, reported results comparing these treatment modalities conflict, with many reports indicating no difference between survival rates in the two patient groups, and others reporting an increased risk of death in PD patients, particularly older diabetics. Habach, Bloembergen, Mauger, Wolfe, and Port (1995) compared hospitalizations between patients treated with PD and HD, using data from the United States Renal Data Systems 1993 Annual Data Report. PD patient hospital admission rates were 14% higher than HD patient admission rates. The authors note additional study is needed to determine causes for hospitalization and the role of dialysis dose and patient selection. Transfer of modality is also more common in PD than in HD (Nissenson, 1994), but this finding may be explainable. In patients unwilling or unable to perform home PD, HD may be the only treatment alternative available. It is not surprising that patients who cannot be maintained on PD may choose and remain on HD rather than choosing no treatment and imminent death.

Death in patients on dialysis is related to a number of factors, including age, race, family history, number and severity of co-morbid conditions, nutritional status, and dialysis modality. Even within a given dialysis therapy, wide variations in dose of dialysis prescribed and patient compliance with prescribed treatment (dose of dialysis delivered) can confound the analysis and affect the outcomes. It is difficult to conclude which of the multiple variables has the major influence in determining the probability of patient death. Although lack of standardization makes comparing results from mortality studies difficult, a few trends are emerging. For PD patients, Avram, Mittman, Bonomini, Chattopadhyay, and Fein (1995) identified four independent predictors of mortality risk: age, diabetes, low serum albumin, and low serum creatinine. Older patients are at a higher risk of death. Diabetic PD patients have an increased risk of death because they have the effects of their diabetes as well as the consequences of CRF affecting their health status. Low serum albumin and other nutritional markers are rapidly becoming the biochemical markers most consistently identified as predictive of mortality in CRF patients, both PD and HD patients. Adequacy of dialysis and its effect on appetite has been postulated to be a factor in protein intake, thus influencing the serum albumin. Teehan, Schleifer, & Brown (1994) propose that the available studies, in aggregate, suggest survival of PD patients may be improved by higher doses of dialysis, noting higher doses of Kt/V are associated with higher protein intake. This information underscores the importance of working together as a multidisciplinary team (nurse, physician, dietitian, social worker, and patient) to address the multifaceted issues influencing patient survival on PD.

Blake (1996) points out that even well designed prospective studies comparing HD and PD will be of limited value, since each treatment is constantly improving. He observes that by the time data is collected, analyzed, and available, changes in efficacy of treatment may make it risky to generalize to the treatment modalities as currently practiced. Blake suggests viewing the two forms of dialysis "as complementary therapies, with many patients using one and then the other at different stages in their course of treatment" (p. 99). Individual patient characteristics, social situations, co-morbid conditions, and geographic factors may outweigh slight differences in mortality rates when considering the renal replacement therapy most appropriate for a given patient.

Summary

PD is a viable treatment option for individuals with CRF. Current challenges for those working in the therapy include finding ways to achieve adequate dialysis for patients with low peritoneal membrane permeability and those large patients whose clearance needs are great. Minimizing infectious complications, particularly those associated with catheter infections and loss, remains a challenge although progress is being made. Nurses need to be in the forefront of research to determine care techniques and educational strategies to encourage compliance in this primarily home patient population. Ongoing research will offer the clinician more information to better assist patients in achieving optimal outcomes with a PD regimen that fits their lifestyle.

References

Akmal, M., Bughi, S., & Kaptein, E. (1995). Endocrine dysfunction in chronic renal failure. In A.R. Nissenson, R.N. Fine, & D.E. Gentile (Eds.), *Clinical dialysis* (3rd ed., pp. 714-743). East Norwalk, CT: Appleton & Lange.

Albee, B. (1995). CAPD catheter exit site healing and clean dressing techniques. *ANNA Journal, 22,* 482-483.

Alexander, S.R., & Honda, M. (1993). Continuous peritoneal dialysis for children: A decade of worldwide growth and development. *Kidney International, 43* (Suppl. 40), S65-S74.

Alpert, M.A., Huting, J., Twardowski, Z.J., Khanna, R., & Nolph, K.D. (1995). Continuous ambulatory peritoneal dialysis and the heart. *Peritoneal Dialysis International, 15,* 6-11.

Anderson, K., & Anderson, L. (1994). *Mosby's pocket dictionary of medicine, nursing, & allied health* (2nd ed.). St. Louis: Mosby.

American Nephrology Nurses Association (ANNA). (1993). *Standards of clinical practice for nephrology nursing.* Pitman, NJ: Author.

Armstrong, S., & Zalatan, S.J. (1992). Microwave warming of peritoneal dialysis fluid. *ANNA Journal, 19,* 535-540.

Ash, S.R. (1993). Peritoneal access devices and placement techniques. In A.R. Nissenson & R.N. Fine (Eds.), *Dialysis therapy,* (2nd ed., pp. 23-27). Philadelphia: Hanley & Belfus.

Ash, S.R., Carr, D.J., & Diaz-Buxo, J.A. (1995). Peritoneal access devices: Hydraulic function and biocompatibility. In A.R. Nissenson, R.N. Fine, & D.E. Gentile (Eds.), *Clinical dialysis* (3rd ed., pp. 295-321). East Norwalk, CT: Appleton & Lange.

Ash, S.R., & Daugirdas, J.T. (1994). Peritoneal access devices. In J.T. Daugirdas & T.S. Ing (Eds.), *Handbook of dialysis* (2nd ed., pp. 274-300). Boston: Little, Brown and Company.

Avram, M.M., Mittman, N., Bonomini, L., Chattopadhyay, J., & Fein, P. (1995). Markers for survival in dialysis: A seven-year prospective study. *American Journal of Kidney Diseases, 26,* 209-219.

Baxter Renal Care. (1996). A look at worldwide use of peritoneal dialysis. *Nephrology News & Issues, 10*(4), 17–18.

Bernardini, J., Holley, J.L., Johnston, J.R., Perlmutter, J.A., & Piraino, B. (1991). An analysis of ten-year trends in infections in adults on continuous ambulatory peritoneal dialysis (CAPD). *Clinical Nephrology, 36*(1), 29-34.

Blake, P.G. (1996). Do mortality rates differ between hemodialysis and CAPD? A look at the Canadian vs. U.S. data. *Dialysis and Transplantation, 25*(2), 75-76, 79-80, 99.

Boeschoten, E.W., Krediet, R.T., Roos, C.M., Kloek, J.J., Schipper, M.E.I., & Arisz, L. (1987). An important complication of CAPD: Leakage of dialysate across the diaphragm. *Peritoneal Dialysis Bulletin, 7*(Suppl. 2), S6.

Brunier, G. (1995). Peritonitis in patients on peritoneal dialysis: A review of pathophysiology and treatment. *ANNA Journal, 22*, 575-584.

Bruno, M., Bagnis, C., Marangella, M., Rovera, L., Cantaluppi, A., & Linari, F. (1989). CAPD with an amino acid dialysis solution: A long-term, cross-over study. *Kidney International, 35,* 1189-1194.

Burkart, J.M. (1994). Adequacy of peritoneal dialysis. In W.L. Henrich (Ed.), *Principles and practice of dialysis* (pp. 111-129). Baltimore: W.L. Williams & Wilkins.

Burkart, J.M. (1995). Avoiding inadequate dialysis in long-term peritoneal dialysis patients. *Seminars in Dialysis, 8,* 336-342.

CANUSA Peritoneal Dialysis Study Group. (1992). Canada-USA (CANUSA) multicentre study of peritoneal dialysis adequacy: Description of the study population and preliminary results. *Advances in Peritoneal Dialysis, 8,* 88-92.

CANUSA Peritoneal Dialysis Study Group. (1996). Adequacy of dialysis and nutrition in continuous peritoneal dialysis: Association with clinical outcomes. *Journal of the American Society of Nephrology, 7,* 198-207.

Coles, G.A. (1995). Towards a more physiologic solution for peritoneal dialysis. *Seminars in Dialysis, 8,* 333-335.

Dasgupta, M.K. (1995). The role of new catheters in avoiding infections in peritoneal dialysis patients. *Seminars in Dialysis, 8,* 362-366.

della Volpe, M., Iberti, M., Ortensia, A., & Veronesi, G. (1984). Erosion of the sigmoid by a permanent peritoneal catheter. *Peritoneal Dialysis Bulletin, 4,* 108.

Devins, G.M., & Binik, Y.M. (1996). Predialysis psychoeducational interventions: Establishing collaborative relationships between health service providers and recipients. *Seminars in Dialysis, 9,* 51-55.

Diaz-Buxo, J.A. (1995). Clinical use of peritoneal dialysis. In A.R. Nissenson, R.N. Fine, & D.E. Gentile (Eds.), *Clinical dialysis* (3rd ed., pp. 376-425). East Norwalk, CT: Appleton & Lange.

Diaz-Buxo, J.A. (1996). Patient selection and the success of peritoneal dialysis. *Nephrology News & Issues, 10*(3), 17-18.

Doyle, C. (1996, May) Peritoneal dialysis catheter exit site infections: A challenge for nursing. In *Integrating research and practice for optimal clinical outcomes.* Symposium conducted at the ANNA 27th National Symposium, Anaheim, CA.

Fine, R.N., & Tejani, A. (1994). Dialysis in infants and children. In J.T. Daugirdas & T.S. Ing (Eds.), *Handbook of dialysis* (2nd ed., pp. 553-568). Boston: Little, Brown, and Company.

Fishman, A., Kroop. I., Leijer, H., & Hyman, A. (1949). Experiences with the Kolff artificial kidney. *American Journal of Medicine, 7,* 15-34.

Fox, L., & Tzamaloukas, A.H. (1994). Infections in patients on continuous ambulatory peritoneal dialysis. In W.L. Henrich (Ed.), *Principles and practice of dialysis* (pp. 437-456). Baltimore: Williams & Wilkins.

Fox, L., Tzamaloukas, A.H., Antoniou, S., Katsoudas, S., Tzouganatou, A., Chisam, G., Goldman, R., Kakavas, J., Dimitriadis, A., Nicolopoulou, N., Symboulidou-Mayopoulou, T., Balaskas, E.V., Kyriazopoulos, G., Voudiklari, S., Dombros, N., & Murata, G.H. (1995). Cross-sectional analysis of erythropoietin use in CPD: Its relation to azotemic index clearances. In R. Khanna (Ed.), *Advances in peritoneal dialysis, Vol. 11* (pp. 243—46). Toronto: Peritoneal Dialysis Publications.

Ganter, G. (1950). About the elimination of poisonous substances from the blood by dialysis. *Munch Med Wchnschr,* 1478-1480.

Gotch, F.A., & Keen, M.L. (1995). Kinetic modeling in peritoneal dialysis. In A.R. Nissenson, R.N. Fine, & D.E. Gentile (Eds.), *Clinical dialysis* (3rd ed., pp. 343-375). East Norwalk, CT: Appleton & Lange.

Gotch, F.A., & Sargent, J.A. (1985). A mechanistic analysis of the National Cooperative Dialysis Study (NCDS). *Kidney International, 28,* 526-534.

Gray, H. (1977). The peritoneum. In T.P. Pick & R. Howden (Eds.), *Gray's anatomy classic collector's edition* (pp. 897-905). New York: Bounty Books.

Graham-Macaluso, M.M. (1991). Complications of peritoneal dialysis: Nursing care plans to document teaching. *ANNA Journal, 18,* 479-483, 491.

Grefberg, N., Danielson, B.G., Nilsson, P., & Berne, C. (1987). Decreasing insulin requirements in CAPD patients given intraperitoneal insulin. *The Journal of Diabetic Complications, 1,* 16-19.

Grodstein, G.P., Blumenkrantz, M.J., Kopple, J.D., Moran, J.K., & Coburn, J.W. (1981). Glucose absorption during continuous ambulatory peritoneal dialysis. *Kidney International, 19,* 564-567.

Growth in PD seen worldwide. (1995). *Nephrology News & Issues, 9*(9), 19.

Guyton, A.C. (1976). *Textbook of medical physiology* (5th ed.). Philadelphia: W.B. Saunders.

Habach, G., Bloembergen, W.E., Mauger, E.A., Wolfe, R.A., & Port, F.K. (1995). Hospitalization among United States dialysis patients: Hemodialysis versus peritoneal dialysis. *Journal of the American Society of Nephrology, 5,* 1940-1948.

Holden, A.L., & Gaumer, G. (1987). Best demonstrated practices program promoting CAPD patients retention in the United States. In R. Khanna, K.D. Nolph, B.F. Prowant, Z.J. Twardowski, & D.G. Oreopoulos (Eds.), *Advances in continuous ambulatory peritoneal dialysis Vol. 3* (pp. 186-191). Toronto: Peritoneal Dialysis Bulletin.

Holley, J.L. (1995). Psychological factors causing technique failure in continuous peritoneal dialysis: The patient and the health care providers. *Seminars in Dialysis, 8,* 395-396.

Holmes, C.J. (1993). Abnormalities of host defense mechanisms during peritoneal dialysis. In A.R. Nissenson & R.N. Fine (Eds.), *Dialysis therapy* (2nd ed., pp. 161-165). Philadelphia: Hanley & Belfus, Inc.

Hospital Infection Control Practices Advisory Committee (HICPAC). (1995). Recommendations for preventing the spread of vancomycin resistance. *Infection Control and Hospital Epidemiology, 16,* 105-113.

Hou, S. (1993). Pregnancy and birth control in CAPD patients. *Advances in Peritoneal Dialysis, 9,* 173-176.

Jindal, K.K., & Hirsch, D.J. (1994). Excellent technique survival on home peritoneal dialysis: Results of a regional program. *Peritoneal Dialysis International, 14,* 324-326.

Keane, W.F., Everett, E.D., Golper, T.A., Gokal, R., Halstenson, C., Kawaguchi, Y., Riella, M., Vas, S., & Verbrugh, H.A. (1993). Peritoneal dialysis-related peritonitis treatment recommendations 1993 update. *International Society for Peritoneal Dialysis, 13,* 14-28.

Keshaviah, P.R. (1995). Technological aspects of hemodialysis and peritoneal dialysis. In A.R. Nissenson, R.N. Fine, & D.E. Gentile (Eds.), *Clinical dialysis* (3rd ed., pp. 46-76). East Norwalk, CT: Appleton & Lange.

Keshaviah, P.R., & Nolph, K.D. (1989). The peak concentration hypothesis: A urea kinetic approach to comparing the adequacy of continuous ambulatory peritoneal dialysis (CAPD) and hemodialysis. *Peritoneal Dialysis International, 9,* 257-260.

Keshaviah, P.R., Nolph, K.D., Prowant, B., Moore, H., Ponferrada, L., Van Stone, J., Twardowski, Z.J., & Khanna, R. (1990). Defining adequacy of CAPD with urea kinetics. In R. Khanna, K.D. Nolph, B.F. Prowant, Z.J. Twardowski, & D.G. Oreopoulos (Eds.), *Advances in Peritoneal Dialysis , 6,* 173-177.

Khanna, R. (1990). Acute management of the patient requiring a chronic peritoneal dialysis catheter. *Seminars in Dialysis, 3*(2), 93-99.

Leehey, D.J., Gandhi, V.C., & Daugirdas, J.T. (1994). Peritonitis and exit site infection. In J.T. Daugirdas & T.S. Ing (Eds.), *Handbook of dialysis* (2nd ed., pp. 338-362). Boston: Little, Brown and Company.

Lefton, C.K. (1995). Fighting infection with new technology applied to catheters. *Nephrology News & Issues, 9*(2), 18-19, 39.

Linblad, A.S., Hamilton, R.W., Nolph, K.D., & Novak, J.W. (1988). A retrospective analysis of catheter configuration and cuff type: A national CAPD registry report. *Peritoneal Dialysis International, 8,* 129-133.

Luzar, M.A., Brown, C.B., Balf, D., Hill, L., Issad, B., Monnier, B., Moulart, J., Sabatier, J.C., Wauquier, J.P., & Peluso, F. (1990). Exit-site care and exit-site infection in continuous ambulatory peritoneal dialysis (CAPD): Results of a randomized multicenter trial. *Peritoneal Dialysis International, 10,* 25-29.

Maiorca, R., Cancarini, G.C., Brunori, G., Camerini, C., & Manili, L. (1992). Morbidity and mortality of CAPD and hemodialysis. *Kidney International, 40* (Suppl.), S4-S15.

Marckmann, P. (1988). Nutritional status of patients on hemodialysis and peritoneal dialysis. *Clinical Nephrology, 29,* 75-78.

McCann, L. (1996). Subjective global assessment as it pertains to the nutritional status of dialysis patients. *Dialysis & Transplantation, 25,* 190, 192-196, 198-199, 202, 225.

Moncrief, J.W., Popovich, R.P., Broadrick, L.J., He, Z.Z., Simmons, E.E., & Tate, R.A. (1993). The Moncrief-Popovich catheter: A new access technique for patients on peritoneal dialysis. *ASAIO Transactions, 39,* 62-65.

Moore, C.G. (1989). Comparison of Blisterfilm® and gauze for peritoneal catheter exit site care. *ANNA Journal, 16,* 475-478.

Nissenson, A.R. (1994). Measuring, managing, and improving quality in the end-stage renal disease treatment setting: Peritoneal dialysis. *American Journal of Kidney Diseases, 24,* 368-375.

Nolph, K.D. (1990). Is residual renal function preserved better with CAPD than with hemodialysis? *AKF Nephrology Letter, 7*(1), 1-4.

Nolph, K.D. (1991). Quantitating peritoneal dialysis delivery: A required stand of care. *Seminars in Dialysis, 4*(3), 139-141.

Nolph, K.D. (1992). What's new in peritoneal dialysis – An overview. *Kidney International, 42* (Suppl. 38), S148-S152.

Nolph, K.D., Miller, RF., Rubin, J., & Popovich, R.P. (1980). New directions in peritoneal dialysis concepts and applications. *Kidney International, 18* (Suppl 10), S111-S116.

Oren, A., Wu, G., Anderson, G.H., Marliss, E., Khanna, R., Pettit, J., Mupas, L., Rodella, H., Brandes, L., Roncari, D., Kakis, G., Harrison, J., McNeil, K., & Oreopoulos, D. (1983). Effective use of amino acid dialysate over four weeks in CAPD patients. *Peritoneal Dialysis Bulletin, 3,* 66-73.

Park, M.S., Lee, E.Y., Cha, M.K., Kim, J.H., Song, K.I., Han, D.C., Hwang, S.D., Moon, C., & Lee, H.B. (1995). Effect of prolonged subcutaneous implantation of peritoneal catheters in peritonitis rate during CAPD. *International Society of Blood Purification, 13* (Suppl 1), S32.

Piraino, B. (1990). A review of *Staphylococcus aureus* exit site and tunnel infections in peritoneal dialysis patients. *American Journal of Kidney Disease, 16,* 89-95.

Piraino, B. (1995). Infections in peritoneal dialysis. In A.R. Nissenson, R.N. Fine, & D.E. Gentile (Eds.) *Clinical dialysis* (3rd ed., pp. 426-449). East Norwalk, CT: Appleton & Lange.

Piraino, B., Bernardini, J., Johnston, J., & Sorkin, M. (1987). Chemical peritonitis due to intraperitoneal vancomycin. *Peritoneal Dialysis Bulletin, 7*(Suppl.), S59.

Piraino, B., Bernardini, J., & Sorkin, M. (1988). Bagless CAPD improves catheter infection rate. *Kidney International, 35,* 275.

Piraino, B., & Faller, B. (1995). The prevention of *Staphylococcus aureus* peritoneal dialysis-related infections. *Seminars in Dialysis, 8,* 355-358.

Ponferrada, L.P., & Prowant, B.F. (1996, May). Enhancing adequacy to promote successful peritoneal dialysis. In *Integrating research and practice for optimal clinical outcomes.* Symposium conducted at the ANNA 27th National Symposium, Anaheim, CA.

Ponferrada, L.P., Prowant, B.F., Schmidt, L.M., Burrows, L.M., Satalowich, R.J., & Bartelt, C. (1993). Home visit effectiveness for peritoneal dialysis patients. *ANNA Journal, 20,* 333-336.

Ponferrada, L.P., & Van Stone, J.C. (1995). Peritoneal dialysis kinetics. *Advances in Renal Replacement Therapy, 2,* 341-348.

Popovich, R.P., Pyle, W.K., Rosenthal, D.A., Alexander, S.R., Balfe, J.W., & Moncrief, J.W. (1981). Kinetics of peritoneal dialysis in children. In J.W. Moncrief & R.P. Popovich (Eds.), *CAPD update* (p. 227). New York: Masson Publishers.

Port, F.K., Held, P.J., Nolph, K.D., Turenne, M.N., & Wolfe, R.A. (1992). Risk of peritonitis and technique failure by CAPD connection technique: A national study. *Kidney*

International, 42, 967-974.

Posen, G.A., & Sachs, H.J. (1979). Treatment of recurrent pleural effusions in dialysis patients by talc insufflation. *American Society of Artificial Internal Organs, 8,* 75.

Powe, N.R., Klag, M.J., Sadler, J.H., Anderson, G.F., Bass, E.B., Bringgs, W.A., Fink, N.E., Levey, A.S., Levin, N.W., Meyer, K.B., Rubin, H.R., & Wu, A.W. (1996). Choices for healthy outcomes in caring for end stage renal disease. *Seminars in Dialysis, 9,* 9-11.

Protic, J., & Hardy, D. (1993). Resurgence of tuberculosis and emergence of multidrug-resistant strains: Implications for healthcare personnel. In *Plant technology & safety management series: Controlling occupational exposure to tuberculosis.* Oak Brook Terrace, IL: Joint Commission on Accreditation of Healthcare Organizations.

Prowant, B.F., & Gallagher, N.M. (1995). Peritoneal dialysis. In L.E. Lancaster (Ed.), *Core curriculum for nephrology nursing* (3rd ed., pp. 281-322). Pitman, NJ: American Nephrology Nurses' Association.

Prowant, B.F., & Schmidt, L.M. (1991). The peritoneal equilibration test: A nursing discussion. *ANNA Journal, 18,* 361-366.

Prowant, B.F., Schmidt, L.M., Twardowski, Z.J., Griebel, C., Burrows, L.M., Ryan, L.P., & Satalowich, R.J. (1988). Peritoneal dialysis catheter exit site care. *ANNA Journal, 15,* 219-223.

Prowant, B.F., & Twardowski, Z.J. (1996). Recommendations for exit care. *Peritoneal Dialysis International, 16*(Suppl 3), S94-S99.

Rodby, R.A., & Korbet, S.M. (1994). Causes, diagnosis, and treatment of peritoneal membrane failure. In W.L. Henrich (Ed.), *Principles and practice of dialysis* (pp. 130-147). Baltimore: Williams & Wilkins.

Ronco, C., Conz, P., Bosch, J., Lew, S., & La Greca, G. (1994). Assessment of adequacy in peritoneal dialysis. *Advances in Renal Replacement Therapy, 1,* 15-23.

Schleifer, C.R., Teehan, B.P., Brown, J.M., & Raimondo, J. (1993). The application of urea kinetic modeling to peritoneal dialysis: A review of methodology and outcome. *Journal of Renal Nutrition, 3,* 2-9.

Schmidt, L.M., & Prowant, B.F. (1991). How to do a peritoneal equilibration test. *ANNA Journal, 18,* 368-370.

Schmidt, R.J. (1995). Residual renal function in peritoneal dialysis patients. *Seminars in Dialysis, 8,* 343-346.

Selgas, R., Bajo, M.A., Del Peso, G., & Jimenez, C. (1995). Preserving the peritoneal dialysis membrane in long-term peritoneal dialysis patients. *Seminars in Dialysis, 8,* 326-332.

Shuler, C.L., & Wolfson, M. (1994). Malnutrition and intradialytic parenteral nutrition in ESRD subjects. In W.L. Henrich (Ed.), *Principles and practice of dialysis* (pp. 277-286). Baltimore: Williams & Wilkins.

Sorkin, M.I., & Diaz-Buxo, J.A. (1994). Physiology of peritoneal dialysis. In J.T. Daugirdas & T.S. Ing (Eds.), *Handbook of dialysis* (2nd ed., pp. 245-261). Boston: Little, Brown, & Company.

Steiner, E.W. (1993). Abdominal catastrophes, peritoneal eosinophilia, and other unusual events in peritoneal dialysis patients. In A.R. Nissenson & R.N. Fine (Eds.), *Dialysis therapy* (2nd ed., pp. 181-185). Philadelphia: Hanley & Belfus, Inc.

Teehan, B.P., Schleifer, C.R., & Brown, J. (1994). Adequacy of continuous ambulatory peritoneal dialysis: Morbidity and mortality in chronic peritoneal dialysis. *American Journal of Kidney Diseases, 24,* 990-1001.

Tenckhoff, H., & Schechter, H. (1968). A bacterial safe peritoneal access device. *ASAIO Transactions, 15,* 181.

Tonshoff, B., & Fine, R.N. (1995). Growth and growth hormone treatment in children with chronic renal insufficiency. In A.R. Nissenson, R.N. Fine, & D.E. Gentile (Eds.) *Clinical dialysis* (3rd ed., pp. 549-573). East Norwalk, CT: Appleton & Lange.

Twardowski, Z.J. (1990). The fast peritoneal equilibration test. *Seminars in Dialysis, 3,* 141-142.

Twardowski, Z.J. (1995). Physiology of peritoneal dialysis. In A.R. Nissenson, R.N. Fine, & D.E. Gentile (Eds.) *Clinical dialysis* (3rd ed., pp. 322-342). East Norwalk, CT: Appleton & Lange.

Twardowski, Z.J., Burrows, L.M., & Prowant, B.F. (1984). Individualization of exchange volume. *Peritoneal Dialysis Bulletin, 4* (Suppl 3), S134-S136.

Twardowski, Z.J., Khanna, R., Nolph, K.D., Scalamonga, A., Metzler, M.H., Schneider, T.W., Prowant, B.F., & Ryan, L.P. (1986). Intraabdominal pressure during natural activities in patients treated with continuous ambulatory peritoneal dialysis. *Nephron, 44,* 129-135.

Twardowski, Z.J., Nolph, K.D., Khanna, R., Prowant, B.F., Moore, H.L., & Nielsen, M.P. (1987). Peritoneal equilibration test. *Peritoneal Dialysis Bulletin, 7,* 138-147.

Twardowski, Z.J., Nolph, K.D., Khanna, R., Prowant, B.F., Ryan, L.P., & Nichols, W.K. (1985). The need for a "Swanneck" permanently bent arcuate peritoneal dialysis catheter. *Peritoneal Dialysis Bulletin, 5,* 219-223.

Twardowski, Z.J., Prowant, B.F., Nichols, W.K., Nolph, K.D., & Khanna, R. (1992). Six-year experience with swan neck catheters. *Peritoneal Dialysis International, 12,* 384-389.

Twardowski, Z.J., & Prowant, B.F. (1996a). Appearance and classification of healing peritoneal catheter exits sites. *Peritoneal Dialysis International, 16*(Suppl 3), S71-S93).

Twardowski, Z.J., & Prowant, B.F. (1996b). Exit-site healing post catheter implantation. *Peritoneal Dialysis International, 16*(Suppl. 3), S51-S70.

Vanholder, R., Van Loo, A., De Smet, R., & Ringoir, S. (1995). Host defense and infection in dialysis patients. In A.R. Nissenson, R.N. Fine, & D.E. Gentile (Eds.), *Clinical dialysis* (3rd ed., pp. 450-482). East Norwalk, CT: Appleton & Lange.

Vas, S.I. (1993). Peritonitis in peritoneal dialysis patients. In A.R. Nissenson & R.N. Fine (Eds.), *Dialysis therapy* (2nd ed., pp. 168-171). Philadelphia: Hanley & Belfus, Inc.

Wadhwa, N.K., Kenward, D.H., Kennedy, B., & Rowe, S.M. (1983). Heating of peritoneal dialysis fluid by a microwave oven in hospital practice – A method of choice. *Peritoneal Dialysis Bulletin, 3,* 187-188.

Walshe, J.J., & Morse, G.D. (1990). Infectious complications of peritoneal dialysis. In A.R. Nissenson, R.N. Fine, & D.E. Gentile, *Clinical dialysis* (2nd ed., pp. 301-318). Norwalk, CT: Appleton & Lange.

Wilkie, D.P.D. (1911). Some functions and surgical uses of omentum. *British Medical Journal, 2,* 1103-1106.

Williams, P.F., Marliss, E.B., Anderson, G.H., Oren, A., Stein, A.N., Khanna, R., Petitt, J., Brandes, L., Rodella, H., Mupas, L., Dombros, N., & Oreopoulos, D.G. (1982). Amino acid absorption following intraperitoneal administration in CAPD patients. *Peritoneal Dialysis Bulletin, 2,* 124-130.

Wiseman, K.C. (1995). Tuberculosis: An old disease with a new face. *ANNA Journal, 22,* 541-554.

Young, G.A., Kopple, J.D., Lindholm, B., Vonesh, E.F., DeVecchi, A., Castelnova, C., Oreopoulos, D.G., Anderson, G.H., Bergstrom, J., DiChiro, J., Gentile, D., Nissenson, A., Sakhrani, L., Brownjohn, A.M., Nolph, K.D., Prowant, B.F., Algrim, C.E., Martis, L., & Serkes, K.D. (1991). Nutritional assessment of continuous ambulatory peritoneal dialysis patients: An international study. *American Journal of Kidney Diseases, 17,* 462-471.

Zabetakis, P.M., Krapf, R., DeVita, M.V., Gleim, G.W., & Michelis, M.F. (1993). Determining peritoneal dialysis prescriptions by employing a patient-specific protocol. *Peritoneal Dialysis International, 13,* 189-193.

Zappacosta, A.R. (1993). Complications of acute peritoneal catheter insertion. In A.R. Nissenson & R.N. Fine (Eds.), *Dialysis therapy* (2nd ed., pp. 28-30). Philadelphia: Hanley & Belfus, Inc.

Zawada, E.T. (1994). Indications for dialysis. In J.T. Daugirdas & T.S. Ing (Eds.), *Handbook of dialysis* (2nd ed., pp. 3-9). Boston: Little, Brown, & Company.

Chapter Highlights

- Many factors influence modality selection, including medical considerations, number and severity of co-morbid conditions, age, cultural and lifestyle issues, self-care ability, financial reimbursement issues and health care delivery systems, and personal preference.

- The peritoneal membrane is a serous membrane consisting of two layers: the visceral peritoneum covering the abdominal organs and the parietal peritoneum lining the outer walls of the abdominal cavity (Guyton, 1976)

- The primary purpose of the peritoneum is to provide a smooth contact surface between the abdominal wall and the intra-abdominal organs, with approximately 100 milliliters (ml) of transudate present under normal circumstances to facilitate movement of the peritoneal layers.

- The permeability of the tissue between the peritoneal capillary lumen and the peritoneal cavity filled with dialysis solution varies among individuals; these characteristics can and should be determined to select an appropriate PD prescription

- The principal barriers to use of amino acid solutions are cost and metabolic acidosis. Thus, alternatives to dextrose as the osmotic agent in PD solution are not in widespread use. This is an area where research may be of significance in the future, to help determine if there is a group of patients for whom the additional cost of amino acid dialysis solution would be beneficial overall, if risk of malnutrition, hospitalizations, or death could be decreased.

- Peritoneal dialysis exchange consists of three phases: (a) *infusion* of dialysis solution into the peritoneal cavity, (b) allowing the solution to remain in the cavity or *dwell*, and (c) allowing the dialysate to *drain* out of the peritoneum.

- When a patient reaches chronic renal failure and a renal replacement therapy is required to sustain life, a number of factors may influence the choice of treatment modality. These include clinical and functional factors, cost considerations, and lifestyle or patient preference.

- Alpert, Huting, Twardowski, Khanna, and Nolph (1995) reviewed 46 studies relating to CAPD and the heart, and concluded that CAPD can decrease left ventricular volume, improve left ventricular function in some patients, and produce symptomatic improvement in patients with refractory congestive heart failure.

- Factors that promote healing include proper positioning of the external cuff, approximately 1 cm–2 cm from the skin (2 cm–3 cm in obese individuals); securing the external segment of the catheter to avoid tension on the cuff; directing the tunnel segment either laterally or downward; and peri-procedural administrating systemic antibiotics (Albee, 1995).

- The elements of the PD prescription include number of dialysis exchanges per day, volume of each exchange, timing of the exchanges (dwell time), dextrose concentrations of PD solution used, and the integration of the dialysis regimen into the patient's lifestyle. Each element of the PD prescription listed can be manipulated to facilitate optimal dialysis.

- *Adequate* refers to the amount of dialysis required to avoid untoward outcomes, while *optimal* dialysis indicates additional dialytic therapy would offer no benefit. Inadequate dialysis has been associated with an increase in morbidity (hospitalizations) and mortality (death).

- Findings recently published (CANUSA Peritoneal Dialysis Study Group, 1996) indicate 680 patients were enrolled; a weekly Kt/V of 2.1 and a weekly creatinine clearance of 70 L per 1.73 meters squared were associated with an expected 2-year survival rate of 78%. A decrease of 0.1 unit Kt/V per week was associated with a 5% increase in the relative risk of death; likewise, a decrease of 5L/1.73 meters squared creatinine clearance was associated with a 7% increase in relative risk of death.

- Burkart (1994) suggests clinical assessment of adequacy of dialysis consists not only of the absence of signs or symptoms of uremia, but also control of blood pressure, anemia and other biochemical parameters, and the patient's subjective sense of well being.

Chapter Highlights (continued)

- Gotch and Sargent (1985) developed the concept of Kt/V, where K is the urea clearance, t the treatment time, and V the volume of urea distribution in the hemodialysis setting. Keshaviah et al. (1990) applied these indices to peritoneal dialysis patients.
- The concept of Kt/V is to determine the removal or clearance (K) of this waste (urea) from the patient's total body water (V) over a period of time (t).
- Individualization of PD therapy has two major goals: (a) to determine what prescription achieved adequate dialysis for the individual patient based on physical factors such as size, dietary intake, residual renal function, and peritoneal membrane characteristics; and (b) to develop a dialysis prescription that the patient is willing and able to carry out on a daily basis.
- In general, patients with highly permeable peritoneal membranes benefit from shorter dwell times and either more frequent exchanges or IPD to maximize clearance while still achieving adequate ultrafiltration for fluid control. A long dwell time for patients with high permeability of the membrane results in small outflow volumes, little clearance (due to the low outflow volume), with no net ultrafiltration or even fluid absorption.
- Patients with low peritoneal membrane permeability need longer dwell times to allow time for solutes to cross the peritoneal membrane and enter the dialysis solution; short dwell times for these patients results in large drain volumes but little solute clearance and potentially inadequate dialysis.
- Over time, residual renal function has been documented to continue to decline. Although this occurs more slowly in patients on PD than those on HD (Schmidt, 1995), it does occur.
- Bio-incompatibility of dialysis solution is thought to contribute to membrane changes over time, as are repeated episodes of peritonitis.
- Infection is the primary complication associated with PD. The most common infections include peritonitis, soft tissue infections of the catheter exit site, and subcutaneous tunnel infections.
- Many advances have significantly lowered the incidence of peritonitis, but it remains the leading cause of catheter loss, transfer to HD (temporarily or permanently), and a major cause of hospitalization for PD patients.
- *Recurrent peritonitis* is reappearance of symptoms within 2 weeks of the completion of antibiotic therapy with the same organism (and same antibiotic sensitivities) on culture.
- Cardiopulmonary compromise in PD patients may occur. A decrease in cardiac output and stroke volume is thought to be related to changes in venous return from the increased intra-abdominal pressure.
- It is important to recall that membrane permeability increases during an episode of peritonitis, with a resulting increased protein losses (from 50% to 100% of baseline), which may persist as long as several weeks following successful treatment of the peritonitis.
- Death in patients on dialysis is related to a number of factors, including age, race, family history, number and severity of co-morbid conditions, nutritional status, and dialysis modality. Even within a given dialysis therapy, wide variations in dose of dialysis prescribed and patient compliance with prescribed treatment (dose of dialysis delivered) can confound the analysis and affect the outcomes. It is difficult to conclude which of the multiple variables has the major influence in determining the probability of patient death.
- Low serum albumin and other nutritional markers are rapidly becoming the biochemical markers most consistently identified as predictive of mortality in CRF patients, both PD and HD patients.

CHAPTER 23

Transplantation: Introduction and Historical Perspectives

Christine Mudge, MS, RN, PNPc/CNS, CNN
Laurie Carlson, MSN, RN
Patricia Brennan, MSN, RN

Chapter Contents

Introduction 663
Historical Perspective 663
National Organ Sharing System 666

Chapter 23A: Immunology
Structure and Function of the Immune System 669
Immunologic Aspects of Organ Transplantation. 684
Immnosuppressive Agents. 688

Chapter 23B: Transplantation
Rejection and Infection: Complications Associated with All Organ Transplants 695
Donor Management and Recovery 707
Kidney Transplantation. 710
Pancreas Transplantation 748
Liver Transplantation 754
Summary 768
References and Readings. 769
Chapter Highlights. 777

Transplantation: Introduction and Historical Perspectives

Christine Mudge, MS, RN, PNPc/CNS, CNN
Laurie Carlson, MSN, RN
Patricia Brennan, MSN, RN

Introduction

Organ transplantation is not just a possibility but a widely accepted treatment option for individuals with end-stage organ failure (Frei, 1992). The purpose of this chapter is to provide a brief overview of the history of transplantation, followed by an indepth discussion of the immunologic therapies of transplantation and immunosuppressive agents. It presents general issues applicable to all organ transplants, including a comprehensive discussion of the clinical patient management of the kidney, pancreas, and liver transplant recipient.

Historical Perspective

The hope of extending life and improving the quality of life through organ transplantation has intrigued and challenged scientists for many centuries. Both Eastern and Western literature records stories of organ transplantation and limb reattachment dating back to the second century (Smith, 1990). While Western medicine tends to view such accounts with suspicion, at the least the literature documents a very long history of fascination with and curiosity over the possibility of transplantation. Scholarship dates the modern era of transplantation during the late 19th and early 20th centuries. To the best of our knowledge, transplantation became a technical possibility in the early 20th century and now is a life-saving reality for thousands of people with organ failure.

In presenting the history of organ transplantation, one needs to acknowledge the achievements and interrelations of three distinct disciplines: surgery, immunobiology, and the law. At different times during the evolution of organ transplantation, each of these disciplines has assumed a leading role, and the accomplishments achieved by one discipline have significantly influenced the progress achieved in the others.

In the late 19th and early 20th centuries, the interest in transplantation was primarily surgical. Experimentation focused on two areas: xenografting and improved vascular surgery techniques. Emerich Ullman experimented with kidney autotransplantation in dogs, dog-to-dog kidney transplant, and interspecies transplants. In 1902, he performed the first successful kidney transplant in a dog. Simultaneously, Alexis Carrel experimented with improved methods of vascular suturing, a prerequisite for solid organ transplantation. He received a Nobel Prize in 1912 for his work in this area (Hamilton, 1984).

These early surgical attempts confirmed that transplantation of solid organs was technically possible; however, its successful realization awaited advances in the areas of immunobiology and the treatment of kidney failure. By the early 1900s (20th century), scientists recognized that the immune system played a crucial role in the rejection of transplanted organs, but it was not until the late 1950s that significant immunologic discoveries moved organ transplantation closer to reality. The most significant of those were the discovery of transplantation antigens, the role they play as a genetic basis for rejection, and the development of immunosuppressive agents. Extensive work in immunology continues to this day.

At the same time, the development of dialysis as a treatment for kidney failure provided a population for which transplantation could be an option. This served as an important impetus to accelerate research efforts in transplantation. In 1946, Hume, Heffnagel, and Landsteiner performed the first successful kidney transplant in a patient with acute renal failure. The transplanted kidney functioned long enough for the patient's native kidneys to regain functioning before ultimately failing. In 1951, Hume attempted cadaveric transplantation; however, without the benefits of immunosuppression, these attempts were unsuccessful. In 1954, Merrill & Murray performed the first successful human kidney transplant between identical twins. But it was not until 1959 that kidney transplants between nongenetically identical persons became possible because of the introduction of azathioprine and prednisone as the immunosuppressive regimen. The introduction of immunosuppressive medications ushered in a new era in the field of transplantation. The ability to use cadaveric donors as well as living related donors with a successful outcome greatly increased the potential donor pool and transformed transplantation from an experimental option to the treatment of choice for kidney

Table 23-1
Historical perspectives of transplantation: Surgical.

	Kidney
1900	Lamber attempts xenografting using the kidneys of a lamb (Rockefeller Institutes, NY).
1902	Ullmann autotransplants a dog kidney from its normal position to the vessels of the neck resulting in some urine flow.
1902	Carrel begins his work on vascular anastomosis, a prerequisite to successful solid organ transplantation.
1906	Jaboulay achieves the first recorded human kidney transplant xenografting goat and pig kidneys to the arm or thigh of patients with chronic renal failure.
1936	Voroney implants human kidney into a patient's groin; patient succumbs in 48 hours.
1946	First clinical success: Hufnagel, Hume, and Landsteiner anastomose human cadaver kidney to the radial artery and cephalic vein of toxemic woman in acute renal failure; the patient recovers (Peter Bent Brigham Hospital, Boston).
1954	Merrill, Murray, and Hume perform first successful living-related transplant between identical twins (Peter Bent Brigham Hospital [Richard Herrick]). Recipient lived 7 years.
1959	Murray performs first successful nonidentical twin transplants (Boston & Hamburger, Paris).
	Liver
1950s	Experimental attempts at liver transplant animal models.
1955	Welch describes unsuccessful heterotopic transplant in dogs.
1956	Cannon describes unsuccessful heterotopic transplant in dogs.
1960	Moore describes the first successful heterotopic transplant in a dog. Moore and Starzl perform the first successful orthotropic transplant in a dog.
1963	Starzl performs the first human orthotropic transplant; patient dies and the survival rate for subsequent patients is poor.
1967	Starzl performed the first successful transplant with survival of 1.5 years.
1983	Consensus Development Conference on Liver Transplantation (sponsored by the National Institute of Health) officially changes status of liver transplantation from an experimental option to an accepted treatment modality for liver failure.
	Pancreas
1966	Kelly and Lillehei perform the first pancreas transplant.
1988	Najarian performs simultaneous kidney-pancreas transplant with a survival rate of more than 1 year.

failure. The combination of advances in surgery and immunobiology resulted in significant achievements in organ transplantation over the next two decades.

As the surgical and immunologic barriers diminished and the development of dialysis became more widely available, a large patient population emerged that could benefit from transplantation. As a result, important economic and legal issues had to be addressed. The two major issues, then and now, concern the cost and accessibility of this technology. Such questions prompted discussion on a federal level resulting in the passage of key legislation. Financial matters were first addressed in 1972 with the Amendment of the Social Security Act. The passage of this amendment provides individuals with chronic renal failure to receive federal support for their treatment through Medicare. Although initially intended to assist patients on hemodialysis, funding for kidney transplantation was also included. This was an unprecedented measure that had enormous positive ramifications for kidney transplantation. However, due to the gross underestimation of the cost of this program and the number of beneficiaries, federal funding for other organ transplantation was denied until the late 1980s.

Even more highly charged and difficult to resolve than the financial questions are issues relating to the acquisition and equitable distribution of donor organs. Some of these issues have been resolved through acts of legislation. Examples of these are the Uniform Anatomical Gift Act, the Uniform Determination of Death Act, and the Organ Procurement and Transplant Act. Others continue to be debated because of their complexity and controversial nature. Examples of these are the use of anencephalic donors, fetal tissue transplantation, and commercialization of organ donation through the buying and selling of organs. The task of achieving equitable distribution and access to transplantation is daunting. This is not surprising since we have difficulty achieving this in other social domains. Nevertheless, recognizing the disparity between supply and demand prompts us to take aggressive measures. In 1995, there were 11,810 kidney transplants, 3,925 liver transplants, and 1,028 pancreas transplants performed (based on donor registration forms received by UNOS Central as of 6/20/94). And yet over 35,000 people are waiting for an organ transplant, and each month 1,000 new names are added to the waiting list. More than 2,500 of those people on the list die while waiting for a transplant. Despite all the progress that has been achieved technologically to this point, these statistics of patients dying remain unacceptable. The major milestones achieved in surgical, immunologic, and legislative activities are listed in Tables 23-1, 23-2, and 23-3.

Table 23-2
Historical perspective of transplantation: Immunology.

1900	Specificity of antigen-antibody interactions (Ehrlich).
1910	ABO blood groups identified (Landsteiner).
1920s	Histocompatibility basis of tumor transplant in mice (Tyzzer and Little). Direct donor to recipient blood transfusions.
1930s	Second set skin graft rejection (Homans).
1940s	Clonal selection theory (Burnet). Isolated organ perfusion (Lindbergh and Carrel). Blood banks, transfusions become common practice. Immunogenetic basis of tumor transplantation (Snell).
1950s	Corticosteriods used in transplantation (Mayo clinic). Lymphocyte cell mediated immunity (Gowans). Red cell chimerism observed in cattle (Owen). Immunologic nature of skin homograft rejection (Medawar). Genetics of H2 locus in the mouse identified (Gorer, Snell). Delayed hypersensitivity (Lanstein and Chase).
1957	Dausett, Payne, Amos etc identify the Human Leukocyte Antigen (HLA).
1960s	Terasaki and Najarian identify antigens and initiate histocompatibility testing.
1959-62	Total Body Irradiation (TBI) first attempted as a form of immunosuppression (Hamburger).
1960	Calne demonstrates effectiveness of 6MP in dog kidney transplant.
1961	Azathioprine (Imuran®) first available for human use.
1962-63	Starzl introduces corticosteroids in combination with Imuran® as an immunosuppressive regimen for transplantation.
1962	First use of tissue matching to select a donor and recipient.
1966	Recognition that positive crossmatching leads to hyperacute rejection.
1970s	Class II antigens defined. HLA locus in man defined biochemically. Immune response genes (McDevitt & Bernacerraf). Mixed lymphocyte interaction (Bach & Amos). Antilymphocyte serum (Woodruff & Anderson).
1973	Opelz describes transfusion effect.
1978	Application of matching for HLADR in renal transplantation.
1978	Borel and Calne introduce cyclosporine.
1980s	Suppressor T cell identified (Gershon). Donor specific transfusions (Newton, Anderson, Salvatierra). Monoclonal antibodies (Kohler and Milstein). Clinical use of cyclosporine A (Calne). Cyclosporine, prednisone and azathioprine use of triple therapy (Goldstein). OKT3 mouse monoclonal antibody for rejection therapy (Goldstein).
1990s	Introduction of Tacrolimus (Prograf®) and mycophenolate mofetil (CellCept®). Toward the development of microchimerism.

Table 23-3
Historical perspective in transplantation: Legislative.

1968	Uniform Anatomical Gift Act: allows a person or next of kin (at time of death) to indicate willingness to become an organ donor.
1972	PL 92603: provides Medicare coverage for patients with chronic renal failure
1980	The Uniform Determination of Death Act provides a comprehensive basis for determining death in all situations.
1984	Organ Procurement and Transplant Act established a task force which ultimately made recommendations for professional and public education regarding organ donation, developing organ procurement standards, established routine inquiry, and Uniform determination of Death Act in all states. The Act provided grants for Organ Procurement Organizations (OPO) and established a national organ sharing system, National Organ Procurement and Transplant Network (OPTN), which included a patient registry and the coordination and allocation of organs.
1986	Omnibus Reconciliation Act: Congress incorporated the Organ Transplant Task Force recommendations into the Omnibus Reconciliation Act. This included 1) Required Request (when a person dies in a hospital, the administrator or designee must ask the deceased's next of kin if they want to make an anatomical gift), 2) transplant centers must belong to OPTN (to participate in Medicare or Medicaid), 3) renal transplantation can only be performed at centers belonging to Medicaid or Medicare programs, and 4) OPOs must meet certification requirements.
Early 1990s	Medicare coverage for immunosuppressive drugs.

Table 23-4
Types of organ transplant grafts.

A transplanted graft is an organ or tissue procured from a donor and transplanted into a recipient with the intent of restoring a failed organ or tissue.

Type of Transplanted Graft	Description of the Transplant
Allograft (homograft)	Organ donor from a genetically non-identical member of the same species (e.g. liver transplant).
Isograft (syngraft)	Organ donor from a genetically identical individual (e.g., monozygotic twins).
Autograft	A part of an individual transplanted from one location of the body to another (e.g., skin grafting).
Heterograft (xenograft)	Organ transplant between species (e.g., pig to human).
Orthotropic graft	Organ transplanted into the normal anatomical location in the body (e.g., heart).
Heterotopic graft	Donor organ placed in a position other than the normal anatomical location (e.g., kidneys are generally placed in the iliac fossa).

National Organ Sharing System

In 1984 the National Organ Transplant Act created the Organ Procurement Transplant Network (OPTN). The OPTN developed a national system for the recovery and distribution of donor organs for transplantation. The OPTN is administered by the United States Department of Health and Human Services through a contract with the United Network for Organ Sharing (UNOS). All transplant centers are required to list all potential recipients within the UNOS computerized system (Hawk et al., 1990). When a local procurement organization identifies a potential donor, UNOS is notified. Information regarding the potential donor is entered into the UNOS computer system, which provides a list of potential recipients based on compatibility with regard to blood type, HLA, sensitization, medical status, and organ size. Organs are then designated to a particular recipient based on match and time on the waiting list. The types of transplanted grafts are outlined in Table 23-4.

CHAPTER 23A

Immunology

Christine Mudge, MS, RN, PNPc/CNS, CNN

Chapter Contents

Structure and Function of the Immune System .669
- **Innate and Adaptive Immunity** .669
- **Cells and Organs of the Immune System** .671
- **Mononuclear Phagocyte System (MPS)** .673
- **Organs of the Immune System** .674
- **Complement** .674
- **Inflammatory Response** .676
- **Immune Response** .679
- **Antigenicity** .680
- **Antigen Processing and Presentation** .680
- **Humoral Immune Response** .680
- **Primary and Secondary Humoral Response** .682
- **Antibodies** .682
- **Cell-Mediated Immune Response** .682
- **Cell Cooperation in the Immune Response** .683

Immunologic Aspects of Organ Transplantation .684
- **Genetic Factors Related to Transplantation** .684
- **ABO Blood Group Antigens** .685
- **Major Histocompatibility Complex** .685
- **Human Leukocyte Antigen (HLA) Inheritance** .687
- **Histocompatibility Testing** .687

Immnosuppresive Agents .688

Immunology

Christine Mudge, MS, RN, PNPc/CNS, CNN

Structure and Function of the Immune System

The word *immune* is derived from the Latin word *immunis*, meaning "free from burden." The major role of the immune system is to prevent the host from the burden of injury, which can be the result of exposure to harmful organisms or environmental substances (Smith, 1990). To accomplish this task, the immune system is composed of a highly complex network of specialized cells and tissues, the goal of which is to protect the host from injury and maintain homeostasis.

To protect the host and prevent injury, the immune system's first goal is to be able to distinguish self from nonself. This crucial discrimination is primarily the responsibility of the major histocompatibility complex (MHC), a gene complex located on the sixth chromosome. In addition to identifying foreign substances, the immune system protects the host by (1) defending the host against invading organisms; (2) removing damaged cells from the circulation; and (3) acting as a surveillance network to recognize and protect against the development, growth, and dissemination of abnormal cells.

Proper immune function is called *immunocompetence*. It occurs when host integrity and homeostasis are maintained during exposure to a foreign stimulus. When the immune response is too weak or too strong, the host's homeostatic balance is disrupted. This is called *immunoincompetence*. Inappropriate responses of the immune system include hyperactive responses against environmental substances (e.g., allergies), inability to defend the host as in immunodeficiency disorders (e.g., acquired immune deficiency syndrome [AIDS]), failure to recognize self from nonself as in autoimmune diseases (e.g., autoimmune hepatitis, systemic lupus erythematosus), and the attack of beneficial foreign tissue, as in organ transplantation. The appropriate responses of the immune system are the ability to recognize self from nonself, respond to foreign invaders, remember the invader, and regulate its action. These responses are referred to as the four "R's": recognize, respond, remember, and regulate (Mudge-Grout, 1992).

Innate and Adaptive Immunity

Immune responses are classified into two major mechanisms of host defense: innate immunity (nonspecific or natural) and adaptive immunity (specific or acquired) (Bellanti, 1985; Smith, 1986). Innate immunity is considered the host's first line of defense. It provides the body with both physical and chemical barriers to invading pathogens. Adaptive immunity further protects the host by providing a specific reaction to each invading antigen. It also has the unique ability to remember the foreign antigen.

> **Antigen**: A substance recognized by the host as foreign and capable of triggering an immune response.

Innate immunity is composed of nonspecific mechanisms that protect the host against foreign antigens. These mechanisms are present at birth. They are both physical and chemical in nature and generally do not require exposure to antigen. Physical barriers include the skin, mucous membranes of the gastrointestinal tract, genitourinary tract and nasopharynx, and the ciliated epithelia of the lungs. These structures not only serve as physical barriers, but they also protect the host by establishing a chemically unsuitable milieu that suppresses microbial growth. Chemical barriers include lysozymes, gastric acid, and lactic acid (see Table 23-5). Lysozymes are mucolytic polysaccharide enzymes located in nasal secretions, saliva, tears, and sweat. These enzymes, in the presence of complement, are capable of disrupting (lysing) the cell wall of many bacteria, thus inhibiting microbial growth. Gastric acid provides a low pH to the gastric mucosa and prevents pathogenic growth in the stomach.

The skin is the primary barrier to microbial invasion. Specific conditions such as pH, temperature, and moisture, alter the potential growth of pathogenic organisms on the skin. Normal flora of the skin and mucous membranes also provides a defense against colonization of pathogenic bacteria. Resident skin flora suppresses the growth of infectious agents by competing for essential nutrients, altering the pH, and by producing growth-inhibit-

Table 23-5
Innate and adaptive immunity.

Innate and adaptive immunity function interdependently to protect the host from foreign invasion.

Characteristics	Innate	Adaptive
Physical Barriers	Physical defense: skin & mucous membranes	None
Soluble Substances	Chemical defense: lysozyme, complement, acute phase proteins, interferon	Antibodies Lymphokines Cytokines
Immune Response	Nonspecific; mononuclear phagocytic system, inflammatory response	Specific; Humoral immunity Cellular immunity
Involved Cells	Phagocytes (granulocytes and monocytes), natural killer cells (NK)	T-lymphocytes B lymphocytes
Specificity	Non specific	Very specific
Memory	No	Yes

Table 23-6
Cells and organs of the immune system.

Cells	Organs and Tissues
Leukocytes (white blood cells) Granulocytes Neutrophils Eosinophils Basophils	Thymus Gland Bone Marrow Lymph Nodes Spleen Tonsils
Mononuclear phagocytes Monocytes` Macrophages	Mucous Associated Lymph Tissue (MALT) Gut Associated Lymph Tissue (GALT) (Peyer's patches)
Lymphocytes T-lymphocytes B lymphocytes	
Platelets	Bronchus Associated Lymph Tissue (BALT) Skin Associated Lymph Tissue (SALT) (Langerhans cells) Genital Associated Lymph Tissue (GALT)

ing substances. Changes in these conditions have the potential to enhance microbial invasion and the development of an infection. There are also non-specific mechanical factors protecting the host, such as the ciliary action in the respiratory tract.

Lack of adequate host protection by innate immunity stimulates the adaptive immune response to provide additional host defense. Adaptive immunity is distinguished from innate immunity by its unique ability to mount a specific response to the invading antigens and to remember the invading antigen (memory) in the event of future invasion.

There are two primary components of adaptive immunity, the cellular immune response (T-lymphocytes) and the humoral immune response (B lymphocytes). Cellular and humoral immunity are responsible for defending the host against a foreign antigen. They do this through a process of clonal selection in which the lymphocytes recognize the antigen as foreign and proliferate, by triggering an immune response against the antigen, and by remembering the antigen in anticipation of future invasion.

Adaptive immunity may be acquired either passively or actively. Passive adaptive immunity requires the administration of preformed antibodies to the host. Examples of passive immunity include the administration of antibody or antitoxin (e.g., gamma globulin, tetanus) and the passage of antibodies from mother to fetus or child via the placenta or colostrum/breast milk (e.g., neonatal IgG and IgA from mother). Passive adaptive immunity provides immediate but temporary immunity. Active adaptive immunity is acquired naturally with exposure to the antigen and subsequent disease (e.g., varicella), and through the inoculation with a variant of antigen (e.g., immunization, attenuated virus). Active adaptive immunity may last for years or be permanent.

Both innate and adaptive immunity are defense mechanisms that function interdependently with the ultimate goal of protecting the host against foreign antigen invasion.

Cells and Organs of the Immune System

All blood cells, through a process of differentiation, are derived from precursor cells in the bone marrow called hematopoietic stem cells. Some of these differentiated cells develop into leukocytes or erythrocytes, while others become platelets. The majority of leukocytes produced remain in the bone marrow until there is an invading antigen and they are summoned to defend the host. Table 23-6 lists cells and organs of the immune system.

Leukocytes are white blood cells (WBCs) associated with both inflammatory and immune responses (see Table 23-7). Leukocytes are one of the most important cellular components participating in host defense. Together they function to maintain host integrity by identifying, attacking, and killing unwanted antigens.

Leukocytes develop from two main lineages, the myeloid lineage and the lymphoid lineage. Myeloid leukocytes are classified into granulocytes and monocytes. Lymphoid leukocytes consist of T and B lymphocytes. These two lineages function collaboratively to protect the host against foreign antigen invasion.

Granulocytes are frequently referred to as polymorphonuclear granulocytes (PMNs) because their nuclei are multilobed and they have intracellular granules. Based on the histologic staining of their granules, granulocytes are further classified into three categories: neutrophils, eosinophils, and basophils (see Table 23-8).

Granulocytes make up 60-80% of the total number of normal blood leukocytes (Roitt, Brostoff & Male, 1985). They are produced at a rate of approximately 80 million a day with an average life span of 2 to 3 days. During episodes of acute inflammation, granulocytes play a key role in conjunction with antibodies and complement to defend the host against microorganisms. Granulocytes are the first cells to reach the site of antigen invasion and provide host defense. Through the process of phagocytosis, granulocytes are able to eliminate foreign invaders and protect the host. Phagocytosis is a process that engulfs and digests dead cells and foreign substances. Thus, granulocytes are considered phagocytes. Although extremely important in protecting the host, granulocytes lack two important attributes typically associated with immunity: antigenic specificity and memory.

One of the primary functions of granulocytes is phagocytosis; therefore they are also called phagocytes. Phagocytosis is a process that engulfs, internalizes, and destroys invading organisms. It is the first event that occurs when a foreign antigen enters the body, and it is the mechanism by which antigen and dead cells are removed from the host.

When a microorganism penetrates the epithelial surface of the skin, it comes in contact with phagocytes strategically located throughout the body. Phagocytes have surface receptors that allow them to seek out, attach, and subsequently destroy damaged cells or foreign antigens (see Table 23-9). Phagocytosis is initiated when phagocytes recognize damaged or foreign substances within the host. Recognition of these substances may occur at nonspecific membrane receptor sites or mediated by opsonic proteins. Opsonization is a process that makes invading organisms or particles more attractive to phagocytes. The process of opsonization coats the foreign substances with certain molecules (e.g., IgG antibody or complement fragment C3b), making them more appealing to phagocytes, thus rendering them readily phagocytized.

When particle attachment is complete, the cell membrane of the phagocyte surface invaginates, engulfs the substance, internalizes it, and forms a phagocytic vacuole (phagosome). The phagosome contains potent hydrolytic enzymes that fuse with the lysosomal granules, damaging and digesting the phagocytosed substance. Finally, the phagocyte releases the digested product and the body subsequently eliminates it.

Phagocytosis causes a number of metabolic changes to occur within the cell. Certain conditions cause lysosomal enzymes and toxic oxygen products to be released from the phagocytic cell. These changes result in the release of toxic oxidative substances, a process called the respiratory burst. These products are responsible for a large portion of tissue damage that occurs in ongoing inflammation.

Lymphocytes are divided into two major cell classes: T-lymphocytes (T cells) and B lymphocytes (B cells). The maturation process of lymphocytes and the lymphoid system begins during fetal development and continues throughout life (Herscowitz, 1985). These cells are primarily responsible for the

Table 23-7
Leukocytes.

Leukocyte	Normal Values	Characteristics & Function
White Blood Cell (WBC)	Children: 4,500-13,000µl Adults: 3,400-10,000µl	Provide host defense; after phagocytosis has taken place, cytoplasmic granules contain potent enzymes that destroy.
Polymorphonuclear Granulocytes	**Percent of Total**	
Neutrophils	60%-80%	First cells to arrive at the site of injury, they participate in host defense by releasing antibacterial substances and digestive enzymes into the site of injury, they remain active in the blood for approximately 7 hours and in the tissue for 48-72 hours.
Eosinophils	20%-25%	Primary host defense against parasites; increased in allergic reactions.
Basophils	2%-3%	Phagocytic action is weak, releases heparin and histamine into surrounding injured tissue, active in allergic responses.
Mast Cells	02% dependent on tissue type	Granules release potent mediators such as heparin, histamine, and others into the target tissue; defend host against parasites.
Mononuclear Phagocytes	2%-10%	Participates in antigen processing and presentation, contains a single large nuclei, and the cytoplasm has few to no granules.
Monocytes Macrophage		Participates in antigen processing and presentation; stimulates T cell maturation and activates T cell response by secreting interleukin-l.
Lymphocytes	20%-40%	
T-lymphocytes	70%-80% of lymphocytes	Participates in cellular immunity; active for months.
B lymphocytes	10%-20% of lymphocytes	Participates in antigen processing and presentation; contact with a specific antigen will cause differentiation of B lymphocytes into antibody-producing plasma cells; plasma cells are active for 3-5 day.

immune response and play a major role in the development of adaptive immunity.

T-lymphocytes (T cells) are responsible for cell-mediated immunity, and they represent approximately 70-80% of the lymphocytes produced. During fetal life, immature T cells (pre-T-lymphocyte) migrate through the blood to the thymus. T cells mature and proliferate under the influence of thymic hormones (thymosin and thymopoietins) in the thymus. In addition, the thymus provides an environment that encourages developing T cells to cultivate the ability to recognize and attach to a specific antigen. T cells are divided into four distinct subsets: helper, cytotoxic, suppressor, and memory T cells. The process of T cell differentiation begins before birth and continues through the first few months of life. If the thymus is removed after about 6 months of life, it will not interfere with T cell

Table 23-8
Granulocytes.

Granulocyte	Morphology Defense	Distribution	Mechanism of Host
Neutrophil	Multilobed nucleus; primary and secondary granules stain purplish pink.	Blood Tissue	Phagocytosis Bactericidal killing
Eosinophil	Bilobed nuclei; many cytoplasmic granules that stain red.	Blood Tissue	Phagocytosis
Basophils	Bilobed or multilobed nuclei; granules are randomly distributed, surrounded by a membrane; granules stain deep violet blue.	Blood	Degradation Phagocytosis

Table 23-9
Characteristics of phagocytes.

Margination or Pavementing	Cells begin to adhere to the capillary endothelium.
Diapedesis	A process that follows margination that occurs when the cell extends a pseudopod between the endothelial cells, dissolving the basement membrane and migrates into the tissues.
Chemotaxis	Process by which a WBC moves to the site of injury or infection.
Phagocytosis	The process of recognition of a foreign substance, engulfment, and digestion.
Degranulation	A process that involves fusion of the intracellular granules within the cellular membrane, followed by the release of granule contents. This reaction is one tactic cells have to utilize their intracellular granular weapons against targets that are too large for phagocytosis.

immunity. This is due to the T cells' capacity to expand by cloning throughout life.

B lymphocytes (B cells) are responsible for humoral immunity and antibody production. They represent the remaining 10-20% of lymphocytes. In birds, B cell maturation takes place in an organ called the Bursa of Fabricius, an outpouching of cloacal epithelium. Stem cells that migrate to this organ differentiate and proliferate into mature antibody-producing cells called bursal or B cells. Although no mammalian bursa-equivalent tissue has been identified, it is thought that B cell maturation and immunocompetence in humans probably takes place in the bone marrow, lymphoid tissues lining the gastrointestinal tract (gut-associated lymphatic tissue [GALT]), or in the liver during the prenatal and neonatal periods. Similar to T cells, B cells are cloned throughout life.

Mature T and B cells circulate in the blood and migrate into the lymphoid tissues, lymph nodes, and the spleen. Lymphatic tissue is strategically located at the body's portals of entry, allowing lymphocytes the advantage of intercepting antigens at the time of host invasion. Most T and B cells circulate in the blood and lymphatic system while a smaller number reside in the lymph tissue.

Mononuclear Phagocyte System (MPS)

The mononuclear phagocyte system (MPS), previously referred to as the reticuloendothelial system (RES), is composed of precursor cells derived from the bone marrow. These precursor cells are phagocytes, specifically monocytes and macrophages.

Table 23-10
Monocytes and macrophages of the mononuclear phagocyte system.

Name	Location
Blood Monocytes	Blood
Granulocytes	Blood
Dendritic Cells	Bone Marrow
Bone Marrow Macrophages	Bone marrow
Osteoclasts	Bone tissue
Microglial Cells	Brain
Histiocytes	Connective tissue
Intraglomerular Mesangial	Kidney
Kupffer Cells	Liver
Alveolar Macrophages	Lung
Lymph Node Sinus Macrophage	Lymph node
Peritoneal Macrophages	Peritoneal cavity
Pleural Macrophages	Pleural cavity
Serosal Macrophages	Serosal space
Langerhans Cells	Skin
Spleen Sinus Macrophage	Spleen
Type A Cells	Synovium

Monocytes tend to be smaller and have fewer phagocytic capabilities than macrophages. Monocytes typically circulate in the blood and within a few days migrate into the tissue to become macrophages. Macrophages are located in a number of tissues throughout the body (see Table 23-10).

There are four primary functions of the mononuclear phagocyte system: (1) protect the host from invading antigens through recognition and phagocytosis; (2) clear tissue debris from sites of injury; (3) serve as a surveillance network, removing cells in an attempt to aid in antitumor host defense; and (4) participate in the immune response.

Participation in the immune response requires macrophages, along with other cells (e.g., B lymphocytes), to function as antigen presenting cells (APC) (Goodman, 1991). Antigen presenting cells act to process and present antigen to specific antigen sensitive lymphocytes. The presentation of antigen by the APC triggers the immune response

The function of macrophages during the immune response is augmented by a number of factors released from T cells (e.g., gamma interferon). Macrophages also act as secretory cells releasing a number of very potent chemicals, enzymes, complement proteins, and regulatory factors (e.g., interleukin-1) that further enhance the immune response.

Platelets (thrombocytes) arise from the myeloid series of the large megakaryocytes in the bone marrow. They contain a number of special factors and enzymes (e.g., histamine). They also have an active role in blood clotting, particularly during inflammation. Following an inflammatory response, platelets aggregate and adhere to the affected endothelial surfaces. They release substances that increase capillary permeability and factors that activate complement, this in turn provides chemotactic stimuli and attracts leukocytes to the injured area.

Organs of the Immune System

Cells involved in the immune system are organized into tissues and organs called the lymphoid system. These structures are classified into two categories, primary and secondary lymphoid tissue (Roitt, Brostoff, & Male, 1985). Primary lymphoid organs are the bone marrow and thymus gland. Secondary lymphoid organs are composed of the spleen, lymph nodes, tonsils, and other lymphoid tissue referred to as the mucosa-associated lymphoid tissue or MALT. Secondary lymphoid organs contain mature T and B cells.

Complement

Complement is a complex of more than 25 enzymatic serum proteins that assist in mediating the inflammatory reaction and augmenting the immune response. Most of these proteins circulate in the plasma and body fluids in an inactive state. The complement system can be activated through two major pathways: the classical pathway, which is initiated by antigen antibody complexes, or the alternative pathway that has no absolute requirement for antibody activation (see Figure 23-1).

The complement system has three main functions: (1) lysis of cells and microorganisms; (2) promotion of particle opsonization and clearance, facilitating the destruction of antigen by neutrophils or antibodies; and (3) the formation of peptide fragments that mediate the inflammatory and immune response. Complement proteins cause vasodilatation at the site of inflammation, chemotactic stimuli to encourage migration of phagocytes to the target area, cell lysis, agglutination of some microorganisms, neutralization of viruses, and assistance in clearing infectious agents from the host (Frank, 1991; Lancaster & Schanbacher, 1991).

Components (C) of the classical and alternative pathways are identified by numbers following the letter "C." C1 activates the classical pathway and C3 activates the alternative pathway. The proteins of each pathway progress in a systematic, sequential manner called the complement cascade. Through a series of enzymatic reactions, the complement cascade leads to the development of a complex enzyme (active enzymes are identified by a bar over the component). This enzyme is capable of binding and cleaving complement component C3, which is common to both pathways. At the junction of C3 both pathways proceed together to form what is called the membrane attack complex

Figure 23-1
Complement cascade.

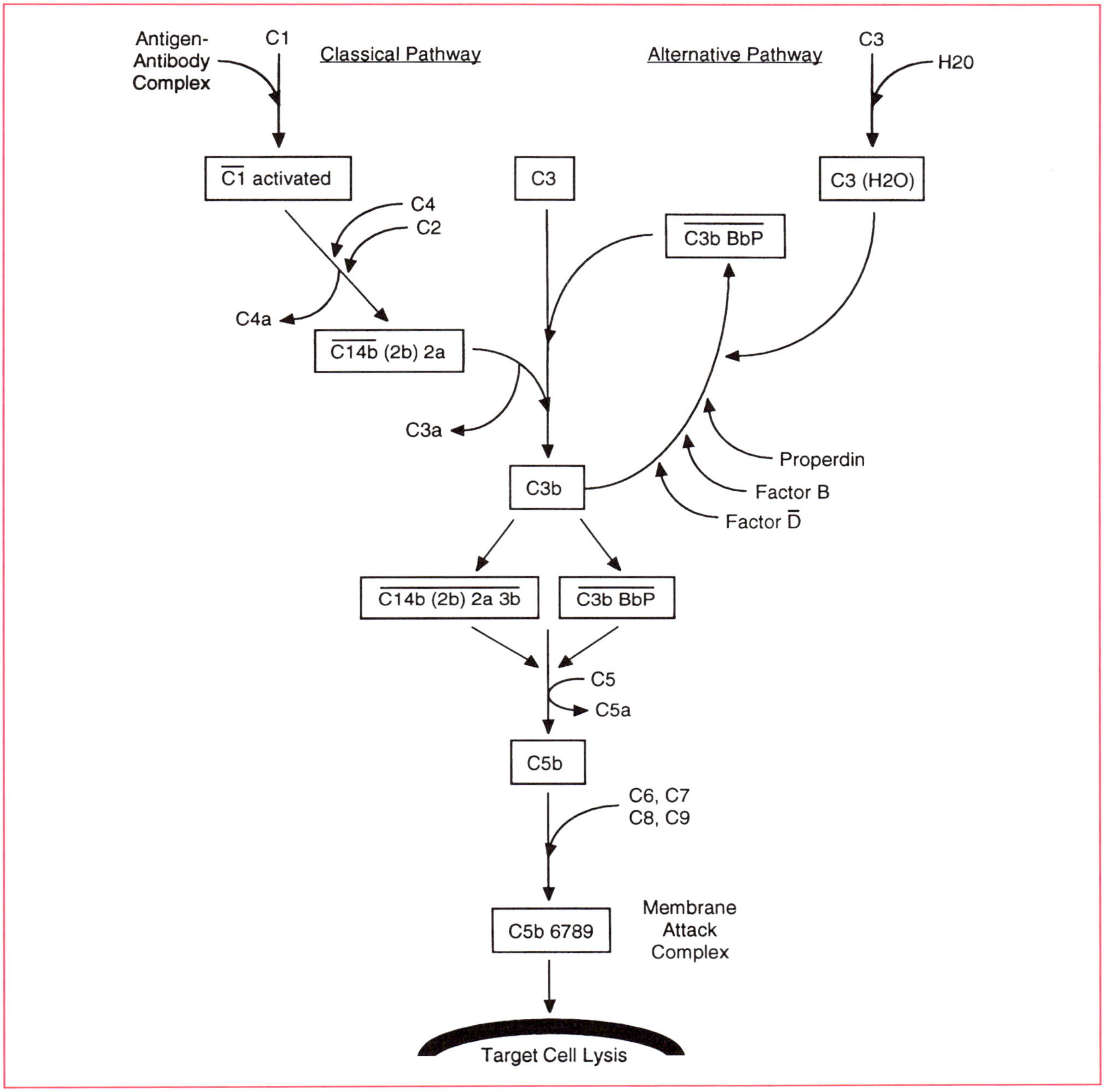

(C5b 6789 on the surface of a target cell). The membrane attack complex is capable of causing cell lysis. Inactivators present in the liver and spleen "turn off" complement activity to prevent injury to normal tissue.

Complement can be activated through either the classical or alternative pathways. Factors responsible for complement activation include the formation of insoluble antigen-antibody immune complexes, aggregated immunoglobulin, release of endotoxins, presence of bacteria, virus, yeast and fungus in the circulation, platelet aggregation, and the release of plasmin and proteases from damaged cells.

Although the complement system protects the host against infectious organisms and may play a role in tumor cell destruction, the uncontrolled activation of this system can result in inflammatory changes and lytic destruction of host tissues.

Figure 23-2
Sequence of major events during the early nonspecific acute inflammatory response to cellular damage and foreign antigens.

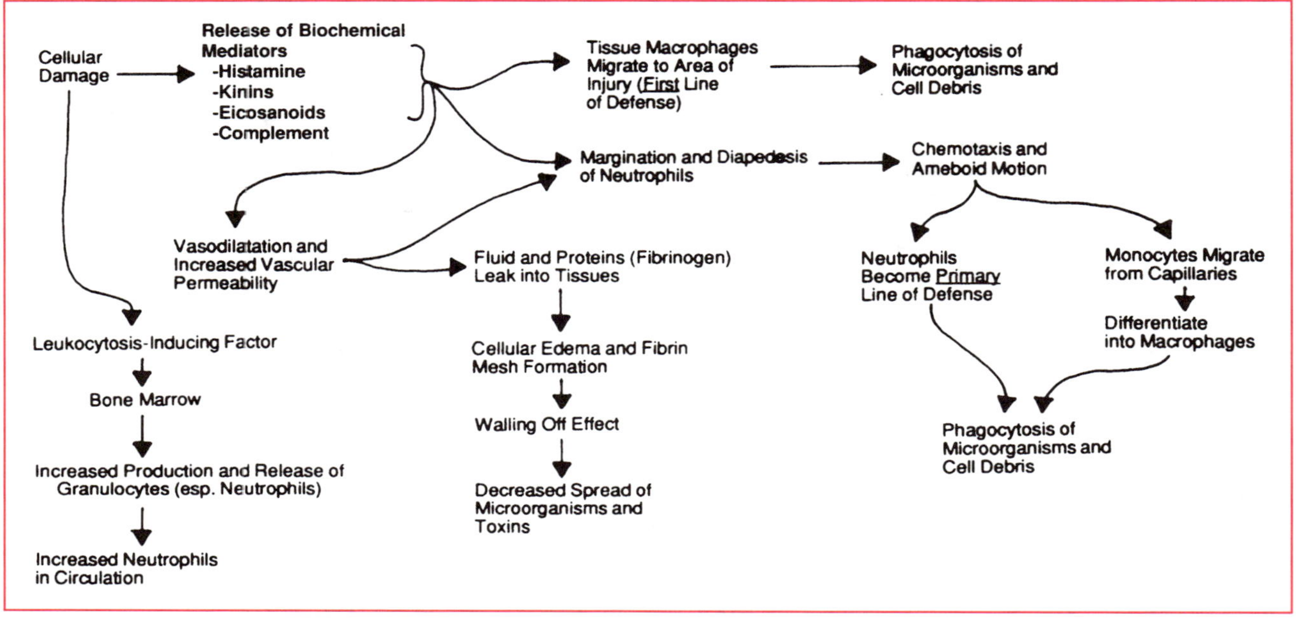

Note: From Lancaster, L.E. & Schanbacher, B. (1995). Renal transplantation. In L.E. Lancaster (Ed.). (1995). *ANNA core curriculum for nephrology nursing* (3rd ed., p. 385). Pitman, NJ: American Nephrology Nurses' Association. Reprinted with permission.

Inflammatory Response

The inflammatory response is a nonspecific reaction that occurs immediately and aggressively by the host in response to cell injury and tissue damage (see Figure 23-2). It is important to both innate and adaptive immunity; the inflammatory response is nonspecific and lacks memory. The inflammatory response performs in exactly the same manner every time it is triggered, regardless of the stimulus or number of exposures to the same stimulus. The aim of the inflammatory process is threefold: (1) to protect the host and prevent further tissue injury, (2) to repair the damage, and (3) to enhance healing. However, inflammation in a transplanted organ is considered an unfavorable response that can lead to subsequent rejection.

There are multiple factors that can trigger the inflammatory process, including mechanical, physical, or chemical injury (e.g., trauma, thrombosis, surgery, malignancies, myocardial infarction, toxins), invasion of microorganisms (e.g., bacteria, fungi, viral), and immunologic alterations (e.g., hypersensitivity reactions). The inflammatory response is triggered by the release of substances from the injured cells and the action of phagocytes, which leads to a cascade of physiologic events.

The major events of the inflammatory process are initiated immediately after cell injury and tissue damage with the release of potent chemical mediators such as histamine, kinins, prostaglandins, cytokines, and complement components (see Table 23-11). These chemical mediators cause the surrounding vessels to dilate, resulting in local hyperemia and increased capillary permeability observed clinically as redness, swelling, and pain. As a result of increased capillary permeability, fluid, fibrinogen, and other proteins and cells leak from the blood vessels into the interstitium. Fibrinogen is activated into fibrin and, in conjunction with platelets, forms a clot. The clot forms a web able to trap microorganisms and provide a framework for healing. The main purpose of this initial process is to wall off the area to protect the host from the further injury or the spread of microorganisms.

Vascular dilation is followed by the migration of tissue macrophages to the site of injury. Macrophages are drawn to the injured area by chemotactic factors released by damaged cells or invading microorganisms. Mast cells and basophils act to secrete inflammatory mediators from their granules such as histamine and heparin, which augment the effects of the phagocytic cells. Also through chemotactic stimuli, other phagocytes, primarily neutrophils, are recruited to the area when damage is extensive. Granulocyte-releasing factor is released from the damaged cells and acts on the

Table 23-11
Mediators of inflammation.

Mediator	Characteristics
Histamine	Stored in granules of basophils, mast cells and platelets; causes vasodilatation, increased vascular permeability, and smooth muscle contraction.
Serotonin	Stored in platelets; causes vasodilatation, increased vascular permeability, and smooth muscle contraction.
Eosinophil chemotactic factor of anaphylaxis (ECFA)	Located in mast cells, chemotactic for eosinophils.
Neutrophil chemotactic factor of anaphylaxis (NCFA)	Located in mast cells, chemotactic for neutrophils.
Complement components (C3a, C5a)	Proteins derived from activation of the complement system; cause mast cell degranulation and histamine release; neutrophil and macrophage chemotaxis; smooth contraction; and increased vascular permeability.
Kinins (e.g., bradykinin)	Substances produced by the kinin system; increase vascular permeability, cause vasodilatation and enhance chemotaxis for neutrophils and macrophages.
Prostaglandins (PG)	Produced from arachidonic acid metabolism, PGI and PGE are potent vasodilators that react with histamine and kinins to increase vascular permeability; promote platelet aggregation; stimulate the hypothalamus to regulate temperature; triggers pain receptors; may have antiinflammatory actions; and may modify immune function.
Leukotrienes (LTB4, LTC4 and LTD4)	Produced from arachidonic acid metabolism; found predominantly as products of mucosal mast cells; promote inflammatory and hypersensitivity reactions; increase vascular permeability and smooth muscle constriction; LTB4 (a type of leukotriene) has chemotactic potency, promotes adherence of leukocytes to endothelial cells, and activates neutrophilic enzymes.
Platelet Activating Factor (PAF)	Located in basophils, neutrophils, and macrophages cell membranes; when released activates platelet aggregation and neutrophils; causes increased vascular permeability, smooth muscle contraction; potent chemotactic stimuli for eosinophils.
Proteinases (lysosomal enzymes)	Enzymes stored in lysosomes of leukocytes, produced in response to inflammation; able to break down bacteria and proteins generated by the inflammatory response.
Clotting System	Interacts with the complement system to produce a number of products essential to the inflammatory response, tissue healing, and repair.
Cytokines	See Table 23-12

Table 23-12
Cytokines.

Adapted with permission from Mudge-Grout, C.L. (1992). *Immunological disorders.* St. Louis: Mosby.

Cytokine	Source	Main Functions
Interleukins (IL)		
IL1 (endogenous pyrogen)	Predominantly Macrophages and other APC	Augments the immune response, inflammatory mediator, activates T cells, activates phagocytes, promotes prostaglandin production, induces a fever.
IL2 (T cell growth factor [TCGF])	Predominantly T Helper Lymphocytes	Activates T-lymphocytes and NK cells, promotes growth and proliferation of T and B cells .
IL3 (multi-CSF)	T-lymphocytes	Hematopoietic growth factor for immature hematopoietic precursor cells.
IL4(B cell growth factor [BCGF])	T-lymphocytes Mast cells	Growth factor for T cells, activated B cells, and mast cells; macrophage activating factor;enhances IgE reactions; inhibits monokine production.
IL5	T helper cells Macrophages Mast cells	Promotes growth and proliferation of activated B cells and eosinophils.
IL6	Monocytes, T and B Lymphocytes, Fibroblasts	B cell stimulatory and differentiation factor; promotes hematopoiesis, enhances the inflammatory response.
IL7	Bone marrow Thymus	Promotes growth of lymphoid cells; stimulates T cytotoxic functions.
IL8 ((monocyte-derived neutrophil chemotactic factor)	Macrophages and Monocytes	Triggers chemotactic activity of neutrophils and lymphocytes.
IL9	T helper cells	T cell and mast cell growth factor, supports maturation of erythroid progenitors.
IL10	T helper cells Cytotoxic T cells B cells Macrophages	Inhibits cytokine production by T cells, NK cells, and APCs, suppresses proliferation and function of T cells, promotes B cell proliferation and antibody function, induces MHC antigen expression.
IL11	Stromal cells	Augments hematopoiesis and thrombopoiesis.
IL12	B cells, macrophages	Stimulates: proliferation and function of activated cytotoxic T cells and NK cells, production of IFN g, induction and suppression of helper T cells, promotion of cell-mediated response.
IL13	T helper cells	Similar to IL4.
Interferons		
αIFN (alpha interferon)	Leukocytes (e.g., macrophages, neutrophils)	Provides antiviral protection, inhibits cell proliferation, stimulates production of IL2, induction of MHC, and activation of macrophages and NK cells
βIFN (beta interferon)	Leukocytes (e.g. macrophages, neutrophils)	Provides antiviral protection, enhances activation of macrophages and NK cells

Table 23-12
Cytokines (continued).

γIFN (gamma interferon)	T-lymphocytes NK cells	Activates macrophages, promotes B cell differentiation and NK cell activity, enhances induction of class I and II MHC, promotes cell medicated immunity, inhibits neoplastic cell proliferation
Tumor Necrosis Factor (TNF)	Macrophages, T cells, fibroblasts, endothelial cells	Promotes the immune and inflammatory responses, kills tumor cells
Colony Stimulating Factors (CSF)		
G-CSF	Monocytes, fibroblasts	Myeloid growth factor
G-MCSF	T cells, fibroblasts, monocytes, endothelial cells	Myelocytic growth factor
M-CSF	Monocytes, lymphocytes, fibroblasts, endothelial and epithelial cells	Macrophage growth factor
Transforming Growth Factor (TGF)	Lymphocytes, macrophages, platelets, bone	Stimulates fibroblasts for wound healing, inhibits the immune response

bone marrow to increase the release of leukocytes, mainly neutrophils, into the circulation (Lancaster, 1991). This is reflected in an elevation of WBCs, particularly neutrophils, on a complete blood count test (CBC). Neutrophils are referred to as the first line of defense because they are produced in large numbers and are the first macrophages present at the site of injury. Occasionally, the demand is so great that immature neutrophils (bands) are released from the bone marrow into the circulation, causing what is known as a shift to the left.

Within 24 hours after the onset of the inflammatory process, monocytes are attracted to the site of injury. Monocytes migrate from the circulating blood into the tissues where they differentiate and transform into macrophages, facilitating the digestion of cell debris, dying neutrophils, and microorganisms.

Macrophages have the capacity to stay in the inflamed area for 2 to 12 months and play a key role in cleaning the affected area of debris in preparation for repair and healing. They also produce interleukin-1, a cytokine that activates T-lymphocytes and promotes the initiation of the immune response.

The hallmark signs of inflammation are swelling, heat, redness, pain, and loss of function of the inflamed area (Lewis, 1992).

Restoration and healing of tissues is the final stage of the inflammatory response, and involves both the processes of regeneration and repair. Regeneration is the replacement of the same type of cells and tissues that were destroyed. Repair is the substitution of damaged cells and tissues with connective tissue.

The involvement of the inflammatory process in organ transplantation is primarily twofold. First, it is the body's initial attempt to destroy the foreign transplanted tissue; however, it is not the specific cause of organ transplant rejection. Second, surgical intervention triggers the inflammatory process to promote wound healing (Lancaster, 1991). In addition, the administration of corticosteroids and other immunosuppressant medications, chronic illness, stress, and advanced age alter the inflammatory response (Smith, 1990).

Immune Response

In contrast to the inflammatory response, which is nonspecific, the immune response is a highly complex, specific reaction that is triggered in response to foreign antigenic stimuli or microorganisms. Although there has been considerable advancement regarding the immune response and the relationship of its numerous components, the exact mechanisms remain unclear (Goodman, 1991).

There are three major cell types involved in the immune response: macrophages, T-lymphocytes (cell mediated immunity), and B lymphocytes (humoral immunity). These cells interact directly with each other under the supervision of a variety of cytokines (see Table 23-12). Complement, kinins, and the clotting and fibrocytic systems are also intimately related to the immune response.

The immune response has four unique characteristics. They include the ability to recognize self from nonself, respond to a nonself invader, remember the invader (memory), and regulate its action. These four characteristics are referred to as the four "R's" (Mudge-Grout, 1992). Recognition of self from nonself is normal. Therefore, under normal circumstances, an immune response is triggered only when the host identifies an invading agent to be foreign. The host response is complex and highly specific to the antigenic stimuli. The ability to remember the antigen is the immune system's memory and allows for a rapid response with subsequent invasion of the same antigen. Regulation allows the immune system to turn on and off when necessary to prevent destruction of host tissue. Inability to regulate may result in damage to host tissue (e.g., systemic lupus erythematosus) or chronic inflammation (e.g., rheumatoid arthritis).

The cooperation of cells in the specific immune response includes antigen processing and presentation, activation of T and B cells, stimulation of nonspecific cells of cell-mediated immunity (e.g., macrophages), and the release of complement.

Antigenicity

An immunogen is any substance capable of inducing an immune response. Examples are lipoproteins and glycoproteins. Antigen is a term frequently used interchangeably with immunogen referring to the capability of a substance to react specifically with components of the immune system, particularly antibodies. Examples are bacteria, viruses, grafted tissue, and pollen. Therefore, all immunogens are antigens, but not all antigens are necessarily immunogens (Goodman, 1991; Benjamini & Leskowitz, 1992). An antigen capable of triggering an immune response generally has a molecular weight of greater than 6,000 Daltons (Benjamini & Leskowitz, 1992)

Antigens are identified by characteristic markers on their cell surface called epitopes. All antigens express a number (some carry hundreds) of different types of epitopes on their cell surface. Antigens and their specific epitopes are the specific markers that allow the host to distinguish self from nonself. Autologous antigens are self-antigens and normally do not trigger an immune response. Modification of autologous antigens by an infectious or inflammatory process may cause the immune system to recognize itself as foreign, evoking an autoimmune response.

Antigen Processing and Presentation

Antigen processing and presentation is a response that allows the host to destroy a particular antigen or render it ineffective. There are a number of cells throughout the body that are thought to be responsible for this process. The major cells are macrophages; others include B cells (lymphoid tissue), Langerhans cells (skin, regional lymph nodes), dendritic leukocytes (most body tissue), Kupffer's cells (liver), follicular dendritic cells (spleen, lymph node follicles), and marginal zone macrophages (spleen, lymph node). Those cells participating in antigen processing and presentation are called antigen presenting cells (APC).

Antigen is recognized as foreign by the host and ingested by APC through phagocytosis. Although the exact mechanism is unclear, the APC alters the antigen through an enzyme-mediated reaction. This is called antigen processing. Processed antigen is reexpressed in conjunction with the major histocompatibility complex (MHC) on the cell surface of the APC in a highly immunogenetic form to T and B lymphocytes. This is called antigen presentation. Therefore, an antigen presenting cell is basically any cell that can internalize and degrade an antigen into fragments and represent these fragments on its cell membrane surface for recognition by lymphocytes. T and B lymphocytes recognize the antigen as nonself through receptors on their cell surface. This recognition triggers a cascade of events that ultimately lead to the destruction of the antigen or rendering it ineffective.

The immune response, a component of adaptive immunity, is triggered when APC process and present antigen to lymphocytes. The major components of the immune response are humoral immunity, directed primarily by B lymphocytes that mature into antibody-secreting plasma cells, and cellular immunity, mediated mainly by T lymphocytes. Humoral and cellular immunity are interdependent and participate collaboratively to protect the host. However, in this discussion, humoral and cellular immunity will be presented separately, concluding with a summary describing the immune response and lymphocyte cooperation.

Humoral Immune Response

Humoral immunity is mediated through the production of antibodies by mature B lymphocytes called plasma cells. Antibodies are antigen receptors present on the cell surface of B lymphocytes. Antibodies are capable of recognizing specific antigens and stimulating proliferation and differentiation of B lymphocytes into antibody-producing plasma cells and memory cells (see Figure 23-3).

Antibody-producing plasma cells are capable of producing only one specific type of antibody. These antibodies appear on the cell surface of plasma cells and bind with antigen in much the same way a key fits into a lock. Production of antibodies and antigen binding protects the host against bacteria, neutralizes viruses, promotes phagocytosis, and triggers the complement cascade (Bartucci & Seller, 1990). Antibody production can also mediate hyperacute rejection of transplanted organs, causing graft destruction and loss (Smith, 1990).

B cell activation may be T cell-independent or

Figure 23-3
The immune response.

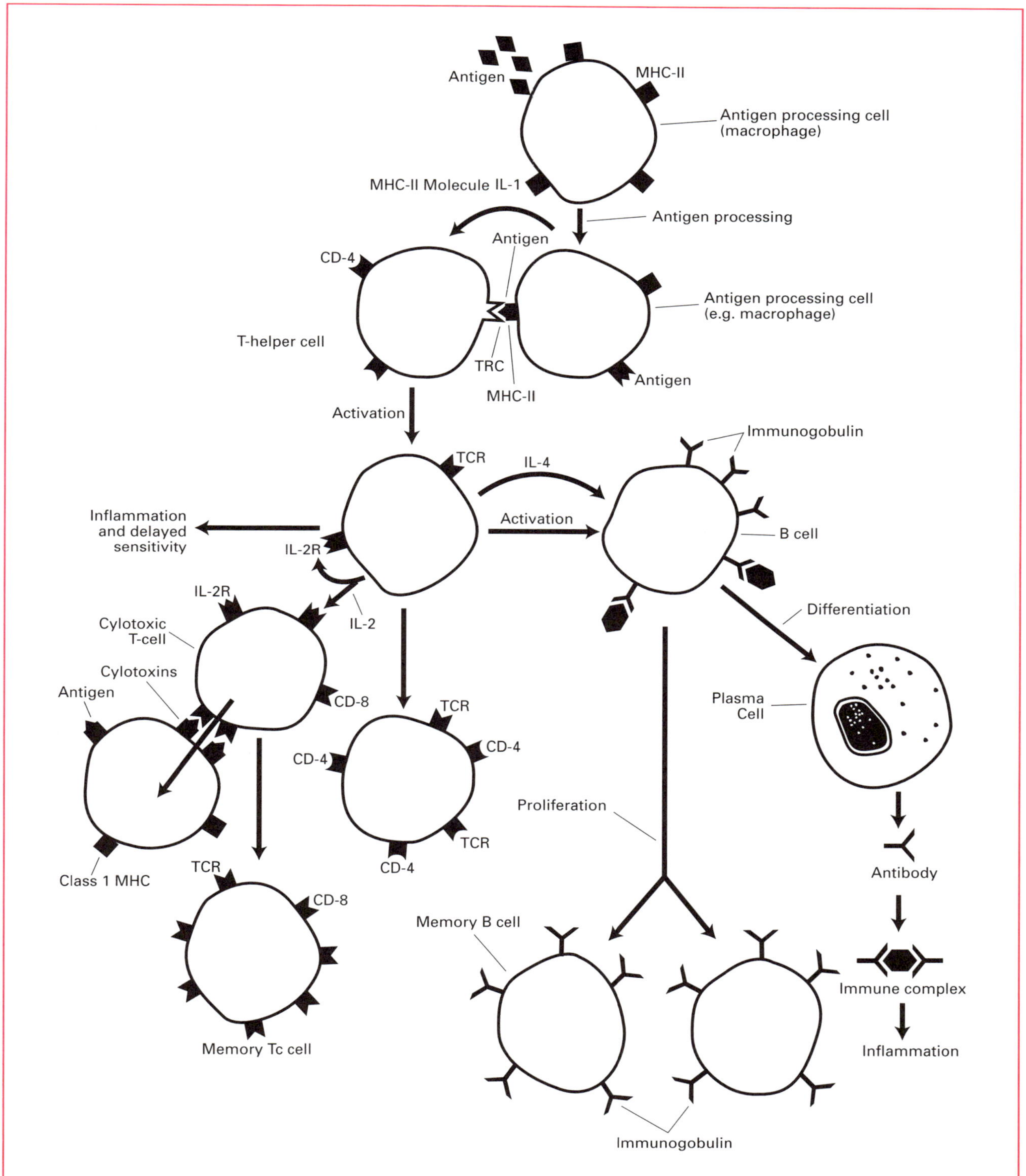

T cell-dependent. A T cell-independent response is when antigen combines with antibody (antigen binding receptor site) on the surface of B lymphocytes and stimulates B cell activity directly. A T cell-dependent response is stimulated when T cells (specifically T helper cells) bind to antigen and release specific substances that deliver signals augmenting B cell proliferation and differentiation. These specific substances are called lymphokines. There are many different types of lymphokines. Cytokines produced by lymphocytes are also known as lymphokines (see Table 23-12). Those lymphokines that are responsible for B cell proliferation and differentiation are referred to as B cell growth factor (BCGF or IL4) and B cell differentiation factor (BCDF) (Goodman, 1991).

Primary and Secondary Humoral Response

The host's encounter with antigen leads to the production of specific antibodies produced by plasma B cells. These antibodies are directed specifically against the invading antigen. Initial exposure to an antigen by the host is called the primary response. During the primary response there is a delay in antibody production. Antibody is not observed in the blood for approximately 2 to 8 days; antibody titers are evident in 10 days; and there is a peak response in 1 to 3 weeks. The first antibody produced is IgM, followed by IgG. Once an individual has responded to an antigen, the immune system will remember the antigen through memory B cells. Subsequent exposure to the same antigen triggers the secondary immune response. Memory B cells are quiescent until there is exposure to a familiar antigen. With recognition of the well-known antigen by the host, there is a rapid (1 to 2 days) rise in antibody titers that is prolific and sustained. The immune system is capable of mounting a secondary response to antigen even if it has been months to years since the initial exposure (Bartucci & Seller, 1990)

Antibodies

Antibodies (immunoglobulins) are a component of humoral immunity that develops in response to an invading organism. They are a group of heterogenous glycoproteins that circulate in body fluids and account for approximately 20% of total plasma proteins. As B lymphocytes mature into antibody-producing plasma cells, they rearrange their genetic material and assemble it into unique antibody regions on their cell surface. As B cells mature and proliferate, all offspring will manufacture this new antibody, and the natural selection of antigen-specific antibodies is formulated. The result of this process is that mature antibody-producing B cells are capable of reacting to an unlimited array of antigens.

The primary function of antibodies is to protect the host. Antibodies protect the host by binding to specific antigens and by initiating a number of immune regulatory activities such as directly attacking antigens through agglutination, neutralization, and lysis; activating the complement system; and triggering components of the inflammatory response.

One or more classes of antibody may participate in a humoral immune response. The exact nature of the response is dependent on the chemical and physical qualities of the antigen, route of antigen entry, and the nature of the host including age, nutritional status, medical and immunization history, metabolic and hormonal factors, and genetics.

Cell-Mediated Immune Response

T-lymphocytes are the mediators of cellular immunity. T cells are identified by antigen-receptor sites (T cell receptors [TCR]) on their cell membrane surface. T cells may have as many as 100,000 receptor sites (Lancaster, 1991). T-lymphocytes are capable of initiating and suppressing the immune response, mediating antigen-specific cytotoxicity and immunity, augmenting T and B cell activation, and cytokine secretion (Lanier, 1991). T cells protect the host from viral and fungal infections and some neoplastic disorders. T-lymphocytes also have the potential to destroy transplanted organs by triggering acute and accelerated graft rejection (Jett & Lancaster, 1983; Roitt, Brostoff, & Male, 1985; Smith, 1990)

When T cells are exposed to antigen, they proliferate into antigen-specific T cell clones in much the same way as B cells produce antibody. However, antigen binding in B lymphocytes is mediated by surface immunoglobulins (antibody). In T-lymphocytes, antigen binding is mediated by T cell receptors (Benjamini & Leskowitz, 1991; Goodman, 1994). Therefore, the capability of lymphocyte antigen binding is extremely diverse, allowing for an enormous, highly varied binding ability. Memory T cells, like memory B cells, are stored in the body. When there is a secondary exposure to a familiar antigen, a rapid activation of T-lymphocytes similar to B lymphocyte activation is triggered.

There are four functionally interactive T cell subsets. They are identified as regulatory cells, called helper T cells, and suppressor T cells, or effector cells, referred to as cytotoxic T cells and memory T cells. Regulatory cells facilitate the activity of other cells in the immune system, whereas effector T cells act directly against antigen.

T cell subsets are differentiated by monoclonal antibodies specific to their cell surface markers or antigens. Cluster of differentiation (CD) is the nomenclature used to identify the characteristic cell surface markers found on human leukocytes. For example, all T cells (T3) express the marker known as CD3, whereas T helper cells express a

CD4 marker, and T suppressor cells express the CD8 marker.

Helper T cells (CD4) and suppressor T cells (CD8) are considered regulatory cells that have a number of specific functions that enhance both cell-mediated and humoral immunity. T helper cells are of principal importance in the immune response because they are needed to activate cytotoxic T cells and antibody-producing B cells. T helper cells stimulate macrophage activating factor (MAF), which stimulates macrophages to release interleukin-1 (IL1).

Activation of T helper cells is dependent on two signals: the release of interleukin-1 (IL1) from APC (e.g., macrophages), and the binding of the T cell antigen receptor to the class II MHC-antigen complex on the APC (see Figure 23-3). The two signals induce T helper lymphocytes to secrete interleukin-2 (IL2), another lymphokine. IL2 amplifies the response of T helper cells and promotes the growth of cells with IL2 receptors, and cytotoxic and helper T cells. Activated T helper cells also produce B cell differentiation factor (BCDF) and B cell growth factor (BCGF), which are important growth factors for clonal stimulation of B cells and antibody formation.

Lymphokines produced by T helper cells also function to facilitate the removal of antigens from the body by promoting B cells and cytotoxic T-lymphocytes to differentiate and proliferate, attracting leukocytes into the target area and enhancing phagocytosis by macrophages. As the lymphokines attract more cells into the target area, the antigen becomes overwhelmed and is subsequently destroyed.

Suppressor T cells (Ts) express CD8 as do cytotoxic T cells. However, they do not appear to have the cytotoxic capability of cytotoxic T cells. Suppressor T cells inhibit the activity of T helper lymphocytes and other immune cells. Although their action is not completely clear, suppressor T cells are thought to release chemicals that indirectly suppress B cell antibody formation and cytotoxic T cell functions. Suppressor T cells are also thought to be responsible for "turning off" the T helper lymphocytes. The balance between T helper (Th) and T suppressor (Ts) cells may contribute to determining the strength and persistence of an immune response. When the delicate balance between Th and Ts cells is disrupted, autoimmune or immunodeficiency diseases may result.

Cytotoxic T cells possess the CD8 marker. Activation of cytotoxic T cells requires two signals, the binding of T cytotoxic cell antigen receptor with the foreign complex and the class 1 MHC on the target cell, and the release of IL2 from activated T helper cells. Once the cytotoxic T cell is activated, it will kill the antigen through the release of lymphokines. Cytotoxic T cells kill any microorganism that is perceived as foreign, for example bacteria or virus infected cells, malignant cells, or allogenic cells introduced in organ transplantation. They also promote phagocytosis at the target site.

Memory T-lymphocytes are T cells that have been sensitized to a specific antigen and have undergone clonal proliferation. Memory T cells promote a more rapid response following a secondary exposure to a familiar antigen. T-lymphocyte memory cells amplify the response to a familiar antigen because clonal augmentation is produced at an accelerated rate during a secondary exposure.

Natural killer (NK) cells are lymphocyte effector cells capable of spontaneous cytotoxicity directed at a variety of target cells that do not require interaction with the major histocompatibility complex (MHC) (Kamani & Douglas, 1991). NK cells are available to kill antigen without prior sensitization and are thought to participate in the immune response by the nonspecific destruction of virally infected cells, tumor cells, and transplanted tissues. They also may have a role in immune surveillance.

Lymphokine activated killer (LAK) cells are lymphocytes that are produced when lymphoid cells are incubated in IL2. They have a nonspecific antigen cytotoxicity against a much wider range of target antigens than NK cells. Clinically, LAK cells have been shown to be effective in combating a number of metastatic malignancies.

Cytokines are a group of extremely potent chemical mediators that are produced by a number of cell types, primarily in response to noxious or physiologic stimuli. Cytokines secreted by lymphocytes are called lymphokines, and those secreted by monocytes or macrophages are called monokines (see Table 23-12).

Cytokines function as regulators of the host's immunologic, inflammatory, and reconstructive responses to injury. In part, they contribute to cell growth and activation, cellular traffic control, stimulation of macrophage function, and the destruction of foreign antigens (see Table 23-12).

Interferons (IFN) are a group of lymphokines that have demonstrated defense against viruses and tumor cell growth. They are also capable of activating and amplifying NK cells cytotoxic capabilities. Three types of interferons have been identified, based on their function and cell origin aIFN, flIFN, and gIFN (see Table 23-12).

Cell Cooperation in the Immune Response

The immune response is an extremely complex, highly regulated series of events that involves a number of cell types (see Figure 23-3). It is triggered when an antigen is introduced into the host and encounters the antigen-presenting cells (APC). Antigens captured by APCs undergo a series of changes called antigen processing. Macrophages are one type of APC that identifies, phagocytizes, and processes foreign antigen. Antigen fragments, called epitopes, are then expressed on the macrophage membrane cell surface together with the class II major histocompatibility complex (MHC) antigen. This is called antigen presentation. The primary purpose for this process is that T cells are the main coordinators of the immune response and generally will recognize antigen only when it is presented by APCs jointly with the class II major histocompatibility complex (MHC) antigens.

The association between APC and antigen-specific T helper cells stimulates the APCs to release IL1, another cytokine. IL1 functions to augment the binding of T helper cells, promote antigen presentation by APC, enhance T helper cell IL2 secretion, and expand T helper cell IL2 receptor expression.

Helper T-lymphocytes are the primary coordinators of the immune response, mainly because they are needed to activate cytotoxic T cells and antibody-secreting plasma (mature B) cells. Activation of T helper cells is the result of two signals that occur during T cell antigen-receptor binding to the antigenic-MHC complex on the surface of the APC. These signals stimulate T helper cells to secrete the cytokine IL2 and express IL2 receptors on their cell surface. In addition to IL2, activated T helper cells secrete other cytokines that subsequently promote the growth, differentiation, and function of B lymphocytes, macrophages, and other cell types (Goodman, 1994). For example, factors released by T helper cells that encourage macrophages to stay in the target area and amplify their phagocytic ability are called macrophage migration inhibition factor (MIF) and macrophage activating factor (MAF).

Cytotoxic T cells are activated by the release of IL2 from T helper cells and by their recognition of foreign antigen in collaboration with class 1 MHC antigens. The activation of cytotoxic T cells results in the release of cytotoxins that cause subsequent target cell (antigen) death. Cytotoxic T cells function to eradicate all cells that express foreign antigen on their cell surface, for example, transplanted tissue or viral infected host cells (Goodman, 1994).

While T cells are undergoing activation, B cells have been trapping antigen in their membrane-bound antibodies. Complete activation of B cells into antibody-secreting plasma cells remains largely dependent on T helper cell activation and the release of B cell growth factor (BCGF) and B cell differentiation factor (BCDF). With the secretion of antibody, antigen-antibody complexes are formed and ultimately destroy or inactivate foreign antigen.

There are a number of mechanisms of antigen elimination. Direct cytotoxic killing of antigen-bearing target cells by cytotoxic T-lymphocytes is a major mechanism and one that does not require antibodies. Other mechanisms of antigen elimination require antibody assistance including neutralization through alteration of the antigen or blocking attachment to target cells, opsonization by antibodies to promote phagocytosis, activation of complement by specific antibodies, resulting in cell lysis, further opsonization by complement components, complement chemotaxis activity for neutrophils, and antibody-dependent, cell-mediated cytotoxicity (ADCC). These antibodies facilitate cells such as natural killer (NK) cells and others to perform ADCC. This is different than T cell cytotoxicity, which attacks and kills target cells independent of antibodies.

The generation of memory B and T cells after the initial exposure to antigen prepares the immune system to provide an augmented response upon subsequent encounters with the same antigen. Regulation of the immune response involves a complex network of interactions between lymphocytes, cytokines, and feedback mechanisms.

Lymphocytes and APCs are the primary cells involved in all immune responses; however, other cells are also recruited. For example, neutrophils may respond to the chemotactic stimuli from cytokines or other products released by activated lymphocytes. Components of the complement cascade may result in increased local vascular perfusion, capillary permeability, accumulation of extravascular fluid, and pain. Other enzymatic pathways may also be triggered, such as the kinin, clotting, and fibrinolytic systems (Goodman, 1994).

The host response involves the immune response and the inflammatory response, which includes a number of factors that trigger the various aspects of inflammation known as inflammatory mediators. Although most aspects of inflammation are generally considered beneficial, excessive, or inappropriate (e.g., organ transplants), inflammatory reactions can cause harm rather than host protection. In these situations, specific medications that suppress the inflammatory and immune responses play a very important role in clinical management, specifically in organ/tissue transplantation and the management of rejection.

Immunologic Aspects of Organ Transplantation

Genetic Factors Related to Transplantation

All human ovum and spermatozoan have 23 chromosomes, 22 autosomes, and one sex chromosome. All chromosomes occur as matched pairs except the sex chromosomes. At the time of fertilization, 46 chromosomes come together to make up the total chromosomal structure for the new individual. Therefore, every individual has 46 chromosomes. Genes are a component of the chromosomal structure and are the functional sites of heredity. It is through the genes that the genetic codes of inheritance are passed from parent to child. Every human cell nucleus carries approximately 30,000 gene pairs, contributing to an almost endless array of genetic combinations. However, since these genes and chromosomes are inherited, similarities within families is possible (Lancaster & Schanbacer, 1991).

Every gene is located in a specific position on a chromosome called a locus. When more than one set of genes is able to occupy any given gene site, it is called an allele (Huffer, Kanapa, & Stevenson, 1986). A pair of alleles is considered homozygous when identical and heterozygous when different. The number of genetic combinations of alleles on a chromosome is called a genotype, and the order in which the genotype is expressed is called a phenotype. The phenotype inherited from one parent is called a haplotype. A haplotype is the combination of alleles at a locus on a chromosome that is inherited as a unit (Schwartz, 1991). For example, one maternal haploid genotype (haplotype) and one paternal haploid genotype (haplotype) make up the unique genetic composition for each individual.

Three variations of expression can occur when a cell has two different alleles at any particular gene site. First, the cell can coexpress (codominant) both alleles as found in the human leukocyte antigen genes. Second, at certain gene sites, one variant allele can suppress the function of another, which is called a dominant trait. Third is a recessive trait, which is not capable of expression unless the allele is carried by both members of a pair of homologous chromosomes.

Genes contain certain codes for specific cell surface antigens that can highly influence transplantation. Two very important antigen systems that must be considered prior to transplantation include the ABO blood group and the major histocompatibility complex (MHC).

ABO Blood Group Antigens

Blood group antigens are expressed on the cell surface of all erythrocytes. Every individual's blood type is determined by inheriting one blood group antigen from each parent. There are three possible alleles that can determine blood type for this locus; A and B which are codominant and O which is recessive (Mudge-Grout, 1992). For example, if an individual is type A, the other inherited gene must be either A or O. Likewise, if the blood type is B, the other gene must be B or O. Since O blood type is recessive, the only instance in which O blood type is expressed is when both inherited genes are O. It is interesting to note that both A and B blood groups can be divided into subgroups. In blood group A, 11 subgroups have been identified, with A1 and A2 being the most important (Donegan & Bossom, 1994).

ABO typing is always performed before a blood transfusion and organ transplantation to ensure compatibility and minimize the risk of transfusion reaction or graft rejection.

Rhesus (Rh) is another blood group antigen present on most erythrocytes. However, it does not appear to be significant in transplantation (Richards, 1986; Smith, 1991).

Table 23-13
Complete list of recognized HLA-A, -B, and -DR specificities (1994).

A1	B5	B49(21)	DR1
A2	B7	B50(21)	DR103
A203	B703	B51(5)	DR2
A210	B8	B5102	DR3
A3	B12	B5103	DR4
A9	B13	B52(5)	DR5
A10	B14	B53	DR6
A11	B15	B54(22)	DR7
A19	B16	B55(22)	DR8
A23(9)	B17	B56(22)	DR9
A24(9)	B18	B57(17)	DR10
A2403	B21	B58(17)	DR11(5)
A25(10)	B22	B59	DR12(5)
A26(10)	B27	B60(40)	DR10(6)
A28	B35	B61(40)	DR14(6)
A29	B37	B62(15)	DR1403
A30(19)	B38(16)	B63(15)	DR1404
A31(19)	B39	B64(14)	DR15(2)
A32(19)	B3901	B65(14)	DR16(2)
A33(19)	B3902	B67	DR17(3)
A34(10)	B40	B70	DR18(3)
A36	B4005	B71(70)	DR51
A43	B41	B72(70)	DR52
A66(10)	B42	B73	DR53
A68(28)	B44(12)	B75(15)	
A69(28)	B45(12)	B76(15)	
A74(19)	B46	B77(15)	
AX80	B47	B7801	
	B48	Bw4	
		Bw6	

UNOS Bylaws, Appendix B, Attachment 1-A

Note: From Lancaster, L.E. & Schanbacher, B. (1995). Renal transplantation. In L.E. Lancaster (Ed.). (1995). *ANNA core curriculum for nephrology nursing* (3rd ed., p. 374). Pitman, NJ: American Nephrology Nurses' Association. Reprinted with permission.

Major Histocompatibility Complex

The major histocompatibility complex (MHC) is a group of genes found in all mammalian species. It is composed of a group of genes located in a specific chromosomal region (Benjamini & Leskowitz, 1991). The MHC is largely responsible for discriminating "self" from "nonself," cell interaction, and immune recognition and response. In mice, where much of the research has been conducted, the MHC is located on the 17th chromosome and is referred

Figure 23-4
The human leukocyte antigen (HLA) is located on chromosome 6. The 6th chromosome is the gene site that encodes HLA antigens.

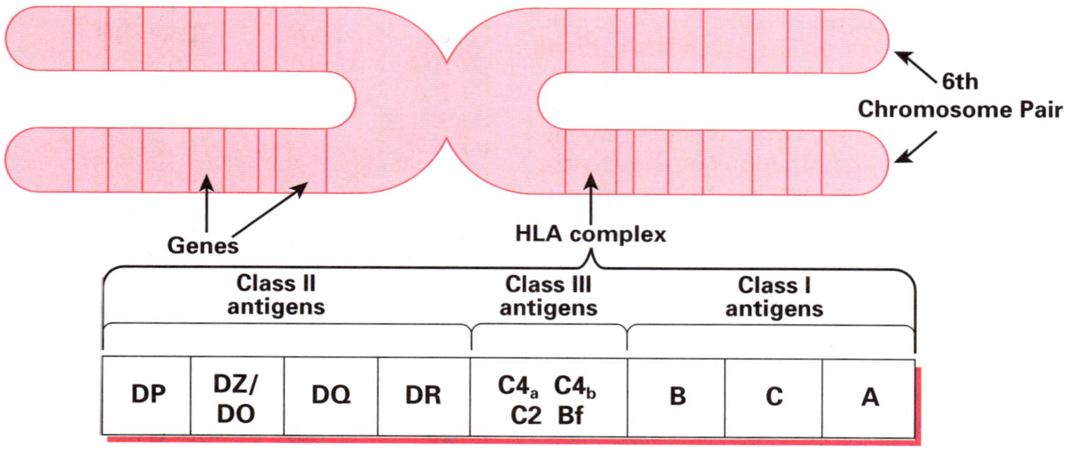

Table 23-14
HLA class I and II antigens.

Characteristics	Class I HLA	Class II HLA
Antigens	HLA A,B, C	HLA D, DR, DQ, DP
Function	Immune recognition, tissue graft rejection, elimination of virally infected cells.	Regulatory communication between T cells, collaboratively present antigen to T helper cells with APC.
Distribution	Surface of all nucleated cells (except sperm) and platelets.	Immunocompetent cells, including B and T-lymphocytes, macrophages, monocytes; some cells be induced to express class II HLA e.g. endothelial cells and resting T cells.

to as H2. In humans, the MHC is called the human leukocyte antigen (HLA) complex and is located on chromosome 6 (see Figure 23-4). Although antigens are considered nonself molecules, the human leukocyte antigens on an individual's leukocytes are the mechanism by which self is determined. For example, the HLA complex on a person's cells become the nonself antigens when injected into another individual.

The HLA genes are present on several loci on the sixth chromosome called HLAA, HLAB, HLAC, HLAD, HLADR, HLADP, HLADQ, and HLA DZ/DO. Well over 120 different HLAs have been identified. The nomenclature of the HLA system has been developed by the Nomenclature Committee of the World Health Organization (see Table 23-13). Every HLA antigen is identified by a letter, which refers to the specific HLA locus, and by number referring to the particular allele. The letter "w" means "workshop" and is dropped when there is a consensus in identification (e.g., HLADRw4 becomes HLADR4).

Antigens on the HLA complex are divided into three categories based on structure, function, tissue distribution, and the specific antigen expressed on their cell surface (see Table 23-14) (Smith, 1990). These categories are called class I antigens (HLAA, HLAB, HLAC), class II antigens (HLAD, HLADR, HLADP, HLA DZ/DO), and class III antigens (complement).

Class I antigens, HLAA, HLAB, and HLAC, are expressed on the surface of all nucleated cells (except sperm) and platelets. These antigens facilitate recognition of a foreign antigen by cytotoxic T cells (CD8). Expressed on the surface of cytotoxic T cells are receptors that recognize class I antigens. For a foreign antigen to be recognized by a cytotoxic T cell, the antigen must be recognized in concert with a class I molecule. Once recognition occurs, the cytotoxic T cell will kill the target cell bound to the foreign antigen. Class I antigens also facilitate elimination of viral infected cells, antitumor activity, and acute graft rejection. During organ transplant rejection, it is the donor (foreign) class I molecules that are recognized by the host cytotoxic T cells and attacked (Schwartz, 1991). In addition, those individuals exposed to class I HLA molecules through blood transfusions, pregnancy, or previous transplants, tend to develop antibodies to donor HLA class I molecules, reducing their potential donor pool.

Class II antigens HLAD, HLADR, HLADP, HLA DZ/DO, are located mainly on immunocompetent T and B lymphocytes, antigen-presenting cells (e.g., macrophages and dendritic cells), and monocytes. The main function of class II antigens is to present processed antigenic fragments to T helper lymphocytes (CD4) during the initiation of the immune response. T helper lymphocytes only recognize antigenic fragments in the context of class II molecules. Therefore, class II antigens contribute to transplant rejection, thus mandating that a negative reaction between donor and recipient must be confirmed prior to transplantation.

Class III antigens are located between class I and class II antigens on chromosome 6. They participate in the alternative and classical complement pathways. They are soluble antigens and facilitate presentation of antigen to T-lymphocytes.

Human Leukocyte Antigen (HLA) Inheritance

Every individual inherits one HLA haplotype from each parent, providing all individuals with two HLA haplotypes. All HLA genes are codominant and expressed. This results in four combinations of HLA haplotypes for all individuals (see Figure 23-5). Therefore, a transplant from a parent to a child or vice-versa is a one-haplotype match. Transplants between siblings provide a 25% chance that the siblings will be a two-haplotype match (identical) or a no-haplotype match (nonidentical), and a 50% chance they will be a one-haplotype match.

Histocompatibility Testing

Histocompatibility is the degree of compatibility between donor and recipient. It is generally performed to identify the potential degree of host acceptance of the donor graft and to avoid or minimize graft rejection. The purpose of histocompatibility testing is to decrease donor foreignness and to reduce donor-specific immune responses to the transplanted organ by the recipient. The exact type and timing of testing varies, depending on the organ to be transplanted. This is because of the difference in the immunogenicity of tissues and the variation in cold ischemia time for different organs. For example, HLA typing is always done before a kidney transplant, whereas in liver transplantation, it may be performed posttransplant or not at all.

Figure 23-5
HLA inheritance.

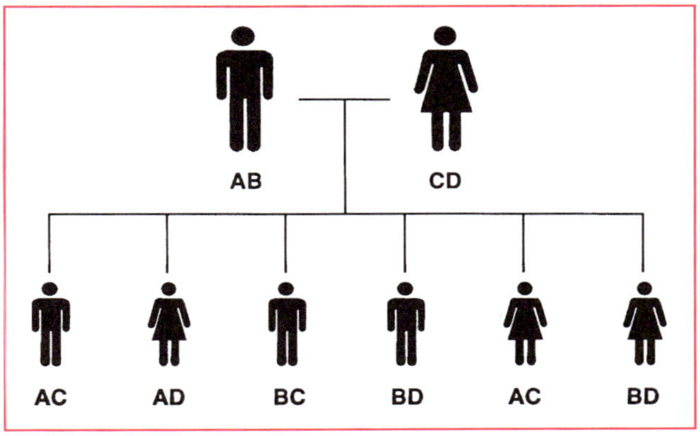

In general, an immunologic evaluation consists of two broad categories: typing and crossmatching. Typing procedures allow for pretransplant identification of specific antigens that could ultimately be responsible for donor-recipient incompatibility. Typing procedures include ABO blood typing, minor red cell antigens, and HLA typing. Matching procedures allow donor and recipient antigens to interact prior to transplantation to ascertain the degree of compatibility. Crossmatching can be performed between a recipient and a specific donor or a panel of random potential donors (Smith, 1991). Matching procedures include white cell crossmatch, mixed lymphocyte crossmatch, and mixed leukocyte culture.

ABO blood type compatibility between donor and recipient is always determined before transplantation. As in blood transfusions, O is the universal donor and AB the universal recipient. An individual with O blood type can receive a kidney only from an O donor, type A from an A or O donor, type B from an B or O, and type AB from an A, B, or O donor. Crossing the ABO barrier during kidney transplantation almost always leads to a rejection (Garovoy et al., 1991). Although ABO incompatibility in liver transplantation does not necessarily lead to rejection, survival rates are considerably lower. Therefore it has been recommended that ABO incompatible liver transplantation be used in emergency situations only and aggressive retransplantation be considered (Reding et al., 1992). Rh factor is not significant in organ transplantation.

Minor red cell antigen systems number over 15; the most important of these is the Lewis system. As a result of multiple blood transfusions, patients who are highly sensitized to minor red cell antigens may experience antibody-mediated rejection (hyperacute or chronic). In these patients, screening for minor cell antigens before transplant can be helpful (Smith, 1991)

Human leukocyte antigen (HLA) testing is known as tissue typing. It needs to be performed only once because an individual's genetic makeup does not change. Since HLAs are present on most tissues, a blood test is all that is necessary. There are a number of assays employed to detect HLA antigens. The primary test used to identify the HLAs is a serologic assay called the complement-dependent cytotoxic test (Colombe, 1994). This test is performed by dispensing lymphocytes into wells filled with anti-HLA antibody (antisera). Approximately 30 minutes are allowed for the anti-HLA antibody to bind to the cell surface of the HLA. Complement is added; if the antibody has bound to the antiserum, complement will be activated and cause cell lysis. A dye is then added to detect cell lysis. If the antibody has bound to the surface of the cell, and complement activation was sufficient to cause cell lysis, the dye will have leaked into the cells and they will appear dark red and swollen. This is considered a positive test. A positive test is one in which 20% or more of the cells have been lysed (dyed) (Colombe, 1991; Colombe, 1994). If the antibody has not bound to the cell surface, the cells will appear clear, round, and intact when observed under the microscope. This is considered a negative test result.

Gene-cloning techniques have allowed a closer look at the genetic structure of HLA. One test is the polymerase chain reaction or PCR. This is an automated method of amplifying a specific known DNA sequence, which can be applied to the HLA complex (Colombe, 1991). Research in this area is continuing and may provide a broader application with regard to the relationship of HLA to transplant and disease in the future.

White cell crossmatch is performed to detect the presence of preformed antibodies in the recipient's serum, directed against the potential donor's HLA antigens (Colombe, 1991). The most common test is the standard cytotoxicity method, which is cell lysis by antibody. In this test, the recipient's serum is incubated with specific donor lymphocytes. If lysis of donor cells occurs, preformed cytotoxic antibodies are present in the recipient serum. This is considered a positive reaction or crossmatch, and the transplant is deferred to eliminate the risk of hyperacute rejection. If lysis does not occur, there are no preformed cytotoxic antibodies in the recipient serum, and transplantation may be considered.

Mixed lymphocyte crossmatch is also performed to detect preformed cytotoxic antibodies in the recipient serum. However, rather than a specific donor, the recipient serum is mixed with a randomly selected panel of donor lymphocytes to determine reactivity. This is called a panel of reactive antibodies (PRA), which is indicative of recipient sensitivity to HLA. Results are calculated in percentages. A high percentage of reactivity suggests that the recipient has a large number of cytotoxic antibodies and poor chance of finding a crossmatch negative donor (Colombe, 1994; Stites, 1994). However, antibodies can change over time; therefore, potential transplant recipients generally undergo this type of testing monthly.

Crossmatches are often performed on multiple occasions between a recipient and a potential living donor. In addition, it is common practice to perform a crossmatch about 24 hours before transplant (Richards, 1986).

Mixed leukocyte culture (MLC) is a test that is used to further identify donor-recipient compatibility. The MLC specifically detects class II (HLA: A-B-C) antigens. The procedure combines lymphocytes of the potential donor and recipient in a tissue culture. If the lymphocytes differ, they will enlarge and proliferate. This type of reactivity of the MLC may be a reflection of the initial step in graft rejection in vivo. If the lymphocytes are similar, they will remain quiescent (Colombe, 1991). The test takes a number of days to perform, and therefore is generally used when attempting to select the most compatible living-kidney donor. The donor who is the least stimulatory to the potential recipient is considered the preferred organ donor (Colombe, 1994).

More recently, the MLC has been eliminated from live kidney donor evaluation, in the interest of cost containment. Matching T and B cell crossmatches, and convenience of donors are considered in selection of donors when multiple ABO compatible donors are available.

Immunosuppressive Agents

The primary function of the human immune system is to protect the host against foreign substances. If the foreign invader is a transplanted organ, this response can lead to rejection of the transplanted graft. Therefore, the success of transplantation is dependent on the alteration of the immune response.

Currently, immunosuppressive medications are administered to alter the immune response and preserve graft function. Immunosuppressive therapy posttransplant is critical to graft survival. However, because immunosuppressive agents alter the immune response, the ability of the host to respond to other invading foreign substances, such as pathogens, is also compromised. As a result, immunosuppressive drugs are often considered double-edged swords, in that they are able to modulate the immune system to prevent rejection, but they can place the host at risk for infection and/or malignancies.

Most clinical protocols for posttransplant immunosuppression employ a combination of corticosteroids, azathioprine, or mycophenolate

Table 23-15
Common medications administered after transplantation.

Immunosuppressives	prednisone, cyclosporine, azathioprine, tacrolimus, cyclophosphamide, mycophenolate, mofetil, ATG, OKT3
Antivirals	gancyclovir, acyclovir
Antifungals	Nystatin, clotrimazole (Mycelex troche)
Antibacterial	trimethoprimsulfamethoxazole, pentamidine, dapsone (specifically *Pneumocystis carinii*)
Antihypertensives	calcium channel blockers, (nifedipine [Procardia])
Antacid or H2 blocker	sucralfate, ranitidine, omeprozole
Diuretics	furosemide, thiazides

mofetil (CellCept®), cyclosporine, tacrolimus (Prograf®), and antilymphocyte preparations (OKT3, antithymocyte globulin [ATGAM]). Each of these agents has advantages and disadvantages, individually and in combination, that must be taken into consideration. Immunosuppressive regimens are often specific to patients, transplant centers, and type of organ transplanted.

Immunosuppressive therapy has always attempted to prevent rejection; however, it has been juxtaposed with the risks of infection and malignancies. Thus, future advances in organ transplantation rest with the ability of immunosuppressive therapy to specifically target local responses of the immune system while simultaneously preserving the host's systemic immune system (Bumgardner & Roberts, 1993). One method for this to become a reality is through immunologic tolerance, which is the induction of immunologic unresponsiveness to a specific antigen (Bartucci & Seller, 1990). Although immunologic tolerance is the posttransplant goal, it has yet to be achieved.

Immunosuppressive medications used in most centers are reviewed in Tables 23-15 and 23-16. See Chapter 12 for a more complete review of these medications.

Table 23-16
Immunosuppressive agents used in transplantation.

*Dosages listed are general guidelines for therapy.
Immunosuppressive management varies between transplant center protocol and organ transplanted.

Immunosuppres- Agent	Primary Mechanism to increase the Action	Use	*Administration Considerations	Major Side Effects (All have risk of infection and malignancies)
azathioprine (Imuran®)	6-Mercaptopurine antimetabolite which interferes with DNA and RNA synthesis; inhibits proliferation of cells (e.g. T lymphocytes)	Induction Maintenance	Intravenous: 1 mg/kg/day Orally: 23 mg/kg/day Preparation: tablet 50 mg solution 10 mg/ml dosed qhs	Bone marrow suppression, leukopenia anemia, thrombocytopenia, alopecia, hepatic dysfunction, gastric upset.
cyclophosphamide (Cytoxan®)	Inhibits cell proliferation through alkylation and DNA crosslinking, inhibits B-cell function.	Maintenance	Oral: 0.25-2 mg/kg/day Preparation 25 to 50 mg tablets	Leukopenia, thrombocy- topenia, gastric disturbance.
prednisone/ prednisolone	Inhibits production of IL-1 and IL-2, inhibits lymphocytes ability to mount an immune response.	Induction Maintenance Treat rejection	Oral and intravenous dosing is the same: Initial 1-2 mg/kg/day Maintenance: 0.1-0.2 mg/kg/day	Early: *cushingoid*, hyper- glycemic, increased appetite, Na+ and water retention, delayed healing, acne, hypertension, pan- creatitis, emotional disturbances. Later: ulcer disease, growth retardation, easy bruis- ing, steroid induced diabetes, avascular joint necrosis, cataracts, skin cancer, cervical cancer.
methylprednisolone (Solu-Medrol®)	Same as prednisone, more potent.	Treat rejection	Intravenous: 10-20 mg/kg/day for 3-5 days	Same as prednisone.
cyclosporine (Sandimmune®) (Neoral®)	Inhibits synthesis of IL-2, prevents gamma- interferon secretion and B cell activating factors	Induction Maintenance	Dosed according to level Intravenous or oral Oral preparation: 100 mg/ml; tablets 25 mg & 100 mg Initial oral dose: 5-10 mg/kg/day Maintenance dose: 2-5 mg/kg/day in 2 divided doses (bid)	Nephrotoxicity, hyperkalemia, hypertension, headaches, gingival hyper hyperplasia, hirsutism, nausea, vomiting, diarrhea, mild anemia, flushing, tremors, seizures, hypomagnesemia
tacrolimus (Prograf® [FK506])	Inhibits IL-2 lymphocyte proliferation cytotoxic T-cell generation, IL-3 and gamma interferon	Induction Maintenance	Dosed according to level and patient response approximately 0.02-0.12 mg/kg/day in 2 divided doses (bid) Oral Preparation: 1 and 5 mg tablets	Nephrotoxicity, diarrhea, nausea, vomiting, hyperglycemia, hyperkalemia, hypertension, hair loss, anorexia, anemia, thrombocytopenia, headache, tremor, insomnia, seizures

Table 23-16 (continued)
Immunosuppressive agents used in transplantation.

Immunosuppres-Agent	Primary Mechanism to increase the Action	Use	*Administration Considerations	Major Side Effects (All have risk of infection and malignancies)
antithymocyte globulin (ATG)	Polyclonal preparation, inhibits activity and number of lymphocytes	Induction Treat rejection	Intravenous: 10-20 mg/kg/day for 5-21 days; Infuse over 4-6 hours via a central line, premedicate with steroids, Benadryl® and Tylenol®	Thrombocytopenia, leukopenia, anemia, hyper-sensitivity response (rash, tachycardia, dyspnea, hypotension, chills, fever, chest & back pain, anaphylaxis) arthralgias, myalgias
muromonab-CD3 (Orthoclone OKT3®)	Monoclonal preparation binds to CD3 complex on the surface of T cells inhibits activity and increases removal of T lymphocytes	Induction Treat rejection	Intravenous 2.5-20 mg/day IV push (usual adult dose 5 mg/day), premedicate with steroids, Benadryl® and Tylenol® monitor CD3 levels; IV preparation 5 mg vials	Flu-like symptoms, fever chills, arthralgias, myalgias, nausea/ vomiting, dyspnea, wheezing, chest pain, pulmonary edema, aseptic meningitis, hypersensitivity response (rash, tachycardia, dyspnea, hypotension, chills, fever, chest & back pain, anaphylaxis)
mycophenolate mofetil (Cellcept®) (RS61443)	Lymphocyte-specific mofetil inhibitor or purine synthesis with antiproliferative effects on both T & B cells. Replaces azathioprine in immunosuppressive regimen.	Induction	23-25mg/kg in 2 divided Maintenance doses; 250mg & 1 gm capsules.	Nausea, vomiting, diarrhea, cramps, gastritis ulcers, leukopenia

CHAPTER 23B

Transplantation

Christine Mudge, MS, RN, PNPc/CNS, CNN
Laurie Carlson, MSN, RN
Patricia Brennan, MSN, RN

Chapter Contents

Rejection and Infection: Complications Associated With All Organ Transplants 695
Rejection Posttransplant 695
Infection Posttransplant. . . . 697
Time Table Approach to Infection Posttransplant 706
Nursing Considerations Regarding Infection Posttransplant 707
Donor Management and Recovery 707
Brain Death 707
Organ Donation 707
Donor Management 707
Donor Recovery 708
Kidney Transplantation. 710
Kidney Transplant Recipient Selection. 710
Kidney Transplant Recipient Evaluation 711
Immunologic Considerations. 714
Kidney Transplant Donor Evaluation and Selection 715
Recipient Considerations Pretransplant 717
Kidney Transplant Surgical Procedure 717
Postoperative Management and Nursing Care of the Kidney Transplant Recipient. 719
Early Complications After Kidney Transplantation 725
Late Complications After Kidney Transplantation 730

Chapter Contents

Pancreas Transplantation 748
Normal Pancreatic Function 749
Diabetes Mellitus 749
Types of Pancreas Transplantation 750
Pancreas Transplant Recipient Selection 751
Pancreas Transplant Recipient Evaluation 751
Pancreas Transplant Surgical Procedure 751
Pancreas Transplant Postoperative Management and Nursing Care 751
Long-Term Management After Pancreas-Kidney Transplantation 754
Liver Transplantation 754
Normal Liver Function 754
Liver Transplant Recipient Selection 754
Controversies in Liver Transplant Recipient Selection 757
Liver Transplant Recipient Evaluation 758
Liver Transplant Surgical Procedure 760
Liver Transplant Postoperative Management and Nursing Care 762
Liver Transplant Complications 765
Summary 768
References and Readings 769
Chapter Highlights 777

Transplantation

Christine Mudge, MS, RN, PNPc/CNS, CNN
Laurie Carlson, MSN, RN
Patricia Brennan, MSN, RN

Rejection and Infection: Complications Associated With All Organ Transplants

Rejection Posttransplant

Rejection after organ transplant is an immunologic response that is not completely understood. It generally does not occur between genetically identical individuals, only in those who are genetically nonidentical (Smith, 1991). Rejection is initiated by the recognition of foreign antigens (histocompatibility) on the membranes of transplanted tissue (Ascher et al., 1989). The host recognizes these foreign antigens expressed on donor cells as nonself by recipient lymphocytes and antibodies. Subsequent to this recognition, the host attacks and damages the antigen-expressing graft, the donor organ.

Rejection is generally classified according to the primary cell type mediating the response and the histopathologic characteristics of the donor organ observed on biopsy. There are three main types of rejection: hyperacute, acute, and chronic (see Table 23-17). An overview of the pathophysiology of rejection is presented. However, since each organ transplanted responds slightly differently, specific attention will be given to the clinical manifestations, diagnosis, and treatment for kidney, pancreas, and liver transplantation in those sections.

Hyperacute rejection is primarily a humoral response with subsequent participation of the complement, coagulation, and kinin cascade systems. It occurs almost immediately following revascularization of the donor organ. Hyperacute rejection is generally the result of recipient preformed antibodies caused by pregnancy, blood transfusions, or previous transplants that react with antigens in the donor organ. Preformed anti-ABO isohemagglutinins or anti-class I HLA antibodies bind to the vascular endothelium of the graft resulting in the activation of complement and the clotting cascade causing microthrombi, ischemia, and subsequent graft necrosis.

Hyperacute rejection usually occurs in the surgical suite and requires prompt intervention. Graft prognosis is poor and frequently results in a transplant graft loss. To prevent hyperacute rejection, the pretransplant evaluation must ensure ABO blood type compatibility and identify donor-specific sensitization to HLA antigens by lymphocyte crossmatch, particularly before kidney transplant.

Table 23-17
Types of transplant rejection.

Type of Rejection	Etiology
Hyperacute	Primary humoral B lymphocyte response caused by preformed cytotoxic antibodies against donor HLA antigens.
Acute	Primary cellular T lymphocyte response with accompanying B lymphocyte response.
Chronic	Primarily humoral B lymphocyte response with accompanying T lymphocyte response.

Hyperacute rejection occurs primarily following kidney transplantation rather than in liver transplant recipients. While ABO compatibility and HLA histocompatibility are important in renal transplantation, HLA typing does not appear to be as significant for liver transplant graft survival. Factors that may be responsible for protecting the liver from hyperacute rejection include the size and structural difference between organs and the proposed possibility that the liver is capable of absorbing circulating antibody. Therefore, hyperacute rejection is less likely to occur after liver transplantation (Snover, 1990).

Acute rejection is primarily a cell-mediated process, and to a lesser degree, humorally mediated. Generally, acute rejection occurs 5 days to 4 months posttransplant. Acute rejection is triggered by antigen presenting cells (APCs) that process and reexpress donor allogenic class I and II HLA antigens on their cell surface. Nonactivated helper T cells encounter specific donor class II antigens and

Figure 23-6
Timetable for the occurrence of infection in the renal transplant recipient. Cytomegalovirus (CMV), Epstein-Barr virus (EBV), varicella zoster virus (VZV), central nervous system (CNS), urinary tract infection (UTI).

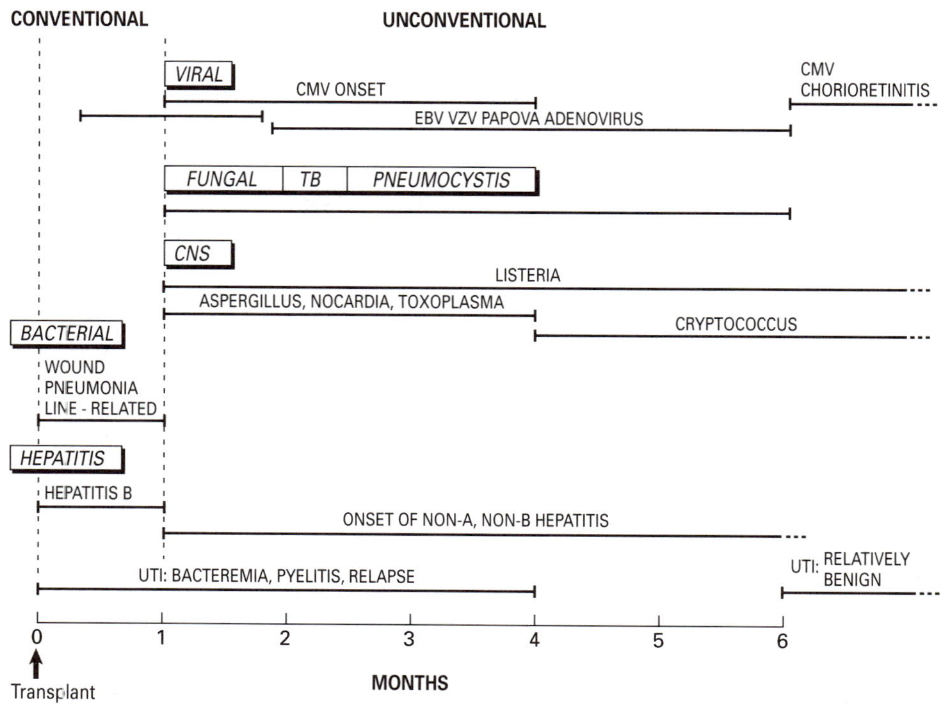

Note: Reprinted with permission from Rubin, R. (1994) Infection in the organ transplant recipient (page 635). In R. Rubin & L. Young (Eds.), *Clinical approach to infection in the compromised host*, 3rd ed. New York: Plenum Publishing Corporation.

become activated cells. Once activated, helper T cells are able to synthesize receptors for lymphokines released from APCs (see Figure 23-6).

Activated APCs (e.g., macrophages) release lymphokine IL-1, causing clonal expansion of activated T helper cells, and assist in the activation of cytotoxic T cells and B lymphocytes. Once T helper (CD4) cells are activated, they release lymphokine IL-2, which is essential in the activation and clonal proliferation of cytotoxic T (CD8) cells and B cells. These activated T and B cells then migrate to the site of the antigen, primarily the transplanted graft, causing damage and destruction.

The exact mechanism of graft destruction remains unclear. Effector cells that participate in graft destruction originate from both CD8 cytotoxic T cells and CD4 T helper cells. CD8 T cells appear to have a greater affinity for recognition of HLA-A and HLA-B antigen bearing cells, and CD4 T cells seem to recognize HLA-DR antigen bearing cells. Both classes of T cells are probably able to directly destroy graft cells by cytotoxic mechanisms. In addition, T cell release of lymphokines contributes to this process. In particular, gamma interferon (IFNg) a lymphokine released by activated T cells, induces the enhanced expression of HLA-A,-B, and -DR on the donor graft, increasing graft vulnerability to T cell activity. IFNg also activates monocytes to mediate a ruinous delayed hypersensitivity response against the graft (Garovoy et al., 1991).

Acute rejection has also been associated with viral infections. Antigens on the viruses may be similar to the donor HLA antigens and stimulate an immune response (Smith, 1991). To minimize the risk of a viral infection during a rejection episode, many centers administer anti-viral (e.g., gancyclovir) agents in conjunction with rejection therapy.

Acute rejection is the most common type of rejection occurring in transplant recipients. Diagnosis generally varies depending on the organ transplanted. However, diagnosis is usually based on graft dysfunction, laboratory findings, clinical manifestations, and biopsy results. Treatment can also vary between organ transplanted, patient, and

Table 23-18
Common infections observed in the posttransplant recipient.

Viral	Bacterial	Fungal	Parasitic
Cytomegalovirus (CMV)	*Pseudomonas*	*Candida*	*Toxoplasmosis*
Epstein-Barr Virus (EBV)	*Escherichia coli*	*Aspergillus*	*Strongyloides stercoralis*
Herpes (HSV1, HSV2)	*Klebsiella*	*Histoplasmosis*	
Varicella Zoster Virus (VZV)			
Hepatitis			
Human Immune Virus (HIV)	*Legionella*	*Coccidioides*	
Influenza A & other RNA viruses	*Clostridium difficile*	*Cryptococcus*	
Papovavirus	Tuberculosis	*Pneumocystis*	*carinii*
Adenovirus	*Streptococcus*	*Nocardia pneumoniae*	
Influenza virus	*Staphylococcus*		

center protocols. However, depending on the severity and organ involved, acute rejection is often initially treated with corticosteroids. Corticosteroids act to halt acute rejection by decreasing expression of class II antigens, reducing the release of IL-1 by APC, and by inhibiting T cell function and consequently the release of IL-2. Diagnosis and management of patients with acute rejection is further discussed in the sections reviewing kidney, pancreas, and liver transplantation.

Chronic rejection is mediated by both humoral responses (B lymphocytes) and cellular responses (T lymphocytes). It generally develops months to years after transplantation. Chronic rejection has an insidious onset that progresses over time. In most cases there is no treatment, and graft failure typically ensues. For extra-renal transplant recipients, this is a life-threatening situation mandating retransplantation. Renal transplant recipients may consider the option of retransplantation or decide to resume dialysis. Chronic rejection is characterized differently in organs transplanted and will be discussed in those sections.

Infection Posttransplant

Although there have been many advances in clinical transplantation, infection continues to be a major problem. Approximately 75% of all organ transplant patients will develop one infectious episode the first year after transplant, and infection remains the principal cause of death in the transplant population (Rubin, 1994). The high incidence of infection posttransplant is largely related to the administration of immunosuppressive therapy.

Immunosuppressive therapy, for the prevention and treatment of rejection, alters the immune system, leaving the host vulnerable to infection. The goal in transplantation is to provide adequate immunosuppression to prevent rejection and simultaneously maintain host defense mechanisms. There is an inverse relationship between rejection and infection, and the balance for each patient must be weighed carefully. For example, the more immunosuppressive therapy administered to prevent rejection, the greater the risk of infection. Less immunosuppressive therapy decreases the chance of infection but promotes the risk of rejection.

Transplant patients are at the greatest risk for acquiring opportunistic infections. Opportunistic refers to the ability of a mildly virulent organism to cause disease in the presence of an altered immune state (Young, 1994). Most of these organisms are naturally present on the skin or in the gastrointestinal tract, or they are innocuous substances in the environment (see Chapter 13). Opportunistic infections result from exogenous organisms (e.g., pneumococcal pneumonia), reactivation of endogenous organisms (e.g., herpes), or endogenous invasion of commensal or saprophytic organisms (e.g., bacterial, viral, fungal, parasitic) (Smith, 1991).

Host protection from infection is provided by adaptive and innate immunity. Innate immunity provides physical barriers (e.g., the skin and mucous membranes) and chemical barriers (e.g., lysozymes and gastric acid). Adaptive immunity provides specific T and B lymphocyte responses.

The risk of infection and the breakdown in protective mechanisms for the organ transplant recipient is based on a number of considerations, the most important being immunosuppressive therapy. Specific factors to consider regarding immunosuppression are the actions of the drug, dosage, length of time receiving the drug, episodes of rejection requiring additional immunosuppression, and number of drugs given simultaneously. Other factors that contribute to the transplant recipient's risk of infection include exposure to microorganisms, the hospital environment, alteration in normal microbial flora, break in the skin or mucous membranes, administration of antibiotics or antacids, decreased gastric motility, poor nutritional status, hyperglycemia, preexisting disease, diminished or absent splenic function, invasive tubes, lines or procedures (e.g., Foley catheter, T-tube, arteriogram, surgery), length of time on a ventilator, and the presence of one of the immune-modulating viruses (Epstein-Barr virus [EBV], cytomegalovirus [CMV], hepatitis B or C, and human immune deficiency virus [HIV]) (Rubin, 1993; Rubin, 1994; Smith, 1991).

Infections in organ transplantation are based on three approaches: type of infection, time of infection, and site of infection (Rubin, 1994). Types of infection are categorized as bacterial, viral, fungal, and parasitic (see Table 23-18). Time of infection is classified as to when the infection is most likely to occur posttransplant, the first month, 1 to 6 months, or more than 6 months (Johnson & Flye, 1988; Rubin, 1988; Rubin, 1994). Frequent sites of infection in transplant recipients include the respiratory tract, gastrointestinal tract, wound, urinary tract, biliary tree, and blood. This section reviews the types of infection observed posttransplant using the timetable approach. Sites of infection for the specific organ transplanted (kidney, pancreas, or liver) will be discussed in those sections.

Bacterial infections are often caused by organisms already present in the host. Specifically, gram negative bacteria are often implicated in causing infection in the transplant recipient (e.g., *Escherichia coli, Pseudomonas, Listeria monocytogenes, Serratia Marcescens,* and *Klebsiella*) (Beckman et al., 1991; Ryan, 1994). Gram-positive cocci such as staphylococcus aureus, normally found on the skin and soft tissue, and streptococcus species which normally colonizes the oropharynx are also frequent offenders. These pathogens typically gain access to the host via a break in the skin or mucous membrane as the result of an invasive procedure (e.g., surgery) or tissue damage.

Bacterial infections vary according to the site of infection; however all present with persistent fever. To determine the causative organism, routine cultures are obtained of the urine, sputum, and blood. If diarrhea is present, stool cultures will also be ordered. If there are prominent pulmonary manifestations, a chest x-ray and possibly a bronchial wash may be indicated. Identification of the causative organism prior to the initiation of antibiotics is the optimum approach to therapy. Since most transplant patients are already taking medications that can adversely affect their kidneys, caution must be taken to avoid nephrotoxic antibiotics.

Clostridium difficile is a common cause of diarrhea and abdominal cramps in posttransplant recipients. Although diarrhea can be the result of many etiologies (e.g., antibiotics, cyclosporine, CellCept®, other infections), *C. difficile* must be considered. Diagnosis is based on a stool specimen for *C. difficile* toxin and culture. Treatment consists of oral vancomycin or Flagyl® for 10 to 14 days with a follow-up stool specimen.

Tuberculosis is a mycobacterial infection. The current incidence posttransplant for active tuberculin infection is approximately 1% (Red Book, 1991). However, with the advent of drug-resistant tuberculosis there is likely to be an increased incidence over the next couple of years.

Tuberculosis (TB) can present in a variety of forms. Early clinical manifestations (1-6 months) of pulmonary TB usually present with one or more of the following manifestations: dry cough, hilar, mediastinal, and cervical lymphadenopathy, chest radiography demonstrating involvement of a segment or single lobe sometimes with consolidation, atelectasis, pleural effusion, and cavitation, or miliary TB. Extrapulmonary infections can affect the bowel, skin, central nervous system, and the bones and joints. Diagnosis is generally confirmed by a positive TB skin test (PPD). However, in the immunosuppressed transplant recipient, a negative TB test can occur in the presence of active disease. Therefore, cultures should be obtained in all suspected cases. Culture specimens include sputum, blood, urine, stool, and tissue as indicated (e.g., liver, lymph node). If positive, therapy usually includes a combination of two bactericidal medications (rifampin, isoniazid, or pyrazinamide). Liver dysfunction can occur as a result from these medications. Therefore, close monitoring of the effects of these drugs on hepatic function is mandatory. In addition, rifampin and isoniazid increase steroid, cyclosporine, and tacrolimus catabolism. Thus, dose adjustment of these drugs is important to prevent hepatic dysfunction and under-immunosuppression.

Legionella pneumophilia is a gram-negative bacillus associated with the development of broncho-pneumonia. It is found only in water sources and can be extremely serious in the posttransplant recipient. Clinical manifestations of Legionella include marked fever, gastrointestinal complaints (e.g., diarrhea, nausea), dyspnea, myalgia, arthralgia, agitation, confusion, and dry, nonproductive cough (Johnson & Flye, 1989). Diagnosis is confirmed by direct fluorescent antibody staining of the bacteria from transbronchial or percutaneous needle biopsies or bronchial washings, and by a fourfold rise in antibody titers over 3 to 4 weeks. Treatment of Legionella infections includes erythromycin, trimethoprim or rifampin. Legionella pneumophilia should be suspected in patients who present with a combination of gastrointestinal and pulmonary symptoms. Care must be taken when administering these medications because they can augment the effects of cyclosporine and tacrolimus (Prograf).

Viral infections can be a serious complication posttransplant. Those viral infections commonly observed posttransplant include the herpes group of viruses, herpes simplex 1 and 2, cytomegalovirus (CMV), varicella-zoster virus, and Epstein-Barr viruses (EBV). Viral hepatitis can also be problematic, and less common is the human immunodeficiency virus (HIV). All these viruses share a number of common characteristics: viral synthesis and replication, type of infection — either primary or secondary (latency), and the risk of being oncogenic.

Viruses enter the host by close cell-cell contact. Once entering the host, viral DNA penetrates host nuclei and begins viral protein synthesis and replication. Viral maturation and proliferation occurs in host nuclei, rendering viruses dependent on host cells for survival.

Viral infections can present as either primary or secondary infections. Primary infections are the first active infection of the virus in an individual who has not been previously infected. Secondary infections are those that are present in the host and are reactivated. Once an individual has had a primary viral infection, he or she is infected for life, even after there is no longer active viral replication or clinical symptoms. Primary viral infections posttransplant usually occur in seronegative individuals as a result of the host's receiving a seropositive donor graft or blood.

Harboring a virus without active infection is called latency. Viruses generally enter the host through the mucous membranes, proliferate, cause active infection, and then set up permanent residence. Viruses usually remain latent in either the lymphocyte pool or sensory ganglia. Viruses are protected from antiviral antibodies because antibodies do not permeate host cells (Smith, 1990).

A latent infection can be determined by drawing blood. If the individual has had a virus and it is in a latent state, the presence of a specific circulating antibody for that virus without active viral replication will be observed. This is called seropositivity. If the individual has not had the virus, antibody for the virus will not be observed; this is called seronegativity.

Table 23-19
Modes of acquiring active CMV infection in the posttransplant recipient.

Latent infection from a seropositive donor
Blood products that harbor latent virus from seropositive donors
Reactivation in a seropositive recipient
Acquisition from the community

Most viral infections posttransplant are due to reactivation of the virus in the host. Viral reactivation in the posttransplant recipient may be related to an alteration in T cell effectiveness secondary to the effects of immunosuppressive therapy (see Chapter 13). For example, the major host defense mechanism against the herpes group of viruses is mediated by virus specific, MHC-restricted, cytotoxic T cells (Rubin, 1993). These cells are susceptible to immunosuppressive agents and are often unable to mount a response to protect the host against the virus.

Cytomegalovirus (CMV) is the most common viral infection affecting organ transplant recipients and is a major cause of morbidity and mortality in this patient population (see Table 23-19). The high incidence of CMV infections can be attributed to two primary factors. First, more than 80% of the adult population is latently infected with CMV, and most latent infections are reactivated after transplantation with the initiation of immunosuppressive therapy. Second, those transplant recipients who are seronegative have a 50% chance or greater of becoming infected de novo (primary infection) from a seropositive or latently infected donor or through leukocyte-containing blood products (Ho, 1990). Additional risk factors for the development of CMV include seropositive donors for seronegative recipients; immunosuppression, particularly the use of monoclonal and polyclonal preparations; allograft reactions (e.g., rejection, graft-versus-host); organ transplanted (e.g., higher incidence in liver than kidney transplantation); and morbidity related to the organ transplanted (e.g., hepatitis in liver transplant) (Ho, 1990; Ho, 1992; Rubin, 1993; Rubin, 1994).

The epidemiologic patterns of CMV acquisition are classified as primary infection, disease reactivation, superinfection, and infection from the general community (Rubin, 1994). Ninety percent of primary (de novo) CMV infections occur as a result of a seropositive latently infected donor to a seronegative recipient (Grundy et al., 1987). The remaining 10% of CMV primary infections are from leukocyte-containing blood products. The incidence of seroconversion is higher in seronegative kidney transplant recipients receiving seropositive cadaveric donors than living-related donors. This may be related to the increased incidence of rejection with cadaveric donors requiring additional immunosuppression. (Rubin et al., 1985). The risk of seronegative recipients developing primary CMV posttransplant and becoming symptomatic is 50% to 60% (Ho, 1991; Rubin, 1990; Rubin, 1994).

Conversely, symptomatic illness as the result of reactivation of latent CMV or secondary infection occurs in approximately 20% of posttransplant recipients (Rubin, 1994).

CMV superinfection occurs when a seropositive recipient receives a seropositive donor and reactivating of the virus is of donor origin. Superinfection is thought to occur in 50% of recipients who develop clinical disease as a result of CMV (Chou, 1986; Grundy, 1988).

Acquisition of CMV infection from the general community is approximately 30% by young adulthood and 60% for those over 50 years of age. The incidence is higher for recipients of blood transfusions, those who are sexually promiscuous, and among lower socioeconomic groups. Therefore, the incidence of CMV is highly variable depending on the location of the transplant center and the population that is cared for (Rubin, 1994; Ho, 1991; Rubin, 1990).

The clinical manifestations of CMV, regardless of epidemiologic classification, develop approximately 1 to 4 months posttransplant. The symptomatology for CMV infections is the same for all organ transplants, except when it affects the transplanted organ itself. CMV has a greater effect on the organ transplanted than on native organs. For example, CMV hepatitis is more serious after liver transplantation than after renal transplantation. The rationale for this observation is unclear. However it may be related to rejection and the effects of the virus on the graft, excessive viral burden in the graft where reactivation occurs, and/or the fact that the graft is the site for viral replication (Rubin, 1990).

Most viral infections, including CMV, present with fever, malaise, fatigue, arthralgias, myalgias, and anorexia. Prolonged unexplained fluctuation in temperature is often the only symptom produced by CMV. On physical exam there is an unusual absence of splenomegaly and lymphadenopathy generally observed during viral illness. Laboratory evaluation may reveal leukopenia (WBC < 1500/mm^3), thrombocytopenia (platelets 30,000-60,000/mm^3), or superinfections. CMV also has suppressive effects on host defense mechanisms that can render the host susceptible to opportunistic superinfections. Although the exact mechanism is not clearly understood, CMV infection may also play a role in the pathogenesis of allograft damage.

CMV can present as a local disease or a disseminated infection. The major organs that are affected by CMV posttransplant that can be life-threatening are the lungs and gastrointestinal tract. CMV pneumonitis occurs in about one-third of the patients who develop a fever as a result of a CMV infection (Rubin, 1994).

Clinical manifestations are dependent on the severity of the disease. Generally pulmonary auscultation is unrevealing in the presence of CMV pneumonia. The degree of respiratory embarrassment is determined by hypoxia assessed by arterial blood gases, respiratory rate, and chest x-ray (Rubin, 1994; Rubin, 1993). One of the primary differential considerations is *Pneumocystis carinii pneumonia*. Pneumocystis presents very similar to CMV pneumonia. It is also possible that the host can be simultaneously infected with CMV and pneumocystis.

CMV infections of the gastrointestinal (GI) tract requiring immediate intervention are not uncommon posttransplant (e.g., CMV hepatitis after liver transplant). Gastrointestinal CMV infection can cause inflammation with functional disturbances, hemorrhage, ulceration, perforation, and possibly pneumatosis intestinalis (Rubin, 1994). CMV of the stomach (CMV gastritis) is a common site of symptomatic CMV infection. It usually presents with complaints of nausea, abdominal fullness and discomfort, anorexia, emesis, and/or dysphagia. Other common sites of upper GI CMV infection include the esophagus and duodenum. Lower GI CMV infection affects the colon, causing inflammation, hemorrhage, and possibly perforation (Mayoral et al., 1991). It has been reported that the incidence of upper GI CMV infections are 28% after liver transplant when the recipient is receiving cyclosporine (Sakr et al., 1992).

Fulminant CMV or the lethal CMV syndrome was first described in the early 1970s (Simmons et al., 1977). It presents with fever and leukopenia, quickly progressing to severe pulmonary and hepatic dysfunction, central nervous system alteration, GI hemorrhage, and death (Rubin, 1994). Although the availability of effective therapy has minimized the incidence of lethal CMV, it is important to be aware of the early manifestations, fever and leukopenia, to initiate prompt and aggressive therapy.

Diagnosis of CMV is often based on clinical manifestations, serologies, and viral cultures. Viremia can be detected several days before clinical symptoms appear. Detection of CMV antigens in the blood or CMV viremia by polymerase chain reaction (PCR) can be observed within 24 hours. Prompt diagnosis of CMV allows for early initiation of therapy, thus minimizing the additional risks of CMV infection. For testing purposes, CMV can be isolated from the blood, urine, breast milk, semen and oropharyngeal, vaginal, and cervical secretions.

Management of CMV in the transplant recipient has two approaches: prevention of infection and disease and treatment of disease. Strategies used to prevent CMV vary considerably among transplant centers. Generally CMV prevention involves one or a combination of the following: the use of CMV seronegative blood products, minimizing the use of seropositive donors in seronegative recipients (more difficult in liver transplantation than kidney), administering prophylactic gancyclovir during the immediate postoperative period and during rejection episodes, high dose (5-10 mg/kg in two divided doses IV depending on renal function) or Cytovene 75 mg/kg in three divided doses orally, acyclovir for 2 to 6 months posttransplant, and administration of prophylactic intravenous immunoglobulin (IV-Ig).

CMV treatment is well established and more clearly delineated than prophylactic therapy. Gancyclovir at 5 mg/kg every 12 hours intravenously (adjustments are made in the dosing schedule in the presence of renal insufficiency) is the primary therapy for CMV disease and has been found to be effective in treating CMV infections (Erice et al., 1987). In some centers, the administration of immunoglobulin is added to the treatment regimen. For those patients with a severe decrease in their WBC and platelets, trimethoprim sulfamethoxazole (*Pneumocystis carinii* prophylaxis) and/or azathioprine are generally held. Occasionally granulocyte colony stimulating factor (GCSF) may be prescribed to enhance cell development.

Epstein-Barr Virus (EBV) is the same virus responsible for infectious mononucleosis. It is harbored in the epithelial cells of the upper respiratory tract, which acts as a natural reservoir for EBV. Transmission of the virus is primarily through exchange of virus-laden saliva. However, the virus may be transmitted through blood transfusions or bone marrow transplantation. Sexual transmission of EBV has yet to be confirmed.

In a normal host, EBV disease is initiated by infecting epithelial cells of the upper respiratory tract and B lymphocytes. EBV entry into the host triggers an intense cytotoxic T lymphocyte response to latently infected B lymphocytes dispersed throughout the body. Generally, a T and B lymphocyte lymphoproliferative response would occur. However in a normal host, EBV mediated lymphoproliferation does not develop. Immunologic surveillance in a normal host provides EBV-specific cytotoxic T cells that prevent lymphoproliferation. In transplant recipients, this immune mechanism has been suppressed, and there is an outgrowth of B lymphocytes, resulting in lymphoproliferation. Thus EBV is not only associated with persistent infection, it is also strongly associated with lymphoproliferative malignancies (lymphoma).

More than 90% of adults are seropositive for EBV. Therefore, since the majority of transplants are performed in adults, most EBV infections posttransplant are reactivation infections. Clinical manifestations vary from being asymptomatic to characteristic symptoms associated with mononucleosis. For example, primary EBV infections posttransplant generally develop in seronegative children who acquire the virus from either the community or the allograft. These infections have clinical manifestations that range from asymptomatic infection to symptoms associated with mononucleosis, to fatal lymphoproliferative disease (Rubin, 1994).

Diagnosis of latent EBV infections can be determined by the presence of a gene product (EBER-1 gene) which is found in abundance in latently infected cells (Rubin, 1994). Diagnosis of viral reactivation is generally based on clinical manifestations, serial increases in antibody titers, and biopsy findings. Primary EBV is diagnosed mainly by the demonstration of a particular gene product (EBER-1 RNA) in mononuclear cells (Randhawa et al., 1992).

Treatment for EBV infection is either gancyclovir or acyclovir. Reactivation of EBV may require only oral therapy, while a primary infection usually mandates intravenous acyclovir or gancyclovir administration. Exact approaches to EBV treatment with acyclovir or gancyclovir vary between organ transplanted and transplant center.

Although all viruses can be considered potentially oncogenic, EBV has specifically been associated with EBV-mediated lymphoproliferative disease (Ho et al., 1988; Nalesnik et al., 1988). EBV mediated lymphoproliferative disease (LPD) can be one of the most devastating complications posttransplant. Approximately 10%-15% of malignancies that develop in posttransplant recipients are a form of lymphoma (Rubin, 1988). The incidence in patients who have received intensive immunosuppressive therapy, including antilymphocyte antibody preparation in conjunction with triple therapy (prednisone, azathioprine and cyclosporine), is approximately 1-2% in renal transplant recipients, and 2.2 % in liver transplant recipients (Malatack et al., 1991; Nalesnik et al., 1988; Stephaman et al., 1991; Straus et al, 1993). The incidence of LPD posttransplant is largely dependent on the number of EBV-infected B lymphocytes and the ability of EBV specific cytotoxic T cells to eliminate these transformed cells (Rubin, 1994). Interruption of EBV replication induced by antirejection therapy could halt the oncogenic process by decreasing the number of infected B lymphocytes. Thus, prophylactic therapy and prevention are key strategies in minimizing the risk of EBV-mediated LPD (Rubin & Tolkoff-Rubin, 1993).

The clinical manifestations of EBV-mediated LPD are highly variable and include one or more of the following: unexplained fever; mononucleosis-like symptoms demonstrated by fever, arthralgias, myalgias, malaise, and lymphadenopathy; persistent upper respiratory congestion similar to allergies; gastrointestinal manifestations (e.g., GI bleeding, abdominal pain/cramps, splenomegaly, perforation, or obstruction); hepatic dysfunction; central nervous symptoms such as seizures, alteration in consciousness; and focal disease (Ho et al., 1988; Rosenthal et al., 1994). Often the allograft is involved, and it is not uncommon for the bone marrow and every other organ to be affected.

Diagnosis of LPD is generally made by biopsy of the affected tissue. Pathologic observations of LPD present in a range of histologic findings. These findings are classified as polymorphic B cell lymphomas and range from nonspecific reactivity to malignancy (e.g., nonspecific reactive hyperplasia, polymorphic B cell hyperplasia, polymorphic B cell lymphoma, and immunoblastic sarcoma). Although CT scanning can be helpful in making the diagnosis of LPD, the absence of adenopathy on scan does not rule out the presence of LPD, since this disease can present completely extranodally (Hanto et al., 1981; Stephaman et al., 1991).

Treatment of LPD usually consists of strictly reducing or withdrawing immunosuppressive therapy. High-dose acyclovir or gancyclovir are typically added to the treatment regimen. Other treatment approaches have included one or a combination of the following: B cell monoclonal antibody, interferon-alpha and intravenous IgG, radiotherapy, surgical resection, and antilymphoma chemotherapy. Emphasis must be placed on prevention, including routine antiviral prophylactic therapy and antiviral therapy during intensive immunosuppression (e.g., rejection episode) to minimize the evolution of EBV-mediated LPD (Fisher et al., 1991; Rubin, 1994).

Herpes simplex (HSV) infection posttransplant is very common. Most HSV infections posttransplant are caused by reactivation of latent virus as the result of immunosuppressive therapy. There are two types of HSV: HSV-I and HSV-II.

HSV-I is responsible for most HSV infections above the waist. By far the most prevalent is herpes labialis (herpetic lesions around the lips, mouth, or face). After the primary infection, the virus is harbored in the dorsal root of the trigeminal ganglion. With the initiation of immunosuppressive therapy, the virus can potentially become reactivated, thus causing an infection.

In the transplant recipient, the lesions usually appear after the first 2 weeks posttransplant, lesion severity peaks at 1 month, and healing occurs over the next 2 to 6 weeks. The development of herpatic lesions may be exacerbated by the administration of immunosuppressive therapy to treat rejection.

HSV lesions appear as large, painful, ulcerated vesicles that can bleed and will eventually crust over. These ulcerations may interfere with normal nutrition and handling of oral secretions. Although aspiration pneumonia is uncommon, the chances of developing herpes pneumonia increases when the patient is unable to handle oral secretions. Primary lower respiratory tract infection with HSV-I is also unusual. However, prolonged intubation in patients with oral HSV can predispose the patient to developing herpetic tracheobronchitis. In addition, the evolution of intraoral and esophageal lesions appear in severely compromised individuals or those with prolonged nasogastric tube placement (Rubin, 1988; Rubin, 1994).

Latent HSV-I infection is determined by serum serial antibodies. Diagnosis of active HSV-I infections is based on the characteristic lesion (vesicle[s] on a erythematous base) and by scraping the lesion and isolating the virus in a cell culture.

HSV-II infections are significantly less common. These anogenital infections are those that occur primarily below the waist. In the transplant recipient, they usually develop 2 weeks posttransplant. Accompanying the characteristic vesicular lesion are prodromal symptoms, including fever, general malaise, itching, soreness, burning, and tingling. Once the lesions erupt, they can be observed anywhere in the genital area or on the buttocks. HSV-II anogenital lesions are characterized as large coalescing ulcerated lesions, or clusters of vesicles, without clearly defined individual vesicles (Rubin, 1994). In addition to the prodromal manifestations, other common symptoms include lymphadenopathy, radiating neuralgia down the buttocks, and erythema on the penis, testes, vulva, vaginal mucosa, or cervix. These lesions can become secondarily infected. Meticulous care must be taken to keep the area clean and protected.

Diagnosis of HSV-II is best obtained with a viral culture or direct immunofluorescence using monoclonal antibodies directed against HSV. Although the Tzanck smear with morphologic evaluation can be helpful, it does not provide a definitive diagnosis since it will also be positive in the presence of herpes varicella and herpes zoster.

The main goals of HSV treatment include: (1) minimize the spread of infection, (2) promote healing, (3) alleviate symptoms, and (4) prevent superinfections. Generally, any strategy employed to prevent CMV and EBV will have an effect against HSV (Rubin & Tolkoff-Rubin, 1993).

Acyclovir is typically the drug of choice in treating HSV infections. It works by penetrating HSV-infected cells and inhibiting HSV DNA synthesis. It may be administered topically, orally, or intravenously. Symptomatic infection generally responds well to oral acyclovir (e.g., 800 mg q.i.d. in adults) for 10 to 14 days. In severe cases, prolonged oral therapy or intravenous administration of acyclovir may be indicated. For those patients with recurrent episodes of HSV, long-term prophylactic therapy may need to be considered. Additional efforts employed to alleviate symptoms include topical anesthetics, analgesics for pain, zinc sulfate to dry the affected area, and antibiotic ointments to prevent superinfections.

Prompt treatment of primary infections can minimize the amount of virus that later will be harbored in the ganglia. Minimizing the amount of shed virus will reduce the viral reservoir for potential reactivations (Rubin, 1994).

Varicella-zoster virus (VZV) is an extremely contagious pathogen. It is also the virus that causes chicken pox. The virus is spread by droplets or contact with infected mucocutaneous lesions. It is harbored in a latent state in the dorsal root ganglia.

The primary infection is varicella (chicken pox), and the secondary or reactivation of latent virus is varicella zoster. Approximately 10% of organ transplant recipients receiving immunosuppressive therapy will develop VZV infection as a result of latent virus reactivation (Rubin, 1994). Reactivation of VZV is manifested by localized dermatomes involving two or three adjoining dermatomes. Usually the thoracic nerve dermatome is involved. This type of infection is often referred to as shingles.

Clinical manifestations of reactivated VZV include extremely painful vesicles that follow a dermatome, low grade fever, fatigue, malaise, and anorexia. Diagnosis is based on clinical manifestations, isolation of VZV from the lesions, and a rise in VZV antibody titers. Treatment is composed of oral or intravenous administration of analgesics and antiviral therapy with high dose intravenous or oral acyclovir (dose varies with renal function).

Disseminated VZV infection is much more severe in the posttransplant recipient and is usually a consequence of a primary VZV infection. It is characterized by skin lesions, hemorrhagic pneumonia, encephalitis, pancreatitis, hepatitis, and disseminated intravascular coagulation. Primary VZV is diagnosed by the development of antibody to VZV and by clinical manifestations. If recognized and treated early with high dose intravenous acyclovir, primary VZV can be effectively managed. Since more than 90% of adults are seropositive for VZV, children are at greatest risk for developing VZV primary infection.

It is generally recommended to screen all patients, particularly children, serologically for VZV pretransplant. Seronegative individuals are taught to promptly report all VZV exposures to allow for the administration of varicella immune globulin (VZIG) within the recommended time frame of 96 hours from time of exposure (Plokin & Peter, 1991). In confirmed exposures, prophylactic oral acyclovir may be initiated. When clinical manifestations develop, the patient is started on high-dose intravenous acyclovir (usually for 7 days, then changed to oral dosing).

Hepatitis has an incidence of 10-20% in the posttransplant population (Rubin, 1994). There are two major etiologies of hepatitis posttransplant: drug-induced hepatotoxicity and virus-induced hepatitis. Two drugs associated with hepatitis in the transplant recipient are azathioprine and cyclosporine. During administration of these medications, close monitoring of hepatic function is recommended. Although the incidence of hepatic damage as a result of these drugs is significantly less in recent years (secondary to decreased dosing), recipients remain at risk and must be closely monitored. In addition to these immunosuppressive agents, transplant recipients receive a number of other agents such as antihypertensives, diuretics, and antibiotics. Of particular concern are the medications used to treat tuberculosis, such as isoniazid or rifampin, which can cause severe hepatic dysfunction.

Viral hepatitis is the predominant cause of hepatitis in the posttransplant recipient. There are five different types of viruses that have been observed, each with the potential of injuring the liver (see Chapter 13). These viruses include hepatitis A virus (HAV), B virus (HBV), C virus (HCV), D virus (HDV), and E virus (HEV). Regardless of the mode of transmission, the hepatitis virus invades the liver, replicates, and causes hepatic injury. Histologic manifestations of hepatic damage is demonstrated by inflammation and mononuclear cell infiltration into the parenchyma and portal ducts, hepatic cell necrosis, proliferation of Kupffer cells, cellular collapse, and accumulation of necrotic debris in the lobulus and portal ducts, all causing a disruption in the hepatic architecture (Grimes, 1991). These viruses are also immunomodulating and contribute to the net state of immunosuppression.

Hepatitis B and C are the viruses primarily responsible for chronic liver disease in transplant recipients. They can both be transmitted by blood products and with the donor organ, and their effects in the host can be significantly modulated by immunosuppressive therapy.

The major problem associated with HBV and transplantation is the persistence of the virus posttransplant and identifying what the optimum approach to management is in patients who are infected prior to transplantation. Effective antiviral therapy for HBV is not yet available. Although recent attempts have been made to treat HBV with ∂-interferon, treatment has focused on alfa-interferon, hepatitis B immunoglobulin, and Lamivudine ® (epivir, 3TC) (Bader 1997; Conjeevaram, 1993; Perrillo et al., 1991). In addition, the administration of corticosteroids posttransplant appears to stimulate viral replication and increase viral levels. With the increase in viral proliferation made possible by immunosuppressive therapy, transplant recipients are placed at further risk for developing hepatocellular carcinoma.

Renal transplant recipients with HBV-associated chronic liver disease have an increased incidence of death from hepatic failure, hepatocellular cancer, and sepsis. They also demonstrate a poorer level of functioning than other recipients afflicted with different types of hepatic dysfunction. However, with the advent of cyclosporine and the use of lower steroid dosing, the prognosis for renal transplant recipients with HBV has improved considerably (Huang et al., 1991; Rao et al., 1991; Wein et al., 1985). However, those individuals who are HBV positive and also hepatitis Be antigen (HBeAg) positive prior to transplantation exhibit a greater risk of progressive hepatic disease with higher rates of mortality posttransplant (Fauley et al., 1991; Rao et al., 1991). Therefore, individuals who are HBeAg positive are considered to have a relative contraindication to transplantation. Other considerations for this population include level of nutrition, presence of other illnesses, quality of life, and patient/family wishes. The risk-benefit ratio regarding transplantation must be heavily weighed in those patients who are HBeAg positive.

Hepatitis C is responsible for more than 80% of progressive hepatic disease that develops posttransplant (Katkov & Rubin, 1991). In the renal transplant population, 80% of individuals who demonstrate abnormal liver function studies suggestive of HCV will do so indefinitely (Rubin, 1994). During the first 1 to 2 years after renal transplant, hepatitis caused by HCV is generally quiescent, with the exception of contributing to the net immunosuppressive state. Two or more years after renal transplantation, progressive liver failure begins, often resulting in end-stage liver disease. In addition, like HBV, HCV is also linked to hepatocellular carcinoma.

Liver transplantation of patients with HBV remains controversial. Posttransplant there is almost a 100% reoccurrence of infection in the allograft despite treatment with hyperimmune globulin or ∂-interferon. There have also been reports of higher mortality rates within the first 6 months in recipients with HBV. However, patients surviving liver transplantation for more than 6 months usually do well for the next 1 to 2 years (Demetris et al., 1990; Levine et al., 1991; O'Grady et al., 1992; Portman et al., 1986; Rubin, 1994; Starzl et al., 1989).

Liver transplant recipients who demonstrate HCV infection prior to transplantation generally reinfect their allograft. As in renal transplantation, the course of HCV is variable. A few patients will develop severe accelerated disease while the majority have minor dysfunction (Katkov & Rubin, 1991).

Occasionally, a posttransplant recipient will present with both HBV and HCV. It is important to note that the combination of HBV and HCV has a greater impact together than either virus does alone (Huang et al., 1992).

HIV seropositive patients who are asymptomatic and would otherwise be satisfactory candidates for transplantation present a very difficult situation. Rubin (1994) suggests, based on current available information, that HIV positive patients undergoing organ transplantation can be divided into three equal groups: one-third will die within 6 months of transplantation from infection, one-third will have a functioning allograft 5 to 7 years posttransplant, and one-third will develop clinical AIDS and have a downhill trajectory 2 to 4 years posttransplant. Since dialysis is available as a life-sustaining therapy, many centers do not recommend AIDS patients with chronic renal failure for transplantation. However, in situations where non-transplant life-sustaining alternatives are not available, HIV positivity is considered a relative contraindication and remains controversial (Rubin, 1993). For those HIV positive patients, minimizing the first group's risk of infection can be performed by thorough screening of patients for history of infection and immune function (CD4 levels). In addition, initiation of antiretroviral therapy and anti-Pneumocystis prophylaxis has been shown to significantly improve well-being and prolong life (Rubin & Tolkoff-Rubin, 1988).

Fungal infections account for a significant number of infections in the transplant recipient. Candidal species are the most common fungi observed in posttransplant recipients with Candida albicans being the most frequently encountered organism. Candida prefers moist warm areas and is ordinarily found on diseased skin, throughout the GI tract, and in the genital area (Rubin, 1994). However, the infection potential depends on the degree of host resistance and number of fungal colonies. Overgrowth of mucosal membrane surfaces develops when there is an elimination of normal bacterial flora secondary to such causes as antibiotics, immunosuppressive therapy, diabetes, and anemia. Therefore, the most frequently observed manifestation of candidal infections in the transplant recipient is from mucocutaneous overgrowth secondary to immunosuppressive therapy. Clinical examples of candidal infections include oropharyngeal thrush, candidal esophagitis, vulvovaginitis, urinary tract candidiases, and disseminated fungal infections.

The most common manifestation of Candida albicans is thrush. Clinically, thrush presents as a white plaque-like covering over the oral mucous membranes, tongue, and pharynx. Surrounding areas, such as the gums, may become erythematous and painful. If severe, thrush can interfere with oral intake and nutritional status, particularly in young children and infants. Thrush is treated with a topical antifungal agent such as nystatin or clotrimazole troche 4 to 5 times daily. It is imperative that the patient be instructed to swish and swallow nystatin or allow the clotrimazole troche to dissolve in the mouth. Swallowing these medications without allowing them to come in contact with the mucous membranes is ineffective treatment. In infants this can be difficult. The use of a nystatin-covered swab rolled directly over the child's mucous membranes can provide adequate therapy. Generally, oral candidiasis (thrush) can be avoided with the prophylactic administration of these antifungal agents during episodes of high-dose immunosuppressive therapy (e.g., immediate posttransplant, during rejection episodes).

Esophageal candidal infections are seen in severely immunosuppressed individuals. Contributing factors include prolonged use of nasogastric or feeding tubes, esophagitis with or without ulcerations, and extended use of antibiotic therapy. Clinical manifestations include the formation of white plaques and erythema along the esophageal mucosa observed on endoscopy, dysphagia, pain, and anorexia. Diagnosis is based on clinical manifestations and cultures taken from the esophagus during endoscopy. Topical antifungal agents are used as initial therapy. If the infection is severe or unresponsive to topical antifungals, systemic therapy with amphotericin B may be indicated.

Vulvovaginal candidiasis is caused primarily by C. albicans. The clinical manifestations include itching, a white clotted and odorous discharge, and perianal irritation with erythema. If severe, perianal edema and excoriations may be present. Diagnosis is based on clinical manifestations, KOH, wet mount, and culture. Primary treatment is clotrimazole (e.g., Gyne Lotrimin®). However, nystatin (e.g., Nilstat®) and miconazole (Monistat-7®) can also be used.

Candidiasis of the urinary tract is usually the result of bladder colonization rather than true infection. It is commonly seen in patients who are severely immunosuppressed and in those with prolonged indwelling urinary catheters. White flecks are often observed during gross examination of the urine. Occasionally patients complain of moderate dysuria. Diagnosis is based on urine culture. Treatment includes intermittent bladder irrigations with amphotericin B and, if possible, removal of the urinary catheter.

Disseminated candidiasis occurs once candidal overgrowth has penetrated the mucocutaneous barrier and invades the blood stream. Contamination is generally the cause of disseminated candidiasis in the posttransplant recipient. Contamination occurs as the result of a complicated liver transplant or intraabdominal kidney transplant from visceral seeding, spillage of candidal organism, and the GI tract into local tissue, hematomas, or ascitic fluid or the placement of intravenous lines. Clinical manifestations of disseminated candidiasis are diverse, ranging from acute sepsis with hemodynamic instability to specific symptoms related to the metastatic site (e.g., hepatic abscess). Diagnosis is based on blood cultures and computerized tomography (CT) scan (e.g., assess for abscess). The initial therapeutic approach is to remove all suspected intravenous access lines and administer intravenous amphotericin B or fluconazole.

Other causes of disseminated fungal infections include *Aspergillus, Cryptococcus, Histoplasmosis,* and *Pneumocystosis carinii. Aspergillus* is found in air, dust, and soil, while *Cryptococcus* is located in the soil, on fruits and vegetables, and in bird feces. In the posttransplant recipient, these fungi enter the host via the respiratory tract. *Aspergillus* can cause brain abscesses, pneumonia, and GI inflammation with bleeding. *Cryptococcus* typically invades the central nervous system, joints, and skin. Treatment includes surgical removal of localized infection if possible and intravenous administration of amphotericin B. Histoplasmosis presents similar to influenza and can progress to the respiratory tract, liver, spleen, lymph nodes, or central nervous system. It is generally diagnosed by biopsy and culture. Intravenous amphotericin B is the usual treatment. Since these infections can be acquired in the hospital, clustering of cases suggests an environmental hazard requiring prompt investigation.

Pneumocystis carinii is now classified as a fungus (Rubin, 1994). Pneumonia caused by *P. carinii* generally presents with fever, a nonproductive cough, dyspnea, interstitial pneumonia observed on chest x-ray, and hypoxia. *P. carinii* pneumonia (PCP) is closely associated with pulmonary CMV infections because of the effects of CMV on alveolar macrophage function, which is important in preventing *P. carinii.* Diagnosis is based on sputum or bronchoalveolar lavage specimens by using monoclonal antibody techniques. Trimethoprim-sulfamethoxazole is the treatment of choice (e.g., Septra®, Bactrim®). If the patient cannot tolerate trimethoprim-sulfamethoxazole, monthly inhaled pentamidine or daily oral Dapsone® can be used. It is generally recommended that all transplant recipients receive prophylactic therapy against *P. carinii* for at least the first 6 months posttransplant, and some centers continue prophylactic therapy for the life of the graft.

Parasitic infections can also be problematic in the transplant recipient. *Toxoplasma gondii*, a protozoan parasite, is one of the more common parasitic offenders. It can be latent and passed to the recipient from the donor, or be reactivated in the presence of CMV (Rubin, 1993; Rubin, 1994). Clinical manifestations are often mild, including fever, malaise, sore throat, and mylagias. Patients who have undergone more intense immunosuppressive therapy may be at greater risk for developing pneumonitis, or severe and occasionally fatal central nervous system toxoplasmosis. (Red Book, 1991). Diagnosis is based on the presence of toxoplasmosis antibody in the serum, seroconversion, and a fourfold rise in antibody titers. Unfortunately, recipients who are extremely immunosuppressed may not demonstrate seroconversion or a rise in antibody titers. In this population, any detectable toxoplasmosis antibody in the serum confirms diagnosis. Treatment of toxoplasmosis is a combination of Pyrimethamine® and sulfonamides which act synergistically to eradicate the infection from the host. Maintenance therapy is recommended in severely immunosuppressed patients to prevent relapse.

Time Table Approach to Infection Posttransplant

Rubin (1994) presents a time table approach to examine the incidence and type of infections that occur posttransplant (see Figure 23-6). The time frames established are the first month, 1 to 6 months, and greater than 6 months posttransplant. The types of infections that develop in these time periods will be reviewed.

During the first month posttransplant, the patient is at risk for developing infections related to (1) an exacerbation of an infection that was present pretransplant, (2) acquiring an infection from the donor allograft, or (3) succumbing to an infection as a result of technical complications.

Pretransplant, all infection is eradicated in potential recipients with the exception of chronic viral infections. Although attempts are made to control active disease, it is not feasible to eliminate viruses such as hepatitis B and C, herpes, CMV, or EBV before transplant. However, the presence of bacterial, fungal, and protozoal infections must be eliminated before transplantation. If active infection is not treated pretransplant, catastrophic events such as septicemia, graft loss, and even death can ensue posttransplant. It is imperative that a complete infectious workup be performed before transplant surgery.

In general, most renal transplant candidates are able to undergo treatment for infection before transplantation. However, liver transplant candidates do not have reliable artificial hepatic support, and eradication of an infection may not always be feasible in circumstances of hepatic failure. In these situations, each case must be evaluated individually based on the risk-benefit ratio.

Strongyloides stercoralis is the most devastating of protozoal infections that can be asymptomatic pretransplant and become life threatening posttransplant. Diagnosis is difficult, and the patient may present with only minor abdominal discomfort. As a result of posttransplant immunosuppressive therapy, the classic eosinophilia is absent, and stool for ova and parasites is positive in only half the cases. It is recommended that individuals coming from endemic areas be completely worked up or undergo treatment based on their epidemiologic history (Rubin, 1993; Rubin, 1994).

Donor acquisition of infection is the second type of infection occurring during the first month posttransplant. To prevent transmission of infection from donor to recipient, potential organ donors (living and cadaveric) undergo an extensive infectious disease workup. Infections that might be acquired from the donor are latent or active viral infections. Hepatitis C is a example of a viral infection that can be passed with the donor organ to the recipient. Hepatitis C is difficult to assay and is not completely identifiable with current testing procedures. The incidence of a recipient developing hepatitis C is 100% when the donor is RNA-hepatitis C positive, and the recipient is negative (Pereira et al., 1992).

Cytomegalovirus (CMV) is an example of a latent viral infection. Latent infections are capable of being reactivated, potentially causing active infection and disseminated disease. Exacerbation of the disease usually takes 4 to 6 weeks posttransplant. It is important to know donor and recipient CMV status to initiate prophylactic therapy immediately postoperatively. Some centers prophylax posttransplant patients for CMV regardless of donor and recipient CMV status with intravenous gancyclovir (DHPG®) for 7 to 10 days, followed by oral gancyclovir (Cytovene) or acyclovir for 2 to 6 months.

Guidelines for minimizing infection in the recipient from the donor include complete cultures of the donor blood, urine, sputum, cultures of the perfusate, administration of prophylactic antibiotics for 2 to 3 days to the recipient, and administration of a 10 to 14 day course of antibiotics to the recipient in the presence of positive donor cultures.

Some potential donors are considered high risk for transmitting infection to the recipient and should be evaluated carefully prior to donation. High risk donors include drowning victims, burn victims, and those who have been on the ventilator for a prolonged period of time (Rubin, 1994).

Technical complications are the third cause of infection during the first month posttransplant. Bacterial infections are the most common cause of infection related to technical difficulties in the transplant recipient. The transplanted organ is often the major source of posttransplant bacteremia. For example, in the renal transplant recipient, the urinary tract is the main portal of entry in 60 to 70% of bacteremias, and in liver transplant recipients, the biliary tree is the primary site (Rubin, 1994).

Wound infections may also be the result of technical complications posttransplant. Causative organisms of wound infections include gram-negative rods, enterococci, staphylococci, and *Candida albicans* (Johnson & Flye, 1989). The incidence of wound infections following transplantation varies: renal 1.8%-56% and liver 5%-15% (Barkholt, 1993; George et al., 1991; Rubin, 1994). These infections generally result from urinary leaks, bile leaks, hematomas, or lymphoceles. In many centers, closed suction drainage (e.g., Jackson-Pratt) is used to remove dead space and fluid collections. Most drains are removed within 5 days posttransplant. If there is concern regarding a leak, indigo carmine dye can be administered intravenously and will turn the drainage blue if a leak is present.

Diagnosis of wound infections is based on clinical manifestations (e.g., fever, purulent exudate from the incision, and pain), computed tomographic (CT) scanning, sterile needle aspirate, and culture of wound drainage. Treatment of wound infections includes antibiotics, periodic debridement of the wound, and surgical evacuation of hematomas.

Other causes of infection during the first month posttransplant include pneumonia and intravenous line sepsis. Pneumonia has a very high mortality rate in transplant recipients. Of all the causative organisms of pneumonia, 80% are bacterial (Rue & Konttra-Buck, 1986). Clinical manifestation are fever, a productive cough, alteration in breath sounds, the feeling of a tight chest, and an abnormal chest x-ray. Diagnosis is based on clinical manifestations, sputum cultures, chest x-ray, and occasionally bronchioscopy. Treatment includes administration of appropriate antibiotics. Further therapy is based on the severity of the disease.

Nursing care of the patient with pneumonia includes frequent pulmonary toiletry, ambulation, administration of antibiotics, education regarding upper airway infections, and smoking cessation.

After the first month, infections posttransplant are relatively similar between organs with regard to incidence, etiology, and clinical significance (see Table 23-18) (Rubin, 1993).

One to 6 months posttransplant is the time of greatest risk for infection in the immunocompromised transplant recipient. Contributing factors that increase the risk of infection during this time include the following: (1) dosage of immunosuppressive therapy remains relatively high and has been administered for a sufficient length of time to enhance the onset of opportunistic infections; (2) most infections occurring during this time are difficult to treat because they are caused by viruses, fungi, or antibiotic resistant bacteria, in particular the presence of immunomodulating viruses (e.g., HSV, CMV, and hepatitis), which can be determining factors in patient and graft survival; and (3) persistent technical complications requiring drains, central lines, catheters, or tubes are innately serious because of the risk of superinfections (Rubin, 1994)

Six months or more posttransplant include infections acquired from the community (e.g., respiratory viruses), opportunistic infections in those recipients who have received excessive acute or chronic immunosuppression, and infections in patients who are afflicted with recurrent problems, such as cholangitis and urinary tract infections (Rubin, 1988; Rubin, 1994).

Nursing Considerations Regarding Infection Posttransplant

One of the primary nursing care goals is to protect the posttransplant patient from infection (see Nursing Care Plan, Table 23-33.) This includes safeguarding the patient from possible sources of infection (e.g., hospital construction, ill visitors), consistent good hand-washing technique, early mobilization, pulmonary toiletry, promotion of good nutrition, maintaining aseptic technique during dressing changes, bladder irrigation and other procedures, initiation of protective isolation for patients with absolute neutrophil counts of less than 500, appropriate collection of ordered specimens, administration of antipyretics and antibiotics as ordered, and monitoring fluid balance to prevent dehydration secondary to fever (particularly in children and infants). Prompt reporting of the signs of infection (fever, swelling, redness, and pain) supports early intervention and management. In addition, circumstances in which the patient has an infection mandates appropriate education for that individual/family. For example, wound infection management may involve teaching the patient/family aseptic care of drain sites, frequent wound irrigation, wet to dry dressing changes, and possibly the use of a shower head directed at the wound to remove debris and improve circulation and wound healing. In some cases, the patient or a family member can be taught to administer intravenous antibiotics at home.

Donor Management and Recovery

Brain Death

Brain death is defined as the irreversible cessation of all brain activity, including that of the brain stem (Hoffman & Malecki, 1990). Prior to organ procurement, brain death must be determined by two physicians independent of the transplant team. Table 23-20 outlines the criteria used to make a brain death declaration.

Organ Donation

Initiation of organ donation should follow hospital policy. Once a potential donor is recognized, a referral is made to the local organ procurement organization (OPO). Referral to the OPO does not commit the family to donation. However, it does allow the OPO to assist the family and staff through the decision-making process and help determine the appropriate plan.

Donor Management

Declaration of brain death and family consent are always obtained before initiating donor management and procurement of organs. A transplant coordinator generally is asked by the intensive care team to help the family make a decision regarding donation of their loved one's organs. The transplant coordinator also provides staff support and assistance in managing the care of the potential organ donor.

The transplant coordinator is generally a registered nurse who assumes clinical management of

Table 23-20
Brain death determination.

Symptom	Assessment Test
Absence of respirations	Apnea test: Administer 100% oxygen to the patient for 15 minutes. Then turn off the ventilator, while closely monitoring vital signs. Arterial blood gases are drawn every minute. Since the stimulus to breath is activated by an increased CO_2 level, if the patient does not breath within 3 to 4 minutes, the ventilator is turned back on. Carefully monitoring of the patient must be ongoing during this test to prevent a cardiac arrest.
No response to painful stimuli.	Deeply pinch the patient's arm or leg and evaluate response.
Fixed and dilated pupils	Check the patients pupils for light reactivity response.
Absent gag or cough reflex	Assess patient for gag reflex during deep suctioning.
Absent corneal reflexes	Gently raise eyebrow and brush each sclera with a cotton wisp and evaluate response.
Absent doll's eye reflex	While holding the eyelids open gently turn the patients head from side to side. If the patient is brain dead the eyes do not move as the head is turned.
No ocular movement	Cold calorics: Inject 20 ml of iced cold water into the tympanic membrane. If the patient is brain dead, there will be no ocular movement.

Note: With thankful permission adapted from Hoffman, M., & Malecki, M. (1990). Organ procurement and preservation. In K.M. Sigardson-Poor & L.M. Haggerty, *Nursing care of the transplant recipient* (p.17). Philadelphia: W.B. Saunders Company.

the donor once brain death has been declared and family consent obtained. Management of donors is based on guidelines and standing orders developed by the transplant physicians affiliated with the organ procurement agency (OPA) involved in the organ recovery. The medical director of the OPA is always available to provide consultation and assistance as needed.

The goal of donor management is to maintain hemodynamic stability as well as viability of organs until the transplant teams arrive for the actual surgical recovery. All donors require ventilatory support in an intensive care unit. The condition of the donor can often become quite unstable, mandating attentive and continuous monitoring by the transplant coordinator.

Hoffman and Malecki (1990) developed an excellent approach to categorizing the principles of donor management. Through the use of nursing diagnosis they clearly outline the major potential problems of donor management and the appropriate nursing interventions. Table 23-21 outlines their approach to donor care.

Donor Recovery

Most recoveries are multiorgan and involve a significant amount of coordination from the OPA local operating room, the procurement surgical teams, and transplant teams. Coordination of this complex process emphasizes the importance of an onsite transplant coordinator.

A full surgical team is required for organ procurement. The local surgical team generally consists of a scrub nurse, circulating nurse, and anesthesiologist who assist separate surgical procurement teams. There can be as many as five separate surgical procurement teams. The procurement teams often arrive from a number of different transplant centers. Therefore, organization of the procurement process is extremely important to facilitate prompt and coordinated donor organ removal.

A multiorgan recovery can include heart, lung, liver, small bowel, kidney, and pancreas. This surgery must occur in a coordinated fashion to preserve function of all organs. The heart team initiates the surgery by opening the chest for assessment and visualization of the heart. The abdomen is then

Table 23-21
Principles of donor management.

Nursing Diagnosis	Predisposing Factors	Signs and Symptoms	Nursing Interventions
Potential fluid volume deficit.	Minimal fluid replacement due to head trauma and risk of increased intracranial pressure. Administration of osmotic diuretics (e.g., mannitol). Administration of steroids. Pituitary gland injury resulting in decreased release of antidiuretic hormone (ADH).	Decreased urine output. Decreased blood pressure. Increased heart rate. Decreased CVP. Initial decrease in urine output followed by an increase in urine output with fluid replacement	Increase IV fluid replacement with initial bolus of fluids (500-1000 cc over 1-2 hr) to maintain CVP 8 to 12 mm Hg Maintain fluid balance with cc for cc plus 100 cc replacement per hour. Monitor accurate I & O. Administer Pitressin as ordered.
Potential alteration electrolyte balance.	Diabetes insipidus secondary to decreased ADH release.	Increased urine output. Increased glucose level. Decreased serum potassium level. Increased serum sodium level.	Monitor serum potassium and sodium levels every 2 hours. Replace with appropriate fluids based on laboratory values. Administer insulin as ordered for increased glucose level.
Potential alteration in hemodynamic status.	Inadequate neurologic response to maintain hemodynamic status. Diabetes insipidus, resulting in increased risk of hypokalemia. Altered fluid and electrolyte balance.	Tachycardia. Frequent premature ventricular contractions. Decreased hemoglobin and hematocrit. Decreased blood pressure.	Monitor ABGs. Adjust ventilatory settings as ordered. Monitor serum potassium levels every 2 hours and prn. Administer potassium bolus as ordered. Maintain systolic blood pressure at 100. Administer vasopressors as ordered (dopamine is the vasopressor of choice).
Potential for infection.	Compromised total body system due to brain death status. Immobility. Ventilator dependence.	Elevated temperature. Increased WBC (these signs may also be secondary to neurologic injury and must be closely evaluated. Cloudy, foul-smelling urine.	Monitor temperature every 2 hours. Provide adequate pulmonary hygiene. Use aseptic technique for all invasive procedures. Maintain patent, aseptic urinary catheter system. Obtain blood, urine, and sputum cultures as ordered.

Note: With thankful permission from Hoffman, M. & Malecki, M. (1990). Organ procurement and preservation. In K.M. Sigardson-Poor & L.M. Haggerty, *Nursing care of the transplant recipient* (p. 30). Philadelphia: W.B. Saunders. Company.

opened by the liver team to visualize and then dissect the liver. At this time, the pancreas surgeon may simultaneously remove the pancreas in conjunction with the liver surgeon. The kidney team then dissects the kidneys. When all organs are anatomically freed, the aorta is clamped, and all organs are flushed with a cold electrolyte solution. The purpose of the solution, specific to each organ, is to cause cellular standstill to decrease warm ischemic damage. Organs are all then removed with the heart and lungs first, followed in order by the liver, pancreas, and kidneys. The order is dictated by the preservation time of each organ (see Table 23-22). The kidneys may be placed in cold storage or on a perfusion pump individually or en bloc with a segment of aorta and vena cava.

The kidney procurement surgeons generally close the chest and abdominal cavity after organ

Table 23-22
Preservation time.

Organ	Preservation Time
Heart	4 to 6 hours
Lung	6 hours
Liver	8 to 12 hours
Pancreas	12 hours
Kidney	24 to 36 hours

recovery is completed. Organ recovery takes approximately 3 to 5 hours. The utmost care and respect are afforded the donor, and no disfigurement takes place. An open-casket funeral is possible, and there is no visible sign that organ and/or tissue donation has occurred (Hoffman & Malecki, 1990).

Kidney Transplantation

Since the first successful renal transplant in 1954, more than 300,000 kidney transplants have been performed throughout the world. Thousands of additional kidney transplants could be performed if more donor organs were available. For example, between 1988 and 1996, the number of patients waiting for kidneys doubled. In the United States, between 1995 and 1996, there were more than 17,500 individuals who underwent kidney transplantation, while 27,000 remained on the waiting list (UNOS, 1996). For those transplanted, 1-year graft survival rates were 90% for live-donor kidney transplant recipients, and 80% for cadaveric kidney transplants. Patient survival was 97% and 93% respectively for living donor and cadaveric kidney transplant recipients (USRDS, 1994; UNOS, 1996).

It is well documented that children with chronic renal failure (CRF) do not tolerate dialysis as well as kidney transplantation (Jordon & Lemire, 1984; Sager & Ettenger, 1993). Therefore, renal transplantation has become well recognized as the optimal therapy for children with CRF (Garcia et al., 1992). The incidence of CRF in children is approximately 11 children per million. In children less than 18 years of age, 1,947 received cadaveric kidney transplants between 1988 and 1993, and 1,856 received living-related kidney transplants. At the end of 1993, there were 624 children under 18 years of age waiting for a cadaveric kidney transplant (UNOS, 1994). Between 1988 and 1993, children under 18 years of age represented 4.5% of all individuals waiting for a cadaver kidney in the United States (Sager & Ettenger, 1993; UNOS, 1991).

Pediatric survival data gathered from the European Dialysis and Transplant Association (EDTA) and the North American Pediatric Renal Transplant Cooperative Study (NAPRTCS) showed pediatric living donor kidney transplant recipients have a 1-year patient survival rate of 96%-97% and a graft survival rate of 87% at 1 year and 80% at 3 years. Pediatric recipients of cadaveric kidneys had a patient survival of 94% at 1 year and 92% at 2 years and a graft survival rate of 74% at 1 year and 62% at 3 years (Alexander et al., 1990; Broyer, 1989; McEnery et al., 1992; Sager & Ettenger, 1993).

With improving success rates for both adults and children undergoing kidney transplantation, the lack of organ donors has become the major problem in transplantation.

Kidney Transplant Recipient Selection

Renal transplantation is a viable treatment option for most patients with CRF, either before or after the initiation of dialysis (Fifueroa, 1992). All patients (families of pediatric patients) with CRF should be informed about kidney transplantation as a therapeutic treatment option at the time of diagnosis. The American Society of Transplant Physicians (1988) confirms this in their Criteria for Selection of ESRD Patients for Kidney Transplantation, which states that "all ESRD patients should be considered as candidates for transplantation unless there is a specific contraindication." Specific contraindications are highly variable between transplant programs and individual patients. Generally accepted contraindications for kidney transplantation include systemic malignancy, active infection, substance abuse, advanced cardiopulmonary disease, marked obesity, seropositive HIV, positive hepatitis B surface antigen, and severe psychosocial instability. However, patients who present with one of these contraindications may be considered a viable transplant candidate with additional screening and evaluation. In each of these cases, the benefits of kidney transplantation must be evaluated with regard to the possibility of complications and the disadvantages of not undergoing transplantation.

The number of diseases that warrant renal transplantation is extensive (see Table 23-23 as well as Chapter 8). The more common causes of kidney disease requiring renal transplantation include diabetes, hypertension, glomerulonephritis (all types), nephropathy, hereditary disorders (e.g., Alport syndrome), congenital disorders (e.g., urinary tract malformation, hypoplastic/dysplastic kidneys), and systemic diseases that result in CRF (e.g., systemic lupus erythematosus) (Perryman & Stillerman; Sager & Ettenger, 1993). The type of renal support or renal replacement therapy an individual is receiving prior to transplantation varies. The range spans from those who are not receiving renal replacement therapy and are being managed medically to those who present with renal insufficiency, or who have been on dialysis for a prolonged period of time (e.g., peritoneal or hemodialysis). Each situation must be

Table 23-23
Overview of disease indications for kidney transplantation.

Congenital Disorders Horseshoe kidney Aplasia Hypoplasia	**Potential Irreversible Causes of Acute Renal Failure** Acute tubular necrosis Cortical necrosis Acute glomerulonephritis Hemolytic uremic syndrome Henoch-Schonlein syndrome
Hereditary Nephropathies Medullary cystic disease Polycystic kidney disease Alport's syndrome	**Inflammatory Disorders** Wegener's disease Chronic pyelonephritis Chronic glomerulonephritis Hypocomplementemic nephritis Goodpasture's disease Systemic lupus erythematous Scleroderma Polyarteritis nodosum
Metabolic Disorders Cystinosis Primary oxalosis Nephrocalcinosis Amyloidosis Fabray's disease	**Tumors necessitating bilateral nephrectomy** Renal carcinoma Wilms tumor Tuberous sclerosis
Obstructive Uropathy Congenital Acquired	**Other** Hypertensive nephrosclerosis Steroid resistant nephrotic syndrome Multiple myeloma Macroglobulinemia
Toxic Nephropathies Lead nephropathy Analgesic nephropathy	
Trauma necessitating bilateral nephrectomy	
Renal Vascular Disease Renal vein thrombosis Renal artery occlusion	

carefully evaluated in collaboration with the patient/family and transplant team. In the event of graft rejection or failure, which may ultimately lead to the urgent need to institute dialytic therapy, it is imperative that dialysis be discussed with those who are not receiving treatment prior to transplantation.

Kidney Transplant Recipient Evaluation

Evaluation of a candidate for kidney transplantation is performed by a multidisciplinary transplant team. The purpose of the evaluation is to confirm CRF and its cause, assess for medical suitability, and evaluate psychosocial status, support systems, and resources of the patient/family. The evaluation consists of a complete history and physical with a review of systems, laboratory and radiologic tests, histocompatibility studies, and a psychosocial assessment (see Table 23-24).

The recipient selection criteria vary among centers. To clarify candidate criteria, The Patient Care and Education Committee of the American Society of Transplant Physicians conducted a survey of all transplant centers in the United States that participate in the United Network for Organ Sharing (UNOS) regarding their evaluation of potential adult kidney transplant recipients (Ramos et al., 1994). In general, they found that (1) university-based centers accept more medically complex patients, (2) most centers feel attendance to dialysis is an indicator of compliance, and (3) pretransplant transfusions are not necessary. Greater than half of the centers participating set no specific age limit; 56% exclude patients with chronic active hepatitis in the setting of hepatitis B antigenemia, and 50% had no specific policy for evaluating hepatitis C antibody-positive patients (Ramos et al., 1994). Although there is variation among centers regarding the evaluation of potential renal transplant recipients, the following provides a general overview of the process.

Age is a major consideration. However, physio-

Table 23-24
Kidney recipient evaluation.

Complete History and Physical Etiology of renal disease Associated disorders Previous illness and surgeries Weight, height, head circumference (pediatrics) Medications Diet history and nutritional evaluation Immunization record (pediatrics) **Routine Lab Tests** Complete blood count with differential, PT, PTT, platelets, electrolytes, calcium, phosphorus, magnesium, BUN, creatinine, uric acid, AST, ALT, GGT, alkaline phosphatase, bilirubin, glucose, amylase, albumin, cholesterol, triglycerides, urinalysis if possible, urine culture, 24-hour urine for creatinine clearance. **Immunologic Procedures** Blood type (ABO) and Rh HLA tissue typing UBC Cross matching to detect preformed cytotic anti bodies and auto antibodies Mixed lymphocyte culture Skin testing (e.g., PPD) Hepatitis B immunization **Infectious Disease Evaluation** Cultures for bacteria, viruses, fungus, parasites as indicated * HIV antibody Hepatitis serologies: A, B, C, B delta Serologies (CMV, EBV, toxoplasmosis, herpes simplex/zoster, varicella) RPR	**Radiologic Procedures** Chest x-ray **Additional Studies** EKG Thallium stress test * Echocardiogram * Pulmonary function tests (for smokers) * Renal biopsy * Colonoscopy/endoscopy * Stool guaiacs **Additional Consults** Anesthesia Transplant Nurse Financial Counselor Social Worker Exercise physiologist/physical therapist Cardiology (age 45 years)* Psychiatrist * Dentist * Child Life Services (pediatrics)* **Provide patient/family education regarding kidney transplantation** * Routine recipient evaluation varies between patient and transplant center.

logic age is a greater determining factor than chronologic age. Patients of all ages are considered viable candidates, and each candidate is considered individually. Although transplants are performed from birth to approximately 70 years of age, those at either end of the age spectrum generally require further evaluation. For children, as previously mentioned, renal transplantation is considered the treatment of choice for CRF, particularly if there is an available living donor (Sager & Ettenger, 1993).

Etiology of renal disease is reviewed for the natural history of the disorder and appropriate timing for transplantation to evaluate the need for pretransplant surgical intervention and to help determine the appropriate type of donor (e.g., cadaveric or living). Patients with type I diabetes should undergo early kidney or kidney-pancreas transplantation to minimize the risk of prolonged dialysis. Those with active autoimmune disorders should wait until there is a period of remission before undergoing transplantation to minimize the risk of immunosuppressive therapy. Pretransplant bilateral nephrectomies may be necessary in patients with (1) polycystic kidney disease to prevent infection and extensive bleeding from the cysts, (2) chronic pyelonephritis, hydronephrosis, or ureteral reflux to minimize the risk of infection, (3) renal tumors, and (4) to control hypertension related to excessive renin production. (Salvatierra, 1987; Haggerty & Sigardson-Poor, 1990). For those disorders that are known to have a high recurrence rate such as focal glomerular sclerosis, membranous glomerulonephritis, and primary oxalosis, in some centers cadaveric donor may be preferred over live donors.

Urinary tract evaluation is highly recommended to determine the functional status of the bladder and ureter patency. It is particularly useful in patients with a preexisting history of urinary tract infections, bladder dysfunction, reflux, or type I diabetes. In patients who continue to urinate, evaluation of the urinary tract may be expanded to cystoscopy or voiding cystourethrogram. Although it is helpful to have a functional bladder, it is not mandatory for kidney transplantation. It is possible to perform other types of urinary tract diversion such as an ileal conduit in those patients without adequate bladder function (Hanto & Simmons, 1987).

Pretransplant surgical intervention may be required for bladder reconstruction and augmentation or correction of strictures. Kidney transplant recipients who have neurogenic (e.g., diabetics) or atonic bladders can be taught to perform intermittent clean self-catheterization posttransplant.

Cardiovascular disease, particularly hypertension, atherosclerosis, and hyperlipidemia, are common in CRF patients (Helderman, 1986). With the addition of corticosteroids and cyclosporine, these problems can be exacerbated. Therefore, it is recommended that an extensive cardiac evaluation be performed on all patients who have a cardiac history, are older than 45 years of age, or have diabetes mellitus. A cardiac evaluation includes an electrocardiogram (EKG) for all candidates. For those individuals at high risk, a comprehensive evaluation by a cardiologist should be completed. This evaluation may include a thallium stress test, an echocardiogram, and possibly a cardiac catheterization if there are positive findings on the noninvasive studies. If treatment is necessary, it should be completed prior to transplantation. In certain situations it may be necessary for the transplant candidate to undergo percutaneous coronary angioplasty or coronary artery bypass surgery before being considered a candidate for transplantation.

Hypertension is a common problem in the CRF population that generally persists posttransplant. Although hypertension can be a major problem, it does not preclude transplantation. Pretransplant hypertension is typically managed with antihypertensive medications and sodium and fluid restrictions. In a few instances, hypertension is the result of renal artery stenosis and excessive renin production. In these cases, a pretransplant nephrectomy may be indicated.

Pulmonary evaluation for all candidates includes a chest radiography, purified protein derivative (PPD) testing, and pneumovax immunization. When a patient has a true positive PPD test and has confirmation of tuberculosis by chest radiography, there is an increased risk for reactivation or progression of TB posttransplant. Tuberculosis is treated with either one or a combination of isoniazid (INH), rifampin, pyrazinamide, and in rare circumstances, streptomycin. Patients generally receive treatment for 6 to 9 months pretransplant depending on their clinical condition.

Individuals with chronic lung disease generally undergo further pulmonary evaluation. Added to the evaluation are pulmonary function tests, arterial blood gases, and a sputum culture. Smokers are encouraged to quit smoking to minimize postoperative complications.

Gastrointestinal (GI) problems may also be present in CRF patients. For example, individuals with peptic ulcer disease, diverticulitis, colitis, or reflux (children) require further evaluation prior to transplantation. It is important to completely assess and manage all GI problems pretransplant because of the risk of bleeding posttransplant secondary to corticosteroid administration, other medications, and stress. Specific types of management might include vagotomy for duodenal ulcers or additional medication for peptic ulcer disease (histamine antagonists [e.g., ranitidine]). Diverticulitis should be monitored, and in rare occasions require surgical intervention. Depending on the severity, patients with gallbladder disease may require a pretransplant cholecystectomy. Liver function tests and hepatitis serologies are also performed. Patients with hepatitis C often undergo liver biopsy to assume there is no cirrhosis.

Endocrine assessment consists of an evaluation of hyperparathyroidism and a gynecologic examination for females. Hyperparathyroidism is a complication of CRF that cannot be overlooked pretransplant. If parathyroid hormone levels are high and not responding to medical management, a subtotal parathyroidectomy may be mandated to prevent hypercalcemia posttransplant (Tilney & Kirkman, 1986). Women should undergo a gynecologic examination, pap smear, and mammogram within 1 year before transplantation. Dental evaluation is performed to assess for periodontal disease, caries, or abscesses that could exacerbate as sites of infection with the onset of immunosuppressive therapy. All periodontal disease must be corrected prior to transplantation to prevent the risk of infection postoperatively.

All active infectious diseases must be treated with antibiotics and eradicated prior to transplant. In addition, a thorough screening of possible infection is performed, including blood, urine, and possibly sputum cultures, viral antibody titers, hepatitis serologies, HIV testing, chest radiography, and follow-up for all elevations in white blood cell count. Individuals who are positive for CMV, EBV, OR HSV-I or HSV-II without active disease are monitored posttransplant for reactivation of these viruses. Those transplant candidates who demonstrate positive hepatitis or HIV tests are considered to

Table 23-25
Time it takes to complete immunologic testing.

Test	Time
HLA	3 hours
MLC	6 days
T & B cell crossmatch	36 hours

have a relative contraindication to kidney transplantation.

Psychosocial assessment is an extremely important component of the evaluation. It provides insight into how the candidate might cope with the immediate and long-term stresses of kidney transplantation. Factors that need to be considered are the patient's history of coping behaviors, available support systems (e.g., family, friends), adjustment to present illness and ability to comply with their medical regimen, past history or active substance abuse, transplant experience and expectations, pre-illness and current lifestyle, quality of life, educational preparation, work status, financial resources, transportation, and live donor availability. In addition, it is important during this time to provide support and appropriate resources for the patient and family.

Education regarding transplantation is initiated during the evaluation process. Aspects of transplantation that are discussed during the evaluation process include donor sources, routine posttransplant course, common complications, immunosuppressive agents, and other medications (purpose, side effects, duration), survival statistics, routine follow-up, and clinic visits.

Immunologic Considerations

The time it takes to complete an immunologic evaluation varies (see Table 23-25). ABO blood grouping, histocompatibility testing (recipient and donor human leukocyte antigens [HLA] and haplotype matching), and level of presensitization to HLA antigens compromises the immunologic evaluation in most centers (Garovoy et al., 1991). Factors that may alter host response are also considered, including previous transplants, number of blood transfusions, and incidence of pregnancy for women.

ABO blood group testing is performed on all transplant candidates. ABO antigens are present on erythrocytes and the vascular endothelium of the graft. Thus transplanting across the ABO barrier can produce hyperacute rejection. In specific situations, it may be possible to overcome the ABO barrier in kidney transplantation. For example, the A2 subtype of blood group A is a weaker antigen, and in some circumstances, organs from donors with blood group A2 can be transplanted across the ABO blood group barrier into recipients who have O or B blood type (Nelson, 1992). This may also be facilitated through the administration of cyclophosphamide (Cytoxan) to prevent antibody formation, and by plasmapheresis to lower the natural titer of anti-A or anti-B antibodies (Garovoy et al.,1991). There have also been attempts to remove anti-A and anti-B antibodies in the recipient by immunoabsorption with varying results (Agishi et al., 1991). As with blood transfusion, blood type O is the universal donor, while AB is the universal recipient.

Human leukocyte antigen (HLA) testing is performed to determine genetic type. All potential renal transplant recipients have complete testing for HLAA, B, C, DR, and DQ antigens found on chromosome 6. This type of testing is particularly useful for living-related kidney transplantation because it is possible to determine each antigen's haplotype assignment. It must be remembered however, that even in unrelated populations. it is still possible for individuals to share components of two HLA haplotypes. The significance of haplotype matching has been demonstrated by improved graft survival. There have been definite improvements in graft survival with better degrees of matching, specifically at the HLA-DR loci (Leivestad et al., 1992). However, matching to the HLA-C antigen does not appear to be significant to kidney transplantation (Garovoy et al., 1987; Perryman & Stillerman, 1991).

In many centers, matching is reported for three loci: A, B, and DR. Since each chromosome is paired, a six-antigen match refers to a perfect match of all three loci. It is generally agreed that matching at DR is the most important in predicting patient and graft survival (Leivestad et al., 1992). However, the degree of acceptable mismatching remains controversial. For example, patients treated with cyclosporine have comparable graft survival regardless of match (Ting, 1988).

Mixed lymphocyte culture (MLC) is extremely helpful in choosing a compatible living-related donor when several are available. Donor and recipient lymphocytes are mixed to determine degree of reactivity between cells. The test measures compatibility between donor and recipient at the HLA-D loci. One-haplotype-matched pairs that demonstrate a low MLC response generally have excellent graft survival, while those with a high MLC response have a poor graft survival (Garovoy et al., 1991). Therefore, those that provoke a low response are considered more compatible as donors immunologically. MLC is useful only in living-related transplants because it takes approximately 6 days to complete (see Table 23-25).

White cell crossmatching is performed to detect the presence of recipient preformed cytotoxic antibodies to donor HLA antigens. It is performed by exposing donor lymphocytes to recipient sera. A positive reaction or crossmatch is determined by cell lysis. Transplantation in the presence of a positive crossmatch would result in hyperacute rejection and possible subsequent graft loss. Therefore, a positive crossmatch is undesirable and precludes transplantation. A negative crossmatch demonstrates a lack of recipient response to donor lymphocytes, indicating transplantation should proceed.

The transplant procedure can take place days to weeks after the evaluation has been completed. Therefore, a final white blood cell crossmatch is always performed just prior to surgery regardless of the type of donor. A white cell crossmatch is performed to determine the presence of preformed anti-HLA antibodies in the recipient sera to donor antigens, thus preventing the risk of hyperacute rejection.

Presensitization is a consequence of exposure to HLA antigens and the development of anti-HLA antibodies. It occurs primarily in response to blood transfusions, previous transplants, and pregnancy. To monitor the number of anti-HLA antibodies produced, monthly screening of all patients waiting for a kidney, transplant is performed. The potential recipients serum is crossmatched with a 40 to 50 cell panel of lymphocytes from a number of different individuals. Each HLA antigen is represented approximately twice, providing the recipient exposure to an entire range of human antigens. The number of individual cells lysed by the potential recipients serum is expressed as a percent (e.g., 20% panel-reactive antibodies (PRA). By using this procedure, it is possible to determine the extent of presensitization. It is also helpful to know the HLA antigens on the lymphocyte panel cells that have been lysed to determine the specific anti-HLA antibodies causing the positive reaction. This knowledge allows for avoidance of donors with these particular HLA antigens. It is much more difficult to identify donors for those patients with high PRA (>50%) levels (Colombe, 1994; Garovoy et al., 1994)

Recipient blood samples are typically frozen and stored until a potential donor becomes available. At that time each sample is tested with the potential donor. A positive crossmatch with peak samples precludes transplantation and the donor is considered for another waiting recipient.

Kidney Transplant Donor Evaluation and Selection

Once the potential recipient is accepted as a transplant candidate, donor sources must be considered and evaluated. There are two donor sources for the potential kidney transplant recipient, living and cadaveric. It is a generally consensus that living-related donors provide the best long-term graft survival (Beckman et al., 1992). However, in an era of cyclosporine, the graft survival of living-unrelated and cadaveric donors is improved and in some cases comparable (Berlocco et al., 1993; Brattstrom et al., 1994; Spital, 1994).

Living-related donors (LRD) provide 15-20% of all donated kidneys (Lewis et al., 1992). These donors are composed of parents, siblings, children, aunts, uncles, cousins, and grandparents (Lancaster, & Schanbacher, 1991). They must be in excellent physical and mental health prior to donation to endure the rigors of the surgical procedure and postoperative course. Kidney donation involves days off from work, physiologic pain, and emotional stress regarding potential rejection of the donor organ. Although the morbidity and mortality of kidney donors is relatively low, the risks of anesthesia and surgery cannot be overlooked.

Life expectancy is not altered by kidney donation, and the mortality rate of a unilateral nephrectomy for donation is less than 0.1% (Garovoy, et al., 1991; Hakim et al., 1984; Spital, 1988; Velsoa, et al., 1985). Three weeks after nephrectomy, renal function, as demonstrated by creatinine clearance, has been shown to be 70.5% of predonation levels (Dunn et al., 1986). Ten to 20-year follow-up reports show no increase in creatinine clearance levels from initial postnephrectomy values (Bay & Herbert, 1987). Most donors feel the benefits of donation outweigh the risks (Konttra-Buck, 1986; Spital, 1988).

The donor evaluation is completed by a multidisciplinary team whose primary responsibility is to ensure that the donor's decision is made without coercion, and that the donor is in acceptable health for surgery. Contraindications to donation generally include kidney disease, advanced cardiopulmonary disease, systemic malignancy, HIV seropositivity, a positive crossmatch, severe hypertension, diabetes as evidenced by proteinuria, and hepatitis B and C seropositivity.

The living-related kidney transplant donor workup is extremely thorough. Donors are generally between the ages of 18 and 65 with the exception of identical twins who may be younger. The evaluation includes an extensive assessment of donor motivation and psychologic well-being, a complete history and physical to determine physical health status, laboratory tests, radiologic procedures, and a number of consults (see Table 23-26). An arteriogram concludes the physical workup. An arteriogram is performed to assess renal arterial structure and rule out any unsuspected abnormalities. The arteriogram also helps the surgeon decide which of the donor kidneys would be most suitable.

The psychologic assessment of the donor focuses on the willingness to donate. Clarification of the intent to donate needs to be identified. For example, is it altruistic or are there other motivating factors (e.g., guilt for previous action, financial). The donor must also be evaluated for their emotional

Table 23-26
Living-kidney transplant donor evaluation.

Complete History and Physical Previous illness and surgeries Current (acute/chronic) illnesses Medications **Routine Laboratory Tests** Complete blood count with differential, PT, PTT, platelets, electrolytes, calcium, phosphorus, magnesium, BUN, creatinine, uric acid, AST, ALT, alkaline phosphatase, bilirubin, glucose, albumin, cholesterol, triglycerides, pregnancy for women, urinalysis with electrolytes, 12- and 24-hour creatinine clearance. **Immunologic Tests** Blood type (ABO) HLA tissue typing Mixed lymphocyte culture (MLC) T and B cell crossmatch **Infectious Disease Evaluation** Cultures* Urinalysis with micro HIV Hepatitis serologies (A, B, C, D, E) Viral serologies (CMV, EBV, toxoplasmosis, herpes simplex/zoster, varicella) RPR	**Radiologic Procedures** Chest x-ray Renal arteriogram Renal tomography * Intravenous pyelogram (IVP) * **Additional Studies** EKG Pulmonary function tests * (particularly with a history of smoking) **Additional Consults** Anesthesia Social Worker Psychiatrist * Transplant Nurse Financial Counselor Exercise physiologist/physical therapist * Cardiologist * Pulmonologist * Gynecologist * **Provide patient/family education regarding living kidney transplantation** * Evaluation varies between patient and transplant center.

and psychologic stability and patterns of coping, their relationship to the potential recipient, family dynamics, and the implication of graft loss or recipient death. Transplant expectations should also be discussed to clarify any misconceptions. The pretransplant evaluation is also an excellent time to initiate or continue the transplant educational process. Aspects to be covered might include the donation and transplant processes, risks and complications, expected outcomes, and financial considerations other than the donation process (e.g., transportation, lodging, child care, and lost work). These are all important issues that must be addressed particularly when considering posttransplant outcomes. When the transplant is successful, there are feelings of satisfactory accomplishment and appreciation. However, if the graft fails, both donor and recipient often experience feelings of failure, disappointment, and depression. These must be addressed before transplantation to assure optimal adaptation regardless of outcome.

Living-unrelated donors are composed of spouses, friends, homosexual couples, significant others, and adoptive parents of children. Due to the shortage of donors and the increased success rate with cyclosporine, even in poorly matched kidneys, many centers have considered living-unrelated individuals as potential donors (Brattstrom et al., 1994; Sankari et al., 1994; Spital, 1994). Some centers report better than an 80% 1-year graft survival rate with living-unrelated donors (Barry, 1985; Berloco et al., 1993).

The evaluation process for unrelated-living donors is the same as for living-related donors with the addition of a more extensive psychosocial assessment. All professionals must be concerned that economic coercion be ruled out as a possible incentive (Onwebalil et al., 1994; Perryman & Stillerman, 1991). The buying and selling of organs in the United States is illegal (NTIS N. HRP0906975).

Cadaveric donors represent 80-85% of kidney

donors. To be considered for organ donation, the individual must be declared brain dead with a functioning cardiovascular system and have family consent. Causes of brain death may include but are not limited to trauma, cerebrovascular accidents, myocardial infarctions, primary brain tumors, and anoxic encephalopathy (e.g., drowning). All potential cadaveric kidney donors must meet brain death criteria, be 0 to 70 years of age, have no preexisting renal disease, no history of malignancy, no evidence of sepsis or transmittable diseases (e.g., HIV positive), no known active substance abuse, and be hemodynamically stable (Hawke et al., 1990). Although the kidneys are generally more resistant to episodes of hypoxia and hypotension, cardiopulmonary stability is important. In situations where the potential donor is unstable, dopamine may assist in maintaining hemodynamic stability. However, it must be remembered that dopamine at high doses for prolonged periods of time can cause damage to the kidneys (Hoffman & Malecki, 1990).

Donors with known infection demonstrated by positive cultures must be treated with the appropriate antibiotics and have negative repeat cultures. All potential organ donors have blood cultures, HIV, hepatitis B and C serologies, and syphilis drawn before the recovery of organs. The main concern is to prevent the transmission of active infection to the recipient from the donor. Recipients of kidneys from infectious donors are treated with antibiotics for 10 to 14 days after transplantation.

During cadaveric kidney procurement, a section of spleen, a few lymph nodes, and a vial of peripheral blood are collected and used to determine the donor's ABO blood group and HLA antigens. Those recipients who are ABO compatible and crossmatch negative are considered further. A second crossmatch is often performed. Recipient selection for the donor is based on ABO compatibility, HLA match, negative crossmatch, time on the waiting list, medical urgency and whether it is a first, second, or third transplant. Cadaveric kidneys are also allocated, based on a point system developed by the United Network for Organ Sharing (UNOS). Although this point system is continually being reviewed, and changes are being implemented, it is generally based on ABO compatibility: immunologic testing, time on the list, number of transplant age, and disease. Children receive additional points depending on their age; younger children receive more points than older children. Specific diseases, such as primary oxalosis which usually requires a liver and kidney transplant, receive additional points.

Recipient Considerations Pretransplant

Blood transfusions have been one of the primary methods of pretransplant conditioning. This includes both donor-specific transfusions in living-related transplantation, and random transfusions for those undergoing cadaveric transplantation. However, in the era of cyclosporine the effectiveness of such therapy has become less clear and more controversial. Whether pretransplant transfusions has an impact on outcome, or if it is the specific number of transfusions that affects graft survival remains unclear (Baatard et al., 1991; Garovoy et al., 1994).

Donor-specific transfusions (DSTs) have been used in recipients who have a potential living donor with the purpose of achieving better graft survival (Salvateirra, 1987). The potential recipient receives small volumes (100-200 ml) of donor blood 2 to 3 times over a period of a few weeks. During this time, the recipient is monitored for cytotoxic anti-HLA donor antibodies which would preclude transplantation. Approximately 10-30% of patients develop antibodies (Garovoy et al., 1991). The mechanisms thought to promote graft survival in patients receiving transfusions include elimination of immunologic respondents who demonstrate cytotoxic antibodies, production of suppressor T cells, and the generation of anti-idiotypic antibodies (Garovoy et al., 1994). Unfortunately, blood transfusions pose several risks to the patients that outweigh the benefits, including hypersensitivity reactions, enhanced presensitization, and transmission of diseases such as hepatitis. Historically, splenectomy, total body irradiation, and thoracic lymph duct drainage were used to reduce the number of circulating lymphocytes. These therapies are rarely used today.

Kidney Transplant Surgical Procedure

Immediately before kidney transplant surgery, a final crossmatch is completed between donor and recipient. If the crossmatch is positive, the surgery is canceled. If negative, the transplant is performed. Recipients are also evaluated regarding their need for dialysis. Generally, most hemodialysis patients undergo one dialysis treatment pretransplant, while those on peritoneal dialysis complete one to two exchanges. Dialysis is performed pretransplant primarily for fluid control and electrolyte management, particularly hyperkalemia.

Living donor nephrectomy usually takes place in an adjoining surgical suite. Before anesthesia is induced, intravenous hydration is initiated to ensure adequate diuresis. If anesthesia is induced before diuresis, the antidiuretic hormone (ADH) effects of the anesthesia may make diuresis more difficult. After induction of anesthesia, the donor is placed in a lateral position with the left or right flank anterior. The patient is typically positioned for a standard retroperitoneal flank approach with or without removal of the distal eleventh and twelfth ribs. The left side is usually preferred because it is technically easier and provides the kidney with a long vein, making the transplant surgical procedure easier (Hanto & Simmons, 1987).

Figure 23-7

Vascular anastomosis techniques in adults. A. end-to-end renal artery to external iliac artery anastomosis and renal vein to external iliac vein anastomosis; B. end-to-end artery to hypogastric artery anastomosis; C. a patch of aorta may be used for an anastomosis to the side of the external iliac artery for cadaver donors with multiple renal arteries; D. entire aorta used for two pediatric kidneys transplanted into an adult.

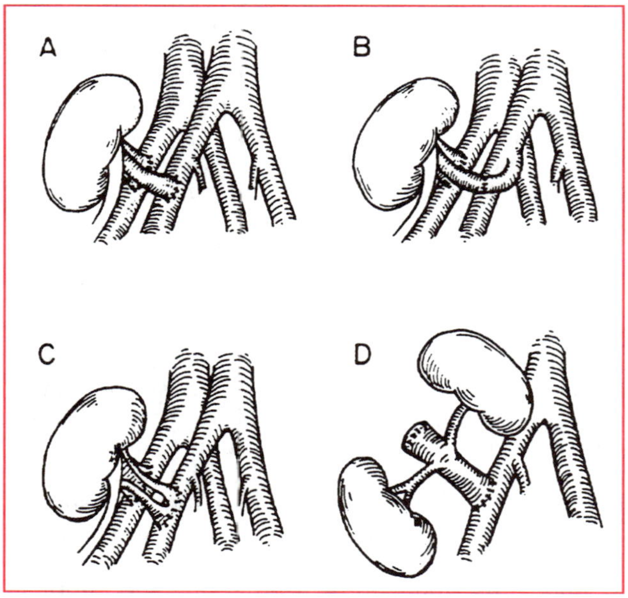

Note: Reprinted with permission from Hanto, D.W. & Simmons, R.L. (1987). Renal transplantation: Clinical considerations, *Radiologic Clinics of North America, 25*(2), 243.

During the surgery, mannitol, other volume expanders, and diuretics may be administered to ensure adequate urine output. During the surgical procedure, it is important to avoid frequent handling of the kidney and arterial vessels. Manipulation of the kidney can stimulate the nerve supply during dissection and lead to vasospasm. Vasospasms can result in poor graft perfusion, inadequate preservation, and ischemia. Subsequent damage to the vessels can result in thrombosis, stenosis, necrosis of the ureter, urinary leakage, and loss of the graft (Diethelm et al., 1987).

The kidney is exposed, and the ureter and vessels are dissected. Often the surgeon will use a heparin solution to perfuse the renal artery and vein prior to excision. The procedure must be performed so that the blood supply to the ureter from the renal vessels is preserved. Ex-vivo renal artery reconstruction is performed prior to transplantation. In cases where there are multiple renal arteries, a carrel patch may be used or the vessels are implanted separately into the recipient's renal vessels (Salvatierra, 1987) (see Figure 23-7).

With completion of the dissection, the kidney is removed and perfused with iced Euro-Collins or University of Wisconsin (UW) solution to remove blood products and reduce the core temperature of the kidney. The kidney is placed in a sterile basin containing lactated Ringer's solution. The surgeon carefully examines and flushes the kidney before it is taken to the recipient's surgical suite. The donor's incision is closed, and the patient remains in the postanesthesia room (PAR) prior to transfer to their hospital room. A nasogastric tube and Foley catheter may be necessary for 24 to 48 hours postoperatively.

Nursing care of the donor is similar to the care of most postoperative patients. Specific attention should be given to good pulmonary hygiene and early ambulation, monitoring for bleeding, prevention of infection, and adequate hydration with particular attention to fluids, electrolytes, and renal function. Pain is often greater in the donor than the recipient since major muscle groups have been disrupted. Postoperative pain is usually controlled with a patient-controlled analgesia (PCA) pump. Support for this patient is extremely important. Donors may experience feelings of loss and demonstrate great concern over the status of the recipient. Most donors are discharged from the hospital 3-5 days postoperatively.

Transplantation of the renal graft has become a fairly standardized procedure. Immunosuppressive therapy may be initiated pretransplant, and patients may receive additional corticosteroids intraoperatively. During the surgical procedure, it is mandatory that blood volumes remain adequate to ensure graft perfusion. Blood pressure is kept slightly elevated to enhance renal blood flow.

Generally the kidney is transplanted extraperitoneally into the recipient's iliac fossa. Advantages to extraperitoneal placement include the close location of the graft to the vessels and bladder and an enhanced ability to assess the graft postoperatively, in the event a biopsy or surgical intervention are necessary (Pattella & Weiskittel, 1991). Intraperitoneal placement is indicated in children when the graft is too large to fit in the extraperitoneal space, in patients with inadequate extraperitoneal access, and in those individuals who have undergone previous kidney transplants (Haggerty & Sigardson-Poor, 1990).

Once the patient has been anesthetized, a large-gauge Foley catheter is inserted into the bladder to monitor urine output and remove clots. In some centers, an antibiotic solution is used to irrigate the bladder to minimize the risk of a postoperative urinary tract infection.

The patient is placed in a supine position, and a curvilinear incision is made in the right or left lower abdominal quadrant between the pubis and iliac crest. The right quadrant is preferred over the left because the sigmoid colon makes it difficult to visualize the vessels on the left side. The abdominal muscles and fascia are divided. The peritoneum is left intact and retracted upward. The epigastric vessels and spermatic cord are retracted. The iliac vessels are dissected and exposed. Lymphatic vessels are ligated to prevent the risk of postoperative lymphocele formation.

Revascularization takes approximately 30 minutes and is of prime importance in preventing prolonged warm ischemic time and tissue injury. Usually an end-to-end anastomosis is performed using the donor renal artery and the recipient's hypogastric artery or internal iliac artery. More common in cadaveric donor transplantation is an end-to-side anastomosis to the iliac artery. In living donors, the hypogastric artery may be the optimal vessel because of the similar size to the renal artery, thus reducing the risk of stenosis. However, with second transplants, there may be an increased risk of sexual impotence in males when the contralateral hypogastric artery is used (Perryman & Stillerman, 1991). If the donor kidney has more than one artery, they may be anastomosed separately, on a patch of aorta together, and then to a recipient vessel.

The kidney is placed in the iliac fossa and the donor vein (vena cava) is anastomosed to the recipient iliac vein. Once blood flow to the kidney is reestablished the kidney becomes pink and firm, and may make urine. If urine production is delayed, it is usually secondary to acute tubular necrosis (ATN) due to prolonged preservation. Often mannitol or diuretics will be administered to promote diuresis.

There are three approaches to ureteral anastomosis. The most widely accepted is the ureteroneocystostomy. This procedure involves tunneling the ureter into an incision in the posterior wall of the bladder and performing an end-to-side suture into the mucosal opening. One feature of the ureteroneocystostomy is that it acts as a one-way valve preventing reflux into the transplanted kidney (Pattella & Weiskittel, 1991). Second is the ureterovesical anastomosis. In this procedure, the ureter is anastomosed through a simple incision directly onto the dome of the bladder. Third and least common is the ureteroureterostomy, which is performed when there have been multiple bladder surgeries or if there is a known bladder contaminant (Perryman & Stillerman, 1991).

In situations where there are severe dysfunction and major anatomic abnormalities of the urinary tract, an intestinal urinary diversion or conduit may be performed. Complications that occur with this type of urinary diversion include urinary leakage, recurrent urinary tract infections, and bleeding from the intestinal loop (Lien et al., 1993).

An antibacterial solution is usually used to irrigate the wound prior to closure. The wound is closed, and the patient is transferred to the postanesthesia room for recovery. Depending on the center, the patient will go either to the intensive care unit or to the transplant unit after recovery from the anesthetic.

Postoperative Management and Nursing Care of the Kidney Transplant Recipient

Nursing care for the postoperative kidney transplant recipient can be challenging and rewarding. Although the care is very similar for any patient who has undergone major surgery, particular attention must be made to renal function and the pretransplant long-term complications of uremia, the impact of immunosuppressive therapy, and the patient's adjustment to the transplant process. Therefore, caring for the kidney transplant recipient mandates advanced nursing diagnosis and assessment skills followed by prompt intervention (see Table 23-33, the Nursing Care Plan). Familiarity with the effects of uremia are helpful in guiding care.

During the postoperative period, patients must be encouraged to become active participants in their own care. Long-term posttransplant care is complex, requiring patients to have a relatively extensive knowledge of their health care management. Therefore, a comprehensive patient/family education program is developed for every recipient.

This section reviews the immediate posttransplant care of the recipient by systems. A comprehensive review of the most applicable nursing diagnosis is presented in the Nursing Care Plan for Kidney Transplant Recipients (see Table 23-33).

Renal function. Assessment of renal function requires diligent monitoring of the color and character of urine flow rate, serum BUN, creatinine, and electrolytes. Renal function is confirmed by the immediate formation of urine, a massive diuresis, a continual decline in serum BUN and creatinine, and the stabilization of electrolytes (see Table 23-27).

Initial graft dysfunction or delay in graft function is fairly common and occurs in approximately 30-40% of transplant recipients. The major causes are acute tubular necrosis, perfusion injury, hyperacute rejection, urologic surgical complication, endogenous donor renal disease (e.g., infection, tumors, renal diseases [IgA nephropathy, microvascular thrombosis]), and coexisting acute rejection (Sanfilippo, 1990).

Acute tubular necrosis (ATN) is the most likely cause of delayed renal function early posttransplant. ATN occurs in approximately 10-30% of all patients after cadaveric transplantation and in less than 3% of those undergoing live donor kidney transplantation (Diethelma et al., 1987). ATN is a reversible condition lasting approximately a few days to weeks. It is caused by changes in the donor kidney secondary to oxygen interruption during renal procurement, prolonged preservation time, or handling during the donor/recipient surgery.

Table 23-27
Differential diagnosis for allograft dysfunction after kidney transplantation.

Delayed Allograft Function
acute tubular necrosis
hyperacute rejection
acute rejection
perfusion injury during procurement
urological complications
Acute Dysfunction
acute rejection
cyclosporine nephrotoxicity
drug reactions
infection
acute transplant glomerulopathy
malignant hypertension
ureteral or vascular complications
intravascular coagulopathy
recurrent disease
Chronic Dysfunction
chronic rejection
chronic cyclosporine nephrotoxicity
chronic transplant glomerulopathy
arterionephrosclerosis
recurrent disease

Note: Adapted from Sanfilippo, R. (1990). Renal transplantation. In G.E. Sale (Ed.), *The pathology of organ transplantation.* Boston: Butterworths.

Prolonged cold and warm ischemic times also contribute to ATN. Cold ischemia time is the length of time the kidney is preserved on ice from donor to recipient. The farther apart the donor and recipient are (e.g., Boston to San Francisco), the greater the cold ischemia time. If the cold ischemia time is greater than 24 hours, there is an increased risk of ATN in the recipient. Warm ischemic time is the length of time between cessation of renal circulation to the achievement of adequate hypothermia in the donor organ. Vascular anastomosis takes approximately 20 to 30 minutes and in some centers is included in the warm ischemia time. Surgical complications related to the vascular anastomosis that can increase warm ischemia time include multiple renal arteries or hypovolemia (Pattella & Weiskittel, 1991).

There are two types of ATN: oliguric and nonoliguric. Oliguric ATN is the most common and is characterized by prolonged oliguria or anuria that can persist for several days to 2 months. Nonoliguric or high-output ATN is demonstrated by a normal or greater than normal urine output without adequate excretion of nitrogenous waste products. In both types of ATN there is an elevation in BUN and serum creatinine with accompanying electrolyte disorders. A renal scan may be performed to evaluate the presence of ATN by assessing renal blood flow and excretion of a radioisotope. If ATN is present, there will be decreased uptake (see Table 23-28) and excretion of the isotope. Renal biopsy will reveal tubular epithelial cell necrosis, mild edema, congestion, and inflammatory cell infiltration.

Although there is no treatment for ATN, gradual improvement in renal function can be observed over time. If ATN is present, close judicious monitoring of fluids and electrolytes is necessary. Temporary dialysis may be needed and is often required in approximately 20% of cadaveric renal transplants secondary to ATN in the early postoperative period (Garovoy, 1994).

Fluids and electrolytes. Monitoring of fluids and electrolytes is of paramount importance in determining renal function. The goal is to attain an evolemic state and maintain renal perfusion. During the initial posttransplant period, there is large diuresis caused by a high osmotic load secondary to pretransplant uremia, high glucose levels (due to steroid induced hyperglycemia, intravenous fluids, or diabetes), and overload from administration of blood and fluid (Flye, 1989). Adequate fluid replacement is given to match urine output, and diuretics are administered if necessary to stimulate continuing diuresis. Fluids are generally replaced with 0.45% normal saline with or without glucose. Inadequate fluid replacement can lead to oliguria and impaired renal function. Conversely, overhydration can result in congestive heart failure or pulmonary edema, promote electrolyte disturbances, or contribute to hypertension. Therefore, it is imperative that the fluid status be closely monitored during the early posttransplant period. Typical assessment parameters include daily weights, total intake and output, urine specific gravity, vital signs, and central venous pressure (CVP) measurement.

Knowledge of the patient's pretransplant dry weight can be helpful in monitoring fluid status. Daily weights (twice daily in infants and children) should be done at the same time every day and on the same scale. Patients undergoing hemodialysis are weighed before and after their treatment (see Chapter 19) and those undergoing peritoneal dialysis are weighed when empty or during their drain cycle (see Chapter 22). Generally, if the patient gains more than 0.03 kg (e.g., 2 kg in a 70 kg individual) in 24 hours, or if the urine output decreases to less than the parameters prescribed, the patient is at risk for becoming volume overloaded.

During the first 24 to 48 hours, intake and output are monitored every hour, and in some centers, every 30 minutes. All fluids (e.g., IV solutions,

Table 23-28
Analysis of diagnostic studies in renal transplantation.

Study	Goal	Interpretation
DTPA Radiology Study	Assess for blood flow to the allograft.	**Normal:** presence of blood flow to the graft. **Absence:** no blood flow; does not differentiate between ATN, rejection, or glomerular nephritis.
Mag-3 Radiology Study	Assess for blood flow & extravasation of isotope indicating anastomotic leak.	**Normal:** prompt uptake to the kidney with rapid clearance of the hippurate isotope from the kidney to the bladder and/or Foley catheter. **ATN:** reduced isotope uptake with cortical retention **Cellular Rejection:** initial changes show a reduction in excretion while later phases (days later) include a progressive reduction in uptake. A single scan can only be characterized as compatible with rejection but not diagnostic. **Rejection Treatment Phase**: the first response to treatment is one of improvement in excretion with subsequent improvement in uptake. **Intrinsic Parenchymal Processes:** reduced uptake and excretion; the tubular luminal flow is fairly well preserved in contrast to the renal blood flow to the allograft.
Renal Ultrasound	Evaluate the allograft for signs indicative of rejection: swelling, prominence of medullary pyramids, pelvic infundibular wall thickening, resistive index (RI), and decreased sinus fat; may also be used to look for obstruction	**Normal:** no dilatation to pelvis or ureters, may have small perinephritic fluid collections, normal sinus fat, and corticomedullary junction appearance and RI < 70%; adequate blood flow. **Acute Rejection:** swelling of allograft, reduced sinus fat (from compression), prominent medullary pyramids, pelvi-infundibular thickening, and RI > 70% (NOTE: these changes are seen when serum creatinine level is > 1 mg%). **Obstruction:** dilated collecting structures (either intraureteral obstruction or periureteral obstruction secondary to lymphocele); changes are usually followed by (a) anterograde pyelogram, (b) intravenous pyelogram, or (c) surgical intervention.

nasogastric secretion, urine, and infants' stool) are measured carefully to assure accurate balance. This is particularly important in children weighing less than 10 kg.

Blood clots are the most common cause of a diminishing urine output in the early postoperative period. If aseptic irrigation is unsuccessful in removing the clots, the catheter should be replaced. If urine volume is high, fluid administration is increased often to 30 ml plus urine output per hour. In addition, a CVP line may be inserted to measure and titrate volume status more closely. CVP readings are usually kept between 6 mm Hg and 12 mm Hg. Persistently low CVP readings may require additional fluid or albumin to ensure graft perfusion and maintenance of an evolemic state. In addition, blood pressure should be maintained at greater than 110/70 in adults to provide adequate blood flow to the kidney.

Evaluation of the patient's volume status is facilitated by the assessment of skin turgor and mucous membranes (fontanelles in infants) for dehydration, palpation, and inspection of the extremities and sacral areas for edema, and the inspection of the neck veins for distention (Perryman & Stillerman, 1991). The development of adventitious breath sounds such as crackles, shortness of breath, and the presence of an S3 on cardiac evaluation are indicative of excess volume (Beckman, et al., 1992).

Table 23-29
Clinical findings in potassium imbalance.

System	Hypokalemia (< 3.5 mEq/L)	Hyperkalemia (> 5.5 mEq/L)
Cardiovascular	EKG changes: depressed ST segment, flat or inverted T wave, presence of a U wave, premature arterial or ventricular progressing to bradycardia, beats, progressing to paroxysmal atrial tachycardia, atrioventricular blocks, and ventricular tachycardia.	EKG changes: spiked T waves, widened QRS complex, hypotension, loss of P waves, idioventricular pattern to systole, and cardiac arrest.
Gastrointestinal	Anorexia, nausea, vomiting, constipation, decreased bowel sounds.	Diarrhea, cramps, colic, increased bowel sounds.
Muscle	Weakness, flabby muscle	Increased muscle irritability, increased tendon reflexes, muscle cramps.
Central nervous system	Lassitude, confusion	Dizziness

Excess volume states may develop as a result of overhydration intraoperatively to maintain renal perfusion, or from ATN. Overhydration is generally treated by administering diuretics (e.g., furosemide). In patients who do not respond to therapy, ATN must be suspected. In these patients, meticulous monitoring of fluid status is crucial. If the patient becomes overhydrated, the physician is notified, and further therapy is promptly instituted. Treatment often includes oxygen and nitroglycerin and morphine sulfate as preload reducers. Morphine sulfate is used to relieve anxiety and relax airway smooth muscles, thus enhancing gas exchange and breathing (Beckman et al., 1992). If treatment is unsuccessful, emergent hemodialysis becomes necessary.

Dehydration can cause a reduction in renal perfusion and subsequent graft damage. Methods of ensuring renal perfusion include maintaining CVP levels above 4 mm Hg, systolic blood pressure greater than 110 mmHg, and monitoring for adequate urine output.

Close monitoring of electrolytes is crucial with fluctuations in fluid status and varying degrees of renal function. Since electrolyte homeostasis is one of the kidney's primary responsibilities (see Chapter 7), disruption in electrolyte balance is not an uncommon problem after kidney transplant. The two most common imbalances are in potassium and glucose.

A normal potassium level is generally considered 3.5 mEq/L to 5.5 mEq/L. Hyperkalemia or hypokalemia may develop after kidney transplant. Hyperkalemia may be observed in the presence of ATN or acute rejection. In these situations, potassium is unable to be excreted by the damaged tubules and accumulates. Other factors that can cause hyperkalemia are potassium administration, blood transfusions, and surgery resulting in cell damage, causing the release of potassium ions. In addition, the initiation of cyclosporine or tacrolimus may increase the risk of hyperkalemia (see Chapter 12 and Table 23-29). The presence of acidosis or hyperglycemia can contribute to hyperkalemia by creating ionic shifts. The clinical findings and electrocardiogram (EKG) changes of hyperkalemia are presented in Table 23-29.

Hyperkalemia is initially treated with diuretics. However, if potassium levels are greater than 6.5 mEq/L, other forms of therapy should be implemented, such as dialysis or sodium polystyrene sulfonate (Kayexalate®) with sorbitol. Both hemodialysis and peritoneal dialysis effectively remove potassium. Kayexalate is an exchange ion that trades potassium ions for sodium ions in a ratio of 1:1 in the small bowel. Sorbitol is administered as an osmotic diarrhea agent to promote evacuation of the potassium from the intestines. A retention enema may be given to patients who have not progressed to oral feeds; however, in many centers this is not recommended because of the pressure the enema can place on the transplanted kidney and surgical site.

Although many dialysis patients have developed a tolerance for elevated potassium levels, it is considered a medical emergency when potassium levels are greater than 6.5 mEq/L or when EKG changes are present. In these situations, administration of Kayexalate® with sorbitol or emergency dialysis are often performed. Intravenous glucose, insulin, and bicarbonate may be employed pending dialysis to move the potassium back into the cells. It must be remembered that the administration of glucose, insulin, and bicarbonate is only a temporary measure and that follow-up hemodialysis or Kayexalate with sorbitol is usually necessary. In severe emergencies, calcium gluconate may be ordered for its inotropic (improved contractility) effects on the heart. However, it must be remembered that calcium gluconate is contraindicated in patients taking digitalis. If hyperkalemia remains a constant problem, dietary adjustment of potassium is considered.

Hypokalemia (< 3.5 mEq/L) develops when potassium losses are greater than intake. In the early postkidney transplant period, hypokalemia is usually the result of massive diuresis, excessive use of diuretics, large gastrointestinal losses, or lack of appropriate potassium replacement. The clinical manifestations and EKG changes caused by hypokalemia are presented in Table 23-29.

Hypokalemia should be treated promptly to avoid EKG changes, particularly in patients receiving digitalis, which potentiates the effects of the drug. Treatment for hypokalemia requires cautious oral or intravenous potassium replacement with EKG monitoring and accurate measurement of gastrointestinal losses, which are high in potassium (e.g., nasogastric, vomiting, diarrhea).

Nursing care for patients with alteration in potassium levels focuses on prevention. This requires astute physical assessment, accurate measurement of gastrointestinal losses, EKG monitoring, and frequent evaluation of serum potassium levels. In the event that alterations in potassium develop, prompt intervention is mandated.

Hyperglycemia is a relatively common problem after kidney transplantation. It is characterized by a blood glucose level greater than 120 mg/dL. Hyperglycemia is generally not treated until glucose levels are greater than 180 mg/dL (Otwell & Leidigh, 1988). Hyperglycemia after kidney transplant is typically associated with the initial high doses of corticosteroids on glucose metabolism, exacerbation of preexisting diabetes mellitus, familial tendency toward diabetes, or the administration of large volumes of dextrose-containing intravenous fluids. Patients with diabetes mellitus account for 30% of all patients with CRF. Those who undergo renal transplantation require particularly close glucose monitoring and assessment for hyperglycemia (Sutherland et al., 1988) (see Chapter 16).

Urinary tract. Depending on the type of anastomosis, a urinary catheter is typically left in place for 3 to 5 days. The purpose of the catheter is to allow for close assessment of urinary flow and urine characteristics, and to decompress the bladder. Once the catheter has been discontinued, the patient is encouraged to void frequently to allow for continued monitoring of urine output, minimize pressure on the suture lines, and promote bladder healing.

Decreased urine flow suggests several causes: ATN, rejection, technical complications, a decrease in circulating volume, or obstruction. Technical complications, such as a bladder leak, require prompt surgical intervention. If other clinical manifestations of hypovolemia are present, a fluid bolus is often administered to improve renal perfusion and urine output.

Obstructive ureteral problems have many causes and may be as simple as a kink in the catheter. One of the major causes of catheter occlusion is blood clots. If the patient is passing large blood clots or has a decrease in urine output, it is usually necessary to aseptically irrigate the catheter. Care must be taken during irrigation not to apply excess stress to the ureterocystostomy. This is particularly true in patients with exceptionally small bladders secondary to disuse, and in children who naturally have smaller bladders. If clots are not removed, bladder distention, pain, and stress on the ureterocystostomy may develop. This may result in a leak at the site of the anastomosis. Occasionally the surgeon will suture a stent to the end of the catheter, passing through the ureter to prevent ureteral stenosis.

Bladder spasms may develop, causing severe lower abdominal pain. Treatment includes belladonna and opium suppositories (B & O), oxybutynin chloride (Ditropan®), and propantheline bromide (Probanthine®). To permit complete bladder emptying, treatment of bladder spasms should be stopped 24 hours before the catheter is removed.

Urinary frequency after the catheter is removed can also be problematic for some patients. However, as the bladder stretches to accommodate larger urine volumes, urinary frequency generally resolves.

Cardiovascular. The goal of nursing care with regard to the cardiovascular system is to maintain circulatory function (Lancaster & Schanbacher, 1991). This requires frequent monitoring of cardiac function, blood pressure, vascular access for dialysis if present, and palpation of peripheral pulses.

Patients with CRF have a number of cardiovascular disorders. These include hypertension, atherosclerosis, left ventricular dysfunction, and/or a history of pericarditis or pericardial effusion (see Chapter 9). With the addition of excess fluid (e.g., development of an S3 or pulmonary edema) and electrolyte imbalances (e.g., hyper/hypokalemia) these patients may develop several additional problems that require monitoring in an intensive care unit (ICU). Indications for ICU monitoring include uncontrolled hypertension, hypotension, dysrhythmias, and ruling out a myocardial infarction.

Blood pressure is frequently monitored postoperatively. The development of hypotension can result from volume depletion or the administration of some immunosuppressive agents (e.g., antithymocyte globulin). Hypotension subsequently leads to decreased renal perfusion, which can exacerbate ATN if present. A single hypotensive episode can also result in loss of the patient's arteriovenous (AV) vascular access, which can be detrimental in the event of graft failure. Frequent monitoring for a bruit and thrill and protection of the involved extremity by eliminating cuff pressures, blood draws, and intravenous line placements are important in maintaining the patient's vascular access.

The development of hypertension is often related to preexisting disease, volume overload, or renal artery stenosis. It is generally initially treated with calcium channel blockers (see Chapter 12). In severe cases, patients are transferred to the intensive care unit for a sodium nitroprusside infusion, possible arterial line placement for frequent blood pressure checks, and EKG monitoring. Diuretics are administered in situations of volume overload. If there is no response to diuretic therapy, dialysis is initiated. Hypertension caused by renal arterial stenosis generally requires surgical intervention.

During the surgical procedure, the kidney is anastomosed to the iliac vessels. Clots or thrombosis of these vessels can occur, causing decreased perfusion to the affected extremity. Frequent assessment of femoral, popliteal, and pedal pulses can allow for early detection and prompt intervention for this problem.

Pulmonary. Prevention of pulmonary compromise is a major concern for patients after kidney transplant. Causes of respiratory problems posttransplant include preexisting disease (see Chapter 9), volume overload, atelectasis, and pulmonary infiltrates. Methods of ensuring sufficient oxygenation and maintenance of pulmonary function include adequate pain management to prevent splinting, early turning, coughing, deep breathing, and ambulation, use of incentive spirometers, and oxygen therapy if indicated. Periodic assessment of breath sounds, respiratory rate and effort, sputum, oxygen saturation, and patient color (e.g., ruddy, pale, cyanotic) can provide the nurse with the necessary information to assure adequate pulmonary function. If there is a change in pulmonary function, arterial blood gases, pulse oximetry, and chest radiography will often be ordered to assess respiratory status. If pulmonary edema or infiltrates are observed on a chest radiography, administration of diuretic medications (e.g., furosemide) and monitoring response is the first line of therapy. In addition, if there is a change in the color and consistency of expectorated sputum, a sputum specimen for culture will be ordered.

Gastrointestinal. The gastrointestinal effects of surgery and general anesthesia secondary to kidney transplantation are akin to those of general abdominal surgery. As in most postoperative patients, gastric motility is delayed. Frequent assessment of the abdomen and knowledge of pretransplant bowel patterns can be helpful. Abdominal assessment includes (1) inspecting for abdominal distention, (2) auscultating for the presence or absence of bowel sounds, (3) palpating for tenderness, and (4) monitoring for nausea, vomiting, diarrhea, constipation, and occult blood in the stool. Nausea and vomiting can develop for a variety of reasons: anesthesia, medications, electrolyte disturbances, and dehydration. The cause should be addressed and treated appropriately. Antiemetics are often prescribed.

Constipation occurs as the result of antacids and decrease motility. Antacids are commonly administered posttransplant to decrease gastric irritation caused by corticosteroids, or as phosphate binders if hyperphosphatemia remains a problem in the early postoperative period. Increased mobility, dietary alterations, stool softeners, or changing medications from phosphate binders to histamine antagonists (e.g., raniditine) are methods of minimizing constipation.

Diarrhea can develop as the result of medications (e.g., cyclosporine and CellCept®), infection, or bleeding. If diarrhea persists, a complete stool workup is performed, including culture for *Clostridium difficile*, rota virus, fecal leukocytes, and occult blood. Gastrointestinal bleeding may be related to corticosteroids or surgical stress. If active bleeding is present, endoscopy or colonoscopy with surgical intervention may be indicated. *Clostridium difficile* is typically treated for 7 to 10 days with antibiotics, usually oral Flagyl® or Vancomycin®.

Psychosocial considerations during the early postoperative period are often related to graft function, the relationship of the recipient to the living donor, and side effects of immunosuppressive therapy. With a successfully functioning graft and steroid administration, recipients often experience a general sense of well-being (Pattell & Weiskittel, 1991). The recipient may also have an improved self-esteem and body image (Thompson et al., 1993). However, for patients who do not experience a successful transplant, the postsurgical period can be an extremely difficult time.

During the early posttransplant period, the recipient can express a wide range of emotional responses secondary to fear of rejection, conflict over the decision to undergo transplantation, incorporation of the graft into their sense of self, fear of taking on characteristics of the donor, coping with feelings about the donor, family functioning, side effects of immunosuppression, pain, and financial worries. It is important that the nurse recognize the recipient's concerns and provide appropriate support. In some situations, consultation with a social worker or financial counselor can be extremely helpful.

Early Complications After Kidney Transplantation

Early complications of kidney transplantation other than the adverse side effects of immunosuppressive therapy can be categorized as rejection, infection, and technical problems related to the surgery. Surgical complications are further classified as urologic, lymphatic, and wound.

The nurse can facilitate early and accurate diagnosis of complications by frequent and exact patient assessments. If complications do occur, appropriate nursing management, support, and education are implemented with regard to the problem.

Rejection. Rejection continues to be one of the major problems in kidney transplantation. Although there is improvement in histocompatibility testing, immune modulating techniques, and availability of new immunosuppressive therapy, most patients experience at least one rejection episode. There are four types of rejection: hyperacute, accelerated, acute, and chronic.

Hyperacute and accelerated rejection episodes are the result of presensitization of the recipient to the donor's class I HLA antigens. The incidence of hyperacute rejection is 0.1-1% (Beckman et al., 1991). Hyperacute rejection occurs within 24 hours of transplantation, whereas accelerated rejection develops up to 6 days posttransplant. Both are humorally mediated rejection episodes.

Clinical manifestation of hyperacute and accelerated rejection are an abrupt cessation of urine output, decreased renal function, pain over the allograft, and a swollen, mottled, and cyanotic kidney.

Diagnosis is made by evaluation of clinical manifestations, renal scan which shows no uptake or excretion by the allograft, and/or surgical exploration (see Table 23-28). Histologic examination of the donor kidney reveals a lymphocyte infiltration in the renal vasculature. There is initial antibody binding to the vascular endothelial cells, which activates complement and the coagulation cascade. This process results in polymorphonuclear leukocyte (PMN) chemotaxis and intravascular glomerular platelet deposition and thrombosis, which leads to congestion and edema, inflammatory injury to the renal vasculature and glomeruli with hemorrhage and necrosis, ischemic tubular injury, and finally frank cortical necrosis (Garovoy et al., 1987; Sanfilippo, 1990). Management and prognosis of hyperacute accelerated rejection is poor, and transplant nephrectomy is frequently necessary.

Hyperacute accelerated rejection can cause emotional trauma for the patient and family. If there is a living donor, the loss of the graft may be even more devastating. Both the recipient and donor are forced to recover from a surgery that neither may feel they have benefited from. This may initiate feelings of failure, guilt, anger, or depression. It is not uncommon that these patients feel neglected postoperatively (Ruse & Kottra-Buck, 1986). It is imperative that both receive support to deal with their loss.

Acute rejection is the most common type of rejection and occurs in 70% of all kidney transplant recipients (Beckman et al., 1991). It is mediated primarily by cellular responses; however, humoral immune responses are observed. It generally occurs between 1 and 4 months posttransplant.

Clinical manifestations of acute rejection can include fever, malaise, weight gain, graft swelling and tenderness, increased blood pressure, elevated serum BUN and creatinine, proteinuria, and a decreased urine output. Cyclosporine treated patients may not experience any of the symptoms associated with rejection, and detection of rejection will be based on laboratory data, radiologic findings, and in some instances, biopsy.

Diagnosis of acute rejection can be facilitated by a renal scan. While not specific, it will show a decrease in the uptake and delayed excretion of the isotope by the graft (Flye, 1989).

Ultrasound will demonstrate swelling of the kidney and blurring of corticomedullary junctions and prominent pyramids in acute rejection and identify fluid collections and other causes of renal dysfunction. Magnetic resonance imaging (MRI) may also be diagnostic, showing loss of corticomedullary differentiation and swelling; however the cost may be prohibitive (see Table 23-28). The differential diagnosis for a decline in renal function with similar abnormalities includes ATN, cyclosporine nephrotoxicity, prerenal azotemia, and obstruction (Garovoy et al., 1987; Garovoy et al., 1994). Therefore, a renal biopsy is the gold standard for a definitive diagnosis to confirm kidney transplant rejection. Histologic examination of acute kidney rejection is characterized primarily by an interstitial infiltration of inflammatory mononuclear cells, mainly lymphocytes, and interstitial edema (Sanfilippo, 1990). In moderate acute rejection, eosinophils or plasma cells can be observed, and in severe rejection, vasculitis of the arterioles or arteries is present (Garovoy et al., 1987; Olsen, 1986).

Management of acute rejection is dependent on the center protocols, degree of renal involvement, and the patient's response to therapy. Generally, most mild rejection episodes are treated with corticosteroids, either as a daily intravenous bolus (e.g., 15 to 20 mg/kg/day) over a few days, or with an oral taper (e.g., starting at 2 mg/kg/day). However, OKT3 has been used for first-time rejection episodes with significant improvement in graft survival (Tesi et al., 1993). Anti-rejection therapy for moderate to severe rejection commonly consists of a 5 to 14 day course of monoclonal antibody OKT3 or polyclonal ATG and/or change to tacrolimus.

Nursing care of the patient with acute rejection requires education and support. Ideally, all patients will have received pretransplant instruction regarding rejection. They will have an understanding of the signs and symptoms, course, and usual treatment. However, even those who have had instruction may feel shocked that a rejection episode is occurring (Kottra-Buck, 1986). Responses to rejection are commonly a compilation of the rejection itself and the side effects of the drugs used to treat it. Emotional responses may include anger, depression, fear, withdrawal, or moodiness. During this time it is important that the patient/family be provided with support. Transplant support groups are most beneficial during rejection episodes.

Patients undergoing treatment for rejection must be closely monitored for drug side effects and episodes of infection. The additional immunosuppressive therapy used to treat acute rejection places the patient at an increased risk for infection. Frequent handwashing can facilitate prevention of infection, and diligent physical assessment will allow the nurse to identify early infection and initiate prompt intervention. Since high-dose steroids are the most common treatment for acute rejection, it is imperative that the patient be monitored for gastric irritation by checking for occult blood in the stool, hyperglycemia, excessive fluid retention, and adjustment to temporary body image changes. Patients will often become cushingoid, gain weight, and develop acne. These side effects are particularly disturbing for adolescents, who should be monitored closely for compliance and be provided additional support. Nursing interventions for patients who are having a difficult time dealing with the changes in their body image during rejection therapy include topical antibacterial medication to help control the acne (e.g., benzol peroxide), a nutritional consult to assist in appetite control and right food choices, physical therapy or exercise physiologist consult to increase activity level, and for young women, different methods of applying their makeup. It is important to have an understanding of the patient's major concerns to appropriately develop an individualized plan of care. Rejection episodes are often an ideal opportunity to provide the patient/family with additional education and resources regarding transplantation.

Chronic rejection is thought to be primarily humoral (B cells) mediated, and to a lesser extent cellular (T cells) mediated. Chronic rejection is a progressive deterioration in renal function. It has an insidious onset that develops over months to years after transplantation. Risk factors predictive of chronic rejection are thought to include an episode of acute rejection, histologic alterations, use of double immunosuppressive therapy rather than triple drug therapy, and lipid abnormalities (Basadonna et al., 1993; Isoniemi et al., 1994; Matas et al., 1994).

Clinical manifestations are highly variable depending on the degree of renal dysfunction. Initial presentation includes proteinuria secondary to increasing glomerular permeability, an increasing serum BUN and creatinine, decreasing urine output, fluid retention, alteration in electrolytes, and increased renin production resulting in hypertension.

Evaluation of chronic rejection by renal scan shows a progressive decreased uptake and excretion of the isotope. Renal biopsy is the most definitive method of diagnosing chronic rejection. Histologically, chronic renal rejection is characterized by the presence of chronic inflammatory mononuclear cells and vascular inflammation (Sanfilippo, 1990). There is narrowing of the vascular arterial lumen with intimal thickening. Eventually, fibrotic changes begin to occur within the blood vessel walls, progressing to glomerular sclerosis and tubular atrophy. Graft ischemia develops and is followed by interstitial fibrosis and subsequent loss of renal function (Garovoy et al., 1994; Isoniemi et al., 1994).

Management of chronic rejection is conservative, focusing on graft preservation and delaying retransplantation or dialysis. Management for chronic rejection is very similar to progressive CRF and includes medications, changes in diet, fluid restriction, monitoring of electrolytes, and blood pressure control (see Chapter 9). As the patient's renal function deteriorates and dialysis becomes necessary, withdrawal of immunosuppressive therapy is recommended.

Transplant nephrectomy is usually not indicated unless the patient develops fever, pain, and swelling over the graft. If such symptoms develop, transplant nephrectomy is recommended. Since the treatment for chronic rejection is usually unsuccessful in maintaining graft function, emphasis is placed pretransplant to secure optimal histocompatibility between donor and recipient.

Care of the patient experiencing chronic rejection requires monitoring for signs and symptoms of CRF (see Chapter 9), administration of medications, and assistance in maintaining activity level, education, and support. As renal function continues to deteriorate, the patient/family will need support and education regarding the addition of new medications, changes in diet and fluids, the status of remaining renal function, and treatment options. For patients who have been previously dialyzed, helping them make the transition back to dialysis is important. This will be highly variable depending on how long it has been since they were last dialyzed. For those who have never been dialyzed, support and education are essential. These patients and families would benefit from a support group and by speaking to other patients who are undergoing dialysis. They often require comprehensive instruction regarding CRF and available treatment options. Many patients will want to be reconsidered for another transplant. For those patients interested in a second transplant, a complete evaluation to determine candidacy must be completed. Early listing for retransplantation or live donor evaluation to avoid dialysis is most desirable.

Infection. There are two major factors that predispose the renal transplant recipient to infection (Chmielewski, 1987). First is the number of factors caused by the preexisting state of uremia that predisposes the recipient to infection (see Chapter 9). Additional risks for infection are complicated by any underlying systemic disease such as diabetes, systemic lupus erythematosus (SLE), scleroderma or malnutrition (see Chapter 8). Second are the alterations in the host's defenses due to the transplant surgery and administration of immunosuppressive therapy. As a result of the surgery the host's first line of defense is broken (e.g., skin, mucous membranes, and changes in body secretions). Further disruption is caused by invasive monitoring, urinary catheterization, central and peripheral intravenous access, and endotracheal intubation. Breakdown of the primary defenses subjects the transplant recipient to infection. In addition, immunosuppressive therapy alters the secondary defense, the immune response, which augments the recipient's risk of infection. Disruption in the host's primary and secondary responses predisposes the postrenal transplant recipient to infection. Other than the infections previously discussed, the renal transplant recipient is primarily susceptible to urinary tract and wound infections.

Urinary tract infections (UTI) after renal transplant are attributed to urinary catheters, bladder atonicity, ureteral reflux, and obstructive abnormalities. The major sites of infection include the urethra (urethritis), bladder (cystitis), ureter (ureteritis) or the renal pelvis (pyelonephritis).

Clinical manifestations of a UTI vary between patients and sites of infection. In general, clinical findings include fever, tachycardia, tachypnea, chills, suprapubic or lower back pain, burning on urination, bladder spasms, frequency, urgency, hesitancy, incontinence, nocturia, hematuria, pyuria, cloudy, foul smelling urine, nausea, and diarrhea (more common in infants).

Diagnosis is based primarily on a urinalysis and urine for culture and sensitivity. The urinalysis will show large quantities of bacteria, pus, red blood cells (RBCs), white blood cells (WBCs), casts, and an increased urinary pH. A complete blood count with differential may reveal an elevated WBC with a shift to the left. If bacteremia is suspected, blood cultures should also be obtained. Other diagnostic tests that may be employed are a computerized tomography (CT) scan or ultrasound to assess the status of the involved kidney and check for enlargement of the kidney, abscesses in the renal tissue, or structural abnormalities.

The management of recipients include treatment with systemic antibiotics (e.g., trimethoprim-sulfamethoxazole, or cephalosporin) and antibiotic bladder irrigations (if the catheter remains in place) for 14 to 21 days. Fluid intake should be increased to 3,000 ml/day for adults to enhance "flushing" of the kidney and urinary tract. Prophylactic therapy may be necessary for recurrent infections. Follow-up cultures should always be performed to assure eradication of the infection. In addition to antibiotics, patients should be given analgesic and antipyretic medications to minimize their pain and lower their temperature.

The nurse can instruct the recipient in five preventive measures to minimize the risk of UTI. First, empty bladder every 2 to 4 hours and drink at least 2 liters of fluid daily. Second, take showers rather than baths (no bubble baths), wash perianal area after every bowel movement, and do not use perfume in the genital area. Third, urinate before and after sexual activity, change tampons frequently, and seek prompt treatment for vaginal discharge. Fourth, avoid tight fitting pants and the use of chlorine bleach when laundering clothes. Fifth, adhere to antibiotic regimen during an infectious episode or as prophylactic therapy (Pattella & Weiskittel, 1991).

Wound infections can be superficial or deep. Those that extend into the perinephric space may result in a transplant nephrectomy. Less severe wound infections lead to prolonged healing and an extended hospital stay. Factors that contribute to the development of wound infections include hypovolemia inducing hypoxia to the wound, obesity, diabetes mellitus, poor preoperative nutrition and the preoperative shave which can lead to microscopic skin lesions where bacteria can colonize (Ahonen, 1987).

Immunosuppressive therapy also has an effect on wound healing. For example, corticosteroids delay wound healing by modifying the initial inflammatory response which transiently diminishes the number of white blood cells available to fight the infection. Azathioprine suppresses cell proliferation and may have a weak effect on inhibiting wound healing (Ahonen, 1987).

The characteristic clinical findings features of a wound infection are purulent wound drainage, pale tissue at the wound site with erythema around the edges, edema of surrounding tissue, fever, pain, nausea, and general malaise.

Diagnosis is based on clinical manifestations and culture of the exudate or purulent drainage from the wound site. Obtaining an accurate culture can be difficult. It must be deep within the wound. Superficial swabbing is generally not helpful and may reflect only skin pathogens.

Management involves systemic antibiotic therapy and meticulous wound management. Some infected wounds may require surgical debridement of necrotic tissue. Less severe wounds can be treat-

Table 23-30
Vascular complications of kidney transplantation.

hemorrhage
spontaneous graft rupture
renal artery thrombosis
renal vein thrombosis
aneurysm
renal artery stenosis

ed with irrigation and packing as ordered. Irrigation may be with normal saline, an antibiotic solution, or a shower head. The shower head is most helpful by providing hydrotherapy which enhances wound healing by removing necrotic debris as well as stimulates the surrounding circulation. Analgesic and antipyretic medications can be administered to minimize pain and reduce fever.

Vascular complications (see Table 23-30). Renal artery thrombosis is an emboli completely blocking the arterial flow to the kidney. Renal artery thrombosis is an early complication that results in graft infarction and failure. Renal artery thrombosis typically occurs in 0.2-1% of patients. It is generally the result of damage related to procurement, preservation, or transplantation, poor alignment of the intima during the anastomosis, especially when there is a disparity in vessel size, and excessive length of the vessels particularly in an end-to-end anastomosis (Diethelm et al., 1987; Salvatierra, 1987).

Sudden anuria may be the first clinical manifestation of renal artery thrombosis, suggesting a lack of blood supply to the graft. There is often accompanying tenderness over the graft and increasing edema of the thigh and leg on the side of the transplant. An elevated serum creatinine is also observed (Beckman et al., 1991).

Diagnosis of renal artery thrombosis should be suspected anytime there is a sudden decrease in urine output during the early postoperative period. Although other causes of acute renal failure are more likely, a misdiagnosis of renal artery thrombosis generally results in graft loss. Diagnosis can be made by ultrasound with Doppler flow studies, renal scan, or arteriogram of renal vessels demonstrating no flow to the graft.

Management includes emergency exploration and revision of the vascular anastomosis as the treatment of choice. If the thrombosis cannot be corrected, transplant nephrectomy is often indicated.

Renal artery stenosis (RAS) is generally a late complication that occurs in 0.6-13.5% of patients (Ruse & Kottra-Buck, 1986; Salvatierra, 1987; Whitten & Toledo-Pereyra, 1992). It is usually the result of vessel size mismatch at the site of the anastomosis, kinking or torsion of the renal artery, or intimal damage during procurement, preservation, or transplantation.

Clinical findings are manifested by moderate to severe hypertension secondary to hypoperfusion of the graft, stimulating increased production of renin (see Chapter 7). Thus, angiotensin-converting enzymes may exacerbate the effects of RAS (see Chapter 12). Other manifestations of RAS include decreased renal function as demonstrated by an increasing serum BUN and creatinine and an arterial bruit over the renal allograft or femoral artery close to the inguinal ligament.

Diagnosis is based on the result of a renal angiogram, which is always performed when renal artery stenosis is suspected. It usually demonstrates poor concentrations of the radioisotope at the site of the stenosis with poststenotic vessel dilatation. The renal angiogram is helpful in that it can also detect the status of the peripheral arteries. In the presence of multiple stenotic lesions, chronic rejection must be considered since the management would not be the same as in RAS and surgical intervention would be contraindicated.

Management of renal artery stenosis is correction by surgical reexploration, resection, and reanastomosis of the vessels. Transluminal angioplasty is an alternative approach but has more risk of injury to the artery with subsequent thrombosis or bleeding.

Renal vein thrombosis (RVT) is the result of an embolism usually in the renal vein and occasionally in the iliac vein. It is usually caused by an irregular intimal surface at the anastomosis site, intimal damage during procurement, preservation or transplantation, and kinking or mechanical occlusion of the donor vein. Clinical findings of RVT are characterized by proteinuria, hematuria, graft enlargement, and decreasing renal function. On occasion, iliac flow will be impaired, causing engorgement ipsilaterally on the affected side. Diagnosis of RVT is by venography. When venous thrombosis is suspected, there is no outflow of the radioisotope from the graft. Management focuses on early surgical intervention with vascular resection and reanastomosis to facilitate graft preservation. Nephrectomy may be indicated if damage is severe. Additional therapy may include the administration of systemic anticoagulation as soon as RVT is suspected.

Graft rupture is very rare, occurring in 0.8%-9.6% of kidney transplants (Witten & Toledo-Pereyra, 1987). Most occur within 2 to 3 weeks of surgery. Causes of graft rupture include swelling of the graft during an acute rejection crisis, renal biopsy, ischemic damage during procurement, urinary obstruction, emboli, lymphatic occlusion, or trauma. Rupture usually starts on the convex border of the kidney along the long axis. Clinical findings of graft rupture include pain and edema over the graft, abdominal swelling and tenderness, bleeding at incisional site, oliguria with declining renal function, hematuria, hypotension, tachycardia, cool and clammy skin, and mental status changes. Care is taken to monitor the patient closely to prevent vascular collapse secondary to blood loss and shock pending surgical intervention. Diagnosis is based on clinical manifestation. It can be confirmed by ultrasonography, computerized tomography (CT) scan, or surgical reexploration. Management mandates immediate surgical intervention. Depending on the extent of the damage, surgical repair of the renal capsule may be attempted. However, in most circumstances, a nephrectomy is the only treatment option.

Urologic complications. Ureteral obstruction is an uncommon complication early posttransplant. It is generally due to a tight submucosal tunnel of the ureter into the bladder or torsion of the ureter. Late ureteral obstruction is more common and is the result of ureteral ischemia secondary to inadequate blood supply to the distal ureter. Lymphocele is often an extrinsic cause of ureteral obstruction. Other causes of ureteral obstruction are outlined in Table 23-31 and may include blood clots, strictures, and stones.

Clinical findings of ureteral obstruction often present with a decrease in urine output, declining renal function as indicated by a rise in serum BUN and creatinine, and local pain or sepsis (Mendez & Vargas, 1987). Accompanying abdominal tenderness or pain and urinary leakage along the suture line may also be present.

Ureteral obstruction is determined by ultrasonography, which demonstrates a marked narrowing at the stenotic or obstructed area and dilatation of the ureter above the stenosis (Mendez & Vargas, 1987). Varying degrees of hydronephrosis may also be observed. A radioisotope renal scan can also be helpful except in patients with only a mild obstruction. In severe ureteral obstruction, the presence of a large hilar defect in the graft and absence of radioisotope in the enlarged renal pelvis are diagnostic. Rejection can be differentiated from ureteral obstruction by the accumulation and stasis of the radioisotope in the enlarged renal pelvis.

Management requires a percutaneous anterograde or cystoscopically placed stent be performed if the obstruction is not complete. The stent is left in place for a number of weeks prior to removal. It is not uncommon for the stenosis to reoccur after stent removal. Surgical intervention is often ultimately required. In the case of distal ureter pathology, reconstruction of the ureter and ureteroneocystostomy is performed. If this procedure is not possible, the native ureter can be anastomosed to the donor ureter or renal pelvis. If there is an inadequate ureter available, the bladder can be directly anastomosed to the renal pelvis. Particular caution must be paid to the latter type of anastomosis to prevent urinary tract infections and subsequent infection of the graft.

Table 23-31
Causes of ureteral obstruction following kidney transplantation.

stricture	periureteral lymphocele
kink	periureteral hematoma
torsion	periureteral inflammation
blood clots	spermatic cord obstruction
stone	ureteral compression
infections (abscess)	periureteral fibrosis
tumor	hematoma

Urinary extravasation (bladder leak) or fistula can be very problematic after kidney transplant. Ureteral fistulas are one of the most serious postkidney transplant complications. Approximately 0.5-10% lead to ureteral necrosis (Mendez & Vargas, 1987). The most common cause of urinary extravasation or fistula is damage to the donor ureter. Damage usually occurs during the donor nephrectomy and results in injury to the donor ureteral blood supply, causing ischemic necrosis of the donor ureter. Insufficient closure of the cystotomy incision during transplant, and preexisting bladder abnormalities can contribute to inadequate bladder emptying and subsequently result in a bladder leak. Patients at particular risk for bladder leaks are insulin-dependent diabetics and those who have small, contracted dysfunctional bladders previously requiring multiple urologic procedures.

Clinical findings are usually present within 5 weeks of transplant. The presenting signs and symptoms of a ureteral extravasation or fistula are pain and swelling over the graft, fever, elevation in serum BUN and creatinine levels, decreased urine output (oliguria, anuria), cutaneous urinary drainage over the surgical incision site, and possibly sepsis.

Diagnosis is made by ultrasonography revealing a periureteral fluid collection or hydronephrosis. A renal scan may demonstrate the isotope extravasating out of the ureter, and in some cases, a cystogram is necessary for diagnosis. Postvoid scintophotographs are often included with the radioisotope renal scans to rule out small bladder extravasation that may not manifest until there is the increased intravesical pressure of voiding. Lower ureteral leaks can be diagnosed once the isotope has been evacuated by the bladder and is retained in an extravasical location.

Management strategies to prevent bladder extravasation include meticulous bladder anastomosis by the surgeon during the transplant procedure, decompression of the bladder with a Foley catheter, and the avoidance of bladder overdistention. It is a nursing responsibility to monitor for adequate urine output and the presence of clots, which may impede urinary drainage and contribute to bladder distention. If a leak does develop, the placement of a ureteral stent may be indicated, or in some circumstances, surgical reanastamosis will be required. Surgical reconstruction is totally dependent on the status of the ureter. If there is extensive necrosis of the ureter, alternate surgical approaches are necessary.

Lymphatic complications. Lymphoceles are a consequence of inadequate ligation of the lymphatics during transplantation. It is the collection of extraperitoneal fluid in the transplant fossa secondary to a leak of lymphatic fluid during the postoperative period. It typically develops 3 to 6 months posttransplant.

Clinical findings of a lymphocele vary depending on their location. In general, clinical manifestations include a rising BUN and creatinine, decreasing urine output, mild lower abdominal discomfort on the affected side, and genital and/or ipsilateral edema of the extremity on the affected side. In extreme situations, the lymphocele may compress the transplanted ureter or iliac vein, causing bladder extravasation or extreme ipsilateral edema of the extremity on the affected side.

Diagnosis of a lymphocele can be confirmed by ultrasonography. A lymphatic fluid collection can be detected on ultrasound and depending on the location, there may be an accompanying dilated ureter with or without hydronephrosis.

Management of a lymphocele may be temporarily treated with percutaneous drainage; however, most require surgical intervention. The definitive treatment is surgical fluid evacuation with the internal marsupialization of the lymphocele cavity into the peritoneal cavity to allow for subsequent drainage of the fluid.

Late Complications after Kidney Transplantation

During the months to years following renal transplantation, several medical problems can develop. Late complications after kidney transplantation are categorized as allograft dysfunction, cardiovascular disease, hypertension, late infections, hepatitis B and C, malignancy, metabolic defects, delayed growth and development in infants and children, sexuality and pregnancy, and psychosocial difficulties. This section provides a brief overview of each of these complications.

Allograft dysfunction after kidney transplant has been reported to be caused by chronic rejection, cyclosporine or tacrolimus nephrotoxicity, recurrent disease, renal artery stenosis, and recurrent urinary tract infections (Braun, 1990). In addition, noncompliance with immunosuppressive medications has been shown to cause allograft rejection 3 months or more after transplantation (Rovelli et al., 1989).

Chronic rejection usually develops months to years after transplantation. It is clinically defined as a gradual but progressive impairment of renal allograft function in the absence of other specific causes. Risk factors predicting chronic rejection in renal transplant recipients have been reported to include elevated triglycerides, elevated low-density lipoprotein cholesterol level, donor age, use of triple immunosuppressive therapy rather than double therapy, low-dose immunosuppression, the occurrence of at least one episode of acute rejection, previous infection, and by the sum of histologic changes taken over time observed on biopsy (Basadonna et al., 1993; Isoniemi et al., 1994; Matas et al., 1994). Typical histologic changes occur in the renal vasculature, and treatment generally involves manipulation of immunosuppressive therapy (Geary et al, 1987; Kirkman et al., 1982; Rosenblum et al, 1988; Rowe et al, 1989). Other therapeutic methods that have been attempted include plasma exchange, dietary protein restriction, and antiplatelet agents (Hendrick et al., 1984; Foster & Dennis, 1992; Kootte & Paul, 1988).

Cyclosporine-treated kidney transplant recipients have demonstrated substantially improved graft survival (Calne, 1987). However, in spite of this improvement, patients often tend to have impaired renal function. The initial effect of cyclosporine (CSA) on renal structure and function is afferent arteriole vasoconstriction. The drug may also cause more permanent changes such as arteriopathy, chronic arteriolar lesions that mimic nephrosclerosis, and interstitial and tubular fibrosis (Mihatsch et al., 1988). Although reducing the dose is generally effective and may be associated with lower toxicity, there is an increased risk of rejection. In general, the majority of renal transplant recipients tolerate long-term cyclosporine therapy without progressively serious nephropathy (Burke et al., 1994).

Recurrent disease depends largely on the original disease and its natural history. Virtually all diseases affecting the native kidney will recur in the kidney allograft with the exception of Alport syndrome, polycystic kidney disease, hypertension, chronic pyelonephritis, and chronic interstitial nephritis (Ramos & Tisher, 1994; Ward & Glassock, 1992). In addition, recurrent nephritis of systemic lupus erythematosus and minimal change disease are also rare (Ward & Glassock, 1992). Table 23-32 outlines common disorders that tend to reoccur after kidney transplant. Fortunately the reoccurrence of original disease has minimal clinical impact and only about 5% of patients lose their graft secondary to recurrent disease (Amend et al., 1987; Ramos & Tisher, 1994). Live donor transplantation is controversial in those patients with disease that is likely to recur, i.e., hemolytic uremic syndrome, focal segmental glomerular sclerosis, membranous glomerulonephritis, Fabray's disease, and primary oxalosis.

Renal artery stenosis (RAS) has been reported in 0.6%-13.5% of postkidney transplant patients (Whitten & Toledo-Pereyra, 1992). However, since the presence of RAS is generally investigated only in patients with hypertension, these figures may grossly underestimate this complication. Three types of renal artery stenosis have been identified based on location and etiology (Lee & Mendez-Picon, 1984). The first type of RAS is localized to the area of the anastomosis and is thought to be related to technical error in approximating the donor and recipient arteries. It is the most common and best treated by resection and reanastomosis. The second type of RAS is a lesion located in the donor artery, evidenced by a smooth tubular lesion probably caused by trauma to the intima during procurement. This type of RAS is managed by resection or bypass of the stenotic segment using a saphenous vein or Dacron graft. In some situations, percutaneous transluminal angioplasty (PCTA) to dilate the stenosis have been used with varying results (Diamond et al., 1979; Sniderman et al., 1980). The third type of RAS is thought to be secondary to immunologic injury and has been associated with rejection. On evaluation of immunofluorescence studies, these lesions are positive for IgM and C3 (Whitten & Toledo-Pereyra, 1992).

Recurrent urinary tract infections can also cause renal dysfunction posttransplant and should be treated promptly. Patients with frequently occurring urinary tract infections should be evaluated for obstruction in the ureteropelvic and ureterovesical junctions. A renal ultrasound or renal scan with furosemide stimulation usually will locate the obstruction if present. If severe, placement of a percutaneous nephrostomy tube may be necessary (Belzer et al., 1988).

Cardiovascular disease (CVD) is responsible for approximately 30-40% of all deaths within the first 10 years after kidney transplant (Kirkman et al., 1982; Washer et al., 1983). Cardiovascular disease generally develops in patients after kidney transplant who are older (49 ± 12 years), predominately male, diabetic, hypertensive, and with left ventricular hypertrophy, who smoke, and have high cholesterol and triglyceride levels (Braun, 1990; Kasiske, 1992). Specifically, hypertension and diabetes are known to accelerate atherosclerotic vascular lesions and undoubtedly contribute to the increased mortality and morbidity from myocardial infarction, transient ischemic attacks, and cerebrovascular accidents (CVA) in these patients. Other contributing factors to CAD and accelerated atherosclerosis may be the synergistic effects of the above risk factors and the accumulation of high-dose prednisone and abnormal lipid metabolism (Braun, 1990; Kasiske, 1992).

Table 23-32
Commonly observed recurrent diseases after renal transplantation.

Membranous glomerulonephritis
Rapidly progressive glomerulonephritis
Anti-GBM glomerulonephritis
Juxtamedullary focal glomerulosclerosis
Focal segmental glomerular sclerosis
Membranoproliferative glomerulonephritis type 1 & 2
IgA nephropathy
Primary hyperotaluria type I
Cystinosis
Fabray's disease
Henoch-Schonlein purpura
Hemolytic uremic syndrome
Diabetes mellitus type I

With the high incidence of arteriovascular disease after kidney transplant, prevention and early treatment must be aggressive. Management measures include rigorous blood pressure control, weight loss and diet control, regular exercise, smoking cessation, and early conversion to an alternate day steroid regimen to lower the incidence of hyperlipidemia and the use of lipid lowering drugs, i.e., fluorestatin (Johnson & Flye, 1989).

Hypertension is the most common complication occurring in renal transplant recipients. The incidence of hypertension is approximately 65%-75% (Doncherwolcke, 1991; Johnson & Flye, 1989). In children, hypertension is almost completely resolved with the reduction of steroid dosage (O'Regan & Yazbeck, 1992). However, in the adult population, approximately 30%-50% of recipients have hypertension 5 to 10 years after transplantation (Kiekman et al., 1982). Several factors contribute to the development of high blood pressure, including cyclosporine, tacrolimus, steroid-related salt and water retention, hypercalcemia, obesity, increased renin and aldosterone levels, recurrent essential hypertension, renal artery stenosis, and chronic rejection (Curtis, 1991; Hiner & Suki, 1987; Johnson & Flye, 1989; Keown et al., 1992; Luke, 1987).

Blood pressure control is critical to prevent complications related to hypertension, particularly those associated with cardiovascular and atherosclerotic disease. In addition, hypertension is also an important contributing factor that may influence long-term graft survival. Treatment of mild hypertension is initiated with a salt-restricted diet with or without diuretic therapy. If the patient is obese, weight loss and increased activity are encouraged. Depending on the clinical situation, tacrolimus, steroids, cyclosporine doses may be decreased (Ingulli et al., 1993). Cyclosporine-related hypertension is best treated with calcium channel blockers (e.g., nifedipine) (Curtis, 1991). Antihypertensive medications are added when the above attempts fail. Antihypertensive agents commonly used include ß2 adrenergic blockers (e.g., propranolol), ß blocker-vasodilators (e.g., Labetalol) or ∂ adrenergic blockers (e.g., prazosin). If unsuccessful in effectively controlling blood pressure, vasodilators (e.g., hydralazine, nifedipine) or angiotensin converting enzyme inhibitors (ACE) (e.g., enalapril) may be administered. Although enalapril may be very effective in managing hypertension, to prevent acute graft failure due to ischemia, care must be taken to avoid administration in patients whose hypertension is secondary to Renal Artery Stenosis (RAS). In general, adrenergic agonists (e.g., methyldopa) are avoided to minimize impotence in men (Curtis, 1991; Johnson & Flye, 1992; Luke, 1982). Assessment of renal renin levels and ateriography to rule out renal artery stenosis are performed on patients who have refractory hypertension.

Late infections occur more than 6 months after transplant. Kidney transplant recipients who are more likely to have late infections are those with poor renal function, higher levels of immunosuppression, leukopenia, and those who have had a splenectomy (Braun, 1990). The most common late infections are community-acquired pneumonias such as influenza or respiratory syncytial virus (RSV) in children, and urinary tract infections (Rubin, 1991; Rubin, 1994). The urinary tract is the portal of entry for 60%-70% of bacteremias in kidney transplant recipients (Rubin, 1994). Although pulmonary and urinary tract infection are responsible for most postkidney transplant infections, it is imperative that the unusual sites of infection be considered. Unusual sites for infection might include the central nervous system, intervertebral disc space, and gastrointestinal tract.

Rubin (1993) categorizes late infections into three groups. The first group represents 75% of patients who have good allograft function and are receiving minimal immunosuppressive therapy. Infection most commonly observed in this group are similar to the general population's influenza, pneumococcal pneumonia, and urinary tract infections. The second group constitutes approximately 10%-15% of patients. These patients often have a chronic viral infection such as CMV, EBV, hepatitis, or HIV, which may lead to graft damage or failure. The third group represents approximately 5%-15% of patients who have relatively poor allograft function and a history of rejection, and receive an excessive amount of immunosuppression. These patients are at highest risk for opportunistic infections, for example, *Pneumocystis carinii, Listeria monocytogenes, Cryptococcus neoformans,* or *Nocardia asteroides.*

Kidney transplant recipients on long-term immunosuppressive therapy should receive prophylaxis against infection. This is particularly true when undergoing dental procedures, surgery, or instrumentation of the gastrointestinal tract. In addition, daily prophylactic administration of penicillin is recommended for splenectomized recipients. Prevention is central to the development of late infection posttransplantation. Avoidance of unnecessarily high doses of immunosuppressive agents can assist in minimizing late infectious episodes.

Hepatitis. The incidence of chronic liver disease after kidney transplant is approximately 10-15%, which is more common than those undergoing dialysis. Eight percent to 28% of individuals surviving kidney transplant for greater than 10 years will die as the result of liver disease (Braun, 1990; Rubin, 1993). The major causes of liver disease after kidney transplant are hepatitis B and hepatitis C (Rubin, 1993).

Hepatitis B virus (HBV) exposure is common among renal transplant recipients. Patients with hepatitis B acquire it pretransplant from hemodialysis, blood transfusions, or during the peritransplant period. Rarely is hepatitis B acquired from a hepatitis B surface antigen (HBsAg) positive donor (Dienstag & Katkov, 1994). Once infected with HBV, recipients are more likely to remain chronically infected, retain high levels of viral replication, and be very infectious to their contacts (Coughlin et al., 1980). High levels of viral replication may be stimulated by immunosuppressive therapy, which may be associated with progressive liver disease. Progressive liver disease secondary to hepatitis is best confirmed by histology obtained from a biopsy, rather than biochemical indicators (Suthanthirn & Strom, 1994).

The clinical effects of HBV infection can be observed in two time frames (Rubin, 1993). During the first 1 to 2 years posttransplant, HBV contributes to the net state of immunosuppression, but there are no obvious clinical manifestations of chronic liver disease. After 2 years, the chronically HBV infected postrenal transplant recipient begins to develop progressive liver disease, hepatocellular carcinoma, or both (Katkov & Rubin, 1991).

The main controversy is the effect of HBV infection on patient survival after kidney transplantation. Some studies have found mortality and morbidity much higher in HBsAg positive patients following renal transplantation (Hillis et al., 1979; Parfrey et al., 1984; Pirson et al., 1977). However, other investigators have found less than a 10% mortality rate in postkidney transplant patients who are HBsAg positive. (Berne et al., 1977; Debure et al., 1988; Fine et al., 1977; Huang et al., 1990; Mani et

Table 23-33
Kidney transplant recipient plan of care.

ASSESSMENT	
Assess	**Potential Observations**
General	Febrile, pain, discomfort, agitated, complains of feeling ill, changes in emotional response, euphoric, depressed.
Renal	Decreased urine output, pain over the graft, weight gain, peripheral edema, hypertensive, increased serum BUN & creatinine, alteration in electrolytes. Decreased blood to the graft demonstrated by renal scan or ultrasound, renal biopsy with inflammation.
Urinary Tract	Urine is cloudy and possibly foul smelling, presence of hematuria with/without clots, complaints of lower abdominal pain (bladder spasms).
Cardiovascular	Hyper/hypotension (check pretransplant B/P); increased or decreased central venous pressure, changes in heart sounds (S3), peripheral edema, vascular access positive for bruit and thrill.
Pulmonary	Decreased breath sounds with crackles in the posterior bases, O_2 saturations 92-94% on room air, slight increase in respiratory rate and effort normal.
Gastrointestinal	Decreased/absent bowel sounds, mild abdominal distention, pain, nausea, vomiting, constipation, decreased or increased appetite. Possible ileus on abdominal radiography.
Immune	Wound site with serosanguineous slightly purulent drainage, elevation in WBC or decrease in WBC secondary to immunosuppressive agents

DIAGNOSE	
Nursing Diagnosis	**Supportive Findings**
Potential for excess fluid imbalance: related to intraoperative & postoperative fluid administration, and/or inadequate urinary elimination.	Decreased urine output, increased respiratory effort, pulmonary infiltrates and congestion on chest x-ray, restlessness, hypertensive, increased central venous pressure, peripheral edema, increased weight, intake > output, may have decreased hematocrit secondary to hemodilution.
Potential for deficit fluid imbalance: related to excessive output, diruetic therapy, inadequate fluid administration, vomiting/diarrhea and/or bleeding.	Orthostatic or hypotensive, decreased central venous pressure, decreased weight, output > intake, elevated BUN, poor skin turgor, dry mucous membranes.

Potential for electrolyte imbalance: related to level of renal function after transplantation, intraoperative blood transfusions, metabolic disorders associated with acidosis and hyperglycemia, side effects of medications (e.g. CSA, steroids).	Elevated BUN & creatinine, elevated potassium, decreased magnesium, decreased urine output, EKG with elevated T-waves, cardiac arrhythmias, hypo-hyperreflexia, seizure activity.
Altered patterns of urinary elimination: related to bladder spasms, anatomical size, or obstruction due to clots, bladder leak, infection, diabetic neurogenic bladder.	Decreased urine output, lower abdominal pain, drainage (urine) from the incision, inability to void spontaneously, hematuria, cloudy, foul smelling urine, pain on urination.
Potential for injury: related to rejection or acute tubular necrosis (ATN).	Increased BUN, creatinine, possible elevation in potassium, decreased urine output, weight gain, fever (not always seen with CSA), complaints of feeling ill.
Potential for infection: related to alterations in the immune system secondary to immunosuppressive therapy, presence of invasive lines and Foley catheter.	Fever, elevation in white blood cell (WBC) count, foul smelling, purulent wound drainage, cloudy foul smelling urine, productive cough, crackles on auscultation.
Potential for constipation or gastroparesis: related to anesthesia immobility, pain medication, fear of straining on defecation, presence of Foley catheter, inadequate dietary intake.	Complaints of abdominal distention and fullness, bloating, nausea/vomiting, inability to defecate, no stool.
Potential for pain: related to incisional pain or bladder spasms.	Complaints of incisional discomfort with mobility, guarding behavior, severe lower abdominal pain that is transient.
Alteration in body image: related to medication side effects and transplantation.	Concern regarding changes in weight (loss or gain), acne, moon faces, facial hair or loss of hair, incorporation of donor organ into sense of self.
Potential for knowledge deficit: related to the short/long posttransplant course, unfamiliar tests and procedures, home management, medications, rejection, and risk of infection.	Patient/family unable to state medications (side effects, dose schedule, purpose), signs of rejection, how to protect themselves from infection, routine procedures and tests (what they are and their purpose, frequency).

Other Related Nursing Diagnoses:
Altered sexual patterns related to body image disturbance; altered family process related to living-related donation; hopelessness related transplant nephrectomy; potential for noncompliance related to physical changes secondary to medication regimen, potential for ineffective breathing related to fatigue and immobility.

PLAN

Patient Goals

The patient will demonstrate normal fluid balance and remain euvolemic.
The patient will obtain adequate fluids to maintain body functions.
Electrolyte balance will be maintained.
The patient will resume normal bladder function.
The patient will have no signs or symptoms of infection.
The patient will resume normal bowel function.
The patient will be without pain and demonstrate effective measures of coping with pain/discomfort.
The patient will have a positive, accepting, realistic body image.
The patient/family will have increased knowledge regarding kidney transplantation and be able to perform all activities required to maintain health posttransplant.

IMPLEMENT

Nursing Diagnosis	Nursing Intervention	Rationale
Potential for excess fluid imbalance: related to intraoperative & postoperative fluid administration, and/or inadequate urinary elimination.	Monitor and measure total hourly intake and output.	Provides fluid balance and status that facilitates early recognition of potential volume overload.
	Daily weights for adults and twice a day for infants and small children. Use the same scale at the same time daily.	To determine changes in fluid status; an increase in weight of greater than 2 kg over 24 hours indicates fluid retention.
	Monitor blood pressure frequently.	Elevation in blood pressure may suggest volume overload. Orthostatic hypotension suggests lack of adequate fluid administration or volume depletion.
	Monitor central venous pressure (CVP).	Elevation suggests volume overload, a decrease suggests a fluid deficit (normal CVP 3 to 6 mm water).
	Assess and monitor jugular vein distention.	Jugular vein distention suggests excess fluid volume.
	Assess and monitor skin turgor; watch for peripheral edema.	Peripheral edema may suggest excess volume or low albumin; dry mucous membranes and poor skin turgor suggest volume deficit.

	Assess and monitor albumin.	Low albumin suggests decreased oncotic pressure allowing for third spacing (leakage of fluid into the interstitial spaces).
	Assess for the presence of S3 heart sounds.	Indicative of fluid overload.
	Frequently auscultate chest for changes in breath sounds.	Presence of crackle may indicate an increase in fluid status and pulmonary edema.
Potential for deficit fluid imbalance: related to excessive output, diuretic therapy, inadequate fluid administration, vomiting/diarrhea and/or bleeding.	Monitor and measure total hourly intake and output.	Provides fluid balance and status that facilitates early recognition of potential volume deficit and dehydration.
	Daily weights for adults and twice a day weights for infants and small children. Use the same scale at the same time daily.	To determine changes in fluid status.
	Monitor blood pressure and heart rate frequently.	Hypotension or orthostatic blood pressures and elevated heart rate may indicate dehydration.
	Monitor central venous pressure (CVP).	Decreased CVP indicates decreased intravascular volume; this can be observed in patients whose weight is increased and have peripheral edema secondary to third spacing.
	Offer fluids frequently if the patient is on an oral diet.	Prevent dehydration.
	Monitor hematocrit and hemoglobin.	Increased hematocrit and hemoglobin may indicate dehydration.
Potential for electrolyte imbalance: related to level of renal function after transplantation, intraoperative blood transfusions, metabolic disorders associated with acidosis and hyperglycemia, side effects of medications (e.g. CSA, steroids).	Monitor changes in serum electrolytes.	To determine electrolyte imbalance, results may vary with changes in renal function and use of diuretics.

	Monitor for EKG changes.	Altered levels of potassium may interfere with cardiac contractility and may be detected by EKG.
	Assess for physical symptoms of electrolyte imbalance (e.g. irritability, hyporeflexia/hyperreflexia, weakness, cardiac arrhythmias, seizure activity.	To assess for the effects of electrolyte imbalance on body systems.
	Administer replacement electrolytes as ordered and/or diuretics.	To maintain normal electrolyte balance (some diuretics remove potassium).
Altered patterns of urinary elimination: related to anatomical size or obstruction due to clots, bladder leak, infection, diabetic neurogenic bladder, bladder spasms.	Measure urine output hourly.	To ensure adequate drainage and appropriate urine output.
	Assess catheter for patency and irrigate as needed for clots (follow unit nursing procedure).	To ensure continuous drainage of urine, avoid distention of the bladder, and identify obstruction.
	Teach personal hygiene and teach/perform Foley care twice daily.	To prevent urinary tract infections.
	Assess wound for urinary leakage; if present, notify the physician.	Indicates a bladder leak.
	Monitor temperature frequently.	Fever indicates infection and may indicate a bladder leak.
	Assess and monitor wound for purulent drainage; if present, notify the physician.	Indication of a wound infection.
	Assess patient's ability to void spontaneously and communicate to physician.	To ensure adequate urine output and prevent bladder distention.

	Instruct patient to void every hour/frequently after Foley is discontinued; if unable to void, patient will need to be recatheterized.	To minimize overdistention of the bladder and stress on bladder incision.
	Check bladder for distention when urine output is decreased.	To determine if decrease in output is functional (e.g. problem with bladder emptying) or is an indicator of changes in kidney function.
	Assess for bladder spasms and medicate as ordered and indicated to minimize spasms.	Bladder spasms can be caused by the Foley catheter and may interfere with continuous urinary drainage. B & O suppositories relax smooth muscle of the bladder and pressure on bladder incision.
Potential for injury: related to rejection or acute tubular necrosis (ATN).	Monitor for signs and symptoms of rejection: fever, decreased urine output, pain over the kidney, general feeling of illness, weight gain.	Promotes early detection of graft dysfunction and facilitates prompt intervention which prevents further complications (e.g. volume overload).
	Monitor BUN and creatinine.	Elevations in BUN and creatinine indicate a decline in renal function requiring further investigation, may indicate rejection.
	Administer immuno-suppressive therapy as ordered and monitor patient response.	To minimize the risk of rejection.
	Prepare patient for diagnostic procedures that may indicate rejection (e.g., biopsy).	To decrease anxiety and facilitate cooperation during procedure.
	Provide emotional support.	Emotional support is essential to assist the patient/family to cope with the unknown and the diagnosis of rejection.
Potential for infection: related to alterations in the immune system secondary to immunosuppressive therapy, presence of invasive lines and Foley catheter.	Monitor for signs and symptoms of infection (steroids may mask symptoms of infection) (e.g., fever, elevated WBC, decreased platelets, redness, swelling, and purulent drainage from incision, pain,	To provide prompt intervention with appropriate treatment.

	Interventions	Rationale
	increased respiratory effort, cough, fatigue).	
	Monitor vital signs frequently.	Fever, hypotension, tachycardia are indications of infection.
	Assess breakdown in integument, including mucosa.	Promotes early detection of infection and facilitates prompt intervention; infection is resisted through the body's defense mechanisms, and the skin is the major mechanical barrier, disruption in wound healing and oral candidal infections are common with high dose steroid administration.
	Monitor and assess complete blood count (CBC) and differential.	Leukopenia and neutropenia increase the risk of infection.
	Initiate protective isolation according to hospital policy (e.g., absolute neutrophil count <500 µL generally requires isolation.	Protect patient from the risk of infection.
	Collect cultures as ordered; pan culture (e.g., blood, urine, drainage) and obtain chest x-ray as ordered for temperature > 38.5 C.	To detect any infection and facilitate proper intervention.
	Instruct and encourage use of incentive spirometer.	To promote lung expansion and decrease the risk of atelectasis or pneumonia.
	Encourage patient to cough, deep breathe, and early physical activity and ambulation.	To prevent respiratory compromise and the risk of pulmonary infection.
	Assess and record presence and characteristics of sputum.	Productive cough may indicate respiratory infection.
	Auscultate lungs every 4 hours and as indicated.	Promotes early detection of changes in respiratory status and allows for prompt intervention to minimize risk of infection/complication.
	Assess and monitor line and tube sites.	Evidence of redness, swelling, heat, or drainage generally indicates an infection; allows for early identification and prompt intervention.

	Maintain sterile technique with dressing and line changes.	To minimize the risk of infection.
	Maintain strict Foley catheter care.	To minimize the risk of infection.
	Administer antimicrobials, antipyretics, and analgesics as ordered and monitor patient's response.	To protect or treat infection in the immunocompromised patient and maintain patient comfort (e.g., decrease fever with antipyretics and minimize pain).
	Practice universal precautions as indicated by procedure and situation.	To prevent transmission of microorganisms while performing care.
	Staff with known infections should not care for immuno-compromised patients.	To minimize the patient's exposure to infections.
	Maintain a clean and safe environment.	To minimize the risk of microorganisms coming into contact with the patient; minimize risk of injury which may promote entry of microorganisms that could cause infection.
Potential for constipation or gastroparesis: related to anesthesia, immobility, pain medication, fear of straining on defecation, presence of Foley catheter, inadequate dietary fiber intake.	Assess abdomen every shift and as indicated for the presence of distention.	Distention may indicate decreased bowel motility or an ileus.
	Auscultate bowel sounds and assess for passage of flatus.	Passage of flatus and bowel sounds indicate GI motility and return of GI function.
	Assess appetite and ability to advance diet as tolerated.	Oral intake should not compensate until GI function has been reestablished to prevent further GI distress; appetite may be an indicator of returning GI function.
	Assess and document episodes of nausea, vomiting, or diarrhea; note character and frequency of emesis and stool; guaiac stool and GI aspirate when appropriate and as indicated.	Nausea and vomiting may indicate postoperative ileus; documentation will help establish level of GI functioning; to assist in the selection of appropriate therapy; to determine the presence of blood in stomach contents and stool, may indicate ulcers secondary to steroids or other GI disturbance.

	Encourage adequate intake of fluid and fiber; and the importance of activity level.	To promote normal stool formation and regulation of bowel habits.
	Assess need for laxatives and document effects every day.	Indicates need or effectiveness of laxative therapy.
	Minimize use of narcotics.	Narcotics decrease GI motility.
Potential for pain: related to incisional pain or bladder spasms.	Assess patient's comfort level and identify sources of pain; use of an established pain scale may be helpful.	To determine need for and specific type of intervention to relieve pain.
	Observe patient for nonverbal expressions of discomfort (e.g., elevated blood pressure and pulse, guarding, grimacing).	To further establish existence of pain, especially if patient is unable or unwilling to verbally communicate pain.
	Identify source of pain, note onset, location, quality, duration, precipitating factors.	To determine appropriate intervention to control pain (e.g., may be related to gas in which case mobilization would be more effective than narcotics which further decrease GI motility).
	Monitor and document patient's response to medications: blood pressure, pulse, respiration, relief of pain.	To evaluate degree and effectiveness of pain medication and to determine if pain relief regimen should be changed.
	Position patient for comfort, anticipate need for medication prior to activity.	To maximize nonpharmaceutical interventions and promote comfort.
	Allow adequate time for sleep and rest between activities.	To promote healing and rest.
	Encourage and teach patient/family to use relaxation, diversional techniques, massage, or other means to minimize patient's discomfort.	To identify additional means to minimize or control pain.

Administer pain medication	To relieve pain. as ordered and indicated.	
Alteration in body image: related to medication side effects and transplantation.	Assess and monitor self-concept in terms of statements and behavior.	To guide therapeutic intervention and referrals.
	Provide a supportive environment for the patient to discuss concerns and anxieties; refrain from negative criticism.	To establish trust and confidence in order to assist the patient to improve self-image.
	Prepare patient for possible side effects of medications that may alter their appearance.	To minimize surprises and facilitate coping and adjustment to physical changes.
	Problem solve with patient methods of minimizing side effects of immunosuppressive medications (e.g., exercise, makeup, hair styles, acne control, food choices).	To facilitate decision making, identify strategies to promote restoration of self-image, and promote a positive body image.
	Acknowledge body changes; assist patient to focus on identifying strengths and accomplishments.	To promote self-image through validation and reinforcement of the patient's positive individual qualities.
	Encourage patient to verbalize concerns or feelings of guilt related to the donor.	Mixed feelings toward the donor are not uncommon; assisting the patient to verbalize their feelings will promote adjustment.
	Direct patient to appropriate resources (e.g., support groups, social worker, psychologist, psychiatrist, counselor, etc.) as indicated.	Use of resources and support groups may facilitate development of a positive sense of self and body image.

Potential for knowledge deficit: related to the short/long-term posttransplant course, unfamiliar tests and procedures, home management, medications, rejection, and risk of infection.	Establish baseline assessment of cognitive/developmental level of patient.	To determine patient's preexisting level of knowledge and development level to establish a realistic, individual, and measurable teaching plan for patient/family.
	Following transplant, assess patient/family readiness to learn.	To determine patient's ability to begin learning about and participating in their own care.
	Initiate discharge teaching per unit protocol.	Patient/family must have a basic understanding of posttransplant care to minimize complications and facilitate early intervention.
	Identify teaching goals and record patient/family response to teaching.	To ensure communication to team members regarding patient/family response to teaching and accomplishment of written goals.
	Assess patient/family ability to manage care at home.	To ensure patient/family ability to provide care at home or identify need for additional support.
	Mobilize appropriate community resources as indicated (e.g., intravenous antibiotic therapy, physical therapy, etc.).	To provide patient/family with additional resources they may need to facilitate transition to home care.

EVALUATE

Expected Outcome	Data Indicating Expected Outcome is Reached
Patient remains euvolemic.	Intake and output are balanced; weight is stable, blood pressure is within normal limits, absence of edema, mucous membranes are moist.
Electrolytes remain normal; there are no complications related to electrolyte abnormalities.	Electrolytes are maintained within normal limits.
Patterns of urinary elimination have returned to normal.	Patient is able to void spontaneously without pain, discomfort, or residual urine and there is no evidence of bladder leak or infection.
Breathing pattern is effective.	Patient is breathing without difficulty, arterial blood gases are normal, oxygen saturation is normal, breath sounds are normal.

Injury related to rejection and acute tubular necrosis (ATN) has been minimized.	Patient exhibits no clinical manifestations of rejection or ATN (fever, decreased urine output, pain over the kidney, general feeling of illness, weight gain) and is tolerating immunosuppressive therapy.
There are no signs or symptoms of infection.	Patient remains afebrile, vital signs, WBCs, and urinalysis are normal, cultures are negative, urine is clear, chest x-ray is clear, patient does not have a productive cough, skin remains intact, line and tube insertion sites are free of redness, swelling, or drainage.
Bowel pattern is regulated; there is no evidence of an ileus.	Patient resumes pretransplant bowel pattern, no evidence of bloating, nausea, or vomiting.
Patient is pain-free and applies alternative methods of pain management.	Patient has no complaints of pain and is able to demonstrate alternative methods of pain management.
Patient has a positive, accepting, and realistic body image.	Patient expresses integration of body image into sense of self, demonstrates an understanding of physical changes, discusses strategies to improve body image, and reports feeling better about physical appearance.
Patient/family are knowledgeable regarding postkidney transplant care.	Patient/family (pediatrics) is able to accurately self-administer medications, states purpose, dose, administration schedule, and side effects of medications, states the signs and symptoms of rejection and appropriate action to take, demonstrates ability to take temperature, weight, blood pressure, heart rate, and blood glucose level as indicated; states posttransplant activities and limitations.

PATIENT TEACHING PLAN

1. Teach all patients and families (especially with regard to pediatric patients) the postkidney transplant routine.
2. Teach patient and family all medications including their purpose, side effects, dosage schedule, and frequency (Chapter 12).
3. Teach patient and family the basic laboratory values that will be monitored (e.g. BUN, creatinine, electrolytes, drug levels, CBC, platelets, and liver function studies).
4. Teach patient and family the signs and symptoms of rejection (decreased urine output, pain over kidney, general feeling of illness, weight gain) and appropriate actions to take.
5. Teach patient and family the signs and symptoms of infection, importance of monitoring these clinical manifestations, and appropriate action to take.
6. Teach patient and family type and purpose of dietary restrictions if any.
7. Teach patient and family the amount and type of fluid to drink.
8. Teach patient and family the importance of skin care, sunscreen, and acne prophylaxis in preventing complications.
9. Teach patient and family the importance of routine dental care, brushing, flossing, and gum care.
10. Teach family planning, use of contraceptives, and risks of pregnancy.
11. Teach the importance of exercise and encourage regular activity.
12. Teach health maintenance skills and encourage a return demonstration (e.g. temperature, weight, pulse, blood pressure, glucose monitoring, incisional/wound care, central line care).
13. Provide the patient and family with information regarding financial, psychological, and rehabilitative resources.
14. Teach patient and family the importance of regular follow-up health care and laboratory tests.
15. Provide the patient and family with information about kidney transplantation and local organizations.
16. Teach the usefulness of keeping a log of the disease course, treatments, and other disease-related information.
17. Teach patient and family the importance of carrying medical alert information at all times.

al., 1993; Rashid et al., 1988; Toussaint et al., 1979).

More recently, Roy et al. (1994) found that HBsAg positive kidney transplant recipients do not convert to a seronegative status after transplantation, 60% develop chronic hepatitis at 36 months, and 75% at 6 years. Mortality due to chronic liver failure was approximately 16% at 3 years. Rao and Anderson (1988) report similar results at 10 years following renal transplantation. In this study, 10 years after transplant 38% of patients developed chronic progressive hepatitis, 38% had chronic active hepatitis, 42% had cirrhosis, and 54% died of liver failure. Those patients who did extremely poorly posttransplant were those who were hepatitis Be antigen positive or who had histologic findings of persistent hepatitis at the time of transplant (Rao et al., 1991).

Other factors that may contribute to hepatic dysfunction after kidney transplant include azathioprine, systemic viral infections (e.g., herpes, CMV), sepsis, and hepatitis C (Dienstag & Katkov, 1994). Since azathioprine may affect hepatic function, withdrawal of this drug as a component of immunosuppressive regimen has become one approach to treatment. Alpha-interferon is another approach to therapy; however, it has not been shown to be successful in the treatment of HBsAg positive patients and may in fact produce adverse effects on allograft function (Rubin, 1993).

Since the data remains controversial, HBsAg positivity should be considered a relative contraindication to kidney transplantation. Other factors to consider include histology results, degree of viral replication (HBeAg, HBV DNA etc.), nutritional status, coexisting illness, quality of life, and the patient's wishes (Rubin, 1993).

Hepatitis C virus (HCV) is the major cause of hepatitis, chronic liver disease, and possibly hepatocellular carcinoma in renal transplant recipients (Rubin, 1993). Early HCV morbidity and mortality (1 to 2 years posttransplant) are more often related to the net contribution of immunosuppression, extrahepatic infection, and subsequent sepsis. Whereas, late (5 to 10 years) morbidity and mortality are caused by hepatic deterioration, demonstrated by elevation in transaminases, ascites, hepatic encephalopathy, and bleeding from varices (Alter et al., 1984; LaQuaglia et al., 1981). In contrast, more than 20% of renal transplant recipients who have evidence of hepatitis C after transplant have been shown to clear the virus over time (Dienstag & Katkov, 1994; LaQuaglia et al., 1981).

It is important to recognize that the subtle and progressive changes of liver disease do develop in patients with HCV, even in the absence of initial symptoms or clinical evidence of hepatic inflammation.

Management of HCV is difficult at best. Withdrawal of azathioprine and effective antiviral therapy, such as interferon, have been shown to be initially effective in treating HCV positive patients. Interferon has been shown to clear HCV RNA and antibody to HCV in the serum, and sustain biochemical, histologic, and virologic responses (Chan et al., 1993; Rubin, 1993). However, this approach to therapy remains in its initial stages, and further research is necessary.

Malignancies remain a serious problem after kidney transplant. Basal-cell carcinoma of the skin and lips, Kaposi's sarcoma, carcinoma of the vulva and perineum, non-Hodgkin's lymphoma, squamous-cell carcinoma, hepatobiliary carcinoma, and carcinoma of the uterine cervix have a higher incidence in transplant recipients then the general population (Hanto et al., 1992). Skin cancers in particular are the most common malignancies after kidney transplantation. Their frequency may be related to sun exposure, skin type, and length of time after transplantation (Eurvrard et al., 1993). High-dose immunosuppression, particularly multiple treatments with antilymphocyte antibodies (monoclonal or polyclonal) augment the risk of malignancies, especially lymphoma (Suthanthiran & Strom, 1994). Triple therapy with cyclosporine or tacrolimus, azathioprine or CellCept, and prednisone have shown an increased incidence of B-cell lymphoma when compared to renal transplant recipients treated with only prednisone and azathioprine (Wilkinson et al., 1989). In addition to conventional treatment of malignancies, reduction or cessation of immunosuppressive therapy is generally indicated (Penn, 1987).

Musculoskeletal disease following renal transplantation includes alteration in calcium-phosphorus metabolism and bone disease (osteomalacia), avascular necrosis, and delay in normal growth and development in children. In general, renal transplantation corrects the calcium, phosphate, vitamin D and parathyroid hormone abnormalities of CRF. However, densitometry and histomorphometry studies have shown impaired bone formation and osteopenia (Suthanthiran & Strom, 1994). Bone loss is further intensified by the use of corticosteroids and prolonged immobilization, which increases bone reabsorption and suppression of osteoblastic activity (Keown & Shackleton, 1992). Management approaches that have been employed include calcitonin, testosterone, estrogens, and a reduction in corticosteroids.

Avascular necrosis occurs in approximately 10% of patients. There is general agreement that steroids are a contributing factor (Johnson & Flye, 1989). Avascular necrosis is described as the death of marrow cells and osteocytes caused by loss of blood supply (Green, 1987). Involvement usually affects the femoral head, femoral condyles, humeral head, or talar dome. Once radiologic changes are present, treatment is initiated with protective weight bearing and antiinflammatory agents. Approximately 42% of patients treated with conservative therapy maintain stability of their hip joint (Andersen & Nielsen, 1981). Surgical intervention and total joint replacement becomes necessary in patients who do not respond to conservative therapy.

Growth and development is impaired in children with severe chronic illness and organ failure secondary to nutritional, metabolic, and endocrine factors. These changes are particularly significant in children with CRF due to metabolic osteodystrophy and the coexistence of osteoporosis, hyperparathyroidism, osteomalacia, and aluminum toxicity (Coburn & Slatopolsky, 1986). In general, successful kidney transplantation corrects these changes and provides the child with an opportunity for normal growth and development. Although growth and development after kidney transplant is superior to dialysis, normal growth patterns are not always attained (Sager & Ettenger, 1993).

Posttransplant growth is influenced by timing of transplantation, physiologic status of the child, growth potential (bone age, stature, and chronologic age), adequacy of the graft, and steroid dosage (Aschendorff et al., 1990; Ohmore et al., 1989; Tsuzuki et al., 1989). For example, growth retardation may be considerable in infants who present with CRF as candidates for kidney transplantation (Jones et al., 1982). Also, children with advanced bone age at the time of transplant do not usually demonstrate catch-up growth. Kidney transplant recipients less than 5 years old have been shown to grow significantly better following transplantation than any other age group. This suggests that transplant in the young child should be expedited to preserve potential growth (McEnery et al., 1992).

Inadequate graft function indicated by a creatinine of greater than 2 mg/dl is also a measure of poor catch-up growth. Linear growth is further retarded by the use of high dose prednisone, which may inhibit somatomedin release and accelerate epiphyseal closure. The use of double immunosuppressive therapy with azathioprine and prednisone demonstrates a delay in bone maturation and lower growth rates resulting in growth retardation for chronologic age that is partially corrected by a longer growing period. Methods of improving growth in these children has been to decrease steroid doses, shift to alternate day doses, or taper and eliminate steroids as a component of the immunosuppressive regimen (Sager & Ettenger, 1993). Children receiving cyclosporine demonstrate growth acceleration approximately 2 to 3 years after transplant with bone maturation occurring at a normal rate when compared to azathioprine and prednisone treated patients (Aschendorff et al., 1990). In addition, monotherapy with tacrolimus shows promise in minimizing growth retardation associated with cyclosporine-based immunosuppressive regimens (Ellis et al., 1994).

Short stature and delay in the development of secondary sex characteristics can be difficult and devastating for some children and teenagers. Psychosocial support and education regarding strategies in managing their altered body image can facilitate coping and social adjustment and minimize noncompliance.

Metabolic defects after kidney transplant include renal tubular defects, obesity, and diabetes mellitus. Distal renal tubular acidosis (RTA) is the most common tubular defect. It is considered an ominous sign since it often indicates chronic rejection. Other renal tubular defects include mainly salt wasting attributed to selective hypoaldosteronism and hyperkalemia related to type IV renal tubular acidosis (see Chapter 7), usually secondary to cyclosporine or tacrolimus.

Weight gain can be quite marked and become a devastating problem to some individuals after transplantation. It is the result of an improved state of well-being, removal of previous dietary restrictions, and steroid therapy. However, severe weight gain can result in the loss of body image and cause significant depression and noncompliance. Early intervention before the problem develops is the best approach to management. Initial instruction regarding eating habits, food choices and exercise is much easier than the subsequent institution of a diet regimen. In some cases, alternate-day steroid therapy or steroid withdrawal may also be helpful.

Steroid-induced diabetes occurs in approximately 10% of patients (Johnson & Flye, 1989). Steroid therapy and a genetic predisposition are the major contributing factors. In general, as the steroid doses are decreased, this problem resolves itself.

Sexuality and pregnancy are concerns of most post-kidney transplant recipients. In general, fertility and reproductive function of both men and women returns to normal following transplantation, making pregnancy and impregnation possible. The possibility of conception emphasizes the need for counseling regarding contraception. Barrier methods are recommended for contraception and the prevention of sexually transmitted diseases (e.g., HIV, herpes, genital warts etc.).

Pregnancy is discouraged for the first 1 to 2 years posttransplant to ensure renal function and promote the outcome of a viable fetus (Davison, 1991). Women who become pregnant following kidney transplantation require specialized care that mandates collaboration between the obstetric and nephrology teams. Management of these patients requires particular attention to immunosuppresion, blood pressure control, renal function, infection, and fetal surveillance (Bumgardner & Matas, 1992; Davison, 1987; Jain et al., 1993; Winkler et al., 1993). Normal vaginal delivery is usually possible; however 40%-50% of infants born to transplant recipients are premature and/or small for gestational age (Armenti et al., 1993; Davison, 1987; Davison & Lindheimer, 1984; Haugen et al., 1991; Penn et al., 1980). Long-term follow-up of women who became pregnant following kidney transplantation demonstrates that pregnancy does not have an adverse effect on patient or graft survival or the development of hypertension or renal insufficiency. The data on the children is encouraging (Sturgiss & Davison, 1992; Whetham et al., 1983).

Psychosocial problems after kidney transplantation are often manifested as noncompliance, particularly among teenagers. In general, risk factors for noncompliance include increased numbers of medications, depression, black race, locus of control given over to others more powerful, unemployment, younger age, low socioeconomic group, and perceived amount of social and family support (Kiley et al., 1993; Schweizer et al., 1990). One retrospective review of 260 kidney transplant recipients who were noncompliant with their medications and follow-up demonstrated that 91% either lost their grafts or died (Schweizer et al., 1990). In another study, 0.6%-13% of 385 renal transplants performed in 365 patients lost their graft secondary to noncompliance (Bittar et al., 1992).

The adolescent's developmental need to "fit in" with peers and not be different is in direct conflict with the continued reminder of their chronic illness that daily medications engender. Teenagers may find their appearance disturbing and stop taking their medications. Consequently, failure to comply with the prescribed immunosuppressive regimen remains a major cause of rejection, especially in teenagers (Ettenger et al., 1991).

Psychologic anxiety and depression can occur as a result of the transplant, immunosuppressive therapy, or changes in family functioning. Glucocorticoids can directly affect the patient's emotional status by causing them to be labile and overreactive. In certain situations, decreasing steroid dose and instituting psychotherapy can be helpful. However, kidney transplantation is generally well recognized as improving one's sense of well-being and quality of life when compared to those on dialysis. Most patients return to their premorbid status and work or attend school.

Pancreas Transplantation

Pancreas transplantation is a viable therapeutic option for insulin-dependent diabetes. The engraftment of a functioning endocrine pancreas into the insulin-dependent patient provides the optimal physiologic means of correcting altered metabolism. The goal of pancreas transplant is twofold: to provide an insulin-independent lifestyle and to prevent the secondary complications associated with diabetes.

It is obvious that pancreas transplantation is not a lifesaving procedure but may greatly improve quality of life and reduce the millions of dollars spent annually on the management of diabetes mellitus and its sequelae (Wills & Post, 1990).

As of November of 1996, there have been 8,845 pancreas transplants performed worldwide, 2,345 of these in the United States. Most non-U.S. cases were reported from Europe.

Of the total number of pancreas transplants reported, 5,505 were simultaneous pancreas/kidney (SPK) transplants. Patient survival rates for SPK transplants were marginally different (p=0.08), with 1 year being 92% for the United States, 91% for Europe, and 86% for other locations. For SPK bladder drainage cases the difference was somewhat less (p<0.09) with a 1-year graft survival in the United States (n=3,989) of 79%, in Europe (n=820) of 73%, and elsewhere (n=120) of 77%. For those undergoing enteric drainage (pancreaticojejunostomy), the graft survival rates were not significantly different with 1 year being 72% in the United States (n=314), 63% in Europe (n=127), and 72% in other locations (n=16) (International Pancreas Transplant Registry [IPTR], 1997).

Preservation time has shown to have minimal impact on outcome in SPK transplant recipients with 1-year graft survival rate for pancreas stored < 12 hours (n=1,400), 12-23 hours (n=2,256) and >23 hours (n=195) being 78%, 80%, and 76% respectively. However, the effects of HLA mismatches on outcome for U.S. SPK cases were significantly higher (p>0.04) with 0 mismatches (n=30) than with higher degrees of mismatches. Zero mismatch graft survival rates were 85% at 1 year versus 69% with 1 mismatch (n=67), 76% with 2-3 mismatches (n=975), and 79% with 4-6 mismatches (n=2,836) (IPTR, 1997; Hiesse et al., 1997).

Currently, pancreas transplantation can be offered to diabetic patients with the same probability of success as other solid organ transplants (Larue et al., 1997). Pancreas transplantation has taken several forms since its inception of the animal model 35 years ago. There are a number of approaches to pancreatic transplantation being evaluated: single pancreas; kidney after pancreas transplant; simultaneous kidney-pancreas; and islet cell transplantation. An SPK transplant is the transplantation of a kidney and a pancreas from the same donor into a known Type I diabetic who also has renal failure. This procedure addresses the increasing number of diabetic patients who present with chronic renal failure. In diabetic uremic recipients, SPK transplants have become progressively successful and have dramatically improved the quality of life for this population (Sutherland, 1996).

Pancreatic graft survival is defined as normoglycemia without insulin. Factors influencing the improved success have been refinement in surgical technique, greater understanding of immunobiology, and wider availability of immunosuppressive therapy.

Table 23-34
Pancreatic cells and their function.

Types of Cells	Cell	Function
Exocrine	Acinar	Produces enzymes needed for digestion of carbohydrates (amylase), protein (trypsin), and fats (lipase).
Endocrine	Islets of Langerhans a) alpha b) beta c) delta	 Produces glucagon Produces insulin Produces somatostatin

Normal Pancreatic Function

The pancreas is located in the posterior aspect of the peritoneum. It is in front of the left kidney, inferior vena cava, and aorta. The pancreas weighs between 100 and 150 grams and is divided into the head, neck, body, and tail. Blood supply to the pancreas is by branches of the celiac trunk and the superior mesenteric artery.

The pancreas has both exocrine and endocrine function. The exocrine or ducted cells of the pancreas are called the acinar cells. These cells produce enzymes that are needed for the digestion of carbohydrates (amylase), proteins (trypsin), and fats (lipase). When foods are eaten, the pancreas secretes and releases digestive enzymes into the duodenum. These enzymes can break down foods into simpler substances to facilitate absorption into the bloodstream. These substances are then transported and ultimately either used or stored as energy.

The endocrine or ductless cells of the pancreas have 1 to 2 million cluster cells, called the islets of Langerhans. The islets contain three types of cells: alpha, beta, and delta. Alpha cells produce glucagon, which increases the blood glucose level. Beta cells produce insulin, which regulates the amount of glucose in the bloodstream and aids in the utilization of glucose as an energy source. When the pancreas does not provide adequate insulin, glucose is not released from extracellular fluid into the cells. Without glucose, the cells become depleted of energy, and the cells begin to oxidize fats and protein from adipose tissue and muscle. Delta cells produce somatostatin, which helps regulate blood glucose levels by inhibiting either insulin or glucagon secretion. Delta cells also reduce the rate of triglyceride absorption from the intestines after a fatty meal (Demayo et al., 1990) (see Table 23-34).

Table 23-35
Manifestations of diabetic complications by system.

System	Clinical Manifestation
Cardiovascular	• accelerated atherosclerosis • increased risk of coronary artery disease • cardiomyopathy • autonomic neuropathy • silent myocardial infarction
Vascular	• diabetic retinopathy potentially causing blindness • potential for cataracts
Renal	• nephropathy manifested by glomerulosclerousm tubular necrosis, or renal failure
Neurologic	• visceral degenerative processes • peripheral nerve degenerative processes • neuropathy resulting in diabetic neurogenic bladder, atrophy of extremities, orthostatic hypotension, neurotrophic foot ulcers, impotence.
Immune	• predisposition for infections
Gastrointestinal	• decreased gastrointestinal motility
Metabolic	• ketoacidosis
Dermatologic	• diabetic dermopathy • necrobiosis lipoidica diabeticorum (NLD)

Diabetes Mellitus

Diabetes mellitus is a syndrome characterized by insufficient insulin secretion, inability to use the insulin properly, and reduced glucose tolerance (Holleroroth, 1986). It leads to the development of universal microangiopathy, neuropathy, and arteriosclerosis (Deckert, 1988). Approximately 40% of patients with insulin-dependent diabetes will develop devastating complications such as renal failure, retinopathy, neuropathy, gastroenteropathy, and peripheral vascular and cardiovascular disease (Demayo et al., 1990). There are two types of diabetes: Type I and Type II. Type I diabetes is often referred to as insulin-dependent diabetes mellitus (IDDM), and is characterized by the absolute defi-

Table 23-36
Pancreas recipient evaluation.

Cardiovascular	• blood pressure close evaluation, EKG, possible echocardiogram and/or stress thallium
Gastrointestinal	• gastric emptying studies
Opthamologic	• slit lamp examination • intraocular pressure measurements • visual acuity determination • stereo color fundus photography • fluorescein angiography
Neurologic	• peripheral nerve conduction studies • autonomic testing • quantitation of sensory loss
Metabolic	• glucose tolerance tests • hemoglobin A1C • urine and serum C-peptide levels • thyroid function studies • serum amylase and lipase
Urologic	• voiding cystourethrogram
Pulmonary	• chest x-ray • pulmonary function tests
Psychologic	• psychiatric evaluation
Financial	• financial counseling

ciency of insulin production. Although Type I IDDM can occur at any age, it is most often diagnosed between the ages of 5 and 20 years. The cardinal symptoms of diabetes are polyphagia, polyuria, polydipsia, and weight loss. Unlike Type I diabetes, Type II diabetes is related more to insulin resistance due to the body's decreased insulin sensitivity and decreased insulin responsiveness. It is generally diagnosed later in life and in many cases can be managed by diet control and oral hypoglycemic medication. The diagnosis of diabetes carries with it the potential for the manifestation of a significant number of secondary complications. Table 23-35 is a systems review of diabetic complications.

Given the potential complications of diabetes, the search for a cure continues. The discovery and use of exogenous insulin in 1921 was found to prolong the life of millions of individuals, but this intervention failed to prevent the development of secondary complications. Pancreas transplantation may prevent or delay the onset of the secondary complications reviewed. What began as an animal model 35 years ago has developed into a therapeutic option for a significant number of diabetic patients. Although the diabetic patient also has insulin therapy as a treatment modality, studies indicate that pancreas transplantation may actually improve the diabetic's quality of life (REF) (Bentley et al., 1990; NaKache et al., 1988)

Types of Pancreas Transplantation

Pancreas transplantation has taken several forms since its inception in the form of an animal model 35 years ago. There are three basic approaches to pancreatic transplantation: single pancreas, islet cell, or combined kidney-pancreas transplant.

Single pancreas transplant or the transplantation of the pancreas alone had been attempted with limited success in the 1970s and early 1980s. This procedure was obviously indicated for the diabetic patient who had not yet developed renal failure. Long-term success rates in this population of pre-uremic diabetics was poor (Kelly et al., 1967; Lillehei et al., 1970; Sutherland et al., 1979; Sutherland et al., 1988). Immunologic barriers were considered the major stumbling block in the success of this procedure. Since the introduction of improved immunosuppressants, single pancreas transplantation is being revisited.

Islet cell transplantation is still in its infancy despite the magnitude of work that has been done in the field to date. Islet cell transplantation involves the meticulous retrieval of cells from a cadaveric source. Retrieval and processing of islet cells remains a cumbersome and labor-intensive task. Once retrieved, the islets are injected into the recipient liver, spleen, or renal capsule or intraperitoneally. The two main problems with islet cell transplantation are the difficulty in islet cell isolation and the long-term viability of these cells (REF) (Sutherland et al., 1996; Zekorn et al., 1996). Islet cell transplant would most certainly be the procedure of choice if these two issues could be resolved. The advantages of avoiding a major surgical procedure would most certainly be desired. Current areas of research that are being tested include the use of islet cells from other animal models and islet cells from human fetal tissue (REF) (Dordevic et al., 1995; Farkas et al., 1995).

Combined kidney-pancreas transplantation is the simultaneous transplantation of a kidney and a pancreas from the same donor into a known Type 1 diabetic who also has renal failure. Controversy still exists regarding whole versus segmental pancreas transplantation. Whole pancreas transplantation is the transplantation of the entire pancreas with or without a duodenal stump. Segmental pancreas transplantation usually involves the transplantation of only the body and tail of the pancreas. At this time it appears to remain physician preference as to which approach is taken.

The clinical future of pancreas transplantation is not completely clear. The trend toward islet cell transplantation may be pursued, or with the increasing scarcity of cadaveric donors, living-related segmental pancreas transplantation may become a more viable option. However, the present procedure of choice is the combined cadaveric pancreas-kidney transplant and, therefore, our discussion will be limited to this approach.

Pancreas Transplant Recipient Selection

Recipient selection is similar to kidney recipient selection but may differ slightly between centers. Criteria for selection includes the presence of type 1 diabetes mellitus, renal insufficiency, imperfect metabolic control of exogenous insulin, and possible evidence of other secondary complications (Trusler, 1991).

Indications for pancreas transplantation is the presence of insulin-dependent diabetes and the potential for developing secondary complications.

Contraindications to pancreas transplantation are similar to those for other solid organ transplants. Absolute contraindications include active systemic infection, extracranial malignancies, and drug addiction. Those disorders that may preclude pancreas transplantation include severe coronary artery disease, incapacitating peripheral and autonomic neuropathies, and psychosocial disorders. The benefits of the procedure must outweigh the risks, and the patient must be willing to accept the uncertainty of both the potential risks and benefits (Wills & Post, 1990) (see Table 23-36).

Pancreas Transplant Recipient Evaluation

Evaluation of a candidate for combined pancreas-renal transplant is performed by a multidisciplinary team. The evaluation consists of a complete history and physical with a review of systems, laboratory and radiologic tests, histocompatibility studies, and a psychosocial assessment. The evaluation of the pancreas candidate is very similar to the evaluation of the kidney transplant recipient (see Table 23-24 earlier in this chapter). However, age is variable, but generally ranges between 15 and 50 years of age. ABO compatibility and a negative crossmatch with the donor are essential. Although some transplant centers are reporting varying degrees of success in reversing some of the reported advanced systemic complications, severe complications are generally considered a contraindication (Kennedy et al., 1990). In addition to the studies in Table 23-24, those in Table 23-36 should be completed.

Pancreas Transplant Surgical Procedure

Pancreas transplant donors are often simultaneous cadaveric kidney donors. The entire pancreas is excised during the procurement. A button of the duodenum (the patch technique) or the intact duodenum (pancreaticoduodenal graft) is also recovered. Vascular components, later used for anastomoses to the recipient, include the portal vein and a Carrel patch of the aorta, encompassing the celiac axis and superior mesenteric artery. Following procurement, the organ is flushed intraarterially and preserved by cold storage using a variety of solutions.

Recipient surgery consists of one of three types of pancreas transplants: (1) islet cell transplants, (2) segmental or whole organ pancreatic transplants, and (3) simultaneous pancreas-kidney transplants. Combined pancreas-kidney transplant is the most common of the procedures. For whole organ transplant, the pancreas is placed first intraperitoneally into the right iliac fossa. The arterial supply of the donor is anastomosed to the common iliac artery of the recipient. The venous drainage of the donor is anastomosed to the common iliac vein. Surgical anastomosis of the kidney follows, and it is generally placed in the left iliac fossa.

Enzymal secretion and management of pancreatic transplantation has proven to be a technical challenge. Two types of exocrine drainage are currently employed: enteric drainage and urinary drainage. Enteric drainage is accomplished by anastomosing the graft to a Roux en Y loop of the jejunum of the recipient. Urinary diversion is accomplished by anastomosing the pancreas to the recipient's bladder by using a segment of the donor duodenum.

There are advantages and potential complications to all three types of enteric drainage. The urinary drainage method is the most common approach to enteric drainage. The advantage of this method is the ability to assess graft exocrine function by measuring urinary amylase levels. These levels have been shown to be early predictors of pancreas rejection (Sollinger et al., 1991).

Pancreas Transplant Postoperative Management and Nursing Care

Postoperative care of the pancreas-kidney transplant recipient is very similar to the care of the patient who receives only a kidney transplant (Trusler, 1991). The goal of the immediate postoperative period is to maintain hemodynamic stability and to prevent complications. If complications occur, early identification to allow for rapid treatment is optimal.

The previous discussion of the postkidney transplant recipient also applies to the postpancreas-kidney transplant recipient. Postoperative management issues specific to the pancreas-kidney transplant patient addressed in this section include metabolic acidosis, urinary tract maintenance, pancreatitis, vascular patency, hemorrhage, rejection, and infection.

Metabolic acidosis and dehydration are frequent occurrences in the pancreas transplant patient whose exocrine drainage is done via urinary diversion. The cause is the loss of pancreatic electrolytes in the urine. In particular, there is a significant loss of bicarbonate from the pancreas into the urine, causing a systemic acidosis. If renal function becomes compromised, there is an obligatory chloride retention augmenting the already present acidotic state. Intravenous supplemental sodium bicarbonate may be required for a short period. In addition, it is not unusual that recipients will require oral supplementation of sodium bicarbonate later in their postoperative course (Wills & Post, 1990).

Urinary tract maintenance is of the utmost importance during both the early and late postoperative periods. An indwelling Foley catheter is used to decompress and drain the bladder. Decompression of the bladder will promote healing of the suture line and bladder and minimize the risk of anastomotic leaks. A urinary leak is diagnosed by a cystogram and may require long-term management of a Foley catheter or surgical repair. Prompt irrigation of the Foley catheter is indicated with any decrease in urine output or suspicion of obstruction. Inability to reestablish an adequate drainage system by irrigating mandates that the Foley catheter be replaced immediately.

Urinary reflux through the duodenal stump to the pancreas graft could also result from an inadequate drainage system. Clinically, urinary reflux produces a rise in serum amylase, indicating pancreatitis.

Graft pancreatitis is demonstrated by hyperamylasemia early or late during the postoperative period. Contributing factors include an inadequately drained urinary tract, damage to the pancreas during organ recovery, rejection, or trauma. Prompt identification of pancreatitis is crucial. Treatment includes administration of intravenous fluids, anticoagulation therapy to prevent thrombosis, early postoperative NPO, late adequate bladder drainage to decompress the pancreas.

Vascular thrombosis continues to be of significant concern in the early postoperative period (first 24-48 hours). Potential causes of thrombosis are mechanical obstruction, trauma to the pancreas during procurement, pancreatitis, thrombogenic effects of immunosuppressants, or microthrombi from the pancreas itself (Soon-Shiang et al., 1988).

Graft thrombosis is manifested by hematuria, a sharp decrease in urine amylase with a simultaneous increase in serum glucose. Severe low abdominal pain is often reported by the patient. In addition, nuclear scans demonstrate lack of blood flow to the pancreas. Treatment is generally a total graft pancreatectomy (Demayo et al., 1990).

Careful monitoring of urinary amylase, serum glucose levels, and anticoagulation factors are all interventions used to monitor and prevent graft thrombosis. It has also been proposed that the avoidance of hypovolemia may help prevent vascular thrombosis after pancreas-kidney transplantation (Sutherland et al., 1988).

Postoperative hemorrhage is associated with any type of surgery and must be monitored and assessed for frequently. Mild hematuria is common in the early postoperative period following pancreas-kidney transplantation. It is particularly common when the surgical approach for exocrine drainage is the urinary diversion. Persistent gross hematuria usually indicates an anastomotic leak at the duodenocystostomy site, ulcerations of the bladder, or duodenal cuff. Bladder irrigation is usually the initial intervention for hematuria. If the patient is receiving anticoagulation therapy, it may need to be temporarily discontinued. Treatment of gross hematuria generally requires either surgical correction of the leak or medical/surgical treatment of the ulcerated duodenum (Wills & Post, 1990).

Rejection is more difficult to diagnose in pancreas transplantation than other solid organ transplant, and thus is a major cause of graft loss (Grundfest-Bronictowski, 1990). Pancreatic transplant rejection is also difficult to differentiate from other types of graft failure, such as vascular thrombosis, recurrent disease, and pancreatitis (Sollinger et al., 1987). Clinical signs of rejection such as fever, ileus, and graft tenderness are often unreliable. A specific example is the elevation in transplant recipient's serum glucose levels, which may be a vague indicator of rejection. Unfortunately, serum glucose levels often remain normal until almost 90% of insulin-producing cells are destroyed. Another unreliable indicator is the elevation in serum amylase levels. The causes of high serum amylase levels vary and include preservation injury of the graft, pancreatitis, infection, and rejection.

Before the bladder drainage technique was instituted, it was difficult to monitor pancreas transplant rejection. As the use of the bladder drainage technique for exocrine drainage has become more universally applied, graft survival rates have improved. Graft survival improved because of the ability to identify and treat pancreas transplant rejection early based on urinary amylase levels. The bladder drainage technique allows for frequent monitoring of urinary amylase levels as an indicator of pancreas graft rejection. Immediately posttransplant, a baseline urinary amylase level is obtained, followed by close monitoring. The diagnosis of rejection can be made if there is a 25%-50% decrease in urine amylase from baseline (Demayo et al., 1990). Other reliable predictors of pancreas graft rejection are a decrease in urinary bicarbonate and pH (Corry, 1987; Prieto et al., 1987).

Other methods that have been used to detect rejection after pancreas transplantation include serum C-peptide levels, radionuclide imaging, open

Table 23-37
Postoperative management of the pancreas-kidney transplant recipient.

System	Expected Outcome	Intervention
Cardiovascular	Normal cardiac output	• monitor blood pressure • auscultate apical pulse • observe skin color and turgor • palpate pulses
Pulmonary	Normal oxygenation and perfusion	• assess breath sounds every shift • monitor oxygen saturations • arterial blood gases as indicated
Renal	Normal fluid and electrolyte balance and removal of waste products	• monitor hourly urine output • hourly total intake and output • maintain urinary catheter patency • irrigate urinary catheter as indicated • daily weights • monitor serum BUN and creatinine • monitor electrolytes
Metabolic	Normal acid-base balance	• monitor electrolytes • administer sodium bicarbonate as ordered
Immunologic	No indication of infection or rejection	• monitor WBC for elevation • inspect and monitor wounds • assess urine for color, clarity and odor • send UA with micro as indicated • assess lung fields • monitor for normal serum glucose levels • monitor urine amylase • report decreased urine amylase levels • monitor urine pH • monitor temperature • assess for complaints of pain
Vascular	No indication of thrombosis	• administer anticoagulants • monitor urine amylase levels • monitor serum glucose levels

wedge or needle biopsy, and aspiration cytology (Grundfest-Broniakosski, 1990). A reversible increase in pancreatic graft size has been observed on computerized tomography (CT) scans during kidney transplant rejection (confirmed by biopsy) in combined pancreas-kidney transplants (Schaapherder et al., 1993). Biopsy of the transplanted pancreas can be performed through cystoscopy. Histologic features that have demonstrated a high correlation with rejection include moderate to severe inflammation of the acinar tissue, acinar tissue loss, and fibrosis and vascular luminal narrowing (Nakhleh & Sutherland, 1992). Classification of pancreatic rejection has been suggested. Mild rejection would include endotheliitis, and vasculitis would define severe rejection (Nakhleh & Sutherland, 1992). Cytologic features of acute rejection have been reported to include hypercellularity with lymphocyoturia, increased numbers of epithelial cells, and a positive staining for HLA-DR antigen (Radio et al., 1993).

A combined pancreas-kidney transplant from the same donor can be beneficial in terms of diagnosing rejection. In this situation, the serum creatinine can be used as a reliable marker for detecting rejection and promptly instituting treatment (Sollinger et al., 1988). In combined pancreas-kidney transplantation, rejection is usually found in the kidney allograft first (Baumgartner et al., 1983). Kidney rejection can occur independent of pancreas rejection. However, it is rare that the pancreas would reject independently. Early detection of kidney transplant rejection often precludes pancreas rejection. Generally antirejection therapy is instituted immediately, thereby protecting the pancreas from an overwhelming rejection episode.

Infection, as with other any organ transplant patient, is a significant cause of morbidity in the pancreas transplant recipient (Chapter 13). Astute nursing assessment for signs and symptoms of infection are crucial (see Table 23-37).

Long-Term Management after Pancreas-Kidney Transplantation

Long-term implications for the diabetic patient after pancreas-kidney transplant remain unclear. Quality of life for the pancreas-kidney transplant patient have improved posttransplant, regarding control over one's life, positive self-image, vocational employment changes, and sexual activity (Bentley et al., 1990). The effect of pancreas-kidney transplantation on secondary complications of diabetes continues to be investigated. Peripheral neuropathy and microcirculation to the extremities have been reported to have improved posttransplant in pancreas-kidney transplant recipients (Abendroth et al., 1989; Kennedy, 1990; Soldiers et al., 1987). Although reports are mixed, the effect of transplantation on retinopathy has not been as promising (Peterson & Vine, 1990). Further investigation into the stabilization of the diabetic process are needed. If regression of diabetic lesions were to occur, the implication for transplanting the nonuremic diabetic patient could be profound (Demayo et al., 1990).

Liver Transplantation

With the advent of cyclosporine during the early 1980s, the 1-year survival rate for orthotopic liver transplantation has soared upward. Prior to the 1980s, the 1-year survival rate was less than 30%. In contrast, many programs now have 1-year survival rates of greater than 85% (Health Resources, 1991). As a result, liver transplantation has become a widely accepted therapeutic treatment option for individuals with end stage hepatic failure and metabolic disorders.

Extended survival rates may be attributed to improved management of end stage liver disease and fulminant hepatic failure, improved recipient selection, enhanced surgical procedures for donor and recipient, availability of increasingly effective immunosuppressive agents, and early recognition and intervention of infection and rejection (Lake, 1993; Riegler & Lake, 1993; Starzl et al., 1989; Stock & Payne, 1990). In addition, the emergence of the transjugular intrahepatic portacaval shunt (TIPS), used to control variceal bleeding and manage ascites while waiting transplantation, has improved the management of patients' pretransplant. Unlike major vessel surgical shunts, the TIPS does not alter the extrahepatic anatomy, avoids surgery, and eliminates the risk of anesthesia (except in the pediatric population). The TIPS is removed with the liver explant at the time of surgery (LaBerg et al., 1993; Lake, 1993; Ring et al., 1992). Other bridges to transplant that promise encouraging results continue in the application of new hepatotropic drugs and the artificial liver device (Riegler & Lake, 1993; Sussman et al., 1994; Uchino & Matsushita, 1994).

Normal Liver Function

Located under the right diaphragm, the liver is the largest organ in the body. It is composed of two lobes, the right and left. The hepatic artery branches from the aorta to deliver oxygenated arterial blood to the liver. The portal vein brings venous blood to the liver from the inferior and superior mesenteric veins and splenic vein. Portal vein blood flow makes up approximately 70% of the blood supply to the liver and carries nutrients absorbed from the gastrointestinal tract.

Hepatocytes are the functional cells of the liver. They produce bile, which empties into small channels known as bile canaliculi that eventually drain into the common bile duct. Between the hepatocytes are small capillaries called sinusoids, which receive both arterial and venous blood. Phagocytic cells identified as Kupffer cells line the sinusoids and remove foreign substances from the blood.

The liver performs over 400 functions that can be categorized as vascular, secretory, metabolic, and storage (Guyton, 1986; Keith, 1985). Vascular functions include blood storage and filtration. Phagocytic Kupffer cells actively participate in filtration. Kupffer cells remove pathogens absorbed from the gastrointestinal tract that are delivered to the liver via the portal vein. This mechanism prevents the entry of the pathogens into the systemic circulation, thereby protecting the host. Secretory functions of the liver include production of bile salts, conjugation, and secretion of bilirubin, and the removal of excess cholesterol. Metabolic functions include the metabolism of carbohydrates, protein and fat; detoxification of drugs, hormones, and other substances; synthesis of clotting factors, and the removal of activated clotting factors from the circulation. Storage functions of the liver include primarily the storage of blood, glucose, fat, vitamins (A, B12, D, E, and K) and minerals, iron, and magnesium. Loss of these functions can be devastating and life threatening (see Table 23-38).

Liver Transplant Recipient Selection

Contraindications to liver transplantation vary between centers and often provoke much controversy (see Table 23-39). Generally, contraindications to liver transplantation are divided into two categories: absolute contraindications where transplantation would not be offered, and relative contraindications where the outcome of transplantation would not be expected to be as good if the condition were not present (Lake, 1993) (see Tables 23-38 and 23-39). Absolute contradictions typically include HIV seropositivity, extrahepatic malignancy, inability to comply with the immunosuppressive regimen posttransplant, active substance abuse, advanced cardiac or pulmonary disease

Table 23-38
Manifestations of liver failure.

Manifestation by System	Physiologic Causes for the Manifestation
Constitutional fatigue, malaise, fever, anorexia, weight loss	Progressive hepatic insufficiency, liver failure
Hepatic varies depending of disease (small retracted liver, enlarged cirrhotic liver (e.g., alcoholic cirrhosis)	Fibrotic scarring
Cardiovascular portal hypertension dysrhythmia peripheral edema and mild hypotension increased left ventricular function	distorted hepatic architecture electrolyte imbalances altered hemodynamics hyperdynamic state
Dermatologic spider angiomata stigmata of cirrhosis palmar erythema jaundice xanthomas pruritus	unable to detoxify estrogens reduction in bilirubin excretion increased serum cholesterol increased serum bilirubin
Gastrointestinal abdominal discomfort/pain enlarged abdomen bleeding/hemorrhage nausea/vomiting/diarrhea fetor hepaticus	hepatic swelling ascites; decreased albumin varices uncleared sulfur compounds decreased fat absorption
Hematologic hypoalbuminemia, hypoprothrombinemia anemia leukopenia thrombocytopenia, ecchymoses	impaired protein synthesis decreased RBCs, hypersplenism hypersplenism impaired synthesis of clotting factors
Endocrin hypo/hyperglycemia gynecomastia, testicular atrophy, decreased libido	increased glucocorticoids, decreased glycogen increased estrogens; diuretic therapy
Neurologic behavioral changes, reversed sleep/wake pattern, confusion, coma asterixis	hepatic encephalopathy
Pulmonary dyspnea	elevated diaphragm secondary to ascites
Renal alternation in sodium/water balance hepatorenal syndrome	portal hypertension/ascites hepatic failure, cause unclear

Table 23-39
Indications and contraindications for liver transplantation.

Indications	Contraindications
severe weakness and fatigue intractable ascites variceal hemorrhage encephalopathy recurrent cholangitis intractable pruritus spontaneous bacterial peritonitis metabolic bone disease with fracture intractable coagulopathy (PT > 5 seconds) serum albumin < 2.5 g/dL cholestasis, serum bilirubin > 10 mg/dL hepatorenal syndrome neurotoxicity manifestation of certain metabolic disorders (e.g., glycogen storage disease)	**Absolute Contradictions** • HIV seropositivity extrahepatic malignancy • inability to comply to immunosuppressive regimen • active substance abuse • advanced cardiac or pulmonary disease • active infection • sepsis • documented anatomic anomalies precluding transplantation **Relative Contraindications** • acute renal failure • advanced malnutrition • primary hepatobiliary malignancy • portal vein thrombosis • previous side-to-side or end-to-side portacaval shunt • chronic hepatitis B virus infection (HBsAg+) • chronic hepatitis C virus infection • psychosocial issues • lack of funding

(ejection fraction < 35%, pulmonary artery pressure > 50, FEV1 < 50%, or PO_2 < 55 mmHg without an intrapulmonary shunt), active infection, sepsis, and documented anatomic anomalies precluding transplantation. Relative contraindications include acute renal failure, advanced malnutrition, primary hepatobiliary malignancy, portal vein thrombosis, previous side-to-side or end-to-side portacaval shunt, chronic hepatitis B virus infection ($HBsAg^+$), chronic hepatitis C infection, or severe psychosocial problems (Lake, 1993; Roberts et al., 1989).

Indications for liver transplantation are continually changing as more knowledge is acquired regarding posttransplant outcomes (see Table 23-39). The most common disease indicators for liver transplantation in adults include primary biliary cirrhosis, primary sclerosing cholangitis, and chronic viral hepatitis (Goldstein, 1991). Extrahepatic biliary atresia is the most common disease indication for liver transplantation in children (Rosenthal, Podesta, Sher, & Makowka, 1994). Most of these children have undergone at least one Kasai procedure (hepatic portoenterostomy), which is successful in approximately 30% of all cases (Barkin & Lilly, 1980; Kasai et al., 1975). For children whose Kasai procedure fails, there is an extremely high mortality rate within the first year. Therefore, early referral and transplantation is indicated for this patient population demonstrates the various disease indications for orthotopic liver transplantation (see Table 23-40).

Lake (1993) divides indications for liver transplantation into two categories, disease-severity indicators and quality of life indicators. Disease-severity indicators threaten the patient's short-term survival. However, in many hepatic disorders, prognostic determination can be difficult since the natural history of these disorders is often unclear. With this in mind, disease-severity indicators for chronic liver disease include hepatorenal syndrome, recurrent spontaneous bacterial peritonitis, serum albumin < 2.5 g/dl, prothrombin time > 5 seconds prolonged, and serum bilirubin > 5 mg/dl. One exception is in cholestatic hepatic disease. In these patients, a higher serum bilirubin (> 10 mg/dl) with jaundice is an indication for liver transplant evaluation.

Quality of life indications for liver transplantation are those indicators that alter the patient's quality of life (from their perspective), but may not put the patient at risk of imminent death. Quality of life indicators for liver transplantation include intractable ascites, encephalopathy, bleeding from esophageal or gastric varices, intractable pruritus, metabolic bone disease with fracture, recurrent episodes of biliary sepsis, exanthematous neuropathy, fatigue, and the correction of nonhepatic manifestations of certain metabolic disease (e.g., Crigler-

Table 23-40
Disease indications for liver transplantation.

Cholestatic disorders Primary biliary cirrhosis Secondary biliary cirrhosis Primary sclerosing cholangitis Biliary atresia (extrahepatic & intrahepatic) Familial cholestatic syndromes Alagille's syndrome Byler's syndrome	**Fulminant hepatic failure** Viral hepatitis (A, B, C, delta) Drug induced (e.g., acetaminophen) Toxins (e.g., amanita mushroom) Metabolic (e.g., Wilson's disease, Reye's syndrome, organic acidurias)
Hepatocellular disorders Chronic viral induced liver disease (hepatitis B/delta, C) Chronic drug induced liver disease Alcoholic liver disease Idiopathic autoimmune liver disease Cryptogenic cirrhosis Carol's disease Angiosarcoma	**Metabolic liver disease** Alpha1 antitrypsin deficiency Amyloidosis Wilson's disease Crigler-Najjar syndrome Erythropoietic protoporphyria Urea cycle deficiencies Glycogen storage disease Tyrosinemia Hemochromatosis Hereditary oxalosis Familial hypercholesterolemia Tyrosinemia Galactosemia
Hepatobiliary malignancy Hepatocellular carcinoma Hepatoblastoma	**Miscellaneous** TPN-induced cirrhosis Cystic fibrosis Congenital hepatic fibrosis
Vascular disease Budd-Chiari syndrome Veno-occlusive disease Hepatic vein occlusion	

Najjar syndrome or hereditary primary oxalosis leading toward renal failure). In children with hepatic disease, delayed growth and development or poor nutritional status are considered indicators for liver transplant.

Although the above manifestations are generally well accepted as indicators for liver transplantation, the decision to transplant must be further evaluated regarding the natural history of the disease and exact timing for transplant, when the patient was referred to the transplant center and their severity of illness, donor availability, patient support system, and ability to comply with the posttransplant regimen (Goldstein, 1991; Lake, 1993; Roberts et al., 1989).

Controversies in Liver Transplant Recipient Selection

Currently there are a number of conditions that prompt controversy regarding patient selection for transplantation. These include alcoholic liver disease (ALD), fulminant and chronic hepatitis B or C (may be related to intravenous drug abuse), and hepatocellular carcinoma (Keeffe & Esquivel, 1993). Poor patient outcome is the major concern for patients with malignancies or hepatitis B. However, for the patient with alcoholic liver disease, the issues are much more complex. The main concerns regarding the patient with ALD include the effect of alcohol on other organs, length of sobriety and risk of recidivism, ability to comply with the posttransplant regimen, insurance coverage criteria, and the general belief that families donating may not want the organs of their loved ones to go to a substance-abusing individual with a substance abuse problem (Lake, 1993). In addition, there has been a lack of consensus whether or not to transplant individuals who are infected with the human immunodeficien-

Table 23-41
Liver transplant recipient evaluation.

Complete History and Physical etiology of liver disease associated disorders previous illness and surgeries weight, height, head circumference (pediatrics) medications diet history & nutritional evaluation immunization record (including hepatitis B and Pneumovax) **Routine Lab Tests** complete blood count with differential PT, PTT, platelets electrolytes, calcium, phosphorus, magnesium, BUN, creatinine, uric acid, protein electrophoresis, AST, ALT, GGT, alkaline phosphatase, bilirubin, serum bile acids, glucose, ammonia, amylase, albumin, serum vitamin A, D, E, levels (pediatrics), cholesterol, triglycerides, urinalysis with electrolytes, alpha-fetoprotein antimitochondrial, antithyroid, and antinuclear antibodies, immunoglobulins (IgG, IgM, IgA) iron, iron binding capacity, and saturation, ferritin, pregnancy for age appropriate women **Special Tests for Specific Liver Disorders*** alpha 1-antitrypsin level and phenotype ceruloplasmin alcohol and other substance abuse **Immunologic Tests** blood type (ABO) tissue typing (living-related liver transplant or done at the time of transplant) cross matching (living-related liver transplant)*	**Infectious Disease Evaluation** blood, urine, throat, sputum, stool, & ascites fluid cultures for bacterial, viral, fungal, and parasitic organisms* HIV hepatitis screen A, B, C /delta serologies (CVM, EBV, toxoplasmosis, herpes simplex/zoster, varicella) RPR (syphilis) PPD **Radiologic Procedures** abdominal ultrasound with Doppler of hepatic vessels chest x-ray magnetic resonance imaging (MRI) of the abdomen* computerized tomography (CT) of abdomen* angiography* cholangiography* **Additional Studies*** EKG; cardiac catheterization echocardiogram; liver biopsy endoscopy/colonoscopy; ERCP pulmonary function test; arterial blood gases PAP smear; mammogram **Additional Consults** Anesthesia Transplant Nurse Financial counselor Exercise physiologist/physical therapist Dental* Cardiology (age $\geq$ 45 years)* Gynecology Social Worker: psychosocial evaluation Psychiatrist* Child life services (pediatrics)* **Provide Patient/Family Education Regarding Liver Transplantation** * Routine recipient evaluation varies between patient and transplant center.

cy virus who are without symptoms (Rosenthal, et al., 1994). Since decisions regarding indications, timing, and appropriateness of liver transplantation are complex and often controversial, most programs use a multidisciplinary selection committee to assist in patient selection decisions (Klintmalm & Moore, 1985).

Liver Transplant Recipient Evaluation

The liver transplant recipient evaluation is a multidisciplinary process. The purpose of the evaluation is threefold: (1) confirm the etiology of liver disease, assess disease progression, and determine whether medical therapy is available; (2) verify indications for liver transplantation and the patient's desire for transplantation; and (3) identify any related disorders or contraindications to transplantation. During the evaluation, it is imperative that time is allotted to provide the patient/family with education and support regarding liver trans-

Table 23-42
A review of liver laboratory tests.

Laboratory Tests	Normal Adult Values	Normal Pediatric Values
AST/SGOT	739 U/L	739 U/L
ALT/SGPT	254 U/L	254 U/L
GGT	male 985 U/L female 658 U/L	male 985 U/L female 658 U/L
Alkaline phosphatase	41133 U/L	240530 U/L
Total bilirubin	0.11.2 mg/dL	newborns 1 to 12 mg/dl
Direct bilirubin	0.1 to 0.3 mg/dl	0.1 to 0.3 mg/dl
Indirect bilirubin	0.2 to 0.8	0.2 to 0.8
Prothrombin time	10.5 to 12.5 seconds	
Ammonia	11 to 35 umol/L	

plantation, long-term management, follow-up, and expectations (see Chapter 27).

The recipient evaluation is broadly reviewed in Table 23-41. A complete history and physical is performed with extensive assessment of cardiopulmonary, renal, and nutritional status. Children are also evaluated for their growth and development.

The degree of hepatic complications related to end-stage hepatic failure (ESHF) are also evaluated, including the presence and degree of portal hypertension, ascites, encephalopathy, variceal bleeding, and the number of episodes of cholangitis or spontaneous bacterial peritonitis. Since patients are unable to receive live vaccines after transplant (e.g., measles, mumps, and rubella [MMR]), pretransplant immunizations are particularly important, especially for children. Patients who have negative hepatitis seriologies should receive the hepatitis B immunization series before transplantation. If the hepatitis vaccine is not given pretransplant, it may still be given posttransplant since it is not a live virus. However, with the addition of immunosuppressive therapy, it may be difficult for the individual to produce antibodies in response to the vaccine.

Extensive laboratory testing is performed which, in part, includes ABO blood type, liver function tests (LFTs), amylase, serum albumin, prothrombin time, ammonia, bilirubin and bile acids, serologies for cytomegalovirus (CMV), Epstein-Barr virus (EBV) and herpes, alpha-fetoprotein levels, toxoplasmosis, syphilis (RPR), HIV antibody, and cultures as indicated. These tests and others (see Table 23-42) are used to facilitate a successful match between donor and recipient, screen for malignancy or other disease, assess for the presence of infection, evaluate current liver function and nutritional status, and monitor for viral infections posttransplant.

Evaluation of the hepatic and abdominal vasculature is very important pretransplant. Doppler ultrasonography is performed to assess patency of the portal vein and hepatic artery. It is also helpful to know the size and direction of flow in the portal vein. If the portal vein is not visualized, routine angiography or magnetic resonance angiography often become necessary. Ultrasound is also a helpful screening tool to assess for a potential malignant mass.

Assessment of potential patient compliance, social issues, family support, and economic status are addressed prior to transplantation by the transplant coordinator, social worker, and financial counselor. In certain situations, it may be necessary for the patient to undergo a complete psychologic evaluation by a psychiatrist.

During the evaluation, attempts are made to optimize the patient's clinical status. For example, the administration of fat soluble vitamins in those patients with cholestatic conditions, paracentesis, adjustment in diuretic therapy, or a TIPS procedure is performed for ascites, and the patient's nutritional status is maximized with supplemental feedings. In children, nasogastric tube feedings may be

Figure 23-8
Surgical anatomy for reduced sized liver grafts.
Review of the surgical anatomy that is the basis for reduced-sized grafts including living-related liver transplantation. A. total liver donor, with segments 2 and 3 being isolated for grafting. B. graft with interposition grafts used to extend the vessels. C. anastomosed liver graft with a Roux en Y jejunal limb.

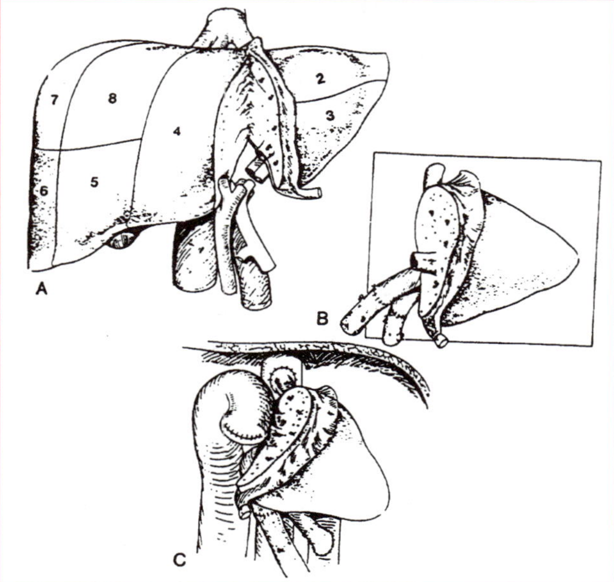

Note: Reprinted with permission from Emond, J. (1993). Clinical application of living-related liver transplantation. In J. Lake (Ed.), Advances in liver transplantation. *Gastroenterology Clinics of North America, 22*(2), 307.

required. Although the evaluation process may be conducted on an outpatient basis, many patients are hospitalized due to the severity of their illness or need for additional testing.

The transplant candidate is presented to a multidisciplinary selection committee after the evaluation is completed. If the committee decides the individual is an acceptable candidate, the patient is activated on the United Network for Organ Sharing (UNOS) transplant list and waits for a donor. Individuals who are stable generally wait for a donor and subsequent transplant as outpatients. These individuals have a higher 1-year survival rate than those who are hospitalized or in intensive care units at the time of transplant (Mora et al., 1992). In addition, other considerations must include the cost incurred due to extended hospitalization, higher cost of transplant, and the greater risk for operative blood loss. Therefore, early referral and evaluation by a liver transplant team is highly recommended.

Patients are listed for transplant based on their clinical status established by the United Network for Organ Sharing (UNOS). The transplant candidate is listed by priority based on blood type, size, and illness severity. Currently, listing criteria for liver transplantation is undergoing reevaluation.

The liver transplant evaluation process is often a very difficult time for many individuals and their families. It is stressful both physically and psychologically and often requires supportive and educational intervention. The type of support and education may vary depending on whether the individual has had a long history of hepatic illness or presents with fulminant hepatic failure. Liver transplant may be viewed as a therapeutic intervention to restore quality of life or diminish it, depending on the circumstances. It is important that the nurse be sensitive to these issues and direct care appropriately.

Liver Transplant Surgical Procedure

Liver transplant donor recovery is generally a very straightforward procedure. Evaluation of a potential cadaveric liver donor is based on the donor's medical/surgical history, type of injury, hospital course and laboratory/serologic results. Donor livers are matched to potential recipients based on blood type and body size. Although it is preferred that the donor and recipient are the same blood type, in cases of urgent need, ABO-incompatible donors have been used (Gordon et al., 1987; Roberts et al., 1989). Donor and recipient weights within 20% of one another are generally considered a likely match (Rosenthal et al., 1994; Shaw & Wood, 1988). If the donor liver is too large, it can result in pulmonary compromise, and if it is too small, there may be hepatic insufficiency or a mismatch in vessel size leading to stenosis or thrombosis. However, with the advancement of surgical techniques in liver transplantation, this is not such a limiting factor as it has been in the past. With the advent of the paired or reduced size graft, the surgeon is increasingly able to accommodate for variation in donor size. General principles for hepatic donor procurement are to ensure stability of the donor's physiologic condition, avoid prolonged warm ischemic time, and rapidly remove the organs in the sequence agreed upon by other transplant teams involved (Shaw & Wood, 1988).

Surgical removal of the donor liver is performed through a midline incision. The major vessels around the liver are dissected, including the celiac truck and branches, portal vein, and the inferior vena cava. The bile duct is transected with attempts to maintain maximum length of the duct for the recipient transplant operation. Cool saline is flushed into the biliary tree via the gallbladder to remove stagnate bile and protect the biliary mucosa. The liver is then flushed in situ with cool heparinized lactated Ringer's solution to remove old blood, and then with University of Wisconsin (UW) solution for preservation. The suprahepatic

Table 23-43
Living-related liver transplant donor evaluation.

Complete History and Physical (performed by an MD not related to the transplant service)
previous illness and surgeries
medications

Autologous Blood Donation (2 units)

Routine Lab Tests
complete blood count with differential
PT, PTT, platelets
electrolytes, calcium, phosphorus, magnesium, BUN, creatinine, uric acid, AST, ALT, GGT, alkaline phosphatase, bilirubin, glucose, ammonia, amylase, albumin, total protein, cholesterol, triglycerides, urinalysis with electrolytes, pregnancy for age appropriate women

Special Tests for Specific Liver Disorders
ceruloplasmin
alphafetoprotein *
iron, iron binding capacity, and saturation, ferritin

Immunologic Tests
blood type (ABO)
tissue typing *
cross matching *

Infectious Disease Evaluation
cultures *
urinalysis with micro
HIV
hepatitis screen A, B, C /delta
serologies (CVM, EBV, toxoplasmosis, herpes simplex/zoster, varicella)
RPR

Radiologic Procedures
chest x-ray
CT of abdomen
hepatic angiography

Additional Studies
EKG
liver biopsy*
pulmonary function test
arterial blood gases *

Additional Consults

Anesthesia	Transplant Nurse
Financial counselor	Exercise physiologist/physical therapist
Dental*	Cardiology*
Pulmonary*	Gynecology *
Social Worker	Psychiatrist*

Provide Patient/Family Education Regarding Living-Related Liver Transplantation

* Routine recipient evaluation varies between patient and transplant center.

cava is transected at the right atrium and the infrahepatic cava just above the renal veins, thus preserving them for possible kidney transplantation. The portal vein is divided at the confluence of the splenic vein and superior mesenteric vein; the abdominal aorta and hepatic artery are excised, preserving the hepatic arterial supply. The liver is packed in UW solution, stored on ice, and transported to the transplant center (Ascher et al., 1984; Smith & Ciferni, 1990; Stock & Payne, 1990).

Reduced-sized grafts have been used to expand the donor pool, primarily for pediatric patients (see Figure 23-8). This surgical technique was initiated in response to the decline in donors for infants and young children less than 2 years old. Children in this age group are generally those in need of liver transplantation, while most available donors for young children are either school-aged children or adolescents who have been victims of automobile accidents (Rosenthal et al., 1994). Since size disparity in this young patient population may prevent transplantation of a whole liver graft, a section of the donor organ may be sufficient. Generally, the left lateral lobe (segments 2 and 3) is used with fairly good results (Broelsch et al., 1988; Broelsch et al., 1990; Emond et al., 1989).

Split liver transplantation is a technique whereby the cadaver donor liver is split between two recipients. This procedure is substantially more complex than a reduced-size graft. It requires two surgical teams, and allocation of structures is often not equal. It also raises the ethical question of organ sharing between children and adults (Emond et al., 1991).

Living-related liver transplantation (LRLTx) evolved from the techniques applied during the reduced-size graft procedure. LRLTx is the donation of the left lateral liver segment by a living-related donor. Initially the primary concern regarding this procedure was the ethical dilemma of placing a healthy donor at risk. However, with increasing experience, LRLTx has now become a well accepted approach to liver transplantation particularly for children (Broelsch et al., 1991; Emond, 1993; Tanaka et al., 1992). Results have been encouraging, and donors have survived without significant complications. Recipient complications and graft function have been comparable to cadaveric liver transplantation, and anecdotally there may be a slightly lower incidence of rejection in recipients (Emond, 1993; Heffron, 1993).

The living-related donor evaluation is performed after informed consent. The specifics of the donor evaluation are outlined in Table 23-43. Computerized tomography (CT) scanning is used to determine donor liver volume and the adequacy of the potential graft. Hepatic arteriography is used to evaluate the anatomy and size of the donor hepatic vasculature in anticipation of the anatamoses during transplantation. The recipient evaluation is the same as for a cadaveric liver transplant.

Living-unrelated liver transplant donors may be a viable option in the future. However, currently, only immediate (parents) and extended family members (aunts, uncles, grandparents) have been living liver donors.

Auxiliary liver transplantation is a surgical procedure in which the liver graft is implanted without removing the native liver. It was originally introduced in 1972 to avoid the morbidity and mortality in total hepatectomy patients (Emond, 1993; Starzl et al., 1989). Although this approach is rarely used, it may have a place in the future, particularly for those individuals with metabolic disorders or fulminant hepatic biliary secondary to toxic ingestion (e.g., acetaminophen).

Combined liver-kidney transplantation has been performed in patients with end-stage hepatorenal disease and hepatorenal syndrome. Primary causes of renal failure have included primary hyperoxaluria, diabetic nephropathy, glomerulonephritis, congenital pyelonephritis, and polycystic disease (Shaked et al., 1993; Taylor et al., 1991). Survival rates of combined liver-kidney transplantation are comparable to the survival rates of liver transplantation alone (Saidman et al., 1994). The surgical procedure is the same for single organ transplantation. In a combined transplant, the liver transplant surgery is performed before the kidney transplant. A pretransplant negative crossmatch is considered optimum, but not mandatory, and it is thought that the liver may protect the kidney from hyperacute rejection (Saidman et al., 1994). Postoperative management is the same for individual liver-kidney transplantation.

Recipient hepatectomy and transplant are performed after the placement of multiple invasive lines. The recipient hepatectomy involves clamping the infrahepatic and suprahepatic inferior vena cava and dividing the portal vein. Venous return from the inferior vena cava is thus momentarily interrupted, and the outflow from the infrahepatic inferior vena cava and portal vein is occluded. Decreased venous blood flow can lead to engorgement of all subdiaphragmatic vessels causing an increase in portal hypertension and bowel congestion. Therefore, it is important to keep the time frame of the anahepatic phase to a minimum (optimally less than 30 minutes). Some centers use a venovenous bypass system to minimize the risks during the anahepatic phase (Griffith et al., 1985), while other centers do not use this procedure because of the risk of air embolism (Khoury et al., 1987).

Once the recipient's hepatectomy has been completed and homeostasis achieved, the donor liver anastomoses are initiated. There are five major anastomoses that are generally completed in the following order: suprahepatic inferior vena cava, infraheptatic inferior vena cava, portal vein, hepatic artery, and biliary anastomosis. After the portal vein anastomosis is completed, the liver is reperfused. The liver is rewarmed, and the hyperkalemic preservation solution is vented through the anterior infrahepatic caval anastomosis. Stagnant splanchnic blood is also flushed. The repercussion phase has been associated with electrolyte imbalances and coagulopathies (Stock & Payne, 1990).

There are two basic approaches to biliary reconstruction: a choledochocholecostomy or choledochojejunostomy. A choledochocholecostomy is an end-to-end anastomosis of the recipient and donor common bile ducts and is used whenever possible (see Figure 23-9). In the presence of biliary disease or a biliary duct-to-duct mismatch, a choledochojejunostomy is performed. This is an anastomosis of the donor bile duct to the recipient's jejunum, also referred to as a Roux en Y (see Figure 23-10).

Liver Transplant Postoperative Management and Nursing Care

The postoperative care of the liver transplant recipient is highly complex. It requires a multidisciplinary approach and collaboration among team members. Close monitoring and frequent assessment are imperative. Recipients and their families often need additional support during the initial posttransplant period.

Early postoperative care is similar to any major abdominal surgery with the addition of close monitoring of the graft, hemodynamics, pulmonary status, and renal function. Immediately posttransplant, laboratory studies are drawn at frequent intervals to assess the patient's clinical status and the function of the graft. A coagulation profile is the most sensitive indicator of graft function and includes a prothrombin time (PT), partial thromboplastin time (PTT), thrombin time (TT), factor V and VIII levels, and fibrinogen levels. Additional routine posttransplant blood work includes a complete blood count with differential, platelets, liver

Figure 23-9
A choledochocholedochostomy.

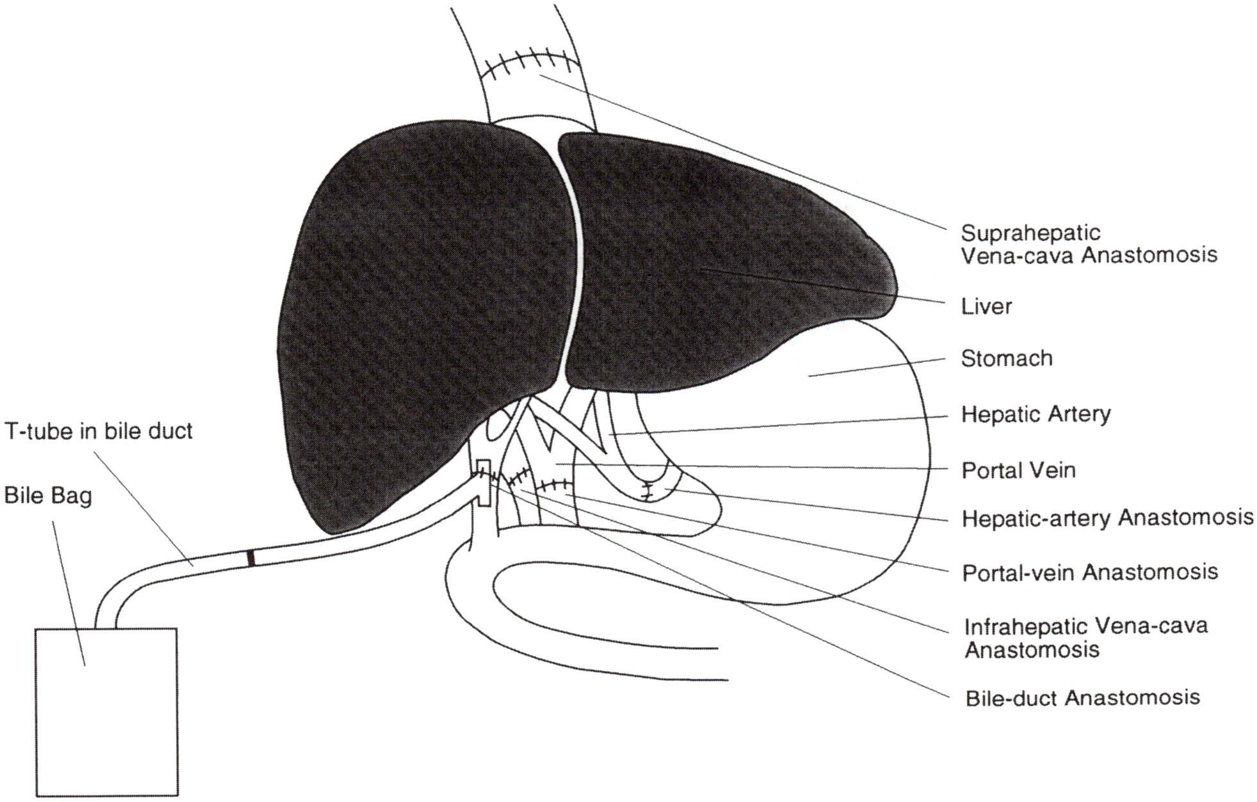

Choledochocholedochostomy

Duct-to-Duct Biliary Anastomosis

function tests (LFTs), electrolytes, calcium, phosphorus, magnesium, blood urea nitrogen (BUN), serum creatinine, urinary creatinine clearance, and arterial blood gases.

Ongoing assessment of graft function is monitored by the production of clotting factors, lactate levels, mental status, and bile production and flow (monitor hourly output if there is a T-tube). If the graft is functioning properly, the prothrombin time and serum lactate should normalize within several hours postoperatively. Elevated lactate levels suggest poor graft function. Frequent mental status evaluations can also be a helpful indicator regarding the liver's ability to clear anesthetic agents and remove toxins associated with hepatic encephalopathy. Therefore, judicious use of narcotic administration should be taken. Fortunately, pain associated with liver transplantation is mild and generally well tolerated, even in children.

Bile production is an indicator of the liver's excretory function and can be measured in patients who have a T-tube. The bile should be thick and range from dark golden yellow to brown. Meticulous care should be taken to keep the T-tube site clean to prevent the risk of ascending cholangitis. T-tube cholangiograms are used to assess the status of the biliary tree and are a common procedure posttransplant. Antibiotics are administered before the procedure to prevent the risk of cholangitis and sepsis. Depending on the patient's clinical status, T-tubes can remain in place up to 6 months posttransplant. Therefore, patients are taught how to care for their T-tube at home.

Within 24 to 48 hours hepatic function can be gauged more closely by alterations in bilirubin, transaminases (AST, ALT) and alkaline phosphatase levels (see Table 23-42). Elevations are generally suggestive of changes in hepatic function. However, low transaminases and prolonged coagulation studies suggest lack of hepatocyte function. This is an ominous sign that generally requires retransplantation. To rule out hepatic vessel thrombosis as a cause of hepatic dysfunction, ultrasonography is performed intraoperatively, on posttrans-

Figure 23-10
A choledochojejunostomy.

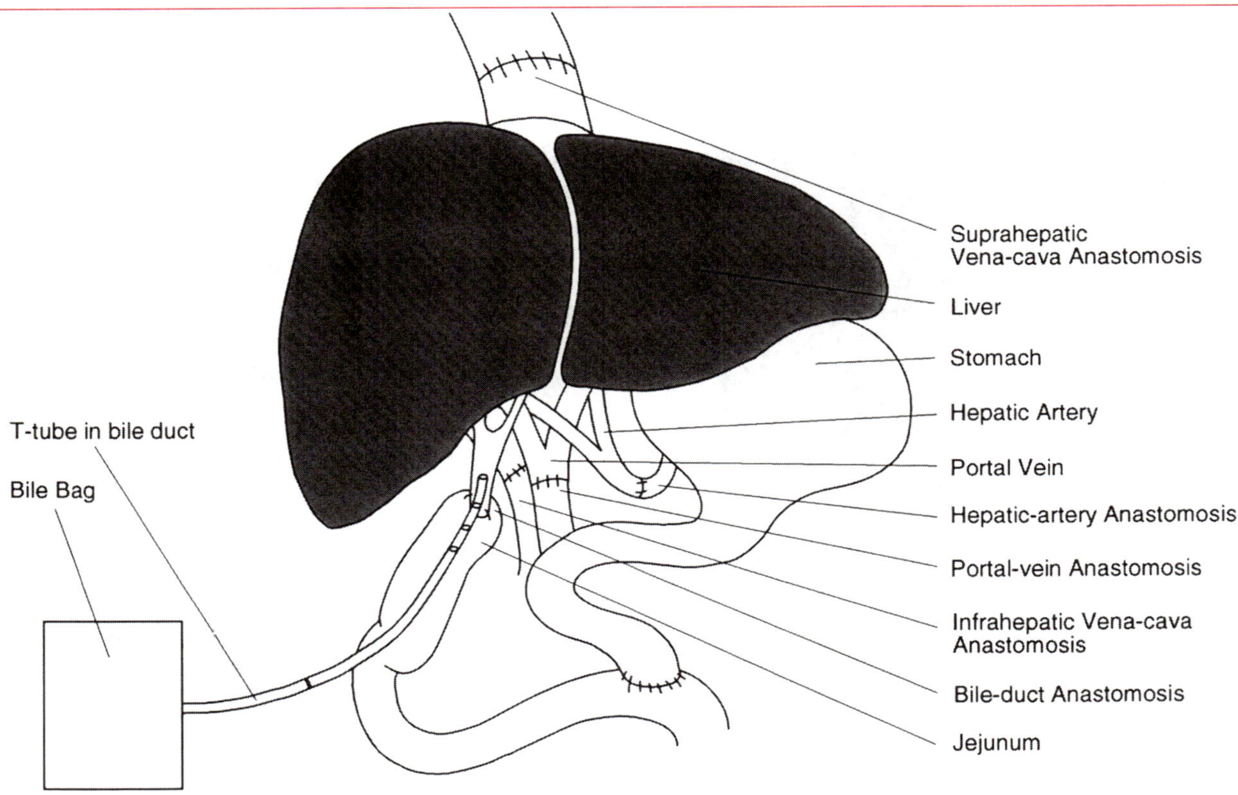

Choledochojejunostomy (Roux "en" Y)

plant day 1, and whenever thrombosis is suspected to confirm vessel patency.

Liver graft function can be further evaluated with a percutaneous biopsy and by radionuclide excretory cholangiography. A liver biopsy can assist in making the differential diagnosis between rejection, infection, ischemia, cholangitis, and obstruction. Biopsy is the gold standard for confirming rejection.

Cholangiography can also assist in clarifying problems associated with graft function. A delay in uptake of the radioisotope can indicate preservation injury, vascular compromise, or rejection of the graft. Delayed excretion by the radioisotope into the biliary system may indicate rejection, ischemia, or infection. Delayed excretion into in the small bowel generally suggests obstruction or deterioration of the biliary anastomosis (Stock & Payne, 1990).

Intraoperative volume and preexisting portal hypertension cause the recipient to normally present with a normal-high cardiac output, normal-low systemic vascular resistance, and an increased preload in the early posttransplant period. Cardiac function is optimized with inotropic support such as low-dose dopamine, and if necessary with preload/afterload reducing drugs such as nitroprusside. A number of recipients develop hypertension postoperatively, which may be related to volume, catecholamines, or a side effect of cyclosporine. Calcium channel blockers such as nifedipine are a very effective first line therapy.

Due to the large volumes of fluid and blood given intraoperatively and the liberal use of furosemide diuresis, hypokalemic metabolic alkalosis is a common problem following liver transplantation (Stock & Payne, 1990). Hypokalemic metabolic alkalosis develops secondary to the citrate in the administered blood products that converts to bicarbonate, and as a result of furosemide diuretic therapy causing renal potassium losses. Occasionally it is necessary to initiate a hydrochloric acid drip to maintain blood pH levels.

Recipients are usually intubated and supported with mechanical ventilation on entry to the intensive care unit. Most patients need pulmonary support for 24 to 48 hours posttransplant. In part, this is due to the increased extravascular fluid volume, which causes a reduction in left ventricular compliance that results in respiratory compromise. Damage to the phrenic nerve causing a right hemidiaphragm may also contribute to the need for mechanical ventilation (Smith & Cifernik 1990). In addition, those patients with a metabolic alkalosis may be difficult to wean from the ventilator because of a reduction in spontaneous respirations. It is worthy to note that patients are often not extubated based on pCO_2, but rather pH and oxygenation. It is important to frequently assess breath sounds and arterial blood gases, suction as needed, provide frequent pulmonary toiletry, encourage early mobilization to minimize respiratory compromise, and monitor chest radiography studies to facilitate extubation. Daily chest radiography is performed on daily unstable posttransplant patients and then as clinically indicated.

Renal function is closely monitored. Indicators of renal function are urine output and electrolytes, creatinine clearance, serum creatinine and electrolytes, and blood urea nitrogen (BUN). During the operative procedure, the kidneys sustain a transient insult and must be evaluated often to assure adequate function. In addition, cyclosporine can be renal toxic, further mandating close renal monitoring and frequent assessment of cyclosporine levels. Occasionally, recipients will need renal replacement therapy (RRT) during the initial postoperative period (see Chapters 20 & 22). However, RRT is generally reserved for those patients who had renal insufficiency pretransplant, such as hepatorenal syndrome (Gonwa et al., 1991).

The risk of a stress ulcer is minimized by frequent assessment of the nasogastric tube aspirate for gastric pH and blood, and with the administration of H_2 blockers (e.g., ranitidine) or antacids (e.g., sucralfate). Bowel sounds are checked routinely, and early mobilization is encouraged to minimize the risk of an ileus. Once bowel function has returned, the nasogastric tube is removed, and the recipient can progress to a regular diet. If the patient is unable to consume adequate calories, supplemental feedings or intravenous hyperalimentation are initiated, depending on the patient's clinical status.

Immunosuppresssive protocols vary between transplant centers and physicians. However, most centers use a combination of the following agents for induction therapy: antithymic globulin (ATG), OKT3, prednisone, azathioprine, cyclosporine, tacrolimus (Prograf®) and Cellcept®. Rejection is typically treated with prednisone, solumedrol, tacrolimus, ATG, or OKT3. Antibiotics, antivirals, and antifungals are also administered posttransplant to prevent the risk of infection (see Chapter 12).

Liver Transplant Complications

Bleeding may develop the first few days postoperatively as a result of coagulopathies, a collapse of one of the anastomoses, or stress ulcers. Coagulopathies develop secondary to preexisting splenomegaly with pancytopenia, the volume of blood required during the transplant, initial hepatic dysfunction due to ischemia, or graft failure. Coagulopathies are managed with a continuous infusion of fresh frozen plasma (1 to 2 cc/Kg/hour), platelet administration to maintain counts greater than 50,000/l, and cryoprecipitated plasma. Posttransplant hemorrhage is demonstrated by a decreasing hematocrit, labile blood pressure and increased heart rate, intravascular contraction despite fluid resuscitation, and a consistent increase in intraperitoneal pressure assessed by frequently measuring the abdominal girth. Reexploration for possible hemorrhage is generally performed in patients who present with normal coagulation parameters and compromised renal or pulmonary function (Stock & Payne, 1990).

Vascular complications following liver transplantation include hepatic artery thrombosis, portal vein thrombosis, and hepatic vein thrombosis. Hepatic artery thrombosis is the most common vascular complication posttransplant (Langnas et al., 1991). In children weighing less than 10 Kg, the small size of the hepatic artery augments the risk of thrombosis and occurs in approximately 10% of these children (Podesta et al., 1993). The clinical presentation of hepatic artery thrombosis depends on the length of time from transplantation to thrombosis (Wiesner et al., 1993). If hepatic artery thrombosis develops early after transplantation, it generally presents with acute hepatic infarct manifested by severe coagulopathy, hemodynamic instability, encephalopathy, hypoglycemic, hyperkalemia, renal impairment, and subsequent liver failure. It is a presentation similar to primary nonfunction. Treatment generally requires prompt retransplantation to prevent imminent death. Occasionally, prompt surgical intervention with declotting and repair of the hepatic artery can save the graft if performed within 24 to 48 of transplantation (Sayage et al., 1989). Thus in many centers, protocol Doppler hepatic ultrasonography has become a common practice within 24 hours posttransplantation and whenever there is a question of hepatic vessel thrombosis.

If hepatic artery thrombosis occurs between 2 weeks and 2 months after transplantation, ischemic necrosis of the bile ducts eventually develops and can cause biliary tree strictures and obstruction with recurrent cholangitis, bile leaks, hepatic abscesses, and sepsis. Diagnosis can be made with Doppler ultrasound. However, hepatic angiography provides a more definitive diagnosis. Treatment often results in retransplantation.

Portal vein thrombosis is the second most common vascular complication after liver transplant. Contributing risk factors for portal vein thrombosis include a preexisting recannulized portal vein thrombosis, previous portacaval shunt, and an interposition vascular graft in the formation of the portal vein anastomosis (Lerut et al., 1987). Clinical presentation is insidious and may include increasing ascites or portal hypertension with variceal bleeding. Diagnosis is based on hepatic ultrasonography or angiography. If the diagnosis is made promptly, early surgical evacuation of the clot and reanastamosis with postoperative anticoagulation therapy may be successful. Treatment may require decompression of the splanchnic system through a splenorenal shunt or retransplantation.

Recurrent hepatic vein thrombosis (Budd-Chiari syndrome) may be successfully managed with anticoagulation after liver transplantation. Caution must be taken to monitor for the risk of bleeding (Wiesner et al., 1993).

Pulmonary complications seen frequently in the early postoperative liver transplant recipient include atelectasis and a right pleural effusion. These problems result in poor ventilation and oxygenation, increasing the risk of pneumonia. Pulmonary complications are attributed to prolonged anesthesia, paralysis of the right diaphragm, ascites, a graft larger than the native liver pressing against the diaphragm, and pain. In addition, metabolic alkalosis and ascites can also interfere with proper ventilation and should be corrected. Vigorous pulmonary toilet, pain management, and early mobilization assist in reversing the effects of a pleural effusion and atelectasis, thus preventing pneumonia.

Renal insufficiency is observed both pretransplant and posttransplant. Pretransplant renal insufficiency is often secondary to hepatorenal syndrome (HRS). These patients generally have the same long-term prognosis as those patients without HRS (Gonwa et al., 1991). Posttransplant renal insufficiency may be due to massive hemorrhage and hypotension, hypovolemia, infection, cyclosporine, antibiotic therapy, or graft failure. Resuscitation with fluid, calculating appropriate antibiotic doses, and reducing intraabdominal pressure through paracentesis can increase renal perfusion, thus preserving renal function.

Primary nonfunction (PNF) is graft failure. It is clinically manifested by lack of bile flow, prolonged coagulation factors, hyperkalemia, and hypoglycemia. In the presence of PNF, there will be an initial elevation in serum transaminases followed by a dramatic decrease and coinciding prolonged coagulation studies. These findings suggest hepatocyte death. Retransplantation is generally necessary for patient survival.

Hepatic allograft rejection has been classified by histologic features, timing, response to therapy, and reversibility (Wiesner et al., 1991). The correlation between the histologic severity of rejection and the degree of biochemical hepatic dysfunction has been poor. Therefore, liver biopsy and histology remain the gold standard for diagnosing alteration in hepatic graft function (Wiesner et al., 1992). In addition, hepatic histology allows rejection to be easily differentiated from viral hepatitis, bile duct obstruction, and other causes of hepatic dysfunction. The major targets of hepatic allograft rejection are the epithelial cells of the bile ducts and the endothelium of the hepatic arteries and veins. The hepatocytes appear to be less vulnerable.

Hyperacute rejection occurs immediately posttransplant and is the result of host preformed antibodies. It is well documented in kidney transplantation and only recently in liver transplantation (Snover, 1993). Histologic findings of hyperacute liver transplant rejection include arteritis, irreversible ischemic damage and thrombosis, and neutrophilic portal infiltrate (Hanto et al., 1987; Snover, 1990). There are three important factors that may be responsible for protecting the liver from hyperacute rejection in liver transplantation. First, the significant "washout" of native antibodies during the operative procedure from blood loss and transfusions. Second, the large reserve capacity of the liver. Third, the sinusoidal structure of the liver, which may protect it from the effects of thrombosis (Hanto et al., 1987; Snover, 1990). Hyperacute rejection after liver transplant can be life threatening. The treatment almost always requires retransplantation.

Acute rejection is generally a cell-mediated process that usually develops within 1 to 6 weeks postoperatively. The incidence of acute cellular rejection after liver transplantation is approximately 50-60% (Wiesner et al., 1991; Wiesner et al., 1993). Clinical manifestations of acute cellular rejection may include fever, malaise, fatigue, a T-tube cessation of bile flow, or a change in bile color from golden yellow or green to colorless fluid. Laboratory manifestations include an elevation in transaminases (AST, ALT, GGT), alkaline phosphatase, and in some situations, total bilirubin. Histologic findings of acute hepatic rejection are portal or periportal inflammation, bile duct damage, and venous endotheliitis (Snover, 1990). Although rejection is treated differently among transplant centers, acute rejection is generally treated with high-dose intravenous corticosteroids. Those patients who experience steroid-resistant rejection are subsequently treated with the murine monoclonal antibody (OKT3®) or tacrolimus (Prograf®).

Chronic rejection after liver transplantation is primarily a cell-mediated response that occurs in approximately 8% of patients (Wiesner et al., 1991). It is often diagnosed 6 weeks or more after liver transplant (Wiesner et al., 1993). It is defined as obliterative endarteritis with ischemic damage that may be accompanied by fibrosis, cirrhosis, and paucity of bile ducts (vanishing bile duct syndrome) with cholestasis (Snover, 1990; Wiesner et al., 1992). Vanishing bile duct syndrome (VBDS) is characterized by loss of bile ducts in the absence of vascular rejection (Ludwig et al., 1987; Snover, 1990). Tacrolimus (Prograf®) has been used as rescue therapy for patients with chronic rejection and VBDS with a relatively favorable response (European FK506, 1994; Klintmalm et al., 1993; McDiarmid et al., 1991; McDiarmid et al., 1993; Roberts et al., 1993). Those patients who fail to respond to medical therapy typically require retransplantation.

Acute rejection typically develops early after transplant and chronic rejection later. However, features of chronic rejection can develop early while features of acute rejection present late. Therefore, the differentiation between chronic and acute rejection is based primarily on histologic findings.

Infection is a common problem after liver transplant. Immunosuppressive therapy and a compromised chronically ill host are contributing factors to infection posttransplant. Transplant recipients are vulnerable to common pathogens as well as opportunistic organisms such as *Candida albicans, Aspergillus,* and *Pneumocystis carinii.* Therefore, most centers prescribe prophylactic antibiotics to prevent and minimize the risk of infection postoperatively. Early postliver transplant recipients are at particular risk for developing bacterial pneumonia or abdominal abscess, and fungal infections with *Candida* and *Aspergillus* being the major pathogens. Viral infections can present anytime but more frequently present 4 to 6 weeks posttransplant (Rubin, 1990). Common viral pathogens that present around this time are the herpes viruses and cytomegalovirus virus (CMV). Herpes is managed with acyclovir, gancyclovir and CMV with gancyclovir.

Epstein-Barr virus (EBV) infection can present anytime posttransplant. It may be asymptomatic, cause infectious mononucleosis syndrome, or result in EBV-mediated lymphoproliferative disease (LPD). Patients with LPD often present with fever, lymphadenopathy, tonsillitis or tonsillar enlargement, splenomegaly, upper respiratory congestion/distress, or abdominal pain (Ho et al., 1988). Diagnosis is confirmed by EBV serology and biopsies. The incidence of EBV-mediated LPD is higher in children than adults because they are more likely to be seronegative for EBV pretransplant and acquire primary infection. Current treatment includes reduction or withdrawal of immunosuppression, intravenous acyclovir or gancyclovir, and if possible, tumor resection or excision (Rosenthal et al., 1994).

Biliary complications after liver transplantation include bile leaks, strictures, and obstruction secondary to stones or biliary sludging caused by the shedding of the epithelial lining of the donor bile duct. Biliary leaks usually occur at the anastomosis within the first 3 weeks posttransplant. If a T-tube is in place the leak can generally be treated by opening the T-tube to drainage. In addition, T-tube removal can result in bile leaks and occurs in approximately 10%-15% of patients (Wiesner et al., 1993).

Bile leaks are often accompanied by peritoneal signs, acute abdominal pain, and fever. Patients who have persistent symptoms within 24 to 48 hours after the T-tube is open, or for those patients without a T-tube, insertion of a nasobiliary tube for 3 to 7 days to drain the biliary tree generally results in resolution of the problem. These patients always receive antibiotic therapy to prevent the risk of infection and abscess. Since the hepatic artery delivers blood to the biliary system, it is important to mention that with all biliary leaks, hepatic artery thrombosis must be ruled out as a potential cause. Doppler ultrasound of the hepatic artery or hepatic angiography can be used to determine hepatic artery patency.

Non-anastomotic strictures can involve both the intrahepatic and extrahepatic biliary tree. They appear to develop in approximately 20% of patients usually 1 to 4 months after transplant (Wiesner et al., 1993). Non-anastomotic strictures have been associated with prolonged donor ischemic time of greater than 12 hours, ABO incompatibility, hepatic artery thrombosis, and ductopenic rejection (Gugenheim, 1990; Sanchez-Urdazpal et al., 1992; Wiesner et al., 1993). These strictures are usually treated with balloon dilatation and stenting either through endoscopy or a transhepatic approach. Although this is generally a successful treatment, it is not uncommon that these patients subsequently require retransplantation, particularly in situations where there are strictures secondary to hepatic artery thrombosis or biliary necrosis. In addition, nonanastomotic strictures that develop within 1 month of transplant have become a predictor of poor graft survival (Langnas et al., 1992).

Hypertension is a common problem posttransplant and is usually related to cyclosporine-based immunosuppression. Treatment is usually initiated with calcium channel blockers, progressing to ß-blockers and finally ACE inhibitors.

Metabolic complications after liver transplant can occur early or late postoperatively. Hyperglycemia is a common complication early posttransplant secondary to high-dose corticosteroids, causing an increase in glucose released from the liver. Cyclosporine and tacrolimus (Prograf®) also contribute to hyperglycemic states. These patients often need initial insulin therapy. However, as the high dose of corticosteroids are tapered, most patients will no longer require insulin.

Hyperlipidemia does occur in postliver transplant recipients. However, the long-term effects on cardiovascular events remains unclear. The cause of hyperlipidemia is multifactorial including high-dose corticosteroids, excessive weight gain, genetic susceptibility, diuretics, and ß adrenergic blockers used to treat hypertension. Treatment involves avoidance of caffeine and alcohol because they tend to increase triglyceride and cholesterol levels, weight control, smoking cessation, and regular exercise. In addition to lifestyle changes, attempts should be made to reduce corticosteroid therapy. If these measures fail, agents that lower serum cholesterol, triglycerides, and low density lipoprotein (LDL) cholesterol levels, such as Lovastatin®, should be instituted.

Hyperuricemia is a common complication for patients receiving cyclosporine A, particularly in those individuals treated with diuretic therapy for hypertension. Patients who develop gout should be treated with colchicine rather than allopurinol, since allopurinol may increase the bone marrow toxic effects of azathioprine.

Metabolic bone disease in the form of osteoporosis and compression fractures are commonly observed in patients with cholestatic forms of hepatic disease such as primary biliary cirrhosis or sclerosing cholangitis. Bone disease is particularly common in patients on prolonged high dose corticosteroids. There is no effective therapy to prevent bone disease posttransplant. However, it has been recommended that early mobilization, regular exercise, calcium supplementation, etidronate (Didronel®), 25-hydroxy-vitamin and vitamin D therapy to maintain D serum levels may reduce bone loss after transplant (Garrel et al., 1988; Horber et al., 1985; Painter & Blackburn, 1988; Wiesner et al., 1993).

Recurrent disease is a major problem for patients with viral hepatitis or hepatic malignancies. In addition, patients with primary biliary cirrhosis and primary sclerosing cholangitis have also been observed to develop recurrent disease, but rarely have significant clinical problems (Dietze et al., 1990; Wiesner et al., 1993).

The incidence of recurrent disease in patients with hepatitis B pretransplant is approximately 85%-95%. Individuals at highest risk are those who are hepatitis E antigen positive or demonstrate high serum levels of hepatitis B virus DNA, which is an indicator of high level viral replication (Davis et al., 1991; O'Grady, 1992).

Individuals with hepatitis C pretransplant have been shown to have a 95% incidence of recurrent disease, and 35% of patients who do not have evidence of hepatitis C pretransplant develop hepatitis C viremia posttransplant. Approximately half of these patients go on to develop chronic active hepatitis observed on liver histology (Wiesner et al., 1993; Wright et al., 1992). Although there is a high incidence of recurrent hepatitis C infection in patients undergoing liver transplantation, the long-term impact on graft survival remains unclear.

Most individuals with biliary cancer pretransplant develop recurrent disease within 1 year of liver transplantation (Ringe et al., 1989).

Summary

The major challenges facing the future of transplantation are graft rejection, the shortage of donor organs, and further management of incurred costs (Jakobsen, 1994). The pragmatic approach to these problems involves building on current research toward isolating a solution. Several new areas of research seem promising. For example, work is underway to develop highly specific immunosuppressive medications that target particular aspects of the immune response and have fewer significant negative side effects (Bumgardner & Roberts, 1993). Progress has been made in modifying the immune response to achieve greater tolerance through gene transfer methods and chimerism (Caldwell, 1992; Starzl et al., 1992). Finally, we have been successful in expanding the donor pool either through xenotransplantation and split grafts or by increasing the options for living-related and nonrelated transplantation (Berloco et al., 1993; Kocoshis et al., 1993). However, particularly in this last instance, we have reason to question whether pursuing a pragmatic approach is sufficient.

Significant progress in augmenting the number of transplants performed has not been achieved despite incredible effort in the past 10 years. These efforts have been devoted to (1) increasing organ donation through education and outreach programs, especially targeted at minority communities, or (2) maximizing the number of organs recovered and minimizing organ waste. Such lack of progress suggests that we may need to shift our focus from expanding current treatments to pursuing more visionary approaches.

Some problems, like suitable distribution and acquisition of resources, are linked to broader issues of social justice over which the medical community has little direct control. Other problems, like organ rejection, may result from restricting our focus too exclusively to the human body and human condition. Perhaps instead of attempting to alter the body's natural response to foreign antigens, we should devise something that the body would not experience as foreign if transplanted into it, like an artificial allograft that simulates the native organ and thus does not cause rejection. To pursue such projects obviously requires the expertise and interaction among several communities: medical, technologic, political, and humanitarian. This means that the medical community must be realistic about the boundaries of our expertise while remaining visionary about what we are working to achieve.

In addition, consideration must be made

regarding who is going to pay for organ transplantation in the future. Currently, over 90% of renal transplants are paid by Medicare, and the question must be raised as to whether the federal government will continue to cover these costs (Eggers, 1988). Innovative approaches to health care, particularly with regard to cost, must be investigated and pursued if organ transplantation is to survive as a treatment option in the years to follow.

References and Readings

Abendroth, D., Landgraff, R., Illner, W.D., & Land, W. (1989). Evidence for reversibility of diabetic microangiopathy following pancreas transplantation. *Transplant Proceedings, 21,* 2850-2851.

Agashi, T., Takahashi, K., Ota, K., & Yagisawa, T. (1992). Comparative evaluation of immunoabsorption and double filtration plasmapheresis for removal of anti-A or B antibody in ABO incompatible kidney transplantation. *Transplant Proceedings, 24,* 557-558.

Ahonen, J. (1987). Kidney transplantation: Wound complications. In L. H. Toledo-Pereyra (Ed.), *Complications of organ transplantation* (pp. 7180). New York: Marcel & Dekker.

Amend, W.J.C., Vincenti, F., Feduska, N., Salvatierra, O., Johnson, W.H., Jackson, J., Tilney, N., Garovoy, M., & Burwell, L. (1987). Recurrence of systemic lupus erythematosus involving renal allografts. *Annals of Internal Medicine, 106,* 444-449.

American Academy of Pediatrics. (1991). *Red book.* Elk Grove Village, IL: Author.

American Diabetes Association. (1987). *Diabetes: Facts you need to know.* Washington, DC: Author.

American Society of Transplant Physicians. (1988). *Statement of criteria for selection of ESRD patients for renal transplantation.* Alexandria, VA: American Counsel on Transplantation.

Andresen, J., & Nielsen, H.E. (1981). Osteonecrosis in renal transplant recipients: Early radiological detection and course. *Acta Orthopaedica Scandinavica, 52,* 475-479.

Armenti, V.T., Ahlswede, M.J., Moritz, M.J., & Garrell, B.E. (1993). National Transplantation Pregnancy Registry analysis of pregnancy outcomes of female kidney recipients with relation to time interval from transplant to conception. *Transplant Proceedings, 25,* 1036-1037.

Ascher, N.L., Simmons, R.L., & Najarian, J.S. (1984). Host hepatectomy and liver transplantation. In R. L. Simmons, M. E. Finch, & N. L. Ascher (Eds.), *Manual of vascular access, organ donation and transplantation* (pp. 255-284). New York: Springer-Verlag.

Ascher, N., Hanto, D.W., & Simmons R.L. (1989). Immunobiology of allograft rejection. In M.W. Flye (Ed.), *Principles of organ transplantation* (pp. 91-104), Philadelphia: W.B. Saunders Company.

Baatard, R., Dantal, J., Hourmant, M., Cantarovich, D., Cesbron, A., Bignon, J.D., & Soulillou, J.P. (1991). Effect of the number of pregraft blood transfusions in kidney graft recipients treated with bioreagents and cyclosporin A. *Transplant International, 4,* 235-238.

Bader, T.F. (1997). Viral hepatitis: Practical evaluation & treatment. Seattle: Hogrefe & Huber.

Barker, R.J., Mayes, J.J., Schulak, J.A. (1991). Wound abscesses following retro peritoneal pancreas transplantation. *Clinical Transplantation, 5,* 403-407.

Barkholt, L., Ericzon, B.G., Tollemar, J., Malmborg, A.S., Ehrnst, A., Wilczek, H., & Andersson, J. (1993). Infections in human liver recipients: Different patterns earlier and later after transplantation. *Transplant International, 6,* 77-84.

Barry, J.M., Hefty, T., Fisher, S.M., & Norman, D.J. (1985). Donor specific blood transfusions and successful spousal kidney transplantation. *Journal of Urology, 133,* 1024-1025.

Bartucci, M.R., & Seller, M.C. (1990). The immunology of transplant rejection. In K.M. Sigardson-Poor & L.M. Haggerty (Eds.), *Nursing care of the transplant recipient.* Philadelphia: W.B. Saunders Company.

Basadonna, J.P., Matas, A.J., Gillingham, K.J., Payne, W.D., Dunn, D.L., Sutherland, D.E.R., Gores, P.F., Gruessner, R.W.G., & Najarian, J.S. (1993). Early versus acute renal allograft rejection impact on chronic rejection. *Transplantation, 55,* 993-995.

Baumgartner, D., Largiader, F., Uhlschmid, G., & Briswanger, U. (1983). Rejection episodes in recipients of simultaneous pancreas and kidney transplantation. *Transplantation Proceedings, 15,* 1330-1331.

Bay, W.H., & Herber, L.A. (1987). The living donor in kidney transplantation in man. *Annals of Internal Medicine, 106,* 719-727.

Beattie, G.M., Otonkoski, T., Lopes, A.D., & Hay, K.A. (1997). Functional beta-cell mass after transplantation of human fetal pancreatic cells: Differentiation or proliferation. *Diabetes, 46*(2), 244-248.

Beckman, N.J., Schell, H.M., Calixto, P.R., & Sullivan, M. (1992). Kidney transplantation: A therapy option. *AACN Clinical Issues in Critical Care Nursing, 3,* 370-384.

Beekman, G. van Dorp, W.T., van Es, L.A., van Bockel, J.H., van Saase, J.L., van der, T. Woude, F.J., & Valentijn, R.M. (1994). Analysis of donor selection procedure in 139 living related kidney donors and follow-up results for donors and recipients. *Nephrology, Dialysis, Transplantation, 9,* 163-168.

Bellanti, J.A. (1985). Introduction to immunology. In J.A. Bellanti (Ed.), *Immunology III.* Philadelphia: W.B. Saunders Company.

Belzer, F.O., Glass, N., & Sollinger, H. (1988). Technical complications after renal transplantation. In P.J. Morris (Ed.), *Kidney transplantation: Principles and practices* (3rd ed., pp. 511-532). Philadelphia: W.B. Saunders Company.

Benjamini, E., & Leskowitz, S. (1991). *Immunology: A short course* (2nd ed.). New York: Alan Liss.

Benenson, E. (Ed.). (1996). United Network for Organ Sharing (UNOS). *November/December Update.*

Bentley, F.R., Jung, S., & Ganser, R.N. (1990). Neuropathy and psychological adjustment after pancreas transplant in diabetics. *Transplantation Proceedings, 22,* 691-695.

Berloco, P., Pretagotini, R., Poli, L., Rossi, M., Caricata, N., Alfani, D., & Cortesini, R. (1993). Living unrelated kidney transplantation: A real source in cyclosporine era. *Transplant Proceedings, 25,* 3085-3086.

Berne, T.V., Ritzgibbons, T.J., & Silberman, H. (1977). The effect of hepatitis B antigenemia on long-term success: An hepatic disease in renal transplantation. *Transplantation, 24,* 412-415.

Bernstein, D.N. (1971). After transplantation: The child's emotional reactions. *American Journal of Psychiatry, 172,* 109-117.

Bittar, A.E, Keitiel, E., Garcia, C.D., Bruno, R.M., Silveira, A.E., Messias, A., & Garcia, V.D. (1992). Patient noncompliance as a cause of late kidney graft failure. *Transplantation Proceedings, 24,* 2720-2721.

Bodmer, J.G., Marsh, G.E., Albert, E.D., Bodmer, W.F., Dupont, B., Erlich, H.A., Mach, B., Mayr, W.R., Parham, P., Sasazuki, T., et al. (1994). Nomenclature for factors of the HLA system, 1994. *Tissue Antigens, 44,* 118.

Brattstrom, D., Wilczek, H., Frodin, L., Claesson, K., Pettersson, E., Backman, U., Lindholm, A., & Groth, C.G. (1994). Experience with genetically unrelated living donors in kidney transplantation: An important but not sufficiently utilized organ resource. *Transplant Proceedings, 26,* 1746-1747.

Braun, W.E. (1990). Long-term complications of renal transplantation. *Kidney International, 37,* 1363-1378.

Broelsch, C.E., Emond, J.C., Thistlethwaite, J.R., Whitington, P.F., Zucker, A.R., Baker, A.L., Aran, P.F., Rouch, D.A., & Lichtor, J.L. (1988). Liver transplantation: Including the concept of reduced size liver transplants in children. *Annals of Surgery, 208,* 410-420.

Broelsch, C.E., Emond, J.C., Whitington, P.F., Thistlethwaite, J.R., Baker, A.L., & Lichtor, J.L. (1990). Application of reduced size transplants as split grafts, auxiliary orthotopic grafts, and living related segmental transplant. *Annals of Surgery, 212,* 368-377.

Broelsch, C.E., Whitington, P.F., Emond, J.C., Heffron, T.G., Thistlethwaite, J.R., Stevens, L., Piper, J., Whitington, S.H., & Lichtor, J.L. (1991). Living transplantation of children from living related donors. *Annals of Surgery, 214,* 428-439.

Bumgardner, G.L., & Roberts, J.P. (1993). New immunosuppressive agents. *Gastroenterology Clinics of North America, 22,* 421-448.

Bumgardner, G.L., & Matas, A.J. (1992). Transplantation in pregnancy. *Transplant Review, 6,* 139.

Burke, J.F., Jr., Pirsch, J.D., Ramos, E.L., Salomon, D.R., Stablein, D.M., Van Buren, D.H., & West, J.C. (1994). Long-term efficacy and safety of cyclosporine in renal transplant recipients. *New England Journal of Medicine, 331,* 358-363.

Cahill, G.F., Etzwiler, D.D., & Freinkel, G. (1976). Blood glucose control in diabetes. *Diabetes, 25,* 237-239.

Calne, R.Y. (1987). Cyclosporin in cadaveric renal transplantation: 5-year follow-up of a multicentre trial [letter]. *Lancet, 2*(8557), 506-507.

Chan, T.M., Lok, A.S.F., Cheng, I.K.P., & Ng, I.O.L. (1993). Chronic hepatitis C after renal transplantation. *Journal of Transplantation, 56,* 1095-1098.

Chantler, C., Broyer, M., Donckerwolcke, R.A., Brynger, H., Brunner, F.P., Jacobs, C., Kramer, P., Selwood, N.H., & Wing, A.J. (1981). Growth and rehabilitation of long-term survivors of treatment for end stage renal failure in childhood. *Proceedings of the European Dialysis and Transplant Association, 18,* 329-342.

Chmielewski, C. (1987). Early recognition of infection after renal transplantation. *ANNA Journal, 14,* 389-391.

Chou, S. (1986). Acquisition of donors strains of cytomegley virus by renal transplant recipients. *New England Journal of Medicine, 314,* 1418-1423.

Colomb, B.W. (1991). Histocompatibility testing. In D.P. Stites & A.I. Terr (Eds.), *Basic and clinical immunology* (7th ed., pp. 29-31). Norwalk, CT: Appleton & Lange.

Colomb, B.W. (1994). Histocompatibility testing. In D.P. Stites, A.I. Terr, & T.G. Parsol (Eds.), *Basic and clinical immunology* (8th ed., pp. 237-255). Norwalk, CT: Appleton & Lange.

Conjeevaram, H., Barlow, J.E., Austin, H., et al. (1993). Longer term follow-up of hepatitis B virus related glomerulonephritis circa alpha-interferon. *Hepatology 18,* 146.

Coughlin, G.P., Van Deth, A.G., Disney, A.P., Hay, J., & Wangel, A.G. (1980). Liver disease and the E antigen in HBsAg carriers with chronic renal failure. *Gut, 22,* 118-122.

Crandal, B. (1990). Immunosuppression. In K.M. Sigardson-Poor & L.M. Haggerty (Eds.), *Nursing care of the transplant recipient.* Philadelphia: W.B. Saunders Company.

Curtis, J.J. (1991). Significant causes and treatments of post transplant hypertension. Nephrology and transplantation: Exploring key issues in long-term patient management. *Nephrology and Transplantation, 1*(2), 19.

Davidson, J.M. (1985). The effect of pregnancy on kidney function in renal allograft recipients. *Kidney International, 27,* 7478.

Davidson, J.M. (1989). Renal transplantation in pregnancy. *American Journal of Kidney Diseases, 9,* 374380.

Davidson, J.M. (1991). Pregnancy after kidney transplantation. *American Journal of Kidney Diseases, 17,* 127.

Davidson, J.M., & Hindheimer, M.D. (1984). Pregnancy in women with renal allografts. *Seminars in Nephrology, 4,* 240-248.

Davies, S.E., Portmann, B.C., O'Grady, J.G., Aldis, P.M., Chaggar, K., Alexander, G.J., & Williams, R. (1991). Hepatic histological findings after transplantation for chronic hepatitis B virus infection, including a unique pattern of fibrosing cholestatic hepatitis. *Hepatology, 13,* 150-157.

Debure, A., Degos, F., Pol, S., Degott, C., Carnot, F., Lugassy, C., Lacombe, M., & Kreis, H. (1988). Liver diseases and hepatic complications in renal transplant patients. *Advances in Nephrology, 17,* 375-400.

Deckert, T. (1988). Insulin dependent diabetes mellitus and its complications. In C.G. Groth (Ed.), *Pancreatic transplantation.* Philadelphia: W.B. Saunders Company.

Demayo, E., Elick, B., & Schanbacher, B. (1990). Pancreas transplantation. In K.M. Sigardison-Door & L.M. Haggerty (Eds.), *Nursing care of the transplant recipient.* Philadelphia: W.B. Saunders Company.

Demetris, A.J., Todo, S., Van Thiel, D.H., Fung, J.J., Iwaki, Y., Sysyn, G., Ming, W., Trager, J., & Starzl, T.E. (1990). Evolution of hepatitis B virus liver disease after hepatic replacement: Practical and theoretical considerations. *American Journal of Pathology, 137,* 667-676.

Diamond, N.G., Casarella, J.J., Hardy, M.A., & Appel, G.B. (1979). Dilation of critical transplant renal artery stenosis by percutaneous transluminal angioplasty. *American Journal of Radiology, 133,* 1167-1170.

Diethelm, A.G., Barger, B.O., Whelchel, J.D., & Barber, W.H. (1987). Organ transplantation. In J.H. Davis (Ed.), *Clinical surgery.* St. Louis: C.V. Mosby Company.

Dienstag, J.L., & Ktkov. (1994). Viral hepatitis in the compromised host. In R.H. Rubin & L.S. Young (Eds.), *Clinical approach to infection in the compromised host* (3rd ed.). New York: Plenum.

Dietze, O., Vogel, W., Margreiter, R., & Mikuz, G. (1990). Early recurrence of primary biliary cirrhosis after liver transplantation [letter]. *Gastroenterology, 98,* 1106-1107.

Donckerwolcke, R.A. (1991). Long-term complications of renal transplantation. *Child Nephrology and Urology, 11,* 179-184.

Donegan, E., & Bossom, E.L. (1994). Blood banking immunohematology. In D.P. Stites, A.I. Terr, & T.G. Parslow (Eds.), *Basic and clinical immunology* (8th ed.). Norfolk, CT: Appleton & Lange.

Dordevic, P.B., Lalia, N.M., Birkic, S., Jotic, A., Paunouc, I., Lalic, K., et al. (1995). Human felt islet transplant in IDDM patients: An 8-year experience. *Transplant Proceedings 27*(6), 31-45.

Dunn, J.F., Nylander, W.A., Rishei, R.E., Johnson, H.K., MacDonnell, R.C., & Sawyers, J.L. (1986). Living related kidney donors: A 14 year experience. *Annals of Surgery, 203,* 637-643.

Eggers, P.W. (1988). Effective transplantation on the Medicare and end stage renal disease program. *New England Journal of Medicine, 328,* 224-229.

Ellis, D., Shapiro, R., Jordan, M.L., Scantlebury, V.P., Gilboa, N., Hopp, L., Weichler, N., Tzakis, A.J., & Simmons, R.L. (1994). Comparison of FK 506 in cyclosporine regimes in pediatric renal transplantation. *Pediatric Nephrology, 8,* 193-200.

Emond, J.C. (1993). Clinical application of living related liver transplantation. *Journal of Gastroenterology Clinics of North America, 22,* 301-315.

Emond, J.C., Whitington, P.F., & Broelsch, C. (1991). Overview of reduced size liver transplantation. *Clinical Transplantation, 5,* 168-173.

Emond, J.C., Whitington, P.F., Thistlethwait, J.R., Alonso, E.M., & Broelsch, C.E. (1989). Reduced size orthotopic liver transplantation: Use in the management of children with chronic liver disease. *Hepatology, 10,* 867-872.

Erice, A., Jordan, M.C., Chace, B.A., Fletcher, C., Chinnock, B.J., & Balfour, H.H., Jr. (1987). Ganciclovir treatment of cytomegalovirus disease in transplant recipients and other immunocompromised hosts. *Journal of the American Medical Association, 257,* 3082-3087.

Ettenger, R.B., Rosenthal, J.T., Marik, J.L., Malekzadeh, M., Forsythe, S.B., Kamil, E.S., Salusky, I.B., & Fine, R.N. (1991). Improved cadaveric renal transplant outcome in children. *Pediatric Nephrology, 5,* 137-142.

European FK 506 Multicentre Liver Study Group. (1994).

Reduced incidents of acute refractory acute and chronic rejection after liver transplantation with FK 506 based immunosuppression. *Transplant Proceedings, 26,* 3260-3263.

Euvrard, S., Schardonnet, Y., Pouteil-Nobel C.P., Kanitakis, J., Thivolet, J., & Touraine, J.L. (1993). Skin malignancies human papilloma viruses in renal transplant recipients. *Transplant Proceedings, 25,* 1392-1393.

Fairley, C.K., Mijch, A., Gust, I.D., Nichilson, S., Dimitrakakis, M., & Lucas, C.R. (1991). The increased risk of fatal liver disease in renal transplant patients who are hepatitis B antigen and/or HBV DNA positive. *Transplantation, 52,* 497-500.

Farkas, A., Degi, R., & Voros, P. (1995). Long-term effects of fetal islet transplant on complications of diabetes as compared with effects of intensive insulin therapy. *Transplant Proceedings, 27*(6), 31-45.

Figueroa, J.E. (1992). Selection of patients for kidney organ transplantation. *Medical Clinics of North America, 76,* 1188-1195.

Fine, R.N., Malekzadeh, M.H., Pennisi, A.J., Uittenbogaart, C.H., Ettenger, R.B., Landing, B.H., & Wright, H.T. (1977). HBs antigenemia in renal allograft recipients. *Annals of Surgery, 185,* 411-416.

Fischer, A., Blanche, S., LeBidois,J., Bordigoni, P., Garnier, J.L., Niaudet, P., Morinet, F., LeDeist, F., Fischer, A.M., Griscelli, C., et al. (1991). Anti B cell monoclonal antibodies and the treatment of severe B-cell lympho proliferative syndrome following bone marrow and organ transplantation. *New England Journal of Medicine, 324,* 1451-1456.

Flye, M.W. (1989). Renal transplantation. In M.W. Flye (Ed.), *Principles of organ transplantation.* Philadelphia: W.B. Saunders Company.

Foster, M.C., & Dennis, N.J.S. (1992). Chronic renal graft rejection. In L.C. Paul & K. Solez (Eds.), *Organ transplantation: Long-term results.* New York: Marcel Dekker.

Frank, M.N. (1991). Complement and kinin. In D.P. Stites & A.I. Terr (Eds.), *Basic and clinical immunology* (7th ed.). Norwalk, CT: Appleton & Lange.

Garcia, C.D., Uhlmann, A., Deboni, L., Keitel, E., Bittar, A.E., Cantisani, G., Vitola, S.P., Guerra, E., Zanotelli, M.L., Goldani, J.C., et al. (1992). Renal transplantation in children. *Transplant Proceedings, 24,* 3092-3093.

Garovoy, M.R., Amend, W.J.C., Vincenti, F., & Feduska, N.J. (1987). *Renal transplantation–The modern era.* New York: Gower Medical.

Garovoy, M.R., Melzer, J.S., Ascher, N., Magilligan, D., & Bozdech, M. (1991). Clinical transplantation. In D.P. Stites & A.I. Terr (Eds.), *Basic and clinical immunology* (7th ed.). Norwalk, CT: Appleton & Lange.

Garovoy, M.R., Stock, P., Bumgardner, G., Keith, F., & Linker, C. (1994). Clinical transplantation. In D.P. Stites, A.I. Terr, & T.G. Parslow (Eds.). *Basic and clinical immunology* (8th ed.). Norwalk, CT: Appleton & Lange.

Garrel, D.R., Delmas, P.D., Welsh, C., Arnaud, M.J., Hamilton, S.E., & Pugeat, M.M. (1988). Effects of moderate physical training on prednisone-induced protein wasting: A study of whole body and bone protein metabolism. *Metabolism, 37,* 257-262.

Geary, D.F., Thurner, P., Baumal, R., Major, M., & Arbus, G. (1987). Cyclosporine A in children with persistent renal transplant rejection and progressively deteriorating graft function. *Pediatric Nephrology, 1,* 140-144.

George, D.L., Arnow, P.M., Fox, A.S., Baker, A.L., Thistlethwaite, J.R., Emond, J.C., Whitington, P.F., & Broelsch, C.E. (1991). Bacterial infection as a complication of liver transplantation: Epidemiology and risk factors. *Review of Infectious Diseases, 13,* 387-396.

Gimson, A.E., White, Y.S., Eddlesdon, A.L., & Williams, R. (1983). Clinical and prognostic differences in fulminant hepatitis type A, B and non-A non-B. *Gut, 24,* 1194-1198.

Gonwa, T., Morris, C.A., Goldstein, R.N., Husberg, B., & Klintmaln, G.B. (1991). Long-term survival in renal function following liver transplantation in patients with and without hepatorenal syndrome experienced in 308 patients. *Journal of Transplantation, 51,* 428-430.

Goodman, J.W. (1991). The immune response. In D.P. Stites & A.I. Terr (Eds.), *Basic and clinical immunology* (7th ed.). Norwalk, CT: Appleton & Lange.

Goodman, J.W. (1994). The immune response. In D.P. Stites, A.I. Terr, & T.G. Parslow (Eds.), *Basic and clinical immunology* (8th ed.). Norwalk, CT: Appleton & Lange.

Gordon, R.D., Makowka, L., Bronsthier, O.L., Lerut, J.P., Esquivel, C.O., Iwatsuki, S, & Starzl, T.E. (1987). Complications of liver transplantation. In L.H.T. Pereyra (Ed.), *Complications of organ transplantation.* New York: Marcel Dekker.

Green, M.M. (1987). Bone and joint complications. In L.S. Toledo-Pereyra (Ed.), *Complication of organ transplantation.* New York: Marcel Dekker.

Grundfest-Broniatowski, S. (1990). Pancreas transplantation: State of the art. *Cleveland Clinic Journal of Medicine, 57,* 564-570.

Grundy, J.E., Lui, S.F., Super, M., Berry, N.J., Sweny, P., Fernando, O.N., Moorhead, J., & Griffiths, P.D. (1988). Symptomatic cytomegalovirus infection in seropositive kidney recipients: Reinfection with donor virus rather than reactivation of recipient virus. *Lancet, 2*(8603), 132-135.

Grundy, J.E., Super, M., Lui, S.F., Sweny, P., & Griffiths, P.D. (1987). The source of cytomegalovirus infection in seropositive renal allograft recipients is frequently the donor kidney. *Transplant Proceedings, 19,* 2126-2128.

Gugenheim, J. (1990). Liver transplantation across ABO blood group barriers. *Lancet, 336,* 519-523.

Gunnarsson, R., Arner, P., Lundren, G., Magnusson, G., Ostman, J., & Groth, C.G. (1977). Steroid diabetes after renal transplantation: A preliminary report. *Scandinavian Journal of Urology and Nephrology, 42*(Suppl.), 191-194.

Gunnarsson, R., Arner, P., Lundren, G., Magnusson, G., Ostman, J., & Groth, C.G. (1979). Diabetes mellitus: A more common than believed complication of renal transplantation. *Transplantation Proceedings, 11,* 1280-1281.

Gunnarsson, R., Lundren, G., Magnusson, G., Ost, G., & Groth C.G. (1980). Steroid diabetes: A sign of over treatment with steroids in the renal graft recipient. *Scandinavian Journal of Urology and Nephrology, 54*(Suppl.), 135-138.

Guyton, A.C. (1986). *Textbook of medical physiology* (7th ed.). Philadelphia: W.B. Saunders Company.

Haggerty, L.M., & Sigardson-Poor, K.M. (1990). Kidney transplantation. In K.M. Sigardson Poor & L.M. Haggerty (Eds.), *Nursing care of the transplant recipient.* Philadelphia: W.B. Saunders Company.

Hakim, R.M., Goldszer, R.C., & Brenner B.M. (1984). Hypertension and proteinuria: Long-term sequelae of uninephrectomy in humans. *Kidney International, 25,* 930-934.

Hanto, D.W., & Simmons, R. (1987). Renal transplantation: Clinical considerations. *Radiologic Clinics of North America, 25,* 239-248.

Hanto, D., Frizzera, G., & Purtillo, D.T. (1981). Clinical spectrum of lymphoproliferative in renal transplant recipients and evidence for role of Epstein Barr virus infection. *Cancer Research, 41,* 4253-4261.

Haugen, G. Fauchald, P., Sodal, G., Halversen, S., Oldereid, N., & Moe, N. (1991). Pregnancy outcome in renal transplant recipients: Influence of cyclosporine A. *European Journal of Obstetrics, Gynecology, and Reproductive Biology, 39,* 25-29.

Hawke, D., Kraft, J., & Smith, S. (1990). Progression of diabetic retinopathy after pancreas transplantation. *Ophthalmology, 97,* 496-502.

Health Resources and Service Administration, Bureau of Health Resources Development. (1991). *Report of center specific graft in patient survival rates.* Rockville, MD: Author.

Heffron, T.J. (1993). Living related pediatric liver transplantation. *Seminars in Pediatric Surgery, 2,* 248-253.

Helderman, J.H. (1986). The role of cardiovascular disease in renal transplantation. In M.R. Garovoy & R.D. Guttman (Eds.), *Renal transplantation.* New York: Churchill Livingstone.

Hendrick, A., Wallin, J.D., & O'Neill, W.M. (1984). Plasma exchange in the treatment of chronic renal allograft rejection. *Transplantation, 37,* 318-319.

Herscowitz, H.B. (1985). Immunophysiology: Cell function and cellular interactions in antibody formation. In J. A. Bellanti (Ed.), *Immunology III.* Philadelphia: W.B. Saunders Company.

Hibberd, P.L., Tolkoff-Rubin, N.E., Cosimi, A. B., Schooley, R. T., Isaacson, D., Doran, M., Delvecchio, A., Delmonico, F.L., Auchincloss, H., Jr., & Rubin, R.H. (1992). Symptomatic cytomegalovirus disease in the cytomegalovirus antibody seropositive renal transplant recipient treated with OKT3. *Transplantation, 53,* 68-72.

Hillis, W. D., Hillis, A, Walker, W. G. (1979). Hepatitis B surface antigenemia in renal transplant recipients increased mortality risk. *Journal of the American Medical Association, 242,* 329-332.

Hiner, H.H., & Suki, W.N. (1987). *Kidney transplantation: Cardiovascular complications.*

Ho, M. (1990). Overview of CMV infections in the immunocompromised transplant patient. *Abstract Brochure Cytomegalovirus Infections in the Immuno Compromise Transplant Patient: Diagnosis and Treatment (XII),* International Congress of the Transplantation Society in San Francisco, California. P. 12.

Ho, M. (1991). *Cytomegalovirus: Biology and infection* (2nd ed.). New York: Plenum.

Ho, M., & Locker, J. (1988). The pathology of posttransplant lymphoproliferative disorders occurring in the setting of cyclosporine A prednisone immunosuppression. *American Journal of Pathology, 133,* 173-192.

Ho, M., Jaffe, R., Miller, G., Breinig, M.K., Dummer, J.S., Makowka,L., Atchison, R.W., Karrer, F., Nalesnik, M.A., & Starzl, T. (1988). The frequency of Epstein Barr virus infection and associated lymphoproliferative syndrome after transplantation and its manifestations in children. *Transplantation, 45,* 719-727.

Hoffman, M., & Malecki, M. (1990). Organ procurement and preservation. In K.M. Sigardson Poor & L.M. Haggerty (Eds.), *Nursing care of the transplant recipient.* Philadelphia: W.B.Saunders Company.

Holleroroth, H. J. (1986). *Diabetes teaching guide.* Boston: Joslin Diabetes Center.

Hooks, M. (1990). Immunosuppressive agents used in transplantation. In S. Smith (Ed.), *Tissue and organ transplantation: Implications for professional nursing practice.* St Louis: C.V. Mosby Company.

Horber, F. F., Scheidegger, J. R., Grunig, B. E., & Frey, F J. (1985). Evidence that prednisone induced myopathy is reversed by physical training. *Journal of Clinical Endocrinology and Metabolism, 61,* 83-88.

Huang, C.C., Lai, M.K., & Fong, M.T. (1990). Hepatitis B liver disease in cyclosporine-treated renal allograph recipients. *Transplantation, 49* 540-544.

Huang, C.C., Liaw, Y.F., Lai, M.K.,Chu, S.H., Chuang, C.K., & Huang, J.Y. (1992). The clinical outcome of hepatitis C virus on antibody-positive renal allograph recipients. *Transplantation, 53,* 763-765.

Huffer, T.L., Kanapa, D.J., & Stevenson, G.W. (1986). *Introduction to human immunology.* Boston: Jones and Bartlett.

Ingulli, E., Sharma, V., Singh, A., Suthanthiron, M., & Tejani, A. (1993). Steroid withdrawal, rejection and the mixed lymphocyte reaction in children after renal transplantation. *Kidney International, 43*(Suppl.), S36-S39.

Isoniemi, H., Nurminen, M., Tikkanen, M. J., von Willebrand, E., Krogerus, L., Ahonen, J., Eklund, B., Hokerstedt, K., Salmela, K., & Hayry, P. (1994). Risk factors predicting chronic rejection of renal allografts. *Transplantation, 57,* 68-72.

Jain, A., Venkataramanan, R., Lever, J., Warty, V., Fung, J., Todo, S., & Starzl, T. (1993). FK 506 and pregnancy in liver transplant patients. *Transplantation, 56,* 751-752.

Jakobsen, A. (1994). State of the art kidney transplantation. *Transplantation Proceedings, 26,* 1704-1705.

Jett, M.F., & Lancaster, L.E. (1983). The inflammatory immune response: The body's defense against invasion. *Critical Care Nurse, 3*(5), 64-86.

Johnson, M., & Flye, N.W. (1989). Infectious complications in renal transplant patients. In M.W. Flye (Ed.), *Principles of organ transplantation.* Philadelphia: W.B. Saunders Company.

Johnson, M., & Flye, N.W. (1989). Long-term follow-up of renal transplant patient. In M.W. Flye (Ed.), *Principles of organ transplantation.* Philadelphia: W. B. Saunders Company.

Jones, R.W.A., Bishti, M., & Chantler, C. (1980). The promotion of annalism in children with chronic renal failure. In B.A. Wharton (Ed.), *Nutrition in childhood.* Tunbridge Wells, England: Pitman.

Jordon, S.C., & Lemire, J.M. (1994). Allograft rejection: Types, mechanism and diagnosis. In N. Fine & A.B. Gruskin (Eds.), *End stage renal disease in children.* Philadelphia: W.B. Saunders Company.

Kahan, B.D., Flechner, S.M., Lorber, M.I., Golden, D., Conley, S., & Van Buren, C.T. (1987). Complications of cyclosporine prednisone immunosuppression in 402 renal allograft recipients exclusively followed at a single center for from one to five years. *Transplantation, 43,* 197-204.

Kamani, N.R., & Douglas, S.D. (1991). The structure and development of the immune system. In D.S. Stites & A.B. Terr (Eds.), *Basic and clinical immunology* (7th ed.). Norfolk, CT: Appleton & Lange.

Kasiske, B. (1992). Atherosclerosis in organ transplant recipients. In L.C. Paul & K. Solez (Eds.), *Organ transplantation: Long-term results.* New York: Macel Dekker.

Katkov, W.N., & Rubin, R.H. (1991). Liver disease in the organ transplant recipient: Etiology, clinical impact, and clinical management. *Transplant Review, 5,* 200-208.

Keeffe, E.B., & Esquivel, C.O. (1993). Controversies in patient selection for liver transplantation. *Western Journal of Medicine, 159,* 586-593.

Keith, J.S. (1985). Hepatic failure: Etiologies, manifestations and management. *Critical Care Nurse, 5,* 60-86.

Kelly, W.D., Lillehei, R.C., Merkel, F.K., et al. (1967). Allo transplantation of the pancreas and duodenum along with the kidney in diabetic nephropathy, *Surgery, 61,* 822-837.

Kennedy, W.R., Navarro, X., Goetz, F.C., Sutherland, D.E.R. & Najorias, J.S. (1990). Effects of pancreas transplantation on diabetic neuropathy. *New England Journal of Medicine, 322,* 1031-1037.

Keown, P.A., & Shackleton, C.R. (1992). Long-term mortality, morbidity and rehabilitation in organ transplant recipients. In L.C. Paul & K. Solez (Eds.), *Organ transplantation: Long-term results.* New York: Marcel Dekker.

Kiley, D.J., Lam, C.S., & Pollak, R. (1993). The study of treatment compliance following kidney transplantation. *Journal of Transplantation, 55,* 51-56.

Kim, M.J., McFarland, D.G, & McLane, A.M. (1991). *Pocket guide to nursing diagnosis* (4th ed.). St. Louis: C.V. Mosby Yearbook.

Kirkman, R.L., Strom, T.B., Weir, M.R., & Tilney, N.L. (1982). Late mortality and morbidity of long term renal allografts. *Journal of Transplantation, 34,* 347-351.

Klintmalm, G.B., Goldstein, R., Gonwa, T., Wiesner, R.H., Krom, R.A., Shaw, B.W., Jr., Stratta, R., Ascher, N.L., Roberts, J.W., Lake, J., et al. (1993). The use of Prograf (FK 506) as rescue therapy for refractory rejection after liver transplantation. U.S. Multicentre FK 506 Liver Study Group. *Transplantation Proceedings, 25,* 679-688.

Klintmalm, G., & Moore, A.E. (1985). Organization of a new liver transplant center. *Seminars in Liver Disease, 5,* 412-417.

Kocoshis, S., Tzakis, A., Todo, S., Reyes, J., & Nour, B. (1993). Pediatric liver transplantation: History, recent innovations, and outlook for the future. *Clinical Pediatrics, 32,* 386-392.

Kootte, A.M.M., & Paul, L.C. (1988). Cyclosporine therapy or dietary protein manipulation in chronic renal allograft rejection. *Transplantation Proceedings, 20,* 821-826.

Kottra-Buck, K. (1986). Renal transplantation. In C.J. Richards (Ed.), *Comprehensive nephrology nursing.* Boston: Little Brown.

LaBerge, J.M., Ring, E.J., Gordon, R.L., Lake, J.R., Doherty, M.M., Somberg, K.A., Roberts, J.P., & Ascher, N.L. (1993). Creation of transjugular intraheptatic portosystemic shunts with the wallstent endoprosthesis: Results in 100 patients. *Interventional Radiology, 187,* 413-420.

Lake, J. (1993). Changing indications for liver transplantation. *Gastroenterology Clinics of North America, 22,* 213-229.

Lancaster, L., & Schanbacer, B.A. (1990). Renal transplantation. In L.E. Lancaster (Ed.), *Core curriculum for nephrology nursing* (2nd ed.). Pitman NJ: American Nephrology Nurses Association.

Langnas, A.N., Marujo, W., Stratta, R.J., Wood, R.P., & Shaw, B.W., Jr. (1991). Vascular complications after orthotopic liver transplantation. *American Journal of Surgery, 161,* 76-82.

Langnas, A.N., Stratta, R.J., Wood, R.P., Ozaki, C.F., Bynon, J.S., & Shaw, B.W., Jr. (1992). The role of intrahepatic cholangiojejunostomy in liver transplant recipients after extensive destruction of the extrahepatic biliary system. *Surgery, 112,* 712-718.

Lanier, L. (1991). Cells of the immune response: Lymphocytes and mononuclear phagocytes. In D.P. Stites & A. I. Terr (Eds.), *Basic and clinical immunology* (7th ed.). Norfolk, CT: Appleton & Lange.

Lee, H.M., & Mendez Picon, G. (1984). Complications of renal transplantation. In L.J. Greenfield (Ed.), *Complications in surgery and trauma.* Philadelphia: J. B. Lippincott Company.

Leivestad, T., Berger, L., & Thorsby, E. (1992). Beneficial effect of DR matching on cadaveric renal graft survival in Scandia transplant. *Transplant Proceedings, 24,* 2447-2448.

Lerut, J., Tzakis, A.G ., Bron, K., Gordon, R.D., Iwatsuki, S., Esquivel, C.O., Makowka, L., Todo, S., & Starzl, T.E. (1987). Complications of venous reconstruction in human orthotopic liver transplantation. *Annals of Surgery, 205,* 404-414.

Levine, J.E., Lake, J.R., Ascher, N.L., Ferrell, L.D., Ganem, D., & Wright, T.L. (1991). Persistent hepatitis B virus following interferon alpha therapy and liver transplantation. *Gastroenterology, 100,* 263-267.

Lewis, S.M., Wood, B., & Seppelt, J. (1992). Nursing role management: Acute and chronic renal failure. In S.M. Lewis & I. C. Collier (Eds.), *Medical and surgical nursing: Assessment and management of clinical problems* (3rd ed.). St. Louis: C.V. Mosby Company.

Lien, B., Brekkle, I.B., Sodal, G., Bentadl, O., Pfeiffer, P., & Jakobsen, A. (1993). Renal transplantation and intestinal urinary diversion: A ten year experience. *Transplant Proceedings, 25,* 1338-1339.

Lillehei, R.C., Simmons, R.L., Najauan, J.S., et al. (1970). Pancreatico-duodenal allotransplantation: Experimental and clinical experience. *Annals of Surgery, 17*(2), 405-436.

Lu, C.Y., Sicher, S.C., & Vazques, M.A. (1993). Prevention and treatment of renal allograft rejection: New therapeutic approaches and new insights into established therapies. *Journal of the American Society of Nephrology, 4,* 1239-1256.

Luke, R.G. (1987). Hypertension in renal transplant recipients. *Kidney International, 13,* 1024-1037.

Malatack, J.F., Gartner, J.C., Jr., Urbach, A.H., & Zitelli, B.J. (1991). Orthotopic liver transplantation, Epstein-Barr virus, cyclosporine, and lymphoproliferative disease: A growing concern. *Journal of Pediatrics, 118,* 667-675.

Malekzadeh, M.H., Pennisi, A.J., Uittenbogaart, C.H., Korsch, B.M., Fine, R.N., & Main. M.E. (1976). Current issues in pediatric renal transplantation. *Pediatric Clinics of North America, 23,* 857-872.

Mani, M.K., Bhaskaran, S., & Prakash, K.C. (1993). The effect of hepatitis B in a dialysis transplant program. *Journal of Transplantation, 55,* 1188-1190.

Matas, A.J., Burk, J.F, DeVault., G.A., Monaco, A., & Pirsch, J.D. (1994). Chronic rejection. *Journal of the American Society of Nephrology, 4,* S23-S29.

Mayoral, J.L., Loeffler, C.M., Fasola, C.G., Kramer, M.A., Orrom, W.J., Matas, A.J., Najarian, J.S., & Dunn, D.L. (1991). Diagnosis and treatment of cytomegalovirus disease in transplant patients based on gastrointestinal tract manifestations. *Archives of Surgery, 126,* 202-206.

McCance, K.L. (1990). Structure and function of the hematological system. In K.L. McCance & S.E. Huether (Eds.), *Pathophysiology: The biological basis for disease in adults and children.* St. Louis: C.V.Mosby Company.

McDiarmid, S.V., Klintmalm, G.B., & Busuttil, R.D. (1993). FK 506 conversion for intractable rejection of the liver allograph. *Transplant International, 6,* 305-312.

McDiarmid, S.V., Klintmalm, G., & Busuttil, R.W. (1991). FK 506 rescue therapy in liver transplantation: Outcome and complications. *Transplantation Proceedings, 23*(6), 2996-2999.

McFarland, G.K., & McFarlane, E.A. (1989). *Nursing diagnosis and intervention: Planning for patient care.* St. Louis: C.V. Mosby Company.

Mendez, R., & Vargas, A.D. (1987). Kidney transplantation: Urological complications. In L.H. Toledo-Pereyra (Ed.), *Complications of organ transplantation.* New York: Marcel Dekker.

Mihatsch, M.J., Thiel, J., & Ryffel, B. (1988). Histopathology of cyclosporine nephrotoxicity. *Transplant Proceedings, 20*(suppl.), 759-771.

Mora, N.P., Klintmalm, G.B., Solomon, H., Goldstein, R.M., Gonwa, T.A., & Husberg, B.S. (1992). Survival after liver transplantation in 300 consecutive patients: The influence of age, clinical status, and pre-transplant disease. *Transplant Proceedings, 24,* 156-157.

Mudge, C. L., & Carlson, L. (1992). Hepatorenal syndrome. *AACN Clinical Issues in Critical Care Nursing, 3,* 614-632.

Mudge-Grout, C.L. (1992). *Immunological disorders.* St. Louis: C.V. Mosby Company.

Nakache, R., Tyden, G. & Groth, C.G. (1988). Quality of life in diabetic patients undergoing combined pancreas-kidney transplant or kidney transplant alone. *Diabetes.*

Nalesnik, M.A, Jaffe, R., Starzl, T.E., Demetris, A.J., Porter, K., Burnham, J.A., Makowka, L., Ho, M., & Locker, J. (1988). The pathology of post transplant lymphoproliferative disorders occurring in the setting of cyclosporine A prednisone immunosuppression. *American Journal of Pathology, 133,* 173-192.

Nelson, P.H., Helling, T.S., Shield, C.F., Beck, M., & Bryan, C.F. (1992). Current experience with renal transplantation across the ABO barrier. *American Journal of Surgery, 164,* 541-544.

O' Regan, S., & Yazbeck, S. (1992). Kidney transplantation complications in children. In L.H. Toledo-Pereyra (Ed.), *Complications of organ transplantation.* New York: Marcel Dekker.

O'Grady, J.G., Smith, H.M., Davies, S.E., Daniels, H.M., Donaldson, P.T., Tan, K.C., Portmann, B., Alexander, G.J., & Williams, R. (1992). Hepatitis B virus reinfection after orthotopic liver transplantation: Serological and clinical implications. *Journal of Hepatology, 14,* 104-111.

Onwubalili, J.K., Obinecheen, J., Assuhaimi, S., & Bassiouni, M. (1994). Outcome of bought living nonrelated donor kidneys followed up at a single center. *Transplant International, 7,* 27-32.

Otwee, J.A., & Leidigh, J.C. (1988). Teaching renal transplant patients with steroid-induced diabetes mellitus. *ANNA Journal, 15,* 295-300.

Painter, P., & Blackburn, G. (1988). Exercise for patients with chronic disease. *Post Graduate Medicine, 83,* 185-195.

Parfrey, P.S., Forbes, R.D.C., Hutchinson, T.A., Beaudoin, J.G., Dauphinee, W.D., Hollomby, D.J., & Guttmann, R.D. (1984). The clinical and pathological course of hepatitis B liver disease in renal transplant recipients. *Transplantation, 37,* 461-466.

Pattella, P.S . & Weiskittel, P.D. (1991). Kidney transplantation. In M.K.G. Norris & M.A. House (Eds.), *Organ and tissue transplantation: Nursing care from procurement through rehabilitation.* Philadelphia: F.A. Davis Company.

Penn, I. (1987). Cancer and transplantation. In H.L. Toledo-Pereyra (Ed.), *Complications of organ transplantation.* New York: Marcel Dekker.

Penn, I., Makowsky, E.L., & Harus, P. (1990). Parenthood following renal transplantation. *Kidney International, 18,* 221-229.

Pereira, B.J., Milford, E.L., Kirkman, R.L., & Levey, A.S. (1991). Transmission of hepatitis C virus by organ transplantation. *New England Journal of Medicine, 325,* 454-460.

Pereira, B.J., Milford, E.L., Kirkman, R.L., Quan, S., Sayre, K. R., Johnson, P. J., Wilber, J. C., & Levey, A. S. (1992). Prevalence of hepatitis C virus RNA in organ donors positive for hepatitis C antibody and in the recipients of their organs. *New England Journal of Medicine, 327,* 910-915.

Perkins, J.D., Fromme, G.A., Nar, B.J., Southorn, P.A., Marsh, C.L., Munn, S.R., Enges, D.E., & Sterioff, S. (1990). Pancreas transplantation at Mayo: II. Operative and perioperative management. *Mayo Clinical Proceedings, 65,* 483-495.

Perrillo, R.P., Schiff, E.R., Davis, G.L., Bodenheimer, H.C., Jr., Lindsay, K., Payne, J., Dienstaf, J.L., O'Brien, C., Tamburro, C., Jacobson, I.M., et al. (1990). A randomized, controlled trial of interferon alpha 2b alone and after prednisone withdrawal for the treatment of chronic hepatitis B. *New England Journal of Medicine, 323,* 295-301.

Perryman, J.P., & Stillerman, P. (1991). Kidney transplantation. In S.L. Smith, (Ed.), *Tissue and organ transplantation: Implications for professional nursing practice.* St. Louis: C.V. Mosby Company.

Petersen, M., & Vine, A. (1990). Progression of diabetic retinopathy after pancreas transplantation. *Ophthalmology, 97,* 496-502.

Pirson, Y., Alexandre, G.P.J., & Ypersele, C. (1977). Long-term effect of HBs antigenemia on patient survival after renal transplantation. *New England Journal of Medicine, 296,* 194-196.

Platz, K.P., Sollinger, H.W., Hullett, D.A., Eckhoff, D.E., Eugui, E.M., & Allison, A. (1991). RS61443: A new, potent immunosuppressive agent. *Transplantation, 51,* 27-31.

Portmann, B., O'Grady, J., & Williams, R. (1986). Disease recurrence following orthotopic liver transplantation. *Transplant Proceedings, 18,* S136.

Ramos, E.L., & Tisher, C.C. (1994). Recurrent diseases in the kidney transplant. *American Journal of Kidney Diseases, 24,* 142-154.

Ramos, E.L., Alexander, S.R., Danovitch, E.L., Kasiske, B.L., Harmon, W.E., Kahana, L., Kiresuk, T., & Neylan, J.F. (1994). The evaluation of candidates for renal transplantation. *Transplantation, 57,* 490-497.

Randhawa, P.S., Jaffe, R., Demetris, H.J., Nalesnik, M., Starzl, T.E., Chen, V.V., & Weiss, L.M. (1992). Expression of Epstein-Barr virus encoded small RNA (by the EBER-1-gene) in liver specimens from transplant recipients with posttransplantation lymphoproliferative disease. *New England Journal of Medicine, 327,* 1710-1714.

Rao, K.V, & Andersen, R.C. (1988). Long-term results and complications in renal transplant recipients: Observations in the second decade. *Transplantation, 45,* 45-52.

Rao, K.V., Kasiske, B.L., & Anderson, W.R. (1991). Variability in morphological spectrum in clinical outcome of chronic liver disease in hepatitis B positive and B negative renal transplant recipients. *Transplantation, 51,* 391-396.

Rashid, A., Senger, D., Couture, R., et al. (1988). Hepatitis in renal transplantation [letter]. *New England Journal of Medicine, 296,* 1170-1171.

Reding, R., Veychemans, F., deVille deGoyet, J., de Hemptinne, B., Carlier, M., Van Obbergh, L., Moulin, D., Reynaert, M., Latinne, D., Vraux, H., et al. (1992). ABO incompatible orthotopic liver allografting in urgent indications. *Surgery, Gynecology and Obstetrics, 174,* 59-64.

Riegler, J.L., & Lake, J.R. (1993). Fulminate hepatic failure. *Medical Clinics of North America, 77,* 1057-1083.

Ring, E.J., Lake J.R., Roberts, J.P., Gordon, R.L., LaBerge, J.M., Read, A.E., Sterneck M.R., & Ascher, N.L. (1992). Using transjugular intrahepatic portosystemic shunts to control variceal bleeding before liver transplantation. *Annals of Internal Medicine, 116,* 304-309.

Ringe, B., Wittekind, C., Bechstein, W.O., Bunzendahl, H., & Pichlmayr, R. (1989). The role of liver transplantation in hepatobiliary malignancy: A retrospective analysis of 95 patients with particular regard to tumor stage and recurrence. *Annals of Surgery, 209,* 88-98.

Roberts, J.P., Forsmark, C., Lake, J.R., & Ascher, N. (1989) Liver transplantation today. *Annual Reviews in Medicine, 400,* 287-303.

Roberts, J.P., Lake, J.R., Hebert, M., Nikolai, B., Ascher, N.L., & Ferrell, L.D. (1993). Reversal of chronic rejection after treatment failure with FK 506 and RS61443. *Transplantation, 56,* 1021-1023.

Roitt, I., Brostoff, J., & Male, D. (1995). *Slide atlas of immunology* (2nd ed.). New York: Gower Medical.

Roitt, I., Brostoff, J., & Male, D. (1985). *Immunology.* St. Louis: C.V. Mosby Company.

Roitt, I., Brostoff, J., & Male, D. (1989). *Immunology* (2nd ed.). New York: Gower Medical.

Rosenblum, N.D., Harmon, W.E., & Levey, R.H. (1989). Treatment of chronic renal allograft rejection with cyclosporine and prednisolone. *Journal of Transplantation, 45,* 232-233.

Rosenthal, P., Podesta, L., Sher, A., & Makowka, L. (1994). Liver transplantation in children. *American Journal of Gastroenterology, 89,* 480-492.

Rovelli, N., Palmeri, D., Vossler, E., Bartus, S., Hall, R., & Schweizer, R. (1989). Noncompliance in organ transplant recipients. *Transplant Proceedings, 21,* 833-834.

Rowe, P.A., Foster, M.D., Morgan, A. J., Burden, R. P. (1989). Effective change to cyclosporine on chronic renal allograft rejection. *Clinical Transplantation, 3,* 70-74.

Roy, D.M., Thomas, P.P., Dakshinamurthy, K.V., Jacob, C.K., & Shastry, J.C.M. (1994). Long-term survival in living related donor renal allograft recipients with hepatitis B infection. *Journal of Transplantation, 58,* 118-119.

Rubin, R. (1988). Infectious disease problems. In W.C. Maddrey (Ed.), *Current topics in gastroenterology transplantation of the liver.* New York: Elsevier.

Rubin, R. (1993). Infectious disease complications of renal transplantation. *Kidney International, 44,* 221-236.

Rubin, R.H. (1990). Impact of cytomegalovirus infection on organ transplant recipients. *Review of Infectious Diseases, 12*(Suppl.), S754-S766.

Rubin, R.H., Tolkoff Rubin, N.E. (1993). Antimicrobial strategies in the care of organ transplant recipients. *Antimicrobial Agents and Chemotherapy, 37,* 619-624.

Rubin, R.H., Tolkoff Rubin, N.E., Oliver, D., Rota, T.A., Hamilton, J., Betts, R.F., Pass, R.F., Hillis, W., Szmuness, W., Farrell, M.L., et al. (1985). Multicenter seroepidemiologic study of the impact of cytomegalovirus infection on renal transplantation. *Transplantation, 40,* 243-249.

Rubin, R.H., Wolfson, J.S., Cosimi, A.B., & Tolkoff Rubin, N.E. (1981). Infections in the renal transplant recipient. *American Journal of Medicine, 70,* 405-410.

Rubin, R., & Young, L. (Eds). (1994). Clinical approached infection and the compromised host. (3rd ed.). *Infection in the organ transplant recipient,* pp. 629-686.

Ruse, L.A. (1986). Nursing care of the renal transplant recipient. In C.J. Richards (Ed.) *Comprehensive nephrology nursing.* Boston: Little Brown.

Ruse, L.A., & KottraBuck, C. (1986). Complications following renal transplantation. In C.J. Richards (Ed.), *Comprehensive nephrology nursing.* Boston: Little Brown.

Russell, P.S. (1989). Prospects for the future. In M.W. Flye (Ed.), *Principles of organ transplantation.* Philadelphia: W.B.

Saunders Company.

Ryan, J.L. (1994). Bacterial diseases. In D.P. Stites, A.R. Terr, & T.G. Parslow (Eds.), *Basic and clinical immunology* (8th ed.). Norfolk, CT: Appleton & Lange.

Sager, S., & Ettenger, R. (1993). Kidney transplantation in children. *Seminars in Pediatric Surgery, 2,* 235-247.

Saidman, S.L., Duquesnoy, R.J., Demetris, A.J., McCauley, J., Ramos, H., Mazariegos, G., Shapiro, R., Starzl, T.E., & Fung, J.J. (1994). Combined liver kidney transplantation and effect of performed lymphocytotoxic antibodies. *Transplant Immunology, 2,* 61-67.

Sakr, M., Hassanein, T., Gavaler, J., AbuElmagd, K., Fung, J., Gordon, R., Starzl, T., & Van Thiel, D. (1992). Cytomegalovirus infection of the upper gastrointestinal tract following liver transplantation: Incidence, location, and severity in cyclosporine and FK 506-treated patients. *Transplantation, 53,* 86-91.

Salvatierra, O. (1987). Renal transplantation. In J.F. Glenn (Ed.), *Urologic surgery* (3rd ed.). Philadelphia: J.B. Lippincott Company.

San Filippo, F. (1990). Renal transplantation. In G.E.Sale (Ed.), *A pathology of organ transplantation.* Boston: Butterworths.

Sanchez-Urdazpal, L., Gores, G.J., Ward, E.M., Maus, T.P., Wahlstrom, H.E., Moore, S.B., Wiesner, R.H., & Krom, R.A. (1992). Ischemic-type biliary complications after orthotopic liver transplantation. *Hepatology, 16,* 49-53.

Sankari, B.R., Wyner, L.M., & Streem, S.B. (1994). Living-unrelated donor renal transplantation. *Urologic Clinics of North America, 21,* 293-298.

Sayhaje, L.H., Husberg, B.S., Klintmalm, G.B., et al. (1989). Vascular complications in adult liver transplant patients: Value of post operative dopler ultrasound surgery and the surgical management of hepatic arterial thrombosis. *Journal of Clinical Transplantation, 3,* 344-348.

Schwartz, B.D. (1991). The human major histocompatibility human leukocyte antigen (HLA) complex. In D.P. Stites & A.I. Terr (Eds.), *Basic and clinical immunology* (7th ed). Norwalk, CT: Appleton & Lange.

Schweizer, R.T., Rovelli, M., Palmer, D., Bossler, E., Hull, D., & Bartus, S. (1990). Noncompliance in organ transplant recipients. *Transplantation, 49,* 374-377.

Shaked, A, Thompson, M., Wilkinson, A.H., Nuesse, E., ElKhoury, G.F., Rosenthal, J.T., Danoviceh, G.M., & Busuttil, R.W. (1993). The role of combined liver-kidney transplantation in endstage hepatorenal disease. *American Surgeon, 59,* 606-609.

Simmons, R.L., Matas, A.J., Rattazzi, L.C., Balfour, H.H., Jr., & Najarian, J.S. (1977). Clinical characteristics of the lethal cytomegalovirus infection following renal transplantation. *Journal of Surgery, 82,* 537-546.

Sketris, I., Waite, N., Grobler, K., West, M., & Gerus, S. (1994). Factors affecting compliance with cyclosporine in adult renal transplant patients *Transplantation Proceedings, 26,* 2538-2541.

Smith, S.L. (1985). Liver transplantation: Implications for critical care nursing. *Heart & Lung, 14,* 617-628.

Smith, S.L. (1986). Physiology of the immune system. *Critical Care Quarterly, 9*(1), 713.

Smith, S.L. (1991). Immunologic aspects of transplantation. In S. Smith (Ed.), *Tissue and organ transplantation: Implications for professional nursing.* St. Louis: C.V. Mosby Company.

Smith, S.L., & Ciferni, S. (1990). Liver transplantation. In S.L. Smith. (Ed.), Tissue and organ transplantation: *Implications for professional nursing practice.* St. Louis: C.V. Mosby Company.

Snover, D.C. (1990). *The pathology of organ transplantation.* G.E. Sale (Ed.). Buttersworth, MA.

Solders, G., Wilczek, H., Gunnarsson, R., Tyder, G., Persson, A., & Groth, C.G. (1987). Effects of combined pancreatic and renal transplantation on diabetic neuropathy: A two-year follow-up study. *Lancet, 2*(8570), 1232-1235.

Sollinger, H., Knechtle, S., Reed, A., D'Alessandro, A., Kalayogu, M., Bezer, F., & Pirsch, J.D. (1991). Experience with 100 consecutive simultaneous kidney-pancreas transplant with bladder drainage. *Annals of Surgery, 214*(6), 703-711.

Sollinger, H.W., Stratta, R.J., D'Alesandro, A.M., Kalayodu, M., Pirsch, J.D., & Belzer, F.D. (1988). Experience with simultaneous pancreas-kidney transplantation. *Annals of Surgery, 208,* 475-483.

Sollinger, H.W., Stratta, R.J., Kalayogul, M., & Belzer, F.O. (1987). The University of Wisconsin experience in pancreas transplantation. *Transplantation Proceedings, 19,* 48-54.

Soon Shiong, D., White, G., Demayo, E., Koyle, M., & Danovitch, G. (1988). Mechanical obstruction of the protal vein as: A cause of vascular thrombosis after pancreas transplantation in man. *Transplantation Proceedings, 20,* 399-402.

Spital, A. (1988). Living kidney donation: When is it justified? *American Kidney Foundation Nephrology Letter, 5*(1), 115.

Spital, A. (1994). Unrelated living kidney donors: An update of attitudes and use among U.S. transplant centers. *Transplantation, 57,* 1722-1726.

Starzl, T.E., Demetris, A.J., Trucco, M., Zeevi, A., Rudert, W.A., Kocova, M., Ricordi, C., Ildstad, S., & Murase, N. (1992). Systemic chimerism in human female recipients of male livers. *Lancet, 340*(8824), 876-877.

Starzl, T.E., Demetris, A.J., & Van Thiel, D. (1989). Liver transplantation: Pt. 1. *New England Journal of Medicine, 321,* 1014-1022.

Starzl, T.E., Demetris, A.J., & Van Thiel, D. (1989). Liver transplantation: Pt. 2. *New England Journal of Medicine, 321,* 1092-1099.

Starzl, T.E., Iwatsuki, S. Van Thiel, D.H., Gartner, J.C., Zittelli, B.J., Malatack, J.J., Schade, R.R., Shaw, B.W., Jr., Hakala, T.R., Rosenthal, J.T., & Porter, K.A. (1982). Evolution of liver transplantation. *Hepatology, 2,* 614-636.

Staschak, S., & Zamberlan, K. (1990). Liver transplantation: Nursing diagnosis and management. In K.M. Sigardson Poor & L.M. Haggerty (Eds.), *Nursing care of the transplant recipient.* Philadelphia: W.B. Saunders Company.

Stephman, E., Gruber, S.A., Dunne, D.L., et al. (1991). Post transplant lymphoproliferative disorders. *Transplant Review, 5,* 120-129.

Stock, P.G., & Payne, W.D. (1990). Liver transplantation. *Critical Care Clinics, 6,* 911-926.

Straus, S.E., Cohen, J.I., Tosato, G., et al. (1993). Epstein Barr virus: Infection, biology, pathogenesis, and management. *Annals of Internal Medicine, 118,* 45-58.

Sturgiss, S.N., & Davidson, J.M. (1992). Effect of pregnancy on long-term function of renal allografts. *American Journal of Kidney Diseases, 19,* 167-172.

Sussman, N.L., Gislason, G.T., Conlin, C.A., & Kelly, J.H. (1994). The hepatic extracorporeal liver assist devise: Initial clinical experience. *Artificial Organs, 18,* 390-396.

Suthanthiran, M., & Strom, T.B. (1994). Renal transplantation. *New England Journal of Medicine, 331,* 365-374.

Sutherland, D.E.R., Moudry, K., & Najarian, J. (1988). Pancreas transplantation. In G.J. Cerilli (Ed), *Organ transplantation and replacement.* Philadelphia: J.B. Lippincott Company.

Sutherland, D.E. Gores, P.E., Hering, B.J., Wahoff, D., McKeehen, D.A., Gruessner, R.W. (1996). Islet transplant: An update. *Diabetes/Metabolism Review, 12*(2), 137-150.

Sutherland, D.E.R., Kendall, D.N., Moudry, K.C., et al. (1988). Pancreas transplantation in non-uremic type I diabetic recipients. *Surgery, 104,* 453-464.

Sutherland, D.E., Moudry, K.C., & Najarian, J.S. (1988). Pancreas transplantation. In G.J. Cerilli (Ed.), *Organ transplantation and replacement.* Philadelphia: J.B. Lippincott Company.

Sutherland, D.E.R., Goetz, F.C., & Najarin, S.S. (1979). Intraperitoneal transplantation of immediately vascularized segmental pancreatic grafts without duct ligation: A clinical trial. *Transplantation, 28,* 485-491.

Tanaka, K., Uemoto, S., Tokunaga, Y., Fujita, S., Sano, K., Nishizawa, T., Sawada, H., Shirahase, I., Kim, H.J., Yamaoka, Y., & Ozawa, K. (1993). Surgical techniques and innovations in living related liver transplantation. *Annals of Surgery, 217,* 82-91.

Task Force on Organ Transplantation. (1995). *Report to the Secretary in Congress on immunosuppressive therapy* (Publication No. HRP0906975). Rockville MD: Health Resources Administration.

Taylor, J.E., Calne, R.Y., & Stewart, W.K. (1991). Massive cystic hepatomegaly in a female patient with polycystic kidney disease treated by combined hepatic and renal transplantation. *Quarterly Journal of Medicine, 80,* 771-775.

Tesi, R.J., Elkhammas, E.A., Henry, M.L., & Ferguson, R.M. (1993). OKT3 for primary therapy of the first rejection episode in kidney transplants. *Transplantation, 55,* 1023-1029.

Thompson, J.M., McFarland, J.K, Hirsch, J.E., & Tucker, S.M. (1993). *Mosby clinical nursing* (3rd ed.) St. Louis: C.V.Mosby Yearbook.

Tilney, M.L., & Kirkman, R.L. (1986). Surgical aspects of kidney transplantation. In M.R. Garovoy & R.D. Guttmann (Eds.), *Renal transplantation.* New York: Churchill Livingstone.

Ting, A. (1988). HLA matching and crossmatching in renal transplantation. In P. Morris (Ed.), *Kidney transplantation: Principles and practice.* Philadelphia: W.B. Saunders Company.

Toledo-Pereyra, L.H. (Ed.). *Complications of organ transplantation.* New York: Marcel Dekker.

Toussaint, C., Cappel, R., Veereerstraeten, P., Kinnaert, P., Dupont, E., & Van Geertruyden, J. (1979). Grafts survival and response to hepatitis B virus in kidney recipients. *Transplant Proceedings, 11,* 89-92.

Trowsdale, J., Ragoussis, J., & Campbell, R.D. (1991). Map of the human MCC. *Immunology Today, 12,* 445-448.

Trusler, L.A. (1991). Simultaneous kidney pancreas transplantation. *ANNA Journal, 18,* 487-491.

Uchino, J., & Matsushita, A. (1994). Artificial liver strategies for liver rescue of patients with liver failure. *ASAIO Journal, 40*(1), 74-77.

United Network of Organ Sharing. (1994). Appendix D1 Cavtary Kidney Transplant Recipient. Appendix D2 Liver Donor Kidney Recipients. Appendix F2 Cadaveric Kidney Waiting List. *OPT and 1994 annual report. UNOS Scientific Registry Data,* July 29, 1994.

UNOS United Network for Organ Sharing. (1995). Pancreas transplantation in the United States as reported to UNOS and analyzed by the International Pancreas Transplant Registry. *Clinical Transplants,* 49-67.

U.S. 1994 annual data report. *Demographics of ESRD population.* Washington, D.C.: Author.

Velosa, J.A., Anderson, C.F., & Torres, V.E. (1985). Long-term renal status of kidney donors calculated small risk of kidney donors. *Transplant Proceedings, 17,* 100-103.

Ward, H.J., & Glassock, R.J. (1992). Glomerular diseases in renal transplants. In L.C. Paul & K. Solez (Eds.), *Organ transplantation: Long-term results.* New York: Marcel Dekker.

Weil, L., Barfield, N., Schroter, G.P., et al. (1985). Children of mothers with kidney transplants. *Transplant Proceedings, 17,* 1569-1570.

Wein, M.R., Kirkman, R.L., Strom, T.B., et al. (1985). Liver disease and recipients of long functioning renal graphs. *Kidney International, 28,* 839-844.

Whetham, J.C., Cardella, C., Harding, M. (1983). Effect of pregnancy on graft function and graft survival in renal cadaver transplant patients. *American Journal of Obstetrics and Gynecology, 145,* 193-197.

Wiesner, R.H. (1992). Acute cellular rejection following liver transplantation incidents: Risk factors and outcome in the NIDDK liver transplant database study. *Journal of Gastroenterology, 102,* 910.

Wiesner, R.H., Ludwig, J., Krom, R.A, Hay, J.E., & van Hoek, B. (1993). Hepatic allograph rejection: New developments in terminology, diagnosis, prevention, and treatment. *Mayo Clinic Proceedings, 68,* 69-79.

Wiesner, R.H., Ludwig, J., van Hoek, B., & Krom, R.A. (1992). Chronic hepatic allograph rejection: A review of ductopenic rejection and advantaging bioduct syndrome. In L.C. Paul & K. Solez (Eds.), *Organ transplantation: Long-term results.* New York: Marcel Dekker.

Wiesner, R.H., Ludwig, J., van Hoek, B., & Krom, R.A. (1991). Current concepts in cell mediated hepatic allograph rejection leading to ductopenia and liver failure. *Hepatology, 14,* 721-729.

Wiesner, R.H., Porayko, M.K., Lake, J.R., Batts, K.P., & Krom, R.A. (1993). Long-term management of liver transplant recipients. *Seminars Gastro Intestinal Disease, 4,* 151-164.

Wilkinson, A.H., Smith, J.L., Hunsicker, L.G., Tobacmin, J., Kapelanski, D.P., Johnson, M., Wright, F.H., Behrendt, D.M., & Corry, R.J. (1989). Increased frequency of post transplant lymphomas in patients treated with cyclosporine, azathioprine and prednisone. *Journal of Transplantation, 47,* 293-296.

Willis, B.G. & Post, L.C. (1990). Pancreas transplantation. In S.L. Smith (Ed.), Tissue and organ transplantation: *Implications for professional nursing practice.* St. Louis: C.V. Mosby Company.

Winkler, M.E., Niesert, S., Ringe, B., & Pichlmayr, R. (1993). Successful pregnancy in a patient after liver transplantation maintained on FK 506. *Transplantation, 56,* 751-753.

Wright, T.L., Donegan, E., Hsu, H.H., Ferrell, L., Lake, J.R., Kim, M., Combs, C., Fennessy, S., Roberts, J.P., Ascher, N.L., et al. (1992). Recurrent and acquired hepatitis C virus infection in liver transplant recipients. *Gastroenterology, 103,* 317-322.

Wrote, N.S. (1990). Alteration in immunity inflammation. In K.L. McCance & S.E. Huether (Eds.), *Path of physiology: The biological bases for disease in adults and children.* St. Louis: C.V. Mosby Company.

Young, L.S. (1994). Opportunistic infections in the immunocompromised host. In D.P. Stites, A.I. Terr, & T.G. Parslow (Eds.), *Basic and clinical immunology* (8th ed.). Norwalk, CT: Appleton & Lange.

Zekorn, T.D., Hordner, A., Mellert, J., Siebers, U., Altua, T., Eume, A., Hahn, H.J., Federlink. (1990). Biocompatibility and immunology in the encapsulation of islets of Langerhans. *International Journey of Artificial Organs, 19*(4), 251-257.

Chapter Highlights: Introduction and Chapter 23A

- In presenting the history of organ transplantation, one needs to acknowledge the achievements and interrelations of three distinct disciplines: surgery, immunobiology, and the law.
- In addition to identifying foreign substances, the immune system protects the host by 1) defending the host against invading organisms; 2) removing damaged cells from the circulation; and 3) acting as a surveillance network to recognize and protect against the development, growth, and dissemination of abnormal cells.
- The involvement of inflammatory processes in organ transplantation is primarily twofold. First, it is the body's initial attempt to destroy the foreign transplanted tissue; however, it is not the specific cause of organ transplant rejection. Second, surgical intervention triggers the inflammatory process to promote wound healing.
- The immune response has four unique characteristics. They include the ability to recognize self from nonself, respond to a nonself invader, remember the invader (memory), and regulate its action.
- Antibodies protect the host by binding to specific antigens and by initiating a number of immune regulatory activities such as directly attacking antigens through agglutination, neutralization, and lysis, activating the complement system, and triggering components of the inflammatory response.
- The amino acid sequence differs between light and heavy chains at the variable region allowing for greater flexibility of antigen binding. The constant region of the heavy chain has five main classes of amino acid sequences that determine the class of antibody (immunoglobulin [Ig]). The five classes are called IgG (gamma), IgA (alpha), IgM (mu), IgE (epsilon), and IgD (delta).
- The exact nature of the response is dependent on the chemical and physical qualities of the antigen, route of antigen entry, and the nature of the host including age, nutritional status, medical and immunization history, metabolic and hormonal factors, and genetics.
- The host response involves the immune response and the inflammatory response, which includes a number of factors that trigger the various aspects of inflammation known as inflammatory mediators. Although most aspects of inflammation are generally considered beneficial, excessive or inappropriate (e.g. organ transplants) inflammatory reactions can cause harm rather than host protection.
- An immunologic evaluation consists of two broad categories: typing and cross-matching. Typing procedures allow for pretransplant identification of specific antigens that could ultimately be responsible for donor-recipient incompatibility. Typing procedures include ABO blood typing, minor red cell antigens, and HLA typing. Matching procedures allow donor and recipient antigens to interact prior to transplantation to ascertain the degree of compatibility. Cross-matching can be performed between a recipient and a specific donor or a panel of random potential donors. Matching procedures include T cell cross-match, B cell cross-match, mixed lymphocyte cross-match, and mixed leukocyte culture.
- The primary function of the human immune system is to protect the host against foreign substances. If the foreign invader is a transplanted organ, this response can lead to destruction of the transplanted graft. Therefore, the success of transplantation is dependent on the alteration of the immune response.
- Immunosuppressive therapy has always attempted to prevent rejection. However, it has been juxtaposed with the risks of infection and malignancies. Thus, future advances in organ transplantation rest with the ability of immunosuppressive therapy to specifically target local responses of the immune system while simultaneously preserving the host's systemic immune system. One method for this to become a reality is through immunologic tolerance, which is the induction of immunologic unresponsiveness to a specific antigen.

Chapter Highlights: Chapter 23B

- Rejection is generally classified according to the primary cell type mediating the response and the histopathologic characteristics of the donor organ observed on biopsy. There are three main types of rejection: hyperacute, acute, and chronic.

- Acute rejection is the most common type of rejection occurring in transplant recipients.

- Approximately 75% of all organ transplant patients will develop one infectious episode the first year after transplant, and infection remains the principal cause of death in the transplant population.

- Infections in organ transplantation are based on three approaches: type of infection, time of infection, and site of infection.

- The symptomatology for CMV infections is the same for all organ transplants, except when it affects the transplanted organ itself. CMV has a greater effect on the organ transplanted than on native organs.

- The significance of haplotype matching has been demonstrated by improved graft survival. There have been definite improvements in graft survival with better degrees of matching specifically at the HLA-DR loci.

- The care is very similar for any patient who has undergone major surgery. Particular attention must be given to renal function and the pre-transplant long-term complications of uremia, the impact of immunosuppressive therapy, and the patient's adjustment to the transplant process. Therefore, caring for the kidney transplant recipient mandates advanced nursing diagnosis and assessment skills followed by prompt intervention.

- In the adult population, approximately 30-50% of recipients have hypertension 5 to 10 years after transplantation.

- Antihypertensive agents commonly used include two adrenergic blockers (e.g., propranolol), blocker-vasodilators (e.g., Labetalol), or adrenergic blockers (e.g., prazosin). If unsuccessful in effectively controlling blood pressure, vasodilators (e.g., hydralazine, nifedipine) or angiotensin converting enzyme inhibitors (e.g., enalapril) may be administered.

- The major causes of liver disease after kidney transplant are hepatitis B and hepatitis C.

- Hepatitis C virus (HCV) is the major cause of hepatitis, chronic liver disease, and possibly hepatocellular carcinoma in renal transplant recipients.

- Weight gain can be quite marked and become a devastating problem to some individuals after transplantation. It is the result of an improved state of well-being, removal of previous dietary restrictions, and steroid therapy.

- The goal of pancreas transplant is twofold: to provide an insulin-independent lifestyle and to prevent the secondary complications associated with diabetes.

- Pancreas transplantation has taken several forms since its inception in an animal model 35 years ago.

- Prior to the 1980s, the 1-year survival rate was less than 30%. In contrast, many programs now have 1-year survivals of greater than 85%. As a result, liver transplantation has become a widely accepted therapeutic treatment option for individuals with end-stage hepatic failure and metabolic disorders.

- Absolute contradictions typically include HIV seropositivity, extrahepatic malignancy, inability to comply with the immunosuppressive regimen posttransplant, active substance abuse, advanced cardiac or pulmonary disease (ejection fraction < 35%, pulmonary artery pressure >50, FEV1 < 50%, or PO2 < 55 mmHg without a intrapulmonary shunt), active infection, sepsis, and documented anatomic anomalies precluding transplantation.

- Relative contraindications include acute renal failure, advanced malnutrition, primary hepatobiliary malignancy, portal vein thrombosis, previous side-to-side or end to side portacaval shunt, chronic hepatitis B virus infection (HBsAg+), chronic hepatitis C infection, and severe psychosocial problems.

- Lake (1993) divides indications for liver transplantation into two categories, disease severity indicators and quality of life indicators. Disease severity indicators threaten the patients short-term survival. Quality of life indications for liver transplantation are those indicators that alter the patient's quality of life (from their perspective), but may not put the patient at risk of imminent death.

UNIT 7

Public Policy and Legislative Issues

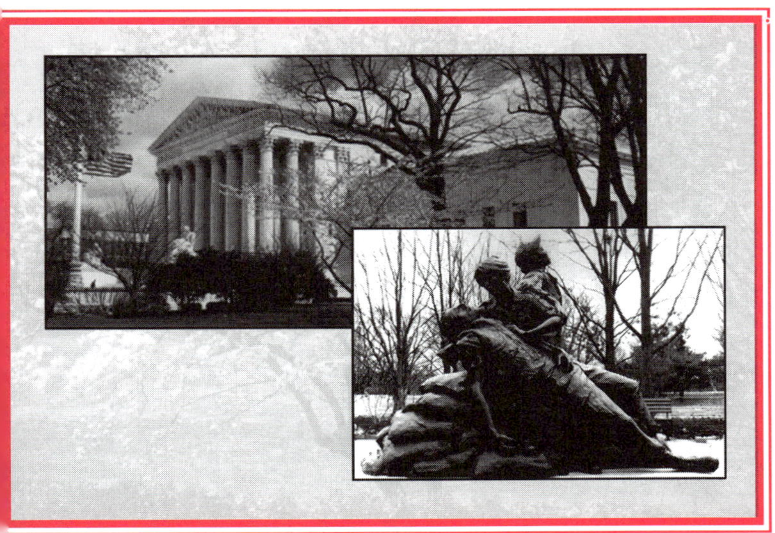

Unit Contents

Chapter 24
The Legislative Process. 781
Kathleen Smith, BS, RN, CNN

Chapter 25
The End Stage Renal Disease (ESRD) Program 795
Janel Parker, MSN, RN, CNN

CHAPTER 24

The Legislative Process

Kathleen Smith, BS, RN, CNN

Chapter Contents

The Importance of Action . . . 783
Structure of the Federal Government . . . 783
Executive Branch . . . 784
Judicial Branch . . . 784
Legislative Branch . . . 784
How a Bill Becomes Law . . . 784
Committee Structure . . . 786
Subcommittee Work . . . 786
Committee Work . . . 787
House and Senate Action . . . 787
The Voting Process . . . 787
Conference Committee . . . 787
Presidential Action . . . 787
Federal Budget Process . . . 787
Federal Regulatory Process . . . 788
Setting the Stage for Legislative Action . . . 788
The Process of Lobbying . . . 789
Nurses and Political Action . . . 789
Becoming Knowledgeable . . . 790
Preparing for Contact . . . 790
Communicating by Letter . . . 790
General Guidelines . . . 791
The Personal Visit . . . 791
Telephone Calls . . . 792
ANNA's Involvement in Legislative Arena . . . 792
1980s Activities . . . 792
1990s Activities . . . 792
Summary . . . 793
Chapter Highlights . . . 794

The Legislative Process

Kathleen Smith, BS, RN, CNN

These are years of rapid change in health care. Nurses face many challenges and have many opportunities to participate in and influence the formation of health care policy. Nurse citizens can become very effective in their lobbying efforts, whether on the federal, state, or local level, when they are armed with information about the key players, the processes, and their belief in what nursing can contribute to the health care system. The purpose of this chapter is to introduce nephrology nurses to the legislative process and the importance of their role in the development of public policy.

The Importance of Action

It has been said that for a democracy to function successfully, its citizens must be willing to participate in their government. The First Amendment of our Constitution, adopted in 1791, guarantees us the freedom of speech, the right to assemble, and the right to petition the government. Therefore, lobbying policy makers to make our interests and concerns heard is a key component of our democratic government.

Participation in government takes many forms. The single most important activity of citizens in a successful democracy is exercising the right to vote. This implies an understanding of the issues concerned and the potential impact brought about by election of the candidates. Other activities that citizens may involve themselves in include participating in campaigns; participating in organizations that promote or oppose certain legislative issues; contacting legislators about issues; and providing testimony at hearings. Citizens can even be involved in helping to originate and encourage the passage of specific legislation.

Much of nurses' professional lives will continue to be influenced by legislation, at both the state and national levels. For this reason, it is imperative that nurses take on these responsibilities of citizenship. For example, the nurse practice act in each state controls nursing education and practice. These laws can be eliminated, amended, or totally rewritten in the legislative process. In addition, any law that involves not only health care, but also general education and social issues, may well have an impact on nursing, sometimes only because they affect the patient populations with which nurses work. On the national level, previous or existing legislation such as Medicare, Social Security, Welfare reform, insurance reform, health professions' education programs, public health service programs, promotion of managed care, health research funding, and labor relations all affect nursing practice.

Keeping in mind that nursing is predominantly a female profession and that women only obtained the right to vote in 1924, it becomes easy to understand that nursing is barely out if its infancy in terms of developing its full potential in this area. Nurses still have a tendency to underestimate their strength in influencing legislation. But over the years there has also been increasing recognition that nurses must become involved in legislative issues. The consequences of nonparticipation are that someone else influences legislative decisions on health care in which nurses should have played a major role, or that nursing issues are overlooked altogether. For example, nurses were not involved in the drafting of Medicare legislation, which, when enacted in 1965, did not include any reimbursement mechanisms for nurses.

In recent years, a number of nurses have successfully run for local, state, and national offices. Eddie Bernice Johnson (D-TX) was the first registered nurse elected to Congress, although this did not occur until 1992.

Since the advent of the 18-year-old vote, nursing students have become increasingly active in legislative affairs, and often their impact has been felt. For example, they have been influential in the passage of state child-abuse legislation and they have been effective in providing testimony on federal funding for nursing education.

While nurses are becoming more sophisticated in the legislative process, they have not yet reached the full potential of their influence as individuals, as members of a profession that numbers over 2 million, and as members of other "power" groups. This is in part due to a lack of knowledge of the process itself and the resultant lack of understanding of the ways they can make their power felt and when they should take action.

The purpose of this chapter is to present an overview of the structure of the federal government and the legislative process and provides basic information needed to get involved in politics and policy making.

Structure of the Federal Government

The three branches of the United States government include the executive, the judicial, and the legislative branches (see Figure 24-1). Each branch

Figure 24-1
Structure of the federal government.

Legislative Branch	Executive Branch	Judicial Branch
CONGRESS: U.S. HOUSE OF REPRESENTATIVES/ U.S. SENATE General Accounting Office Congressional Budget Office Library of Congress - Congressional Research Service	WHITE HOUSE President Vice President Cabinet Federal Departments and Agencies Office of Management and Budget Council of Economic Advisors National Security Council	SUPREME COURT Courts of Appeal District Courts

has specific roles and functions and each participates in a system of checks and balances that is provided by the due process of law in a democratic government.

Executive Branch

Included in the executive branch are the office of the president and the vice president and the federal departments and agencies. The duties of the executive branch include recommending legislation, such as President Clinton's sweeping health care reform proposal, the Health Security Act of 1993, administering laws, and signing or vetoing legislation. Current executive branch policy is usually presented to a joint session of Congress and to the nation by the president in the State of the Union address each January. Within the executive branch of government, responsibility for health policy lies with the Department of Health and Human Services (DHHS).

Judicial Branch

The judicial branch of the government, the court system, has as its chief function the interpretation of laws and sometimes the changing of laws within its jurisdiction. One of the checks and balances in our system of government gives Congress the authority to supersede an unpopular Supreme Court decision by enacting new legislation. This has often been talked about in relation to the 1973 Roe vs. Wade abortion decision, but to date, the Supreme Court's ruling remains intact.

Legislative Branch

The legislative branch of government consists of the Congress and its primary responsibility is to make laws. It is called the "heart of the government" because of its responsibility to listen and respond to the needs of the people. Our federal legislature is bicameral, meaning it has two chambers, the House of Representatives and the Senate. While the House has the constitutional responsibility to originate legislation that deals with raising revenue and spending it, sole authority rests in the Senate to approve the ratification of treaties, nominations by the president, and federal circuit court and Supreme Court nominations.

How a Bill Becomes Law

Nurses have long been involved in the drafting of policy and the procedures to carry them out within their employer organizations. In much the same way, national health policy is crafted. At the federal level, however, such policies are written in the form of laws passed by the Congress (see Figure 24-2). The procedures for carrying out these laws are expressed in federal regulations and published in the *Federal Register.*

A bill faces difficult odds in wending its way through the House and Senate. For example, in the 103rd Congress, which was in session during calendar years 1993 and 1994, 9,822 measures were introduced, while only 2,037 were made law (20%) (see Figure 24-3). The only measures assured of passage are those that provide annual funds that keep the government operating. Otherwise, it takes strong White House support or the support of a substantial number of lawmakers for a bill to survive.

A bill can be introduced in either house of Congress, or it can be introduced in both houses simultaneously. Anyone can initiate a bill. It is a citizen's demand for action and it can originate from an individual, who takes his complaints or ideas to a legislator, or it can originate within and be put

Figure 24-2
The path of legislation.

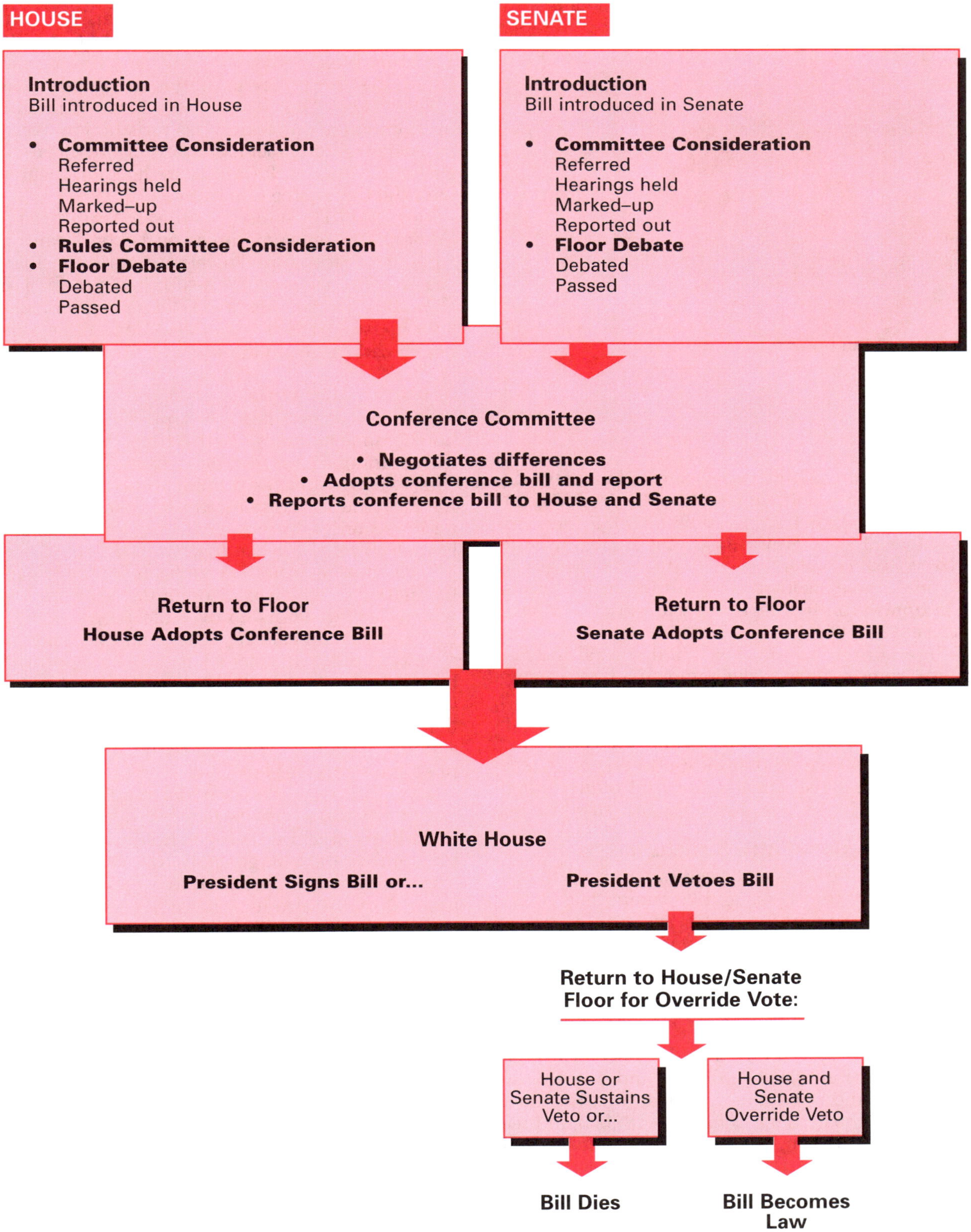

Figure 24-3
How many bills become law?

Percentage of Bills Introduced That Became Law In the 103rd Congress

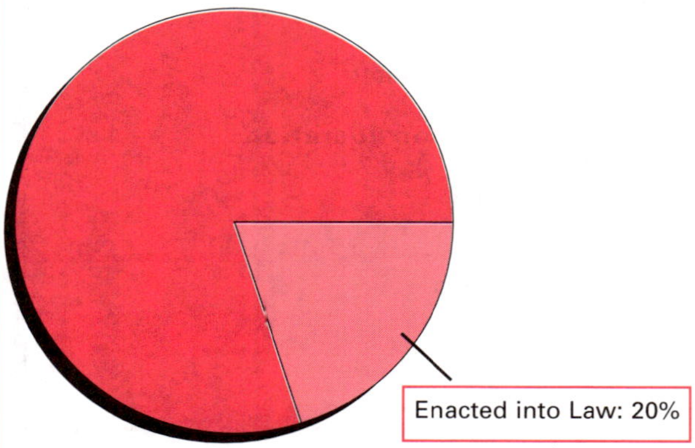

forth by a special interest group. Obviously, the larger and more politically active the group is, the better chance they have of being heard. If there are a number of such groups, representing even more citizens (that is, voters) with an interest in the issue, they may come together as a coalition in support of or in opposition to a legislative proposal and have even more clout.

In addition to individuals and special interest groups, some common originators of bills are a governmental administrator, agency or department, a delegation of citizens in a legislator's district, a legislative committee, or the legislator himself. Many more citizens involve themselves in responding to legislation that has already been introduced than are involved in the initial introduction of a bill.

Committee Structure

Much of the work of Congress occurs in the 20 committees of the House and 20 committees of the Senate. Each committee has jurisdiction over certain areas of public policy. Committees are further divided into subcommittees; 32 in the House and 26 in the Senate. Virtually all bills are sent to these panels after introduction, and many die there as a result of inaction.

The two major committees in the Senate that have jurisdiction over health care and oversee the activities of the Department of Health and Human Services are the Finance Committee, Subcommittee on Health, with jurisdiction over Medicare and Medicaid, and the Labor and Human Resources Committee, which authorizes programs under the Public Health Service Act, including federal funding of nursing education and research, National Institutes of Health programs, the Centers for Disease Control and Prevention, and the Food and Drug Administration.

In the House of Representatives there are also two major committees that are primarily responsible for health issues. The Commerce Committee, Subcommittee on Health and the Environment, authorizes the programs under the Public Health Service Act. The Ways and Means Committee, Subcommittee on Health, has jurisdiction over the physician reimbursement part of Medicare and shares jurisdiction for Medicare hospital insurance with the Commerce Committee.

In both houses, the Appropriations Committees, Subcommittees on Labor, Health and Human Services, and Education, are responsible for yearly appropriations for health items in the federal budget, except Medicare. Other committees in both houses, such as the Budget Committees, affect health care issues in their work.

Subcommittee Work

Once a committee takes up a bill, it usually holds public hearings. At this time, the members of the committee hear testimony from the bill's sponsors, expert witnesses, administration officials, and interest groups. Written testimony can be submitted for the record if the group or individual is not asked to participate at the hearing.

The next step in the process is for the bill to go to "markup," which is a committee session during which the legislators go over the proposal line by line and vote on changes. The committee then considers the bill. The outcome is either to approve the bill (report it out to the full committee) with or without amendments, some of which can change the nature of the bill completely; to "kill," or stop action on the bill; or to draft a new bill to accomplish the same goal but in a different manner.

The subcommittee to which a bill is referred is the first place where its fate can be influenced. If the bill is never put on the committee agenda or is not approved, it will generally not proceed further. The chairman has the power to keep the bill off the agenda, or to introduce it early or at a favorable time.

To get the desired action, which may be any of the above, interested persons/groups begin their legislative action at this point. All members of the subcommittee, and especially the chairman, are important targets for the individuals or organizations that want to see the bill move forward. Individual members of these organizations whose legislators sit on the subcommittee may be asked to contact their legislator because of the influential position he or she has over the fate of the legislation at this point. Letters, phone calls, telegrams, fax messages, and personal contact are used to reach the chairman and other committee members.

Committee Work

The same process outlined for subcommittees takes place at the full committee level, the next step in the legislative process for a bill that is reported out of the subcommittee. Opportunity for citizen/organization action occurs in the same way, focusing this time on the chairman and members of the full committee.

A bill that survives committee action is then scheduled for action "on the floor," meaning the total membership of the body. Under certain circumstances, amendments may be proposed at this stage and are approved or rejected by the majority of those assembled.

House and Senate Action

In the House, most bills approved by committee proceed to the Rules Committee to determine how the bill will be handled on the House floor, how much time will be allotted for debate and whether amendments will be permitted. The Majority Leader, who is chosen by the party controlling a majority of seats, decides when to call-up a bill for action. Members are given a limited amount of time to speak for or against the measure. Most issues are dealt with in a few hours.

In the Senate, bills approved by committees go directly to the calendar and are taken up whenever the Majority Leader of that body decides to call them. There are fewer limits on debate in the Senate than in the House and rules allow members to speak twice for as long as they want on any issue before the Senate.

In light of this, to speed action on a bill, the majority leader may seek "unanimous consent" to vote at a certain time. If a member objects to this, a motion to limit debate (and therefore prevent a bill's opponents from "filibustering," may be offered. The procedure, called cloture, requires 60 affirmative votes. This is often difficult to obtain on closely divided issues. The Majority Leader rarely proceeds on an issue that he wants to succeed until he is assured of at least 60 votes.

The Voting Process

Roll-call votes in the House are cast electronically, each member using a plastic card and inserting it in terminals located throughout the chamber. The Senate still votes by voice; each Senator replies "aye" or "nay" as the roll is called. After a bill passes one chamber, it is sent to the other for a complete repetition of the process it went through in the first chamber.

Conference Committee

If the bill passed by the House and the one passed by the Senate are not the same, or if the bill has been amended by the second house after passing the first, and the first house does not agree with the amendments, the bill is sent to a conference committee.

This committee consists of an equal number of members of each house and usually includes members from the committees that originally handled the bills. Once the members of the conference committee are named by the leadership, opportunity for citizen action begins again.

The conference committee attempts to work out a compromise that will be accepted by both houses. Sometimes, however, the two houses are not able to arrive at a compromise and the bill dies, but usually an agreement is reached. The conference report, issued by the committee when it achieves a compromise, is sent to both chambers for vote. The compromise bill must be approved by each chamber before it is sent to the White House for signing by the President.

Presidential Action

After passing both houses, the bill goes to the President. If he approves it or fails to take action within 10 days, the bill becomes law. If Congress adjourns before the 10 days in which the President should sign the bill, it does not become law. This is known as a "pocket veto." The President may veto the bill and return it to the house of origin. A two-thirds affirmative vote in both houses for repassage is necessary to override the veto. Voting on a veto is often along party lines.

With such a complicated system of checks and balances provided by the due process of law in a democratic government such as the United States, often accompanied by extreme political pressure from within the government and influence of lobbyists, it is easy to understand why it is so difficult and time-consuming to translate an idea for legislation into statutory law.

Federal Budget Process

In early February each year, the president is required to submit his budget request to the Congress. This document represents a year of work by agency officials, who channel their budget requests up to the cabinet level and through the Office of Management and Budget. It is their responsibility to reconcile the requests with the president's programs. Within 6 weeks after receiving the president's proposed budget, all standing House and Senate committees submit their views and estimates of expenditures for the coming year for programs under their jurisdiction to their respective budget committees. The House and Senate budget committees set economic priorities and make spending recommendations to the appropriations and tax committees.

Each spring, Congress is required to pass a concurrent budget resolution that limits the level of funds that the appropriations committees can approve. The resolution establishes a number of things, including targets for and ceilings on total federal spending and budget authority, targets for appropriations and other forms of spending in the budget, and a floor on total revenues. Once approved by Congress, the resolution serves as a guide to the appropriations and other spending committees on the amount of funding available for programs within their jurisdiction.

The annual congressional budget cycle is composed of three main processes: authorization, appropriations, and budget resolution. An authorization bill is a prerequisite for an appropriation bill. Passed through the process described above, authorizing legislation specifies the substance of federal programs and the agency that will implement them, and establishes program policies and the program's budget limit. A program may be authorized annually or less frequently. Renewal or modification of such programs is known as reauthorization. Responsibility for authorizing most health care programs rests with the Ways and Means and Commerce Committees in the House and with the Finance and Labor and Human Resources Committees in the Senate.

Once an authorization bill is enacted, Congress must also pass yearly appropriation bills to determine the actual amount of funds that will be available for the authorized program. The appropriations process also determines how much funding each department or agency receives for a specific fiscal year. If zero funds are appropriated, the program is essentially dead for that fiscal year.

Within the appropriations committees there are 9 subcommittees in the Senate and 7 subcommittees in the House. The House and Senate subcommittees on Labor, Health and Human Services and Education appropriate the funds for most health programs. Because the Constitution requires all revenue measures to originate in the House of Representatives, it initiates all appropriations and taxation bills. Therefore, the House Appropriations Committee plays a major role in crafting spending bills. Interest groups and agencies appeal to the Senate Appropriations Committee when they disagree with the funding decisions made in the House.

As the federal fiscal year begins on October 1, it is expected that all appropriations bills for the new fiscal year will be enacted by that date. When this is not the case, to avoid a shutdown of the federal government, a continuing resolution may be passed by Congress that permits federal agencies to continue to operate at their current funding level until their regular appropriations bills are enacted.

The Budget Enforcement Act of 1990 established "pay-as-you-go" entitlements and revenues, which means that any changes Congress makes in taxes and mandatory spending, such as entitlement programs, must be budget neutral. That is, they cannot contribute to the deficit by reducing taxes or increasing spending without corresponding offsets. With few exceptions, tax increases or cuts in entitlement programs would be necessary to pay for tax cuts or increases in spending.

Federal Regulatory Process

Action on a bill does not end with its passage. Laws are usually written very generally, as too much specificity makes them quickly obsolete. After a law is passed, it is sent to the particular federal agency that is responsible for writing the regulations to implement the law. These regulations are as important as the law itself; they have the force of law and they spell out the specifics of how it will be carried out.

It is possible to influence policy at this point also and to strengthen or weaken the intent of the law. The opportunity to contribute to the development of regulations is available to interested organizations, which may make recommendations for individual appointments on advisory committees or offer informal participation and cooperation. The American Nephrology Nurses' Association (ANNA) has such a relationship with the Health Care Financing Administration, the agency within the Department of Health and Human Services that is responsible for managing the federal Medicare and Medicaid programs.

Setting the Stage for Legislative Action

Influencing legislation cannot occur unless there is clear understanding of how our government works, how a bill becomes law, and how the legislative branch of government interacts with the executive and judicial branches. The congressional leadership is of critical importance; they are elected by their colleagues, they guide bills through the legislative process, and they act as chief advocates for the legislative agendas of their parties. A primary example of this is Speaker of the House Newt Gingrich's (R-GA) masterminding and spearheading of the 10-point Republican agenda contained in the Contract with America through the House during the first 100 days of the 104th Congress, as promised during the campaign of 1994.

Most legislators are elected on platforms, either their own or their party's, and on promises for action that they make to their constituents. These platforms set their goals, the fulfillment of which comes with successful passage of appropriate legislation. However, they must also vote on other legislation to the satisfaction of their constituents. Most legislators want to be reelected to the same or higher office; many of their actions while in office reflect this desire.

As mentioned previously, during each 2-year Congress, lawmakers wade through thousands of bills, many of them on very intricate issues, only a small fraction of which are enacted into law. Obviously, not all of the bills introduced are brought to a vote, and certainly not all are of interest to nurses, but legislators need information on at least those bills that are of importance to their interests and constituents. On a typical workday, members of Congress scurry between committee hearings and meetings and sessions in the House or Senate chamber while trying to squeeze in meetings with constituents, lobbyists, and visiting dignitaries.

To help cope with their expanded workload, lawmakers have grown increasingly dependent on their staffs, a diverse group of lawyers, accountants, clerks, and others who act as secretaries, aides, assistants, researchers, and policy analysts. In short, they keep the legislative machinery informed. These individuals review the issues and summarize background information on key bills and brief the legislators on the issues. They are very influential individuals in that the legislators generally use this information to decide how they will vote. These individuals get information from numerous sources; organization representatives, individuals, and lobbyists usually become acquainted and maintain good relationships with them, providing information about the issues with which the legislator must deal. When nurses are not involved in this process they find that the legislator may have received information about nursing that is either inaccurate, incomplete, obsolete, or skewed in another group's favor.

Placement on committees, where most preliminary action on bills takes place, is a measure of the influence a legislator has. Committee appointments are made by party leaders in each chamber of the Congress, that is, House and Senate. Committee chairmanships are particularly powerful positions; the chairmen are usually members of the majority party with seniority in their respective chambers. Some committees are more prestigious than others and are sought after eagerly. It is extremely important for citizens to know the committees on which their legislators sit because the action of committees affects the future of bills.

Congress is usually slow to act on controversial issues. The majority of lawmakers want to avoid the forefront of change for many reasons, including the wide diversity in political views that exists, regional interests, and general political caution. Congress seems more comfortable following trends than creating them such that it often takes a groundswell of public pressure or a national crisis to shape consensus.

As a rule, the Senate is less reactive than the House, primarily because the senators are elected only every 6 years as opposed to House members who must be reelected every 2 years. Also, House members are much closer to their constituents geographically as there is one Congressional representative for a specific number of citizens. This is very different from the Senate, where there are two senators from each state, regardless of size. This structure, purposefully designed by our founding fathers, makes the Senate less compelled to react immediately to issues.

One example of a national crisis providing the driving force for change is the obsession of the 104th Congress with the federal budget deficit. Lawmakers have been preoccupied with this issue for many years while at the same time they seem to have ignored the rising tide of red ink by enacting tax-and-spend programs. Only now are members talking and acting seriously about getting the budget under control.

The Process of Lobbying

The increasing complexity of public issues has forced lawmakers to rely heavily on the expertise and opinions of professional and trade associations, as well as business, labor, and industry groups. Such expertise is provided by lobbyists, who are paid representatives of interest groups, many of which, depending on the size and contribution power of their constituencies, wield considerable power in legislative bodies.

It is important to remember that individual citizens can also "lobby" for or against legislation. Although there is a certain mysticism about the process of lobbying, it is quite simply an attempt to legitimately influence legislators to promote or suppress proposed legislation.

Influencing the lawmaking process involves educating the legislators and staff members who decide what issues to consider in a given congressional year and who vote on those issues as they move through the legislative process. This process of influencing, or lobbying, is nothing more than educating, marketing, and selling. These are not foreign concepts to nurses who spend their days educating patients and colleagues, marketing ideas to physicians to get appropriate orders written, and selling good health habits or practices to patients. There is no special skill set required of nurses who decide they want or need to involve themselves in the legislative process.

There are numerous ways in which lobbyists attempt to influence legislators. Much is on the basis of direct contact in personal meetings and semisocial gatherings. Lobbyists provide information to the legislators and their staff, and introduce resource people to them. They are also valuable in that they keep their interest group informed about any pertinent legislation and aid the group in effective action.

Nurses and Political Action

From the foregoing, it can be seen that nurses and nursing students are major stakeholders in legislation. Whether acting as individuals or as part of groups, such as ANA and ANNA, they can make an impact on the political scene.

Learning to effectively communicate with legislators is essential to achieving positive results.

While legislators want, and often need, to hear from their constituents, their time is limited. Carefully planned and organized contacts are usually the most effective means of communication with One way that individuals 'lobby" is through membership in a professional association that establishes a legislative agenda and works as a group, and in coalitions with other like groups, to advance the agenda. For nurses, supporting these organizations with dues and making their opinions heard through various available mechanisms are some ways of indirectly influencing the legislative process.

However, to effectively influence a specific piece of legislation, multiple lobbying strategies need to be employed. ANNA's Board of Directors typically prepares a letter outlining the association's official position with regard to a specific piece of legislation that it is interested in. The letter is distributed to all members of the subcommittee or full committee to which the measure has been referred.

However, the individual members of those committees are more strongly influenced by what their own constituents tell them about a bill than they are by any other factors. This is where individual citizens become critical to the process and to their specialty association's ability to truly influence legislation. At this point, more direct lobbying techniques are necessary, such as communicating with legislators. This communication can take several forms, such as letters, phone calls, and/or personal visits.

Becoming Knowledgeable

A number of ways exist for nurses to become more knowledgeable in matters of legislation. The American Nurses' Association and its constituent state groups take a very active role in legislation, as does the National Student Nurses' Association. A number of specialty nursing organizations devote significant resources to get involved in the legislative issues that affect their membership and its specific patient population. The major legislative activities of the nursing associations are discussed in the local chapters of these organizations. In addition, members are kept informed about legislation through the written materials of organizations. All major nursing journals routinely report key national legislative efforts and even those on the state level that have particular significance.

Another way for nurses to become more informed is by reading the newspaper. Feature articles, news stories, and editorials may not cover narrow pieces of legislation of special interest to nurses, such as reauthorization of the Nurse Education Act or funding for the National Institute for Nursing Research, but broader bills will be reported on, such as changes in the Medicare and Medicaid programs and welfare reform. Some newspapers list the major bills in the state legislature and in Congress, the action taken on those bills, and their current status. The votes of legislators on particular bills is also occasionally reported. This information enables readers to follow the path of a bill and to see how their legislators vote in general. The League of Women Voters and other political action groups can also be a source of such information.

One of the first pieces of information that nurses need to become familiar with is the names of their own legislators. One way to begin is to call the local municipal building or the County Clerk's office. A local or state League of Women Voters branch is also a good source, as is the district and state nurses' association. The state nurses' associations are usually headquartered in the state capital. Registration and voting are, of course, important, since voters are more influential than their nonvoter counterparts.

Preparing for Contact

Prior to contacting legislators, it is important to do some preparation on the issue at hand *and* on your legislators. With regard to the latter, make sure you are aware of your legislators' party affiliations and whether they have an interest in or any prior knowledge about the issue in question.

Legislators' local offices can be contacted, and are usually listed in the blue pages of the telephone book. Simply tell the staff what the issue is and ask if the legislator has taken a position on it or not. To call legislative offices in Washington, dial (202) 224-3121 for the Senate information operator and (202) 225-3121 for the House operator. Callers will be connected directly to their legislator's office, and operators will provide the direct phone number for future reference.

Communicating by Letter

While this section focuses on writing a letter to a Congressional representative, it applies as well to writing state assembly representatives, city council members, the governor, the mayor, or even the President of the United States. The essentials of developing a letter to influence a policy maker are the same regardless of the intended recipient.

For members of Congress, letters can be mailed or sent via facsimile to the legislator's office. This is especially helpful if time is critical, and fax numbers are available from the legislator's offices.
The Inside Address and Salutation should look like this...

The Honorable Full Name
United States Senate
Washington, DC 20510
Dear Senator ___________:

U.S. House of Representatives
Washington, DC 20515
Dear Representative ______________:
or
Dear Congressman/Congresswoman _______:

The writer should identify herself immediately in the opening paragraph as (a) a constituent, by indicating residence; (b) as a health care professional, including any relevant information that may be helpful, such as place of employment and the nature of work done, the patient population affected, etc.; and (c) as a member of a large group or coalition, such as ANNA or state nurses' association, which suggests strength in numbers. It may be important at times, however, to differentiate between issues that are of personal interest from those of any associations you belong to. Enough background should be provided to establish the writer as knowledgeable and credible in the specific area or issue of interest At the end of the paragraph, state the issue and the purpose for the writing.

General Guidelines

In terms of discussing the issue there are several rules of thumb:

Rule #1: Be specific. Use the actual bill number if you know it. Share your position on the issue and why you have come to that position. Ask for your legislator's position on this issue. If you can, include information on the local impact of a specific proposal. Tell the Member what you want done, for example do you want the Member to cosponsor the bill to add support to it, do you want to urge hearings on the matter, or do you want a particular vote? Look for the Member to make a commitment and ask for a response.

Rule #2: Be brief and to the point. Legislators and their staff have very little time, and long letters and documents will not be read. Limit letters to one page and focus on one issue per letter. Pare down support material to a concise fact sheet, double-spaced, with bullets and good statistics and information that can easily be seen "at a glance;" such material will be kept and referred to as necessary.

Rule #3: Be constructive. If you think a particular bill is the wrong approach, explain what you think the correct approach would be.

Rule #4: Be persistent. One contact probably will not be enough. Call the office a week or so after you have sent a letter to ask if it was received and to discuss it further with the appropriate staff member. (The staff members are assigned different types of issues. Typically, you will want to speak to the legislative assistant [LA] for health.) Ask for an appointment to discuss it with the legislator when he or she is in town. Keep the heat on!

Rule #5: Be courteous. It is not wise to threaten any kind of action if you don't get what you want from the legislator. If a vote is contrary to your position, let the Member know politely how you feel.

Rule #6: Keep in regular contact. This need not be time-consuming and is important in relationship building. Send a note of thanks for a specific vote or for some activity that was held locally. Such behavior makes asking for something later a lot easier.

Rule #7: Report back. Let your organizations know what you have done. If you receive a reply letter from your Member that indicates support, the association leadership can use that letter in Washington to ensure that support. Sometimes Members say they cannot support a measure because they haven't heard from their constituents. Knowing that letters were sent and having copies of them can be very helpful.

Rule #8: Say Thank You. Always thank your legislator for time spent in a meeting or on the phone, or for a vote on your issue.

In closing the letter, establish yourself as a source of information and offer your assistance as a resource for more information. Prepare to be called if your issue becomes a hot topic. Invite the Member or the staff to your workplace if that would help illustrate your point.

In terms of the form your letter takes, typed personal letters are more suspect than handwritten ones. Members say handwritten letters are the only way to ensure that a personal letter is, in fact, personal. The next best thing would be to print the letter on personal stationery.

It cannot be stressed enough how much *your letter counts!* Sometimes specific letters are read by the Members on the floor of the House or Senate; some letters are shared with colleagues if they illustrate a point particularly well. Members are told every day how much correspondence came in to both the district and Washington offices on a particular topic. Your voice will be heard. Don't forget to spread the word to others with whom you work or network. Urge them to write as well.

The Personal Visit

Personal visits with legislators and staff members are a very effective means of grassroots lobbying. It is generally wise to be on time and to stick to the agreed-upon time frame, to be friendly and polite, to greet the legislator with a firm handshake, and to keep the visit short. As with letter writing, it is important to identify yourself as a nurse and to offer to be a resource in the area of health care with which you are most familiar. Also identify early in the meeting the purpose of your visit. Present the facts in an orderly manner, be succinct, and avoid jargon or too many statistics.

It is thoughtful to comment on any of the legislator's bills or votes of which you approve and it is appropriate to ask if the legislator has taken a position on the issue you are there to discuss. Most of the guidelines for letter writing are also applicable to personal visits, including telling the legislator or staff member what you want the legislator to do and asking when you might have an answer on the legislator's position on your issue. If you are asked a question you cannot answer, do not lie; simply promise to get the information and provide it to them at a later date. This is one way to establish yourself as a reliable source of information that could improve your access to your legislator in the future.

At the end of the meeting, establish agreement on when you should follow-up and with whom, and then do so. Leave a one or two-page fact sheet that summarizes the issue and your position and one that includes the name and phone number of a contact person if there should be a need for further information. Leave behind your business card as well. Remember the value of saying thank you and follow-up after the meeting with a letter thanking the legislator or staff member. Take this opportunity to reiterate your position, and include any information requested during the meeting.

Telephone Calls

Telephone calls are best for obtaining information. Lobbying calls should be kept very short. When making the call, ask for the legislative assistant who handles health issues since this person can give you the best indication of the Member's position on the issue. If you do not know your legislator's Washington office telephone number, call the Capitol switchboard at (202) 225-3121 (House) or (202) 224-3121 (Senate) and ask to be connected.

ANNA's Involvement in Legislative Arena

The American Nephrology Nurses' Association (ANNA) began its involvement in the legislative and regulatory arenas under the leadership and direction of Nancy Sharp during her tenure on the Board of the Directors and as the association's president in 1981-1982. The association established a Government Relations Committee to formally begin its journey into these arenas.

1980s Activities

When it was still known as the American Association of Nephrology Nurses and Technicians (AANNT), the association's first Legislative Policy Statement appeared in November 1983 (see Appendix E). It was a bold and visionary statement that addressed topics such as open physician staffing in dialysis facilities, the use of advanced practice nurses with reimbursement for their services under Medicare, elimination of certificate of need, and support for cost containment efforts in the ESRD program. This marked the first time the association had taken a public position on these issues. Many of the tenets, such as support for efforts to increase organ donation and the development of national standards and guidelines for the reprocessing of disposables and for water treatment safety, remain appropriate well into the 1990s (see Appendix F).

The 1983 document supported concepts such as access, quality, patient responsibility, data collection and reporting, cost effectiveness, and research. It even called for coverage of immunosuppressive drugs under Medicare. Given the contents of this document, it is clear that ANNA's Government Relations Committee was off to a very strong start.

Some of the early committee activities included two Head Nurse Surveys (one in 1984 and one in 1987) to evaluate the impact of the ESRD prospective payment regulations/reductions in reimbursement on the delivery of care in dialysis facilities. In 1983 and 1984, the committee was very involved with then-Congressman Albert Gore and his staff as they were beginning to research the issues involved in organ transplantation. These activities resulted in the passage of the National Organ Transplant Act and the establishment of the Division of Organ Transplantation in the Health Resources and Services Administration of the Public Health Service, the Organ Procurement and Transplantation Network, and the Scientific Registry. Over the years, the committee has provided written and oral testimony to major House and Senate committees on such as topics as reuse, organ transplantation, the composite rate, and immunosuppressive drug coverage, and has responded to all proposed regulations that would affect the ESRD program.

In 1985 the association took a major step and hired a part-time legislative consultant. Years later, this became a half-time position, further demonstrating ANNA's commitment in this area.

Although the appointment of the state legislative representatives began during 1986-1987, it was during 1988-1989 that the State Legislative Representative Program was established to provide ANNA with a grassroots lobbying network and to provide the committee with information about state legislative activities. A Legislative Handbook was published and distributed for use by these state representatives, and the committee was reorganized with its members — regional advisors — coordinating the legislative activities within their regions. In 1993 the number of regional advisors was increased to two, with a legislative representative in almost every ANNA chapter.

1990s Activities

In 1990-1991, the Government Relations Committee became the Legislative Committee, and its first meeting was held in Washington, DC. During the following year, the first Legislative Workshop for 50 ANNA legislative representatives was held in Washington; a chapter-level continuing education program was developed, entitled "Influencing the Legislative Process;" the legislative handbook was revised; and four reading packets were distributed to chapter legislative representatives.

In 1992-1993, to further increase grassroots participation in the legislative process, a section for legislative representatives was added to the *ANNA Chapter Officer Orientation Manual*, and the number of legislative representatives continued to grow. The Second Legislative Workshop was held in March 1994 in Washington, DC, with nearly 50 legislative representatives in attendance lobbying their elected officials on Capitol Hill.

One of the objectives of this committee has been to encourage more nurses to learn about and to incorporate legislative activity and public policy information into their professional activities. To that end, the committee and the legislative consultants have kept the membership informed through numerous articles in both the *ANNA Update* and the *ANNA Journal*; publishing the Legislative Agenda and Legislative Policy Statement each year after they are revised (see Appendix F); and sharing all formal letters, testimonies, and responses to proposed regulations in these publications. Since 1985, the year of the first Nurse in Washington Internship, ANNA members have participated in the planning of the event, have served as faculty, and have supported it with their attendance.

ANNA continues to stay involved with other nephrology organizations, including the National Renal Administrators Association (NRAA), the American Association of Kidney Patients (AAKP), the Renal Physicians Association (RPA), the National Association of Nephrology Technicians (NANT), and the more inclusive Renal Coalition as we anticipate the impact of various health care reform measures. Work continues in lobbying for appropriate funding levels for the National Institute for Nursing Research, and the Nurse Education Act. Collaboration continues with the Health Care Financing Administration and the ESRD Networks in support of quality initiatives in the ESRD program.

ANNA's Board of Directors, Legislative Committee, and legislative consultant continually monitor and respond to issues affecting nursing, Medicare, and the ESRD program, providing information to policy makers on Capitol Hill, regulatory agencies, and those who influence policy decisions on various government boards and commissions. This is done based on ANNA's Legislative Agenda, which is updated and approved by the Board of Directors each year. The legislative agenda is to a large extent based on the association's Long-Range Strategic Plan.

Summary

As nursing activist Peggy Chinn has said, "For the remainder of this century, the most worthy goal that nurses can select is that of arousing their passion for a kind of political activism that will make a difference in their own lives and in the life of society."

References/Readings

American Nephrology Nurses' Association. (1996) *ANNA legislative handbook*. Pitman, NJ: Author.

Smith, K. (1994). ANNA's involvement in legislative arena targets all levels of government. In *ANNA: Celebrating 25 years of service to the Nephrology Community* (p. 20). Pitman, NJ: Author.

Chapter Highlights

- The First Amendment of our Constitution, adopted in 1791, guarantees us the freedom of speech, the right to assemble, and the right to petition the government. Therefore, lobbying policy makers to make our interests and concerns heard is a key component of our democratic government.
- Much of the professional lives of nurses is, and will continue to be, influenced by legislation at both the state and national levels. For this reason, it is imperative that nurses take on these responsibilities of citizenship.
- Nurses still have a tendency to underestimate their strength in influencing legislation.
- Over the years there has been increasing recognition that nurses must become involved in legislative issues or they find, after the fact, that someone else has made legislative decisions on health care in which they should have had a major voice.
- While nurses are becoming more sophisticated in the legislative process, they have not yet reached the full potential of their influence as individuals, as members of a profession that numbers over 2 million, and as members of other "power" groups.
- The Legislative Branch of government consists of the Congress and its primary responsibility is to make laws. It is called the "heart of the government" because of its responsibility to listen and respond to the needs of the people.
- After a law is passed, it is sent to the particular federal agency that is responsible for writing the regulations to implement the law. These regulations are as important as the law itself; they have the force of law and they spell out the specifics of how it will be carried out.
- Influencing legislation cannot occur unless there is clear understanding of how our government works, how a bill becomes law, and how the Legislative Branch of government interacts with the executive and the judicial branches.
- It is extremely important for citizens to know the committees on which their legislators sit because actions of committees affect the future of bills.
- The increasing complexity of public issues has forced lawmakers to rely heavily on the expertise and opinions of professional and trade associations, as well as business, labor, and industry groups.
- Although there is a certain mysticism about the process of lobbying, it is quite simply an attempt to legitimately influence legislators to promote or suppress proposed legislation.
- This process of influencing, or lobbying, is nothing more than educating, marketing, and selling. These are not foreign concepts to nurses, who spend their days educating patients and colleagues, marketing ideas to physicians to get appropriate orders written, and selling good health habits or practices to patients.
- ANNA's Board of Directors, Legislative Committee, and legislative consultant continually monitor and respond to issues affecting nursing, Medicare, and the ESRD Program, providing information to policy makers on Capitol Hill, regulatory agencies, and those who influence policy decisions on various government boards and commissions.

CHAPTER 25

The End Stage Renal Disease (ESRD) Program

Janel Parker, MSN, RN, CNN

Chapter Contents

Genesis of the Medicare ESRD Program 797
History of the ESRD Program 798
Legislative and Regulatory History of the ESRD Program 798
  Social Security Amendments of 1972 798
  ESRD Program Amendments of 1978 803
  OBRA 1981 803
  National Organ Transplant Act of 1984 804
  COBRA 1985 804
  OBRA 1986 804
  OBRA 1987 805
  OBRA 1989 806
  OBRA 1990 806
  Transplant Amendments Act of 1990 807
  OBRA 1993 807
  Medicare Amendments of 1993 and 1994 808
  Miscellaneous Regulatory Activity 808
The Continuance of the Medicare ESRD Program 809
  Past Considerations 809
  Current Considerations 810
  Future Considerations 812
Summary 812
References 812
Chapter Highlights 813

The End Stage Renal Disease (ESRD) Program

Janel Parker, MSN, RN, CNN

The End Stage Renal Disease (ESRD) Program is the only federal program that entitles people of all ages to Medicare coverage on the basis of their diagnosis. Any American who is either eligible for Social Security or is the dependent of someone who is eligible, is entitled to Medicare coverage for most, and occasionally all, of the costs of their treatment regardless of age, race or sex.

In the Social Security Amendments of 1972 (HR-1, Title XVIII), Public Law No. 92-603, Congress created this authorization to Medicare in support of persons with the diagnosis of chronic renal failure who were eligible for benefits under Social Security, and for the spouses or dependent children of these persons. These Medicare benefits, effective on July 1, 1973, provided access to dialysis treatments and kidney transplantation, inpatient and outpatient care from physicians as well as renal treatment centers.

The Medicare ESRD Program has provided financial support for life-saving treatments for hundreds of thousands of Americans. During the first year, 8,000 patients were treated at a cost of approximately $220 million. During 1995 22 years later, 262,760 patients were treated at a cost of approximately $13.06 billion dollars (United States Renal Data System, 1997). The purpose of this chapter is to present an overview of the legislative and regulatory histories of the ESRD Program and a discussion of issues that affect Medicare ESRD entitlements.

On an individual level, the ESRD program has been and remains important to each of the hundreds of thousands of individuals and their loved ones whose lives have been saved by it. A broader perspective on its impact must recognize that the existence of a federal program spurred the further development of kidney disease treatment in this country, and influenced the rest of the world.

Genesis of the Medicare ESRD Program

The roots of the program date back to the 1960s and the development of two forms of treatment for ESRD, hemodialysis and transplantation. Prior to this time, treatment for people suffering from this disease was not possible.

During the 1950s, it became possible to transplant kidneys between genetically nonidentical donors and recipients (Levinsky, 1993; Plough, 1986). In the early 1960s, the first patient was initiated on chronic dialysis therapy (Scribner, 1990). With these advances in science, the federal government began to engage in a number of public policy efforts before creating the ESRD Program. The first facility for long-term dialysis, the Seattle Artificial Kidney Center located at Swedish Hospital in Seattle, was established in 1962 as part of a 2-year trial program to test the clinical and economic feasibility of chronic dialysis therapy (Albers, 1989). In 1963, the Veterans' Administration announced the establishment of dialysis centers in its hospitals throughout the country. The National Institutes of Health (NIH) began to fund kidney research in 1965, and the Public Health Service (PHS) supported a small number of dialysis centers as part of federally funded demonstration projects (Iglehart, 1993). With these exceptions, no systematic methodology had been established in the 1960s to fund dialysis and transplantation services.

In the early 1960s, renal failure was claiming 100,000 victims in the United States annually (Scribner, 1990), but there were not enough dialysis machines available to meet the demand. It is estimated that treatment costs were $15,000 per year (Scribner, 1990). Often a small number of patients were accepted into the few maintenance programs in existence based on social criteria. The social criteria included age (adults less than 45 years old were preferred), emotional stability and maturity, and the potential for return to a useful and productive role in society (Murray, Tu, Albers, Burnell, & Scribner, 1962; Schupak & Merrill, 1965). The psychiatric criteria used were criticized for mixing psychosocial evaluation with moral judgment (Abram, 1972).

The membership of these early selection committees reflected the demographic features of the medical profession and the values of the middle class, rather than those of the population of potential beneficiaries. In 1967, well-educated white men with stable marriages were represented among those chosen to receive treatment (Evans, Blagg, & Bryan, 1981), while today more members of minorities, women, and persons with less education are represented in the ESRD population.

In 1966, the President's Bureau of the Budget established an expert committee, under the chairmanship of Dr. Carl Gottschalk, to analyze the public policy issues related to ESRD. The following year, the committee concluded that dialysis and transplantation were established therapies for chronic renal failure and that the institution of a nationally funded clinical program was justified (Committee on Chronic Kidney Disease, 1967). This report is considered to have been most instrumental in the subsequent establishment of a federal policy for ESRD (Plough, 1986, p. 118).

After the report was issued, the idea of a federal program for ESRD simmered in the Congress until December 1971. At that time, Arkansas Representative Wilbur D. Mills brought the idea forward by formally proposing the formation of such a program in the House of Representatives. This action followed 1 month after a patient underwent hemodialysis on the floor of the House of Representatives during a hearing of the House Ways and Means Committee, which Rep. Mills chaired.

History of the ESRD Program

Every year, thousands of bills are introduced in Congress, but only a few hundred pass the Senate and the House of Representatives and are signed into law by the President of the United States. Legislation authorizes the Health Care Financing Administration (HCFA) as the agency with administrative responsibility to formulate regulations that implement the public laws governing the Medicare ESRD Program. Oversight of these regulations is retained by Congress.

The regulatory process is a two-step procedure including a notice of proposed rule making (NPRM) and final regulations or rules. A NPRM is a text of the proposed regulation, history of the issue, description of the impact, and other related issues announced in the *Federal Register*. The public is invited to comment on the NPRM when specific instructions and deadlines are followed. Consideration is given to all comments in issuance of final regulations. Final regulations or rules include a statement of purpose and the basis for the regulation. All final regulations are published at least 30 days prior to the effective date. (Bocchino & Burrows-Hudson, 1995).

Although the legislation was never formally considered by the appropriate House or Senate committees, Indiana Senator Vance Hartke successfully attached the measure as a floor amendment to the Social Security Amendments of 1972, after only 30 minutes of discussion. This amendment was adopted in the context of a broader provision of legislation that extended Medicare coverage to the disabled regardless of age.

On October 30, 1972, President Richard Nixon signed into law Public Law (P.L.) 92-603. Section 299I of that law altered Title XVIII of the Social Security Act, declaring that chronic renal disease constitutes a disability. As a result, those suffering from ESRD would be covered for medical costs in the same ways as all other disabled individuals under Title XVIII. It is estimated that between 92% and 93% of the U.S. population is covered for treatment for ESRD through this entitlement. These Medicare benefits, effective on July 1, 1973, provided access to dialysis treatments, kidney transplantation, and inpatient and outpatient care from physicians as well as renal treatment centers.

The growing cost of the ESRD Program has made it an increasingly visible part of the Medicare program. The cost to Medicare of maintaining a patient on chronic dialysis is currently about $45,000 per year. (These figures do not include additional costs for copayments and deductibles not covered by Medicare.)

The national expenditures for the ESRD Program have been much higher than initial estimates, which predicted expenditures of about $250 million by the end of 1977. Annual expenditures were $229 million in 1974, and had risen to $3.7 billion by 1988. Part of the increase in cost is due to inflation; the cost per treatment of dialysis has actually fallen in constant dollars, from 1974 to the present. The growth in the number of beneficiaries, which has far outpaced initial expectations, accounts for much of the rising cost of the program.

Congress and the Health Care Financing Administration (HCFA), the agency within the Department of Health and Human Services (DHHS) responsible for the management of the Medicare program, have periodically addressed various aspects of the ESRD Program. This action has resulted from the progressive increase in expenditures of the ESRD Program in an increasingly constrained Medicare system and allegations that the quality of care of dialysis patients deteriorated as reimbursement decreased both in constant dollars and due to Congressional action.

Table 25-1 is a legislative and regulatory history of the public laws and regulations managing the ESRD Program since its inception.

Legislative and Regulatory History of the ESRD Program

Social Security Amendments of 1972

Legislative activity: Public Law 92-603 extended Medicare benefits to patients suffering with chronic renal failure. Section 2991 created the ESRD Program. Effective date for Medicare coverage was July 1, 1973.

Regulatory action: Following enactment of P.L. 92-603, interim regulations implementing the law were published in the *Federal Register* on June 29, 1973, titled "Interim Conditions of Participation

Table 25-1
Legislative and regulatory histories.

Legislative History	Regulatory History
Public Law *P.L. 92-603 Social Security Amendments, October 1972* Extended Medicare benefits to patient suffering with end stage renal disease.	Interim regulations, June 29, 1973: interim conditions of participation and payment rates for dialysis and transplant services.
Section 2991 created the End Stage Renal Disease (ESRD) Program. Effective date for Medicare coverage was July 1, 1973.	Interim regulations, April 22, 1975: minor modifications to and republication of initial interim regulations concerning coverage of services. *NPRM: July 1, 1975.* a. specifies conditions of coverage that facilities must meet to qualify for Medicare reimbursement. b. includes health and safety requirements. c. directs the organization of the ESRD Network System. Final rule, June 3, 1976: finalized condition of participation as ESRD provider/supplies and coverage.
P.L. 95-292 ESRD Program Amendments of 1978, June 1978 Early entitlement for self-dialysis training and reimbursement for home patient equipment and supplies. These amendments were designed to encourage self-dialysis and transplantation and provide financial incentives to medically appropriate self-dialysis.	Final rule, August 11, 1978. a. authorized temporary approval as renal transplantation centers for pediatric hospitals. b. allows for Medicare approval/reimbursement without meeting the required minimal utilization for number of kidney transplants performed. Final rule, September 28, 1978: implemented early entitlement to ESRD benefits for patients entering a program of self-dialysis training or transplantation. Final rule, October 19, 1978. a. defined self-dialysis services, training, and facility. b. revised minimal utilization rates and rate provisions for self- dialysis services. Final rule, October 19, 1979. a. provided target rate reimbursement for facilities providing home dialysis services, equipment, and support services. b. developed incentives to allow providers to retain differences in actual cost and target rate. c. encouraged more cost-effective services.
P.L. 96-499 Omnibus Budget Reconciliation Act (OBRA) of 1980 *Section 94* Amends regulation concerning reasonable charge for services furnished under Part B of the Medicare Program.	
P.L. 97-35 Omnibus Budget Reconciliation Act of 1981 *Section 2145* Designed to increase the cost-efficiency of the ESRD Program by developing incentive reimbursement rates for dialysis treatments. Designated Medicare as the secondary payer to other insurance coverage for the first 12 months of a course of dialysis.	*NPRM: January 15, 1981.* a. specified conditions of coverage for training-only facilities. b. provided limited approval of special purpose facilities on time- limited basis for vacation and emergency purposes.

Table 25-1 (continued).

Legislative History	Regulatory History
Revised methodology for determining the composite rates for prospective payment proposal by Health Care Financing Administration (HCFA).	Prospective composite rate payment system. a. NPRM. February 12, 1982. b. final rule: May 11, 1983. c. established a payment rate per treatment adjusted for geographic wage differences. d. separate rates for hospital-based and independent dialysis facilities. e. exception process developed based on atypical patient mix, extraordinary circumstances, education costs, or as an isolated essential facility. f. physician payment modified to a single monthly prospective capitation payment (MCP). Final rule: April 5, 1983. a. services furnished to ESRD beneficiaries who are covered under employer group health insurance. b. Medicare became secondary payor for initial 12-month period. c. effective May 5, 1983.
P.L. 98-507 National Organ Transplant Act of 1984 Created task force on organ transplantation.	
P.L. 99-272 Consolidated Omnibus Reconciliation Act of 1985 (COBRA) *Section 9214* Maintains renal networks; disallows merger of networks to other organizations or entities but allows the Secretary to consolidate to not less than 14.	
P.L. 99-609 Omnibus Budget Reconciliation Act of 1986 (OBRA) *Section 9335* Requires establishment of 17 networks and defines responsibilities of the Network organization.	*NPRM: May 13, 1986.* a. proposed current composite rate reduction and methodology for determining the rate. b. proposed reduction never implemented due to legislative mandate to reduce rate by $2.00.
P.L. 99-609 Omnibus Budget Reconciliation Act of 1986 *Section 9335K* Establishes protocol on standards and conditions for reuse of hemodialyzer filters for those facilities voluntarily electing to reuse. *P.L. 99-609* *Section 9318* *Omnibus Budget Reconciliation Act of 1986* Specific organ procurement protocols are a requirement for hospitals or organizations involved in procuring organs or transplantation.	Final rule: August 26, 1986. a. authorized the Secretary of DHHS to designate the ESRD Network areas. b. delineated 14 network areas and criteria used to determine these areas. c. OBRA of 1986 required modification to at least 17 Network organizations.
P.L. 99-609 Omnibus Budget Reconciliation Act of 1986 *Section 9335* Payment Rates for Renal Services and Improvements in Administration of ESRD Networks and Program. Facility Composite Rate for dialysis treatments. Coverage of Immunosuppresive drugs. Study of the potential effect of payment reductions on access and quality of care. Establishes a National ESRD Registry by January 1, 1988. Develops and promulgates standards/conditions for safe and effective dialyzer reuse. Hospital protocols for organ procurement. Modification and Funding of ESRD Network Organization.	

Table 25-1 (continued).

Legislative History	Regulatory History
P.L. 100-203 Omnibus Budget Reconciliation Act of 1987 *Section 1881* Requires the Secretary of Department of Health & Human Services (DHHS) to direct a study of the ESRD Program to be conducted by the Institute of Medicine (IOM). *Section 4036d* Requires the 10M to examine the following issues: (1) access to treatment by Medicare-eligible beneficiaries and those individuals not eligible. (2) quality of care provided to beneficiaries as measured by clinical indicators, functional status of patients, and patient satisfaction. (3) effect of reimbursement on quality of treatment. (4) major epidemiologic and demographic changes on the ESRD population that may affect access, quality care, or resource requirements. (5) adequacy of existing data systems to monitor such matters on a continuing basis.	*NPRM: April 9, 1987.* a. revised Network area designations for 17 areas, set forth geographic areas of each Network and criteria for each designated area. b. proposed evaluation criteria and performance indicators for monitoring the performance of these organizations. Final rule, October 2, 1987, 18 Network areas designated. *NPRM: April 9, 1987.* Final rule: September 19, 1988 a. alternate sanctions for suppliers of ESRD services. b. effective October 19, 1988. c. failure to participate in the activities and pursue the goals of the ESRD Network. Final rule: October 1, 1987. a. standards for the reuse of hemodialyzers, filters, and other dialysis supplies. b. reuse involves the cleaning, disinfecting, and preparation of disposable hemodialyzer devices for subsequent use for the same patient. *NPRM: July 31, 1987.* Final rule: March 1, 1988. a. conditions of coverage for the approval of organ procurement agencies (OPAs) for participation in the Medicare or Medicaid programs. b. strengthen organ procurement agencies by establishing criteria to be certified. c. written protocols required for each hospital to identify potential organ or tissue donors. d. required transplant providers to be members of and abide by rules of the Organ Procurement and Transplantation Network (OPTN). e. only one OPA designate per defined service area. *NPRM: July 17, 1988.* a. protocol for the reuse of dialysis bloodlines. b. subject to FDA regulation under authority of the Medical Device Amendments of 1976. c. manufacturer requested to submit reuse protocol for approval by FDA.
P.L. 101-239 *Omnibus Budget Reconciliation Act of 1989 (ESRD Provisions)* Maintains current composite rate until October 1, 1990. Capped Method II reimbursement as the median composite rate. Requires a written agreement between beneficiaries and suppliers providing supplies/services directly, inclusive of all supplies and equipment. Requires all supplies and equipment be provided by one supplier. All suppliers must accept Medicare assignment. All suppliers must maintain a written agreement with an approved provider of services (dialysis facility) to furnish home support services. Reallocates funds for Network organizations as necessary to carry out previously defined responsibilities. Extends provisions that currently apply to Peer Review Organizations (PROs) regarding protections against liability. Requires the Secretary of DHHS to submit a report on the methodology and rationale used to establish a Medicare payment rate for erythropoietin.	*NPRM: February 13, 1989.* Inherent Reasonableness for Home Dialysis Supplies and Equipment. a. HCFA attempted to reduce Method II reimbursement to composite rate via inherent measurableness ruling. b. resulted in court action by a major supplier against HCFA/DHHS. c. court case remains undecided. d. resolved via legislation (OBRA, 1989).*NPRM: May 30, 1989.* Occupational exposure to bloodborne pathogens. a. infection control plan must be designed and implemented by each employer to minimize or eliminate employee exposure. b. plan shall be reviewed and updated as needed. c. universal precautions shall be observed inclusive of: (1) handwashing as frequently as needed. (2) use of personal protective equipment. (a) gloves.

Table 25-1 (continued)
Legislative and regulatory histories.

Legislative History	Regulatory History
	(b) masks, eye protection, and face shields. (c) gown, eye protection, and other protective body clothing (fluid-resistant, if needed). (d) shoe coverings. (3) needles and other sharp objects shall be shared, bent, or broken. (4) eating, drinking or smoking prohibited in potential exposure area. d. equipment/environmental surfaces must be cleaned and disinfected after exposure. e. work surfaces shall be decontaminated with appropriate disinfectant. f. equipment and environmental surfaces should be protected with coverings (plastic wrap, foil, or absorbent paper). g. all receptacles intended for reuse are inspected, cleaned, and disinfected regularly. h. potentially infectious materials, such as blood, shall be placed in a closable, leak-proof container. i. infectious waste shall be disposed of in closable, leak-proof containers. j. laundry from potentially contaminated workplaces shall be bagged separately, labeled or color-coded, and transported in leak-proof bags. k. HIV and HBV research laboratories and production facilities shall meet standard microbiological practice and other specialty defined practices. l. hepatitis B vaccination shall be made available to all employees who have occupational exposure one or more times per month. m. biohazard signs shall be posted in these work areas. n. all employees with occupational exposure shall participate in a training program. *Interim rule: June 12, 1989.* a. payment for erythropoietin (EPO). b. paid for dialysis patients by an add-on amount to the ESRD facility composite rate. (1) add-on amount is set, nationally, by HCFA. (2) $40 per administration of EPO for doses up to 10,000 units. (3) if 10,000 units or more are required per patient, an additional $30 is reimbursed. c. medical documentation is required. (1) iron deficiency with or without need for iron supplements. (2) concomitant conditions (infection, inflammation, or malignancies) affecting EPO. (3) unrecognized blood loss. (4) concomitant hemolysis, bone marrow dysplasia, or refractory anemia. (5) folic acid or vitamin B_{12} deficiencies. (6) patient's weight, current dose, historical record, or cumulative dosage to date, and hematocrit response (reported monthly). *Interim rule: November 1989.* a. EPO covered as an incident to a physician's service. b. must be furnished in a nonfacility setting (i.e., outpatient clinic or physician's office). c. reimbursed at cost plus administrative fee deemed reasonable by local Medicare carrier. **Key** NPRM — Notice of proposed rule making * *For a brief history on miscellaneous regulatory activities, see text.*

and Payment Rates for Dialysis and Transplant Services." Additional regulations were published on April 22, 1975, making minor modifications to and republication of the initial interim regulations concerning coverage of services. A Notice of Proposed Rulemaking (NPRM), published July 1, 1975, specified the "conditions of coverage" that facilities would be required to meet to qualify for Medicare reimbursement. It also included health and safety requirements of providers and directed the organization of the ESRD Network system. A Final Rule was published on June 3, 1976 that finalized the conditions of participation for ESRD providers/suppliers.

ESRD Program Amendments of 1978

Legislative activity: On June 13, 1978, P.L. 95-292 was enacted, amending the Social Security Act by including several new provisions for the ESRD Program to encourage home dialysis and transplantation.

Financial incentives were used to promote the use of lower cost, medically appropriate self-dialysis (primarily home dialysis) as an incentive to the more costly in-center dialysis, and to eliminate some of the existing financial disincentives to transplantation. The law provided for early Medicare entitlement for patients beginning self-dialysis or transplantation during the first 3 months following the initiation of chronic dialysis treatment.(Normally, Medicare entitlement begins 3 months *after* initiating treatment for chronic dialysis.)

The law also provided for the implementation of a prospective reimbursement method for dialysis payment, with incentives to assure more cost-effective delivery of services to patients dialyzing in facilities or at home. Medicare transplant benefits were extended from 12 to 36 months; that is, an individual with a functioning transplant would remain covered by Medicare under the ESRD benefit for 36 months posttransplant. The amendments included a mandate to develop a long-range national objective with respect to the most effective use of resources for treating renal disease and clarified the scope and responsibilities of the ESRD Networks.

In terms of background, Medicare's payment policy for outpatient dialysis services from 1973 to 1983 reimbursed independent renal facilities on a reasonable *charge* basis and hospital-based facilities on a reasonable *cost* basis, for both incenter and home dialysis services. Under the Interim Regulations, effective July 1, 1973, reimbursement for outpatient dialysis services was limited by a screen or payment ceiling of $138 per treatment (*Federal Register*, 1973). Home dialysis was paid for separately, and facilities managing home patients were reimbursed on a reasonable *cost* basis. Although home dialysis was the most economical modality in terms of overall program cost, it was simultaneously the least lucrative for facilities and physicians.

Congressional hearings on the ESRD Program were held in 1976, prompted by the rapid growth of ESRD expenditures and a concurrent decline in the proportion of patients treated by home dialysis (Rettig, 1980). These led to the ESRD Program Amendments of 1978.

Regulatory action: A final rule published on September 28, 1978, implemented the early entitlement to ESRD benefits for patients entering a program of self-dialysis training or transplantation. Another final rule, published October 19, 1978, defined self-dialysis services, training and facilities, and revised the minimal utilization rates and rate provisions for self-dialysis services. An October 19,1979, the final rule provided target rate reimbursement for facilities providing home dialysis services, equipment, and support services; developed incentives to allow providers to retain the difference between actual costs and the target rate reimbursement level; and encouraged more cost-effective services.

OBRA 1981

Legislative activity: The ESRD provisions in Section 2145 of the Omnibus Budget Reconciliation Act (OBRA) of 1981 (P.L. 97-35) again directed the Secretary of the Department of Health and Human Services (DHHS) to establish a prospective reimbursement system for outpatient dialysis to promote home dialysis, and revised physician payment to provide an incentive for home dialysis. To reduce the financial burden of the ESRD Program on total Medicare expenditures, the provisions also modified Medicare, making it the secondary payer to other private insurances for the first 12 months of Medicare entitlement.

Regulatory action: A NPRM published on February 12, 1982, with a subsequent final rule published on May 11, 1983, established the prospective composite rate payment system for dialysis in fulfillment of the requirements imposed by the ESRD Program Amendments of 1978 and the ESRD provisions of OBRA 1981. These regulations established a per-treatment payment rate adjusted for geographic wage differences, with slightly separate rates for hospital-based and independent dialysis facilities. The regulations also included a process for dialysis facilities to obtain an exception to the composite rate based on atypical patient mix, extraordinary circumstances, education costs, or designation as an isolated essential facility. Physician payment was modified to a single monthly prospective capitation payment (MCP) that was inclusive of all routine medical care provided to ESRD beneficiaries.

For the first time, payments for home and center dialysis treatments were consolidated into a single base composite rate. Since providers would be reimbursed at the same per treatment rate whether the patient dialyzed in-center or at home, the composite rate was intended to be an incentive to encourage dialysis providers to promote home dialysis among their patient populations.

Also, pursuant to the 1981 legislation, a final rule published on April 5, 1983, and effective May 5 of that same year, specified that Medicare would become the secondary payer for the first 12 months of Medicare entitlement for ESRD beneficiaries who are also covered under employer group health insurance.

National Organ Transplant Act of 1984

Legislative activity: The National Organ Transplant Act (P.L. 98-507) authorized the creation of the National Task Force on Organ Transplantation. It also amended the Public Health Service Act to address the acquisition and distribution of whole organs (including kidneys) through the Organ Procurement and Transplantation Network (OPTN) (Rettig & Levinsky, 1991). Kidney transplantation was covered by Medicare as a treatment for chronic renal failure as stated in the Social Security Amendments of 1972. Under these provisions, Medicare reimburses for organ procurement, the transplant surgical procedure, and related physician fees.

Regulatory action: A NPRM was published on July 31, 1987, with a subsequent final rule on March 1, 1988, that identified the conditions of coverage for the approval of organ procurement organizations (OPOs) for participation in the Medicare and Medicaid programs, and specified that there could be only one OPO for a defined service area. These regulations strengthened the OPOs by establishing the criteria by which they would be certified. The regulations required that each hospital participating in the Medicare/Medicaid programs must have written protocols for the identification of potential organ or tissue donors. They also required transplant providers to be members of and abide by the rules of the OPTN.

COBRA 1985

Legislative activity: In COBRA 1985 (P.L. 99-272, Section 9214), Congress directed the Secretary of the DHHS to consolidate the 32 existing ESRD Networks into not less than 14 networks. The law also disallowed the merger of ESRD Networks to other organizations (Bocchino & Burrows-Hudson, 1995).

Regulatory action: A final rule was published on August 26, 1986, that delineated 14 Network areas and identified the criteria used to determine these areas.

OBRA 1986

Legislative activity: OBRA 1986 authorized the Secretary of DHHS to set the composite rate for dialysis services provided between October 1, 1986, and October 1, 1988, at a level equal to that in effect as of May 13, 1986, reduced by $2.00. It further reduced the composite rate by an additional $.50 to finance the ESRD Networks.

OBRA 1986 also required a study to evaluate the effects of the payment reductions on access and quality of care. HCFA contracted with the Urban Institute in Washington, DC, to conduct the study. The report, "Review of the Impact of the Reduction of the Composite Rate for Renal Dialysis on Access and Quality of Care," submitted in December 1987, concluded that reductions in the payment rates had made no impact on access to dialysis treatments and no deleterious effect on the quality of care provided (Bocchino & Burrows-Hudson, 1995).

OBRA 1986 established the U.S. Renal Data System (USRDS), a national ESRD registry, to assemble and analyze data on the ESRD Program. The USRDS originated from discussions involving the renal community, Congress, and the National Institute of Diabetes and Digestive and Kidney Diseases (NIDDK)at the National Institutes of Health (NIH). Data are reported to the USRDS by Network organizations, transplant centers, and all other sources collecting information on ESRD patients. The registry was to:

1. Prepare an annual ESRD report to Congress;
2. Identify the economic impact, cost-effectiveness, and medical efficacy of alternative modalities of treatment;
3. Evaluate the most appropriate allocation of resources for the treatment and research into the causes of chronic renal failure;
4. Determine patient mortality and morbidity rates, and trends in such rates, and other indices of quality of care; and
5. Conduct other analyses to assist the Congress in evaluating the ESRD Program.

The establishment of USRDS represented a major commitment by the NIH to kidney disease and related epidemiologic research. Since its inception, the USRDS has made a substantial contribution to the renal community by allowing researchers and clinicians to use its published data to explore a variety of unanswered questions regarding the care of ESRD patients (Rettig & Levinsky, 1991).

The 1986 legislation further modified and reorganized the ESRD Networks. OBRA 1986 required a reorganization of the Networks to establish 17 Networks; this was later increased to 18 (see Figure 25-1). The legislation also defined the responsibilities of the Network organization as follows: (a) establishment of a medical review board to conduct on-site reviews and report on facilities and providers utilizing criteria and standards related to the appropriateness of patient care established by the Network organization; (b) review of medical records that fail to meet approved standards with local facility personnel and opportunities for the

Figure 25-1
The ESRD Networks.

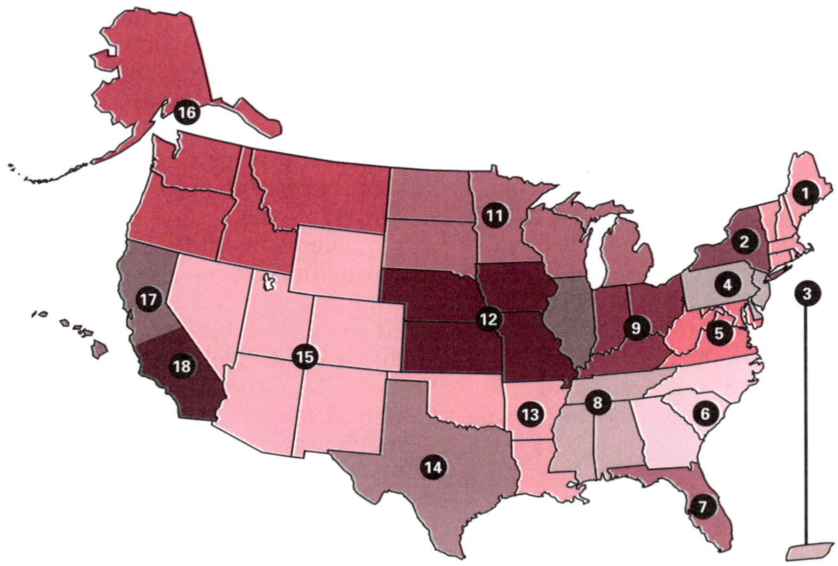

facility for discussion, written comment, the development of a Corrective Action Plan, specific educational activities, or sanctions; and, (c) data collection for annual census, population estimates, and population characteristics to be incorporated in the USRDS annual reports.

Payment was authorized for 1 year of immunosuppressive medications on an outpatient basis following transplantation. (This authorization was mainly in response to the high cost of cyclosporine.) The legislation also required standards and conditions for the safe and effective reuse of dialyzers, and required organ procurement protocols as a requirement for hospitals and organizations involved in procuring organs for transplantation.

Regulatory action: On April 9, 1987, a NPRM outlined the revised 17 Network area designations; these were then published in a final rule on October 2 of that same year. Also in the April 9 notice, alternate sanctions were identified for suppliers of ESRD services and the requirement for such suppliers to participate in the activities and pursue the goals of the ESRD Networks was stated. These became effective October 19, 1988. In an October 1, 1987, final rule, the standards for the reuse of hemodialyzers, filters, and other dialysis supplies were published.

OBRA 1987

Legislative activity: OBRA 1987 (P.L. 100-203) required the Secretary of DHHS to direct a study of the Medicare ESRD Program by the National Academy of Sciences, Institute of Medicine (IOM). The study would examine the following issues:

1. Major epidemiologic and demographic changes in the ESRD patient population that may affect access to treatment, quality of care, or the resource requirements of the program;
2. Access to treatment by individuals with chronic renal failure, whether eligible for Medicare benefits or not;
3. Quality of care provided to ESRD beneficiaries, as measured by clinical indicators, functional status of patients, and patient satisfaction;
4. Effect of reimbursement on quality of care, and;
5. Adequacy of existing data systems to monitor these matters on a continuing basis (P.L. 100-203, Section 4036d).

The final report, entitled *Kidney Failure and the Federal Government*, was published by National Academy Press in 1991, edited by Rettig and Levinsky. The authors published a "special report" entitled "The Medicare End Stage Renal Disease Program: A Report from the Institute of Medicine" in the *New England Journal of Medicine* (see volume 324, pages 1143-1148, April 18, 1991 issue). The report includes a number of recommendations related to access to treatment for all for whom it is medically appropriate; provision of quality care that achieves desirable health outcomes consistent with patient health status and current professional knowledge; the development of policies that steadily improve patient well-being and patient outcomes; and prudent program management at the lowest cost compatible with adequate care.

OBRA 1989

Legislative activity: The ESRD provisions of OBRA 1989 (P.L. 101-239) maintained the existing base composite rate, for both hospital-based and independent dialysis facilities, including in-center and home dialysis patients, as those established in 1983 (and reduced by $2 in 1986) until October 1, 1990.

OBRA 1989 addressed the Method II form of reimbursement for home dialysis equipment and supplies and stipulated certain restrictions on Method II suppliers. It limited that reimbursement to the median national composite rate, with an exception for continuous cycling peritoneal dialysis (CCPD), which was set at 130% of the median national composite rate.

The Method II provisions in this legislation were largely in response to controversy surrounding Home Intensive Care, Inc. (HIC), a supplier of dialysis equipment and supplies to home patients. HIC saw the advantages to patients of the Method II billing methodology, as this rate was sufficient enough to allow the company to provide staff assistants to dialyze patients in their homes who would otherwise not have been able to do so (Rettig & Levinsky, 1991). Prior to this legislation, in February 1989, HCFA published a NPRM attempting to reduce Method II reimbursement to the composite rate level through an inherent reasonableness ruling. This resulted in court action, which necessitated the inclusion of these provisions in the OBRA 1989 legislation.

OBRA 1989 reallocated funds for the 18 ESRD Network organizations to "report on facilities and providers that are not providing appropriate care" and "conduct on-site reviews of facilities and providers... utilizing standards of care established by the Network organization" (OBRA 1986). In addition, the legislation extended the provisions that applied to Professional Review Organizations (PROs), regarding protection of their liability for medical review to ESRD Networks. Following their reorganization, Networks existed in administrative oblivion until the issue of liability was resolved. The Networks now follow HCFA quality assurance efforts (Rettig & Levinsky, 1991).

OBRA 1989 required the Secretary of DHHS to submit a report on the methodology and rationale used to establish a Medicare payment rate for erythropoietin. Recombinant human erythropoietin (EPO) was the first recombinant DNA-based biological for use in clinical practice. In June 1989, the Food and Drug Administration (FDA) approved EPO (Amgen, Inc.'s Epogen or Epoetin-alfa) for treatment of anemia in dialysis patients (FDA, 1989). HCFA responded immediately with a decision to provide coverage and an interim reimbursement policy (HCFA, 1989).

The interim rule was published on June 12, 1989, and specified that EPO for dialysis patients was to be paid for by an add-on amount to the ESRD facility composite rate (set nationally by HCFA). Reimbursement was initially set at $40 per administration of EPO for doses up to 10,000 units; an additional $30 was reimbursed if the patient required greater than 10,000 units per dose. The rule required certain documentation to be provided for payment.

The payment for EPO was not incorporated into the composite rate because all patients were not expected to receive it, nor were all patients expected to receive the same dose. Only the cost of the medication itself was recognized for reimbursement. Supplies, nursing care, medication administration, and laboratory services were absorbed by the facilities (Rettig & Levinsky, 1991).

In another interim rule published in November 1989, EPO was covered "incident to" a physician's service for patients on home dialysis. The rule specified that the EPO must be furnished in a nonfacility setting (i.e. outpatient dialysis clinic or physician's office). In these cases, it was to be reimbursed at cost plus an administrative fee (to be deemed reasonable by local Medicare carrier).

Regulatory action: A NPRM published on December 26, 1990, and a final rule published on November 17, 1992, carried out the provisions of OBRA 1989 related to Method II reimbursement.

OBRA 1990

Legislative activity: OBRA 1990 was enacted as P.L. 101-508. It extended and expanded waivers for social health maintenance organizations (SHMOs). SHMOs consolidated the acute and chronic care delivery systems and managed care across a full range of services (acute care, postacute care, and expanded community care). Four innovative projects, created to refine methodologies and benefit design, were approved and in addition, four existing SHMO sites were extended (Bocchino & Burrows-Hudson, 1995).

The President's budget for fiscal year 1991 (FY91), submitted to Congress in January 1990, recommended extending the second-payer provision from 12 to 18 months if the patient is covered by both Medicare and employer group health insurance. Congress adopted the provision in OBRA 1990 to become effective on February 1, 1991. Several organizations in the renal community supported this provision because: (a) providers generally received higher reimbursement from private insurers than they did from Medicare, (b) private insurers have a limited ability to track expenditures for ESRD patients in their claims processing systems, or (c) private payers were more reasonable payers than Medicare (Bocchino & Burrows-

Hudson, 1995; Rettig & Levinsky, 1991).

In 1990 the General Accounting Office (GAO) examined options to provide home dialysis aides for some dialysis patients. Some accepted "hardship case" criteria were patients who were confined to a bed or wheelchair, those unable to transfer without assistance or with no available transportation to the dialysis center, or those at risk while traveling (GAO, 1990). Several legislative proposals to implement payment for home partners resulted in Congress authorizing, in OBRA 1990 (Section 4202), a 3-year demonstration project to evaluate the safety and cost-effectiveness of staff-assisted home dialysis.

OBRA 1990 directed the Prospective Payment Assessment Commission (ProPAC) to study "the costs, services, and profit associated with dialysis treatment modalities," to recommend the method of payment for the facility component of outpatient dialysis services for fiscal year 1993, and the methodology for updating payments in subsequent years. (ProPAC was a federal commission that was responsible to advise Congress and the Secretary of DHHS on the Medicare Prospective Payment System [PPS]).

Section 4201(c) of OBRA 1990 made two changes in the EPO policy. Self-administration of EPO by competent home dialysis patients who do not require medical supervision became effective on July 1, 1991, and the payment for EPO administered to patients became $11 per 1,000 units.

Regulatory action: An interim rule published on September 4, 1991, and a subsequent final rule published on January 10, 1994, addressed the Medicare coverage of EPO used by competent home patients. The rule revised the conditions of coverage for these services furnished to ESRD beneficiaries to include patient selection; assessment of the patient's ability to administer the drug and the patient's compliance; the physician-supervised plan of care, including training to give the injection; monitoring of the drug's effectiveness; and the patient's ability to assess side effects.

Transplant Amendments Act of 1990

Legislative activity: Transplant Amendments Act of 1990 (P.L. 101-616) reauthorized the National Organ Transplant Act of 1984 for 3 years. In this legislation, Congress expanded the authority of the Health Resources and Services Agency (HRSA) within DHHS to make grants related to organ procurement and factors affecting access, outcomes, and organ donation, to nonprofit private organizations other than organ procurement organizations (OPOs). OPOs shifted from being hospital-based to being independent entities, and multiple OPOs in a single statistical metropolitan area (SMA) were consolidated to assure "sufficient size, maximum effectiveness, and equitable distribution of organs." The minimum qualifications of the OPTN contractor, the composition of the OPTN Board of Directors, and the responsibilities of the OPTN were changed. The Secretary of DHHS was required to establish criteria to assure that an OPO meets target effectiveness regarding the number of organs procured each year.

The Transplant Amendments Act of 1990 called for a study by the GAO to determine the extent to which the procurement and allocation of organs had been equitable, efficient, and effective; the difficulties that were encountered in the procurement and allocation of organs; and the effect of state required-request laws.

Regulatory action: A NPRM published on June 21, 1991, and an interim final rule published on September 8, 1994, addressed the conditions of coverage for OPOs. The rules set the eligibility requirements and procedures for OPOs to receive Medicare and Medicaid reimbursement, clarified certification and designation, and redefined OPO service area. To obtain first time designation as an OPO, an organization must demonstrate that its service area has the potential to produce 50 donors or comprises an entire state; must procure a minimum of 24 donors per calendar year over a 2-year period; and maintain an average ratio of three organs per donor. The performance standards to evaluate OPO effectiveness became more quantitative on January 1, 1996.

In addition, the regulations specified that HCFA approval would be necessary for change of OPO ownership or service area; that OPOs must have a system in place for the equitable allocation of organs; and that OPOs must ensure that tests are done on all donors for the presence of communicable diseases, including AIDS.

Regulatory action: A NPRM, published on September 8, 1984, addressed the operation of the OPTN. The rules put forth the guidelines for OPTN functions, membership and the governing board; addressed federal oversight of the allocation of organs to ensure fairness and equity; stated compliance requirements for participation in Medicare and Medicaid; and established minimum requirements to improve the outcome of transplantation and minimize the waste of donated organs. As of October 1997, no final rule has been published.

OBRA 1993

Legislative activity: The ESRD provisions of OBRA 1993 (P.L. 103-66) extended coverage of immunosuppressive drug therapy from 12 months to 36 months.

The extension period was phased in to reduce the impact on the federal budget. Effective in 1995, immunosuppressive drug therapy was covered for 18 months; during 1996, reimbursement was extended to 24 months; and during 1997, immunosuppressive drug therapy was extended to 30 months. Any year following 1997, the benefits will be extended to 36 months (Bocchino & Burrows-Hudson, 1995, p. 429).

OBRA 1993 included physician self-referral limitations. Effective January 1, 1995, physicians were barred from referring patients for designated health services to any business entity with which that physician has a financial relationship if payment is to be made by Medicare or Medicaid. Eleven designated health services were specified as applicable for the self-referral ban. Such dialysis-related services included bone densitometry or other nonroutine tests, durable medical equipment, parental and enteral nutrients, equipment and supplies, outpatient prescription drugs, and inpatient hospital services.

In OBRA 1993, Congress reduced payment for EPO to $10 per 1,000 units from $11 (OBRA, 1990). In addition, self-administration of EPO was reimbursed for all dialysis patients and no longer limited to just those patients who dialyze at home.

The Social Health Maintenance Organization (OBRA, 1990) waivers were extended under OBRA 1993 for 2 years, and one new site was authorized for an ESRD capitation demonstration project.

Medicare Amendments of 1993 and 1994

Legislative activity: These Medicare amendments were legislated as the Social Security Act Amendments of 1994 (P.L. 103-432). Known as technical amendments, they amended and corrected sections of OBRA 1986-1990 and 1993. Some of the provisions related to the ESRD Program included the following:

1. Conditions were defined under which a hospital could have an agreement with an OPO other than its designated OPO, including the waiver process and the criteria for granting waivers;
2. Eligibility criteria were defined for the staff-assisted home dialysis demonstration project, and clarified that an individual could be a resident of a nursing facility and/or a skilled nursing facility; and
3. The extended coverage of immunosuppressive drug therapy was clarified to achieve budget neutrality and prevent gaps in coverage.

Miscellaneous Regulatory Activity

Transplant: A final rule published on August 11, 1978, authorized temporary approval of renal transplantation centers for pediatric hospitals and allowed for Medicare approval and reimbursement for transplant facilities without the required minimal utilization for number of kidney transplants performed.

Dialysis: A NPRM published on January 15, 1981, specified the conditions of coverage for training-only dialysis facilities and provided limited approval of special purpose dialysis facilities on a time-limited basis for vacation and emergency purposes.

Dialysis: A NPRM published on July 17, 1988, declared the reuse of hemodialysis blood tubing to be subject to regulation by the FDA under the authority of the Medical Device Amendments of 1976. Blood tubing manufacturers were required to submit reuse protocols to the FDA for approval.

Dialysis and transplantation: A NPRM was published on May 30, 1989, addressing the occupational exposure to and transmission of bloodborne pathogens. The final rule was published on December 6, 1991, and became effective March 6, 1992. These regulations defined employer requirements to protect health care workers and member of other occupations who had exposure to blood and potential bloodborne pathogens through their employment. These regulations required that Hepatitis B vaccination be made available to all employees who have occupational exposure one or more times per month.

Dialysis: A NPRM published on January 6, 1994, revised the definition of ESRD and clarified the resumption of entitlement for individuals who return to a regular course of dialysis treatments after one course is ended and if a second transplant occurs after a beneficiary loses eligibility due to the 3-year rule.

Dialysis: A NPRM published on February 14, 1994 revised the guidelines on the reuse of hemodialysis filters (dialyzers) and addressed the standards for the quality of water used in dialysis. The 1993 Association for the Advancement of Medical Instrumentation (AAMI) guidelines on "Recommended Practice for Reuse of Hemodialyzers" were incorporated by reference in these regulations.

Dialysis: A NPRM published on June 17, 1997, addressed the updating and revising of HCFA's policy on coverage of ambulance services, including such services for ESRD beneficiaries. The current regulation limits ambulance transportation for ESRD beneficiaries living at home to the nearest hospital-based dialysis facility only. The proposed rule adds a provision that would cover medically necessary ambulance services for an ESRD beneficiary living at home to the nearest dialysis facility capable of furnishing the necessary dialysis services without regard to whether that facility is hospital-based.

Dialysis: A NPRM published on August 26, 1994, with a final rule published on August 15, 1997, specified the criteria HCFA uses to determine if a facility that furnishes dialysis services to Medicare patients with ESRD qualifies for a payment rate higher than the prospectively determined payment rate, and the procedures HCFA uses to evaluate ESRD payment exception requests. It also addressed and revised the way HCFA computes acquisition costs for organs that are transplanted into Medicare beneficiaries.

The Continuance of the Medicare ESRD Program

Past Considerations

The IOM, in response to a request by Congress (OBRA, 1987, Section 4036d of P.L. No. 100-203), conducted a study of the Medicare ESRD Program. The study was conducted by an IOM expert committee. The individuals brought expertise to the study from internal medicine, nursing, nephrology, geriatrics, transplant surgery, economics, epidemiology, ethics, the social sciences, social work, and the perspective of a dialysis patient.

The committee submitted a report to Congress and the Secretary of the DHHS. It was published as *Kidney Failure and the Federal Government* by the National Academy Press, Washington, DC, in 1991. There is no question that the objectives for the Medicare ESRD program and recommendations based on the objectives set forth in the IOM report will have a profound impact on the ESRD Program for years to come (Klahr, 1990).

The IOM committee endorsed four objectives for the Medicare ESRD program:

1. Guarantee access to treatment for all in which it is medically appropriate;
2. Provide care of high quality that achieves desirable health outcomes consistent with patient health status and current professional knowledge;
3. Develop policies that steadily improve patient well-being and patient outcomes; and,
4. Manage the ESRD program prudently at the lowest cost compatible with adequate care.

Based on the four objectives set forth in the IOM report, the following recommendations were made by the committee:

- As a matter of equitable treatment of all individuals with chronic renal failure, the committee finds no justifiable basis for restricting Medicare eligibility other than citizenship or resident alien status. It recommends that Congress modify the Medicare eligibility criteria for individuals with chronic renal failure and extend the entitlement to all US citizens and resident aliens.
- Congress should eliminate the 3-year Medicare eligibility limit for successful transplant patients and thereby authorize a lifetime entitlement comparable to that of dialysis patients.
- Coverage for payment of immunosuppressive medications for kidney transplant patients should be made coterminous with the period of entitlement.
- The donation of kidneys should receive high priority.
- Patients and clinicians in adult and pediatric nephrology, and bioethicists should develop guidelines for evaluating patients for whom the burdens of renal replacement therapy may substantially outweigh the benefits. These guidelines should be flexible and encourage the physician to use discretion in assessing an individual patient. Guidelines should be developed specifically for children and should describe the role of the parents in the decision making process.
- Nephrologists and other clinicians should discuss with all ESRD patients, their wishes about dialysis, cardiopulmonary resuscitation, and other life-sustaining treatments and encourage documented advance directives.
- ESRD clinicians should be encouraged to participate in continuing education in medical ethics and health law. Some specialists in the medical ethics of renal disease should be available to educate clinicians, to train members of the ethics committee, and to do research on ethical issues in dialysis and transplantation.
- Assess the shift of providers from not-for-profit to for-profit providers and the implications for access and quality.
- There is no persuasive reason for the application of state certificate-of-need (CON) regulations on dialysis treatment capacity that is regulated mainly by the Medicare payment level. The committee strongly favors the elimination of CON as applied to dialysis facilities, but recognizes that this requires state government rather than federal government action. It recommends that HCFA review with each of the relevant states the effect of CON regulations on ESRD patient access to care.
- Follow general Medicare payment policies in setting dialysis payment policies: update the rate, yearly; rebase the rate only when HCFA rebases the other parts of Medicare governed by the Prospective Payment System (PPS); ultimately, rebasing outpatient dialysis reimbursement from efficacy and quality studies that determine the components needed for appropriate dialysis care. Because these components will change as clinical and technical knowledge advance, HCFA should establish an expert advisory body to review periodically the services that Medicare should reimburse; and, ProPAC, consistent with its charge to examine Medicare outpatient as well as inpatient reimbursement, should periodically review ESRD payment policy.
- The following ESRD reimbursement policies should be adopted: evaluate the justification for the rate differential between hospital-based and independent facilities, especially in terms of patient complexity, and retain or eliminate the differential based on that analysis; establish a separate rate for hospital back up units that treat both inpatients and outpatients that provide support to independent units in the care of

complex outpatient cases; establish a separate rate for ESRD pediatric patients; and, evaluate the need for a separate rate for rural facilities.

- HCFA should review the monthly capitation physician payment policy (MCP) regarding its exclusion from the Medicare Fee Schedule and the impact of this policy on the quality of care provided.
- The Medicare ESRD state survey system should be improved by HCFA to develop uniform training and certification requirements for surveyors and integrating the state survey system with other ESRD quality assurance (QA) efforts.
- In an effort to improve quality assessment and assurance, HCFA QA oversight of ESRD providers could be exercised by coordination within the HCFA of all relevant bureaus (Health Standards and Quality Bureau [HSQB], Bureau of Policy Development, and Office of Research and Demonstrations), linking existing data bases to provide a systematic examination of the relation between cost of treatment and the quality of care, and integrate the ESRD networks and state surveys in a coherent national QA strategy; adequate financial support should be provided to facilities for quality assurance activities by incorporating facility QA costs in reimbursement for both dialysis and transplantation; evaluate all policies, including reimbursement policies for their quality impacts on patients; establish an advisory group of nephrology professionals and experts in QA to design and develop ESRD-specific QA systems; support the regional and national data systems necessary for an effective QA system, and support a continuing program of ESRD QA research.
- A strong ESRD data acquisition and analysis capability should be maintained by HCFA to: modify the acquisition of patient information to include the periodic collection of data on comorbid conditions, risk factors, functional status, and other factors bearing on treatment and outcomes; identify data needs for systematically analyzing the relations among resource use, treatment, and patient outcomes; fund research pertinent to these questions; and provide public use tapes for research on all aspects of the ESRD program to the interested research community.
- The USRDS should be authorized to conduct research linking epidemiologic and economic data on the ESRD patient population and, the special studies approach should be exploited to its full potential.
- The Secretary of the DHHS should take all steps necessary to fully implement all functions of the National ESRD Registry called for in OBRA 1986, within the next 2 years.
- The Renal Data System should be continued another 5 years when the current USRDS contract expires and that the contract be renegotiated at that time.
- NIDDK should expand its support for basic research that has the promise to prevent or to reduce the progression of kidney disease that leads to chronic renal failure.
- Clinical research on dialysis, supported by NIDDK or HCFA, should be resumed.
- Epidemiologic research should be supported to identify risk factors for renal failure and its clinical outcomes, the value of various interventions to prevent and treat chronic renal failure, and factors influencing access to care. Special attention should be given to racial and ethnic differences in the incidence and causes of renal failure and in transplantation (access, outcomes, and organ donation).
- Health services research be supported to determine which components of medical care lead to better outcomes and to identify and validate quality measures for structure, process, and outcomes.

Current Considerations

As the Medicare ESRD program continues to provide financial reimbursement for the treatment of patients with chronic renal failure in the midst of current debates regarding health care reform, the nephrology community sets forth the following considerations for further legislation and regulations.

Transplantation. According to the UNOS Research Department, as of January 31, 1997, of the 50,496 patients waiting for organs, 34,766 patients were on the national waiting list for kidney transplants. An additional 1,462 are in line for kidney/pancreas transplants. Those waiting for livers placed a distant second, at only 7,618 followed by potential heart recipients (3,695). Males waiting for kidneys comprised 57% of the total ("Kidney Transplant Waiting List," 1997).

- Demonstration projects on "rewarded gifts" and "presumed consent" and other strategies that could improve our knowledge and the role of the federal government with regards to increasing organ donation.
- The nephrology community and transplant community establishing a consensus on meaningful transplant public policy to create a more cohesive force.
- There should be at least as much focus on donation as on allocation in any future NOTA bill.
- A request for removal of Medicare's 3-year cap on immunosuppressive medication coverage or preferably, extension of Medicare coverage for immunosuppressive medication for the life of the transplant.
- Elimination of the preexisting condition barrier for transplant recipients who are not currently employed, but who, upon recovery, wish to

Table 25-2
NKF-DOQI project goals.

Process Objectives	Outcome Objectives
• Develop and promulgate outcome goals for patients with chronic renal failure.	• Improve patient survival.
• Provide a road map on how to improve outcomes for these patients.	• Reduce patient morbidity.
• Facilitate adoption and use of practice guidelines within the renal community.	• Increase efficiency of care.
• Establish a mechanism for evaluating compliance with such standards of care.	• Improve quality of life for ESRD patients.

reenter the workforce, and the prohibition of excessive health insurance coverage costs for transplant recipients (Smith, 1996; "Continuous Quality Improvement", 1997).

Dialysis composite rate. In mid-January 1997, ProPAC approved a 2.8% increase in the amount paid to dialysis units for performance of the dialysis treatment and ancillary services. On the average, the increase will translate into approximately 3 dollars per dialysis treatment. If the increase is approved by Congress, it will represent only the second time in the history of the Medicare ESRD program that an increase in the composite rate has been granted (ProPAC, 1997).

Managed care. The renal community has concerns related to the access of patients with renal insufficiency and renal failure to specialists and therapies that can delay their need for dialysis, reduce their hospitalizations, and improve their health outcomes. The federal government should proceed with caution in expanding access to managed care plans to this patient population at this time ("Statement of principles..., 1997).

National Kidney Foundation-Dialysis Outcomes Quality Initiative (NKF-DOQI). The advent of DOQI was March 1995. The purpose of the DOQI is to develop practice guidelines in the areas of vascular access, peritoneal dialysis adequacy, and anemia. Additionally, DOQI will develop educational materials to improve implementation of the Renal Physicians' Association (RPA) practice guidelines for hemodialysis adequacy. A fifth group, focusing on nutrition, was later added to the project. The goal of the DOQI guidelines is to assist in increasing life expectancy and to improve overall health and quality of life for the more than 220,000 people in the United States on chronic dialysis therapy (see Table 25-2).

The DOQI project started as a joint renal community effort organized by the NKF and supported by Amgen, Inc. This initiative will build on and complement the work that has already been accomplished by other organizations and professionals by improving quality of care in dialysis. The NKF-DOQI project represents an unprecedented effort to develop evidence-based clinical practice guidelines for patients with chronic renal failure.

The areas selected for practice guidelines development are based on criteria similar to those recommended by the AHCPR. These criteria include: a high degree of variability in practice; high level of controversy or uncertainty; significant benefits or risks associated with the practice in question; significant number of patients affected; availability of sufficient information; and lack of contemporary practice guidelines.

The Work Groups will apply a formal structured review of the findings and methodology of each clinical study or paper. Draft guidelines will be developed by the Work Groups and presented for review the Advisory Council. The draft guidelines will also be presented to every organization of nephrology professionals for their review and critique. All feedback will be used to make the appropriate changes in the draft copies.

Final DOQI Clinical Practice Guidelines Draft review copies were distributed by NKF in Spring 1997 and final guidelines will be released later in the year. Many professionals in the nephrology community believe that - with the effort expended by the DOQI work group members as well as the commitment to educate both the patient and the public and the widespread dissemination/implementation plans-the guidelines could play a major role in improving patient care and reducing the mortality rate ("Continuous quality improvement...," 1997; Price, 1996a; 1996b).

Future Considerations

The Medicare ESRD Program provides 92.5% of the necessary funds to maintain the lives of patients with chronic renal failure requiring either dialysis treatments or kidney transplantation (USRDS Annual Report, 1996). Additional funding sources include Medicaid, private insurances, Veterans Administration, state kidney programs, and supplemental Medicare insurances. The continued financial support of the government and third party payers must be based on reimbursement models that are created from standards of care, established practice guidelines, and measurable patient health care outcomes.

As the patient population continues to increase, a greater number of geriatric patients, high-risk patients with co-morbid conditions, and minorities which usually require more consideration of socio-economic problems will enter the program. Advances in surgical procedures and medical management of transplantation will continue to improve renal transplantation and long term graft survival. Aggressive organ donation efforts will promote public awareness and increase the number of available organs. Technological improvements will enhance hemodialysis treatments by providing no-needle access and insuring a dialysis prescription that is precise and reliable, and that assures adequacy of treatment. Peritoneal dialysis treatments will be augmented by connecting devices to alleviate contamination, equipment capable of perfusing the peritoneal membrane with in situ generated fluid, and kinetic modeling to enhance effectiveness.

Increased mergers leading to larger dialysis provider corporations; continuing government interest in capitation models; and enhanced collaboration between hospitals, dialysis facilities, transplant centers, and medical groups will promote cost effectiveness, prevention and early intervention, consumer satisfaction, and increased quality improvement techniques and expertise (Bocchino & Burrows-Hudson, 1995). The ESRD health care team must collaborate to coordinate patient care and enhance the patient's role as a decision maker.

Summary

Nephrology nurses have participated in the development of the clinical, legislative, and regulatory management of the ESRD Program since its inception. As we consider the environment in which the ESRD Program enters a new millennium, the nephrology nurse's greatest challenge will be to adapt to his/her expanded role in delivering care to the patient with renal disease.

References

Abram, H.S. (1972). Psychological dilemmas of medical progress. *Psychiatry Medicine, 3,* 51-58.

Albers, J. (1989). Reflections on the first dialysis nurse training program. *ANNA Journal, 16*(3), 230-231.

Bocchino, C., & Burrows-Hudson, S. (1995). Other salient issues related to ESRD and its treatment. In L.E. Lancaster (Ed.), *Core curriculum for nephrology nursing* (3rd edition) (pp. 423-446). Pitman, NJ: American Nephrology Nurses' Association.

Committee on Chronic Kidney Disease. (1967). *Report of the Committee on Chronic Kidney Disease* (GPO publication No. 933-491). Washington, DC: Government Printing Office.

Continuous quality improvement: HCFA plans important new patient-specific data collection initiative to improve CQI at the dialysis facility level. (1997). *Contemporary Dialysis & Nephrology, 18*(7), 17, 28.

Evans, R.W., Blagg, C.R., & Bryan, F.A. Jr. (1981). Implications for health care policy: A social and demographic profile of hemodialysis patients in the U.S. *Journal of the American Medical Association, 245,* 487-491.

Federal Register. (1973, June 19). 38, 17210. Washington, DC.

Food and Drug Administration. (FDA). (1989). *Summary basis of approval: Drug license name: Epoetin alfa.* Washington, DC: Author.

General Accounting Office. (1990). *Medicare: Options to provide home dialysis aides* (GAO/HRD-90-153). Washington, DC: Author.

Health Care Financing Administration (HCFA). (1989). Reimbursement for ESRD and transplant services. In *Medicare provider reimbursement manual: Transmittal No. 11.* Baltimore, MD: Author.

Iglehart, J.K. (1993). The American health care system: The End Stage Renal Disease Program. *New England Journal of Medicine, 328*(5), p. 367.

Kidney waiting list statistics are announced. (1997). *Contemporary Dialysis & Nephrology, 18*(5), 8.

Klahr, S. (1990). Rationing of health care and the end stage renal disease program. *American Journal of Kidney Disease, 16/*(4), 392-395.

Levinsky, N.G. (1993). The organization of medical care: Lessons from the Medicare end stage renal disease program. *New England Journal of Medicine, 329*(19), 1395-1399.

Murray, J.S, Tu W.H., Albers, J.B., Burnell, J.M., & Scribner, B.H. (1962). A community hemodialysis center for the treatment of chronic uremia. *Transcript, American Society for Artificial and Internal Organs, 8,* 315-320.

Plough, A.L. (1986). *Borrowed time* (p. 25). Philadelphia: Temple University Press.

Price, C. (1996a). President-Elect's message: Now is the time to get prepared for DOQI. *ANNA Update, 26*(1), 4, 6.

Price, C. (1996b). President's message: DOQI guidelines to be released to the renal community. *ANNA Update, 26*(6), 3.

ProPAC approves 2.8% increase in the composite rate. (1997). *Dialysis & Transplantation, 26*(3), 124.

Rettig, R.A. (1980). The politics of health cost containment: End-stage renal disease (Editorial). *Bulletin of the New York Academy of Medicine, 56,* 115-138.

Rettig, R., & Levinsky, N.(Eds.).(1991). *Kidney failure and the federal government/Committee for the study of the Medicare ESRD program, Division of Health Care Services, Institute of Medicine.* Washington, DC: National Academy Press.

Scribner, B. (1990). A personalized history of chronic hemodialysis. *American Journal of Kidney Diseases, XVI*(6), 512.

Schupak, E., & Merrill, J.P. (1965). Experience with long-term intermittent hemodialysis. *Annals of Internal Medicine,* 62, 509-518.

Smith, K. (1996). Representatives from the transplant community convene in Washington. *ANNA Update, 26*(5), 8.

Statement of principles on managed care and the ESRD population. (1997). *ANNA Update, 27*(3), 28.

United States Renal Data System (USRDS). (1990). *Annual Report. National Institute of Diabetes and Digestive and Kidney Diseases.* Bethesda, MD: Author.

Chapter Highlights

- In the Social Security Amendments of 1972 (HR-1, Title XVIII), Public Law Number 92-603, Congress created authorization to Medicare in support of persons with the diagnosis of chronic renal failure who were eligible for benefits under Social Security, and for the spouses or dependent children of these persons.

- The membership of the early selection committees reflected the demographic features of the medical profession and middle class values rather than those of the population of potential beneficiaries.

- In the 1960s and 1970s, the cost of health care represented a much lower percentage of the gross national product (GNP) than it does today, therefore, to deny life-saving treatment to Americans exclusively because of financial cost was given only cursory consideration.

- Legislation authorizes the Health Care Financing Administration (HCFA) as the agency with administrative responsibility to formulate regulations that implement the public laws governing the Medicare ESRD program.

- A national ESRD registry to assemble and analyze data, known as the United States Renal Data System (USRDS), was established by the Secretary of the DHHS, as directed by Congress. The USRDS originated from discussions involving the renal community, Congress, and the National Institute of Diabetes and Digestive and Kidney Diseases (NIDDK).

- The IOM committee submitted a report to Congress and the Secretary of the DHHS and the report was published as *Kidney Failure and the Federal Government* through the National Academy Press, Washington, DC, 1991. There is no question that the objectives for the Medicare ESRD Program and recommendations based on the objectives set forth in the IOM report will have a profound impact on the ESRD Program for years to come (Klahr, 1990).

- The NKF-DOQI project represents an unprecedented effort to develop evidence-based clinical practice guidelines for patients with chronic renal failure.

- As the patient population continues to increase, a greater number of geriatric patients, high-risk patients with co-morbid conditions, and minorities, which usually require more consideration of socio-economic problems, will enter the program.

UNIT 8

Communication and Collaboration

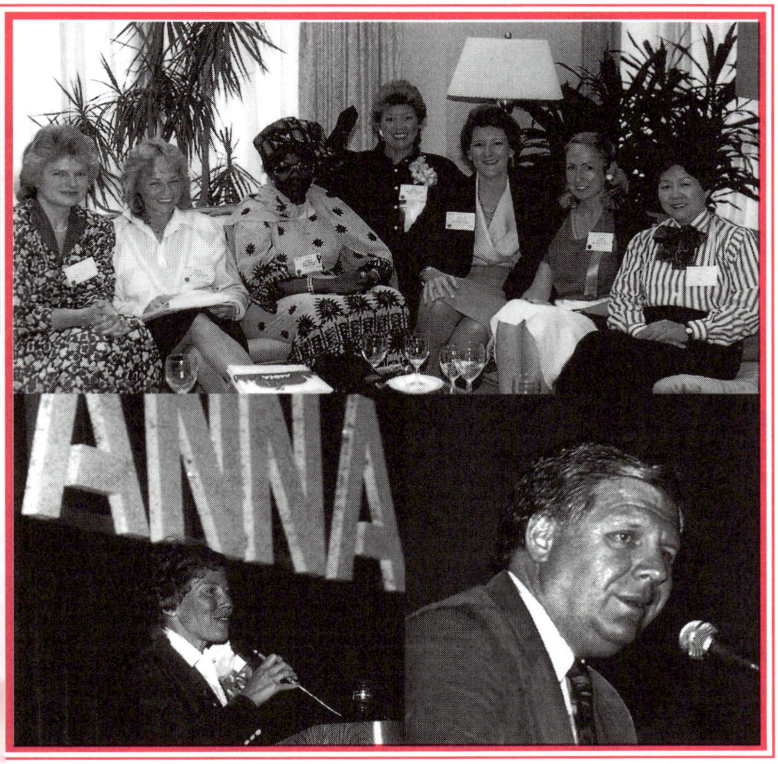

Unit Contents

Chapter 26
Maintaining and Documenting Standards of Care: Using the Nursing Process. 817
Eileen Peacock, MSN, RN, CNN, CIC, CPHQ
Barbara Bednar, MHA, RN, CNN

Chapter 27
Patient Education 837
Karen C. Robbins, MS, RN, CNN
Gail S. Wick, BSN, RN, CNN

Chapter 28
The Nephrology Community . . 853
Evelyn Butera, MS, RN, CNN
Nancy Gallagher, BSN, RN, CNN

CHAPTER 26

Maintaining and Documenting Standards of Care: Using the Nursing Process

Barbara Bednar, BSN, MHA, RN, CNN
Eileen Peacock, MSN, RN, CNN, CIC, CPHQ

Chapter Contents

Standards 819
Historical Background 820
Standards of Professional Performance 820
Standards of Care 821
Benefits Derived From Using Standards 822
Clinical Practice Guidelines 822
Historical Background 823
Application of Practice Guidelines 823
Summary 823
Documentation and The Nursing Process 824
Step 1 825
Step 2 825
Step 3 829
Step 4 829
Step 5 831
Legal and Risk Management Aspects 833
Quality Assurance/Continuous Quality Improvement Aspects 833
References 834
Chapter Highlights 835

Maintaining and Documenting Standards of Care: Use of the Nursing Process

***Barbara Bednar** BSN, MHA, RN, CNN*
***Eileen Peacock** MSN, RN, CNN, CIC, CPHQ*

Nephrology nurses have both an ethical and legal duty to practice nursing according to a professional nursing standard of care (Cournoyer, 1989). Like all professional nurses, nephrology nurses are required to use the same degree of knowledge and skill as reasonably prudent nurses would under similar circumstances. If nurses fail to provide appropriate care, they may be held liable. The American Nurses Association (ANA) *Standards of Nursing Practice*, standards that are published by the specialty professional nursing organizations, and the Joint Commission on the Accreditation of Healthcare Organizations' standards are types of documents that are usually used in a court of law to prove standards of care. For example, the Joint Commission's *Standards for Documentation of Nursing Care* state that the nursing process (assessment, planning, intervention, and evaluation) shall be documented for each hospitalized patient from admission through discharge (Cournoyer, 1989).

It is vital for nephrology nurses to become familiar with the profession's standards of care; the benefits of these standards such as the promotion of quality care; the difference between standards and practice guidelines; the benefits of practice guidelines such as reducing the incidence of inappropriate care; and the standards of nursing practice that require nursing documentation to reflect accurate and appropriate observations, assessment, interventions, and evaluation.

The purpose of this chapter is to help nursing students and nephrology nurses to document their practice within the framework and context of the nursing process while communicating legally relevant information about patient status, medical care, and nursing care, and compliance with established standards of care (Fischbach, 1991).

Standards

Standards are criteria for professional practice that serve as a model to facilitate and evaluate the quality of nursing service provided to nephrology patients. As a profession, nursing has a responsibility to guarantee the quality of nursing care to a society that calls for self-regulation. The foundation for this guarantee are the standards of the nursing profession that provide a means for professional nurses, individually and collectively, to accept responsibility and accountability for their practice. In dealing with the issue of accountability for nursing practice, Donabedian (1988) notes that,

> There is a social contract between society and the professions. Under its terms, society grants the professions the authority over functions vital to itself and permits them considerable autonomy in the conduct of their own affairs. In return, the professions are expected to act responsibly, always mindful of the public trust. Self-regulation to assure quality in performance is at the heart of this relationship. It is the hallmark of a mature profession (p. 1743).

Nephrology nursing is directed toward assessing the health needs of adult and pediatric patients and their families who are experiencing the real or threatened impact of acute or chronic renal failure, as well as diagnosing and treating their responses to these problems. Within this context, nephrology nurses are committed to helping each individual to achieve an optimal level of functioning (American Nephrology Nurses' Association [ANNA], 1986). In order to provide nursing care that meets these goals, nephrology nurses must have a defined practice base to guide the delivery of nursing care. Many components of the practice base for nephrology nurses have been developed by ANNA. *The Scope of Practice for Nephrology Nursing* (ANNA, 1986) was published in 1986 to define the role of the nephrology nurse. *The Core Curriculum For Nephrology Nursing* (Lancaster, 1987), first published in 1987, delineated the knowledge base required for nephrology nursing practice. *Nephrology Nursing: A Guide to Professional Development* (Jordan, 1993) was published in 1993 to promote clinical expertise through the professional growth and development of registered nurses entering the field of nephrology or currently practicing in this specialty. *The Standards of Clinical Practice for Nephrology*

Table 26-1
Standards of clinical nursing practice.

Standards of Professional Performance		Standards of Care	
I.	Quality of Care	Assessment	Nursing Process
II.	Performance Appraisal	Diagnosis	
III.	Education	Outcome	
IV.	Collegiality	Planning	
V.	Ethics	Implementation	
VI.	Collaboration	Evaluation	
VII.	Research		
VIII.	Research Utilization		

Note: From American Nurses Association. (1991). Standards of clinical nursing practice (1991). Washington, DC: Author.

Nursing (Burrows-Hudson, 1993), revised and expanded in 1993, serves as a framework for developing and monitoring nephrology nursing practice and represents the remaining components of the practice base for nephrology nurses.

Historical Background

The first publication of *Standards of Nursing Practice* was developed by the American Nurses' Association (ANA) Congress for Nursing Practice in 1973. In the introduction, nursing is identified as a profession with responsibilities for evaluating its service to the public through the development of standards. These generic *Standards of Nursing Practice* (ANA, 1973) were written within a nursing process framework that provided a basis for both the provision and evaluation of nursing care. ANA recognized that ongoing revision of standards was necessary to reflect the enlarging scope of practice upon which nursing practice rests.

In keeping with the nursing agenda to address quality, appropriateness, and effectiveness, in 1991 ANA issued a revision of the *Standards of Nursing Practice*. While some nursing organizations have collaborated with ANA to develop clinical standards, other clinical standards have been developed by specialty nursing organizations.

In 1977, The American Association of Nephrology Nurses and Technicians (AANNT) published *Standards of Clinical Practice for the Nephrology Patient*. The four separate documents addressed hemodialysis, transplantation, peritoneal dialysis, and acute renal failure. These were not strictly nursing standards. In 1982, AANNT published *Nephrology Nursing Standards of Clinical Practice* using a nursing process format. In 1984, the title of the standards was changed to reflect the association's name change, the *American Nephrology Nurses' Association (ANNA) Standards of Clinical Practice.* Although the standards focused on nursing process, structure standards were minimally addressed, and outcome standards were not included. In 1988, the *ANNA Standards of Clinical Practice for Nephrology Nursing* were published and identified desired patient outcomes based on nursing management. The document included two major sections, structure standards and process standards. Structure standards defined the environment within which care is provided and included organizational and management characteristics, qualifications of the nurse, physical plant, and equipment. Process standards outlined the action or behaviors necessary to implement nursing care.

In 1993, the *Standards of Clinical Practice for Nephrology Nursing* (Burrows-Hudson, 1993) were published and incorporated ANNA's acceptance of the revised ANA format for standards of practice and standards of care, regulatory changes in the End Stage Renal Disease Program (ESRD), and health care since 1988, as well as advances in technology, pharmacology, and nephrology nursing practice. As a result, the new standards include standards of professional performance, standards of care for nursing practice, and universal nephrology nursing standards of care. These standards are defined as authoritative statements that describe a level of care or performance common to the nursing profession by which the quality of nursing practice can be judged (Burrows-Hudson, 1993). Standards of clinical nursing practice include both standards of care and standards of professional performance (see Table 26-1).

Standards of Professional Performance

Standards of care reflect the activities and

behaviors included in the nursing process while standards of professional performance reflect other role activities and behaviors essential to the role of professional nursing.

Standards of professional performance include activities that may not be directly evident in providing care to patients but are integral to the professional nursing role and are indirectly reflected in the provision of direct nursing services to patients. These standards of professional performance describe the competency level of professional behavior and include quality of care, performance appraisal, education, collegiality, ethics, collaboration, research, and resource utilization. Although these behaviors are universally expected, attainment depends on education, current position, and practice environment. The standards include measurement criteria that identify a range of activities that may demonstrate compliance with a particular standard. The expected professional behaviors form a foundation for incorporating the established standards into day-to-day practice by serving as the foundation for role description and performance appraisals for nephrology nurses (Jordan, 1993).

The eight standards for professional performance include:

Standard I: Quality of Care

The nephrology nurse systematically evaluates the quality and effectiveness of nursing practice.

Standard II: Performance Appraisal

The nephrology nurse evaluates his/her own nursing practice in relation to professional practice standards and relevant statutes and regulations.

Both the quality of care and the performance appraisal standards focus on participating in quality of care activities while using the results of such activities to identify benchmarking opportunities to initiate change in nursing practice. These standards include possible activities such as a clinical benchmarking program designed to use comparative data to develop policy, procedures, and practice guidelines.

Standard III: Education

The nephrology nurse acquires and maintains current knowledge in nephrology nursing practice.

The Education Standard permits flexibility for nephrology nurses to participate in formal or informal education activities. It includes possible activities that range from regularly reading professional journals to attending educational seminars.

Standard IV: Collegiality

The nephrology nurse contributes to the professional development of peers, colleagues, and others.

The collegiality standard is closely related to the performance appraisal and education standards. This standard places an emphasis on nephrology nurses sharing skills and knowledge while contributing to an environment that is conducive to the clinical education of nursing students.

Standard V: Ethics

The nephrology nurse's decision and actions on behalf of patients are determined in an ethical manner.

This standard reinforces that nursing care must be delivered in a nondiscriminating manner that protects patient autonomy and dignity.

Standard VI: Collaboration

The nephrology nurse collaborates with the patient, significant others, and health care providers in providing patient care.

This standard underscores the increasing need for collaborating with others through consultation, referral, and communication.

Standard VII: Research

The nephrology nurse uses research findings in practice.

Standard VIII: Resource Utilization

The nephrology nurse considers factors related to safety, effectiveness, and cost in planning and delivering patient care.

Standards of Care

Standards of care describes nursing care competency within the framework of the nursing process; that is, assessment, diagnosis, desired patient outcome, planning, implementation, and evaluation (see Table 26-2). Nursing practice in all settings must possess the characteristics identified by these standards if patients are to receive a high level of quality nursing care (Leddy & Pepper, 1985).

Standard I: Assessment

The nephrology nurse performs an accurate and continuous assessment of the patient.

Standard II: Diagnosis

The nephrology nurse analyzes the assessment data to formulate nursing diagnosis.

Standard III: Outcome Identification

The nephrology nurse identifies expected outcomes individualized to the patient.

Standard IV: Planning

The nephrology nurse formulates a written comprehensive care plan that prescribes interventions based on identified nursing diagnosis and expected outcomes.

Standard V: Implementation

The nephrology nurse implements the interventions identified in the plan of care.

Standard VI: Evaluation

The nephrology nurse evaluates the client's progress toward attainment of outcomes and modifies the plan of care.

Table 26-2
Relationship between nursing process and standards of care.

Steps of Nursing Process	Standards of Care
Assessment	Standard I
Diagnosis	Standard II
Planning	Standards III & IV
Implementation	Standard V
Evaluation	Standard VI

Note: Adapted from Leddy, S., & Pepper, M. (1985). Conceptual basis of professional nursing. Philadelphia: J.B. Lippincott Company.

Benefits Derived from Using Standards

Implementation of standards of care serve to improve care, make managers' jobs easier, and make nurses' jobs more satisfying. Benefits derived from using standards include:

- *Facilitates clear role description, expectations and evaluations.*
  Role descriptions based on standards provide clear expectations. In addition, standards can be used to evaluate the nursing care provided by individual nurses. Use of standards when writing job evaluations results in a more objective appraisal of nurses. The use of standards in performance appraisals also provides a mechanism for direct feedback to nurses for future improvement strategies.
- *Outline for orientation and staff development programs.*
  Standards may be used in orientation as a basis for nursing practice in a renal unit or department, and delineate the content, skills, and competencies expected from clinical nurses. They can provide a systematic approach to provide information to employees. Educational staff programs and inservices, based on standards, provides a consistent framework from which to work and can serve as a mechanism of quality control.
- *Promotes quality and improves the delivery of health care.*
  The use of standards promotes continuity and consistency of care. Continuity implies that clinical practice does not vary among practitioners or different shifts. In addition, the use of standards facilitates collaboration opportunities among peers and physicians. All nephrology nurses should participate in clinical practice patterns that reflect the appropriate standard of care. With standards of care, nurses can establish the minimal level of competence to ensure quality of care. In continuous quality improvement, standards may assist in the development of criteria for evaluating the environment, professional practice, and patient outcomes.

In summary, the *Standard of Clinical Practice for Nephrology Nursing* focuses on the process of providing nursing care and performing professional role activities. ANNA (1991) proposed that these standards for nursing practice, along with the development of practice guidelines, could be used by health care providers for the basis of quality assurance, health care reimbursement, agency policies and procedures, and educational offerings.

Clinical Practice Guidelines

Clinical practice guidelines are systematically developed statements designed to help caregivers and their patients make decisions about appropriate care for specific health conditions. Guidelines reflect current scientific knowledge of practices and the best professional judgment used to prevent, diagnose, treat, or manage diseases and disorders.

While standards of care are generally accepted *principles* for patient management, guidelines are recommendations that may identify a particular management strategy or a range of management strategies (Hirshfeld, 1990). While standards are intended to be followed *all* the time, guidelines should be followed in *most* cases. However, depending on the patient, setting, and other factors, guidelines can and should be tailored to fit individual needs (Eddy, 1990). Deviations from guidelines will be fairly common and can be justified by differences in individual circumstances because they are strategies of patient management. The following example should clarify the difference between a standard and a guideline. The outcome Standard on Vascular Access for the Hemodialysis Client states as a patient outcome, "The patient will be free of vascular access complication." This is a principle of care to be applied in all cases for all patients. A practice guideline would include treatment or procedure strategies to manage, prevent, diagnose, and treat vascular access complications applicable to individual clients.

The goals of practice guidelines include the following:

- Provide guidance to clinicians based on the best available scientific information and clinical judgment and to enhance the quality of care received by clients with renal disease.

- Combine the science and art of the practice of nephrology to provide a structure for nursing judgment.
- Reduce the incidence of inappropriate care in the treatment of clients with renal disease.
- Reduce the wide variation of practice patterns among practitioners who care for clients with renal disease.

Historical Background

Research during the past two decades has identified major variations in practice patterns. Studies by researchers have documented large inconsistencies in the rate with that specific procedures are performed in different geographic areas. Because these variations may be caused by clinician uncertainty about proper indications for procedures, some have argued that providing guidelines might reduce the magnitude of practice variation and inappropriate care. There also is concern that health dollars spent by patients or their families, insurers, employers, and federal and state programs such as Medicare and Medicaid are being wasted on ineffective care. Prominent health leaders suggest that one-quarter to one-third of all medical care may be unnecessary.

In Spring 1989, Congress introduced a series of bills calling for expanded federal funding for effectiveness research and the creation of a formal Public Health Service (PHS) agency with responsibility for the development and dissemination of practice guidelines. This legislation received wide political support (Woolf, 1990).Therefore, in 1989, Congress established the Agency for Health Care Policy and Research (AHCPR) to improve the quality, appropriateness, and effectiveness of health care in the United States.

AHCPR commissioned guidelines recommend ways of diagnosing, treating, managing, and where possible, preventing complications. The guidelines are based on a comprehensive review of the scientific literature, on valid evidence presented at open meetings, and on the professional judgments of panel members and other experts in the field. In contrast to other guidelines developed by the National Institutes of Health (NIH), the Centers for Disease Control (CDC), and the Food and Drug Administration (FDA), those developed under AHCPR sponsorship are the product of many different types of health providers (primary care physicians, specialists, nurse and allied health care providers) and consumer representatives. The AHCPR is a full Public Health Service agency, which was authorized to receive $221 million in 1992.

AHCPR considers a number of factors in selecting guidelines topics, including:

- Adequacy of science-based evidence.
- Number of individuals affected by the clinical condition.
- Expected potential for reducing inappropriate variations in the prevention, diagnosis, management, or outcomes associated with the condition.
- Specific needs of Medicare and Medicaid populations.
- Cost of the condition to all payers, including patients.
- As guidelines are completed, AHCPR promotes wide dissemination to consumers, practitioners, policy makers and researchers.

Application of Practice Guidelines

The future implications of practice guidelines are far reaching. For practitioners, although there is a general agreement that guidelines can contribute to medicine as an educational tool and as a source of guidance to aid clinical decision-making, it is unclear whether rigid enforcement will improve the quality of care (Woolf, 1990). It has become evident that some third-party payers, malpractice courts, utilization reviews, and regulators are monitoring compliance with practice guidelines and as a result, it may be possible that patients may be denied access to necessary services mislabeled as inappropriate (Brook, 1989; Hirshfeld, 1990; Sandrick, 1993; Kenkel, 1993). This debate is focusing increased attention on the clinical and scientific validity of guidelines, the process by which they are developed, and who develops them.

In summary, practice guidelines present a promising strategy to define appropriate medical care. Guidelines are intended to be flexible strategies to assist both customers and practitioners in clinical decision-making. Properly developed, guidelines are supported by scientific evidence and achieve the objectives of accuracy, accountability, predictability, defensibility, and usability. The future use of clinical guidelines is still uncertain, however, alterations in policy making, consumer selection of health plans, licensing bodies credentialing activities, and third-party payer reimbursement practices could be expected. (See Table 26-3 for a current list of AHCPR Clinical Practice Guidelines.)

Summary

Standards of clinical nursing practice include both standards of care and standards of professional performance. Standards of professional performance reflect role activities and behaviors essential to the role of professional nursing. Standards of care set minimum criteria for nursing proficiency. These standards describe the activities for which nurses are accountable. Standards of care also provide direction for evaluating practice. ANA standards apply to all registered nurses in clinical practice regardless of their specialty

Table 26-3
AHCPR sponsored clinical practice guidelines.

1. Acute Pain Management: Operative or Medical Procedures and Trauma.
2. Urinary Incontinence in Adults*
3. Pressure Ulcers in Adults: Prediction and Prevention
4. Cataract in Adults: Management of Functional Impairment
5. Depression in Primary Care: Detection, Diagnosis and Treatment
6. Sickle Cell Disease: Screening, Diagnosis, Management, and Counseling in Newborns and Infants
7. Early HIV Infection: Evaluation and Management
8. Benign Prostatic Hyperplasia: Diagnosis and Management
9. Management of Cancer Pain
10. Unstable Angina: Diagnosis and Management.
11. Heart Failure: Evaluation and Care of Patients with Left Ventricular Systolic Dysfunction
12. Otitis Media with Effusion in Children
13. Quality Determinants of Mammography
14. Acute Low Back Problems in Adults
15. Treatment of Pressure Ulcers
16. Post-Stroke Rehabilitation
17. Cardiac Rehabilitation

**These guidelines were originally released in 1992 and updated in 1996*

and outline a competent level of nursing care using six standards that correspond to a specific step of the nursing process. To meet the ANA standards, nurses must provide for and document evidence that a competent level of care has been provided for each stage of the nursing process; assessment, diagnoses, planning, implementation, and evaluation (see Table 26-2).

Documentation and The Nursing Process

Accepted national standards are becoming increasingly important in how courts rule on issues of nursing malpractice or negligence (Springhouse Corporation, 1993). Nursing documentation not only relays information, it records how well nurses have met the established standards of care. Nursing documentation provides evidence that the care rendered meets the accepted standards of nursing care that are mandated by law, the profession, and the health care institution in which you practice (Springhouse Corporation, 1995). Cournoyer (1989), author of *The Nurse Manager and The Law,* reports that of the 20 deficiencies most frequently cited during Joint Commission Accreditation visits, 3 involve nurses' responsibility for documentation. One of these three documentation deficiencies pertained to documentation of the nursing care that should address patients needs, problems, capabilities, and limitations as well as nursing interventions and patient responses to the nursing interventions. Knowledge and correct use of the nursing process improves documentation and aids in ensuring that your contributions as nephrology nurses to patient well-being are recognized (Springhouse Corporation, 1993).

Leddy and Pepper (1985), authors of *Conceptual Bases of Professional Nursing*, noted that the focus of nursing — when based on a model of autonomous professional practice — is support of patients with the goal of improving the patients' well-being, status, and potential. In order to achieve this goal, nurses need knowledge about the patient from which nursing interventions will be developed. The rationale for nursing goal development and intervention is knowledge based on assessment, planning, and feedback from evaluation, also known as the nursing process (Leddy & Pepper, 1985).

The nursing process provides a systematic approach to nursing practice and documentation of the delivered care. The nursing process can also be seen as a set of actions leading to a particular goal or more simply, as a problem solving process used to identify your patient needs and the nursing interventions to be utilized.

Table 26-4
Examples of NANDA taxonomy - classification system for nursing diagnosis.

Pattern 1	**Exchanging** - Fluid volume excess - Fluid volume deficit - High risk for injury
Pattern 2	**Communicating** - Impaired verbal communication
Pattern 3	**Relating** - Impaired social interaction - Altered family process
Pattern 4	**Valuing** - Spiritual
Pattern 5	**Choosing** - Ineffective denial - Noncompliance
Pattern 6	**Moving** - Impaired physical mobility - Fatigue
Pattern 7	**Perceiving** - Body image disturbance - Sensory-perceptual alternative
Pattern 8	**Knowing** - Knowledge deficit - Altered thought processes
Pattern 9	**Feeling** - chronic pain - anxiety

Step 1: Assessment (Standard of Care I)

The collection of data about the health status of patients must be systematic, continuous, and include both subjective and objective data about patients. This step of the nursing process involves obtaining a health history, making general observations, and performing a physical assessment. The quality of the data collected during the assessment will determine the appropriateness of the nursing diagnosis and the subsequent plan of care. Documentation during this phase provides a record of what was seen, heard, and felt during the assessment. This record may be later used by other members of the health care team who may not have access to the recorder, rendering the data subject to interpretation. It is important therefore, that the recorded assessment be objective, complete and concise as possible (Malasanos, Barkauskas, & Stoltenberg, 1986).

Documentation during Step 1 of the nursing process should include:

- Recording subjective data as just that, using patients' own words whenever possible.
- Avoid using subjective terms such as "large" or moderate" when recording objective data. Use measurements whenever possible. For example, instead of describing urinary output as moderate in amount, document the actual number of milliliters of urine.
- Avoid interpreting the data and reflecting your opinion. For example, don't write "patient in fluid overload." Instead document your findings of +4 peripheral edema, blood pressure of 180/100, 10 pounds above estimated dry weight, rales on auscultation, shortness of breath, respirations 32.

Cournoyer (1989) provides the following as examples of appropriate observations and assessments:

- Routine observations of the patient's condition with normal findings.
- Changes in the patient's status, especially the initial and ongoing assessments that may indicate that the patient's condition is improving or deteriorating.
- Description of the patient's behavior, appearance, and symptoms.
- Statements by patients and family that are relevant to the nurse's assessments and observations.

Step 2: Nursing Diagnosis (Standard of Care II)

Nursing diagnosis, which are obtained from assessment data, identify problems that nurses are qualified and licensed to treat. Nursing diagnoses, focus on patients' responses to illness and have three components: (a) clients' actual or potential health problems, combined with (b) etiologic factors, and supported by (c) signs and symptoms (Leddy & Pepper, 1985).

Nurses either use standardized diagnoses or develop their own diagnoses. The most widely used taxonomy of nursing diagnoses, which are organized around 9 human response patterns, has been developed by the North American Nursing Diagnosis Association (NANDA). Table 26-4 lists the 9 response patterns and provides examples of nursing diagnosis taxonomy for each pattern. Readers should refer to Table 26-5 for the complete list.

Table 26-5
NANDA Taxonomy I, Revised

The North American Nursing Diagnosis Association (NANDA) endorsed its first nursing diagnosis taxonomic structure, NANDA Taxonomy I, in 1986. In 1989, this taxonomy was revised. Organized around nine human response patterns, the revised taxonomy represents the currently accepted classification system for nursing diagnoses. The nine patterns and their definitions are:

1. Exchanging: Mutual giving and receiving
2. Communicating: Sending messages
3. Related: Establishing bonds
4. Valuing: Assigning worth
5. Choosing: Selection of alterations
6. Moving: Activity
7. Perceiving: Reception of information
8. Knowing: Meaning associated with information
9. Feeling: Subjective awareness of information.

The complete taxonomy appears below. Taxonomy II is under development.

Pattern 1: Exchanging

1.1.2.1	Altered nutrition: More than body requirements
1.1.2.2	Altered nutrition: Less than body requirements
1.1.2.3	Altered nutrition: Potential for more than body requirements
1.2.1.1	High risk for infection
1.2.2.1	High risk for altered body temperature
1.2.2.2	Hypothermia
1.2.2.3	Hyperthermia
1.2.2.4	Ineffective thermoregulation
1.2.3.1	Dysreflexia
1.3.1.1	Constipation
1.3.1.1.1	Perceived constipation
1.3.1.1.2	Colonic constipation
1.3.1.2	Diarrhea
1.3.1.3	Bowel incontinence
1.3.2	Altered urinary elimination
1.3.2.1.1	Stress incontinence
1.3.2.1.2	Reflex incontinence
1.3.2.1.3	Urge incontinence
1.3.2.1.4	Total incontinence
1.3.2.2	Urinary retention
1.4.1.1	Altered (specify type) tissue perfusion (renal, cerebral, cardiopulmonary, gastrointestinal, peripheral)
1.4.1.2.1	Fluid volume excess
1.4.1.2.2.1	Fluid volume deficit
1.4.1.2.2.2	High risk for fluid volume deficit
1.4.2.1	Decreased cardiac output
1.5.1.1	Impaired gas exchange
1.5.1.2	Ineffective airway clearance
1.5.1.3	Ineffective breathing pattern
1.5.1.3.1	Inability to sustain spontaneous ventilation

1.5.1.3.2	Dysfunctional ventilatory weaning response
1.6.1	High risk for injury
1.6.1.1	High risk for suffocation
1.6.1.2	High risk for poisoning
1.6.1.3	High risk for trauma
1.6.1.4	High risk for aspiration
1.6.1.5	High risk for disuse syndrome
1.6.2	Altered protection
1.6.2.1.1	Altered oral mucous membrane
1.6.2.1.2.1	Impaired tissue integrity
1.6.2.1.2.2	High risk for impaired skin integrity
Pattern 2: Communicating	
2.1.1.1	Impaired verbal communication
Pattern 3: Relating	
3.1.1	Impaired social interaction
3.1.2	Social isolation
3.2.1	Altered role performance
3.2.1.1.1	Altered parenting
3.2.1.1.2	High risk for altered parenting
3.2.1.2.1	Sexual dysfunction
3.2.2	Altered family processes
3.2.2.1	Caregiver role strain
3.2.2.2	High risk for caregiver role strain
3.2.3.1	Parental role conflict
3.3	Altered sexuality patterns
Pattern 4: Valuing	
4.1.1	Spiritual distress (distress of the human spirit)
Pattern 5: Choosing	
5.1.1.1	Ineffective individual coping
5.1.1.1.1	Impaired adjustment
5.1.1.1.2	Defensive coping
5.1.1.1.3	Ineffective denial
5.1.2.1.1	Ineffective family coping: Disabling
5.1.2.1.2	Ineffective family coping: Compromised
5.1.2.2	Family coping: Potential for growth
5.2.1	Ineffective management of therapeutic regimen (individual)
5.2.1.1	Noncompliance (specify)
5.3.1.1	Decisional conflict (specify)
5.4	Health-seeking behaviors (specify)
Pattern 6: Moving	
6.1.1.1	Impaired physical mobility
6.1.1.1.1	High risk for peripheral neurovascular dysfunction
6.1.1.2	Activity intolerance
6.1.1.2.1	Fatigue
6.1.1.3	High risk for activity intolerance

6.2.1	Sleep pattern disturbance
6.3.1.1	Diversional activity deficit
6.4.1.1	Impaired home maintenance management
6.4.2	Altered health maintenance
6.5.1	Feeding self-care deficit
6.5.1.1	Impaired swallowing
6.5.1.2	Ineffective breast-feeding
6.5.1.2.1	Interrupted breast-feeding
6.5.1.3	Effective breast-feeding
6.5.1.4	Ineffective infant feeding pattern
6.5.2	Bathing or hygiene self-care deficit
6.5.3	Dressing or grooming self-care deficit
6.5.4	Toileting self-care deficit
6.6	Altered growth and development
6.7	Relocation stress syndrome

Pattern 7: Perceiving

7.1.1	Body image disturbance
7.1.2	Self-esteem disturbance
7.1.2.1	Chronic low self-esteem
7.1.2.2	Situational low self-esteem
7.1.3	Personal identity disturbance
7.2	Sensory-perceptual alterations (specify as visual, auditory, kinesthetic, gustatory, tactile, olfactory)
7.2.1.1	Unilateral neglect
7.3.1	Hopelessness
7.3.2	Powerlessness

Pattern 8: Knowing

8.1.1	Knowledge deficit (specify)
8.3	Altered thought processes

Pattern 9: Feeling

9.1	Pain
9.1.1.1	Chronic pain
9.2.1.1	Dysfunctional grieving
9.2.1.2	Anticipatory grieving
9.2.2	High risk for violence: Self-directed or directed at others
9.2.2.1	High risk for self-mutilation
9.2.3	Posttrauma response
9.2.3.1	Rape-trauma syndrome
9.2.3.1.1	Rape-trauma syndrome: Compound reaction
9.2.3.1.2	Rape-trauma syndrome: Silent reaction
9.3.1	Anxiety
9.3.2	Fear

Documentation during Step 2 of the nursing process should include:

- Each nursing diagnoses should include a diagnostic label or problem and a related etiology or cause (Springhouse Corporation, 1993). For example, a diagnostic label for patients on continuous ambulatory peritoneal dialysis (CAPD) could be high risk for injury; infection. The etiology could be expressed as related to insertion and maintenance of peritoneal catheter, and compromised immune system of the ESRD patient (see Figure 26-1.)
- Documentation of the nursing diagnosis must facilitate identification of expected outcomes and formulation of the plan of action or care. In other words, individualized expected outcomes and a plan of care prescribing interventions must be derived from the nursing diagnoses that has been derived from analysis of the assessment data (Springhouse Corporation, 1993; Jordan, 1993).

Step 3: Planning (Standards of Care III and IV)

The third step of the nursing process, which corresponds to Standard of Care III "Outcomes" and Standard of Care IV "Planning," involves identifying expected outcomes and developing a plan of care that includes nursing interventions designed to achieve expected outcomes (Springhouse Corporation, 1993). This plan of nursing care includes goals that state the criteria for what observable behavior or expected outcomes will occur as a result of the interventions and the time frame within which it will occur. Expected outcomes can either specify an improvement in the patient's ability to function or the resolution of a problem. For example, the expected outcomes for a renal failure patient with a nursing diagnoses of "alteration in tissue perfusion; decreased, secondary to intermittent hypovolemia," might include achieving and maintaining a BP > 110 mmHg systolic and reduction in the number of/or elimination of orthostatic hypotension episodes by a specified date.

Jordan (1993) noted that nephrology nurses identify expected outcomes individualized to patients that are:

- derived from the diagnoses,
- documented as measurable goals,
- mutually formulated with patients and the health care team when possible,
- realistic in relation to patients' present and potential capabilities,
- attainable in relation to resources available to patients,
- including a time estimate for attainment, and
- providing direction for continuity of care.

The plan of nursing care includes priorities and the prescribed nursing approaches or measures to achieve the goals derived from the nursing diagnoses. A good nursing care plan is the blueprint for concise, meaningful documentation (Springhouse Corporation, 1995) (see Figure 26-2).

There are two basic types of nursing care plans: (a) the traditional plan of care and (b) the standardized plan of care. Traditional plans are written from scratch for each patient with the form and style varied. Standardized plans provide a set of interventions for patients with similar diagnoses. No matter what type of plan you choose to use, documentation during Step 3 of the nursing process must include a nursing plan of care that (Springhouse Corporation, 1993, 1995):

- provides direction, guidance, and meaning to nursing care,
- consists of patient problems identified during the assessment phase,
- is realistic with goals that are not too difficult for patients to achieve,
- utilizes quantitative, precise terms, and measurable expected outcomes, and
- provides for continuity of care that includes all nursing care from admission to discharge.

Step 4: Implementation (Standard of Care V)

The fourth step of the nursing process, "implementation," corresponds to Standard of Care V and consist of nursing actions that provide for patient participation in health promotion, maintenance, and restorations as well as nursing actions that assist patients to maximize their health capabilities. For example, nursing interventions for the previously mentioned patient with a nursing diagnosis of "alteration in tissue perfusion; decreased, secondary to intermittent hypovolemia" might include:

- monitoring sitting/standing BP every a.m.,
- instructing patient to alter fluid intake according to daily weights and absence/presence of signs/symptoms of fluid volume excess,
- minimizing use of high % dextrose peritoneal dialysis solutions to prevent excessive ultrafiltration and fluid loss with dialysis exchanges, and
- monitoring fluid intake and output.

Documentation of nursing interventions may be completed using different formats. Progress notes, open narrative notes, flow sheets and other specialized documentation forms such as the hemodialysis treatment record, may be used for documenting nursing interventions. Documentation during Step 4 of the nursing process must include a description of the intervention, the time

Figure 26-1.
Sample nursing care plan (Adapted from Nuttal, 1990).

Patient:____________________

Date	Nursing Diagnosis	Rational/Data Collection	Goals Expected Outcomes	Target Date	Nursing Intervention	RN Signature	Evaluation	RN Signature	Resolution Date
	High risk for injury; infection	Potential for injury; infection Secondary to: • Insertion and maintenance of peritoneal catheter • Compromised immune system of ESRD patient • Lapses in aseptic technique when patient is fatigued Data Collection: • Complaints of chronic fatigue & weakness • Indwelling peritoneal dialysis catheter • Ashen skin color • Serum album less than 3.5 mg/dl. • Documented history of recurrent peritonitis • Documented periods of confusion	1. Exit site will remain free of signs/symptoms of infection 2. Patient will remain afebrile 3. Patient will remain free of signs/symptoms of peritonitis 4. Patient will report breaks in aseptic technique immediately and acquire appropriate prophylaxis 5. Signs and symptoms of infection will be recognized early and complications avoided/minimized		1. Instruct patient to recognize sign/symptoms of tunnel/exit site infections 2. Instruct patent to monitor daily signs/symptoms of peritonitis 3. Instruct patient to monitor temperature daily 4. Monitor WBCs closely 5. Culture any cloudy effluent 6. Culture any drainage from exit site 7. Instruct patient on daily catheter care procedures 8. Instruct patient in proper procedure for administration of intraperitoneal medications 9. Assess patients ability to complete exchange procedure without the use of a UV assistive device 10. Assess patients ability to complete exchange procedure without the use of a partner				

Table 26-6
Purposes of recording nursing care.

1.	Documents patient assessment and care.
2.	Assists in planning patient care.
3.	Evaluates the patient's condition in response to treatment.
4.	Contributes to consistency of practice among practitioners.
5.	Assists in the determination of whether hospital resources are used appropriately.
6.	Provides data for quality of care review.
7.	Records of nursing care form the basis of evaluation by federal, state, and voluntary agencies.
8.	Provides data for billing and reimbursement.
9.	Constitutes a legal record for use by the institution, other providers of care, and the patient.

Note: From Gross, K. (1987). Legal, financial, and risk management aspects of documentation for nurses. Madison, WI: Professional Education Systems, Inc.

it occurred, and the patient's response. Examples of appropriate interventions include (Cournoyer, 1989):

- identification or description of treatment, therapy, or teaching and the patient's response;
- description of the intervention made in response to the observation of the patient's change of status and/or condition;
- identification of actions taken in response to a change in the physician's orders; and
- identification of patient and family teaching activities and discharge information and instructions.

Documentation reflecting each step of the nursing process is one way to demonstrate that the nursing standard of care was met. Table 26-6 list specific purposes of recording the nursing care that nurses provide. There are many formats of the nursing record that may be used for such documentation, including the open narrative and the problem-oriented notes. Each format has advantages and disadvantages as noted in Table 26-7.

Whether you document using open narrative notes or problem-oriented notes, your documentation should reflect the nursing process. Although nurses are pressed for time and must deliver patient care before they write on the chart, they must develop a charting style that uses concise, specific terminology, describing reported symptoms accurately (Hapster & Veach, 1990).

Step 5: Evaluation (Standard of Care VI)

The fifth step of the nursing process, "evaluation," corresponds to Standard of Care VI and consists of selecting evaluation criteria, reassessing the patient's status, documenting the evaluation statement, and revising the plan of care as appropriate. The goal of this step of the nursing process is to judge the effectiveness of those nursing actions chosen to treat human responses to health problems or to prevent problems from occurring.

Data collection and the development of a conclusion statement are two necessary steps in evaluation documentation (Fischbach, 1991). Documented data collection is necessary before formulating a summary statement. Data collection documentation may include a statement such as "Blood Pressure 120/80, weight stable at 145 lbs., and no episodes of orthostatic hypotension after 3 days of utilizing lower percent dextrose peritoneal dialysis solutions." Conclusion or summary statements such as "exhibiting hemodynamic stability" are not meaningful without such associated substantiating data. Conclusive statements may reflect both ineffective or effective outcomes (Fischbach, 1991).

Griffith and Christensen (1982) have suggested the following questions that still apply today to assist with the evaluation process:

1. Was the assessment complete and appropriate?
2. Was the planning complete and sufficient?
3. Were the nursing diagnoses complete and appropriate?
4. Were the objectives appropriately stated?
5. Were the objectives met? Does the data collection support the conclusion? Were all participants satisfied?
6. Was the intervention effective and efficient? Does

Table 26-7
Nursing record formats.

Open Narrative Notes

Format:
- The format is blank, lined, with no per-printed prompts or cues.
- The form is labeled with the agency's name.

Advantages:
- Factual, unprompted data are entered.
- Chronology is preserved.

Disadvantages:
- The nurse must re-think and format the notes.
- Specificity can be lost and this format is very time consuming.

Problem-Oriented Notes

Format:
- The format is semi-blank and multiple forms may be needed. A Problem List is kept where health problems are identified and recorded, using a chronological order to number the problem. Open format note paper is used and acronyms such as SOAP ([S] Subjective Symptoms, [O] Objective Symptoms, [A] Assessment, [P] Plan]), are established for observations regarding specific numbered problems.

Advantages:
- Nursing records focus on problems not tasks.
- Communication with members of health care teams is improved.
- Continuity of care is recorded.
- Problem resolution is clearly documented.

Disadvantages:
- Routine care may be omitted.
- This approach may produce redundant charting.
- The use of narrative format makes the approach time consuming.
- Problem lists may not be updated to reflect current needs.

the data collection support this conclusion?
7. What changes were desirable in planning and intervention?
8. Were all steps communicated effectively?
9. What changes have occurred in the patient's needs, health status, or coping ability? Are additional changes desirable?
10. How does the patient feel about the outcomes?
11. What could have been done differently?

Depending on the outcome of the evaluation the following may be necessary:
- modification of the goals and/or interventions,
- a continuation of the planned strategies with a modified timetable, and
- termination of the relationship if the goals have been met and no new ones have emerged.

In outpatient dialysis settings, where patients may continue their care until transplant, transfer, or death, the nurse-patient relationship will continue and will include the monitoring of patient status to assist with sustained improvement while developing a plan of care and reinitiation of the nursing process to address emerging health care needs.

Legal and Risk Management Aspects

As stated in the beginning of this chapter, nephrology nurses have both an ethical and legal duty to practice nursing according to a professional nursing standard of care. Nursing malpractice or professional negligence is the failure of nurses to provide the standard of care that is provided by reasonably prudent nurses acting under the same or similar circumstances (Cournoyer, 1989). Although each state has laws that define malpractice, they all recognize that malpractice occurs when patients suffer because of health care professionals' wrongful conduct, improper discharge of duties, or failure to meet the standards of care (Springhouse Corporation, 1995). Documentation that fails to provide evidence that the standard was met will only serve to aid the plaintiff's case.

Patients' medical records constitute the legally recognized health care document for patients and are almost universally allowed as evidence during trial proceedings (Fischbach, 1991). Accurate nursing documentation based on the assumption that certain guidelines can direct documentation to reflect legally relevant data serves several purposes:

1. Documentation of obvious adherence to established standards of nursing care.
2. Maintenance of a legal record of adherence to accepted standards of care.
3. Provision of pertinent and useful data regarding the patient's condition as well as the medical and nursing regimen employed in the care of the patient.
4. Provision of self-protection against litigation when documentation complies with established standards of care (Fischbach, 1991).

Effective use of the nursing process for directing and documenting nursing care provides such guidelines. Cournoyer (1989) noted that the nursing process is a clinical management system that provides individualized goal-directed nursing care to patients. The author goes on to further state that most of the litigation involving nursing negligence focuses on the assessment and intervention stages of the nursing process. The author also explains that failure to plan or evaluate the care provided will usually result in inadequate or inappropriate assessments and interventions that can be identified by the plaintiff as a breach of the standard of practice that caused or significantly contributed to the plaintiff's injuries (Cournoyer, 1989). Proper and effective use of the nursing process along with cogent accurate documentation addressing each step of the nursing process may serve as a protectant against litigation.

Quality Assurance/Continuous Quality Improvement Aspects

Quality assurance (QA) and continuous quality improvement (CQI) relate to specific programs of standard setting and ongoing evaluation process designed to continually improve the quality of care. There are several models for monitoring and improving the quality of care. The model most nurses in hospital-based institutions will experience is from the Joint Commission on the Accreditation of Healthcare Organizations (JCAHO) (Fischbach, 1991). This process is widely recognized as a model for the process of CQI.

"Improving performance is the essence of JCAHO's agenda for change " (Harbert & Wick, 1995). Performance is the service rendered and how well it is accomplished to provide health care. The "Nine Dimensions of Performance" are:

- the degree to which care is rendered to the patient (treatment/test/procedure) is *efficacious,*
- the degree to which care is rendered to the patient (treatment/test/procedure) is *appropriate,*
- the *availability* of the needed treatment/test/procedure focuses on the performance of care in a timely fashion,
- the *effectiveness* with which the treatment/test/procedure is provided to the individual patient,
- the *continuity* of the services provided to the patient, focusing on the coordination that exists between departments as well as the interdisciplinary team,
- the *safety* of the patient/staff/visitors in the environment where care is rendered, and
- the treatment/test/procedure rendered to the patient being performed in an *efficient, caring, and respectful* manner (Harbert & Wick, 1995).

Fischbach (1992) noted that QA/CQI programs are built upon the foundation of standards. These standards reflect the structures needed to support quality care, the processes that define how care is to be delivered, and the patient outcomes to be achieved that demonstrate that quality patient care has been delivered.

An effective quality improvement program is critical to validating nursing practice while comparing nursing performance to practice standards. In addition, quality management programs often provide nurses with real opportunities to evaluate the quality of nursing care and improve professional practice with a positive effect on patient outcomes (Harbert & Wick, 1995).

Nephrology nurses, like other nurses must deliver quality care that meets established standards, community standards, as well as patient and employer expectations. Comprehensive sound nursing documentation that demonstrates a logical approach to problem solving provides one mechanism by which this quality care be measured. In fact, the patient's record is the *primary* source for QA/quality improvement information and often provides evidence that acceptable and appropriate care has been delivered in compliance with the established standards of nursing practice and the nursing process (Fischbach, 1991). In summary, nursing documentation is often used with quality monitoring activities and as such should be a systematic, accurate meaningful account of nursing practice.

References

American Association of Nephrology Nurses and Technicians (AANNT). (1977). *Standards of clinical practice for the nephrology patient.* Park Ridge, IL: Author.

American Association of Nephrology Nurses and Technicians (AANNT). (1982). *Nephrology nursing standards of clinical practice.* Pitman, NJ: Author.

American Nephrology Nurses' Association (ANNA). (1984). *ANNA standards of clinical practice.* Pitman, NJ: Author.

American Nephrology Nurses' Association (ANNA). (1986). *Scope of practice for nephrology nursing.* Pitman, NJ: Author.

American Nephrology Nurses' Association. (1988). *Standards of clinical practice for nephrology nursing.* Pitman, NJ: Author.

American Nurses' Association. (1973). *Standards of nursing practice.* Kansas City, MO: Author.

American Nurses' Association. (1991). Certification helps RNs achieve their goals. *American Nurse, 23*(2) 28-29.

American Nurses' Association. (1991). *Standards of clinical nursing practice.* Kansas City, MO: Author.

Brook, R. (1989). Practice guideline and practicing medicine. *Journal of the American Medical Association, 262*(21),3027-3030.

Burrows-Hudson, S. (1993). *Standards of clinical practice for nephrology nursing* (revised edition). Pitman, NJ: American Nephrology Nurses' Association..

Cournoyer, C.P. (1989). *The nurse manager and the law.* Rockville, MD: Aspen Publishers.

Donabedian, A. (1988). The quality of care. How can it be assessed? *Journal of the American Medical Association, 260,* 1743-1748.

Eddy, D. (1990). Designing a practice policy. *Journal of the American Medical Association, 263*(22), 3077, 3081-3084.

Fiesta, J. (1983). *The law & liability: A guide for nurses.* New York: John Wiley and Sons, Inc.

Fischbach, F.T. (1991). *Documenting care: Communication, the nursing process, and documentation standards.* Philadelphia: F.A. Davis Company.

Griffith, J.W., & Christensen, P.J. (1982). *Nursing process: Application of theories, frameworks, and models.* St. Louis: C.V. Mosby Company.

Gross, K. (1987). *Legal, financial and risk management aspects of documentation for nurses.* Madison, WI: Professional Education Systems, Inc.

Hapster, L. & Veach, M. (1990). *Risk management handbook for healthcare facilities.* Chicago: American Hospital Publishing, Inc.

Harbert, G., & Wick, G. (1995). Introduction to the total quality movement. In G. Wick & E. Peacock (Eds.), *Continuous quality improvement: From concept to reality,* (pp. 5-10). Pitman, NJ: American Nephrology Nurses' Association.

Hirshfeld, E. (1990). Practice parameters and the malpractice liability of physicians. *Journal of the American Medical Association, 262*(11), 1556-1562.

Jordan, P. (Ed.). (1993). *Nephrology nursing: A guide to professional development.* Pitman, NJ: American Nephrology Nurses' Association.

Kenkel, P. (1993, November). Illinois blues will require specialist to follow clinical practice rules. *Modern Healthcare, 15,* 70.

Lancaster, L.E. (Ed.). (1987). *Core curriculum for nephrology nursing* (1st ed.) Pitman, NJ: American Nephrology Nurses' Association.

Lancaster, L.E. (Ed.). (1991). *Core curriculum for nephrology nursing* (2nd ed.) Pitman, NJ: American Nephrology Nurses' Association.

Leddy, S., & Pepper, M. (1985). *Conceptual basis of professional nursing.* Philadelphia: J.B. Lippincott Company.

Malasanos, L., Barkauskas, V., Moss, M., & Stoltenberg-Allen, K. (1986). *Health assessment.* St. Louis: C.V. Mosby Company.

National Center for Health Services Research and Health Care Technology Assessment. (1989, September 11.) *Research Activities: DHHS Secretary Sullivan Announces NCHSR grants totaling $4 million for patient outcome research assessment teams* (Publication No. 241-274-00054). Rockville, MD: Author.

Nuttal, A. (1990). Nephrology nursing consult: Case study - ESRD and cardiovascular instability. *ANNA Journal, 17*(2), 192-193.

Sandrick, K. (1993, May 5). Out in front: Managed care helps push clinical guidelines forward. *Hospitals,* pp. 30-31.

Springhouse Corporation. (1993). *Nursing process in clinical practice.* Springhouse, PA: Author.

Springhouse Corporation. (1995). *Matering documentation.* Springhouse, PA: Author.

Woolf, S. (1990, September). Practice guidelines: A new reality in medicine. *Archives of Internal Medicine,* 1811-1818.

Chapter Highlights

- It is vital for nephrology nurses to become familiar with the profession's standards of care; the benefits of these standards such as the promotion of quality care; the difference between standards and practice guidelines; the benefits of practice guidelines such as reducing the incidence of inappropriate care; and the standards of nursing practice that require nursing documentation to reflect accurate and appropriate observations, assessment, interventions, and evaluation.

- *The Standards of Clinical Practice for Nephrology Nursing* (Burrows-Hudson, 1993), revised and expanded in 1993, serves as a framework for developing and monitoring nephrology nursing practice.

- Implementation of standards of care serve to improve care, make managers' jobs easier, and make nurses' jobs more satisfying.

- While standards are intended to be followed *all* the time, guidelines should be followed in *most* cases. However, depending on the patient, setting, and other factors, guidelines can and should be tailored to fit individual needs (Eddy, 1990).

- In 1989, Congress established the Agency for Health Care Policy and Research (AHCPR) to improve the quality, appropriateness, and effectiveness of health care in the United States.

- Guidelines are intended to be flexible strategies to assist both customers and practitioners in clinical decision-making. Properly developed, guidelines are supported by scientific evidence and achieve the objectives of accuracy, accountability, predictability, defensibility, and usability.

- Standards of clinical nursing practice include both standards of care and standards of professional performance. Standards of professional performance reflect role activities and behaviors essential to the role of professional nursing. Standards of care set minimum criteria for nursing proficiency. These standards describe the activities for which nurses are accountable. Standards of care also provide direction for evaluating practice.

- Nursing documentation not only relays information, it records how well nurses have met the established standards of care. Nursing documentation provides evidence that the care rendered meets the accepted standards of nursing care that are mandated by law, the profession, and the health care institution in which you practice.
- The nursing process provides a systematic approach to nursing practice and documentation of the delivered care

- Nurses either use standardized diagnoses or develop their own diagnoses. The most widely used taxonomy of nursing diagnoses, which are organized around 9 human response patterns, has been developed by the North American Nursing Diagnosis Association (NANDA).

- The plan of nursing care includes priorities and the prescribed nursing approaches or measures to achieve the goals derived from the nursing diagnoses. A good nursing care plan is the blueprint for concise, meaningful documentation.

CHAPTER 27

Patient Education

Gail S. Wick, BSN, RN, CNN
Karen C. Robbins, MS, RN, CNN

Chapter Contents

Nurses and the Nephrology Health Care Team 839
Patient Education 840
  Goals of Patient Education 840
  The Process of Patient Education 840
  Assumptions for Patient Education 841
  Considerations in Adult Patient Education 842
Patient Learning 844
  Theories of Learning 844
  Goals of Patient Learning 844
  Assumptions for Patient Learning 846
  Literacy Skills and Learning 847
Nurses as Successful Teachers/Educators 847
  Planning the Teaching Strategy 847
  Barriers to Teaching 849
  Planning Steps for Written Material 849
Summary 850
References and Readings 850
Chapter Highlights 852

Patient Education

Gail S. Wick, BSN, RN, CNN
Karen C. Robbins, MS, RN, CNN

When individuals enter the health care system to receive any services, they become patients, and may be subjected to events and needs never before experienced. Information, skills, and behavioral changes are often required for successful adaptation to change and to avoid the loss of control, which is often experienced when appropriate learning does not occur (Bille, 1981). Hence, the need for patient or health education occurs throughout the health care system; the nephrology settings are no exception. All health professionals who work with the public are educators in that they teach, inform, advise, and counsel others in health-related matters. The importance of health education and teaching as a tool of nursing has been recognized since the early days of nursing. Although the centrality of health education and patient teaching varies with formal philosophies of nursing leaders, patient education as a goal of nursing is well recognized (Kovner, 1990; Bille, 1981). Over the years, nurses have taught, counseled, and advised patients on a wide variety of topics ranging from sanitation, cleanliness, and basic care of the sick, to highly technical home care treatments. With the increasing focus on maintaining and promoting health, rather than merely treating illness or responding to disease, health education has become a central theme of health care efforts. Because of the profession's knowledge base, practice locations, and frequent contact with consumers of health care services, nursing is one of the health care disciplines that is well-positioned to provide quality health education services.

Patient education is seen as both a basic human right and responsibility. Patients have the right to knowledge and skills, which can influence behavior in such a way as to affect health status and promotion. The role of the nurse as health education teacher is included in nurse practice acts and establishes the legal basis for patient education as one of the basic nursing functions (Rankin & Stallings, 1990; Redman, 1993, p. 5). The *Standards of Clinical Practice for Nephrology Nursing* (Burrows-Hudson, 1993), published by the American Nephrology Nurses' Association (ANNA), address patient education throughout all clinical modalities as a basic standard of practice. The American Hospital Association has also developed and approved the Patient Bill of Rights, which includes patient education as both a right and responsibility (Redman, 1993, p. 5). Recognized benefits of patient education are numerous and include improved quality of care, improved patient-family satisfaction, improved staff satisfaction, and more efficient use of resources (Redman, 1980).

Patient education is defined as "the process of influencing behavior and producing changes in the knowledge, attitudes, and skills required to maintain and improve health" (Rankin & Stallings, 1990) and, as such, involves teaching and learning. Teaching is defined as "the intentional structuring of content and environment to enhance human interactions in order to facilitate learning," while learning is defined as "a change in behavior" (Baer, 1995). Education is a process that may begin with imparting information, but must also include interpretation and integration of information by learners with the goal of bringing about attitudinal or behavioral changes that benefit individuals' health status (Rankin & Stallings, 1990). Because patient education is a process, not an event in itself, it occurs over time and is influenced by a number of factors involving learners and significant others, educators, and the environment. Many factors within each of these variables ultimately determine the effectiveness of health care teachings. Skills, ability, motivation, values, age, and gender of both teachers and learners combine with an environment conducive to learning to determine the success of the teaching-learning process. Health education, therefore, presents ongoing challenges to even the most experienced and skilled practitioners. The purpose of this chapter is to explore the knowledge, structure, and skills necessary for effective patient education.

Nurses and the Nephrology Health Care Team

Nurses work closely with physicians, social workers, renal dietitians, physical therapists, occupational therapists, and a host of others in caring for nephrology patients. The partnership of these professionals offers a comprehensive approach to patients and those around them. Each brings a unique perspective to meet the complex needs of renal patients. However, it is often nurses who have the greatest amount of contact with patients and thus have more interaction and potential for planned and spontaneous teaching opportunities than other health care workers. This places nurses in the unique position of having the opportunity to influence patients' behaviors and enhance their adaptation to illness. In so doing, patients are ultimately able to assume more active roles in their care and regain or retain control over their future.

Patient Education

Goals of Patient Education

The primary goal of patient education is to affect changes in health-related behaviors that will optimize health through prevention, promotion, maintenance, or modification (Redman, 1993, p. 5). In the face of illness, the desired behavioral changes include the integration of the illness into one's life experience and/or prevention of regression or dissociation of the event (Redman, 1980). Specific goals are to assist patients in the following:

- to adapt behaviors that maintain health and prevent illness;
- to adapt to and follow treatment programs once illness occurs;
- to return to the previous level of health or the maximum level possible;
- to minimize complications from illness or disease;
- to make informed decisions;
- to improve quality of life; and
- to carry out the basic tasks of living.

A review of these goals demonstrates that patient education is both necessary and appropriate anywhere health care services are provided, including nephrology settings. Whether the recipient of conservative management, dialytic therapy, transplantation, or related therapies, patients and their families experiencing real or potential renal insufficiency need to modify behavior in order to optimize health. Although the site of the teaching and content may vary depending on the nature of the illness, phase of health care, and focus of the intervention, the need to develop appropriate behavioral changes that maintain health, minimize morbidity, and improve quality of life exists. Active participation in their own education allows patients to feel as though they have regained some control over their situation, may influence a faster recovery, and encourage a more rapid adjustment upon returning home (Christopher & Lajkowicz, 1993).

The Process of Patient Education

The goal of patient education and the teaching-learning process is to help patients process the messages and skills presented during the encounter in order to make appropriate decisions; thus, an understanding of the process and principles of education is important. First and foremost, presenting information is not teaching, and receiving information does not ensure that learning has occurred. Health education has a far broader meaning than simply providing patients with information or demonstrating skills. Education includes a wide variety of actions such as instructing, advising, explaining, listening, leading discussion, and helping patients make decisions. Teaching can be described as "activities that allow the teacher to help students learn" (Redman, 1993, p. 8).

The actual process of patient education is very similar to the nursing process, and includes:

1. completing an assessment on patient need and readiness.
2. identifying learning needs and readiness to learn.
3. mutually establishing outcomes by the learner and teacher through development of behavioral objectives.
4. planning interventions in the form of a teaching plan based upon objectives and desired outcomes.
5. implementing the plan as education or training occurs.
6. receiving feedback and evaluating the feedback.

This process then allows for possible revision of the plan and perhaps return to the first step.

Assessment and diagnosis. The assessment includes patients' need to learn as well as readiness to do so. In describing this phase, Baer (1995) indicates that careful observation of patients' behavior and questions to assess knowledge base, attitudes, and beliefs are appropriate approaches to identification of learning needs and approaches necessary for meeting these needs. The questions asked by patients can be good indicators of what they do or do not know, or if they even recognize what they do not know. Baer describes readiness to learn as a function of physical, psychological, and maturational states. More specifically, physiologic state, previous life and health care experiences, attitudes toward health care, motivation, mental state and coping mechanisms, vocabulary, and problem-solving abilities will influence patients' readiness and ability to learn. These factors must be included in the assessment.

Patients' cultural and religious beliefs about health and disease can be determined in the assessment process. Grossman (1994) suggests some questions that might assist in this process. These include patients' understanding of the etiology and severity of the illness and why it started at the time it did. If patients believe that an illness resulted from such things as a punishment, or disharmony of energy, this will directly affect their understanding of the disease and how willing they will be to embrace modern, scientific interventions. Fears about the illness, ideas about the types of treatment they should receive, and expectations of the treatment can be key elements in determining what approach(es) might be necessary in formulating a plan.

Planning and outcomes identification. Much of the success of the educational process will depend upon the plan that is developed. The plan is perhaps the most tedious part of the process, and identifies the types of activities that are to be used, including clear purpose of the needs and desired outcome. It is here that the approaches best suited to meet patients' needs are identified, with the inclusion of pertinent religious or cultural beliefs. Is the purpose for patients merely to understand that they have kidney failure and recognize the implications for their care during conservative management? Or are they ready to go beyond conservative management and begin to make decisions about possible choices for replacement therapy? As this is determined, the desired outcomes will be articulated by behavioral objectives. The clarification of these objectives leads to the development of the content to be presented and the specific activities that will be employed to achieve those objectives.

Education/implementation. Table 27-1 suggests appropriate alternatives for specific levels of learning. Alternate approaches might be identified at this point in the event that the initial approach chosen may not be achieving the desired outcomes. Remembering that a number of factors can influence the interaction, contact should not overwhelm patients. Reinforcement of information via a variety of sources augments the experience. The more resources used and the greater the sensory input, the greater the outcome will be. Hearing, seeing, reading, and restating represent different sensory input and participation, and serve to reinforce learning.

Evaluation. While teaching is occurring, nurses must continually assess if the established behavioral objectives are being met. Observation of behaviors accompanied by carefully thought-out oral and written questions are effective methods of evaluating if desired changes in behavior are occurring. If objectives are not being met, it may be necessary to use one of the previously identified alternate approaches. When a planned approach is not working, having previously identified alternate approaches will facilitate moving from one approach to another with ease.

Behavioral objectives are then an integral part of the evaluation process. The behaviors identified are measured to determine if a desired behavioral change has, in fact, occurred. If it has, then the behavior should be reinforced. If not, the process is begun again with a return to the assessment phase to determine what the learning needs are at that point, and to establish a new teaching plan with possible alternate approaches to implementation.

Table 27-1
Teaching methods and media appropriate for producing specific levels of learning.

Level of Learning	Appropriate Methods and Media
1. Signal learning	lecture, still pictures, motion pictures, television, audio recordings, texts
2. Stimulus-response learning	still pictures, motion pictures, models, television, demonstration
3. Chaining	motion pictures, programmed instruction, demonstration, still pictures, television
4. Verbal association	motion pictures, programmed instruction, television, texts, lecture, still pictures
5. Multiple discrimination	motion pictures, programmed instructions, still pictures, television, texts, lecture
6. Concept learning	motion pictures, television, still pictures, programmed instruction, texts, lecture
7. Principle learning	motion pictures, television, still pictures, programmed instruction, texts, lectures, simulation
8. Problem solving	lecture, motion pictures, television, texts, simulation

Assumptions for Patient Education

Nurses and patients interact during the education process, thus making it a shared experience. When considering patient education in the context of illness, certain assumptions can be made: (a) motivation is present because a crisis such as illness exists; (b) learning needs will be communicated; and (c) complex factors affect the readiness to learn, ability to learn, and the speed in which knowledge and skills are acquired. Motivation is an important aspect of the learning experience because patients who are not motivated to learn will be resistant to attempts to educate and to change behavior. Motivation, an internal phenomenon, is generally assumed to be present in illness because the illness or change in health status gives patients a reason and need to learn. If one considers Maslow's Hierarchy of Needs (5-Self-Actualization; 4-Self-Esteem; 3-Social; 2-Safety; 1-Physiological), the stage and extent of the change in health status will determine what patients are motivated to learn (Bille, 1981). For example, physiological needs are the most basic needs, and if patients are experiencing a life-threatening illness such as renal failure, they will initially focus on immediate survival, rather than planning for the future. Once the immediate challenge to physiology and safety are met, patients might be motivated to learn about rehabilitation and self-care.

When a change in health status is present and motivation is lacking, the reasons should be sought. Common reasons for lack of motivation include the severity of and adaptation to the illness, differences in value systems between patients and health care professionals, and the role of health behaviors in lifestyles (Redman, 1993, pp. 18-19, 23-26). Culture and socioeconomic status have a strong influence on value systems that may vary and often negate the motivation to learn created by a decline in or challenge to health. The nursing assessment will provide an understanding of patients' beliefs, values, and culture. Teaching efforts will be enhanced by integrating them into the teaching plan.

To succeed in the teaching role, nurses must be cognizant of their own beliefs and value systems, as well as those of patients and families. Difficult as it may be, nurses must avoid imposing their own standards upon patients and/or expecting them to adopt one's own personal beliefs and attitudes. For example, dietary management education is imperative for the patient following renal transplantation. If the patient's culture values obesity, it is incumbent upon the nurse to approach the issue of obesity with an awareness of the cultural worth, while attempting to teach the health risks associated with obesity, for example, risks of cardiovascular disease, hypertension, and increased potential for wound infection in the postoperative period.

It is important to appreciate patients' socioeconomic status and resources to the extent that they influence living conditions and the ability to obtain medications, prescriptions, or other treatment requirements. Patients may be motivated to adhere to the prescribed regime, but lack the resources to do so. The incentive to follow the prescribed regime must be strong enough to offset disincentives (Green & Frankish, 1994). If nurses are aware of the problem, they can explore alternatives that may help patients receive medications or support services.

Considerations in Adult Patient Education

For the educational process to be successful and to occur in a time and cost-efficient manner, the theories of learning must be translated into principles or considerations that can be applied in health care delivery settings. Established principles of adult learning are as follows:

- Adults learn more readily when the information and skills are meaningful or life-centered. In other words, adults are more open to the learning process and more motivated when they perceive that there is a need to learn and the information and skills presented are problem centered to their needs, not necessarily the needs of the teacher.
- When adults know what to expect and are mentally ready to learn, the learning process is expedited. Before the learning experience begins, learners should be active participants in identification of the need for acquisition of new information and/or skills and in planning the learning experience. A common way of doing this is to use the methods of teaching identified by learners as the best ones for them and to involve them in setting realistic goals and objectives. Assessment of emotional status is necessary to ensure that learners are psychologically or emotionally adjusted to the situation, teachers, and settings and are ready to learn.
- Because adults mimic those they respect or those who exemplify the achievements that they desire, role models often facilitate new behavior.
- Because adult learners have limited attention spans of approximately 20 minutes and are easily distracted if learning methods and tools are boring, presentations must be novel, creative, different, and varied to facilitate learning. Important points to keep in mind include the following:
  -opening paragraphs or comments must "grab" the attention of the audience immediately and the high priority information should be contained in these openers.
  -attention is retained if information is perceived as relevant by learners and if learners are actively involved in the learning activities, that is, reports, discussion, practice sessions, and use of visual aids.
- The setting for patient education should be pleasant and comfortable and the climate supportive, accepting, free, spontaneous, and person centered. Adults generally will resist learning when they feel uncomfortable with either the environment, fellow students, teachers, or teaching style. They must feel free to make errors, to explore the problem, generate solutions, and weigh alternatives, as well as to help organize and set the tone of the learning experience.
- A number of conditions facilitate the transfer of knowledge. These conditions include the skills, interests, and attitudes of teachers, as well as good instructional media, time to learn, practice, and review, and a logical sequence of learning. For these reasons, each learning experience must be individualized within acceptable standards.
- Individuals can generally learn approximately seven new pieces of information at

Table 27-2
An overview of the major classifications of learning theories.

Classification	Definition	Major Tenets	Major Theorists	Example of the Learning
Behaviorist or Connectionist	Interprets human behavior as connections between stimuli and responses under the influence of reinforcement.	Respondent behavior results from a specific stimulus (S-R). Operant behavior is emitted as an instrumental act (R-R). Reinforcement increases the possibility of operant behavior recurring. Most human behaviors are operant in nature. Punishment decreases the possibility of a response recurring. Continuous reinforcement leads to faster learning. Intermittent reinforcement leads to longer retention of that which is learned.	Skinner Watson Thorndike Guthrie	Programmed instruction for skill development such as administering an insulin injection.
Cognitive, Organismic, or Gestalt	Interprets human behavior in terms of cognitive processes such as insight, intelligence, and organizational abilities.	Concerned with the process of decision making, cognitive structure, understanding, perception, and information processing. The emphasis is on the how of learning rather than what.	Bruner Paiget Ausubel	Exploring relationships such as those that exist between risk factors and the tendency to develop certain diseases.
Humanistic	Interprets human behavior as being self-centered and directly related to the process of self-actualization.	Learning is an individual internal process. People learn what they perceive to be helpful to maintaining their own structure. Self-actualization is the motivation for learning. Self-actualization and learning involve creative functioning. The organization of the self must not be threatened in order for new learning to occur.	Rogers Kohl	Exploring specific health promotion behaviors in order to stay healthy.

one time.

- Individuals learn better when information is put into meaningful context, sometimes called "chunking" (Redman, 1993, p. 57). For example, it is much easier to remember the 13 words "the, salad, grapes, colorful, the, red, melons, yellow, and, purple, make, bananas, orange" when put into a sentence - "The red and orange melons, purple grapes and yellow bananas make the salad colorful," rather than taught randomly. Chunking helps the learner process the information and increases recall by approximately 50%. An application in the clinical setting would be to list symptoms in complete sentences, rather, than phrases. An example might be as follows:

  "When you drink more fluid than you should, your legs and feet may swell. You may not be able to breathe easily."

Smaller "chunks" are appropriate for patients with low literacy skills. They may be most effective if limited to 3 to 5-item lists (Doak, Doak, & Root, 1996, p. 57).

- New information is learned more slowly than familiar information and may require more repetition before it is remembered.
- Sequential learning requires the use of appropriate teaching tools. Concrete information - such as facts - is lower on the learn-

ing hierarchy than abstract thinking and is easier to learn than abstract thinking and problem solving. Practice, repetition, and increasing insight in the form of case studies, problem solving, and discussions facilitate more advanced cognitive learning.

- For comprehension to occur, the information must be seen as logical, relevant, doable, and understandable.
- Stress, suppression, and distraction are factors in forgetting information and skills taught.
- Satisfaction must occur for learning to continue; therefore, it is important to set small goals initially, progressing toward the major goals of the learning process. For example, if the primary goal is for the patient to perform a successful and safe home dialysis, smaller successive goals such as setting up the equipment and supplies, initiating dialysis, monitoring the procedure, and ending dialysis will be set and achieved. The culmination of each of these steps is the performance of dialysis in the home.
- Learning is facilitated when standards of performance in the form of goals and objectives are mutually set by the learner and the teacher, accomplishment of the goals is recognized, and correction of possible problems occurs in a timely fashion.

Patient Learning

Theories of Learning

There are three major classifications of learning — behaviorist, cognitive, and humanist. The major tenets and examples of types of learning represented are shown in Table 27-2. Because learning is a process involving a hierarchy, certain levels of learning are required to achieve certain outcomes. Table 27-3 shows Gagne's hierarchy of learning, which is useful in developing teaching-learning tools and activities that result in effective patient education. These theories will be discussed indepth later in the chapter as they relate to learning objectives.

Goals of Patient Learning

There are a number of different learning/teaching goals in health care settings, and all are applicable to nephrology patients. These goals include awareness of health issues, knowledge and understanding, clarification of health values, attitudes that promote positive health-related activities, informed decision making, and active involvement in health matters (Ewles & Simnett, 1985). Education and training activities are aimed at achieving these goals. Educational activities guide learners, helping them to increase their awareness of options, alternatives, and appropriate behaviors with the goal of taking control of their care through informed decision making. Training, in contrast, manipulates the learning process so that specific behaviors and skills are developed. The tasks and procedures necessary for the maintenance or restoration of health or treatment of disease fall into these categories.

The goals or objectives of patient education are the behaviors desired at the conclusion of the teaching-learning process. These outcomes are stated as behavioral objectives and are determined by the learning needs assessment. When stated clearly and concisely, they facilitate an efficient approach to the process and lay the foundation for the related activities. The four elements present in a goal/objective/outcome are as follows:

1. **Behavior:** a verb indicates what is to take place or be accomplished.
2. **Content:** indicates the area in which the behavior will occur.
3. **Single idea:** articulates only one expected outcome to facilitate its evaluation.
4. **Measure:** specifically defines the time or expectation that will be measured. The more clear and concise the objectives, the more efficient the process can be.

Learning can be classified into three types: cognitive, affective, and psychomotor (Anderson, 1990, p. 107). Educational activities focus more on the cognitive and affective domains while the training activities focus on psychomotor skills.

Cognitive learning involves objectives that focus on giving and explaining information, helping patients to understand and integrate the information, and increasing their knowledge. These outcomes can be measured by paper and pencil tests or by verbally expressing an understanding of the information. Cognitive objectives are hierarchal as the synthesis of information becomes more complex. A comparison of lower and higher level objectives demonstrates this progressive concept through the cognitive domain:

1. *Lower level:* "Describes collection of clean catch urine sample."
2. *Higher level:* "Evaluates the procedure for collecting a clean catch urine sample using aseptic technique."

The first example simply requires that patients recount the procedure with no understanding of the specific processes of the procedure necessary to satisfy the objective. Conversely, for the second objective to be met, an understanding of aseptic technique and its application is required, that is, an understanding of the concept must be present in order to achieve the stated outcome. The following offer other examples of cognitive objectives.

- Name at least five foods high in potassium.
- List three problems with vascular access that should be reported to a

Table 27-3
Gagne's hierarchy of learning.

Level of Learning	Definition	Example of the Learning
1. Signal learning	Learning to respond to a signal or developing a conditioned response.	Generating anxiety at the sight of a hypodermic needle.
2. Stimulus-response learning	Voluntary learning that involves making a specific response to a specified stimulus.	Responding "dialysis machine" when the stimulus of "artificial kidney" is given.
3. Chaining	Learning to connect sequentially, two or more stimulus-response situations.	Performing each of the steps necessary to implement home dialysis.
4. Verbal association	Learning to attach names or labels to objects or to translate words into other languages.	Translating medical terminology into lay terms for easy understanding.
5. Multiple discrimination	Learning an extensive series of simple chains and differentiating between similar stimuli.	Recalling the specific name of each medication when several different tablets or capsules are presented.
6. Concept learning	Learning to make a common response to a number of stimuli that may differ in appearance.	Recognizing that even though the substances presented are tablets, capsules, and elixirs, that they are all medications.
7. Principle or rule learning	Learning a chain of two or more previously and separately learned concepts.	Recognizing that the concept of compliance represents a relationship between the concepts of adherence to a therapeutic regimen and feelings of being better.
8. Problem solving	Learning that requires considering previously learned principles in order to develop new, higher level principles.	Deciding how frequently to institute home dialysis based on previously agreed upon parameters.

doctor or nurse.

- Describe how an infected fistula or graft looks and feels.
- State at least four signs of a possible rejection episode.

Affective or feeling objectives focus on attitudes, beliefs, values, and opinions and address clarifying, forming or changing attitudes, beliefs, values and opinions (Ewles & Simnett, 1985). These objectives may also focus upon acceptance or rejection. They are not easily measured and are not as precise as cognitive objectives. In fact, they cannot be measured as right or wrong. Examples of affective objectives are listed below:

- Agrees that a restricted potassium diet has merit;
- Regularly adheres to a restricted potassium diet; and
- Is aware of different feelings about transplanting an organ from one person to another.

The first two address acceptance of the concept of a restricted diet as evidenced by adherence to the prescribed diet (described in the second objective). The third outcome speaks to the emotions and psychological acceptance of incorporating an organ from one person to another. Such issues can be discussed, but do not lend themselves to quantification.

A feeling objective that may be perceived as more vague than the others is illustrated by the following:

- Is sensitive to changes one experiences that are suggestive of a rejection episode.

While a concrete demonstration of these objectives cannot be observed, patients would need to be able to articulate some of the symptoms they might experience with a rejection episode: tenderness around the kidney, flu-like syndrome, general malaise, etc.

Psychomotor learning activities, the third domain, focus on skills acquisition, including physical, coordination, and/or manipulation activities. These activities most often involve an action but may also involve thinking and feeling, and are generally easier to evaluate as they entail action. Some examples of psychomotor objectives include the following:

- Takes blood pressure accurately 100% of time; and
- Consistently cannulates vascular

Table 27-4
Vascular access: Patient teaching objectives, outcomes.

Outcome: The patient will have a functioning external vascular access.

Objectives:

- The patient demonstrates the proper technique in exercising his/her native arteriovenous fistula.
- The patient states understanding of appropriate hygienic care of vascular access.
- The patient knows not to wear constrictive clothing, watch, or jewelry over vascular access.
- The patient preps the vascular access using proper technique prior to cannulation.
- The patient applies sufficient pressure to achieve hemostasis when the needles are removed without totally obstructing blood flow through the access.
- The patient knows appropriate interventions if the vascular access bleeds at any time.

Self-Care Patients:

- The patient performs proper cannulation technique.
- The patient tapes the needles securely in place.

access without difficulty.

These activities can be evaluated to determine if individuals successfully meet the objectives. The latter example illustrates that most learning needs involve more than one type of objective; in order to successfully cannulate an access (psychomotor), there must first be an understanding of the access itself (cognitive), the use of a particular needle, the steps involved, and perhaps, how comfortable one feels about using a large bore needle for the first time (affective).

Each domain presented responds best to particular methods of teaching, although no one method has been proven to be superior to others in many cases (Redman, 1993) (see sample in Table 27-4). Cognitive learning encompasses facts and concepts and is often taught by written materials, use of audiovisual aids, lectures, and discussions. In fact, some have used critical pathways as a guide to develop pictorial teaching tools for patients (DeLong, 1995, p. 45). Attitudinal changes do not respond successfully to knowledge of facts and, therefore, are most often achieved through discussion and exploration of options. Development of motor skills requires demonstration of the skills accompanied by an explanation of the "whys" of the steps, followed by practice with periodic refresher sessions.

Assumptions for Patient Learning

Learning needs are communicated either verbally or nonverbally and change with time and conditions. For this reason, ongoing assessment of learning needs must occur while nursing care is rendered. Verbal communication of learning needs is a direct form of needs identification and can include questions asked or comments made. More often, needs are communicated nonverbally and must be identified through observation. Examples include adherence or nonadherence to treatment programs, physical condition, and emotional state. Additional learning needs may be common to certain disease conditions and their treatment.

An assessment of the patients' degree of uremia and its effect upon his mentation should be part of the assessment of patients with renal impairment or renal failure as an indication of their readiness and ability to learn. A brief teaching interaction with a subsequent evaluation of patients' comprehension and retention are simple means of assessing patients' readiness to learn. Renal failure patients often cannot concentrate more than 10 to 15 minutes, so teaching efforts should consider this limitation. Repetition will enhance learning and can take many forms, for example, written materials and audio or visual tapes (Baer, 1995, p. 150). If patients are unable to retain or comprehend very basic pieces of information, further educational opportunities should be postponed until patients indicate an ability to integrate information presented, so that among other things, adherence will be enhanced.

What learners can and will learn depend on a number of factors. Readiness and ability to succeed at the learning experience are determined by such diverse factors as stage of illness, medical status, anxiety level, literacy level, maturity, importance of health and its restoration, probability of success in learning, freedom from the expectations of failure, and sense of control in the decision-making process.

Knox (1986) has described some general concepts about the learning process. In addition to those factors listed above, previous life experiences influence learning. The differences or similarities can be effectively used to enhance the learning experience. The relevance of the information and the immediate need for applying the knowledge will also promote learning. For example, patients undergoing training for automated peritoneal dialysis might be able to apply previous mechanical experience to the use of the equipment. The need to understand and apply the knowledge has immediate application, that is, patients must perform the treatment procedure successfully at home. This procedure draws upon a readiness to learn using previous experiences with the need for immediate application of the material.

Literacy Skills and Learning

Several facts and myths about literacy in the United States are relevant to patient education. Twenty-seven million American adults may not be able to comprehend what they are being taught by health care providers. That is, nearly 1 of every 5 adults lack the literacy skills needed to perform in society while about 30% are only marginally competent (Doak et al., 1996, pp. 1, 3). The approximate reading levels of adults in the United States are as follows (Doak et al., 1996, p. 3): (a) 18% of adult population are at a 5th grade reading level or below; (b) 32% are at a 5th to 10th grade reading level; and (c) 50% are above a 10th grade reading level.

In spite of low literacy levels, many of these people have average IQs and are found in all walks of life and income levels. It is important to note that years of school do not correlate to reading level because students may be advanced in grade for social reasons even if academic standards and criteria have not been met (Doak et al., 1996, p. 6).

Doak et al. (1996, p. 6) describe myths about literacy. They include some of the following:

- *Illiterate individuals are dumb and incapable of learning.*

Some illiterate individuals can be quite intelligent but failed to learn how to read and write.

- *The number of years spent in school is a good indicator of one's literacy.*

Articulate people who present themselves professionally may have never learned to read or write but have been advanced in school for social reasons. Rather, the years in school reflect what they have been exposed to, not their literacy level. Thus the presentation and articulation alone are not accurate indicators of literacy.

- *Those who are illiterate are usually from a foreign country or minority group.*

People from another country for whom English is a second language may have difficulty with the language, although that has no relevance to intellect. More minorities and immigrants have difficulty reading, proportionally speaking. Enunciation and socioeconomic class are not accurate predictors of literacy.

- *Someone will tell you if he cannot read or write.*

In fact, just the opposite may be true. Low literacy or illiterate individuals may simply agree with any information presented. They may not ask questions for fear of having to describe that which they do not understand and, therefore, may not be able to articulate. This situation could be embarrassing, and people may even offer other reasons for their inability to read, such as having forgotten their glasses.

The facts and myths of literacy are important factors in developing teaching strategies that enhance learning and desired behavior changes (see sample in Table 27-5).

Nurses as Successful Teachers/Educators

To succeed as teachers of health care, nurses must possess or develop certain qualities and characteristics that positively influence the teaching-learning experience. Knowledge of the subject matter and the principles and practice of teaching is a key to success, as well as a strong belief in and commitment to patient teaching as a right and responsibility (see Table 27-6).

Planning the Teaching Strategy

The teaching strategy involves creating a specific teaching plan based on the assessed needs and learning level of patients, put into behavioral objectives. The information presented must be relevant to patients' situations and should be presented as such. In devising the teaching methods to be used, it is imperative for nurses to be aware of the facts associated with the national literacy level and not assume that all adults have high comprehension and literacy. The factors that must be considered in planning the teaching strategy include core information to be covered, patient literacy, and methods to be used in presenting the information to patients.

Because the health care setting and change in health status is so often overwhelming, it is important to teach patients only what they need to know in the initial stages of the teaching-learning process. Initially, they need core or "bottom line" informa-

Table 27-5
Examples of writing and verbalizing on the fifth to sixth grade levels.

Original Text	Revised
Every cell in the body needs a constant supply of energy to do its work. This energy is obtained from food that you eat, which is absorbed by the stomach and small intestines into the blood. In the constant metabolic processes that support life, waste materials are created.	Your body needs energy to do its work Your body digests the food that you eat. You get energy from the food. Your body uses what food it needs. The parts of the food that it does not need are called waste products. Your kidneys should remove these waste products.
Dialysis: A process of osmosis, diffusion, and ultrafiltration used to restore electrolyte and fluid balance and remove waste products from the blood. (Nurse's thought process)	Dialysis: A way to clean my blood now that my kidneys have failed. (Patient's thought process)
Fistula: An internal connection between an artery and a vein in an arm or leg.	Fistula: A hole is made by the surgeon between an artery and a vein in your arm or leg. Some of the blood in the artery goes to the vein. Your vein gets big enough for needles to be used for hemodialysis.
The critical stage occurs following surgery when there is the possibility that the newly implanted kidney will be rejected. Since the body's immune system is set up to attack any foreign element, it will attempt to do its work. Lymphocytes, a type of white blood cell, and antibodies, which the body makes to combat invaders like bacteria and viruses, will be mobilized immediately to attack the newly implanted kidney.	After surgery, there is a chance that special cells in your body might attack your new kidney. This is called rejection. We will give you medications to help prevent this. *Copyright 1996 Fresenius USA, Inc.*

tion provided in such a way as to gain their attention immediately and to stimulate their interest. Adults often respond best when challenged with relevant questions. Using medication information as an example, the usual approach and a more innovative approach are shown in Table 27-7.

The points must be made vividly to enhance learning. Words used should be short, precise, and have a common meaning for both teachers and learners. The active voice, "you," is preferred. Information should be logical, condensed, summarized, and reviewed frequently. Illustrations may be used if appropriate and easily related to the information presented. During evaluation of the learning process, comprehension is confirmed when learners can repeat the information in their own words or demonstrate the skill. Frequent feedback checks the correction of the short-term memory and facilitates transfer of the knowledge or skill into the long-term memory. For desired behaviors to stay in the long-term memory, they must be reviewed and reinforced on a regular basis.

The use of audiovisual aids can supplement and reinforce written information. In the example of medications (see Table 27-7), flash cards with a word or a few words to familiarize patients with the terms and what the words look like are useful. The use of pictures of medications or the medicines themselves actually taped to an index card can be a very effective approach. Next to the pill itself can be the name of the pill, for example, hydrochlorothiazide, followed by "water pill," and the time(s) of day the medication is to be administered. This approach can be effective with patients of different literacy levels and can be individualized to the learning needs of patients. For patients with a greater understanding, or potential of same, "diuretic" may be written following hydrochlorothiazide rather than "water pill."

Special instructions can also be illustrated for low literacy patient. For example, high potassium foods can be shown next to the diuretic if hyperkalemia is not anticipated, but there is a need to avoid hypokalemia. If hyperkalemia is thought to be a potential risk, then a red line can be drawn through the foods to indicate they are to be avoided. The development of general information tools that can be individualized for the learning needs of patients allow for generally accessible teaching aids, while maintaining the ability for individualization.

Words should be chosen carefully and medical jargon avoided. A statement such as to "hook the patient up to dialysis" or "string a dialysis machine" will have no meaning to patients and can serve to increase anxiety. The former example could generate greater fear of being "hooked up to dialysis," without an understanding that this simply means initiating a hemodialysis treatment. If the hemodialysis machine is "strung," what might that mean to patients? Will they be tied to the machine or "strung out"? The opportunity for misunderstanding is high in either of these cases if concise, easy-to-understand terminology is not used.

Barriers to Teaching

In spite of being well recognized as a tool and a standard of nursing practice, barriers to effective patient education exist. Nurses often have misconceptions about teaching, miss or ignore teaching opportunities, and/or fail to correctly assess learning needs and use appropriate approaches and instructional media. Failure to provide effective education is documented by surveys that show that patients, physicians, and nurses feel that of the essential categories of nursing care, teaching is the least well accomplished compared to other categories (Redman, 1980). Some reasons for a lack of success in patient education may include the following:

- real or perceived time restraints;
- confusion among members of the health care team as to where the responsibility for education lies;
- lack of communication among members of the health care team, and lack of continuity in the teaching-learning process;
- failure of employers to hold employees accountable for education and to provide resources;
- lack of appropriate knowledge and skills for effective patient education; and
- attitudes and values that do not recognize the right and responsibility for education of patients.

Patient factors may also present barriers in the teaching-learning process. There is a perceived motivation to learn when change in health status occurs, but patients' lack of response to the teaching-learning encounter is often frequent. Bergevin states that adult learning is limited by two factors: (a) the individual's intellectual capacity and (b) the psychologic restrictions placed on the self (Bille, 1981). A change in health status compounds difficulties in learning. Patient factors are often complicated and range from fear of asking questions, cultural influence in the form of a passive role in health care, and a desire to not know the true facts. Regardless of the reasons for failure to provide adequate and effective patient education, nurses in all health care settings face the challenge of developing proficiency in adult education and principles of patient teaching. Nurses specializing in pediatrics face the added challenge of gaining knowledge and skills in teaching children.

Table 27-6
Qualities and characteristics that positively influence the teaching-learning experience.

Positive attitude	Motivation
Optimism	Trustworthy
Sensitivity	Positive self-concept
Discipline	Goal oriented
Determination	Consistency
Knowledge	Good communicator
Responsible	Frank and honest
Kinetic	Creative
Good listener	Imaginative
Natural	Efficient
Understanding	Professional

Planning Steps for Written Material

The illiteracy factor need not be a drawback in the planning process for written material if certain steps are followed in devising the materials. Although effective learning can occur without the use of written material, written material with verbal reinforcement often enhances learning. To prepare written material that addresses the learning needs of patients with all levels of literacy, the following steps should be followed:

- List the desired behavioral changes or skills in the form of behavioral objectives.
- Decide what specific information is needed to achieve each objective.
- Select the best method (written, written with visual, demonstrations, models, etc.) to present the information.
- Organize the material in a logical sequence, starting with the most important point first, and summarize the point again at the end. If information is of equal importance, start with the more

Table 27-7
Usual approaches and more innovative approaches in teaching-learning process.

Example: Medication Information

Usual Approach	More Innovative Approach
1. Purpose	"What do I take"
2. Dosage	"How much do I take?"
3. Side effects	"What problems can it cause?"
4. Specific information	"What will it do for me?"
	"When do I take it?"

general information and progress to the specific information.

- Use short words and sentences and the active voice "you."
- Limit sentences to one main idea and support information per sentence. The topic or main sentence should open each paragraph.
- Build reviews and feedback into the written material and summarize the main points often.
- Write the information on the appropriate reading level. Eighth grade or below is the mean literacy level in the United States (Redman, 1993, p. 141). Print size should be at 14-point and print should be double or triple spaced. Various models for verifying readability are available, with the Fry readability graph being one of the most well known.
- Use illustrations or visual aids as appropriate if they enhance the learning and are easily understood.
- Pilot the material before instituting it in the general patient population.

By basing the teaching experiences on the principles listed above, nurse educators will ensure a positive learning experience. When materials are easy to read and understand (see Table 27-8) and the teaching processes employed are interesting and innovative, the learning environment is conducive to success for patients and nurse educators.

Summary

The role of nurses as health educators and teachers is one of the functions of nursing described in many nurse practice acts. The process of patient education follows the nursing process of assessment, diagnosis, outcome identification, planning and subsequent identification of behavioral objectives and outcomes, implementation and intervention, and evaluation.

Nurses must determine the most appropriate approach to patient education based upon a number of factors. Patients with renal impairment and renal failure require a great deal of education in order to alter behaviors as a result of the pathophysiological changes that result. Nurses, in concert with other members of the health care team, are responsible for preparing patients for the physiologic and therapeutic changes that follow. This role can be one of the most challenging, yet fulfilling and rewarding, for nurses.

References and Readings

Anderson, C. (1990). *Patient teaching and communicating in an information age.* Albany, NY: Delman Publishers, Inc.

Baer, C.L. (1995). Principles of patient education. In L.E. Lancaster (Ed.), *Core curriculum for nephrology nursing* (2nd edition). Pitman, NJ: American Nephrology Nurses' Association.

Bille, D.A. (1981). *Practical approaches to patient teaching.* Boston: Little, Brown and Company.

Burrows-Hudson, S. (Ed.). (1993). *Standards of clinical practice for nephrology nursing* (revised edition). Pitman, NJ: American Nephrology Nurses' Association.

Christopher, M., & Lajkowicz, C. (1993). Patient teaching by the book. *RN, 56*(7), 48-50.

Cunningham, D. (1993). Improving your teaching skills. *Nursing 93, 23*(12), 24J.

DeLong, R.L. (1995). This path has pictures. *RN, 58*(9), 44-45.

Doak, C.C., Doak, L.G., & Root, J.H. (1996). *Teaching patients with low literacy skills* (2nd edition.). Philadelphia: J.B. Lippincott Company.

Ewles, L., & Simnett, I. (1985). *Promoting health: A practical guide to health education.* Chichester, England: John Wiley & Sons.

Green, L.W., & Frankish, C.J. (1994). Theories and principles of health education applied to asthma. *Chest, 106*(12), 2195.

Grossman, D. (1994). Enhancing your 'cultural competence.' *American Journal of Nursing, 94*(7), 58, 60, 62.

Kovner, A.R. (1990). *Health care delivery in the United States* (4th edition). New York: Springer Publishing Company.

Lancaster, L.E. (Ed.). (1995). *Core curriculum for nephrology nursing* (3rd edition). Pitman, NJ: American Nephrology Nurses' Association.

Rankin, S.H., & Stallings, K.D. (1990). *Patient education* (2nd edition). Philadelphia: J.B. Lippincott Company.

Redman, B.K. (1980). *The process of patient teaching in nursing* (4th edition). St. Louis: C.V. Mosby Company.

Redman, B.K. (1993). *The process of patient education.* St. Louis: Mosby-Year Book.

Redmond, M.C. (1993). The importance of good communication in effective patient-family teaching. *Journal of Post Anesthesia Nursing, 8*(2), 109-112.

Table 27-8
Sample peritonitis home instruction sheet.

We have just placed very large doses of two different kinds of antibiotics (called "loading doses") into your bag. This exchange is to dwell for at least 6 hours. You may do your next exchange at _________. Continue to add the medication until it is all gone. Do not stop just because the symptoms disappear and you feel better.

Your physician has ordered medication to be administered into your new bag before every exchange for the next ____ days. You have been given written instructions on how to mix the dry medication and inject it into your bag of solution for each exchange.

You have come to the PD unit with symptoms of peritonitis. We have sent samples of your solution to the lab. The first report should be back within 24 hours. We will then be able to decide what medicine you need. We will call within 48 hours if you need new medicine. Continue to take the same medication if we do not call.

Any symptoms you are experiencing today (pain, nausea, vomiting, cloudy bags) should stop within 1 to 3 days. If the symptoms do not improve, you may be on a medication that is not working. There may be something more seriously wrong also. Call us if you still have symptoms after 3 days. Call us, also, if you have any new symptoms.

There is a chance that your medication may need to be changed or another one added. You may want to purchase just one bottle of the medication until the bacteria has been identified.

I, ________________________, hereby state that I have been given both verbal and written instructions on my care and how to add the medication to my bags. I know that I will be asked to return to the unit 2 days or the first working day after I have finished the antibiotics. This will be _________. I understand that I am to bring the drainage bag from my morning exchange with me.

If you have any questions or think something is not right, call us!

Chapter Highlights

- All health professionals who work with the public are educators in that they teach, inform, advise, and counsel others in health-related matters.
- Over the years, nurses have taught, counseled, and advised patients on a wide range of topics ranging from sanitation, cleanliness, and basic care of the sick, to highly technical home care treatments.
- With the increasing focus on maintaining and promoting health, rather than merely treating illness or responding to disease, health education has become a central theme of health care efforts.
- Patients have the right to knowledge and skills that can influence behavior in such a way as to affect health status and promotion.
- Skills, ability, motivation, values, age, and gender of both teachers and learners combine with an environment conducive to learning to determine the success of the teaching-learning process.
- Knowledge of the subject matter and the principles and practice of teaching is a key to success, as well as a strong belief in and commitment to patient teaching as a right and responsibility.
- The primary goal of patient education is to affect changes in behavior that will optimize health through prevention, promotion, maintenance, or modification.
- There are a number of different learning/teaching goals in health care settings and all are applicable to nephrology patients. These goals include awareness of health issues, knowledge and understanding, clarification of health values, attitudes that promote positive health-related activities, informed decision making, and active involvement in health matters.
- The goals or objectives of patient education are the behaviors desired at the conclusion of the teaching-learning process. These outcomes are stated as behavioral objectives and are determined by the learning needs assessment.
- Learning can be classified into three types: cognitive, affective, and psychomotor. Educational activities focus more on the cognitive and affective domains while the training activities focus on psychomotor skills.
- The teaching strategy involves creating a specific teaching plan based on the assessed needs and literacy level of patients.
- The role of the nurse as health educator and teacher is one of the functions of nursing described in many nurse practice acts.
- The process of patient education follows the nursing process of assessment, diagnosis, outcome identification, planning, and subsequent identification of behavioral objectives and outcomes, implementation and intervention, and evaluation.

CHAPTER 28

The Nephrology Community

Evelyn Butera, MS, RN, CNN
Nancy M. Gallagher, BSN, RN, CNN

Chapter Contents

Nephrology Nursing in the United States 855
Roles for Nephrology Nurses: Diversity of Practice 855
  Types of Practitioners 855
  Functional Roles 855
Working With the Health Care Team 855
The Nephrology Community 856
  Regional 857
  National 857
  International Community 859
Summary 859

The Nephrology Community

Evelyn Butera, MS, RN, CNN
Nancy M. Gallagher, BSN, RN, CNN

Nephrology nursing within highly developed countries has evolved beyond its initial boundaries, while nephrology nursing in developing countries continues to define its place in the larger health care community. Nephrology nursing reflects the dynamic, rather than static nature of the specialty, which is continually evolving and expanding its knowledge, phenomena of concern, and societal changes. The purpose of this chapter is to describe professional nephrology nurses as members of the nephrology community in local, regional, national, and international contexts.

Nephrology Nursing in the United States

Nephrology nursing is a holistic, caring-based practice in which the processes of diagnosis and treatment are applied to manage the health care needs of individuals experiencing the impact of acute or chronic renal disease. Nephrology nursing in its broadest sense is concerned with both the prevention of disease and the care and assessment of the health needs of patients and families across the life cycle.

Nephrology has been recognized as a specialty for more than 40 years. In 1973, hemodialysis, peritoneal dialysis, and transplantation were funded by the federal government and these treatments became more common. Nephrology nurses worked with other health care professionals as the specialty emerged. Since then, the role of nephrology nurses has expanded and its practice boundaries broadened.

Nephrology nurses care for a diverse patient population in the roles of direct caregiver, educator, coordinator, administrator, consultant, and researcher. The broad scope of nephrology nursing practice is a reflection of the characteristics of the diverse and challenging patient groups that are encountered by nurses in the specialty. These patients include pediatric, adult, and geriatric individuals from diverse ethnic, cultural, and socioeconomic backgrounds.

Roles for Nephrology Nurses: Diversity of Practice

Nephrology nursing practice occurs in primary, secondary, and tertiary care settings and in the home. The depth to which individual nephrology nurses engage in the scope of nephrology nursing practice is dependent upon their educational preparation, experience, role, health care setting, and the nature of the patient group(s) they serve.

Types of Practitioners

The American Nephrology Nurses' Association (ANNA) has described two categories of nurse providers in the specialty of nephrology nursing. These are the nursing generalist, who practices within the field of nephrology, and the nephrology nursing specialist, who has demonstrated expertise in advanced practice in the care of renal patients. Areas of specialized care include conservative management (pretreatment), hemodialysis, peritoneal dialysis, renal transplantation, and continuous renal replacement therapies.

Functional Roles

Nephrology nurses are active in the areas of clinical practice, education, management, research, quality improvement, and corporate and government activities.

Working With the Health Care Team

Nephrology nursing is an integral part of an interdisciplinary group of health care workers providing care for patients with chronic renal failure (CRF). Although interdisciplinary care was specifically defined by the federal government in the 1996 rules of coverage for funding of the End Stage Renal Disease (ESRD) program, the complex nature of renal disease and its effect on all aspects of the patient's life, require a multifaceted plan of care. More recently, the increasing age and frequency of co-morbid conditions in the CRF population such as age, hypertension, diabetes, and peripheral vascular disease, have complicated care delivery. This often results in more devastating and declining physiologic abilities, as well as greater changes in life style and role function.

Figure 28-1
Characteristics of the scope of nursing practice for nephrology nursing.

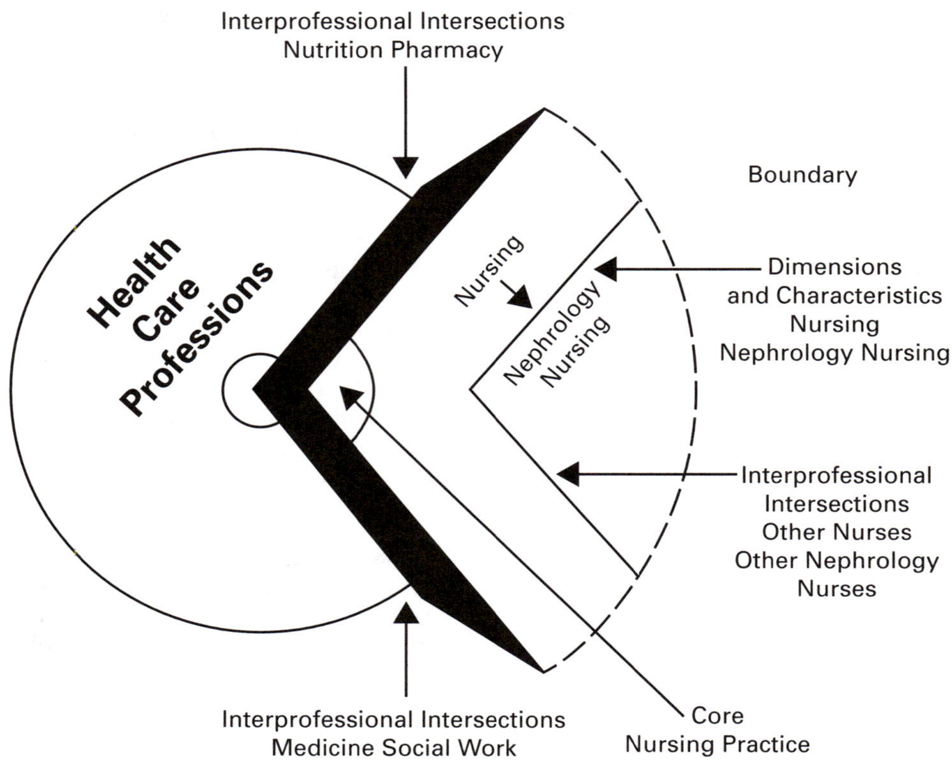

Note: Jordan, P.J., Parker, J., & Butera, E. (1993). Role of the Nephrology Nurse. In P. Jordan (Ed.), *Nephrology Nursing: A guide to professional development* (p.25). Pitman, NJ: American Nephrology Nurses' Association. Reprinted with permission.

The team approach in this coordinated care effort usually includes nurses, technicians, nephrologists, dieticians, social workers, and patients and their families. The roles of nurses, technicians, and nephrologists in providing direct care are well elaborated upon elsewhere in this textbook. The renal dietician's focus is patient education related to good nutrition and emphasizing those aspects of nutritional intake that need adjustment in the presence of renal dysfunction, for example, potassium, sodium, and fluid restriction and the need for adequate protein and caloric intake. Nephrology nurses working with dieticians are in a position to reinforce dietary education, answer or direct questions, and refer patients for further nutritional counseling as necessary.

Renal social workers attend to issues of support and adjustment. Psychological assessment plays a major role in patient treatment plans and outcomes of care. Input from nurses and other interdisciplinary team members assists social workers in developing a family and community resource base in which patients can draw support.

As identified by individual patient care facilities or patient assessment, other members of the interdisciplinary team may include pharmacists, physical therapists, clergy, physician assistants, financial counselors, and psychologists. Although the interdisciplinary team may vary in its total composition, nursing provides a vital link for collaboration and communication in assuring delivery of high quality and individualized care. Many others are involved in providing care to CRF patients, including nurse educators, business administrators, technical services vendors, and their nurse representatives who provide education and guidance in the use of the technology necessary to deliver treatment.

The boundary of nephrology nursing practice is flexible and responsive to changes in the health care needs of the patient group served, technological changes, and collaborative practice with other disciplines (see Figure 28-1).

The Nephrology Community

The practice of nephrology has always been

interdisciplinary due to the complexity of the patients we care for. Chronic illness is manifested by total system disease with significant changes in life style and societal roles, requiring a team of highly skilled caregivers, with a wide scope of expertise. Nephrology nursing practice has also traditionally overlapped the boundaries of other specialty practitioners, requiring a more diverse and expanded practice knowledge base for nephrology nurses.

The renal community is comprised of patients, professionals, providers, manufacturers, organizations, and companies who respond to the needs surrounding dialysis and transplantation. The community often works together to address many problems that inevitably arise in a program as complex and sensitive as CRF.

The support of interdisciplinary members of the CRF health team on the local level is promoted by a network of facility communication; local chapters of professional associations such as ANNA, the Council of Nephrology Social Workers, and the Council On Renal Nutrition. State affiliates of the National Kidney Foundation and other independent Kidney Foundations support the interdisciplinary team through educational activities and direct funding of fellowships. Industry also plays an important role as a link between technology and caregivers through service-linked education, development of algorithms and treatment guides, and financial support for local educational sessions. Beyond individual providers, the interdisciplinary approach to care extends to a regional, national, and international base.

Regional

The Network System. Dialysis treatment was approved for payment by Medicare in 1972. As the number of dialysis facilities grew, a system to provide oversight and to bring together the various dialysis providers was needed. In 1978, the End Stage Renal Disease (ESRD) Network system was developed to provide an active means of monitoring the care of patients at the regional level. Today, the United States and its territories are divided into 18 Networks, each overseeing local facilities within their region. The ESRD Networks provide a mechanism to monitor quality of care indicators and maintain a timely and complete data base on the ESRD program. The primary focus of the Networks is quality improvement, patient satisfaction, data collection, and to serve as a clearinghouse for the exchange of information on a variety of issues important to the care of patients. These functions are administered at a regional level, providing direct and immediate access from the local treatment provider to the Health Care Financing Administration (HCFA) through the ESRD Network. Each Network is under contract with HCFA. Networks are required to meet a set of defined requirements whose ultimate goal is to ensure the quality of care to Medicare patients with chronic renal failure.

The 18 Networks are in immediate contact with over 2,900 dialysis providers and greater than 240 transplant centers, serving over 260,000 patients. Each Network is administered by a governing body made up of representatives from local dialysis providers. A Medical Review Board, also made up of dialysis provider representatives, serves as the advisory group on clinical issues. Networks benefit from the expertise and leadership of renal professionals, representing providers across the country. In addition to meeting specific goals as set by HCFA, each Network conducts special studies that address the needs of its own providers of care, that will result in improved outcomes of care.

Nephrology nurses play an active role in their respective ESRD Networks. Nurses may be employed by the Networks as an Executive Director, or in a role involving continuous quality improvement (CQI) educational activities. Nurses working at individual facilities participate in data collection and may also sit on various committees, such as the Medical Review Board or the Board of Directors.

National

Health care reform and quality improvement must focus on patient outcomes. In turn, the assessment of the outcomes must be closely linked to the process of patient care. A CQI model was developed by HCFA called the Health Care Quality Improvement Program (HCQIP). This CQI model examines the process of providing patient care at the facility level and provides an opportunity for facilities to self-assess and make changes to improve the patient outcomes demanded by patients, providers, and payers. Under HCQIP, Networks perform professional reviews of patterns and outcomes of patient care, coordinate and educate providers and consumer communities, and develop collaborative clinical projects with communities to improve the process and outcomes of care. Individual dialysis providers will use the data to compare current practice to professional standards and develop a process of improvement specific to their facility needs. Together the Networks and providers will build a partnership for analyzing and improving performance.

Currently, the three major projects of HCQIP are the National Core Indicators Project, that is collecting data annually on patient nutritional status, adequacy of hemodialysis, anemia, and blood pressure; the National Cooperative Anemia Project, which focuses on hematocrit and the development of a CQI process with ongoing monitoring, analysis, plans of improvement, and intervention for anemia; and facility-specific indicators, interventions that are developed at the Network and facility level.

Nephrology nurses are actively involved in the

Table 28-1
Professional nephrology organizations.

American Association of Kidney Patients (AAKP)
100 S. Ashley Drive
Suite 280
Tampa, FL 33602
Executive Office (813) 223-7099
Fax (813) 223-0001

American Diabetes Association (ADA)
1660 Duke Street
Alexandria, VA 22314
National Office (800) 232-3472

American Kidney Fund (AKF)
6110 Executive Boulevard
Suite 1010
Rockville, MD 20852
Executive Office (301) 881-3052
Fax (301) 881-0898

American Nephrology Nurses Association (ANNA)
East Holly Avenue/Box 56
Pitman, NJ 08071
Executive Office (609) 256-2320
Fax (609) 589-7463
E-Mail http://www.iNurse.com/~ANNA

American Society of Nephrology (ASN)
Judith Thomas, Executive Director
1200 19th Street NW
Suite 300
Washington, DC 20036
Executive Office (202) 857-1190
Fax (202) 223-4570

National Association of Nephrology Technologists and Technicians (NANT)
PO Box 2307
Dayton, OH 45401-2307
Executive Office (937) 586-3705
Fax (937) 586-3699
E-Mail nant@nant.meinet.com

National Kidney Foundation Inc. (NKF)
30 East 33rd Street
New York, NY 10016
Executive Office (212) 889-2210
Fax (212) 689-9261
Customer Service (800) 622-9010

National Renal Administrators Association (NRAA)
11250 Roger Bacon Drive
Suite 8
Reston, VA 20190
Executive Office (703) 437-4377
Fax (703) 435-4390

Renal Physicians Association (RPA)
2011 Pennsylvania Avenue NW
Suite 800
Washington, DC 20006-1808
Executive Office (202) 835-0436
Toll Free (800) RPA-7525
Fax (202) 835-0443

United Network For Organ Sharing (UNOS)
Walter Graham, Esq., Executive Director
Douglas J. Norman MD, President
PO Box 13770
1100 Boulders Parkway
Suite 500
Richmond, VA 23225-8770
Executive Office (804) 330-8500
Fax (804) 330-8517

CQI initiative. Nursing participates on the ESRD Quality Consensus Committee, which acts in an advisory role in identifying elements of care for the National Core Indicators Project. While nurses are integral in the collection of data, they play an even more important role in the process of facility self-assessment and implementation of interventions to improve care.

The emphasis on CQI in nephrology patient care has lead to the creation of several other interdisciplinary renal community efforts involved in examining process and outcomes of care, including the Dialysis Outcomes Quality Initiatives (DOQI) Clinical Practice Guidelines for Vascular Access, Adequacy of Hemodialysis and Peritoneal Dialysis, Anemia and Nutrition.

Renal Coalition. Nephrology nurses participate in local, regional, and national renal community activities that address both professional and care delivery issues. The Renal Coalition provides a forum to address major public issues that impact patients with renal failure. Formed in the mid-1980s in response to proposed changes in reimbursement for dialysis therapy, the coalition continues to meet on an informal basis as issues concerning the renal community arise.

Individuals attending the meetings represent national patient and professional nephrology organizations. Professional organizations represented are found in Table 28-1.

The Renal Coalition addresses global issues of concern to the ESRD community. Currently, the major focus has been on developing and/or responding to legislative regulatory and organizational initiatives that affect the Medicare ESRD program and the care of patients with organ failure.

Industry. Historically, nephrology nursing and industry have been partners in the evolution of the technology that plays such an important role in the improvement of patient outcomes. Care of dialysis patients includes the use of highly technical equipment and supplies that have a direct impact on care delivery. The partnership between the renal community and industry enhances the opportunities for the development of new technology that is both safe for patients and user friendly for staff to operate. Without good communication and a sense of community and commitment to patients, these technologies would be slower in development and appropriateness of use. Industry provides the nephrology community with product development, service and product education, support of CQI activities, research grants, and financial support for organizational programming. Nephrology nursing is involved in all aspects of these activities.

International Community

Nephrology nursing is an international specialty. It is essential that we develop and maintain links to our colleagues in other nations across the world. Sharing common issues and potential solutions is the natural evolution of our new global community. Although we are of different cultures and societal norms, we share a common experience -- the care of patients with renal failure.

Nephrology nursing has been active through its professional association, ANNA, and in conjunction with other professional associations, has developed links to the international nephrology community. International nephrology organizations have recognized the need to form and support an international charitable foundation, the World Council of Renal Care (WCRC), to provide ongoing educational information and materials to our colleagues in developing countries.

The mission of the WCRC is to teach and share collective knowledge and expertise in the prevention, care, and treatment of renal diseases in the developing world. Its vision is to improve the care provided to individuals with disease of the kidney and urinary tract through promotion of internationally recognized standards of patient care, education of practitioners, dissemination of new ideas throughout the field, and promotion of interdisciplinary communication and cooperation. To accomplish its mission, the WCRC will seek partnerships with the World Health Organization, the International Society of Nephrology, and other apolitical organizations with similar objectives. ANNA has endorsed the concept of the WCRC and is a member of its Advisory Board. Nephrology nurses have participated in the formation of the WCRC and sit on the WCRC's Board of Directors.

In addition to working with the WCRC, delegates from ANNA attend the annual meetings of the Canadian Association of Nephrology Nurses and Technicians and the European Dialysis and Transplant Nurses Association/European Renal Care Association. These organizations in turn send representation to the annual ANNA meeting.

Just as nephrology nursing works within an interdisciplinary community, locally, regionally and nationally, they work within an interdisciplinary international community. The international nephrology community has responded to natural disasters around the world by sending dialysis equipment, personnel, and supplies to support emergency care, such as in the 1985 earthquake in Armenia that saw a large number of victims with crush injuries who developed acute renal failure and required dialysis therapy. This international team set up emergency dialysis and trained local health care providers to carry on the dialysis treatments after the team left the area.

In 1995 and 1997, international teams of physicians, nurses, technicians, social workers, and dieticians visited Russia, the Baltic States, China, and Turkey to present nephrology workshops to local health care providers. These workshops provided a means to share information, to improve nephrology patient care, and to develop a communication system that will provide ongoing support to the international community in their efforts to develop the health care systems in their communities.

Nephrology nursing will continue to support the efforts of the international community toward eliminating barriers that impede professional education and standards that negatively affect quality of patient care.

Summary

Nephrology nurses in the United States care for a diverse patient population in multiple roles. In the past 40 years, the role of nephrology nurses has expanded and its practice boundaries broadened. Nephrology nurses are active in many functional roles, as described earlier, and are an integral part of an interdisciplinary group of health care workers providing care for patients with renal failure.

Because of the complexity of patients cared for, the nephrology community has always been interdisciplinary in nature. The nephrology community and its members are active on the regional, national, and international levels with nephrology nurses able to participate in a broad range of community activities that address both professional and care delivery issues.

Appendices

Contents

Appendix A: A Chronological History of the American Nephrology Nurses' Association 863

Appendix B: Nursing Management of the Patient with Renal Failure 869

Appendix C: Nursing Management of the Patient with Renal Failure 876

Appendix D: Nursing Management of the Patient with Renal Failure 878

Appendix E: AANNT Legislative Policy Statement – November 1983 885

Appendix F: ANNA's Health Policy Statement 888

Appendix A
A chronological history of the American Nephrology Nurses' Association.

The growth of the American Nephrology Nurses' Association (ANNA) as the voice of nephrology nursing practice has its roots in the 1950s when nurses began to provide dialysis and transplant care in a new specialty practice.

A common bond emerged to share information on nephrology nursing practice and to network with colleagues, eventually leading to the formation of the American Association for Nephrology Nurses (AANN) in 1969 in Atlantic City, New Jersey.

Today, ANNA reaps the rewards of its rich heritage. With the highest membership and strongest financial base in its history, future leaders have the opportunity and challenge to achieve the association's mission. That mission is to "advance the professional development of registered nurses practicing in nephrology, transplantation, and related therapies, and to promote the highest standards of patient care."

This appendix chronicles association activities and highlights year-by-year over the past three decades, from the struggles of the early pioneers of nephrology nursing to the steady growth of an association.

The 1950s

1950s:

- Nurses began working as part of renal research teams providing dialysis and transplant nursing care.

1955:

- Nurses attended meeting of the American Society for Artificial Internal Organs (ASAIO), the only forum for exchange of ideas and information at that time related to nephrology practice issues.

The 1960s

1966:

- About 100 nephrology nurses met informally in Boston for an educational offering at Peter Bent Brigham Hospital.

1968:

- A 1-day meeting, "Dialysis Symposium for Nurses," was held at the ASAIO meeting in Philadelphia with over 200 nurses in attendance. A core group of nurses pursued the idea of forming a specialty nursing organization dedicated to nephrology practice.

1969:

- A second nursing symposium was held at ASAIO in Atlantic City, New Jersey, where the American Association for Nephrology Nurses (AANN) was formed and officers elected. Bernice Hinckley was elected as the new association's first president, serving in 1969-1970.

The 1970s

1970:

- AANN changed its name to the American Association of Nephrology Nurses and Technicians (AANNT), allowing LPNs and technicians full membership.

- The First National Symposium was held in conjunction with ASAIO in Washington, DC, attracting 450 registrants.
- Beth Cameron served as AANNT president.

1971-1972:
- Five regions were formed, and the first regional meeting was held in the Southeast in conjunction with the Southeast Dialysis and Transplant Association (SEDTA).
- The AANNT logo was approved, and quarterly newsletters were initiated.
- Mary O'Neill served as association president until the Spring of 1973.

1972-1973:
- The first *Standards of Clinical Practice* were published.
- A liaison was established with the European Dialysis and Transplant Nurses' Association (EDTNA).
- AANNT representatives first attended meetings of the National Federation for Specialty Nursing Organizations (NFSNO).

1973-1974:
- A process to approve programs for continuing education was implemented.
- Medicare coverage was extended to end stage renal disease.
- Betty Preston and Lois Bernbeck served as association presidents.

1974-1975:
- The *AANNT Journal* was initially published with Margery Fearing serving as the first editor.
- Membership reached 1,600 nurses and technicians.
- Lois Bernbeck served as president.

1975-1976:
- AANNT sponsored a summer camp for children undergoing hemodialysis at Frost Valley in upstate New York.
- AANNT's first co-sponsored meeting, "Laboratory for Leadership," was held in Nashville, Tennessee.
- Membership reached 2,000 under President Martha Leonard Orr.

1976-1977:
- Management functions were centralized in a national office.
- AANNT sponsored conferences on hepatitis in addition to the "Basic Learning Institutes."
- The three existing sets of the *Standards of Clinical Practice* were revised.
- Membership surpassed 2,200 under President Marcia Clark.

1977-1978:
- Twenty chapters were chartered at the Ninth National Symposium in Chicago.
- AANNT was approved as a provider of continuing education by ANA.
- Membership held steady near 2,200 under President Susan Hopper.

1978-1979:
- Chapter growth continued as 12 new chapters were chartered.
- An education director was hired to oversee continually expanding education opportunities.
- The milestone 10th Anniversary National Symposium was held in New York City.
- Lois Foxen served as the association's president.

1979-1980:
- A decision was made to change association management firms.
- A monograph on hepatitis was published.
- A Policy and Procedure Manual was initiated.
- Susan Yuhas served as the association's president.

The 1980s

1980-1981:
- In a transition year, AANNT's management firm changed twice. Anthony J. Jannetti, Inc. was hired in 1980 and still serves as the association's management firm today.
- The association's first National Symposium was held under the direction of its new management firm with a successful meeting in Anaheim, CA.
- The first AANNT awards were presented to members.
- The position paper, "Role of the Registered Nurse in Dialysis," was published.
- The *AANNT Journal* began publishing bimonthly instead of quarterly.
- Carmella Bocchino served as the association's president.

1981-1982:
- The Government Relations Program began as association leaders regularly met with federal and state representatives regarding nephrology nursing issues and care of the ESRD patient.
- AANNT hosted the NFSNO Annual Meeting.
- The 13th National Symposium in Chicago attracted 1,000 registrants.
- Membership grew to 3,237 under President Nancy Sharp.

1982-1983:
- The association led a delegation of specialty nurses to the White House for National Nurses' Day.
- The association bylaws changed to limit full membership to registered nurses only, a step toward development of a professional nursing organization.
- Despite the bylaws change, membership held steady at nearly 3,000 under President Dawn Brennan.
- The First National Meeting separate from ASAIO was held in Philadelphia in June 1983.
- The First Congress of Chapters was held at the National Symposium in Philadelphia.
- An International Workshop on Nephrology Nursing followed the 14th National Symposium.

1983-1984:
- The organization approved a new name – The American Nephrology Nurses' Association (ANNA).
- Attendance at the 15th National Symposium in Hollywood, FL reached 1,000.
- Special Interest Groups (SIGs) became an official subcommittee of the Clinical Practice Committee.
- The *ANNA Journal* published a monograph on rehabilitation.
- Mary Baker served as the association's president.

1984-1985:
- The slogan, "ANNA: Protecting the Future of Quality Care," was adopted for the association.
- The position statement, "Use of Unlicensed Personnel in Dialysis," was published.
- The monograph, *Protecting the Future of Quality Care: An Understanding of Hemodialysis Principles*, was published.
- The association hosted the First Assembly of Nephrology Organizations.
- ANNA contributed significantly to the passage of organ procurement legislation.
- Membership held steady at 3,000 and chapters numbered 55 under President Beth Ulrich.

1985-1986:
- The position of education director was reinstituted after being vacant since 1981.
- Planning took place to publish the *Scope of Practice for Nephrology Nursing*.
- The development of the *Core Curriculum for Nephrology Nursing* was established as a major priority.
- Foundation was laid for the development of nephrology nursing practice base.
- New directions for nephrology nursing certification were defined.
- Regional educational programming was redefined with the First Clinical Concerns in Nephrology Meetings planned for the Fall of 1986.
- Geraldine Biddle served as the association's president.

1986-1987:
- The Nephrology Nursing Certification Board (NNCB) was established and development of a certification examination took place.
- A pilot certification examination was administered at the 18th National Symposium in New York City.
- The *Scope of Practice for Nephrology Nursing* was published.
- The *Core Curriculum for Nephrology Nursing* was published.
- Linda Smith was hired as the ANNA education director.
- The First Clinical Concerns in Nephrology Meetings were held in Chicago and San Diego.
- The 18th National Symposium in New York City attracted 1,335 participants.
- Membership reached an all-time high of 3,690 while chapters increased to 65 under President Janel Parker.

1987-1988:
- Association income officially reached the $1 million mark.
- The first Nephrology Nursing Certification Exams were administered by the NNCB in conjunction with the National League for Nursing (NLN) Test Service.
- The *Standards of Clinical Practice for Nephrology Nursing* were revised and published.
- The association chaired a task force with the FDA and HIMA that developed a videotape on infection control in dialysis units.
- A pilot research project studying nephrology care in the U.S. was conducted.
- Membership surpassed 4,000 for the first time under President Gail Wick.

1988-1989:
- The association celebrated its 20th anniversary with a successful National Symposium in Dallas that attracted a record 1,355 registrants.
- A nursing shortage survey was conducted and published in the *ANNA Journal*.
- The ANNA staffing survey was distributed to ESRD facilities with the HCFA Facility Report.
- The *Quality Assurance Manual for Nephrology Nurses* was developed.
- The association established a legislative office in Washington, DC.
- A bylaws change extended the term of office for regional vice presidents from 1 to 2 years, eliminated the regional secretary position, and established the positions of chapters coordinator and chapters coordinator-elect.
- A standing Research Committee was established.
- Membership surpassed 5,000 under President Patricia S. Jordan.

1989-1990:
- ANNA received 6-year reaccreditation by the American Nurses' Association Board of Accreditation.
- ANNA participated as a member of HCFA's Medical Review Indicators Committee.
- ANNA became committed to the development of a Patient Classification System.

- The association served as chair of the Health Care Policy Committee of NFSNO.
- The first ANNA-sponsored research grants were awarded at the 21st National Symposium in Washington, DC.
- A 5-year strategic plan for the association was developed by the Strategic Planning Task Force in Philadelphia.
- ANNA chapters grew to an all time high of 70!
- Association membership reached 5,745 under President Evelyn Butera.

The 1990s

1990-1991:

- ANNA Career Mobility Scholarships were established.
- ANNA provided representation for the FDA/HIMA tape on the safe and effective use of hemodialysis devices.
- "For Chapters Only" programs were established.
- Audio-conferencing was initiated as a new education offering for chapters.
- The first Management/Education 2-day seminar was held in La Jolla, CA.
- ANNA established a task force to examine the role of the dialysis technician.
- The Staffing Pattern Survey was sent to all acute, chronic, and transplant facilities.
- Membership grew to over 6,500 under President Sally Burrows-Hudson.

1991-1992:

- Association revenues exceeded the $2 million mark, and the cash reserve fund exceeded $1 million.
- Leadership Workshops: The Regional Connection were held in eight cities.
- The 10th Annual Congress of Chapters was held during the National Symposium in Chicago.
- The Board of Directors supported NNCB's change in eligibility requirements to include the requirement of a BSN degree after January 1, 2000.
- The Conceptual Models Task Force was developed to explore the use of conceptual models in nephrology nursing.
- ANNA began a disaster registry for provision of acute nephrology care to disaster victims.
- The association endorsed *Nursing's Agenda for Health Care Reform.*
- ANNA endorsed the *ANA Standards of Clinical Nursing Practice.*
- Membership grew to over 7,500 under President Marilyn Neff.

1992-1993:

- The *Standards of Clinical Practice for Nephrology Nursing* were revised.
- ANNA's *Certification Review Course* was published.
- "The Directory of Nephrology Nurse Researchers" was published in the *ANNA Journal*.
- Thirteen research grants became available to members.
- ANNA became a charter member of the Coalition for Organ Donation.
- Membership surpassed 8,000, and ANNA chapters grew to 99 this year under President Barbara Bednar.

1993-1994:

- The association celebrated its 25th anniversary.
- Involvement in the National Health Care Reform movement was very strong, including representation at the National Nursing Summit on Health Care Reform.
- The association released a Patient Classification System.
- ANNA conducted a 1-day workshop entitled "Diabetes & Renal Disease" in collaboration with the American Association of Diabetes Educators and two practice groups of the American Diabetic Association.
- ANNA hosted two Renal Coalition Meetings.

- The association provided representation for the First UNOS/DOT Public Forum on Transplantation.
- ANNA initiated a revision and expansion of the *Quality Assurance Guide for Nephrology Nursing* and initiated a third edition of the *Core Curriculum for Nephrology Nursing*.
- The association conducted a 2-day Strategic Planning Think Tank in Philadelphia.
- ANNA held a 2-day "Team Think" session with all ANNA committees in Dallas.
- The *ANNA Journal* published a monograph, "Ethical Dilemmas in Nephrology."
- Membership grew to an all-time high of over 9,000 under President Terran Warren Sims.

1994-1995:

- *Continuous Quality Improvement: From Concept to Reality* was published in January 1995.
- The *Core Curriculum for Nephrology Nursing* was revised in the Third Edition in June 1995.
- The Awards Committee oversaw the selection process for over $60,000 in awards and scholarships.
- The Board of Directors approved the position of research consultant.
- The 26th National Symposium in Philadelphia attracted nearly 1,200 registrants.
- Membership surpassed 10,000 under President Karen Schardin.

1995-1996:

- ANNA established a national 800 number at the National Office for association leaders.
- An Advanced Practice Special Interest Group was formed.
- A major effort was made to take the scope of legislative activities into state government in an effort to promote and support the role of RNs in the delivery of patient care.
- A successful 27th National Symposium was held at the Anaheim Convention Center in Anaheim, California.
- Under President Nancy Gallagher ANNA membership continued to increase to 10,500 members.

1996-1997:

- National educational programming included two CORE Learning Institutes, an Advanced Practice Conference, the Management/Education Seminar, and the National Symposium.
- Forty nephrology nurses participated in responding to the PEW Health Professions Commission Report, while nephrology nurses also contributed formal responses to new JCAHO standards and the DOQI Guidelines.
- ANNA issued a joint position with NANT on unlicensed personnel in dialysis.
- ANNA and Sigma Theta Tau secured a joint research grant that focused on investigation of clinical practice outcomes related to treating chronic illnesses.
- The 28th National Symposium was held at the Minneapolis Convention Center in Minneapolis, Minnesota.
- Membership surpassed 11,000 under ANNA President Christy Price.

Note: Portions of this appendix are reprinted from Brennan, D.T., & Jordan, P.S. (1994). *Celebrating 25 years of service to the nephrology community.* Pitman, NJ: American Nephrology Nurses' Association. Used with permission.

Appendix B
Nursing management of the patient with renal failure.

Alterations in Fluid, Electrolyte, and Acid-Base Balance

Problem and Clinical Manifestations	Nursing Intervention	Rationale
Hypervolemia Laboratory findings • Decreased hematocrit • Decreased urine specific gravity • Edema • Weight gain • Hypertension • Hypotension (if there is a decrease in EABV) • S_3 gallop • Pulmonary rales • Pleural effusion • Cough • Ascites • Hepatic congestion • Elevated jugular venous pressure • Peripheral edema • Periorbital edema	Identify patients at risk for the development of hypervolemia.	All patients with compromised renal function are at risk. Close observation of these patients can help prevent acute complications.
	Weigh the patient daily or more often if indicated.	A rapid weight gain usually reflects fluid retention.
	Monitor 24-hour fluid intake and urine output. Also assess urine for presence of abnormal sediment.	As the GFR decreases the kidney loses the ability to excrete fluid and concentrate urine. Abnormalities may be present in urine (see Tables 9-8 and 9-9).
	Maintain accurate records of intake and output (I&O). Compare findings. • Administer prescribed IV medications in the smallest amount of fluid possible. • Distribute the oral intake evenly throughout 24 hours. • Maintain the prescribed fluid restriction and sodium restriction. • Plan fluid intake schedule with the patient.	I&O records are important in evaluating the fluid status; however, weight is the *most accurate* indicator of volume status.
	Monitor BP and pulse in lying, sitting, and/or standing positions (if possible). Wait approximately 5 minutes between each reading. Note the rate and rhythm of the pulse. Monitor hemodynamic parameters if applicable, including CVP and PCWP.	Hypervolemia is frequently accompanied by an increase in BP and P, elevations of central venous, and pulmonary capillary wedge pressures. However, hypotension and a decrease in CVP and PCWP and an increase in P may be seen in patients with volume excess accompanied by a decreased EABV.
	Assess the neck veins with the patient sitting at a 45-degree angle. Measure the vertical distance in centimeters between the level of venous pulsation and sternal angle. An elevation of 3 cm or more is consistent with volume overload.	Intravascular fluid volume excess is associated with venous congestion and engorged neck veins. In fluid volume excess associated with decreased EABV, the neck veins may be "flat," even in the supine position.
	Monitor the heart sounds. Note the rate, rhythm, and presence of an S_3.	The onset of an S_3 is associated with heart failure and is an important clinical finding.
	Monitor the respiratory status. Assess the respiratory rate, characteristics of the respirations, and breath sounds. Note the quantity and character of sputum.	Tachypnea may be associated with fluid volume excess. The presence of crackles and wheezes indicates pulmonary congestion. Fluid can also accumulate in the pleural cavity and cause pain on respiration and decreased breath sounds over the area.
	Note periorbital, pedal, pretibial, and sacral areas for edema. If ascitic fluid is also accumulating, measure the circumference of the abdomen. Check tissue turgor. Provide meticulous skin care to prevent breakdown.	Edema is usually first noted in dependent areas.
	Administer prescribed medications including diuretics and dopamine. Monitor patients on dialysis and CRRT closely.	A diuretic may be prescribed to assist in fluid elimination. In ARF, dopamine may be used to increase renal blood flow and enhance diuresis.

Problem and Clinical Manifestations	Nursing Intervention	Rationale
Hypervolemia (continued)	Monitor the serum and urinary sodium, serum osmolality, fractional excretion of sodium, and hematocrit.	A patient with fluid retention may have a "dilution hyponatremia" and a drop in serum osmolality and hematocrit directly related to the excess fluid. Urinary electrolytes are important in the evaluation of tubular function.
	Consult with the physician about any changes that may indicate a deterioration of renal and/or cardiovascular function.	The following are reported promptly: • Weight gain greater than 5 lbs. in 24 hours • Development of wheezes and crackles or decreased breath sounds • Development of S_3 • Sudden decrease in urine output
	Encourage compliance with low-sodium diet. Educate patient regarding foods to avoid and fluid restriction.	Sodium promotes fluid retention.
	Provide psychologic support to the patient and family.	Fluid retention can precipitate anxiety and cause changes in body image.
Hypovolemia Laboratory Findings • Increased hematocrit • Increased BUN • Increased urine specific gravity • Weight loss • Hypotension • Thirst • Tachycardia • Decreased jugular venous pressure • Poor skin turgor • Dry skin and mucous membranes • Fatigue • Fever	Identify patients at risk.	Volume loss can be seen in early CRF and during the diuretic phase of ARF. Patients receiving diuretics are also at risk.
	Monitor weight daily or more often if indicated. Assess for volume losses from vomiting, diarrhea, drainage, etc.	Weight will assist in identifying insensible fluid losses.
	Monitor the blood pressure and pulse using the same procedure outlined under "Hypervolemia."	Orthostatic changes increase as volume decreases. Hypotension is usually seen in volume depletion.
	Assess for signs of hypovolemia: dry skin, decreased skin turgor, dry mucous membranes, sunken eyeballs, flat neck veins. Provide good skin care and oral hygiene.	Fluid volume deficit depletes intravascular, interstitial, and intracellular volume stores.
	Monitor laboratory studies, including hematocrit, sodium, BUN, creatinine, BUN: creatinine ratio, and urinary electrolytes. Consult with the physician about significant findings.	In hypovolemia, the hematocrit may increase. Depending on other factors, serum sodium levels are variable. The BUN may increase disproportionately to serum creatinine (normal ratio 10:1).
	Administer prescribed fluids, either orally or intravenously, or by both routes. • Monitor 24 hour intake and output	If nausea and vomiting are not present, the best way to replace fluids is orally. If fluids and electrolytes need to be replaced rapidly, the intravenous route is used.
	Provide psychologic support and education to the patient and family.	The patient and family are frequently anxious about the patient's current and future health status. They need to be instructed to increase fluid intake in situations where losses may increase.

Problem and Clinical Manifestations	Intervention	Rationale
Hyponatremia Laboratory Values • Serum Na^+ < 135 mEq/L Gastrointestinal • Anorexia • Nausea • Vomiting Neurologic • Confusion, apprehension, anxiety • Stupor • Seizures • Coma • Weakness • Muscle cramps	Monitor serum Na^+ levels. Assist in preventing hyponatremia. • Use normal saline instead of distilled water for irrigations • Avoid tap water enemas in bowel management • Replace fluid losses with fluid similar in composition • Monitor renal sodium losses • Monitor volume status closely Assess patient for signs and symptoms of hyponatremia. Monitor serum Na^+ levels. Assist with treatment which may include: • Water restriction • PO and IV sodium replacement • Discontinuing diuretic Monitor the neurologic status of the patient closely during treatment. Teach patient the importance of compliance with fluid restriction.	ARF and CRF patients may develop hyponatremia depending on urinary sodium loss and free water intake. Also free water can easily be absorbed during enemas and irrigations. Hyponatremia can occur with normal, increased, or decreased volume. Signs and symptoms develop because of increased water content in brain and nerve cells. Goal of treatment is to restore normal serum Na^+ and osmolality. Rapid correction of hyponatremia can cause shrinkage of brain tissue resulting in severe neurologic signs and symptoms. Excess water intake is a common cause of chronic hyponatremia in the CRF patient.
Hypernatremia Laboratory Findings • Serum Na^+ >146 mEq/L General • Fever • Dry mucous membranes • Thirst • Flushed skin Neurologic • Lethargy • Altered mental status • Seizures Renal • Oliguria	Identify patients at risk and prevent problems if possible. Administer appropriate amounts of water. Monitor volume status closely. Identify sources of free water loss. Monitor serum and urinary sodium levels and serum osmolality and urine specific gravity. Monitor patient for manifestations hypernatremia Monitor correction of volume status. Follow: • Vital signs • Neurologic status • Muscle strength Educate patient and family regarding sodium restriction.	Most commonly occurs in patients with limited access to water. Hypernatremia can occur in hyper-, hypo-, or euvolemic status. Hypernatremia depletes ICF volume and leads to severe neurologic abnormalities. Volume replacement and/or diuretics may be used in an effort to restore normal osmolality. Rapid correction of osmolality may lead to cerebral edema, seizures, and death. Dialysis can assist in correcting hypernatremia. Usual diet is 2g Na^+/day. Renal failure patients should not use salt substitute as these contain potassium.
Hypokalemia Laboratory Values • Serum K^+ < 3.5 mEq/L • Alkalosis Neurologic • Confusion • Depression	Monitor serum K^+ levels. Assess patient for signs and symptoms of hypokalemia. Assess renal and non-renal causes of potassium loss.	In renal insufficiency, significant potassium can be lost in the urine if the patient is on diuretics. Patients can also lose potassium via the GI tract, skin, or wound drainage. Patients on CAPD receiving insulin in the fluid may become hypokalemic since insulin facilitates movement of K^+ into the cells.

Problem and Clinical Manifestations	Nursing Intervention	Rationale
Hypokalemia (continued) Cardiovascular • Hypotension • Increased sensitivity to digitalis • Arrhythmias • ECG changes - see Figure 9-9 Skeletal-Muscular • Weakness • Cramps • Paralysis Gastrointestinal • Anorexia • Vomiting • Diarrhea	Administer potassium supplements, monitoring potassium levels carefully. If possible, encourage intake of high K^+ foods such as fruits and vegetables. • Monitor for GI irritation if using oral K^+ supplementation. • Administer IV K^+ slowly—monitor for phlebitis. Monitor patients who are receiving digitalis closely. Elevate K^+ content of dialysate if indicated.	Patients in renal failure are at high risk for developing hyperkalemia. Patients on dialysis who are receiving digitalis may require an increased K^+ concentration in the bath to prevent manifestations of digitalis toxicity.
Hyperkalemia Laboratory Values • Serum $K^+ > 5.5$ mEq/L • Acidosis Neuromuscular • Weakness • Paresthesias • Muscle cramps • Flaccid paralysis Cardiac • EGG changes (see Figure 9-9) • Cardiac arrest Gastrointestinal • Nausea • Vomiting • Abdominal pain • Ileus	Monitor serum K^+ levels. Report elevations to physician. Assess patient for signs and symptoms of hyperkalemia. Administer treatment for hyperkalemia (see Table 9-27). • Potassium restriction, kayexelate administration, diuretics, dialysis. • Administration of glucose and insulin or sodium bicarbonate. • Administration of calcium salts. Educate patient and family regarding K^+ dietary restriction, importance of dialysis and severe, life-threatening complications of hyperkalemia.	In renal failure, potassium excretion decreases placing patients at high risk for the development of hyperkalemia. Hyperkalemia increases the resting membrane potential and causes increased neuronal excitability. Treatment for hyperkalemia may include these interventions which: • Reduce body K^+ content • Shift K^+ into cells • Antagonize the effects of hyperkalemia on the heart muscle Diet compliance and regular dialysis treatments can prevent hyperkalemia.
Hypocalcemia Laboratory Values • Serum $Ca^{++} < 8.5$ mg/dl Neuromuscular • Circumoral and acral paresthesias • Skeletal muscle cramps • Muscle cramps • Chvostek's/Trousseau's sign • Laryngeal stridor • Tetany • Weakness • Fatigue • Seizures Cardiovascular • Hypotension • ECG changes (see Figure 9-12) • Cardiac arrhythmias • Cardiac arrest	Monitor serum Ca^{++} levels. Assess patient for signs and symptoms of hypocalcemia. • Monitor albumin levels • Monitor serum pH	Patients in renal failure have decreased intestinal absorption of Ca^{++} because of decrease Vitamin D levels. Hypocalcemia causes partial depolarization of neurons and increases neuromuscular excitability. Correct Ca^{++} level for albumin level and ph level. • A decrease of 1 g/dl in albumin is associated with an increase in serum Ca^{++} of 0.8 mg/dl. • A drop in ph of 0.1 units results in a reciprocal rise in ionized Ca^{++} of 0.1 mEq/L.

Problem and Clinical Manifestations	Intervention	Rationale
Hypocalcemia (continued) Other (chronic) • Rickets • Osteomalacia • Cataracts • Dry Skin • Dental Caries	Prevent hypocalcemia. • Administration of oral or IV Ca^{++} supplements and vitamin D as required. • Monitor patients carefully if on digitalis or if hypomagnesemia or hypokalemia are present. • Instruct patient in importance of keeping phosphate levels within normal limits.	Calcium and Vitamin D supplement are given as therapy. High phosphate levels promote the formation of calcium/phosphate complexes which precipitate out of solution and decrease ionized calcium.
Hypercalcemia Laboratory Values • Serum $Ca^{++} > 10.5$ mg/dl Neuromuscular • Personality changes • Acute psychosis • Weakness • Lethargy • Confusion and coma Cardiovascular • Hypertension • Shortening of the QT interval (see Figure 9-12) Gastrointestinal • Anorexia, nausea, vomiting • Constipation Renal • Polyuria • Nephrolithiasis Skeletal • Bone pain • Pathologic fractures Metabolic • Metastatic calcifications	Monitor serum Ca^{++} levels. Monitor patient for signs and symptoms of hypercalcemia. • Monitor albumin levels • Monitor serum pH Monitor serum phosphate levels closely. Follow calcium and phosphate product Administer appropriate therapy. A. In ARF or insufficiency • Saline and diuretics (if renal function permits) • Pamedronate - 30 mg over 4 to 6 hours • Calcitonin • Mithramycin B. In CRF or insufficiency • Withdrawal of Ca^{++} supplements and vitamin D therapy • Dialysis • Mithramycin • Surgical removal of parathyroid tissues	Major causes of hypercalcemia in ARF are bone destruction secondary to malignancy or release of Ca^{++} intracellular stores from injury or catabolism. In CRF, hypercalcemia is most often seen with calcium administration or Vitamin D therapy and secondary hyperparathyroidism. Hypercalcemia causes decreased neuronal excitability. When calcium $\times$ phosphate > 70, metastatic calcification can occur. • enhances renal excretion of Ca^{++} • reduces osteoclastic activity • inhibits PTH activity • slows bone resorption • decreases intestinal absorption of Ca^{++} • removes ionized Ca^{++}
Hypophosphatemia Laboratory Values • Serum $PO_4^{=} < 2.5$ mg/dl in adults and 4.5 mg/dl in children Neuromuscular • Encephalopathy • Parenthesis • Hyporeflexia • Seizures • Weakness Gastrointestinal • Anorexia • Dysphagia Hematologic • Impaired oxygen finding capacity • Hemolysis • Impaired leukocyte function • Impaired platelet function	Monitor serum $PO_4^{=}$ levels. Monitor patient for signs and symptoms of hypophosphatemia. Replace phosphate • IV supplementation may be necessary for severe causes. • Dietary supplement, such as milk • Oral phosphate supplement • Neutraphos Instruct RF patients in appropriate use of phosphate binders.	Although hyperphosphatemia is more common in the renal failure patient, hypophosphatemia can occur with malabsorption syndrome and other abnormalities causing shifts of $PO_4^{=}$ into cells. Hypophosphatemia can also develop during TPN administration or when excess phosphate binders are given. Symptoms are caused by decreased ATP synthesis in most cells and decreased 2, 3 DPG synthesis in red blood cells. Excessive use of phosphate binders is a cause of hypophosphatemia in CRF patients.

Problem and Clinical Manifestations	Nursing Intervention	Rationale
Hyperphosphatemia Laboratory Values • Serum $PO_4^=$> 4.5 mg/dl • Associated with a decrease in serum Ca^{++}	Monitor serum $PO_4^=$ and Ca^{++} levels. Monitor patient for signs and symptoms of hyperphosphatemia.	As renal function declines, phosphate excretion decreases. When the $Ca^{++} \times PO_4^=$ is greater than 70, there is a drop in serum ionized calcium because of the formation and precipitation of calcium phosphate complexes.
Metabolic • Metastatic calcification • Secondary hyperparathyroidism Renal • Deteriorating renal function Gastrointestinal • Abdominal cramps • Nausea • Diarrhea	Administer treatment which may include: • Dietary restriction of phosphate • Phosphate binders are best given with meals • Aluminum antacids • Calcium carbonate • Calcium acetate • Dialysis	These interventions decrease intestinal absorption of PO_4. Use aluminum antacids only for initial control. Effective in removing limited amounts of phosphate.
Neurological • Muscular cramps • Flaccid paralysis • Increased reflexes	Prevent hyperphosphatemia • Educate patient and family regarding dietary restrictions, use of phosphate binders, and long-term consequences of hyperphosphatemia • Never give RF patients phosphate-soda enemas	
Hypomagnesemia Laboratory Values • Serum Mg^{++} < 1.7 mg/dl (1.4 mEq/L)	Monitor serum Mg^{++} levels.	Hypomagnesemia usually occurs in malnourished dialysis patients or those receiving TPN.
Neuromuscular • Personality changes • Tremors • Asterixis • Myoclonus • Seizures • (+) Trousseau's or Chvostek's sign Cardiovascular • Ventricular tachycardia • Increased risk of digitalis toxicity • Cardiac arrest	Monitor patient for signs and symptoms of hypomagnesemia. Treatment includes oral, IM, or IV Mg^{++} supplementation.	Hypomagnesemia increases release of acetylcholine at neuromuscular junctions which increases neuromuscular irritability.
Hypermagnesemia Laboratory Values • Serum Mg^{++} > 2.6 mg/dl (2.1 mEq/L)	Monitor serum Mg^{++} levels.	In the RF patient, hypermagnesemia is usually caused by intake of magnesium containing laxatives, enemas, or antacids.
Neuromuscular • Lethargy • Confusion • Respiratory paralysis • Hyporeflexia	Assess patient for signs and symptoms of hypermagnesemia.	Hypermagnesemia decreases the release of acetylcholine at the neuromuscular junction, which causes decreased neuromuscular excitability.
Cardiovascular • Hypotension • Arrhythmias • Bradycardia • Arrest • EKG abnormalities (tall T-waves)	Treatment is to discontinue magnesium containing compounds. Hemodialysis or peritoneal dialysis are also effective in removing magnesium. Administer prescribed medications • Calcium gluconate • IV insulin and glucose	Magnesium is in many antacids. • Calcium is a magnesium antagonist. • Promotes movement of magnesium into the cells.
Gastrointestinal • Nausea • Vomiting	Instruct patient to avoid use of magnesium containing medications such as in some multivitamins, antacids, enemas, and laxatives.	

Problem and Clinical Manifestations	Nursing Intervention	Rationale
Metabolic Acidosis Laboratory Values • Serum pH ¬ • Serum HCO_3- ¬ Respiratory • Hyperventilation Neurological • Headache • Lethargy • Coma Gastrointestinal • Anorexia • Nausea and vomiting • Diarrhea Cardiac • Arrest • Dysrhythmias	Monitor arterial blood gases and serum HCO_3- levels. Monitor patient for signs and symptoms of metabolic acidosis. Treatment includes: • Reduction of dietary protein • Supplemental sodium bicarbonate - oral or IV • Dialysis Educate patient regarding the importance of protein restriction.	As functional renal mass declines, the kidney is unable to excrete hydrogen and ammonium ions. Changes in serum pH alter cellular functioning. • Decreased acid loads of sulfates • Increase bicarbonate load • Removes H^+ and adds buffers
Metabolic Alkalosis Laboratory Values • Serum pH • Serum HCO_3 Respiratory • Hypoventilation Neuromuscular • Confusion • Tetany • Convulsions Gastrointestinal • Nausea • Vomiting • Diarrhea	Monitor arterial blood gases and serum HCO_3^- levels. • Assess for sources of H^+ loss, vomiting, NG suction • Assess for bicarbonate load, i.e. antacids Monitor patient for signs and symptoms of metabolic alkalosis. Treatment includes correction of cause. Dialysis can assist in correcting the abnormality.	Metabolic alkalosis is uncommon in renal failure patients. However, it may occur as a result of vomiting, nasogastric suctioning, or when diuretics are used.

Expected Outcomes

1. Balanced intake and output with maintenance of patient volume states within established parameters.
2. Physical findings indicate optimum volume, electrolyte, and acid-base status as evidenced by:
   A. Normal vital signs (including hemodynamic parameters, if indicated)
   B. Good skin turgor without edema
   C. No signs and symptoms of electrolyte/acid-base balance alterations
3. Laboratory values are within normal limits. If abnormalities develop, they are promptly identified and treated.
4. Patient and family understand the importance of compliance with fluid and dietary prescription.
5. Patient and family understand the nature and use of medications used to treat fluid, electrolyte, and acid-base alterations.

Appendix C
Nursing management of the patient with renal failure.

Metabolic and Endocrine Disturbances

Problem and Clinical Manifestations	Nursing Intervention	Rationale
Glucose Intolerance Laboratory Values • Elevated glucose levels in some patients. (However, fasting serum glucose levels are usually normal in non-diabetic hemodialysis patients. In patients on CAPD, fasting levels rarely exceed 160 mg/dl).	Monitor blood glucose levels—periodic fasting levels may be indicated. Assess insulin requirements of diabetic patients. Prevent hypoglycemia after dialysis. • Adequate oral intake prior to dialysis • Dialysate glucose bath of 200 mg/dl Consult with dietician to plan appropriate diet. • Develop a dietary plan that will fit in with patient's lifestyle • Teach patient to incorporate diet into lifestyle	Urine testing is inaccurate in RF patients. Patients in renal failure have resistance to the peripheral utilization of insulin. However, there is also decreased excretion and metabolism of insulin. Thus, insulin dependent diabetics may require decreased doses of insulin. These patients may also have a blunted response to hypoglycemia. Although carbohydrate excess may contribute to hyperglycemia and development of obesity, patients need adequate caloric intake to prevent catabolism.
Abnormal Protein Metabolism Laboratory Values • Low serum albumin • Low serum transferrin • Low serum complements • Elevated BUN General • Weight loss • Muscle wasting	Monitor weight and anthropometric measurements. Monitor appropriate laboratory values - albumin, transferrin, and BUN. Consult dietician and nutritional support team to conduct a nutritional assessment. Instruct patient to eat high biologic value protein foods. Provide patients with adequate protein intake: • Oral, enteral, or parenteral feedings Monitor patient for GI problems which might interfere with eating, appetite - diarrhea, abdomen distention, cramping. Provide adequate dialysis or CRRT. • Monitor KT/V and PCR (see Chapter 19) Educate patient and family regarding the importance of appropriate protein intake	Patients in ARF and CRF have altered protein metabolism which places them at high risk for development of a protein wasting state. Nutritional assessment and history is important in determining nutrient needs. Protein foods of high biologic value such as meats and eggs provide essential amino acid. Adequate nutrition may help improve outcome of patient in ARF. On-going nutritional assessment is important to prevent catabolism and muscle wasting It is important to provide adequate removal of metabolic wastes in order to decrease uremic symptoms.
Abnormal Lipid Metabolism Laboratory Values • Elevated triglyceride levels > 200 mg/dl • Normal or slightly elevated serum cholesterol	Monitor cholesterol and triglyceride level. Consult dietician and/or nutritional support team. Administer prescribed medications • Monitor liver function tests. • Avoid medications known to elevate lipid levels especially beta-blockers. Encourage patient to exercise. Assess patient for other risk factors which could accelerate arteriosclerosis. • Hypertension • Obesity • Smoking • Stress	Hypertryglyceridemia is believed to be caused by a deficiency of lipoprotein lipase. Lowering dietary intake of fats and carbohydrates can help in decreasing triglyceride levels but may be very difficult in view of other dietary restrictions. As cardiovascular disease is a major cause of death in the CRF patient, some physicians may prescribe antilipemic medications. Exercise can assist in decrease in triglyceride levels.

Problem and Clinical Manifestations	Intervention	Rationale
Endocrine Disorders Hypothyroidism • Hoarseness • Goiter • Weight gain • Dry skin • Cold intolerance	Assess CRF patient for signs and symptoms of endocrine-related disorders (see Table 9-32) • Glucose intolerance • Hypertension (renin-dependent) • Hyperparathyroidism • Decreased gonadal function • Hypothyroidism	CRF patients have a variety of endocrine abnormalities related to changes in the synthesis, secretion, and metabolism of various hormone. Some endocrine abnormalities have been described in ARF patients, but these problems generally resolve after recovery of renal function.
Decreased gonadal function - male • Atrophic testes • Decreased sperm count and mobility • Impotence • Decreased libido • Gynecomastia • Galactorrhea • Sluggishness	Monitor T_3, T_4, and TSH levels. • Assess patient for signs and symptoms of hypothyroidism • Administer thyroid supplements if needed	There is an increase in incidence of hypothyroidism in CRF patient. T_3 and T_4 levels are usually normal, but TSH levels are reliable in diagnosing hypothyroidism. Propylthiouracil (thyroid supplement) has increased half life in RF.
Decreased gonadal function - female • Amenorrhea • Dysmenorrhea • Decreased libido • Galactorrhea	Assess sexual functioning. A thorough history and physical is essential in work-up of sexual dysfunction. • Monitor appropriate laboratory values FSH Testosterone Prolactin	Sexual problems are wide spread in dialysis patients. It is important to rule out vascular insufficiency and autonomic neuropathy.
Glucose intolerance	Patient and partner should receive sexual counseling to explore alternative methods of sexual satisfaction if impotence is not treatable.	Dialysis patients endure a wide variety of emotional stresses.
Hypertension	Provide emotional support for patient and partner.	Correction of anemia with erythropoietin may improve sexual functioning.
Hyperparathyroidism	Administer prescribed medications • Bromocryptine • Testosterone • Zinc • Erythropoietin	Hyperprolactinemia can be treated with bromocriptine. Zinc supplements have been reported to increase plasma testosterone levels.

Expected Outcomes

1. Patient's dry weight is appropriate for age, height, weight, and body frame.
2. Caloric intake is appropriate for energy demands and for the prevention of acceleration of catabolism.
3. Glucose levels are normal in non-diabetic dialysis patients. Glucose levels of diabetic patients are within established parameters.
4. Anthropometric measurements are appropriate for patient's size.
5. Laboratory values used to assess nutrition as status are at optimal levels.
6. Endocrine-related disorders are identified and treated appropriately.
7. Patients will express satisfaction regarding their sexuality.

Appendix D
Nursing management of the patient with renal failure.

The Uremic Syndrome

Problem and Clinical Manifestations	Intervention	Rationale
Neurologic Manifestations Central • Headache • Lassitude • Apathy • Drowsiness • Insomnia • Emotional lability • Memory deficits • Somnolence • Confusion • Coma • Seizures • Sleep disturbances • Asterixis	Educate patient and family regarding neurologic effects of uremia and provide emotional support.	The patient and family may become anxious regarding memory or behavioral changes. The psychosocial stresses associated with renal failure can aggravate neurologic symptoms.
	Assess patient's ability to think and reason. Baseline cognitive function testing may be helpful in planning care.	Cognitive abilities are decreased in uremia.
	Allow patient adequate time to think about and respond to discussion.	The patient may require additional time to process information.
	Conduct patient teaching according to patient's level of readiness. Provide frequent reinforcement.	
	Observe for changes in general neurological status. • Perform baseline neurological exam and assessment of premorbid personality • Exam should be repeated as indicated	
	Assess for other causes of CNS deficits: • Alcoholism • Drug abuse • B_{12}/folate deficiency	Metabolism of drugs is altered in renal failure. Patients may respond to stress with drug abuse.
	Monitor patient for signs and symptoms of disequilibrium syndrome during dialysis. • Encephalopathy • Seizures • Headache • Blurred vision • Muscle cramps	Sodium modeling can help prevent this complication.
	Assess sleep patterns. Instruct patient in sleep hygiene. • Retire and awaken at regular times • Have a relaxation period before going to bed • Avoid long day-time naps • Get at least one-half hour of sunlight within 30 minutes of out-of-bed time	Sleep disturbances can increase fatigue and worsen cognitive deficits. Sleep thrives on the "routine."
Peripheral • Paresthesias • Dysthesia • Decreased tendon reflexes • Muscle twitching • Restless leg syndrome • Gait abnormalities • Asterixis • Hearing loss • Facial asymmetry	Perform complete assessment of peripheral nervous system including cranial nerves.	Assessment may also include nerve conduction studies. Auditory studies may be indicated if hearing loss develops. Cranial nerve abnormalities can also occur.
	Maintain optimal fluid, electrolyte, and acid-base balance.	Metabolic abnormalities can aggravate peripheral neuropathies.
	Provide vitamin supplements.	Pyridoxine and B_{12} deficiencies can cause peripheral neuropathies.

Problem and Clinical Manifestations	Intervention	Rationale
Peripheral (continued)	Restless leg syndrome may cause great discomfort and interfere with sleep.	Benzodiazepines, opiates, and L-dopa can be used to treat this condition. Although tricyclics are frequently used to treat peripheral neuropathies, they can *worsen* 1eg movements at night.
	Educate patient regarding prevention of trauma to extremities: • properly fitting shoes • thermal precautions	Trauma can lead to infection and possible loss of limb.
Autonomic • Orthostatic hypotension • Depressed cough reflex • Decreased sweating	Assess patient for orthostasis. Take blood pressure and pulse in sitting and standing position. Use of TED stockings may help prevent orthostatic hypotension.	ANS abnormalities occur in renal failure, particularly in diabetic patients. Stockings help increase venous return to the heart.

Expected Outcomes

1. Neurologic complications which occur are promptly recognized, evaluated, and treated.
2. Patient's comfort and safety is maintained.
3. Patient is maintained in optimum metabolic state.
4. Patient and family will understand the neurologic manifestations of the uremic syndrome.

Problem and Clinical Manifestations	Intervention	Rationale
Cardiovascular Manifestations • Hypertension • Congestive heart failure • Cardiac arrhythmias pericarditis • Cardiac tamponade • Accelerated atherosclerosis	Monitor BP, P, and weight. Instruct patient to take hypertensive medications.	Most hypertension is volume dependent but may also be related to excess production of renin.
	Monitor fluid and electrolyte status. Auscultate heart sounds for rate, rhythm, gallops, and murmers. • Observe for distended neck veins • Palpate for enlarged liver • Check PMI placement	Fluid and electrolyte disturbances can cause changes in heart rate and rhythm. In addition, gallops (S_3 and S_4) may occur in congestive heart failure and hypertension. Murmers develop with anemia, placement of vascular access.
	Assess for symptoms of pericarditis including tachycardia, ECG changes, pericardial friction rub (heard best when the patient is setting up and leaning forward), fever, and leukocytoses.	Pericarditis frequently occurs in uremic patients and may indicate the need for more aggressive dialysis. Pain of pericarditis is aggravated by movement, breathing, coughing, and lying down. The pain is relieved by sitting up and leaning forward.
	Monitor patient for signs and symptoms of effusion and tamponade i.e., paradox in the BP, distended neck veins, engorged liver, hypotension, displaced PMI, tachycardia, and enlarged heart on physical examination, CXR, and/or echocardiogram.	Effusion is the collection of fluid in the pericardial sac. Cardiac tamponade is a medical and/or surgical emergency.

Problem and Clinical Manifestations	Intervention	Rationale
	Assess for signs and symptoms of atherosclerosis: • angina • decreased peripheral pulses • claudication Educate patient and family regarding cardiac complications associated with renal failure and the roles that diet, medications, and dialysis play in their prevention. Educate patient regarding cardiac risk factor reduction.	Accelerated atherosclerosis in CRF may be related to abnormalities in glucose and lipid metabolism.

Expected Outcomes

1. Blood pressure is within normal limits.
2. Adequate cardiac output is maintained as evidenced by:
   A. stable vital signs
   B. ability to maintain consistent activity level
   C. strong peripheral pulses
3. Cardiac complications are promptly recognized, assessed, and treated.
4. Patient and family understand possible cardiac complications of uremia and can verbalize appropriate information regarding diet, medications, and signs and symptoms to report.

Problem and Clinical Manifestations	Intervention	Rationale
Respiratory Manifestations • Kussmaul's respiration • Pulmonary edema • Pneumonitis • Increased susceptibility to infections	Monitor respiratory rate and rhythm.	Respiratory rate may increase in compensation for metabolic acidosis.
	Auscultate lung fields for: a. decreased breath sounds b. rales c. rhonchi d. pleural friction rub	Rales and rhonchi develop in pulmonary edema. Decreased breath sounds occur with pleural effusion. Pleural friction rub is a sign of pleuritis.
	Monitor character and amount of sputum.	Pulmonary infections are characterized by increased, tenacious sputum production.
	Follow arterial blood gases and CXR as indicated.	Respiratory compromise may cause decreased oxygenation.
	Instruct patient to avoid those with respiratory infections.	Patients in renal failure have increased susceptibility to infection.
	Ensure patient receives appropriate vaccinations.	Vaccination against the influenza virus is recommended annually. Pneumococcal vaccination is given according to antibody response.

Expected Outcomes

1. Respiratory rate less than 24/min. without dyspnea.
2. Absence of adventitious breath sounds.
3. Normal $p0_2$ and $pC0_2$ within limits of existing pathology.
4. Normal CXR.
5. Negative sputum culture.

Problem and Clinical Manifestations	Intervention	Rationale
Hematologic Manifestations Anemia • Fatigue • Decreased appetite • Increased angina • Cold intolerance • Hypotension • Reduced exercise tolerance • Dyspnea on exertion • Pallor • Tachycardia	Monitor hematocrit, iron studies, and bleeding time.	Anemia develops in RF secondary to erythropoietin deficiency. Bleeding time is the most reliable test to evaluate bleeding tendency.
	Administer recombinant human erythropoietin (r-HuEPO) as ordered.	r-HuEPO causes an increase in hematocrit within 8 to 12 weeks.
	Administer oral and/or IV iron and folate supplements as ordered. Keep iron saturation > 20%.	Adequate iron and vitamin stores are necessary for RBC production.
Increased bleeding tendency • Petechiae • Ecchymosis • Epistaxis • Hematochezia	Monitor patient for blood loss. • Check stool for occult blood • Bleeding from skin and mucous membranes • Bleeding from access or around IV lines	Platelet count may be only slightly ¬ but they do not function normally in uremic environment.
	Protect patient from trauma. Instruct patient in ways to prevent bleeding and bruising, i.e., avoid trauma, vigorous nose blowing, constipation, injury to gums during tooth brushing. • Administer appropriate medications if uncontrolled bleeding occurs.	• Cryoprecipitate, DDAVP, and estrogens may help control uremic bleeding. Dialysis also can improve bleeding time.
Impaired leukocyte function • Increased susceptibility to infections • Lymphopenia • Suppression of cellular and humoral immunity	Avoid penetration of skin/mucous membrane barriers. • Discontinue IV lines if possible • Avoid urinary catheter • Monitor WBC	Uremic patients have impaired leukocyte function.
	Teach patient good oral hygiene and skin care.	
	Assess patient for viral, fungal, and parasitic infections.	Infections are the major cause of death in ARF.

Expected Outcomes

1. Hematocrit is maintained at optimal level for patient (30%-35%).
2. Iron saturation is $\geq$ 20%.
3. Folate levels are within normal limits.
4. Blood losses are kept to a minimum.
5. Patient and family are knowledgeable regarding ways to prevent infection and bleeding.
6. Appropriate actions are taken to prevent infection.

Problem and Clinical Manifestations	Intervention	Rationale
Dermatologic Manifestations • Pruritus • Dry skin • Skin color changes • Pallor • Nail changes • Uremic Frost	Asses skin for dryness, signs of scratching, poor turgor, and changes in color. Consult dermatologist if necessary.	Pruritus is a frequently described problem in acute chronic real failure. Possible causes indicate urochrome and metabolic waste retention, deposition of calcium phosphate crystals in skin, hyperparathyroidism, and histamine release.
	Avoid use of drying soaps and use lanolin-based soaps. After bathing, patient should apply emollient while still wet and then pat dry.	Applying emollient while wet helps seal moisture in skin.
	Instruct patient and family in good skin care. Advise patient to keep nails short and to avoid scratching. Explain nature of skin changes in renal failure.	Trimmed nails can aid in preventing skin trauma from scratching.
	Instruct patient in control of phosphorus and calcium.	See Appendix A.
	Administer medications or treatments as ordered (see Table 9-36). • Diphenhydramine • Oral charcoal • UV light	 • antihistamine • may bind with toxic substances in GI tract
	Assess nail for changes and signs of fungal infection.	Nail changes do not occur in all uremic patients. Patients are susceptible to cutaneous infection.

Expected Outcomes

1. Patient's skin will remain intact and free from infections.
2. Patient will verbalize understanding of the dermatologic changes which occur in renal failure and importance of good skin and nail care.

Problem and Clinical Manifestations	Intervention	Rationale
Gastrointestinal Manifestations • Unpleasant taste in mouth • Gingival hyperplasia • Caries • Stomatitis • Anorexia • Nausea • Vomiting • Constipation • Diarrhea • Gastritis • Duodenitis • Colitis	Assess oral status. Examine gums, tongue, and mucous membranes. Assess for alterations in taste.	Oral membranes become pale. Metallic taste, halitosis, and stomatitis are caused by high urea concentration.
	To alleviate dry mouth, patient can be instructed to: • brush teeth frequency • chew gum • suck on hard candy • maintain daily fluid allotment	Fluid losses can reduce salivary flow and cause dry mouth.

Problem and Clinical Manifestations	Intervention	Rationale
Gastrointestinal Manifestations (continued)	Teach patient the importance of good oral hygiene or perform oral care for patient. Instruct patient to have regular dental check-ups every 3-6 months. Dental prophylaxis is recommended for invasive procedures: • Penicillin VK 1 gm 1 hour prior to procedure then 500 mg every 6 hours for 2 days. • Erythromycin - 1 gm 1 hour prior to procedure then 500 mg every 6 hours for 2 days.	Good oral hygiene habits and regular dental check-ups can help prevent morbidity.
	Assess patient for nausea, vomiting, anorexia and abdomen for pain, tenderness, distention and bowel sounds. • Plan food so that it is appealing • Small, frequent feedings may decrease nausea • Antiemetics can be used in small doses • Metaclopromide can enhance gastric emptying	Gastropathy is related to high levels of urea. As renal function deteriorates, GI symptoms may worsen.
	Assess patient for constipation/diarrhea • Stool softeners and bulk laxatives can be used to establish normal bowel habits. • Avoid excessive use of harsh laxatives • Saline enemas can provide relief • Diphenoxlate hydrochloride can be used to treat diarrhea.	Constipation may be due to decreased gastric motility and is a side effect of aluminum-based phosphate binders. Never administer a phosphate-soda enema to a renal failure patient as it will increase serum phosphate.
	Periodically, check stools for occult blood. • Prophylactic use of antacids and H_2 blockers can help prevent ulcer formation in the ARF/CRF patient	Ulcerative lesions and platelet dysfunction predispose the renal failure patient to GI bleeding.
	Educate patient and family in the gastrointestinal manifestations of uremia.	

Expected Outcomes

1. Patient will maintain a good program of oral hygiene.
2. Patient will establish a desired bowel elimination pattern.
3. Gastrointestinal complications will be prevented. If problems develop they will be promptly recognized and treated.
4. Patient and family will verbalize an understanding of the GI manifestations of uremia and know how to best manage them.

Problem and Clinical Manifestations	Intervention	Rationale
Skeletalmuscular Manifestations Renal osteodystrophy • Bone pain • Pathological fractures • Metastatic calcifications	Monitor serum phosphate and calcium and the calcium phosphate product (calcium × phosphate) • Instruct patient and family in dietary phosphate restriction	As functional renal mass decreases, normal calcium and phosphate balance are disturbed. Hypocalcemia develops secondary to reduced Vitamin D levels. Hyperphosphatemia occurs from reduced renal phosphate excretion.
	Administer phosphate binders with meals. Calcium binders should be used instead of aluminum binders if calcium phosphate product is less than 70 to prevent aluminum toxicity. • Assess patient for constipation	The calcium phosphate product should stay below 70 to prevent metastatic calcifications. Phosphate binders bind with phosphate in the GI tract.

Problem and Clinical Manifestations	Intervention	Rationale
Skeletalmuscular Manifestations (continued)	Administer calcium supplements and Vitamin D therapy as indicated. Evaluate response to therapy.	Vitamin D (calcitriol) enhances intestinal absorption of calcium and suppress PTH secretion. Calcium and Vitamin D therapy should not be given if hyperphosphatemia is present as metastatic calcifications will occur.
	Follow PTH, alkaline phosphatase, aluminum levels in addition to bone biopsy results and hand and clavicle films.	Elevated PTH and alkaline phosphatase levels are consistent with hyperparathyroidism. A bone biopsy will assist in diagnosing the presence and type of renal bone disease.
	Assess patient's ability to ambulate, range of motion, muscle strength, coordination, and bone pain. • Assess patient's environment for potential hazards.	These symptoms are associated with hyperparathyroidism. Changes in gait and muscle strength predispose patient to injuries.
	• Assess for soft tissues calcification • Joint pain • Pruritus • Conjunctivitis	Calcium phosphate complexes can be deposited in soft tissues.
	Educate patient and family regarding: • Manifestations of renal osteodystrophy. • Signs and symptoms to report to health care team. • Methods to minimize disability and enhance current mobility.	

Expected Outcomes

1. Phosphate, calcium, PTH, aluminum, and alkaline phosphatase levels will remain within established parameters.
2. Patient will remain free of disability related to renal osteodystrophy.
3. Patient and family will verbalize an understanding of the importance of phosphate control in the prevention of renal osteodystrophy.

Appendix E
AANNT Legislative Policy Statement – November 1983.

Preamble

AANNT is a national organization of 3500 members who are involved in the supervision and delivery of care to adult and pediatric patients with end stage renal disease (ESRD) in all modalities of care.

AANNT has established a Government Relations Committee and has become actively involved in legislative issues affecting the ESRD Program. The committee has provided oral and written testimony before congressional committees and federal agencies.

The positions expressed by this committee have been developed based on comments from the AANNT Board of Directors, committee chairpersons, and direct membership input. This Legislative Policy Statement represents the views of AANNT regarding the ESRD Program as it currently exists. The committee will utilize this document in formulating future comments relating to the following issues.

I. Delivery of ESRD Health Care

1. AANNT believes that appropriate treatment of high quality must be available to all ESRD patients. AANNT supports the view that patients must be provided with complete and accurate information about methods of treatment available and their associated benefits and risks and become active participants in the decision-making process regarding choice of therapy and treatment setting.

2. As a component of health promotion, AANNT endorses the principle that patients assume as much responsibility for their overall care as they are willing and able to take, with the goal of optimal rehabilitation.

3. AANNT supports the development of national standards and guidelines for the reprocessing of disposables. AANNT believes that ESRD facilities must be required to adhere to such standards.

4. AANNT strongly supports efforts to increase organ donation through public education programs and increased awareness of the need for organs among the health professions. In addition, AANNT endorses the development of a national data bank and coordination system to improve the effectiveness of the organ distribution system.

II. Nursing

1. AANNT supports a minimum of one Registered Professional Nurse, experienced in rendering care (including dialytic therapy) to ESRD patients, to be on site for direct supervision of patient care personnel during dialysis treatments.

2. AANNT believes the Registered Professional Nurse must be a major participant in the decision-making process to determine appropriate staffing ratios for facilities providing care to ESRD patients.

3. AANNT supports the improved utilization of Master's prepared Registered Professional Nurses with advanced clinical nephrology expertise, and licensed nurse practitioners in the provision of more individualized patient care, which should reduce morbidity and mortality among patients. We support the recognition of and compensation for such specialized services in the Medicare payment system. We believe such payments would be cost-effective.

4. AANNT encourages the development of a standardized program for the education and training of licensed and unlicensed patient care personnel for the management of ESRD patients as a condition of Medicare participation.

III. Health Care Planning/ESRD

1. AANNT supports "open" staffing within dialysis units. Open staffing is defined as the opportunity for any qualified physician who meets medical criteria set forth by the governing body of a certified ESRD facility to admit and treat his or her patients in that unit. This policy will promote access to and selection of the physician and facility of the patient's choice.

2. AANNT favors the establishment of minimum utilization rates for transplant centers. Home dialysis training programs should include a sufficient number of patients in-training to maintain appropriate skill levels for the training staff. Such standards should be incorporated in the Medicare conditions of participation.

3. AANNT supports elimination of certificate of need approval for the establishment of renal dialysis services as a means of promoting competition among providers.

IV. ESRD Networks

1. AANNT has long recognized the need for accurate and complete tracking of ESRD patient data. AANNT supports, therefore, adequate funding to continue Network involvement in collecting and reporting such critical data.

2. AANNT supports professional peer review and quality assurance activities at the Network-wide level. AANNT encourages active ESRD nursing participation in such peer review activities and the opportunity for patients to have input into the peer review process. AANNT supports adequate funding for Network Medical Review Board activities which have included:
   - questionnaires to determine patient knowledge and/or satisfaction with treatment modality;
   - interdisciplinary team site visits of ESRD facilities;
   - research into the reasons for nursing shortages in ESRD facilities;
   - development of uniform ESRD definitions for levels or types of care provided for acute and chronic patients;
   - development of guidelines for water treatment safety; and
   - development of guidelines for training new ESRD staff, including development of new staff role definitions.

V. ESRD Program Management

1. AANNT supports the concept of cost containment in the provision of high quality ESRD care. AANNT supports studies by qualified health professionals, in conjunction with knowledgeable consumers, to determine the quality and cost effectiveness of ESRD services.

2. AANNT endorses policies and payment regulations to prevent inappropriate and exorbitant profit margins in the provision of ESRD services at the expense of taxpayers and consumers.

3. AANNT urges HCFA to analyze and disseminate data and information from its evaluation of the paid-aide demonstration projects (1978-1981). These data include input from patients concerning factors that influence their choice of treatment modality and setting.

4. AANNT believes the provision of paid home dialysis aides and family partners may influence patient selection of a long-term treatment method and, if proven, should be incorporated into HCFA's reimbursement structure.

5. AANNT encourages HCFA to analyze other studies conducted within the renal community, such as patient acuity studies, morbidity/mortality studies, and CAPD studies.

6. AANNT believes the evaluation of ESRD units should be continued on an annual basis and that members of the site team must have experience in the delivery of ESRD services.

7. AANNT supports the rapid dissemination of the results of studies concerning improvements in renal transplantation and recommends the costs of chronic immunosuppressive drug therapy be covered under the program.

Networks Remain

Key staff persons on the Senate Finance and House Ways and Means Committees report that the section of the House and Senate bills that calls for the elimination of Networks has been dropped from both bills.

In July when the Senate and House Appropriations committees marked up the DHHS budget, the $4.5 million budget for the 32 collective networks remained in the budget.

Note: From ANNA Legislative Policy Statement. (1983, November/December). *ANNA Update,* p. 12. Used with permission.

Appendix F
ANNA's Health Policy Statement

Preamble

ANNA is a national organization of registered nurses practicing in nephrology, transplantation, and related therapies, who are involved in the supervision and delivery of care to adult and pediatric patients in all modalities of treatment for renal disease and other organ system failure states. ANNA supports the multidisciplinary approach to health care and believes that registered nurses must be major participants in the planning, delivery, and evaluation of that care.

ANNA, as a professional organization, has the obligation to set forth and update high standards of patient care, educate practitioners, stimulate research, disseminate new ideas throughout the field, promote interdisciplinary communication and cooperation, and address issues encompassing the practice of nephrology nursing.

The opinions expressed in this document have been developed based on comments from ANNA members, officers, and committee chairpersons, with final approval of the ANNA Board of Directors. In conjunction with ANNA's Legislative Consultant, the Board of Directors reviews and revises this document as necessary on at least an annual basis. This Health Policy Statement represents the views of ANNA regarding the major public policy issues related to the treatment of patients with renal disease and the practice of professional nursing in nephrology. This document will be used to provide direction as the Association addresses legislative and regulatory issues on a local, state, and national level.

Nursing

A. ANNA believes the practice of nephrology nursing is directed toward assessing the health needs of adult and pediatric patients and their families who are experiencing the real or threatened impact of compromised renal function, acute or chronic renal failure, or other organ system failure states, as well as to diagnose and treat their responses to these problems.
Within this context, the Association believes that nephrology nurses must be committed to helping each individual and his/her family to achieve an optimal level of functioning and that they must establish high standards of patient care that are routinely updated.

B. ANNA believes that every patient has the right to professional nursing care and that the registered nurse experienced in dialytic therapy must be present for the direct supervision of patient care activities and personnel during dialysis treatments.

C. ANNA believes that a registered nurse must be actively involved in establishing staff-patient ratios in facilities providing care to patients with renal disease, and that such ratios should be determined based on some measure of patient acuity and need.

D. ANNA believes that care for patients with renal disease is provided effectively and responsibly by registered nurses. Further, the use of advanced practice registered nurses in the management of patients with renal disease can be cost effective and of high quality, which is of benefit to the health care delivery system in general and the ESRD program in particular. ANNA therefore supports the recognition of and compensation for advanced practice registered nurses by all payers.

E. ANNA endorses the certification of qualified nephrology nurses as defined by the Nephrology Nursing Certification Board. Further, the Association supports the process of continuing certification in an effort to define the knowledge of nephrology nurses required to provide quality care and appropriate therapies to patients in all stages of renal compromise across the life span.

F. ANNA supports the development of a standard national program of education and training for unlicensed patient care personnel in dialysis. Such education and training is ideally done in a formal setting, with standardized competency testing immediately upon completion of the program, and with annual continuing education requirements.

G. ANNA believes that all licensed patient care personnel must complete a standardized nephrology education program reflecting the ANNA Standards of Clinical Practice for Nephrology Nursing. The Association believes that a sound education program is necessary to develop, maintain, and augment competence in practice.

H. ANNA supports any nurse's right to refuse to perform an act or take an assignment that in the nurse's judgement is not safe or is not within that nurse's skill, experience, qualifications, or capability.

I. In accordance with our commitment to compassionate end-of-life care, ANNA believes that nurses should not participate in assisted suicide or active euthanasia and that such acts are in direct violation of the American Nurses Association (ANA) Code for Nurses with Interpretive Statements and the ethical traditions of the profession. The ANA statement asserts that, "Nurses individually and collectively have an obligation to provide comprehensive and compassionate end-of-life care which includes the promotion of comfort and the relief of pain and, at times, foregoing life-sustaining treatment." ANNA acknowledges, however, that refusal to participate in assisted suicide or euthanasia does not constitute abandonment of patients.

ANNA believes that nephrology nurses should continue to advocate for health care environments that provide humane and dignified patient-centered care. Nephrology nurses have been at the forefront of promoting quality of life as an essential component of nephrology patient care. The Association supports continued dialogue on the issues of assisted suicide, euthanasia, and appropriate decision making related to withdrawal of treatment, and it recognizes the critical need for reform of end-of-life care.

J. ANNA supports the inclusion of registered nurses at the policymaking level and on all boards, commissions, task forces, and other groups setting policies that affect nursing practice.

K. ANNA supports the promotion of nursing's role in patient advocacy.

L. ANNA believes personnel must be protected from occupational or environmental health hazards related to dialytic therapy and that standards should be developed that identify these hazards and recommend protective measures.

M. ANNA believes that any efforts to detect or test for substance abuse or communicable diseases must be consistent with good medical practice and shall not violate the civil rights of nurses and others.

N. ANNA opposes the licensing of assistive personnel and supports the least restrictive approach to the direct regulation of such personnel, such as registration of personnel who meet specific educational or experiential requirements and who have demonstrated some level of competency. The Association supports that the term "certification" should be reserved for voluntary private sector programs that attest to the competency of individual health professions and occupational groups.

Elements of Care

A. ANNA is committed to assuring and protecting the access of patients with renal disease, and those undergoing transplantation and other related therapies, to professional nursing care delivered by experienced registered nurses.

B. ANNA believes that appropriate, quality treatment must be available to all patients with renal disease and those undergoing transplantation and other related therapies. ANNA supports that patients must be provided with complete and accurate information about alternative forms of therapy, including their associated risks and benefits, and without regard for their cost. The Association believes that patients must be active participants in the decision-making process regarding choice of therapy and treatment.

C. As a component of health promotion, ANNA endorses the concept that patients assume as much responsibility for their overall care as they are physically and mentally able to assume to achieve the goal of optimal rehabilitation. This includes continuing support for all home and self-dialysis modalities, with patient training and supervision under the direction of a qualified registered nurse.

D. ANNA believes that continuing research is indicated in the area of dialyzer reprocessing that addresses the potential risks and benefits or all aspects of reprocessing, including sterilants, and other environmental hazards that may affect patients and personnel.

E. ANNA believes that all patients must be protected from the possible threat of communicable diseases related to dialytic, transplant, and other extracorporeal therapies and that access to testing for such diseases be available to all patients as defined by state health policies.

Transplantation

A. ANNA supports public and private sector efforts that promote organ donation and increase transplantation. The Association believes this can be accomplished by:
   1. Continued support for education programs for the public and for health professionals concerning the lack of available donor organs and the appropriate identification of potential donors. One activity to be considered is:

   a. Inclusion in state statute that requestors must have documentation of completion of a course in medical record review by the OPO, tissue bank, or eye bank.
2. Continued support for a national system of organ procurement and allocation.
3. Implementation of uniform state codes and laws regarding organ donation, procurement, and transplantation. Some possible alternatives that could be considered include:
   a. Routine referral legislation which would mandate that hospitals adopt a routine referral policy within their institutions with mandatory notification of OPOs of potential candidates and automatic death notification. Such legislation could also include that OPOs, tissue banks, and eye banks collectively be allowed to perform hospital medical record reviews as an education mechanism for hospital personnel. This could also include that a hospital can participate in death record reviews if it chooses.
   b. Legislation to amend the Anatomical Gift Act to support that a donor card cannot be revoked by the next of kin and that if there is evidence that the individual did not want to donate, the family would not be approached.
   c. To add organ/tissue donation language in each of the following categories in any existing or future legislation: advance directives, living wills, and durable powers of attorney.
4. Continued federal support of transplant activities including medical research and coverage of immunosuppressive drug therapy.
5. Removal of incentives or statutory language to prevent insurers from denying access to transplantation to their members.
6. Requirements that states provide access to transplantation in their Medicaid coverage policies.

   ANNA remains opposed to coercive behavior in the solicitation of organs for transplantation from living donors if the donor's decision is based primarily on financial gain.

ESRD Network Organizations

A. ANNA has long recognized the need for accurate and complete tracking of ESRD program data. The Association supports the continuation of federally funded Network organizations and the United States Renal Data System (USRDS) to assure the continuation of collecting and reporting such critical data.

B. ANNA believes that each dialysis facility must assess patient outcomes on a regular and ongoing basis and participate in independent quality improvement activities. Further, ANNA believes that these activities can best be coordinated and monitored by the ESRD Network organizations, as is currently being done through Medicare's Health Care Quality Improvement Program (HCQIP). ANNA supports the continuation and expansion of the HCQIP to eventually include every dialysis facility in the country, including non-Medicare providers.

ESRD Program Management

A. ANNA supports the concept of cost containment in health care while maintaining quality. The Association therefore supports measures designed to assure appropriate cost containment in the ESRD program and to prevent excessive profit margins at the expense of consumers. To that end, the Association encourages studies by qualified professionals, in conjunction with knowledgeable consumers, to determine cost effectiveness in relation to the quality of health care proposed and delivered.

B. ANNA is concerned that some cost containment measures negatively affect patient access to care or lead to compromised quality of care delivery. ANNA does not support regulatory changes in the ESRD program or any prospective payment system that will undermine the standards of professional nephrology nursing established by ANNA.

C. ANNA encourages the Health Care Financing Administration (HCFA) to analyze studies conducted within the renal community addressing such issues as patient acuity, morbidity/mortality, and alternative therapies that frequently reflect changing practice patterns and a constantly revised state of the art. The Association therefore endorses the implementation of the recommendations of the federally commissioned Institute of Medicine (IOM) study, Kidney Failure and the Federal Government, 1991, including those regarding the initiation and withdrawal of dialysis.

D. ANNA believes the evaluation of ESRD facilities should be continued annually and that members of the on-site survey team be knowledgeable about the various aspects of the delivery of care to patients with renal disease. Controls to assure that adequate patient care and treatment are delivered to all patients must be included in the monitoring process.

Principles of Medicare and Medicaid Reform

ANNA has developed a statement of principles for Medicare and Medicaid reform as it relates to the federal End-Stage Renal Disease (ESRD) program and the access of patients with ESRD to needed services.

Over 230,000 Americans suffer from ESRD, meaning they must receive dialysis or a kidney transplant in order to maintain life. Given that health care for kidney patients is literally a matter of life or death, ANNA strongly supports inclusion of the following principles in any proposal to restructure Medicare and Medicaid.

A. The Medicare ESRD program entitlement and services MUST BE MAINTAINED in its current form until the results of the ESRD capitation demonstration project are evaluated and specific recommendations are made to improve the program.
   1. Coverage for all dialysis and transplantation services as specified in Medicare ESRD regulations, including physical, vocational, nutritional, and psychosocial rehabilitation.
   2. Funding for the ESRD network organizations, including data collection for the United States Renal Data System (USRDS), oversight activities for quality assurance and continuous quality improvement, and patient grievance procedures. All ESRD patients, whether covered by Medicare or by another health insurance system, must be included in the ESRD network programs and the USRDS data system.
   3. Appropriate funding for the USRDS to ensure timely analysis and availability of data to guide good clinical practice.
   4. Disincentives, such as disproportionately higher premiums, deductibles, and coinsurance, will create unacceptable financial burdens for ESRD beneficiaries and increase bad debt for providers and, therefore, should not be used for individuals who select the fee-for-service Medicare program.
   5. Exemption of ESRD beneficiaries from voucher and medical savings accounts proposals. Appropriate risk adjusters for this population must first be determined.
   6. As the ESRD program is already a form of managed care with a prospective payment for dialysis services, a monthly capitated payment for physician outpatient dialysis services and the DRG payment system for hospital care, we support continuation of the prohibition on new ESRD enrollees in Medicare risk HMOs unless they are already enrolled when their kidneys fail. The ESRD population has experienced high levels of dissatisfaction and poor quality of care in HMOs as documented in a March 1995 Inspector General's report entitled "Beneficiary Perspectives of Medicare Risk HMOs."

B. All U.S. citizens and legal resident aliens with ESRD must be given the opportunity of choosing available health insurance options, including Medicare and Medicaid (if eligible).

C. Coverage for immunosuppressives for all transplant patients shall be assured for the duration of the transplant. The Association does not oppose measures that would require patients to pay a means-adjusted copayment.

D. Simultaneous with any restructuring of Medicare, insurance reform must be adopted to prohibit exclusion of coverage for preexisting conditions and to require portability of coverage, community rating, and guaranteed renewability.

E. Quality-of-care initiatives, including outcomes measures for the ESRD population, should receive high priority for funding and evaluation, with input from the ESRD community and other experts in the field.

F. The funding formula for Medicaid block grants should be based on a per capita basis to take into account states projected to have high growth and high poverty rates in the future and to account for recessionary periods. The funding formula should take into account the incidence and prevalence of individuals with ESRD.
   1. ESRD services shall be covered under Medicaid.
   2. The Qualified Medicare Beneficiary (QMB) program shall be required to continue to pay the Medicare Part B premium and Medicare's other cost-sharing requirements for low income ESRD Medicare beneficiaries.

G. Inclusion of advanced practice nurses as independent health care providers of services which they are legally authorized to perform under state law.
H. Public disclosure of staffing and quality data when federal dollars are spent.
I. Elimination of the current Medicare and Medicaid disincentives that ESRD beneficiaries face in seeking gainful employment, in order to reduce dependency of beneficiaries on these programs.

Principles on Managed Care and the ESRD Population

A. Each health plan must develop a process to ensure access of members with renal insufficiency or ESRD to relevant specialists, without gatekeeper approval prior to each visit once diagnosed.
B. Each health plan must develop a protocol for screening their members for specific indications of renal disease and early referral of those members to nephrologists for evaluation.
C. Each health plan must have a mechanism for providing its members who are children or adolescents access to a pediatric nephrologist in the geographic area of coverage. If none is available, the guidelines for care delivery to the childhood and adolescent patients with renal disease must be developed by a committee involving a pediatric nephrologist.
D. Each health plan must have a mechanism for providing members with ESRD access to a dialysis and a transplant provider who are geographically accessible to the patients, whose outcomes and waiting times are known to meet acceptable national standards and averages, and who are able to provide the ESRD patients with all forms of dialytic therapy currently available, including peritoneal dialysis, home dialysis, and a dialysis schedule that conforms with the members' employment or other rehabilitation needs.
E. Each health plan must develop mechanisms for rapid response to nephrology personnel requests for referral of a member with renal disease to specialists for evaluation.
F. Each health plan must involve nephrologists, nephrology nurses, renal social workers, and renal nutritionists in the development of guidelines for care delivery for members with renal insufficiency or ESRD.
G. Each health plan must have an ongoing patient education program for those members who have been diagnosed with renal insufficiency or who are at risk for developing renal disease (i.e., those with diabetes, hypertension, hereditary diseases, etc.). This program is, ideally, managed by experienced nephrology nurses or, in their absence, other experienced nephrology professionals.
H. Each health plan must develop literature specific to the ESRD population that outlines the limits and extent of coverage to that patient population.
I. Each health plan must develop mechanisms to ensure the inclusion of members with ESRD in the ESRD network programs and the United States Renal Data System (USRDS) database.
J. Each health plan must conduct periodic evaluations of all contractors (e.g., dialysis facilities and transplant programs) providing care to members with ESRD.
K. Each health plan must provide coverage for dialysis services for members who travel outside the health plan's normal coverage area.
L. Each health plan must provide coverage for immunosuppressive agents for all transplant recipients for the duration of the transplant.
M. No health plan may discriminate in any way against a member on the basis of a diagnosis of ESRD.

Approved 3/97
Revised/approved 11/97

Glossary of Terms

A

Absorption: the uptake of fluid or other substances by the tissues of the body.

Aberrant: unusual or deviant.

ABO compatibility: compatibility of the factors in the major blood grouping system in humans.

Abscesses: localized collections of purulent material in the body surrounded and walled off by damaged and inflamed tissue.

Access patency: open lumen of vascular access for dialysis.

Accountability: the obligation and structures to act with responsibility, authority, and autonomy.

Acetate: an organic compound commonly found in dialysis concentrate that releases bicarbonate when broken down by the liver.

Acidemia: high concentrations of acids in the blood.

Acquired cystic disease (ACD): a disease of the kidney characterized by the development of renal cysts in the kidneys of patients with CRF originating from a noncystic renal disease.

Acromial: related to the acromion, that is the lateral triangular projection of the spine of the scapula forming a point of the shoulder and articulating with the clavicle.

Activated clotting time (ACT): a measure of the adequacy of heparinization on dialysis using an activated process to speed clotting in the test tube.

Acute rejection: the reaction that occurs in the first few weeks after transplantation of an allogeneic or xenogeneic organ.

Acute tubular necrosis (ATN): an acute onset of renal failure due to ischemia and/or toxins; the pathology is not necessarily limited to the renal tubules.

Acute interstitial nephritis (AIN): an inflammatory process of the kidney usually associated with a sudden deterioration in renal function resulting from inflammation and edema in the renal interstitium.

Acute renal failure (ARF): a sudden loss of kidney function that is often reversible.

Acute diffuse glomerulonephritis: an inflammatory process of sudden onset that primarily affects the glomeruli of the kidney and involves all glomeruli to some extent.

Acute pyelonephritis: an infection of the kidney of sudden onset.

Acute bacterial cystitis: an infection of the bladder of sudden onset caused by invasion of bacteria into the tissue.

Acyclovir: an anti-viral agent with a high degree of specificity for herpes simplex and varicella zoster.

Adaptive responses: those responses that meet the individual's goals for survival, growth, and mastery.

Adaptive (specific or acquired) immunity: immunity that develops as a result of exposure to an antigen.

Adenocarcinoma: a malignant adenoma arising from epithelium of a glandular organ.

Adenosine: a compound containing adenine and the sugar ribose; it is found in ATP.

Adipocytes: fat cells.

Affective: pertaining to the affect or emotions.

Afferent: blood vessels that feed a capillary network in an organ or part.

Age-appropriate: appropriate, suitable, or usual for chronological age.

Ageusia: an absence or impairment of the sense of taste.

Air detector: a monitor on hemodialysis machines that detects minute amounts of air in the extracorporeal circuit.

Air embolism: an air lock that obstructs the outflow of blood from the right ventricle of the heart.

Albumin: the most abundant group of plasma proteins.

Albuminuria: the presence of albumin, a protein, in the urine, indicating renal dysfunction.

Aldosterone: hormones that increase renal absorption of sodium.

Allele: one of two or more alternative forms of a gene, only one of which can be present in a chromosome. If two alleles are the same, the individual is homozygous for the gene; if they are different they are heterozygous.

Allergies: disorder in which the body becomes hypersensitive to particular antigens. Exposure to the antigen or allergen will provoke characteristic symptoms.

Alloantibodies: antibodies found against tissues that arise from members of the same species.

Allograft (homograft): organ donor from a genetically non-identical member of the same species.

Alpha cells: polypeptide chains associated with the CD3 complex that are part of the T-cell receptor.

Alpha-adrenergic receptor: plasma membrane receptor for epinephrine and norepinephrine that, when activated, opens a calcium channel in the membrane.

Alport syndrome: an inherited renal disease characterized by loss of hearing as well as renal dysfunction.

Amenorrhea: absence of menses.

Aminoglycosides: a group of antibiotics used against serious infections caused by gram negative bacteria.

Amyloidosis: a metabolic disorder marked by deposition of amyloid in organs and tissues.

Amyotrophy: muscular wasting.

Anabolism: cellular synthesis or organic molecules.

Analgesic nephropathy: damage to the kidney as a result of ingestion of analgesics or pain medications.

Analytical observational studies: those studies characterized by the existence of a control or comparison group and the absence of allocation of patient to control or treatment groups by the investigator. Quasi-experimental studies fit into this category.

Anaphylactic dialyzer reaction: a sudden acute allergic reaction resulting in hypotension and shock on exposure to an antigen, in this case an artificial kidney.

Anastomosis: a surgical connection or communication often created by joining of two blood vessels without any intervening capillary network.

Andragogy: the theoJ3

ry of how and why adults learn.

Anemia: a reduction in the quantity of oxygen carrying pigment, hemoglobin, in the blood. The major symptoms are fatigue, tiredness, breathlessness on exertion, pallor, and poor resistance to infection.

Aneurysm: a balloon-like swelling in the wall of an artery.

Angiodysplasia: a formation of abnormal cells in the blood vessels.

Angiotensin II: a hormone important in the regulation of blood pressure. It is released by the action of an enzyme, renin, from the kidney, causing an increase in the output of aldosterone from the adrenal cortex. Angiotensin is capable of causing constriction of blood vessels, thus raising blood pressure.

Angiotensin-converting enzyme (ACE) inhibitors: drugs used to treat hypertension that prevent the conversion of angiotensin I to angiotensin II, therefore controlling blood pressure.

Anion: negatively charged ion.

Anorexia: lack of appetite.

Anthropometric: pertaining to measurement of the human body, its parts and functional capacities.

Antibiotics: drugs that destroy or inhibit the growth of microorganisms such as bacteria and fungi.

Antibodies: blood proteins synthesized by lymphoid tissue in response to exposure to a particular antibody. They serve to attack the antigen and render it harmless.

Antibody-dependent cell-mediated cytotoxicity (Adcc): immunity that is dependent principally on the presence of T-lymphocytes.

Anticoagulant: an agent that prevents the clotting of blood.

Antidiuretic hormone: a peptide hormone synthesized in the hypothalamus and released from the posterior pituitary; it increases water permeability of the kidney's collecting ducts (also known as ADH and vasopressin).

Antigen: any substance that the body regards as foreign or potentially dangerous and against which it produces an antibody.

Antigenic specificity: selective reactivity; the ability to distinguish among different determinants or sections of antigens.

Antihistamines: a drug that inhibits the action of histamine in the body by blocking the receptors for histamine (H1 and H2 receptors).

Anuria: absence of urine formation.

Aortofemoral: pertaining to the aorta and femoral artery.

APD (automated peritoneal dialysis): peritoneal dialysis (i.e., the process of removal of fluids and wastes from the body using the semi-permeable membrane of the peritoneum for diffusion and osmosis) that employs use of a cycler, that is a machine that automates the infusion, dwell, and drainage periods.

Apheresis: a process of removal of selected blood components for the purposes of treating selected diseases through membrane technology and an extracorporeal circuit.

Apical membrane: the layer of cells lining (facing) the lumen of the tubule in the nephron.

Appropriation: the second phase of the annual congressional budget cycle.

Apraxia: an inability to perform certain purposive movements without loss of motor power, sensation, or coordination.

Arcuate: at the cortical medullary border, the arteries that travel parallel to the renal capsule are termed arcuate (arc-shaped); the arcuate arteries branch further into the interlobular arteries and travel into the cortex, where they further subdivide into the afferent arterioles.

Arterial pressure: pressure exerted on the walls of arteries.

Arterial and venous blood tubing: tubing that carries blood to the dialyzer (arterial) and back to the body (venous).

Arteriosclerosis: a nonspecific term used to describe calcium or fatty deposits in the arteries as part of the aging process and thickening of the arterial walls due to aging of hypertension.

Arteriovenous (AV) graft: a vascular access for hemodialysis created by surgically implanting a vascular graft between an artery and a vein.

Arteriovenous fistula (AVF): a vascular access device for hemodialysis that is created by anastomosing an artery and vein together.

Arthralgia: pain in joints.

Ascites: the accumulation of fluid in the peritoneal cavity causing abdominal swelling.

Asterixis: involuntary abnormal jerking muscular movements induced by dorsiflexion of the wrist and extension of fingers (or other joints/muscle groups).

Asystole: the condition in which the heart no longer beats, accompanied by the absence of complexes in the electrocardiogram.

Atelectasis: a failure of part of the lung to expand.

Atheroembolic renal disease: dysfunction of the kidneys caused by obstruction of a blood vessel by an atheroma.

Atheromatous: pertaining to atheroma, which is a fatty degeneration or thickening of the wall of larger arteries.

Atrial natriuretic peptide (ANP): a peptide hormone that is secreted by atrial cells in response to atrial distension and causes decreased renal sodium reabsorption.

Atrophy: wasting, decrease in size.

Attitudes: feelings toward or about a person, object, idea, or situation that involve cognitive, affective, and behavioral components. Attitudes are considered to be rather constant feelings and are made up of many beliefs and values

Authorization: the first phase in the annual congressional budget cycle. Authorizing legislation specifies the substance of federal programs and the agency that will implement them and establishes program policies and the program's budget limit.

Autoantibodies: antibodies to normal self-antigens.

Autograft: a part of an individual, such as skin, transplanted from one location of the body to another (e.g., skin grafts in the case of burns).

Autoregulation: the ability of an individual to control its vascular resistance independent of neural and hormonal influence.

Autosomal dominant polycystic kidney disease (ADPKD): the most common hereditary renal disease characterized by multiple cysts in the kidneys. It affects approximately 500,000 adults and children in the United States and is the third most common cause of CRF in the United States.

Autosomal: pertaining to paired chromosomes, other than the sex chromosomes.

Avascular: lacking blood vessels or having a poor blood supply.

B

B lymphocytes: cells derived from the bone marrow that respond to antigen stimulation by producing antibodies.

Bacterial infection: invasion of the body or part of the body by bacteria.

Baroreceptors: a group of sensory nerve endings, located primarily in the carotid sinuses, aortic arch, the walls of large arteries and veins, and the heart, which are specialized to monitor changes in blood pressure.

Base line value: the level at which an activity or function is at, before an intervention or change.

Basilic vein: the large vein in the arm, extending from the hand along the back of the forearm, then passing forward to the inner side of the arm at the elbow.

Basolateral membrane: the membrane where the side of the epithelial cell is facing away from the lumen.

Basophils: a variety of white blood cells distinguished by coarse cytoplasmic granules that stain purple-black with Romanovsky stains. They are capable of ingesting foreign particles.

Batch system: a system of producing dialysate that involves mixing water and chemicals in a cistern.

Behavioral adaptation: an adjustment in the way of conducting oneself.

Beliefs: a proposition thought to be true where there is some evidence, although not conclusive evidence, for the truth. Beliefs are related to knowledge and may be characterized as stronger than an opinion, but weaker than knowledge.

Beta cells: polypeptide chains associated with the CD3 complex that are part of the T-cell receptor.

Beta-blocker: a drug that prevents stimulation of the beta adrenergic receptors of the nerves of the sympathetic nervous system and therefore decrease the activity of the heart; used to control blood pressure, control arrhythmias, and treat angina.

BFR (blood flow rate): the rate at which blood flows, for example, through an extracorporeal circuit or through a vascular access, measured in ml/minute.

Bicarbonate: a salt resulting from the incomplete neutralization of carbonic acid; an alkali.

Bicarbonate generation: the process of conversion of carbon dioxide and water to bicarbonate and hydrogen ions.

Bicarbonate reclamation: the process of returning filtered bicarbonate to the plasma.

Biocompatibility: the extent to which there is compatibility as measured by reaction between blood and the membrane in a dialyzer.

Blood: a fluid tissue that circulates throughout the body through the arteries and veins in order to distribute oxygen to the body and carry wastes to their site of excretion.

Blood circuit: the extracorporeal path of blood held in the tubing for hemodialysis therapy.

Blood detector: a monitor on a hemodialysis machine that detects minute amounts of blood leaking into the dialysate fluid.

Blood lines: the tubing attached to a dialyzer that carries blood from the individual to the dialyzer and from the dialyzer back to the individual on dialysis.

Blood pump: a pump (usually a roller pump) on a dialysis machine that moves the blood through the extracorporeal circuit at a set rate.

Bloodletting procedure: removal of blood.

Bolus: a quantity of a substance for ingestion or injection.

Bone demineralization: reduction in the mineral (calcium, phosphate) concentration of the bone.

Bone marrow: the tissue contained in the internal cavities of bones involved in the formation of blood.

Bowman's capsule: the cup-shaped end of a nephron that holds the glomerulus. It is the site of primary filtration of blood before entering the kidney tubules.

Bowman's space hydrostatic pressure (P_{BS}): pressure exerted by fluid in Bowman's space, which surrounds the glomerular tuft in the nephron.

Bowman's space colloid osmotic pressure (Π_{BS}): pressure created by large molecules, mainly protein, to which capillaries are relatively impermeable that results in preventing the osmotic flow of water across the membrane from a compartment of solution of lower density.

Brachial artery: the artery that extends from the axillary artery (at the armpit) down the side and inner surface of the upper arm to the elbow where it divides into the radial and ulnar arteries.

Bruit: a noise, heard on auscultation over an artery.

C

Calcification: the deposition of calcium salts in tissue.

Calcitriol: 1,25-$(OH)_2D_3$ - a metabolically active form of Vitamin D that aids in the absorption of calcium.

Calcium: an element that is essential for the normal development and functioning of the body, particularly the bones and teeth.

Calcium channel blockers: drugs that inhibit influx of calcium ions into cardiac and smooth muscle cells, reducing the strength of heart muscle contraction, reducing conduction of impulses in the heart, and causing vasodilation.

CAPD (continuous ambulatory peritoneal dialysis): an ongoing continuous dialysis process that involves infusion of fluid into the peritoneum, a prolonged dwell period for dialysis, and drainage. The procedure typically involves four exchanges of fluid daily.

Cardiac output (CO): the blood volume pumped by each ventricle per minute.

Cardiocytes: cells in the heart.

Cardiomegaly: a morbid condition characterized by enlargement of the heart with localized deposits of glycogen in the heart muscle.

Caries: decay and crumbling of the substance of a tooth or bone.

Carnitine: a quaternary amine that plays an important role in lipid metabolism and has been shown to be of some benefit in lowering serum lipids.

Carpal synovial: pertaining to the membrane surrounding the joints in the hand.

Carpal tunnel syndrome: compression of the median nerve as it enters the palm of hand. This causes pain and numbness in the index and middle fingers and weakness in the thumb.

Carpopedal: pertaining to both the wrist and foot.

Cascade: a chain of events in which proteins are converted in sequence from an inactive to active form. The term is used in relation to AMP and complement activation.

Catabolic: pertaining to the cellular breakdown of organic molecules.

Catabolism: cellular breakdown of organic molecules.

Catecholamines: a group of physiologically important substances with roles in the functioning of sympathetic and central nervous systems.

Cation: positively charged ion.

Caval: pertaining to the vena cava.

CAVH (continuous arteriovenous hemofiltration): an extracorporeal continuous renal replacement therapy involving use of a highly permeable hemofilter.

CAVU (continuous arteriovenous ultrafiltration): an extracorporeal continuous renal replacement therapy that involves removal of blood from an arterial blood supply through a highly permeable filter to remove fluid from the circulatory system and return it through a venous access.

CCPD (continuous cyclic peritoneal dialysis): a peritoneal dialysis procedure that involves use of a cycler during the night to regulate infusion, dwell, and drainage periods. The cycler typically operates continuously during the night, leaving the patient free during the day.

Celiac: relating to the abdominal region.

Cellular immunity: specific immunity that is dependent on the presence of T-lymphocytes.

Cellular immune response: the immune response that relates to the role of T-lymphocytes.

Cellulose: the most commonly used semi-permeable membrane used in dialyzers.

Cellulose acetate: a membrane used in artificial kidneys.

Central and individual proportioning systems: machines that mix a concentrated solution consisting of electrolytes with water for the dialysis treatment. Individual proportioning systems prepare enough dialysate for one patient, while a central proportioning system prepares dialysate solution for a group of patients in a unit.

Central line dual lumen catheter: a small tubing or catheter, with two paths or lumens, that is inserted into a major central vein in the body. The two lumens can be used to remove and return blood during extracorporeal therapies.

Centrifugal force: on rotation, the force that keeps the body away from the center.

Centrifugation: the process of separating solids from liquids by rotating the substance at very high speeds.

Cerebral embolism: a blood clot lodged in the brain.

Cerebral edema: swelling of the cerebrum with fluid.

Certificate of Need: a certification made by a state that a certain health service is needed and authorizes a specific operator, at the operator's request, to provide that service.

Chemical mediators: chemicals or substances in the body that facilitate the action of one substance on another.

Chemotactic: pertaining to the chemical attraction of phagocytic cells to the site of inflammation or infection.

Cholangitis: an inflammation of the bile ducts. It usually occurs when the ducts are obstructed, especially by stones.

Chronic renal insufficiency: dysfunction of the kidney, developing gradually and considered to be irreversible.

Chronic rejection: the rejection of a transplanted organ that occurs months and years after transplantation which can eventually cause graft failure.

Chronic interstitial disease: a disease of the kidney characterized by tubulointerstitial fibrosis, atrophy, and in certain forms, papillary necrosis. It is most commonly associated with analgesic nephropathy, sickle cell disease, and obstructive uropathy.

Chvostek's sign: a facial twitch occurring when the facial nerve is tapped, commonly associated with hypocalcemia.

Class I antigens: genes of the major histocompatibility complex responsible for compatibility of tissues and organs; HLA-A, B, and C loci encode for the class I HLA molecules in humans.

Class II antigens: genes of the major histocompatibility complex that participate in the immune response; HLA-D loci encode for the class II HLA molecules.

Class III antigens: genes of the major histocompatibility complex that contribute to the complement system and tumor necrosis factor.

Clearance (Cl): a quantitative measure, expressed in ml/minute, of the rate at which waste products are removed from the blood by the kidneys.

Clinical practice guidelines: suggested practices relating to patient care that are based upon research/ best knowledge available about an area. Clinical practice guidelines are useful resources to practitioners in identifying the more appropriate interventions or strategies for problems.

Clot: a mass of coagulated blood.

Cloture: procedure used to speed action on a bill; the majority leader may seek "unanimous consent" to vote at a certain time. If a member objects to this, a motion to limit debate (and therefore prevent a bill's opponents from "filibustering," or talking it to death) may be offered. Cloture requires 60 affirmative votes.

Cluster of differentiation (CD): a nomenclature system that categorizes cell surface molecules of human leukocytes; it is also used to categorize monoclonal antibodies according to the antigens that they recognize.

Cognitive: pertaining to knowing, perceiving, or conceiving.

Collecting tubule: a portion of the nephron found distal to the convoluted tubules.

Colloids: a solution containing protein.

Comorbidity: an associated illness or disease condition that exists at the same time as a primary disease condition.

Complement: a substance in the blood, consisting of nine different fractions, that aids the body's defenses when antibodies combine with antigens. Complement is involved with the lysis, agglutination, and opsonization of foreign cells.

Complement activation: a process that can lead to cell lysis, when stimulated, where a group of plasma proteins go through a series of steps.

Complement cascade: a series of steps involving activation of complement that will lead to cell lysis.

Compliance: adherence to a regimen.

Condyles: rounded protuberances that are found at the end of some bones and form an articulation with another bone.

Concentration gradient: the relative difference in molecular concentration between solutions on both sides of a membrane.

Conceptual model: a set of abstract and general concepts and propositions that present a particular perspective about the phenomena of interest to a discipline. Conceptual models of nursing present perspectives regarding the nursing recipient/client/patient, the environment, health, and nursing.

Conservative management: management with diet and medications, avoiding more invasive therapy.

Continuous flow techniques: therapies that involve the continuous slow movement of blood through an extracorporeal circuit for the purposes of dialysis, fluid removal, or removal of other toxins.

Continuous quality improvement (CQI): a process of monitoring, reviewing, and striving to improve or better a situation. Many health care institutions have implemented CQI programs to assess their situation, make changes, and reevaluate to assure quality and high standards of care.

Contralateral: on or affecting the opposite side of the body, particularly applied to brain lesions where symptoms are on the opposite side of the lesion.

Convective transport: occurs as a result of the frictional forces between the solvent (water) and the solute.

Cortex: the outer part of an organ, situated immediately beneath its capsule or outer membrane.

Creatinine: a substance excreted in the urine, which is derived from creatinine and creatine phosphate in muscle.

Crescentic glomerulonephritis: a disease of the kidney that typically exhibits the nephritic syndrome, for which crescents can been seen in kidney tissue when examined histologically.

Crescents: represent accumulations of cells and other materials that create a disruption in the glomerular capillary wall, resulting in direct contact between plasma and cells in the circulation and elements in Bowman's capsule.

Crohn's Disease: Regional enteritis or ileitis.

Crossmatch: a test used to determine the compatibility of blood groups or histocompatibility.

Cryoprecipitate: a concentrated derivative prepared from fresh frozen plasma of multiple donors, containing factor VIII.

Crystalloids: a solution that consists of water and crystals, typically minerals or electrolytes.

Cuprophan: a membrane commonly used in artificial kidneys.

CVVH (continuous venovenous hemofiltration): an extracorporeal continuous renal replacement therapy that runs from vein to vein involving use of a highly permeable hemofilter.

CVVHD (continuous venovenous hemodiafiltration): an extracorporeal renal replacement therapy, with vascular access from one vein to another. It employs diffusion, as with dialysis, and convective transport with ultrafiltration.

Cyanosis: a bluish discoloration of the skin and mucous membranes resulting from an inadequate amount of oxygen in the blood.

Cytapheresis: a therapeutic procedure for the removal of cells, typically white blood cells, through the use of membrane technology and an extracorporeal circuit.

Cytotoxic agents: pharmaceuticals that have the effect of destroying cells and that are used to treat malignancies.

Cytotoxic T-cells: a subclass of T-cells, which are lymphocytes, that are involved in killing cells.

D

Daltons: a measure of molecular weight.

Deferoxamine (DFO): an iron and aluminum chelating agent used to treat high levels/overload of iron or aluminum.

Deionization: a process of water treatment that involves the removal of ions.

Delivery system: A system to deliver dialysate to a dialyzer.

Delta cells: a polypeptide chain associated with the CD3 complex on the T-cell receptor.

Dementia: a chronic or persistent disorder of the mental processes due to organic brain disease, manifested by memory disorders, changes in personality, deterioration in personal care, impaired reasoning, and disorientation.

Descriptive studies: studies in which there is no comparison or control group. Some examples include: studies of the incidence, prevalence, or frequency of a disease or clinical characteristic; studies of the natural history of a disease; and studies to establish normal values of a parameter in a population.

Desmopressin: an antidiuretic hormone analogue, known as DDAVP, that reabsorbs water in the renal tubule. It also improves the bleeding time by supplying or inducing other forms of factor VIII.

Diabetes mellitus (DM): a disorder of carbohydrate metabolism in which sugars in the body are not oxidized to produce energy due to the lack of the pancreatic hormone insulin or the resistance of insulin.

Diabetic glomerulosclerosis: a disease of the kidney, specifically the glomerulus, caused by diabetes, commonly manifested with the nephrotic syndrome.

Diabetic nephropathy: renal disease and dysfunction caused by diabetes, which now is the leading cause of CRF in the United States, accounting for approximately 30% of all patients entering dialysis programs.

Dialysate: the fluid used in dialysis, typically with a lower solute concentration than the blood, into which wastes and excess electrolytes diffuse.

Dialysate concentrate solutions: the mixture of chemicals that is mixed with water to make dialysate solution, (i.e., the solution of lower concentration used) to create a concentration gradient with the blood for the purposes of dialysis therapy.

Dialysate delivery system: typically referred to as the hemodialysis machine, the dialysate delivery system is the equipment that mixes water with a concentrated solution of electrolytes in order to make and provide a solution of lower concentration than the blood through the artificial kidney.

Dialysate flow rate: the rate at which dialysate fluid moves through the dialyzer.

Dialysate lines: the lines that carry dialysate fluid to the dialyzer for dialysis and the expended dialysate to the machine for discharge.

Dialysis: the process of separating colloids and crystalline substances in solution by the difference in their rate of diffusion through a semi-permeable membrane.

Dialysis disequilibrium syndrome: a condition resulting from disproportionate rates of urea clearance from the brain and plasma, resulting in cerebral edema. It may occur in initial dialysis treatments when dialysis is too rapid.

Dialysis encephalopathy: a dysfunction of the brain, associated with dialysis therapy, sometimes thought to be related to aluminum.

Dialysis solution flow: the rate at which dialysate solution flows through the dialyzer and down the drain. Typical flow rates are 500 to 600 ml/min.

Dialyzer: a device used to separate components of a liquid mixture, such as blood, as in an artificial kidney.

Dialyzer blood compartment: the part of the dialyzer, or artificial kidney, which holds blood.

Dialyzer clearance (K): the rate of clearance by an artificial kidney of various substances from the blood.

Diaphoresis: excessive sweating.

Diffuse nephritis: a widespread disorder of the kidney causing symptoms associated with nephritis, such as hematuria and hypertension.

Diffusion: the tendency of molecules of a substance to move from a region of higher concentration through a semi-permeable membrane to a region of lower concentration.

Digitalis: a medication used to correct cardiac arrhythmias, by slowing and strengthening the heart beat.

Disability: the inability to engage in substantial gainful activity by reason of a physical or mental impairment.

Disease-specific: symptoms relating specifically to a particular disorder.

Distal: farthest from the center from a medial line.

Distal sensory: pertaining to sensation away from the central part of the body.

Distal tubule: portion of the renal tubule between the loop of Henle and collecting duct/tubule.

Diuresis: increased excretion of urine

Divalent: having a double electrical charge

Diverticulitis: inflammation of diverticula, small sacs, or pouches in the wall of the colon.

Dominant trait: a trait that appears in offspring even though other corresponding opposite traits are also passed on.

Dorsiflexion: a backward flexion of the foot or hand or their digits, (i.e., bending toward the upper surface).

Dorsiflexors: muscles involved in dorsiflexion.

Double lumen catheter: a catheter, or narrow tubing, that has two interior lumens or tubes; for dialysis, double lumen catheters include one lumen for removal of blood and one for return of blood. This ensures that only one (rather than two) catheter/line/needle is required.

Dry weight: the ideal body weight, without excess fluid volume.

Dual lumen catheter: a narrow tubing that has two paths or lumens; typically, one is used to remove blood while the other is used to return blood or fluids.

Duodenitis: an inflammation of the duodenum, the first part of the small intestine.

Dysarthria: pain in joints.

Dysgeusia: difficulty swallowing.

Dyspnea: difficulty breathing.

Dysthesias: an impairment of sensation.

E

E. coli: a gram negative rod-like bacterium of the Escherichia family.

Ecchymosis: bruising.

ECF (extracellular fluid): the fluid situated outside of cells, including the blood and lymph fluid.

Effector cells: cells that directly function to achieve the end result, as opposed to regulatory cells.

Effluent: the used dialysate fluid that is carried to the drain.

Eicosanoids: a general term used to describe products of arachidonic acid metabolism such as prostaglandins, prostacyclin, thromboxanes, and leukotrienes.

Electrical gradient: a force determining the direction and magnitude of net electrical charge movement.

Electrogenic pump: an active transport system that directly separates electric charges, thereby producing a potential difference.

Electrolyte: a hormone, produced by the kidney, that is necessary for the production of red blood cells.

Electrolyte imbalance: deviation from the normal levels of electrolytes or ions in the body.

Electroneutral: a balance of positive and negative ions, resulting in a neutral solution.

Ellipsoid: a solid figure, all plane sections of which are ellipses or circles.

Embolization: the obstruction of a blood vessel by a foreign substance or a blood clot.

Empiric: based on observation or experiment, not on theory; deriving knowledge from experience.

Encephalopathy: any dysfunction of the brain.

Endarteritis: an inflammation of the inner (intimal) portion of the wall of an artery.

Endemic disease: the constant presence of a disease or infectious agent within a given geographic area or population group; may also refer to the usual prevalence of a given disease within such area or group.

Endocarditis: inflammation of the lining membrane of the heart.

Endocrine gland: a gland that manufactures one or more hormones and secretes them directly into the bloodstream.

Endocytosis: a process in which the plasma membrane folds into the cell, forming small pockets that pinch off to produce intracellular, membrane-bound vesicles.

Endogenous: produced or arising from within a cell or organism.

Endogenous biosynthesis: the process of development of chemical substances within the body.

Endometriosis: ectopic endometrium (lining of the uterus) located in various sites throughout the pelvis or in the abdominal wall.

Endothelium: a lining of flat cells that line the blood and lymphatic vessels, heart, and various other body cavities.

Endothelium-derived relaxing factor (EDRF): substances secreted by vascular endothelium that relax smooth muscle and cause dilation of arterioles.

Endotoxin: a poison harmful to all body tissues, contained within certain gram negative bacteria and released only when the bacterial cell is broken down or dies and disintegrates.

Endotracheal: within the trachea.

Enteral: within the intestines.

Enteric: relating to or affecting the intestine.

Environmental factors: variables or factors that relate to the world around us.

Eosinophils: polymorphonuclear granulocytic leukocytes whose granules take up the red dye eosin; they are involved in allergic responses and parasite destruction.

Epidemic: the occurrence in a community or region of cases of an illness, specific health-related behavior, or other health-related events clearly in excess of normal expectancy. The community or region, and the period in which the cases occur, are specified precisely. The number of cases indicating the presence of an epidemic varies according to the agent, size, and type of population exposed, previous experience or lack of exposure to the disease, and time and place of occurrence; epidemicity is thus relative to usual frequency of the disease in the same area, among the specified population, at the same season the year. A single case of a communicable disease long absent from a population or first invasion by a disease not previously recognized in that area requires immediate reporting and full field investigation; two cases of such a disease associated in time and place may be sufficient evidence to be considered an epidemic.

Epidemiology: the study of the distribution and determinants of health-related states or events in specified populations, and the application of this study to control of health problems.

Epistaxis: nosebleeds.

Epithelial: pertaining to the tissue that lines hollow structures and covers the outside of the body.

Epoetin: a hormone involved in the production of red blood cells (also known as erythropoietin).

Epstein-Barr virus (Ebv): a virus similar to the herpes virus that is the causative agent of glandular fever.

Equilibrium: the body's attempt to maintain balance or homeostasis.

Eradication (of disease): termination of all transmission of infection by extermination of the infectious agent through surveillance and containment. Eradication, as in the instance of smallpox, was based on the joint activities of control and surveillance.

Erythrocyte sedimentation rate (ESR): the rate at which red blood cells settle out of suspension in blood plasma, measured under standardized conditions. The ESR rises with certain inflammatory disorders.

Erythropoietin: a hormone secreted mainly by the kidney that stimulates red blood cell production.

Essential amino acid (EAA): an amino acid (molecular subunit of protein) that cannot be synthesized and as a result must be obtained from food sources.

Ethical problem/dilemma: a situation that occurs when a person or a group is faced with a conflict between ethical principles, both of which are accepted, or when persons or groups are faced with a decision and do not know what is the best/right approach to make a decision.

Ethylene glycol poisoning: poisoning from the ingestion of ethylene glycol, commonly known as antifreeze.

Euthyroid: normal thyroid functioning.

Euvolemic: normal state of extracellular fluid volume.

Evertors: muscles involved in turning outwards.

Excretion: refers to the process by which unwanted substances are eliminated from the body through the passage of urine.

Exocrine gland: a gland that discharges its secretion by means of a duct, which opens onto an epithelial surface.

Experimental studies: studies in which the investigator manipulated the factor under investigation, in which his/her intent was to examine the direct effects of that factor. Some examples include: randomized clinical trials with concurrent controls and studies in which the investigator allocates patients to control or treatment groups.

Exsanguination: the process of expressing blood from a part, or near total loss of blood.

External arteriovenous shunt: a vascular access device consisting of silastic that shunts blood between an artery and vein.

Extracorporeal circuit: the circuit outside the body through which the blood is carried, as in dialysis circuit.

F

Fc region: the region that relates to the cystallizable fragment, the portion of an immunoglobulin that binds to macrophages, lymphocytes, and mast cells.

Feeling: sensation.

Femoral: pertaining to the thigh bone or femur.

Femoral-popliteal: the area between the femoral and popliteal arteries, which runs from the upper thigh to behind the knee.

Femoral vein catheter: a catheter or small tubing inserted into the femoral vein.

Ferritin: an iron-binding protein that stores iron in the body.

Ferrous fumarate: an iron supplement used to treat iron-deficiency anemia.

Fiber bundle volume test: a test used to test the patency and continuing effectiveness of a dialyzer.

Fibrin: a whitish filamentous protein formed by the action of thrombin on fibrinogen.

Fibrinogen: a coagulation factor present in blood plasma that is acted upon by the enzyme thrombin to produce the insoluble protein fibrin in the final stage of blood coagulation.

Fibrinogen level: the amount of the coagulation factor, fibrinogen, in the plasma. The normal level is 2-4 g/l (4 - 6 g/l in pregnancy).

Fibroblasts: cells in the renal cortex that secrete collagen and fibrils.

Fibrosarcoma: malignant tumor of the kidney usually arising from the renal capsule. Rapid growth of the tumor is characteristic with abdominal pain as the presenting symptom. Five-year survival rates are poor and may be as low as 10%.

Fibrosis: abnormal formation of fibrous tissue.

Filibuster: talking a subject to death.

Filtration: the shift of fluid from one area to another.

Fistulogram: an X-ray/diagnostic procedure, involving injection of a dye to check the patency of an AV fistula.

Flaccid: relaxed, flabby, having defective or absent muscular tone.

Fluid imbalance: an abnormal level of fluid in the body, either too high or too low.

Focal nephritis: localized disorder of the kidney causing nephritic symptoms.

Fogarty catheter: a catheter with an inflatable balloon on one end used to remove clots from vascular access devices.

Folate: folic acid, a B complex vitamin that is necessary for normal erythropoiesis and nucleoprotein synthesis.

Fragment of antigen binding (FAB): the single antigen-binding site of an antibody formed by the cleaving of the antibody to fragments with papain.

Fresh frozen plasma: the part of blood remaining when the red blood cells are removed, containing serum, clotting factors, and white blood cells. It is frozen to preserve it for future administration.

Fulminant: a rapid rise in serum creatinine and consequent renal failure as in rapidly progressive glomerulonephritis.

Function: a mode of activity or action by which a purpose is fulfilled.

Functional limitation: an inability to perform specific actions or functions.

Functional outcome: a visible effect or result that relates to function or ability to perform various activities.

Functional status: an individual's ability to perform various activities or actions in life.

Fungal: infectious agent.

Fungal infection: invasion of the body by a microorganism in the fungus family.

Fungas: a general term used to encompass the diverse morphological forms of yeasts and molds.

G

Galactorrhea: continuation of lactation or flow of milk at intervals after cessation of nursing.

Gallop rhythm: refers to a heart rhythm heard on auscultation, an extra heart sound.

Gastritis: an inflammation of the stomach.

Genes: basic units of genetic material, consisting of DNA or RNA, which are carried at a particular place on the chromosome.

Genotype: the genetic constitution of an individual or group as determined by the particular set of genes it possesses; or, the genetic information carried by a pair of alleles, that determines a particular characteristic.

Glomerular basement membrane: the structural support for the glomerular capillary cells that is composed primarily of collagen and glycoproteins. It participates in filtration and repels negative substances such as proteins.

Glomerular capillary endothelium: the layer of flat cells lining the capillaries of the glomerulus.

Glomerular capillary hydrostatic pressure (P_{GC}): pressure created due to the presence of fluid and solutes in the glomerular capillaries.

Glomerular capillary osmotic pressure (GC): pressure created in the glomerulus that is related to the osmotic flow of water across the membrane from a compartment of solution of lower density.

Glomerular capillary tuft: the structure at the beginning of the kidney nephron consisting of the vasculature (tuft of capillaries).

Glomerular filtration: the process of movement of an essentially protein-free plasma from renal glomerular capillaries into Bowman's capsule.

Glomerular filtration rate (GFR): the rate at which blood is filtered through the glomerulus of the nephron, measured in ml/min, which is a measure of renal clearance and function.

Glomerulopathy: pathology or disease of the glomerulus of the nephron, commonly manifested with the nephrotic syndrome.

Glomerulosclerosis: a diffuse condition, affecting most of the glomeruli that consists of thickening of the basement membrane, expansion of the mesangial matrix, and mesangial cell proliferation. It is commonly seen in diabetes.

Glucagon: a hormone produced by the pancreas that causes an increase in blood sugar level and thus has an effect opposite to that of insulin.

Gluconeogenesis: the formation of glucose by the liver from pyruvate, lactate, glycerol, or amino acids.

Glutamate: a major excitatory CNS neurotransmitter formed from the amino acid glutamic acid.

Glycoproteins: a group of compounds consisting of a protein combined with a carbohydrate. Examples of glycoproteins are certain enzymes, hormones, and antigens.

Glycosides: a substance derived from plants which upon hydrolysis yields a sugar and one or more additional products.

Gram negative organism: organisms or bacteria that do not retain the gentian violet stain, but retain the counterstain.

Granulocytes: any of a group of white blood cells when stained with Romanovsky stains, are seen to contain granules in their cytoplasm. They can be subclassified on the basis of the color of the stained granules into neutrophils, eosinophils, and basophils.

Guidewire: a rigid wire that guides insertion of a catheter, over which a catheter is inserted, and which is removed when the catheter is in place.

Guillain-Barre syndrome: a disease of the peripheral nerves in which there is numbness and weakness in the limbs, which develops 10-20 days after a respiratory condition that provokes an allergic response in the peripheral nerves.

H

Habilitation: to qualify for an office or role or activity.

Halitosis: bad breath.

Haplotype: a complete set of HLA antigens inherited from either parent.

Health-related quality of life: an assessment of an individual's or group's satisfaction or happiness in life, particularly as it relates to health or illness.

Health status: the state of an individual's health or well-being, as measured through objective or subjective means.

Hematopoietic: pertaining to the production of blood cells and platelets.

Hematuria: blood in the urine.

Hemochromatosis: a hereditary disorder in which there is excessive absorption and storage of iron. This leads to damage and functional impairment of many organs and a bronze color of the skin.

Hemodialysis: a process of removal of chemical substances and water from the blood by passing it through an artificial kidney composed of semipermeable membranes.

Hemodilution: an increase in the volume of blood plasma resulting in reduced concentration of red blood cells.

Hemodynamic: the study of the circulation of blood.

Hemofilter: a highly porous device for removal of fluid and small molecular weight plasma contents.

Hemolysis: the destruction of red blood cells with the liberation of hemoglobin that leaks into the surrounding tissue.

Hemoperfusion: a process of running blood through a charcoal filter for the purposes of removing poisons, drugs, and toxins.

Hemostasis: the arrest of bleeding involving the physiological processes of blood coagulation and the contraction of damaged blood vessels. The term is also used to refer to surgical means to stop bleeding.

Heparin pump: a medication pump that infuses heparin, an anticoagulant on a regular basis.

Heparin rinse: a rinse of an artificial kidney with a saline/heparin solution.

Hepatectomy: the surgical operation of removing the liver.

Hepatobiliary: pertaining to the liver and bile ducts.

Heterotopic graft: donor organ placed in a position other than the normal anatomical location.

High biologic value (HBV): proteins that have most of the essential amino acids.

High-density lipoproteins (HDL): plasma lipid protein aggregate having low proportion of lipid, which promotes removal of cholesterol from cells.

High flux dialysis: dialysis that is conducted using a dialyzer with a highly permeable membrane, capable of removing fluids and toxins at a higher rate than conventional dialyzers.

High-output congestive heart failure: heart failure that is related to fluid overload (rather than cardiac dysfunction).

High permeable dialyzers: artificial kidneys with higher ultrafiltration coefficients and generally larger pore size, making them better able to remove fluid and particles at faster rates.

Hilar region: the hollow region or area on the surface of an organ, such as the kidney, at which structures such as blood vessels, nerve fibers, and ducts enter or leave it.

Hirsutism: condition characterized by the excessive growth of hair in unusual places.

Histamine: a compound derived from the amino acid histidine. Histamine has pronounced pharmacological activity, causing dilation of blood vessels and contraction of smooth muscle. It is an important mediator of inflammation and is released in large amounts after skin infection or in allergic conditions and anaphylactic reactions.

Histocompatibility: the form of compatibility that depends on tissue components, mainly glycoprotein antigens in cell membranes. A high degree of histocompatibility is necessary for a tissue or organ transplant to be successful.

Histologically: pertaining to microscopic tissue anatomy.

Historical studies: investigations to determine what happened in the past to gain greater understanding of the present.

Hollow fiber dialyzer: a dialyzer, or artificial kidney, in which the semipermeable membranes are arranged as numerous hollow fibers, resulting in higher surface area.

Homeostasis: the relatively stable condition of extracellular fluid that results from regulatory system actions.

Human leukocyte antigen (HLA): a series of four gene families (labeled A, B, C, D) that code for polymorphic proteins expressed on the surface of most nucleated cells. Successful transplantation requires a minimal number of HLA differences between donor and recipient tissues.

Humoral immune response: specific immunity mediated principally by immunoglobulins that are secreted from plasma cells.

Humoral immunity: immunity that involves circulating antibodies in the blood stream.

Hydralazine: an antihypertensive agent that acts by causing peripheral vasodilation.

Hydrocarbon solvents: a compound made up only of hydrogen and carbon that is in solution.

Hydronephrosis: collection of urine in the kidney pelvis due to obstructed outflow.

Hyperacute rejection: an immediate reaction to the transplantation of an incompatible organ.

Hypercalcemia: higher than normal concentrations of calcium in the blood.

Hypercapnia: the presence of an abnormally high concentration of carbon dioxide in the blood.

Hypercholesterolemia: high levels of cholesterol in the blood.

Hyperemia: an unusual amount of blood or congestion in a body part.

Hyperfiltration: higher than normal rates of filtration.

Hyperglycemia: high concentrations of sugars in the blood.

Hyperkalemia: high levels of potassium in the blood.

Hyperlipidemia: presence in the blood of abnormally high concentrations of fat.

Hyperlipoproteinemia: high levels of lipoproteins in the blood.

Hyperoxaluria: high levels of oxalates in the urine.

Hyperparathyroidism: excessive production of parathyroid hormone by the parathyroid gland, often causing hypercalcemia.

Hyperphosphatemia: the presence of an abnormally high concentration of phosphates in the blood.

Hyperplasia: an increased production and growth of normal cells in a tissue or organ.

Hyperpolarization: the situation when a cell's resting membrane potential becomes extremely negative, which may lead to difficulty in reexcitation of cell membranes.

Hyperreflexia: increased action of reflexes.

Hypertensive nephropathy: damage to the kidney as a result of the chronic hypertension (essential or secondary) in which the small intrarenal arteries and arterioles are affected, leading to renal insufficiency and possibly to CRF.

Hypertriglyceridemia: high levels of triglycerides in the blood.

Hyperuricemia: abnormally high concentrations of uric acid in the blood.

Hyperuricosuria: high levels of uric acid in the urine.

Hypervitaminosis: an excessive level of vitamin.

Hypoalbuminemia: a low amount of albumin in the blood, which causes decreased plasma oncotic pressure, facilitating the movement of fluid by osmosis into the interstitial spaces, resulting in edema.

Hypoglycemia: low levels of sugar in the blood.

Hyponatremia: lower than normal levels of sodium in the blood.

Hypophosphatemia: low levels of phosphate concentration in the blood.

Hyposmolar: low osmotic concentration caused by higher numbers of water molecules in the solution.

Hypotension: low blood pressure, causing light-headedness, fainting, dizziness, sweating, and possibly impaired consciousness with shutdown of peripheral vascular circulation.

Hypothermia: reduction in body temperature below the normal range.

Hypothyroidism: a condition due to deficiency of the thyroid secretion, resulting in a lowered basal metabolism.

Hypoxic: referring to a deficiency of oxygen in the tissues.

I

ICF (intracellular fluid): the fluid located in cells.

Icteric: relating to or marked by jaundice.

Idiopathic membranous nephropathy: a disease of the kidney of unknown origin most commonly associated with the nephrotic syndrome in adults.

Idiopathic thrombocytopenic purpura (ITP): a condition of unknown etiology with low platelet counts resulting in bleeding into the skin and from various orifices.

IgA nephropathy: a common form of glomerulonephritis, or disease of the glomerulus, which can be benign or severe.

Immune-complex: antigen-antibody complex.

Immune-mediated: reactions that are immune-mediated take place when circulating immune complexes are deposited on endothelial surfaces or when the immunoglobulin is directed to a tissue antigen.

Immunocompetence: proper immune function.

Immunogen: a substance that causes a detectable immune response.

Immunogenicity: the extent to which an antigen causes an immune response.

Immunoglobulins: a group of structurally related proteins that act as antibodies.

Immunoincompetence: the inability of the body to provide an adequate immune response.

Impairment: a situation where something has been damaged or weakened.

Impetigo: an inflammatory skin disease marked by isolated pustules, which become crusted and rupture.

Impotence: inability and/or difficulty of the male to copulate.

Incidence: the number of instances of illness commencing, or of persons falling ill, during a given period in a specified population. More generally, the number of new events, e.g., new cases of a disease in a defined population, within a specified period of time.

Incidence rate: the rate at which new events occur in a population. The numerator is the number of new events that occur in a defined period; the denominator is the population at risk of experiencing the event during this period, sometimes expresses as person-time.

Industrial quality management science (IQMS): a study of variables and programs that function to improve quality in industrial or business settings.

Ineffective responses: those responses that are not effective, satisfactory, or do not meet the goals. Ineffective responses may, therefore, signal a need for nursing intervention.

Infection: invasion of the body by harmful organisms such as bacteria, fungi, protozoa, rickettsiae, or viruses.

Inferior vena cava: the largest vein in the body that is situated to the right of the aorta and receives blood from the common iliac veins.

Inflammatory response: the natural nonspecific response of a body to the presence of a foreign protein or antigen in order to protect itself and maintain homeostasis.

Infrahepatic: below the liver.

Infusate: solution that is infused into the extracorporeal circuit during hemofiltration.

Innate (nonspecific or natural) immunity: naturally occurring defense mechanisms present in the body that are not directed to a specific antigen.

Inotropic: affecting the contraction of heart muscle.

Insulin dependent diabetes mellitus (IDDM): diabetes mellitus that is controlled through regular injections of insulin.

Integumentary: related to the integument or skin.

Intercalated disk: the thickened end of cardiac muscle cell where the cell is connected to the adjacent cell.

Interdependence mode: a concept in Roy's Adaptation Model that refers to a way or method of doing or acting according to a system of interdependence in seeking help, attention, and affection.

Interdialytic: between dialyses.

Interferons (IFN): substances produced by cells infected with a virus that have the ability to inhibit viral growth.

Interleukin 1: in the family of proteins involved in hemopoiesis and the immune response.

Interlobar: between lobes.

Interlobular: between lobules.

Intermittent therapies: therapies with gaps of time between treatments (as opposed to continuous therapies).

Internal jugular veins: large paired veins running vertically down the side of the neck and draining blood from the brain, face, and neck. It ends behind the sternoclavicular joint, where it joins the subclavian vein.

Interstitial: surrounding the tissue/cells.

Interstitium: cells separating the nephrons, found in greater number in the renal medulla than in the cortex.

Intracellular: within the cells.

Intradialytic parenteral nutrition (IDPN): nutritional supplementation by means of adding amino acids to peritoneal dialysis solution.

Intraglomerular: inside the glomerulus.

Intraluminal: within the interior of

any tubular structure.

Intramitochondrial: inside mitochondria, which are the energy-producing areas of cells.

Intramural: within the walls of a hollow organ or cavity.

Intraperitoneal: inside the peritoneum.

Intravascular: within the vascular compartment.

Introducer: a wire or other rigid material that is used to aid in the introduction of catheters or tubings.

In-vitro: a Latin term used to describe biological phenomena that are made to occur outside the living body, (e.g., in a test tube or laboratory).

In vivo: a Latin term describing activities or phenomena that occur or are observed occurring within the bodies of living organisms.

IPD (intermittent peritoneal dialysis): a process of intermittent dialysis, several times during the week, where a prescribed number of exchanges (e.g., 10-12) are performed with a relatively short (20-minute) dwell phase. IPD can be performed manually or with the assistance of a cycler.

Ipsilateral: on or affecting the same side of the body.

Islet cells: small groups of endocrine cells located in the pancreas producing glucagon, insulin, and somatostatin.

Isograft (syngraft): organ donor from a genetically identical individual (e.g., monozygotic)

Isosmotic: having the same osmotic pressure, thus the same concentration of solutes or particles.

J

Jaundice: a yellowish staining of the integument, sclerae, and deeper tissues and the excretions with bile pigments, which are increased in the plasma.

Johnson's Behavioral Systems Model: a conceptual model for nursing that focuses on efficient and effective behavioral functioning. This is a systems model that posits that the behavioral system performs many tasks to maintain its own integrity.

Jugular vein catheter: a catheter, or small tube, placed in the internal jugular vein for infusion of fluids or access to the circulatory system.

Juxtamedullary apparatus: the renal structure consisting of the macula densa and granular cells that is the site of renin secretion and the sensor for renal homeostatic responses.

K

Ketosis: raised levels of ketone bodies in the body tissues. Ketone bodies are normal products of fat metabolism and can be oxidized to produce energy. Ketosis may result in severe acidosis.

Kidneys: the pair of organs, situated below the diaphragm at the back of the abdomen, responsible for the excretion of nitrogenous wastes and excess fluids from the body.

Kinetic model of Kt/V: a measure of dialysis adequacy calculated by dividing the product of time on dialysis by clearance over volume cleared.

King's General Systems Framework: a conceptual model for nursing, based on systems theory, which includes a goal-oriented nursing record (GONR). The GONR, which contains space for demographic and health data, problem list, goal list, nursing care plan, and progress notes, can be used to document nursing care.

Kinins: a group of naturally occurring polypeptides that are powerful vasodilators, which lower blood pressure and cause contraction of smooth muscle. They are there to play a role in inflammatory response.

Klebsiella: a gram negative bacillus bacterium in the Enterobacteriaceae family.

Kt/V: a measure of adequacy of dialysis reflecting clearances, time, and volume of urea distribution.

Kupffer cells: phagocytic cells that line the sinusoids of the liver. They are involved in the formation of bile and often contain fragments of red blood cells and pigment granules derived from the breakdown of hemoglobin.

Kussmaul's respirations: a pattern of breathing of deep rapid respirations that accompanies metabolic acidosis.

L

Latency: a brief period with little or no activity.

Leukocytes: white blood cells associated with both inflammatory and immune responses.

Lactic acidosis: a high level of lactic acid in the blood caused by breakdown of glycogen in the absence of oxygen.

Lassitude: weariness and exhaustion.

Leachable allergens: foreign proteins capable of generating an allergic response that can be leached or rinsed out (e.g., leached out from dialyzer membranes).

Learning: the process of attaining knowledge, attitude, and skills.

Lee white clotting time (LWCT): a test of adequacy of heparinization that reflects the time it takes for blood, at body temperature, to clot in a test tube.

Lethargy: a condition of functional sluggishness and stupor.

Leukemia: a disease characterized by rapid and abnormal proliferation of leukocytes and the presence of immature leukocytes in the peripheral circulation.

Leukopenia: a reduction in the number of white blood cells in the blood.

Leukotrienes: lipoxygenase metabolites of arachidonic acid with multiple biologic activities.

Libido: sexual desire or drive.

Lipase: an enzyme that acts on triacylglycerols to form 2-monoglycerides and free fatty acids.

Lipogenesis: the process by which glucose and other substances, derived from carbohydrate in the diet, are converted to fatty acids in the body.

Lipoprotein lipase: an enzyme, produced by the pancreas and glands of the small intestine, that breaks down fats into glycerol and fatty acids during digestion.

Locus: position on the chromosome where a specific gene is found.

Loop of Henle: a part of the nephron, specifically a tubule, situated between the proximal and distal tubules.

Low-density lipoproteins (LDL): a protein-lipid aggregate that is a major carrier of plasma cholesterol to the cells.

Lymph nodes: small swellings found at intervals along the lymphatic system.

Lymphadenectomy: disease of the lymph nodes, typically characterized by enlargement.

Lymphocytes: a type of leukocyte

(white blood cell) that is responsible for specific immune defenses.

Lymphokine activated killer (LAK) cells: a heterogenous population of cells, primarily natural killer cells and T-cells that become cytotoxic in the presence of interleukin-2. They appear to be more selective for tumor cells than for normal cells.

Lymphoma: a type of malignancy that refers to growth of new tissue in the lymphatic system (e.g., Hodgkin's disease, lymphosarcoma, and malignant lymphoma).

Lysis: the destruction of cells through damage or rupture of the plasma membrane, allowing escape of the cell contents.

M

Macronutrients: the major nutrients required in the body, including protein, fat, and carbohydrate.

Macrophage: a large scavenger cell present in connective tissue and many major organs and tissues including the bone marrow, spleen, lymph nodes, liver, and central nervous cells.

Macrophage activating factor (MAF): agents that activate macrophages and attract them to the area of the tumor; they are produced by antigen-stimulated T-cells.

Magnesium: a metallic element essential to life, necessary for functioning of muscle and nervous tissue.

Major histocompatibility complex (MHC): also known as HLA or human leukocyte antigen complex and refers to factors that can facilitate the matching of donor and recipient tissue for transplantation.

Malaise: a vague feeling of bodily discomfort.

Malignancies: Tumors that invade and destroy the tissue in which they originate and can spread to other sites of the body via the blood and lymphatic system.

Malnutrition: a condition caused by an improper balance between what individuals eat and what they require to maintain health.

Marsupialization: a surgical technique for curing a cyst. The cyst is opened, its contents removed, and the edges stitched to the skin incision. The wound is then kept open until it has healed by granulation.

Mast cells: large cells in connective tissues with many coarse cytoplasmic granules. These granules contain heparin, histamine, and serotonin, which are released during inflammation and allergic responses.

Maximal transport capacity (TM): the maximal rate of mediated transport of a substance across the renal tubule wall.

Mean arterial pressure (MAP): the average blood pressure during the cardiac cycle; approximately diastolic pressure plus one-third pulse pressure.

Medial: relating to or situated in the central region of an organ, tissue, or the body.

Medulla: the inner region of any organ, as distinguished from the cortex or outer region.

Medullary sponge kidney (MSK): a disease of the kidney characterized by dilated intramedullary collecting ducts, imparting a sponge-like appearance to the kidney. MSK is often an asymptomatic, benign condition, or it may present with nephrolithiasis, hematuria, and urinary tract infection.

Membrane resistance: a term used to describe the flexibility or rigidity of a semi-permeable membrane in a dialyzer.

Membrane surface area: the total area or space for exposure of blood or other fluids to a semi-permeable membrane. Surface area is related to clearance.

Membranous glomerulopathy: a disease of the kidney most commonly associated with the nephrotic syndrome in adults. It is usually idiopathic or in some cases, the consequence of infections, systemic autoimmune disease, or medication administration.

Memory: the property of evoking a more vigorous specific immune response upon reexposure to a particular antigen.

Memory T-lymphocytes: T-lymphocytes that upon later exposure to the same antigen, greatly augment the specific immune response. Upon reexposure, the development of antibodies is much quicker and more intense.

Meningitis: an inflammation of the meninges, the membranes covering the brain.

Mesangium: one of four layers of cells found in the glomerular capillaries. They are irregularly shaped cells with dense nuclei and little cytoplasm found beneath the endothelium and separated by a matrix. It is thought that the mesangium is phagocytic, helps preserve the basement membrane, participates in regulation of glomerular flow and is associated with production of collagen fibrils.

Metastatic calcification: deposits of calcium in areas outside bone.

Method I: payment for home dialysis under the composite rate.

Method II: Medicare authorization for patients to obtain supplies and equipment directly from a supplier on a reasonable charge basis as determined by the Medicare carrier. Medicare pays 80% of the reasonable charge and the patient is responsible for the remaining 20%. This was done for the convenience of patients and was not required by law.

Methodologic studies: studies involving the development of diagnostic procedures or techniques of measurement, including new instrumentation, comparison of various modes of measurement, development of screening techniques, studies dealing with reliability and validity of various instruments or diagnostic techniques, and studies that pertain to observer error and variation.

Microalbuminuria: microscopic amounts of albumin in the urine.

Microvilli: microscopic hair-like structures projecting from the surface of epithelial cells. They serve to increase the surface area of the cell and are seen on absorptive and secretory cells.

Migratory polyarthropathy: dysfunction of multiple joints that will migrate or shift to other joints.

Minimal change disease (MCD): dysfunction of the kidney characterized by minor histological changes, often with few symptoms.

Miosis: abnormal contraction of the pupils; also refers to a method of cell division which allows each nucleus to receive half the number of chromosomes present in the cells.

Mitochondria: structures in the cytoplasm of cell that are the site of the cell's energy production.

Mixed lymphocyte cross-match: a test where serum from the recipient is incubated with lymphocytes from the potential donor for 30 minutes. If no cytotoxic antibodies are present, the crossmatch results would be negative.

Molecular size: the weight or size of a group of atoms in a molecule, as measured in daltons.

Molecules: groups of atoms of which material substances consist.

Monoclonal proteins: an antibody produced artificially from a cell clone and therefore consisting of a single type of immunoglobulin.

Monocytes: white blood cells with a single large nucleus that serves to ingest foreign particles such as bacteria.

Monokines: substances such as interleukin-1 and tumor necrosis factor that are secreted by monocytes and macrophages.

Mononuclear phagocytes: monocytes, a type of white blood cells involved in phagocytosis.

Monooxygenase: a vasoactive substance produced in the kidney by glomeruli, vascular endothelium, and interstitial cells. Some monooxygenases produce vasoconstriction.

Moral dilemmas: those situations where the individual must choose between two mutually compatible choices related to right and wrong which prove to be difficult and/or troublesome.

Moral reasoning: the cognitive and developmental process of reasoning about moral choice. Moral reasoning is often described as moral judgment or moral development and refers to the mental process that occurs between recognition and the reaction to a moral dilemma.

Morals: that which is concerned with conduct, character, intentions, and social relations insofar as they are appraised as being excellent, right, deserving, virtuous, just, or proper.

Morbidity: evidence of disease or illness.

Morbidity rate: a term used indiscriminately to refer to incidence or prevalence rates of disease.

Mortality: pertaining to death or loss of life.

Mortality rate: death rate.

Motivational factors: factors whose presence lead to satisfaction; also called satisfiers.

Motor deficits: dysfunctions or limitation in movement.

Multiple myeloma: a neoplastic disease characterized by infiltration of bone and bone marrow by myeloma cells forming multiple tumor masses.

Myalgia: muscular aches and pains.

Myasthenia gravis: a chronic disease marked by abnormal fatigue and weakness of selected muscles, which is treated by rest or anticholinergic drugs.

Myelinolysis: destruction of myelin, the sheath covering nerve fibers.

Myocardial contractility: the force of heart contraction that is independent on fiber length.

Myoclonus: a sudden spasm of the muscles, typically flexing and lifting the arms.

Myogenic: originating in muscle.

Myoglobinemia: the presence of myoglobin in the blood. Myoglobin is released with the destruction of muscle cells.

Myopathy: pathology or dysfunction of the muscles.

N

Na/K ATPase pump: the primary active transport carrier protein that splits ATP and releases energy that is used to transport sodium out of the cell and potassium into the cell.

Natriuresis: the excretion of sodium in the urine.

Natural killer (NK) cells: lymphocytes that preferentially kill virally infected or malignant cells in the absence of prior immunization.

Negative pressure: a suction pressure applied to a dialyzer membrane by a dialysis machine for the purposes of removal of fluid.

Nephritis: a disease of the kidneys classically associated with a nephritic syndrome that includes hematuria as its distinguishing component. Other classic symptoms include hypertension, renal insufficiency, volume overload, edema, and in some cases, mild proteinuria.

Nephroblastoma: Also known as Wilm's tumor, it is one of the more common tumors of childhood comprising from 6% to 30% of malignant solid tumors in children. An early symptom is abdominal pain.

Nephrolithiasis: stones in the kidney.

Nephron: the active functioning unit of the kidney.

Nephropathy: pathology or dysfunction of the kidney.

Nephrosclerosis: damage to the small arteries and arterioles in the kidney, often caused by chronic hypertension, leading to renal insufficiency and possibly to CRF.

Nephrotic: pertaining to, resembling, or caused by nephrosis.

Nephrotic syndrome: a clinical entity having multiple causes characterized by increased glomerular permeability resulting in proteinuria, hypoalbuminemia, edema, hyperlipidemia, and hypercoagulability.

Nephrotoxic: damaging to the kidneys.

Nephrotoxicity: damage to the kidneys primarily as a result of direct toxic effects on the renal tubules, with hemodynamic mechanisms possibly contributing to dysfunction.

Net filtration pressure (NFP): the pressure exerted by passage of fluid through a semipermeable membrane as a result of a difference in hydrostatic pressures.

Net ultrafiltration: volume of water drawn into the peritoneal cavity less the volume reabsorbed (into the peritoneal vasculature or by the lymphatic system).

Neuman Systems Model: a conceptual model for nursing that is based on an individual's, group's, or community's response to stressors. It describes primary, secondary, and tertiary prevention.

Neutralization: process in which antibodies either with or without complement neutralize the infectivity of microorganisms.

Neutrophil: a type of white blood cell that is distinguished by a lobed nucleus and the presence in its cytoplasm of fine granules that stain purple with Romanovsky stains. It is capable of ingesting and killing bacteria and provides an important defense against infection.

Nodular: pertaining to nodules, or small swellings or aggregations of cells.

Nomogram: graphical presentation of relationships between quantities whereby value of one variable may be found by examining another.

Non-insulin dependent diabetes mellitus (NIDDM): diabetes mellitus that does not require the use of insulin; it may be controlled by diet and/or oral hypoglycemic agents.

Nonoliguric: not related to low volume of urine excretion.

Nonstreptococcal postinfectious

acute glomerulonephritis: an inflammation of the glomeruli, which can follow infection by a variety of bacteria, viruses, and parasites.

Normal saline: a solution often used for intravenous therapy consisting of 0.9% sodium chloride.

Normochromic: blood possessing normal color and hemoglobin content.

Normocytic: a normal average-sized red blood cell.

Normoglycemic: normal levels of blood glucose.

Nursing intervention: an action that is planned to manage stimuli or problems to achieve nursing care goals.

Nystagmus: constant involuntary cyclical movement of the eyeball.

O

Orem's Self-Care Framework: a conceptual model for nursing that posits that the goal of nursing is self-care. Individuals or patients have universal self-care requisites and, in the situation of health problems, health deviation requisites that are addressed through self-care actions.

Obesity: a condition in which excess fat has accumulated in the body, mostly in the subcutaneous tissues. Obesity is usually considered to be present when a person is 20% above the recommended weight for his/her height and build.

Obstructive nephropathy: damage to the kidney caused by impaired or blocked flow of urine through the urinary tract.

Obstructive uropathy: the structural or functional impediment to the normal flow of urine.

Obtundation: blunted or decreased sensitivity.

Occult blood: blood in such minute quantities that it can only be recognized by microscopic or chemical means.

Olecranon: the area of the ulna that projects behind the elbow joint.

Oliguric: pertaining to low levels of urine output.

Oncogenic: pertaining to things that are capable of causing neoplastic transformation of cells.

Opinion: a conclusion or judgment held with confidence that falls short of positive knowledge.

Opportunistic infection: infections with organisms that would not necessarily be dangerous to a healthy person, but that are harmful to immunosuppressed or vulnerable individuals.

Opsonization: the process by which particles, microorganisms, or immune complexes become coated with complement or antibodies that make them more easily phagocytosed.

Optimal function: an ideal or best possible level of activity given the circumstances.

Organic factors: variables that relate to the structure of the body or part of the body.

Orthopnea: respiratory condition in which breathing is only possible in an upright position.

Orthotopic: in the normal anatomic location.

Orthotopic graft: organ transplanted into the normal anatomic location in the body (e.g., heart).

Osmolality: the osmotic concentration, that is the characteristic of a solution determined by the ionic concentration of the dissolved substance per unit of solvent.

Osmoreceptors: a group of cells in the hypothalamus that monitor blood concentration.

Osmosis: The movement of a solvent (liquid) through a semi-permeable membrane from an area of lower concentration to an area of higher concentration of the solute.

Osmotic pressure: pressure of fluid created by different strengths of solution separated by a semi-permeable membrane.

Osteoblastic: pertaining to osteoblasts, which are cells responsible for the formation of bone.

Osteoblasts: a type of cell responsible for laying down the protein matrix of bone.

Osteoclasts: a large multinuclear cell found in depressions on the surface of a bone causing resorption of bone substance.

Osteodystrophy: a generalized bone disease resulting from a metabolic disorder, such as chronic renal failure.

Osteomalacia: a softening of bone caused by deficiency of Vitamin D and/or calcium.

Osteomyelitis: an inflammation of bone marrow due to infection often caused by compound fractures.

Outcome standards: the degree of excellence or quality expected for the results of care.

Outflow pressure: the pressure leaving or flowing from a source.

Oxalate: a salt of oxalic acid.

Oxalosis: an inborn defect of metabolism that causes deposition of oxalate in the kidneys and other organs, resulting in renal failure.

P

Pallor: lack of color or paleness of skin.

Palmar arch: the arterial blood supply to the hand.

Pamidronate: a medication used to regulate bone metabolism that inhibits osteoclast bone resorption.

Pancreas: a compound gland about 15 cm long that lies behind the stomach. It secretes the hormones insulin and glucagon into the blood stream and is also responsible for secretion of pancreatic juices required for digestion.

Papillary necrosis: damage to the kidney caused by vascular ischemia in the papilla that leads to generalized vasculopathy and ultimately to glomerulosclerosis, atrophy, and CRF.

Papilledema: edema and inflammation of the optic nerve at the point of entrance into the eyeball.

Paracellular: located near a cell.

Parallel plate dialyzers: artificial kidneys in which the semi-permeable membranes are arranged in flat sheets rather than coiled or organized in fibers.

Parasitic: pertaining to parasites.

Parasitic infection: an invasion of the body by a parasite, (i.e., a living organism that lives in or on another organism). Human parasites include bacteria, viruses, fungi, protozoa, and worms.

Parathyroid hormone (PTH): a peptide hormone secreted by parathyroid glands, that regulates calcium and phosphate concentrations of the internal environment.

Parenchymal: the body, or working functioning part of an organ.

Paresis: partial or incomplete paralysis.

Paresthesia: abnormal sensations such as numbness, prickling, tingling, and heightened sensitivity.

Partial prothrombin time: a measure of coagulation of blood used to indicate effectiveness of coagulation or anticoagulation.

Passive transport: movement through a semipermeable membrane that does not involve the expenditure of energy.

Pathogenesis: the postulated mechanisms by which the etiologic agent produces disease. The difference between etiology and pathogenesis should be noted: The etiology of a disease or disability consists of the postulated causes that initiate the pathogenetic mechanisms; control of these causes might lead to prevention of the disease.

Patient education: the process of systematic instruction of patients.

Percutaneous: denoting the passage of substances through unbroken skin, as in abosorption by inunction; also passage through the skin by needle puncture, including introduction of wires and catheters by Seldinger technique.

Percutaneous transluminal angioplasty (PCTA): a procedure involving introduction of a catheter with an inflatable balloon into a major central artery for the purposes of widening an area of stenosis or narrowing.

Pericardial tamponade: a constriction of the heart by the pericardium due to a collection of fluid or scar tissue.

Pericardiectomy: surgical removal of the pericardium.

Pericardiocentesis: perforation/incision into the pericardium, generally by needle, for the purposes of drainage.

Pericardiostomy: formation of an opening into the pericardium for drainage.

Pericardium: the membranous fibroserous sac enclosing the heart and the bases of the great vessels.

Periodontal: pertaining to or relating to the tissues surrounding the teeth.

Periorbital: around the eyes.

Peripheral vascular system: the parts of the vascular system, outside the central cardiac area, responsible for distributing nutrients to cells and tissues throughout the body and for transporting waste products from the tissues to the organs of elimination.

Peripheral vascular resistance (PVR): the resistance of all the peripheral blood vessels in the systemic vascular system.

Peristalsis: a wave-like involuntary movement of muscles that progresses along some of the hollow tubes of the body.

Peritubular: closely associated with a tubule (as in peritubular capillary, which is around the renal tubule).

Peritoneal dialysis: the process of removal of fluids and wastes from the body using the semi-permeable membrane of the peritoneum for diffusion and osmosis.

pH: a measure of the concentration of hydrogen ions in a solution, and therefore, of its acidity or alkalinity. pH decreases as acidity increases.

Phagocytic: pertaining to the engulfment and digestion of particles by a cell.

Phagocytosis: the engulfment and digestion of bacteria and other foreign particles by a cell.

Phagosome: a vesicle that forms around a particle within the phagocyte that engulfed the particle.

Phenomenology: a philosophy and research approach that involves developing an understanding of human experience holistically as it is actually lived.

Phenotype: a description of all the alleles detected in a given individual.

Phimosis: a stenosis or narrowing of preputial orifice so that the foreskin cannot be pushed back over the glans penis.

Phosphate binders: a medication that binds phosphate commonly given to people with chronic renal failure to prevent bone disease.

Phosphorus: a nonmetallic element mostly concentrated in bone.

Phosphorylation: addition of a phosphate group to an organic molecule.

Physiological mode: a concept in Roy's Adaptation Model that refers to the way in which an individual adapts to physiological needs.

Plasma clearance: a hypothetical volume of plasma that is completely cleared of a given solute per unit of time.

Plasma exchange: an extracorporeal therapy that involves removal of plasma from the blood and replacement with plasma substitutes.

Plasma membrane separators: membranes used in the process of plasma exchange (much like the dialyzer in hemodialysis).

Plasma replacement fluids: fluids used to replace removed plasma in the process of plasma exchange.

Plasmapheresis: a therapy used to remove plasma from blood in order to remove selected blood components from the body.

Platelet count: the number of platelets present in the blood; the normal count is 150-400 million per liter of blood.

Platelets: disk-shaped structures present in blood required for clotting (Also called thrombocytes).

Pleural effusion: an accumulation of fluid in the pleural space (between the layers of pleural covering the lungs).

Pneumothorax: the presence of air in the pleural cavity resulting in collapse of the lung.

Pocket veto: a veto in which a bill – after passing both Houses of Congress and sent to the President – does not become law if Congress adjourns before the 10 days in which the President should sign the bill. Normally, a bill goes to the President after passing both Houses; if he approves it or fails to take action within 10 days, the bill becomes law.

Podocytes: the layer of cells found in the inner wall of Bowman's capsule and the outer layer of the capillaries with footlike processes that radiates from the cell body. This layer functions as the final filter in the glomerular filtration process.

Polyacrylonitrile: a highly permeable semi-permeable membrane used in some dialyzers for high flux dialysis.

Polydipsia: extreme thirst.

Polymerase chain reaction (PCR): a process that enables the amount of a particular DNA sequence or gene to be greatly amplified.

Polymethyl methacrylate: a synthetic material used in dialyzer membranes.

Polymorphonuclear granulocytes: a type of white blood cell that is distinguished by a lobed nucleus and the presence in its cytoplasm of fine granules that stain purple with Romanovsky stains. It is capable of ingesting and killing bacteria and provides an important defense against infection (also known as a neutrophil).

Polytetrafluoroethylene (PTFE): a teflon-like material used to create internal arteriovenous grafts for vascular access for dialysis.

Polyuria: passing large volumes of

urine.

Porosity: the extent to which a material is porous.

Porous: full of minute openings in a surface through which fluids can pass.

Positions: classifications of people and of status.

Post-infectious glomerulonephritis: dysfunction of the glomerulus of the kidney that results after infection (often streptococcal).

Pressure monitor: a monitor on the dialysis delivery machine that is used to assess the pressure of the circulating blood.

Prevalence: the number of instances of a given disease or other condition in a given population at a designated time; sometimes used to mean "prevalence rate." When used without qualification the term usually refers to the situation at a specified point in time (point prevalence).

Prevalence point: the number of persons with a disease or an attribute at a specified point in time.

Prevalence ratio: the total number of all individuals who have an attribute or diease at a particular time (or during a particular period) divided by the population at risk of having the attribute or disease at this point in time or midway through the period.

Primary infection: the major or first infection in a body.

Principles: a set of rules of personal conduct or moral standards collectively.

Process: the progress or course of events.

Process standards: the degree of excellence or quality expected for the provision of care.

Prodromal: a term characterizing the initial stage of a disease from the time of the earliest symptoms to the appearance of major symptoms.

Productivity: the quality or state of being productive; often described as a measurement of production per unit of effort.

Progenitor: a precursor, ancestor, one who begets.

Prolactin: a peptide hormone secreted by the anterior pituitary that stimulates milk secretion by mammary glands.

Propositions: statements that describe or link concepts.

Prospective Payment: 1. A method of payment for health care services in which the amount of payment for services is set before the delivery of those services and the hospital (or other provider) is at least partially at risk for losses or stands to gain from surpluses that accrue during the payment period. Prospective payment rates may be per-service, per-capita, per-diem, or per-case rates. 2. Payment for medical care on the basis of rates set in advance of the time period in which they apply. The unit of payment may vary from individual medical services to broader categories, such as hospital case, episode of illness, or person capitation.

Prostaglandin E2 (PGE2): one of the prostaglandins that serves as a vasodilator.

Prostaglandins: lipid substances metabolized from fatty acids, mainly arachidonic acids, that influence renal hemodynamics by regulating blood flow to the kidney. The kidney plays an important role in synthesizing and degrading prostaglandins.

Proteinases: enzymes that break down protein.

Protein catabolic rate (PCR): the rate of breakdown of protein, particularly in the case of disease or injury.

Proteins: a group of organic compounds with a complex structure made up of one or more amino acids linked by peptide bonds. They form the structural material of muscles, tissues, and organs and form enzymes and hormones.

Proteolytic: breaks down protein.

Proteus: a genus of the family Bacteriaceae found in intestines and decaying material.

Prothrombin time: a laboratory measurement estimating prothrombin activity that involves mixing a citrated sample of blood with standardized amounts of thromboplastin and calcium ions and reporting the time required for this plasma to clot.

Proximal: close to the central part of the body.

Proximal tubule: first tubular component of a nephron after Bowman's capsule.

Pruritis: itching.

Pseudoaneurysm: areas of weakening and outpouches of AV fistulae and grafts usually caused by repeated needle punctures in one location.

Pseudohyperkalemia: false elevation of potassium ions in the blood.

Pseudohyponatremia: false readings for low levels of sodium in the blood.

Psychomotor: pertaining to physical skills or activities that need to be performed.

Psychosis: disorder of psychogenic origin characterized by delusions and hallucinations.

Psychosocial factors: variables or things that pertain to psychological or social phenomena.

Pulmonary edema: an accumulation of fluid in the lungs caused by fluid overload.

Pyridoxine (B_6): Vitamin B_6, a vitamin of the B complex that is a constituent of the coenzyme pyridoxal phosphate B_6 and is involved in the transamination of amino acids.

R

Radial artery: the artery that continues from the brachial artery down the lateral aspect of the forearm and carries blood to the hand. It is the artery typically used to measure pulse.

Rales: an abnormal sound heard on auscultation of the chest produced by passage of air through bronchi that contain secretions or exudate. Rales may be heard on either inspiration or expiration.

Rapidly progressive glomerulonephritis (RPGN): an idiopathic primary glomerular disease characterized by a rapid deterioration in renal function with distinctive glomerular crescent formation on renal biopsy.

Rate of blood flow: the speed at which blood runs through the artificial kidney.

Reabsorption: in the kidney, reabsorption refers to the transport of substances from the tubular lumen into the interstitium and blood.

Recessive trait: a chromosome for a trait that does not appear in an offspring.

Recidivism: the rate of readmission to an institution.

Reflux nephropathy: the term used to denote the renal scarring that occurs as the result of vesicoureteral reflux (VUR).

Refractory: a term applied to a condition that fails to respond satisfactorily to a given treatment.

Regeneration: the process of generating again; bringing into renewed existence.

Regenerative (Sorbent) dialysate systems: a dialysate delivery system in which a small quantity of water is used to create an initial dialysis bath, and the used dialysate solution is recycled and reused; rather than discarded. This type of system is typically used for patients while they are traveling.

Regional citrate anticoagulation: dialysis in which citrate, rather than heparin, is used as the anticoagulant. Citrate is broken down quickly by the body, so there is less likelihood of bleeding as a result of the therapy.

Regulatory cells: helper and suppressor lymphocytes.

Rehabilitation: a process that mobilizes an individual's residual capacity for optimal function in his or her usual environment.

Rejection: the reaction that occurs after transplantation of an allogeneic or xenogeneic organ. Antibody, complement, clotting factors, and platelets are involved in the failure of the graft to survive.

Renal threshold: the plasma concentration of a substance at which the transport system becomes saturated, and the substance is excreted by the kidney.

Renal artery stenosis: a narrowing of the renal artery, that results in hypertension.

Renal system: the body system pertaining to kidneys.

Renin: A proteolytic enzyme that catalyzes the splitting of a decapeptide (Angiotensin I) from a plasma protein known as angiotensinogen that is produced mainly by the liver and is present in the plasma in high concentration.

Renovascular hypertension: a secondary elevation of blood pressure produced by various conditions that interfere with the arterial circulation to kidney tissue, causing ischemia.

Repair: to restore to good condition.

Residual capacity: the remaining ability or capacity to perform activities or tasks.

Resource allocation: the distribution of resources among a range of uses or activities.

Respiratory acidosis: increased arterial hydrogen ion concentration due to carbon dioxide retention.

Retinopathy: pathology or disorder of the retina (the light sensitive layer of cells inside the eye) resulting in impairment or loss of vision.

Retrocaval: behind the vena cava.

Retroperitoneal: behind the peritoneum (the membrane that covers the abdominal cavity).

Retroperitoneal fibrosis: a disease of unknown origin that results in fibrosis and inflammation of the retroperitoneal abdominal cavity, which can result in compression anywhere along the course of one or both ureters.

Rickettsial: a disease caused by an organism of the genus Rickettsia.

Reverse osmosis: a system of water treatment that selectively removes ions and organic material by use of a membrane and pressure.

Rhabdomyolysis (myoglobin): injury of skeletal muscle tissue with release of intracellular substances including myoglobin, often resulting in acute renal failure.

Rhonchi: a continuous low pitched sound with a snoring quality heard in the chest on auscultation when air flows through the bronchi are reduced.

Right pleural effusion: an accumulation of fluid or exudate in the pleural space, between the pleura, on the right side.

Rinse volume: the volume of fluid (usually saline) used to rinse a dialyzer.

Rogers' Science of Unitary Human Beings: a conceptual model for nursing that is based on existential philosophy and includes many sophisticated concepts and linkages. It includes the concepts of energy fields, openness, pattern and organization, and four-dimensionality, as well as describing the complex linkages among nursing, unitary man, health, and environment.

Role function mode: a concept in Roy's Adaptation Model that refers to one of the four adaptive modes. The role function mode refers to the performance of duties based on given positions within society (e.g., mother role).

Role: a set of learned behaviors.

Role ambiguity: the experience of having to deal with single or multiple roles that have not been clearly articulated in terms of expected behavior or performance levels.

Role conflict: contradictory role expectations.

Role overload: the situation that occurs when too much work expected in the allotted time or the role becomes too complex.

Role strain: an internal response or emotional reaction to role stress.

Role stress: the challenges and difficulties that are encountered when roles and role obligations are vague, irritating, conflicting, or unrealistic.

Roy Adaptation Model: a conceptual model for nursing that can be viewed primarily as a systems model, where the patient is viewed as having elements linked in such a way that force on linkages can be increased or decreased. There are four subsystems (adaptive modes) described in the model and they are faced with constantly changing environmental, focal, contextual, and residual stimuli.

S

Sarcoidosis: a chronic granulomatous disease characterized by the formation of tubercle-like lesions in organs such as the skin, lymph nodes, lungs, and bone marrow.

Screening: was defined in 1951 by the US Commission on Chronic Illness as, "The presumptive identification of unrecognized disease or defect by the application of tests, examinations or other procedures which can be applied rapidly. Screening tests sort out apparently well persons who probably have a disease from those who probably do not. A screening test is not intended to be diagnostic. Persons with positive or suspicious findings must be referred to their physicians for diagnosis and necessary treatment."

Scribner shunt: a silastic tubing, one side of which is inserted into an artery and the other side which is inserted into a vein, through which blood flow can be diverted to dialysis. It is also known as an arteriovenous cannula or shunt and was named after its founder, Belding Scribner.

SCUF (slow continuous ultrafiltration): an extracorporeal renal replacement therapy that slowly and continuously removes fluid. It can be done from artery to vein or vein to vein.

Sebaceous: containing or pertaining to sebum, an oily fatty matter secreted by the sebaceous glands.

Secondary infection: invasion of the body by microorganisms at a time when the immune system of the body is already weakened by another infection or disease.

Secretion: the release of organic molecules, ions, and water by cells in response to specific stimuli.

Secretory: pertaining to secretion, which is the process by which a gland isolates constituents of the blood or tissue fluid and chemically alters them to produce a substance that it discharges for use by the body or excretes.

Self-concept mode: a concept in Roy's conceptual model, specifically, one of the four modes of adaptation that reflects a person's self-concept, or ways of thinking about him/herself, as determined by interactions with others.

Semipermeable membrane: a membrane with pores that are permeable to some (smaller molecules) but not to larger molecules.

Semi-recumbent: sitting up.

Septic catabolism: breakdown of tissue due to infectious agents.

Seronegativity: a negative result indicative of absence of a disease or virus detected in serum.

Seropositivity: a positive result indicating presence of a disease, detected in serum.

Serotonin: a compound widely distributed in tissues that is thought to play a role in inflammation similar to histamine. It acts as a neurotransmitter and is involved in the process of sleep.

Severity: the extent of or harshness of a disease or illness.

Sialoproteins: proteins in saliva.

Sickle cell disease: a genetic disease causing anemia in which abnormal, sickle, or crescent-shaped erythrocytes are present. The sickle cell becomes deoxygenated and can obstruct blood flow in the microcirculation.

Single lumen catheter: a small tube with a single path, or lumen, inserted into a blood vessel.

Single needle devices: a device used to regulate blood flow with dialysis when only one needle is used. The device alternates between removing blood from the patient and returning blood to the patient.

Sinusoidal: pertaining to sinusoids.

Sinusoids: a small blood vessel found in certain organs such as the adrenal gland and liver.

Societal limitation: a barrier or limit imposed by the customs and organizations of a community.

Sodium modeling: the process of adjusting sodium concentrations in the dialysate solution in order to attain patient-specific goals.

Solute: any substance that dissolves in a solvent (liquid) to form a solution.

Solvent: the fluid in which a solute is dissolved.

Somatomedin: a protein hormone responsible for stimulating protein synthesis and promoting growth that is produced by the liver in response to stimulation by growth hormone.

Somatotropin: growth hormone secreted by the anterior pituitary, which stimulates somatomedic release thereby enhancing body growth by acting on carbohydrate and protein metabolism.

Somnolence: the feeling of being sleepy.

Spermatogenesis: the formation of sperm.

Spleen: a large oval organ on the left hand side of the body, behind the stomach, which is part of the reticuloendothelial system and is involved in producing lymphocytes in newborns and containing phagocytes.

Splenomegaly: enlargement of the spleen.

Squamous cell: flat epithelial cells lining the body.

Standards of care: the degree of excellence or quality expected for the care of an individual or group. Standards of care are typically described as structure, process, and outcome standards.

Standards of professional performance: the degree of excellence or quality expected of professionals functioning in their roles.

Staphylococcus epidermidis: a gram positive coccus (bacteria) commonly found on the skin.

Steal syndrome: a situation caused by shunting of blood from the artery to the vein in side-to-side anastamosis fistulae, resulting in arterial insufficiency and ischemia of the hand.

Stem cells: cells capable of self-replication and differentiation into various kinds of secondary cells.

Steroid-induced diabetes: a metabolic disorder of carbohydrate metabolism, resulting from inadequate production or utilization of insulin, caused by the therapeutic use of glucocorticoids.

Steroids: a group of compounds having a common structure consisting of three six-membered carbon rings and one five-membered carbon ring. Naturally occurring steroids include male and female sex hormones, hormones of the adrenal cortex, progesterone, bile salts, and sterols.

Stomatitis: inflammation of the mouth caused by a range of factors or conditions.

Streptokinase: an antithrombolytic agent used to dissolve clots in vascular access devices.

Stridor: a harsh sound during respiration caused by obstruction of air passages.

Stroke volume: blood volume ejected by a ventricle during one heartbeat.

Structure standards: the degree of quality or excellence expected in terms of the environment or setting in which care is provided.

Subclavian: a major artery and vein running in the area of the clavicle.

Subclavian vein catheter: a small tube inserted into the subclavian vein, that drains the veins from the arms.

Subperiosteal: below the periosteum.

Sulfadiazine: an antibacterial agent used in combination with another agent often prescribed for urinary tract infections.

Suppressor T-cells: a subclass of T-lymphocytes responsible for suppressing the immune response to a stimulus.

Suprainfection: a secondary infection following closely after a primary infection.

Supraoptic: above the eye.

Surveillance: ongoing scrutiny, generally using methods distinguished by their practicability, uniformity, and frequently their rapidity, rather than by complete accuracy. Its main purpose is to detect changes in trend or distribution in order to initiate investigative or control measures.

Surveillance of diease: scrutiny of all aspects of occurrence and spread of a disease that are pertinent to effective control.

Syncope: dizziness.

Synsitium: a mass of protoplasm with many nuclei but no clear cell boundaries.

Synthetic graft: a graft made of artificial rather than human materials.

T

T-lymphocytes: cells that are derived from the bone marrow and that differentiate within the thymus; they play a major role in the activity of the cell-mediated immune system.

Tamponade: a condition resulting from accumulation of excess fluid in the pericardium causing constriction.

Teaching: the process of providing instruction.

Tetany: a set of symptoms including intermittent tonic spasms, nervousness, and muscular irritability induced by changes in calcium or pH.

Therapeutic apheresis: the removal of selected blood components or cells for the treatment of selected diseases, thought to have autoimmune components, through use of membrane technology and an extracorporeal circuit.

Therapeutic plasma exchange (TPE): an extracorporeal therapy that involves removal of plasma from the blood and replacement with plasma substitutes.

Thiazides: a category of diuretics that act on the loop of Henle to prevent reabsorption of water.

Thoracentesis: surgical puncture of the chest wall usually with a needle for removal of fluids from the pleural space.

Thrill: the vibrating sensation felt at the site of anastomosis between an artery and a vein for creation of an arteriovenous fistula. The thrill is an indication of patency of the fistula.

Thrombocytopenia: a reduction in the number of platelets in the blood resulting in bleeding into the skin, spontaneous bruising, and prolonged bleeding after injury.

Thrombolytic agent: a medication or pharmaceutical agent that assists in breaking down clots.

Thrombophlebitis: an inflammation of a vein caused by a blood clot.

Thrombotic thrombocytopenic purpura (TTP): a skin rash resulting from bleeding into the skin from capillaries caused by a deficiency of platelets and clotting in small vessels.

Thromboxanes: an eicosanoid closely related to prostaglandins.

Time on dialysis (t): a measure of length of the dialysis treatment used to calculate adequacy of dialysis.

Total quality management (TQM): a process and program of monitoring and improving quality.

Toxemia: toxins in the blood.

Toxins: substances that have a poisonous or toxic effect on the body.

Trajectory: a path or course often used to describe a process uncovered using grounded theory research.

Transcellular: across cells.

Transferrin: an iron-binding protein carrier for iron in plasma.

Transmembrane pressure (TMP): the total pressure across the dialyzer membrane including both negative pressure created by the machine and positive pressure of the blood.

Trendelenburg position: a position used for some surgical procedures and for patients with shock where the patient is laid on his back with the pelvis higher than the head, inclined at an angle of about 45 degrees with the knees bent.

Triglycerides: a subclass of lipids composed of glycerol and three fatty acids.

Trousseau's sign: muscular spasm resulting from pressure applied to nerves and vessels of the upper arm, indicative of latent tetany.

TSH: thyroid-stimulating hormone, which is a glycoprotein hormone secreted by the anterior pituitary that induces secretion of thyroid hormone (also called thyrotropin).

Tubuloglomerular: pertaining to tubules and the glomerulus.

Tubulointerstitial fibrosis: development of fibrous tissue around the renal tubules and interstitial spaces.

Type A reaction: a severe and acute reaction to a dialyzer that occurs within the first few to 30 minutes of dialysis and is manifested by symptoms such as dyspnea, feeling of warmth, a sense of impending doom, and possibly followed by anaphylaxis.

Type B reaction: a reaction to a dialyzer thought to be caused by complement activation, occurring in the first hour of dialysis and manifested by chest pain.

U

Ulnar artery: a branch of the brachial artery arising at the elbow and running deep within the muscles of the medial side of the forearm. It passes into the palm of the hand, where it unites with the arch of the radial artery and gives off branches to the hand and fingers.

Ultrafiltrate: plasma water removed during dialysis or extracorporeal treatment that is free of formed cells and protein.

Ultrafiltration: filtration under pressure. In hemodialysis, ultrafiltration refers to the removal of fluid using pressure.

Ultrafiltration coefficient: the indicator of permeability of a dialyzer to water. This coefficient can be used to calculate fluid removal during dialysis.

Ultrafiltration (UF) controller: a device on a dialysis machine used to regulate fluid removal.

Ultrafiltration controls: the controls on a dialysis machine that regulate the amount of water to be removed.

United States Renal Data System (USRDS): created in 1988, provides an important source of data about ESRD patients' mortality and treatment modality experience. The USRDS is not the clinical information system called for by the Rehabilitation Task Force and does not routinely collect rehabilitation-relevant data on variables such as patients' educational or employment status.

Urease: an enzyme that catalyzes the hydrolysis of urea to ammonia and carbon dioxide.

Uremic pericarditis: an inflammation of the pericardium, or lining around the heart, caused by uremia.

Urochrome: the substance, derived from urobilin that gives urine its characteristic color.

Urokinase: an enzyme produced in the kidney that is capable of breaking up blood clots. It activates plasminogen directly to plasmin, which dissolves fibrin thrombi.

Uropathy: any pathologic change in the urinary tract.

Usual environment: the typical or normal surroundings or conditions of the community.

V

Value: an affective strongly motivational disposition towards a person, object, or idea. Values are usually organized in a hierarchical manner and form the basis for decision making.

Variable sodium: the device on a dialysis delivery system that provides the opportunity to adjust the proportioning rate so that the dialysate solution can have varying levels of sodium depending on patient requirements at different times of the dialysis treatment.

Vasa recta: straight collecting tubules of the kidney.

Vascular access: the devices used to gain access to the circulation on a repeated basis for dialysis. The term is inclusive of internal and external devices.

Vasculopathy: any disorder of blood vessels.

Vasoactive: functioning to constrict or dilate blood vessels.

Venipuncture: the puncture of a vein for any therapeutic purpose, such as to extract blood for laboratory tests.

Venous monitor: a monitor on the hemodialysis machine that measures venous pressure.

Venous pressure: the pressure of the venous blood circuit during dialysis.

Venous stasis: the stagnation or reduction in blood flow through the veins caused by obstruction.

Ventricular fibrillation: a cardiac arrhythmia where the muscle fibers of the ventricles beat rapidly and chaotically resulting in cardiac arrest.

Very low density lipoproteins (VLDL): a lipid-protein aggregate having a high proportion of fat.

Vesicoureteral reflux (VUR): the situation when urine and any bacteria in the bladder are able to flow backward into the ureter and kidney.

Viral: pertaining to, caused by, or of the nature of virus.

Visceral: pertaining to organs in the thoracic and abdominal cavities.

Visceral layer: the layer of the peritoneum that surrounds the viscera (i.e., the inside layer).

Volume dependent: dependent on extracellular fluid volume.

Volume of urea distribution: the concentration of urea throughout the body considering fluid volume status of the individual. For instance, the volume of urea distribution will be higher (or more concentrated) in dehydrated states and lower when the individual is edematous.

W

Water softening: an inexpensive method of water treatment that involves exchange of calcium and magnesium for sodium.

Weight: a measure of body mass.

Wheezing: production of whistling sounds during difficult breathing that occurs with asthma, croup, and other respiratory conditions.

Whole blood partial thromboplastin time (WBPTT): a measure of the coagulation factors in a person's blood often used to monitor the effect of heparinization.

Z

Zirconium oxide: a compound used in sorbent dialysis to remove phosphate and fluoride.

INDEX

Note: Page numbers followed by **f** indicate figures; page numbers followed by **t** indicate tables.

A

AANNT Journal, 37
AANNT Legislative Policy Statement, 879-881
AANNT Update, 37
Abdominal pain, peritoneal dialysis and, 648-649
ABO blood group antigens, in renal transplantation, 685
ABO blood group testing, in renal transplantation, 714
ABO blood typing, 687
Absorption
 of cyclosporine, 334
 of pharmacologic agents, rate of, factors affecting, 310t, 311
 in water purification, 536-537
Accelerated rejection, posttransplant, 725
Acceptance committees, history of, 1960-1972, 29, 30f
Accountability, described, 46
Acetaminophen
 renal damage due to, 317
 in renal failure patients, 319
Acetylsalicylic acid (ASA), in renal failure patients, 319
Acid-base balance
 alterations in, 246-247
 nursing management of, 9
 maintenance of, 162
 in potassium secretion regulation, 149
 systemic, maintenance of, 163
Acid-base homeostasis, maintenance of, renal mechanisms in, 162-163
Acid-base physiology, principles of, 158-160
Acidemia, in renal failure, 521
Acidification, renal, 157-164, 158f-161f
Acid-load, changes in magnitude of, adaptations to, 163-164
Acidosis, metabolic, 246-247, 247t
 nursing management of, 9
Ackerman, T., 88
Acquired cystic disease (ACD), 185
 Acquired immunodeficiency syndrome (AIDS), 362-367. *See also under* Human immunodeficiency virus (HIV) infection
 history of, 362-363, 362t
 nursing management of, 383-384, 384t
 opportunistic infections in patients with, 383-384, 384t
 in renal patients, 188-189, 189t, 349-350
 in women *versus* men, 363
Activated clotting times (ACTs), in hemodialysis of pediatric renal patients, 447
Active diluting segment, described, 143
Activity level, renal failure effects on, 318t
Acute cystitis, 188
Acute interstitial nephritis (AIN), 182-183
 drug-induced, 316
Acute rejection
 following liver transplantation, 766, 767
 posttransplant, 695-697, 695t, 696f, 725-726
Acute renal failure (ARF), 214-229
 in AIDS, 188-189, 189t
 anemia in, 254
 cardiac failure associated with, 216, 216f
 CAVH for, 581
 defined, 201, 214
 described, 214
 dialysis with, mortality associated with, 214
 drugs and, 316-317
 fluid, electrolyte, and acid-base disturbances in, 234-247
 health care professional's responsibilities related to, 582
 hypovolemia associated with, 216, 216f
 incidence of, 214
 intrarenal failure, 221-229. *See also* Intrarenal failure
 laboratory findings in, 216-217, 217t
 metabolic and endocrine disturbances in, 247-249, 249t
 mortality associated with, 214
 outcome of, 214
 postoperative, mortality associated with, 214
 postrenal failure, 20-23. *See also* Postrenal failure
 in pregnancy, 192
 prerenal failure, 214-218. *See* Prerenal failure
 risk factors for, clinical settings associated with, 220t
 SCUF for, 581
 systemic manifestations of, 234-260
 treatment of, 226-228, 227t, 229t, 582
  historical review of, 577
 uremic syndrome in, 250-260. *See also* Uremic syndrome, in ARF and CRF
Acute tubular necrosis
 drugs and, 316-317
 intrarenal failure due to, 221-224, 221t, 222f, 224t
 ischemic, intrarenal failure due to, 221-223, 222f
 nephrotoxic, intrarenal failure due to, 223-224, 224t
 posttransplant, delayed renal function due to, 719-720
Acute uncomplicated pyelonephritis, 188
Acyclovir
 for herpes infections, 366
 in renal failure patients, 323
Adaptation, to dialysis, stages of, 270
Adaptation level, defined, 62
Adaptive immunity
 active, 671
 components of, 670-671
 versus innate immunity, 670-671, 670t
 passive, 671
Adenine nucleotides, for ARF, 227t
ADH. *See* Antidiuretic hormone
Administration of nursing services, described, 51
Administrators, nurse, described, 51
ADPKD. *See* Autosomal dominant polycystic kidney disease
Adult learning, theory of, 44
Advance directives, 277-279, 278t, 283t
 uses of, 283
Advanced practice nurses, 50
 described, 50
 issues related to, 50-51
 roles of, 50
Advanced practice nursing, nursing opportunities in, 40
Advanced practitioners, responsibilities of, 51
Advocacy
 interdisciplinary, 91
 in nursing, 90-91
Affective learning, 845, 845t
Age
 as factor in blood volume, 444t
 as factor in hypertension, 184
 as factor in renal failure treatment in children, 439
 as factor in renal transplant recipient evaluation, 711-712
 renal failure effects on, 316t
Aging. *See also* Elderly patients
 developmental demands of, 488-489
 expected changes related to, 486t-487t
 perspective on, 483-484, 484t
 physical changes associated with, research implications of, 508t
 physiology of, sexuality responses related to, 489
 population of, demographics of, 483, 484t
 renal patients and, 481-513
 stressors of, 489
AIDS. *See* Acquired immunodeficiency syndrome
Air embolism, hemodialysis and, 559t, 566-567
Akinsanya, J.A., 67
Alanine, for ARF, 227t
Albers, J., 34-35
Albumin
 drugs that bind to, 312t
 molecular weight of, 609t
Alcohol
 effect on sexuality in the elderly, 490
 moonshine, renal insufficiency due to, 191
Aldosterone
 in potassium secretion regulation, 149
 in sodium reabsorption, 167
Alexander, S., 29
Alfa-interferon
 for hepatitis B virus, 358
 for hepatitis C virus, 361
 for hepatitis D virus, 362
Alkalosis, metabolic, 247, 247t
 nursing management of, 9
Allergy(ies), OTC medications for, 340t
Allis Chalmers Company, 31
Allograft, described, 666t
Allograft dysfunction, posttransplant, 730
 differential diagnosis of, 720t
Allograft rejection
 acute, following liver transplantation, 766, 767
 chronic, following liver transplantation, 766, 767
 following liver transplantation, 766
 hyperacute, following liver transplantation, 766
Allopurinol, for ARF, 227t
$Alpha_1$ acid glycoprotein, drugs that bind to, 312t
$Alpha_1$-receptor blockers, in renal failure patients, 320

Alpha$_2$-agonists, centrally acting, in renal failure patients, 330-321
Altered dynamic responsiveness, described, 316
Altered receptor binding, described, 316
Altered responsiveness to receptor stimulation, described, 316
American Association for Nephrology Nurses (AANN), 5
American Association of Kidney Patients (AAKP), address for, 858t
American Board of Nursing Specialties (ABNS)
  history of, 5
  standards and criteria of, 10t-12t
  standards for recognition and approval of nursing specialties, 13-21, 16f, 17t-19t
American Diabetes Association (ADA), address for, 858t
American Kidney Fund (AKF), address for, 858t
American Nephrology Nurses' Association (ANNA)
  history of, 5
  members by state, 15, 16f
  mission statement of, 9t
  objectives of, 9, 9t
  position statements of, 18, 18t
  research-based practice promotion by, 14-15
  address for, 858t
  chronologic history of, 882-888
  history of, 35f, 36-38
    development of government relations program in, 37-38
  development of publications in, 36-37
  in organizing of nephrology nurses, 35f, 36
  in legislative arena, 791-792
  members in, 36, 37f
  nurses' role in
    certification in nephrology nursing, 38
    educational offerings, growth in, 38
  purposes of, 36
  research agenda, 115t, 119
  significant events in, 36-38
American Nephrology Nurses' Association (ANNA) Conceptual Model Task Force, accomplishments of, 70
American Nephrology Nurses' Association (ANNA) Health Policy Statement, 888-892
American Nephrology Nurses' Association (ANNA) Standards of Clinical Practice, assessment tool and intervention typology linkage to, 76
American Society for Artificial and Internal Organs (ASAIO), history of, 7
American Society of Nephrology (ASN), address for, 858t
American Society of Superintendents of Training Schools for Nurses, described, 6
Amino acids, for ARF, 227t
Aminoglycoside(s), in renal failure patients, 322
Amphotericin B
  renal damage due to, 317
  in renal failure patients, 323
Amyloidosis, 180
  hemodialysis-related, 561t, 570
  systemic, 180
Analgesic(s), in renal failure patients, 319
Analgesic nephropathy, described, 317
Andragogical model, theory of, 44
Andragogy, 44
Anemia
  in chronic renal failure, iron metabolism and, 290
  control of, in renal failure management, 521
  in renal failure, 254
    causes of, 521
    in children, 441
    drugs for, 325-326
Angiotensin converting enzyme (ACE) inhibitors, renal damage due to, 316
Angiotensin II
  in renal blood flow, 139f, 140
  in sodium reabsorption, 167
Angiotensin-converting enzyme (ACE) inhibitors
  in diabetic nephropathy management, 471
  for hypertension in renal failure, 520
  in renal failure patients, 320
Anion(s), non-reabsorbable, distal delivery of, in potassium secretion regulation, 149
ANNA. *See* American Nephrology Nurses' Association
ANNA Scope of Practice, 13
ANNA Standards of Clinical Practice for Nephrology Nursing, 14
Annas, G., 90
ANP. *See* Atrial natriuretic peptide
Antacids, in renal failure patients, 322
Anthropometric measurements
  described, 294
  nutritional assessment in renal patients, 294, 294f, 295f
Antianemic(s), in renal failure patients, 325-326
Antibiotic(s)
  antituberculosis, in renal failure patients, 324
  in peritoneal dialysis, 632, 632t
Antibody(ies)
  core, 355
  in humoral immune response, 682
  monoclonal
    in kidney transplantation, 338
    purpose, dose, administration, and side effects of, 333t
  polyclonal
    in kidney transplantation, 338
    purpose, dose, administration, and side effects of, 333t
Anticoagulation, during hemodialysis, 552-555. *See also* Hemodialysis, anticoagulation during
Antidiabetic agents, 324
Antidiuretic hormone (ADH)
  in renal blood flow, 140
  in urinary concentration and dilution, 144-145
Antifungal agents
  oral, for transplant recipients, 340
  in renal failure patients, 323
Antigen(s)
  ABO blood group, in renal transplantation, 685
  described, 680
Antigen elimination, mechanisms of, 684
Antigen processing and presentation, 680
Antigenicity, 680
Antigen-presenting cells (APCs), in immune response, 683-684
Antihypertensive(s)
  classes of, 320
  for hypertension in renal failure, 520
  in renal failure patients, 319-321
  for transplant recipients, 341
Anti-inflammatory drugs, nonsteroidal (NSAIDs)
  renal damage due to, 316
  in renal failure patients, 319
Antimicrobial agents, in renal failure patients, 322-323
Antioxidants, for ARF, 227t
Antiprinciplism period, of ethical theory development, 85t, 87-89
Antithymocyte globulin (ATG), in renal transplantation, 691t
Antituberculosis antibiotics, in renal failure patients, 323
Antiulcer medication, for transplant recipients, 340
Antiviral agents, in renal failure patients, 323-324
Anuria, conditions associated with, 203t
Anxiety, posttransplant, 748
APD. *See* Automated peritoneal dialysis
Apheresis
  continuous centrifuge, 592f
  therapeutic, historical review of, 590-591
Applegate, W.B., 418
ARF. *See* Acute renal failure
Arrhythmia(s), hemodialysis and, 560t, 568
Arterial pressure, during hemodialysis, monitoring of, 556-557
Arteriovascular disease, posttransplant, 731
Arteriovenous fistulas
  primary, in hemodialysis, 542-545, 542f, 544t
  sites of, 542f
Arteriovenous grafts, in hemodialysis, 545-548, 546f
Arteriovenous Teflon shunt, history of, 31
Artificial clearance, of pharmacologic agents, 315, 315t
Artificial kidney, history of, 28
Assessment
  in patient education, 840
  in standards of care, 825
Assist devices, in peritoneal dialysis, 617
Atherosclerosis, systemic, renal disease and, 183-184
Atrial natriuretic hormone, in sodium reabsorption, 167
Atrial natriuretic peptide (ANP)
  for ARF, 227t
  in renal blood flow, 141
Autograft, described, 666
Automated peritoneal dialysis (APD)
  described, 614t, 615
  for renal failure in children, 450, 452
Autonomic system, uremic syndrome effects on, nursing management of, 13
Autonomous practice, described, 46
Autonomy
  in care of elderly patients, 503-504
  defined, 86
Autoregulatory mechanism, in renal blood flow, 138-139

Autosomal dominant polycystic kidney disease (ADPKD), 184-185
Avascular necrosis, posttransplant, 746-747
Azathioprine
  in kidney transplantation, 337
  history of, 337
  purpose, dose, administration, and side effects of, 332t
  in renal transplantation, 690t
  side effects of, 335t, 337
Azidothymidine (AZT), for HIV infection, 366
Azotemia, prerenal, 214-218. *See also* Prerenal failure
Aztreonam, in renal failure patients, 323

B

B cells. *See* B lymphocytes
B lymphocytes (B cells), 671, 673
  values, characteristics, and function of, 672t
Bacille Calmette-Guérin (BCG) vaccine, for tuberculosis, 369-370
Back pain, peritoneal dialysis and, 649
Bacterial infections, posttransplant, 697t, 698-699
Baldree, K.S., 274
Barnett, R.C., 48-49
Basophil(s), values, characteristics, and function of, 672t
Batch system, dialysate, 534-535
Baxter Corporation, 32
BCG vaccine. *See* Bacille Calmette-Guérin (BCG) vaccine
Beach, D., 506
Beanlands, H., 276
Beauchamp, T., 86
Beecroft, P.C., 69
Beery Developmental Test of Visuomotor Integration, 442
Behavior
  nursing, patterns of, 47-48
  patterns of, 46-48, 46t
  professional, patterns of, 46-47, 46t
Behavioral adaptation, rehabilitation for, 423-424
Belenky, M.F., 116
Beneficence, defined, 86
Benner, P., 47
Bergum, V., 89
Berk Enamel Company, 31
Beta-adrenergic blockers, in renal failure patients, 318
Bicarbonate reclamation, described, 162-163
Bicarbonate reclamation process, 160f
Bicarbonate regeneration, described, 163
Bicarbonate regeneration process, 161f
Bile leaks, following liver transplantation, 767
Biliary complications, following liver transplantation, 767
Bill, how it becomes law, 783-785, 784f, 785f
Biochemical data, nutritional assessment in renal patients, 294
Bioethics
  birth of, 84-85
  principles of, 86-87, 86t
Bladder, examination of, in renal failure assessment, 207
Bleeding
  following liver transplantation, 765
  gastrointestinal, in uremic syndrome, factors contributing to, 257f
Blegen, M.A., 49
Blood, analysis of, following hemodialysis, 561-562
Blood analyses, in renal failure assessment, 206t, 207t, 208
Blood circuit, in hemodialysis, 532-533, 532f
  blood lines in, 532, 532f
  blood pump in, 532-533
  monitoring devices in, 533
  monitoring of, 556-557
Blood clots, posttransplant, in renal transplant recipient, 721
Blood flow
  hepatic, drug metabolism effects of, 312t, 313
  renal. *See* Renal blood flow
Blood glucose, control of, in diabetic nephropathy management, 471
Blood lines, in hemodialysis, 532, 532f
Blood pressure
  control of
    in diabetic nephropathy management, 471
    posttransplant, 731-732
    in renal failure management, 519-520
  elevation of, peritoneal dialysis and, 649
  posttransplant, in renal transplant recipients, 724
Blood pump, in hemodialysis, 532-533
Blood pump speeds, estimation of, 445, 445f
Blood urea nitrogen (BUN), in diabetic nephropathy diagnosis, 470
Blood volume, by age, in children, 444t
Bloodborne pathogens, exposure to, nursing management of, 382-383
Board of Directors, of nonprofit organizations, role of, 52-53, 52t
Body cell, 145f
Body fluid, classification of, 235t
Body fluid compartments, ionic composition of, 234f
Body image, in CRF patients, 273
Body size, renal failure effects on, 318t
Body temperature
  during hemodialysis, monitoring of, 557
  renal failure effects on, 318t
Bone disease, metabolic, following liver transplantation, 768
Bowel medications, for transplant recipients, 340
Bowman's capsule
  described, 131-132
  visceral layer of, described, 135f, 136
Boyle, R., 89
Brain death
  defined, 707
  determination of, criteria for, 708t
Bramlet, M., 91
Brazelton Scale for Infant Development, 442
Breckenridge, D.M., 69
Brenner, P., 53
Brequinar, in kidney transplantation, 337
Brett, J.L., 118
Briggs, M., 89
Bright, R., 28
Budd-Chiari syndrome, following liver transplantation, 766
Buffer pairs, 158f, 159
Buffer systems
  described, 158f, 159-160
  extracellular, 159f, 160-162
  intracellular, 159f, 160-162
Bumetanide, in renal failure patients, 317
BUN/creatinine ratio, in diabetic nephropathy diagnosis, 470

C

Cadmium, renal insufficiency due to, 191
Calcitonin, calcium transport and, 154
Calcitriol, in renal failure patients, 320-321
Calcium
  calcitonin and, 154
  in collecting tubule, 153
  in dialysate, 550
  in dialysis patients, 290
  in distal tubule, 152-153, 152f
  effects on membrane excitability, 240f
  excretion of, regulation of, 153-154, 153f
  functions of, 150-151
  imbalances of, 151
  in loop of Henle, 152
  in proximal tubule, 152
  PTH in regulation of, 152f, 153
  renal control of, 150-154
  renal handling of, 151-153, 151f
  role in, metabolic and physiologic processes, 241
  vitamin D3 and, 153-154
Calcium balance
  alterations in, in acute and chronic renal failure, 241-244, 242f, 242t, 243f
  hormonal regulation of, 242f
Calcium carbonate, in water, 536
Calcium channel blockers
  for ARF, 227t
  for hypertension in renal failure, 520
  in renal failure patients, 320
  in transplant recipients, 341
Calcium homeostasis, 150f, 151
Calcium levels, alterations in, ECG abnormalities associated with, 243f
Camp(s), as factor in children with renal failure, 460-461
Campaniello, J.A., 48
Candida albicans
  peritonitis due to, 641
  thrush due to, 704-705
Candidiasis, posttransplant, 704-705
CAPD. *See* Continuous ambulatory peritoneal dialysis
Capillary endothelium, described, 135f, 136
Cardenas, D.D., 409
Cardiac arrest, hemodialysis and, 560t, 568
Cardiac evaluation, in renal transplant recipient evaluation, 713
Cardiac failure, ARF and, 216, 216f
Cardiotonic(s), in renal failure patients, 321
Cardiovascular disease, posttransplant, 731
Cardiovascular system
  changes in, in elderly patients with renal disease, 485-487, 486t
  diabetic effects on, 749t
  disorders of, posttransplant, of renal transplant recipient, 724-725
  renal failure in children effects on, 440
  uremic syndrome effects on, 251f, 252-254, 252t
    nursing management of, 13-14
Care ethic, 88
Career opportunities, for nephrology nurses, 39-40

Caregivers, of the elderly, 506
Carlson, L., 410
Carnitine, in dialysis patients, 291-292
Carper, B.A., 116
Carrel, A., 663
Cascade (secondary) plasma filtration, 594, 594f
Cascade (secondary) plasma filtration circuit, 594f
Case management
  described, 51
  nursing opportunities in, 40
Casts, in urine, 211
Casuistry, described, 88
Cates, D.S., 48
Cathartic(s), in renal failure patients, 321
Catheter(s)
  acute, in access to peritoneal cavity for peritoneal dialysis, 620
  chronic
    in access to peritoneal cavity for peritoneal dialysis, 620-625
    care of, 622-625, 624t, 625t
    extraperitoneal cuffs in, 620-621
    insertion of, 621-622
    segments of, 620
    types of, 621f
  cuffed double-lumen silastic, in hemodialysis, 548-549, 548f
  femoral vein, in hemodialysis, 540
  in hemodialysis in pediatric renal patients, 448
  jugular vein, in hemodialysis, 541
  in peritoneal dialysis management, complications associated with, 646-648
  subclavian vein, in hemodialysis, 538-540, 538f
  vein, in hemodialysis, 540
Cation-exchange resins, for non-life-threatening hyperkalemia, 323-325
CAVH. *See* Continuous arteriovenous hemofiltration
CAVU. *See* Continuous arteriovenous ultrafiltration
CCPD. *See* Continuous cyclic peritoneal dialysis
Cell(s)
  body, 145f
  epithelial, described, 135f, 136
  lymphokine activated killer, function of, 683
  mast, values, characteristics, and function of, 672t
  mesangial, of glomerulus, 136
  natural killer, function of, 683
  pancreatic, function of, 749, 749t
  regulatory, function of, 682
Cellcept. *See* Mofetil
Cell-mediated immune response, 682-683
Cellular immune response, 670-671
Central hemodialysis delivery systems, 445
Cephalosporin(s), in renal failure patients, 321
Certified Nephrology Nurses (CNNs), members by state, 15, 16f
Chalmers, H., 68
Champion, V., 118
Charitable corporations, laws related to, 52
"Chemical" peritonitis, described, 640
Chemotaxis, described, 673t
Chest pain, hemodialysis and, 558t, 564-565
Chest x-rays, in tuberculosis detection, 373
Children. *See also under* Pediatric
  growth and development in, posttransplant, 747
  rehabilitation for, 415-417, 416t
  renal failure in, 435-465
    acquired, 440
    anemia due to, 441
    camp experiences for, 460-461
    CAPD for, 438
    cardiovascular effects of, 440
    causes of, 439-440
    congenital, 439-440
    cutaneous effects of, 440
    diabetes and, 439
    effects of, 440-444
    epidemiological data, 438t, 439
    family relationships and, 458
    gastrointestinal effects of, 440
    genitourinary effects of, 441
    growth and development effects of, 442-444
    hematologic effects of, 441
    hemodialysis for, 437-438
    hemolysis due to, 441
    hypertension and, 439
    ICU care for, 437
    immune effects of, 442
    intermittent peritoneal dialysis in, 437
    metabolic effects of, 441
    $\beta_2$microglobulin deposition in, 441
    neuromuscular effects of, 441
    normal life of, 458-461
    nursing opportunities related to, 39
    peritoneal lavage for, 438
    play in life of, 459-460
    prevalence of, 439
    programs assisting families of, 461-462
      financial, 461
      in foreign countries, 462
      information sources, 461-462
    psychosocial care in, 458-459
    renal transplant surgery for, 438
    respiratory effects of, 441
    school placement for, 460
    skeletal effects of, 441
    special occasions of, 460-461
    travel of, 460
    treatment for, 437, 444-458
      age as factor in, 439
      CRRTs, 453-455, 454f
      environment during, 457-458
      hemodialysis, 444-450, 444t, 445f, 446t, 449t. *See also* Hemodialysis, for renal failure in children
      measuring adequacy of dialysis in, 455
      nursing interventions in, 456
      nutrition needs in, 456
      peritoneal dialysis, 450-453, 451f, 452f. *See also* Peritoneal dialysis, for renal failure in children
      pharmacologic concerns in, 456-457
      transplantation, 455
  renal insufficiency in, growth retardation due to, 651
  renal transplantation in, 710
Childress, J., 86
Chills, hemodialysis and, 558t, 565
Chloride reabsorption
  in early distal tubule, 171-172, 171f
  in early proximal tubule, 169-170, 169f
  in late distal tubule and collecting ducts, 172, 172f
  in thick ascending limb of Henle, 170f, 171
Choledochocholedochostomy, 762, 763f
Choledochojejunostomy, 762, 764f
Choosing, in NANDA taxonomy classification system for nursing diagnoses, 825t, 827t
Chronic illnesses
  described, 270
  prevalence of, 270
  sexuality among the elderly and, 489-490
Chronic interstitial disease, 183
Chronic obstructive pulmonary disease (COPD), as contraindication for pulmonary dialysis, 619
Chronic rejection
  following liver transplantation, 766-767
  posttransplant, 695t, 697, 726-727, 730
Chronic renal failure (CRF), 230-234. *See also* Psychosocial issues, in renal disease
  body image in, 273
  causes of, 230-233
  clinical features of, 233, 234f
  compliance in, 272-273
  coping strategies for, 274
  costs of care for, 230
  depression related to, 274
  described, 230, 270
  diabetes and, drugs for, 324
  in the elderly, education related to, 501
  fluid, electrolyte, and acid-base disturbances in, 234-247
  hypertension in, 319-320
  illness trajectory of, 270-271
  impact on family, 276-277
  infertility due to, 651
  intrusiveness in, 272
  laboratory findings in, 233
  lack of control due to, 271-272
  metabolic and endocrine disturbances in, 247-249, 249t
  noncompliance in, 272-273
  pathophysiology of, 230-233, 231f, 232t, 233f
  powerlessness due to, 271-272
  prevalence of, 230
  prevention of, 233-234
  progression of, mediation of, risk factors for, 232t
  psychosocial impact of, 269-283
  sexuality and, 273-274, 274t, 275t
  social support for, 274-276
  stressors associated with, 271, 271t
  systemic manifestations of, 234-260
  treatment of, 233-234
    government's role in, 32-33
    restrictions imposed by, 272-273
  uremic syndrome in, 250-260. *See also* Uremic syndrome, in ARF and CRF
Chronology, renal failure effects on, 318t
Church, J., 118
Chvostek's sign, 243
Chyatte, S., 407
Cimetidine, in renal failure patients, 322
Circulation, renal, described, 134f, 135-136

Clark, C.C., 118
Clearance
  creatinine
    defined, 612
    formulas for, 613, 613t
  estimation of, 445, 445f
  in hemodialysis, 530
  of pharmacologic agents, 315, 315t
  plasma, defined, 612
  in solute removal and transport, 612-613, 613f, 613t
  urea, defined, 612
Clinchy, B.M., 116
Clinical nurse specialists (CNSs), described, 51
Clinical practice guidelines, 822-824
  AHCPR-sponsored, 824t
  application of, 823
  described, 822
  goals of, 822-823
  historical background of, 823
  selection of topics, 823
Clinical roles, of nephrology nurses, 49-51, 50t
Clostridium difficile infection, posttransplant, 697t, 698
Clotting system, characteristics of, 677t
CMV. *See* Cytomegalovirus
CNNs. *See* Certified Nephrology Nurses (CNNs)
CNSs. *See* Clinical nurse specialists
COBRA 1985, 804
Cockcroft and Gault equation, 212
Codeine, in renal failure patients, 319
Cognitive development, renal failure in children effects on, 443-444
Cognitive learning, 844-845
Cold, OTC medications for, 340t
Coleman-Wysocki, B., 33f, 34, 34f, 35
Colic, renal, conditions associated with, 203t
Collaboration, in ethical decision making, 99-100
Collecting ducts, sodium and chloride reabsorption in, 172, 172f
Collecting tubules, 133
  calcium transport in, 153
  filtrate composition of, 143
Colloid oncotic pressure, described, 610
Colloid osmotic pressure, described, 610
Colony stimulating factors (CSF)
  functions of, 679t
  types of, 679t
Committee for the Organization of a
National Association for Nurses, described, 6
Communicating, in NANDA taxonomy classification system for nursing diagnoses, 825t, 827t
Communication
  in assessment of elderly patients, 492
  in ethical decision making, 99-100
  importance of, 49, 49t
  in legislative process, 789-791
Competency, defined, 53
Complement, 674-675, 675f
Complement activation, hemodialysis and, 561t, 569-570
Complement cascade, 674, 675f
Complement components, characteristics of, 677t
Complement system, functions of, 674
Complement-dependent cytotoxic test, 688
Compliance
  in CRF patients, 272-273
  defined, 272
Concentration gradient, defined, 609
Concept(s), defined, 62
Conceptual Bases of Professional Nursing, 824
Conceptual framework. *See* Conceptual models of nursing
Conceptual models of nursing, 61-83
  defined, 62
  described, 62-67, 63t-66t
  functions of, 67-68
  future directions in, 76
  and nephrology nursing practice, 68
  overview of, 63t-66t
  review of literature, 68-70
  value of, 68
Conceptual Models Task Force, of ANNA, accomplishments of, 70
Conceptual system. *See* Conceptual models of nursing
Conductivity, during hemodialysis, monitoring of, 557
Congenital anomalies, renal failure in children due to, 439-440
Congestion, sinus, OTC medications for, 340t
Congestive heart failure, uremic syndrome and, 252
Connective tissue, aging effects on, 486t
Consequentialists, described, 86
Constipation
  OTC medications for, 340t
  posttransplant, of renal transplant recipient, 724
Consultation, ethics, 100-101
Content of nursing, 47
Contextual ethics, 88
Continuous ambulatory peritoneal dialysis (CAPD)
  described, 614, 614t
  for renal failure in children, 438, 450
  stressors associated with, 271, 271t
  treatment of, 298t
Continuous arteriovenous hemofiltration (CAVH). *See* Continuous renal replacement therapy
  for ARF, 581
  for renal failure in children, 453-454
  uses of, 580
Continuous arteriovenous ultrafiltration (CAVU). *See* Continuous renal replacement therapy
Continuous centrifuge apheresis, 592f
Continuous cyclic peritoneal dialysis, for renal failure in children, 450, 452
Continuous cyclic peritoneal dialysis (CCPD)
  described, 614, 614t
  treatment of, 298t
Continuous flow centrifugation, development of, 592, 592f
Continuous quality improvement (CQI), 832-833
  in patient care, 857-858
Continuous renal replacement therapy (CRRT), 577-587
  components of, 578, 579f
  diagrams of, 583f
  equipment for, 578-582
  hemofilters in, 578-582
  monitoring of, formulae and calculations for, 580, 580t
  nursing care during, 583f-584
  nursing care following, 584
  nursing care prior to, 582-583, 583f
  nursing literature related to, 584-585
  for renal failure in children, 453-455
    access issues in, 455
    CAVH, 453-454
    complications of, 455
    CVVH, 454
    hemodiafiltration, 454-455, 454f
    techniques, 453-455, 454f
  research related to, 584-585
  technologies associated with, 578-582
  uses of, 580
Continuous venovenous hemofiltration (CVVH), for renal failure in children, 454
Control loss, CRF-related, 271, 271t
Convective transport, in solute removal and transport, 612
COPD. *See* Chronic obstructive pulmonary disease
Coping strategies, for CRF patients, 274
Coping with life, among the elderly, 491
Core antibodies (anti-HBc), 355
Corporate/government arena, nursing opportunities in, 40-41
Cortex, described, 130-131, 131f
Corticosteroid(s)
  in kidney transplantation, 335t, 337-338
  for minimal change disease, 180
Cough, OTC medications for, 340t
Cramp(s), muscle, hemodialysis and, 558t, 564
Creatinine
  in diabetic nephropathy diagnosis, 470
  molecular weight of, 609t
Creatinine clearance
  calculation of, 137
  defined, 612
  in diabetic nephropathy diagnosis, 469
  formulas for, 212, 469-470, 613, 613t
  in peritoneal dialysis adequacy, 637
  in renal failure assessment, 212
CRF. *See* Chronic renal failure
Criteria for Approval of Specialties, 9
Crixivan, for HIV infection, 366
Crossmatch(es)
  mixed lymphocyte, 688
  white cell, 688
CRRT. *See* Continuous renal replacement therapy
Cruz catheter with coiled intraperitoneal segment, 621f
Crystals, in urine, 211
Cuffed double-lumen silastic catheters, in hemodialysis, 548-549, 548f
Cultural diversity in renal patients, 300
Cupit, M.C., 69
Cycler(s), in peritoneal dialysis, 618
Cyclophosphamide
  purpose, dose, administration, and side effects of, 333t
  in renal transplantation, 690t
Cyclosporine
  absorption of, 334
  administration of, 332t
  described, 334
  dosage of, 332t
  drug interactions with, 334
  in kidney transplantation, 332-334
    history of, 333
  monitoring levels of, 334-336, 336t

primary action of, 334
purpose, dose, administration, and side effects of, 332t
purpose of, 332t
in renal transplantation, 690t
side effects of, 332t, 334, 335t
Cyclosporine G, in kidney transplantation, 339
Cyst(s), renal, 184-185
Cystitis, acute, 188
Cytapheresis, described, 590
Cytokine(s), 678t-679t
characteristics of, 677t
function of, 683
Cytomegalovirus (CMV)
from general community, 700
fulminant, posttransplant, 700
posttransplant, 697t, 699-701, 699t
causes of, 699
clinical manifestations of, 700
diagnosis of, 700-701
epidemiologic patterns of, 699-700
of gastrointestinal tract, treatment of, 700
incidence of, 700
management of, 701
organs affected by, 700
presentation of, 700
prevalence of, 699
risk factors for, 699
Cytomegalovirus (CMV) superinfection, 700
Cytotoxic T cells
function of, 683
in immune response, 684
Cytoxan. *See* Cyclophosphamide

D

Dane particle, 355
Death and dying, in care of elderly patients, 504
Decision making
in care of elderly patients, 503-504
ethical, 91-93, 92t
Deferoxamine, for ARF, 227t
Degranulation, described, 673t
Deionization, in water purification, 537, 537f
Delivery systems, for peritoneal dialysis, 615-618, 615f, 616f, 617t
Dementia, dialysis, 250-251
Denver Developmental Screening Test, 442
Deontological theory, of ethical theory development, 86
15-Deoxyspergualin, in kidney transplantation, 339-340
Depression
in CRF, 274
in the elderly, 491
posttransplant, 748
Dermatologic system, uremic syndrome effects on, 256-257, 256t
nursing management of, 16
Dextran, iron, for anemia of renal failure, 326
Dextrose, in dialysate, 550
Diabetes
insulin-dependent, pancreas transplantation for, 748
renal failure due to, drugs for, 324
renal failure in children due to, 439
steroid-induced, posttransplant, 747
Diabetes Control and Complications Trial (DCCT), 468
Diabetes mellitus, 465-479, 749-750. *See also* Diabetic nephropathy
complications of, 467
control of, in renal failure management, 520
described, 467
dialysis for, survival following, 467
extrarenal disease due to, 471-472
forms of, 467
insulin in, dosage determinants, 468
insulin-dependent, described, 467
macroangiopathy due to, 472
metabolic complications of, 472
microangiopathy due to, 472
nephrology nurses' role in, 477
non-insulin-dependent, described, 467
peritoneal dialysis for patients with, insulin requirements for, 651-652
pregnancy effects of, 472
rehabilitation for, 415
risk factors for, 468
screening for, 468
systemic manifestations of, 749t
type I, described, 467
type II, described, 467
types of, 750
Diabetic nephropathy, 188, 467. *See also* under Diabetes mellitus
chronic renal failure due to, 520
clinical features of, 470-471
management of, 471-477
ACE inhibitors, 471
contraindications for, 474
control of blood glucose levels, 471
control of blood pressure, 471
hemodialysis, 474-475
indications for, 474
medical assessment in, 472-473
patient assessment in, 472
patient education, 471
peritoneal dialysis, 475-476
protein restriction, 471
social-family issues in, 473-474
transplantation, 476-477
clinical history of, 469
diagnosis of, 469-470
laboratory tests in, 469-470
physical examination in, 469
physiological changes leading to, 467
stages of, 467-468
structural and functional abnormalities in, 468-469
Diabetic patients, 465-479. *See also* under Diabetes mellitus
Diagnosis
described, 46
in patient education, 840
Diagnostic tests, in renal failure assessment, 206t, 207-214, 207t-211t, 213t
Dialysate
calcium in, 550
dextrose in, 550
in hemodialysis, 533-534, 533t
potassium in, 550
sodium in, 550
Dialysate circuit, 534-535, 534f
dialysate lines in, 534f, 535
in hemodialysis, monitoring of, 557
monitoring devices in, 535
Dialysate delivery systems, types of, 534-535, 534f
Dialysate lines, in dialysate circuit, 534f, 535
Dialysis
in acute renal failure, mortality associated with, 214
adaptation to, stages of, 270
defined, 606
for diabetic patients, survival following, 467
diet for, 288-292
calcium in, 290
carnitine in, 291-292
energy requirements in, 291
fluid in, 288
hyperlipidemia in, 291
iron in, 290
phosphorus in, 290
potassium in, 288, 289t
protein in, 291
sodium in, 288
vitamin C in, 290
Vitamin D in, 290
zinc in, 290
drug elimination by, 314
first procedure of, in U.S., 28, 28f
for glomerulonephritis, survival following, 467
heparin-free, 553
history of, 27-42
HIV infection in patients on, 349
home, 5
malnutrition and, 294, 296t, 296-298, 297t
IDPN for, 296-298, 297t
nutritional supplementation for, 296
peritoneal, 603-657. *See also* Peritoneal dialysis
intermittent. *See* Intermittent peritoneal dialysis
regulatory activity related to, 808-809
requirements for, 606
Dialysis dementia, 250-251
Dialysis disequilibrium syndrome, hemodialysis and, 559t, 565-566
Dialysis encephalopathy, 560t, 569
Dialysis solution. *See also* Dialysate
in hemodialysis, 533-534, 533t, 550
in peritoneal dialysis prescription, 629-631, 629t, 630t
Dialysis unit, size of, stress related to, 49
Dialyzer, structure of, 530-531, 530f
Dialyzer(s). *See also* Hemodialysis system
design of, general scheme for, 527f
hoop form, history of, 28
membrane composition of, 531-532, 532t
reuse of, 572-573
structure of, 530-531, 530f
types of, 531-532, 532t
Dialyzer reactions, hemodialysis and, 559t, 567-568
Diapedesis, described, 673t
Diarrhea
OTC medications for, 340t
posttransplant, of renal transplant recipient, 724
Didanosine, for HIV infection, 366
Dideoxycytidine, for HIV infection, 366
Dideoxyinosine, for HIV infection, 366
Diet
for dialysis, 288-292. *See also* Dialysis, diet for

as factor in renal failure progression, 287-288
in renal failure management, 520-521
Dietary potassium intake, in potassium secretion regulation, 148
Dietitians, in nutritional care of renal patients, 287
Diffusion
defined, 608
factors affecting, 608-610, 610t
in hemodialysis, 527-528, 529f
in solute removal and transport, 608-610, 609t, 610t
Digoxin, in renal failure patients, 321
Diminished renal reserve, defined, 201
Disability, classification for, 407
Disciplinary matrix. *See* Conceptual models of nursing
Disconnect systems, in peritoneal dialysis, 615-616, 615f, 617t
Distal tubule(s)
calcium transport in, 152-153, 152f
described, 132-133
filtrate composition of, 143
reabsorption in, 171-172, 171f, 172f
Distal tubule flow rate, in potassium secretion regulation, 148-149, 148f
Distribution, drug, factors affecting, 311-312, 311t
Diuretics
for ARF, 227t
potassium-sparing, in renal failure patients, 317
in renal failure patients, 315, 317
Diverticular disease, as contraindication for pulmonary dialysis, 619
Documentation, and nursing process, 824-833
Docusate sodium, for transplant recipients, 340
Donor evaluation
living-kidney transplant, 715-717, 716t
in renal transplantation, 715-717, 716t
Donor management, in transplantation, 707-708, 709t
Donor recovery, in transplantation, 708-710, 710t
Donor-specific transfusions (DSTs), in renal transplant recipients, 717
Dopamine
for ARF, 227t
in renal blood flow, 140
Dossetor, J., 89
Double-cuff Swan Neck catheter with straight intraperitoneal segment, 621f
Double-cuff Tenckhoff catheter with coiled intraperitoneal segment, 621f
Double-cuff Tenckhoff catheter with straight intraperitoneal segment, 621f
Dow Corporation, 31-32
Dribbling, conditions associated with, 203t
Drucker, P., 52
Drug(s). *See* under Pharmacologic agents
Drug actions, time course of, 313, 313f
Drug activity, normal, process of, 309, 309f
Drug distribution, factors affecting, 311-312, 311t
Drug elimination, through artificial clearance, 315, 315t
Drug overdose, during hemodialysis, treatment of, 572
DTPA radiology study, in renal transplantation, goal and interpretation of, 721t
Durable Power of Attorney for Health Care, 504
Dysfunctional organ systems, renal failure effects on, 318t
Dysrhythmia(s), hemodialysis and, 560t, 568
Dysuria, in renal failure assessment, 203t

E

EBV. *See* Epstein-Barr virus
Eddy, D., 102
Edema
conditions associated with, 203t
pulmonary, uremic syndrome and, 254
EDRF. *See* Endothelium-derived relaxing factor
Education
defined, 1675
for elderly renal disease patients, 501-502, 502f
ethics, in ethical decision making, 100
nursing opportunities in, 40
patient, 837-852. *See also* Patient education
in psychological stability of the elderly, 493
in rehabilitation of elderly patients, 505
transplantation-related, 714
Educational background, sexuality among the elderly and, 490
Educators, nurse, 51-52
Egalitarians, theory of justice, 86t, 87
Eicosanoid synthesis, in renal blood flow, 139-140
Elderly patients, 481-513. *See also* Aging
assessment of, 491-495
biological data in, 493
communication techniques during, 492
environmental setting during, 492
nursing strategies and adaptations in, 492
psychological/emotional data in, 493-494, 494f
social/functional data in, 494-495
timing of, 492
tools and interventions in, 492-495, 494f
care of
ethical aspects of, 502-504
quality of life in, 503
resource allocation in, 503
caregivers of, 506
comprehensive nursing assessment and interventions for, 491-495
coping with life among, 491
depression in, 491
dietary restrictions in, 497-498
drug therapy for, 498-501, 500t
compliance issues related to, 499-500
nursing interventions for, 500-501
pharmacodynamics of, 499
pharmacokinetics of, 499
education of, 501-502, 502f
CRF-related, 501
environmental conditions related to, 501
in the elderly
instructional systems design in, 501-502, 502f
outcomes following, 502
psychological stability of, interventions for, 493-494, 494f
rehabilitation for, 417-420, 418t, 419t
rehabilitation in, 504-506
renal disease in
cardiovascular system effects of, 485-487, 486t
holistic care for, 484
incidence of, 483
issues related to, 484-491
medical treatment for, goal of, 484
nursing home placement for, 484
physiological/functional changes related to, 484-488, 486t-487t
prevalence of, 483
psychosocial challenges and realities related to, 488-491, 490t
renal system effects of, 487t, 488
respiratory system effects of, 487t, 488
sensory changes with, 485, 486t
renal replacement therapies for, 495-497
research on, 506-507, 508t, 509t
sexuality of, 489-491, 490t
spirituality among, 491
Electrolyte(s)
monitoring of, posttransplant, in renal transplant recipients, 720-723, 722t
urinary, in renal failure assessment, 211-212, 211t
Electrolyte supplements
in renal failure patients, 321
for transplant recipients, 340
Elimination
described, 313
of pharmacologic agents, 313-314, 313f
ELISA (enzyme-linked immunosorbent assay), in HIV infection detection, 365
Embolism, air, hemodialysis and, 559t, 566-567
Employment, in rehabilitation of elderly patients, 505-506
Empowerment, in psychological stability of the elderly, 493
Enabling, in psychological stability of the elderly, 493
Encephalopathy, dialysis, 560t, 569
End Stage Renal Disease (ESRD) Network system, 857
End Stage Renal Disease (ESRD) Program, 795-813
Amendments of 1978, 803
COBRA 1985, 804
continuance of, 809-812, 811t
current considerations related to, 810-811, 811t
described, 467, 797
future considerations related to, 812
genesis of, 797-798
history of, 798
legislative and regulatory history of, 798-809, 799t-802t
Social Security Amendments of 1972, 798-803, 799t-802t

Medicare amendments for 1993 and 1994, 808
National Organ Transplant Act of 1984, 804
OBRA 1981, 803-804
OBRA 1986, 804-805, 805f
OBRA 1987, 805-806
OBRA 1989, 806
OBRA 1990, 806-807
OBRA 1993, 807-808
past considerations related to, 809-810
percentage of patients in, 467
Transplant Amendments Act of 1990, 807
End Stage Renal Disease (ESRD) Program of Medicare, 404
Endocrine assessment, in renal transplant recipient evaluation, 713
Endocrine disorders
in acute and chronic renal failure, 248-249, 249t
nursing management of, 11
Endocrine system
aging effects on, 487t
peritoneal dialysis effects on, 651-652
Endothelin, in renal blood flow, 140
Endothelium, capillary, described, 135f, 136
Endothelium-derived relaxing factor (EDRF), in renal blood flow, 140-141
End-stage renal disease (ESRD)
health outcomes database for, 422-423
malnutrition in, causes of, 296, 296t
peritoneal dialysis for, 603-657. *See also* Peritoneal dialysis
pre-, treatment of, 298t
quality of life associated with, 277
End-stage renal disease (ESRD) treatment modality, and rehabilitation, 414-415
Energy, in dialysis patients, 291
Enterococcus(i), vancomycin-resistant, 392, 394-395
Environment, effects on renal failure treatment in children, 457-458
Environmental conditions, in education of elderly renal disease patients, 501
Environmental issues, in dietary restrictions in the elderly, 498
Environmental setting, in assessment of elderly patients, 492
Enzyme(s)
in drug metabolism, 312, 312t
lysosomal, characteristics of, 677t
Enzyme-linked immunosorbent assay (ELISA), in HIV infection detection, 365
Eosinophil(s), values, characteristics, and function of, 672t
Eosinophil chemotactic factor of anaphylaxis (ECFA), characteristics of, 677t
Epidemiology
analytic, 351
descriptive, 351
methods in, 351-352
nurse's role in, 352-353
overview of, 350-353
Epidermal growth factor (EGF), for ARF, 227t
Episode of peritonitis, described, 640
Epithelial cells, described, 135f, 136
Epivir, for HIV infection, 366
Epoetin alfa (EPO), for anemia of renal failure, 325
Epstein-Barr virus (EBV) infection
following liver transplantation, 767
posttransplant, 697t, 701-702
Equilibration, defined, 609
Erickson, P., 412, 420
Erythromycin, in renal failure patients, 323
ESRD. *See* End-stage renal disease
ESRD Rehabilitation Task Force, 404-405
Essential hypertension. *See* Hypertension
Ethambutol, for tuberculosis, 375-377, 376t
Ethic(s)
care, 88
contextual, 88
defined, 84
described, 84
principle-oriented, basis of, 87-88
virtue, 88
Ethical decision making, 91-93, 92t
strategies in enhancement of, 99-102
collaboration, 99-100
communication, 99-100
ethics at bedside, 100
ethics consultation, 100-101
ethics education, 100
research, 101
resource allocation, public and health care provider dialogue about, 101-102
Ethical issues, 83-109
in care of elderly patients, 502-504
autonomy, 503-504
death and dying, 504
decision making, 503-504
quality of life, 503
resource allocation, 503
case studies, 93-98
future directions in, 102-103
in gerontological research, 507
levels of professional responsibility, 89-91, 89t
Ethical theories, 85-89, 85t, 8787t
antiprinciplism period of, 85t, 87-89
development of, 85-89, 85t
Hippocratic period of, 85t, 86
period of principlism in, 85t, 86
Ethics consultation, in ethical decision making, 100-101
Ethics education, in ethical decision making, 100
Ethics of strangers, 88
Ethics resources, 91-93, 92t
Ethics rounds, in ethical decision making, 100
Evaluation
described, 54
in patient education, 841
as process to improve medical practice, 421
in rehabilitation of elderly patients, 506
in standards of care, 830-832
Evans, R.W., 412
Exchange(s)
dialysis, in peritoneal dialysis prescription, 628-629, 628t
peritoneal dialysis, 614
Exchanging, in NANDA taxonomy classification system for nursing diagnoses, 825t, 826t-827t
Excretion, described, 134-135
Executive branch, of federal government, 783, 783f
Exercise, in rehabilitation process, 409-410
in elderly patients, 505
Exit site infections, peritoneal dialysis and, 643-645, 645t
Exsanguination, hemodialysis and, 560t, 569
External arteriovenous shunt, in hemodialysis, 541-542, 541f
Extracellular fluid volume, renal regulation of, 164-173
Extracorporeal dialysis, drug elimination by, 314

F

Family, CRF effects on, 276-277
Family history, in renal failure assessment, 202
Family issues, in diabetic nephropathy management, 473-474
Family relationships, of children in renal failure, 458
Fawcett, J., 69-70
Federal budget process, 786-787
Federal government
committee structure in, 785-786
committee work in, 786
conference committee in, 786
executive branch of, 783, 783f
House and Senate action in, 786
judicial branch of, 783, 783f
legislative branch of, 783, 783f
presidential action in, 786
structure of, 782-783, 783f
subcommittee work in, 785-786
voting process, 786
Federal government hemodialysis grants, in CRF treatment, 32-33
Federal regulatory process, 787
Feeling, in NANDA taxonomy classification system for nursing diagnoses, 825t, 828t
Fellows, B., 34
Femoral vein catheters, in hemodialysis, 540
FENa. *See* Fractional excretion of sodium
Fever
with bacterial infections, 698
hemodialysis and, 558t, 565
Filtration, in water purification, 536
Filtration fraction, described, 137
Fistula(s), arteriovenous
primary, 542-545, 542f, 544t
sites of, 542t
FK506. *See* Tacrolimus
Fluid(s)
in dialysis patients, 288
monitoring of, posttransplant, in renal transplant recipients, 720-723, 722t
Fluid and electrolyte balance
in acute and chronic renal failure, 234-247
alterations in, nursing management of, 3-8
Fluid balance, alterations in, in acute and chronic renal failure, 236
Fluid removal, in hemodialysis, 550
calculation of, 446t
Fluid volume, alterations in, peritoneal dialysis and, 649-650, 650t
Fluorescence polarization immunoassay (FPIA), in cyclosporine monitoring, 334-335, 336t
Focal glomerulosclerosis, 189
Fowler, M., 90, 91
Fox, D., 101-102

Fractional excretion of sodium (FENa), 211
Frank, D.I., 69
Freeman, R., 91
Frequency, conditions associated with, 203t
Fry, S., 90
Function(s), defined, 53
Functional changes, in elderly patients with renal disease, 484-488, 486t-487t
Functional roles, of nephrology nurses, 49-51, 50t
Fungal infections, posttransplant, 697t, 704-705
Furosemide, in renal failure patients, 317

G

Gadow, S., 90
Gagne's hierarchy of learning, 845t
Ganciclovir, in renal failure patients, 323
Ganter, G., in peritoneal dialysis, 605
Gardner, D.L., 49
Gastrointestinal bleeding, in uremic syndrome, factors contributing to, 257f
Gastrointestinal (GI) problems, evaluation of, in renal transplant recipient evaluation, 713
Gastrointestinal system
  aging effects on, 487t
  diabetic effects on, 749t
  monitoring of, posttransplant, in renal transplant recipients, 724-725
  renal failure in children effects on, 440
  uremic syndrome effects on, 257-259, 257f
    nursing management of, 16-17
Gender
  as factor in nursing profession, 47
  renal failure effects on, 318t
Gene-cloning techniques, 688
Genetic factors
  renal failure effects on, 318t
  in renal transplantation, 684-685
Genital system, aging effects on, 487t
Genitourinary system, renal failure in children effects on, 441
Geriatric patients. *See* Aging; Elderly patients
Gerontological research, 506-507, 508t, 509t
  ethical issues related to, 507
  future implications in, 507
  methodological considerations in, 507
GFR. *See* Glomerular filtration rate
Gillies, D.A., 118
Gilligan, C., 88
Gillon, R., 88
Glomerular basement membrane
  described, 135f, 136
  injury to, glomerular disease due to, 178
Glomerular diseases, 178-182
  causes of, 178
  classification of, 178, 178t
  nephritic syndrome, 180-181
  nephrotic syndrome, 179-180
  pathology of, 179
  primary, 178, 178t
  renal failure due to, 178
  secondary, 178, 178t
Glomerular filtration
  described, 134, 135, 135f, 136-138
  and filtration fraction, 136-138, 137f
  pressures influencing, 137-138, 137f
Glomerular filtration rate (GFR)
  calculation of, 136-137
  conditions altering, 138
  in continuum of renal function, 201, 201t
  described, 136-137
Glomerular mass, loss of, renal response to, 231f
Glomerulonephritis
  dialysis for, survival following, 467
  postinfectious acute, 181-182
    nonstreptococcal, 182
  poststreptococcal, 181-182
  rapidly progressive, 182
Glomerulopathy, membranous, in nephrotic syndrome, 180
Glomerulosclerosis, focal, 189
Glomerulus
  anatomy of, 135f, 136
  described, 131, 135-136
Glucose
  blood, control of, in diabetic nephropathy management, 471
  molecular weight of, 609t
Glucose intolerance
  in acute and chronic renal failure, 247-248
  nursing management of, 10
  in renal failure, 520
Glycine, for ARF, 227t
Glycoprotein, alpha, acid, drugs that bind to, 310t
Goal-oriented nursing record, 68
God Squad, 85
Goldberger, J.M., 116
Goodenough Draw-A-Man test, 442
Gottschalk, C., 33
Gottschalk Committee on Chronic Kidney Disease, 33
Gottscho, I., 32
Gottscho Packaging Company, 32
Government
  federal. *See* Federal government
    participation in, 782
Graft(s)
  arteriovenous, in hemodialysis, 545-548, 546f
  transplant, types of, 666t
Graft rupture, posttransplant, 728-729, 728t
Graham, T., 28
Granger, C., 505
Granulocyte(s)
  described, 671, 673t
  function of, uremic syndrome and, 255
  polymorphonuclear, values, characteristics, and function of, 672t
Greater omentum, described, 608
Growth and development
  cognitive development, renal failure in children effects on, 443-444
  physical development, renal failure in children effects on, 442-443
  posttransplant, 747
  psychosocial development, renal failure in children effects on, 443-444
  renal failure in children effects on, 442-444
  sexual maturation, renal failure in children effects on, 442-443
Growth factors, for ARF, 227t
Growth retardation, in infants and children with renal insufficiency, 651
Gueldner, S., 91
Guideline(s), *versus* standards, 822
Gullberg, M.T., 45
Gurklis, A., 274
Gutman, R.A., 404

H

Hadorn, D., 102
Half-life, 313
Hand, position of, in hypocalcemic tetany, 243f
Handicapped Children's Assistance, for children with renal failure, 461
Harvey, Sir W., 27
Hathaway, D., 69
Havinghurst, R.J., 488-489
Havrix, for hepatitis A virus, 354
Hayne, Y., 68
Hayward, M.B., 69
Headache, OTC medications for, 340t
Health Care Financing Administration (HCFA), 404-405
Health Care Quality Improvement Program (HCQIP), 857
Health care workers, HIV infection in, risk factors for, 366-367
Health outcomes assessment, strategies for, 421-422, 422t
Health outcomes database, for ESRD, 422-423
Hearing, aging effects on, 486t
Heart. *See also* under Cardiac
  evaluation of, in renal transplant recipient evaluation, 713
Heart failure, ARF and, 216, 216f
Heffnagel, H., 663
Helper T cells
  function of, 683
  in immune response, 684
Hematologic system, uremic syndrome effects on, 254-256, 255t
  nursing management of, 15
Hematology tests, in diabetic nephropathy diagnosis, 470
Hematopoietic system, aging effects on, 487t
Hematuria
  conditions associated with, 203t
  in nephritic syndrome, 180-181
Hemodiafiltration, for renal failure in children, 454-455, 454f
Hemodialysis, 525-576
  acute hemolysis due to, 559t, 566
  air embolism due to, 559t, 566-567
  amount of time for, 549-550
  amyloidosis due to, 561t, 570
  anticoagulation during, 552-555
    assessment of, 554-555
    heparin in, 551t, 552-554. *See also* Heparin, during hemodialysis
    regional citrate, 553-554
  arrhythmias due to, 560t, 568
  arterial pressure monitoring during, 556-557
  basic principles of, 527-530
  blood work following, 561-562
  cardiac arrest due to, 560t, 568
  chest pain due to, 558t, 564-565
  chills due to, 558t, 565
  clearance in, 530
  complement activation due to, 561t, 569-570
  complications of, 558t-561t, 562-571

conductivity monitoring during, 557
delivery of treatment, 551-552
in diabetic patients, 474-475
advantages of, 473t
disadvantages of, 473t
dialysis disequilibrium syndrome due to, 559t, 565-566
dialysis solution in, 550
dialyzer reactions due to, 559t, 567-568
dialyzers in. *See* Dialyzer(s)
diffusion in, 527-528, 529f
drug overdose in, treatment of, 572
in the elderly, 495-496
encephalopathy due to, 560t, 569
equipment and supplies for, 595
equipment care following, 562
exsanguination during, 560t, 569
fever due to, 558t, 565
fluid removal in, 550
calculation of, 446t
heparin prescriptions for, 596
heparin-free, 553
high-flux, for renal failure in children, 447
history of
1900-1959, 28
1960-1972, 29
1973-present, 30
hyoptension during, 550
hypotension due to, 558t, 562-564
hypoxemia due to, 561t, 570
indications for, 594
interleukin-1 stimulation due to, 561t, 570-571
intradialytic monitoring during, 556-557
isolated ultrafiltration with, 571-572
muscle cramps due to, 558t, 564
for neonatal renal failure, 449
neutropenia due to, 561t, 569-570
nursing opportunities in, 39
patient assessment following, 557, 561
patient monitoring during, 557
versus peritoneal dialysis, comparison of, 606-607, 607t
postprocedural nursing care, 597
predialysis equipment preparation for, 555
predialysis patient assessment and preparation, 555-556
prescription for, 549-550
pretreatment nursing assessment in, 594
procedure of, 555-562
for renal failure in children, 437-438, 444-450
access issues in, 448-449
catheters in, 448
complications of, 449, 449t
cost of, 449
heparinization in, 447
incenter *versus* home, 449-450
techniques, 444-448, 444t, 445f, 446t
as risk factor for hepatitis C virus, 360
Roy Adaptation Model assessment tool for, 72t-75t
Roy Adaptation Model-based typology of nursing interventions for, 77t-79t
seizures due to, 560t, 568-569
semipermeable membrane for, described, 527, 527f
sorbent, 571, 571f
special procedures related to, 571-573, 571f
stressors associated with, 271, 271t
temperature monitoring during, 557
termination of, 557
therapeutic plasma exchange and, comparison of, 594-597, 595t
treatment of, 298t
initiation of, 556
water, 536-537, 537f. *See also* Hemodialysis, water treatment of
ultrafiltration in, 528-530, 529f
vascular access in, 537-549, 594-595
arteriovenous grafts in, 545-548, 546f
assessment and preparation, 556
cuffed double-lumen silastic catheters in, 548-549, 548f
external arteriovenous shunt in, 541-542, 541f
femoral vein catheters in, 540
jugular vein catheters in, 541
permanent, 542-549, 542f, 544t, 546f, 548f
primary arteriovenous fistula in, 542-545, 542f, 544t
subclavian vein catheters in, 538-540, 538f
temporary/acute, 538-542, 538f, 541f
water treatment for, 536-537, 537f
absorption, 536-537
deionization, 537, 537f
filtration, 536
purification methods, 536-537, 537f
reverse osmosis, 537, 537f
water softening, 537
Hemodialysis system
blood circuit in, 532-533, 532f
components of, 530-536, 532f
diagram of, 532f
dialysate circuit in, 534-535, 534f
dialysis solution in, 533-534, 533t
dialyzer in, 530-532. *See also* Dialyzer(s)
heparin pump in, 535
optional components in, 535-536
single needle devices in, 536
sodium in, 535-536
ultrafiltration controller in, 535
Hemofilters, in CRRT, 578-582, 579f, 580t
Hemolysis
acute, hemodialysis and, 559t, 566
during hemodialysis, 596-597
renal failure in children and, 441
during therapeutic plasma exchange, 596-597
Hemoperfusion
described, 572
drug elimination by, 314
Hemorrhage, renal hemodynamic factors in, integration of, 141-142, 141f
Heparin
during hemodialysis, 551t, 552-554, 596
routine heparin, 551t, 552-553
tight or minimal heparin, 551t, 553
during peritoneal dialysis, 631, 632t
Heparin pump, in hemodialysis, 535
Heparinization, of pediatric renal patient, 447
Hepatic artery thrombosis, following liver transplantation, 765
Hepatic blood flow, drug metabolism effects of, 312t, 313
Hepatitis, 353-362
defined, 361
described, 353
hepatitis A, 352t, 353-355
described, 353
diagnosis of, 353-354
incubation period for, 352t, 353
laboratory findings with, 353
mode of transmission of, 352t, 354
prevention and treatment of, epidemiology of, 354-355
symptoms of, 353
hepatitis B, 352t, 355-359
clinical course of, 355-356
described, 355
incubation period for, 352t, 355
laboratory findings with, 355
mode of transmission of, 352t, 357
posttransplant, 703, 732, 746
prevention and treatment of, epidemiology of, 357-359, 358t
structure of, 354f
symptoms of, 355
hepatitis C, 352t, 359-361
complications of, 360
described, 359
diagnosis, 359
hemodialysis and, 360
incubation period for, 352t, 359
mode of transmission of, 352t, 359
posttransplant, 703, 704, 746
prevention and treatment of, epidemiology of, 360-361
symptoms of, 359-360
hepatitis D, 352t, 361-362
clinical course of, 361
described, 361
diagnosis of, 361
mode of transmission of, 352t, 361
prevention and treatment of, epidemiology of, 361-362
structure of, 361f
hepatitis E, 352t, 362
clinical features of, 362
described, 362
diagnosis of, 362
incubation period for, 352t, 362
modes of transmission of, 352t, 362
prevention and treatment of, epidemiology of, 362
nursing management of, 383
posttransplant, 697t, 703-704, 732, 746
viruses causing, 352t, 353-362
Hepatitis B surface antigen (HBsAg), 354f, 355
Hepatitis E antigen (HBeAg), 355
Hepatocyte(s)
described, 754
in drug metabolism, 312
Hepatocyte growth factor, for ARF, 227t
Hepavax, for hepatitis B virus, 357
Herald, P.A., 69
Herpes simplex virus (HSV) infection, posttransplant, 697t, 702-703
Herzberg, F., 44
Hesitancy, conditions associated with, 203t
Heterograft, described, 666t
Heterotopic graft, described, 666t
High performance liquid chromatography (HPLC), in cyclosporine monitoring, 334-335, 336t
Hinckley, B., 32, 35
Hippocratic period of ethical theory development, 85t, 86
Histamine

characteristics of, 677t
in renal blood flow, 140
Histamine H_2 receptor antagonists, in renal failure patients, 322
Histocompatibility testing, 687-688
History
of nephrology nursing, 25-42
ANNA, 36-38. *See also* American Nephrology Nurses' Association, history of
nephrology nurses today, 38-40
1900-1959, 28-29, 28f
nurses' roles in, 33-36
Albers, 34-35
Coleman-Wysocki, 33f, 34, 34f
Fellows, 34
Hinckley, 35
Lewis, 34
Shebelski, 35
Smyth, 34, 35f
organizing of nephrology nurses, 35f, 36, 37f
roles of early nephrology nurses, 35-36
of transplantation, 661-666
HIV infection. *See* Human immunodeficiency virus (HIV) infection
HIVID, for HIV infection, 366
HLA testing. *See* Human leukocyte antigen (HLA) testing
Hoffart, N., 113, 114, 116
Holistic care, for elderly patients with renal disease, 484
Hollow fiber hemodialyzer, 530-531, 530f
Home dialysis, nurses' role in, 35
Home management, of peritoneal dialysis patients, 632-634, 633t, 635t
Homograft, described, 666t
Hoop form dialyzer, history of, 28
Hospitals, in 1870s, 27
Host response, described, 684
House of representatives, in federal government, action of, 786
Houston, B.K., 48
HSV infection. *See* Herpes simplex virus (HSV) infection
Human growth hormone, for children with chronic renal failure, 443
Human immunodeficiency virus (HIV) infection, 362-367
clinical manifestations of, 363-364
described, 363
diagnosis of, 365
in dialysis settings, 349
ELISA for, 365
epidemiology of, 363
incubation period for, 363
nursing management of, 383-384, 384t
opportunistic infections with, 364
prevention of, 387t-388t
pathophysiology of, 363
renal disease in, 188-189, 189t
risk factors for, 364-365, 365t
risk to health care workers, 366-367
transmission of, 364-365, 365t
treatment of, 365-366, 366t
tuberculosis and, treatment of, 377
vaccine for, 365
Human immunodeficiency virus-associated nephropathy, 188-189, 189t
Human leukocyte antigen(s) (HLAs), class I and II, 686-687, 686f
Human leukocyte antigen (HLA) complex, 686, 686f
Human leukocyte antigen (HLA) genes, 686-687, 686f
Human leukocyte antigen (HLA) inheritance, 687, 687f
Human leukocyte antigen (HLA) testing, 688
in renal transplantation, 714
Humoral immune response, 670-671, 680-682, 681f
primary, 682
secondary, 682
Hydrothorax, peritoneal dialysis and, 649
Hygiene factors, 44-45
Hyperacute accelerated rejection, complications following, 725
Hyperacute rejection, 725
following liver transplantation, 766
posttransplant, 695, 695t
Hypercalcemia
defined, 244
neuropsychiatric manifestations of, 244
nursing management of, 7
treatment of, 244
Hyperimmune hepatitis B immunoglobulin (HBIG), for hepatitis B virus, 357-358
Hyperkalemia
cation-exchange resins for, 323-325
causes of, 239t
dietary, 289t
nondietary, 289t
defined, 239
described, 239
insulin for, 324
nursing management of, 6
posttransplant, infection following, 722-723, 722t
treatment of, 241t
Hyperlipidemia
in dialysis patients, 291
following liver transplantation, 768
Hypermagnesemia
causes of, 246t
defined, 246
nursing management of, 8
symptoms of, 246
treatment of, 246
Hypernatremia
causes of, 238t, 242t
defined, 237
nursing management of, 5
symptoms of, 237
treatment of, 237-238
Hyperparathyroidism, in renal failure, development of, 258f
Hyperphosphatemia
causes of, 245t
defined, 245
nursing management of, 8
treatment of, 245
Hypertension
in ADPKD, 185
age and, 184
causes of, 184
in chronic renal failure, 319-320
in diabetic patients, 475
evaluation of, in renal transplant recipient evaluation, 713
following liver transplantation, 767
nephrosclerosis due to, 519-520
posttransplant, 731
racial predilection for, 184
in renal failure, treatment of, 520
renal failure in children due to, 439
renovascular, 183
treatment of, 184
uremic syndrome and, 252
Hypertensive nephrosclerosis, 184
Hypertonic medullary interstitium, in urinary concentration and dilution, 143-144
Hypertonic saline, for anemia of renal failure, 326-327
Hypertriglyceridemia, 248
Hyperuricemia, following liver transplantation, 768
Hypervolemia
causes of, 222t
nursing management of, 3-4
Hypnotic(s), in renal failure patients, 320
Hypocalcemia
causes of, 242t
clinical features of, 243-244
defined, 243
nursing management of, 6-7
treatment of, 244
Hypocalcemic tetany, position of hand in, 243f
Hypoglycemic(s), 324
Hypokalemia
causes of, 239t
clinical manifestations of, 238-239, 240f
defined, 238
nursing management of, 5-6
posttransplant, infection following, 722t, 723
treatment of, 239
Hypomagnesemia
causes of, 246t
clinical manifestations of, 245
defined, 245
nursing management of, 8
treatment of, 245
Hyponatremia
causes of, 238t
defined, 236
nursing management of, 5
symptoms of, 236-237
treatment of, 237
Hypophosphatemia
causes of, 245t
clinical manifestations of, 244
defined, 244
neurologic manifestations of, 244
nursing management of, 7
treatment of, 244
Hypotension
during dialysis, 550
hemodialysis and, 558t, 562-564
Hypovolemia
ARF and, 216, 216f
causes of, 222t
nursing management of, 4
Hypoxemia, hemodialysis and, 561t, 570

I

Ideal rehabilitation opportunity, 407
IDPN. *See* Intradialytic parenteral nutrition
IgA nephropathy, 180-181
Illness trajectory, 270
IMM-125, in kidney transplantation, 337
Immune, defined, 669
Immune response
cell cooperation in, 683-684
cell types involved in, 678t-679t, 679
cell-mediated, 682-683

cellular, 670-671
characteristics of, 680
described, 679-680
humoral, 670-671, 680-682, 681f
mechanisms of, 669
Immune serum globulin (ISG), for hepatitis A virus, 354
Immune system. *See also* under Immunity
aging effects on, 487t
antibodies in, 682
antigen processing and presentation in, 680
antigenicity of, 680
cells of, 670t, 671-673
complement in, 674-675, 675f
diabetic effects on, 749t
inflammatory response in, 676-679, 676f, 677t
mononuclear phagocyte system, 673-674, 674t
organs of, 670t, 671-673, 674
purpose of, 329
renal failure in children effects on, 442
role of, 669
structure and function of, 669-684
tissues of, 670t, 671-673
Immunity
adaptive, 670-671. *See also* Adaptive immunity
humoral, 680-682, 681f
innate, 669-671, 670t
Immunocompetence, defined, 669
Immunoglobulin(s)
in humoral immune response, 682
hyperimmune hepatitis B, for hepatitis B virus, 357-358
IgA nephropathy, 180-181
Immunoincompetence, described, 669
Immunologic evaluation, in renal transplantation, 714-715, 714t
Immunology
in renal transplantation, 667-683. *See also* Immune system
in renal transplantation history, 663-664, 665t
Immunosuppressant(s)
history of, 793t-795t, 331-333, 329-331, 329t-331t
infection due to, 697, 698
in renal transplantation, 688-689, 689t, 690t-691t. *See also* specific agents, e.g., Methylprednisolone
in transplant patients, 331-344
azathioprine, 335t, 337
brequinar, 339
cyclosporine, 333t, 334-336, 335t, 336t
cyclosporine G, 339
15-deoxyspergualin, 339-340
IMM-125, 339
monoclonal antibodies, 338
mycophenolate mofetil, 335t, 338
new, 339-340
OKT3, 338-339
polyclonal antibodies, 338
rapamycin, 339
side effects of, 331
steroids, 335t, 337-338
tacrolimus, 335t, 336-337
Implementation, in standards of care, 829-830, 830t, 831t
Imuran. *See* Azathioprine
Incontinence, conditions associated with, 203t
Indinavir sulfate (IDV), for HIV infection, 366
Industry, contribution to nephrology, 31-32
Ineffective renal plasma flow, increase in, during pregnancy, 191
Infant(s), renal insufficiency in, growth retardation due to, 651
Infection(s). *See also specific types, e.g.,* Peritonitis
exit site, peritoneal dialysis and, 643-645, 645t
following liver transplantation, 767
latent, posttransplant, 706
opportunistic
in AIDS patients, 383-384, 384t
described, 364
posttransplant, 697-698
peritoneal dialysis and, 639-646
posttransplant, 697-707, 727-728. *See also* specific infection, e.g., Tuberculosis
pretransplant, 706
in renal patients
causes of, 522
management of, drug therapy complications, 522
prevention of, 522
in renal transplant recipients, treatment of, 713-714
tunnel, peritoneal dialysis and, 645-646
Infectious diseases
analytic
intervention, 351-352
observational, 351
epidemiology of, 350-353
methods of, 351-352
natural history of, 350-351, 350t
pathogenesis of, 350-351, 350t
prepathogenesis of, 350, 350t
prevention of, 350, 350t
in renal patients. *See also Human immunodeficiency virus (HIV) infection; specific infections, e.g.,* Hepatitis
AIDS, 362-367
causes of, 349
control of, 349-402
OSHA's Bloodborne Pathogens Regulations in, 379-381
strategies in, 378-381
drug-resistant organisms and, control of, 389-395
hepatitis, 353-362
history of, 349
HIV infection, 362-367
nursing management of, 381-389
in outpatient dialysis unit, control of, 393
prevention of, 393-395
screening for, 378
significance of, 393
surveillance of, 378-379
tuberculosis, 367-368
Inference, described, 46
Infertility, chronic renal failure and, 651
Inflammation
mediators of, 677t
signs of, 679
Inflammatory response, 676-679, 676f, 677t
Innate immunity, 669-671, 670t
Insulin
for diabetics on peritoneal dialysis, 651-652
dosage of, determinants of, 468
for hyperkalemia, 324
in peritoneal dialysis, 631, 632t
Insulin-dependent diabetes mellitus (IDDM), described, 467
Insulin-like growth factor (IGF-1), for ARF, 227t
Intensive care unit (ICU), for renal failure in children, 437
Interdependence mode, of Roy Adaptation Model, 70
Interdisciplinary advocacy, 91
Interferon(s)
functions of, 678t-679t, 683
types of, 678t-679t
Interleukin(s)
functions of, 678t
types of, 678t
Interleukin-1 stimulation, hemodialysis-related, 561t, 570-571
Intermittent flow centrifugation, development of, 591
Intermittent peritoneal dialysis (IPD)
described, 614-615, 614t
for renal failure in children, 437
techniques, 450
Interpersonal domain, roles in, 45
Interstitial diseases, 182-183
Intra-abdominal pressure, increased, peritoneal dialysis and, 648
Intra-abdominal vascular graft, as contraindication for pulmonary dialysis, 619
Intradialytic parenteral nutrition (IDPN)
administration procedure for, 297t
for malnutrition in dialysis patients, 296-298, 297t
Intraperitoneal medications, in peritoneal dialysis, 631-632, 632t
Intraperitoneal nutrition, for malnutrition in dialysis patients, 298
Intrarenal failure, 221-229
causes of, 221-224, 221t, 222f, 224t
clinical features of, 224-226, 225t
laboratory findings in, 224-226
pathophysiology of, 221-224, 221t, 222f, 224t
prevention of, 228
treatment of, 226-228, 227t, 229t
Intrusiveness, CRF-related, 272
Inulin, described, 137
IPD. *See* Intermittent peritoneal dialysis
IPDN. *See* Intradialytic parenteral nutrition
Iron
for anemia of renal failure, 325-326
metabolism of, in anemia of chronic renal failure, 290
Iron dextran, for anemia of renal failure, 326
Irwin, S.C., 419
Ischemia, renal, acute tubular necrosis due to, 221
Islet cell transplantation, described, 750
Isograft, described, 666t
Isolated ultrafiltration, hemodialysis with, 571-572
Isoniazid, for tuberculosis, 375-377, 376t

J

Job expectations, contradictory, of nephrology nurses, 48
Job satisfaction, 48
Johnson, D.E., 67-68, 76
Johnson, E.B., 782
Johnson's Behavioral System Model, overview of, 63t
Judicial branch of federal government, 783, 783f
Jugular vein catheters, in hemodialysis, 541
Justice
 defined, 87
 theories of, 86t, 87
Juxtaglomerular apparatus, described, 131f, 133-134, 133f

K

Kallikrein-kinin synthesis, in renal blood flow, 140
Kant, I., 86
Kant's theory, 86
Kelly, K.E., 48
Ketoconazole, in renal failure patients, 321
Kidney(s). *See also* under Renal
 aging effects on, 487t, 488
 anatomy of, 130, 130f
  circulatory, 134f, 135-136
  glomerulus, 135f, 136
 juxtaglomerular apparatus, 131f, 133-134, 133f
  macroscopic, 130-131, 131f
  microscopic, 131-133, 131f
  renal processes, 134-135
 artificial
  history of, 28
  Kolff-Brigham, history of, 31
 blood flow into, rate of, 135
 diabetic effects on, 749t
 examination of, in renal failure assessment, 207
 neoplasms of, 192-193
 physiology of, 287
 rotating drum, history of, 31
 vascular supply to, 130, 130f
Kidney disease, 177-197. *See also* Chronic renal failure
 acquired cystic disease, 185
 AIDS and, 188-189, 189t
 atheroembolic, 183-184
 classification of, 178
 congenital, obstructive uropathy due to, 187t
 cystic diseases, 184-185
 developmental diseases, 184-185
 diabetic nephropathy, 188
 drug-induced, 316-317, 318t
 in the elderly, 481-513. *See also* Aging; Elderly patients
 glomerular diseases, 178-182. *See also* Glomerular diseases
 history of, treatment of, 1960-1972, 29-30, 30f
 HIV and, 188-189, 189t
 hypertensive nephrosclerosis, 184
 infectious, 188-189, 189t
 interstitial diseases, 182-183
 medullary sponge kidney, 185
 nutritional care for, 285-303. *See also* Nutrition, for renal patients
 obstructive disorders, 185-188, 186f, 187t
 pharmacologic agents in, 307-327. *See also* Pharmacologic agents
 polycystic, 184-185
 preexisting, pregnancy and, 191-192
 in pregnancy, 191-192, 191t
 psychosocial impact of, 269-283
 radiologic studies in, 212, 213t
 renal artery disorders, 183-184
 systemic atherosclerosis and, 183-184
 toxic nephropathies, 189-191, 190t
 treatment of
  history of
   1900-1959, 28-29, 28f
   1973-present, 30-31
   prior to 20th century, 27-28
  industry's contributions to
   early to mid-20th century devices, 31
   historical perspectives on, 31-32
   1950s and 1960s, 31-32, 33f
 vascular diseases, 183-184
Kidney disease control program (KDCP), 32
Kidney failure, glomerular diseases and, 178
Kidney transplantation. *See* Renal transplantation
Kidney-islet cell transplantation, in diabetic nephropathy management, 477
Kidney-pancreas transplantation
 described, 750-751
 in diabetic nephropathy management, 477
Kikuchi, J., 276-277
Kim, H.S., 116
King's General Systems Framework, 68
 overview of, 63t
Kinin(s), characteristics of, 677t
Knowing, in NANDA taxonomy classification system for nursing diagnoses, 825t, 828t
Knowledge, defined, 53
Knowles, M., 44
Kohlberg, 88
Kohlberg's Model of Moral Development, 88
Kohnke, M., 90
Kolff, W., 28, 31
 in peritoneal dialysis, 605
Kolff-Brigham artificial kidney, history of, 31
Korniewicz, D.M., 69
Kt/V, defined, 636-637, 636t
Kurtin, P.S., 414
Kutner, N.G., 412t

L

Laboratory tests, in diabetic nephropathy diagnosis, 469-470
Lack of control, CRF-related, 271-272
Lamivudine, for HIV infection, 366
Lapp, C.L., 69
Lasix, for ARF, 227t
Latency, described, 699
Latent infections, posttransplant, 706
Law
 how bill becomes, 783-785, 784f, 785f
 in renal transplantation history, 664, 665t
Leach, A., 118
Learning. *See also* Patient learning
 adult, theory of, 44
 affective, 845, 845t
 cognitive, 844-845
 Gagne's hierarchy of, 845t
 levels of, 841, 841t, 845t
 literacy skills and, 847, 848t
 patient, 844-850. *See also* Patient learning
 principles of, 842-844, 843t
 psychomotor, 845-846, 846t
 roles in, 855, 856f
 theories of, classification of, 843t
Legal issues, in standards of care, 832
Legionella infection, posttransplant, 697t, 698-699
Legislation, path of, 784f
Legislative action, setting stage for, 787-788
Legislative branch of federal government, 783, 783f
Legislative process, 781-794
 action in, importance of, 782
 ANNA's involvement in, 791-792
 committee structure, 785-786
 federal budget process, 786-787
 federal regulatory process, 787
 legislative action, setting stage for, 787-788
 lobbying, 788
 nurses' role in, 782, 788-791
  becoming knowledgeable, 789
  communication by letter, 789-790
  personal visit, 790-791
  preparing for contact, 789
  telephone calls, 791
Leichter, H., 101-102
Lethal CMV syndrome, 700
Leukocyte(s)
 described, 671, 672t
 function of, impaired, uremic syndrome effects on, nursing management of, 15-16
 source of, 671
 values, characteristics, and function of, 672t
Leukotriene(s), characteristics of, 677t
Levels of Certification, 19
Levine's Conservation Model, overview of, 64t
Levy, N., 270
Lewis, C., 34
Libertarian conception of justice, 86t, 87
Life span issues, in rehabilitation process, 405f, 408
Lipid metabolism
 abnormal, nursing management of, 10
 alterations of, in acute and chronic renal failure, 248
Liquid chromatography, high-performance (HPLC), in cyclosporine monitoring, 334-335, 336t
Lister, P., 76
Literacy skills, and learning, 847, 848t
Lithium, chronic renal dysfunction due to, 317
Liver
 blood flow from, drug metabolism effects of, 312t, 313
 normal, function of, 754
Liver failure, manifestations of, 755
Liver grafts, reduced-sized, 760f, 761
Liver transplantation, 693-778, 754-768
 ABO blood group antigens in, 685
 complications associated with, 695-707
 complications following, 765-768
  biliary complications, 767
  bleeding, 765
  Budd-Chiari syndrome, 766
  hepatic allograft rejection, 766

hepatic artery thrombosis, 765
hyperlipidemia, 768
hypertension, 767
hyperuricemia, 768
infection, 767
metabolic, 767
metabolic bone disease, 768
non-anastomotic strictures, 767
portal vein thrombosis, 766
primary nonfunction, 766
pulmonary, 766
recurrent disease, 768
renal insufficiency, 766
vascular, 765
contraindications to, 754, 756, 756t
disease indications for, 756, 757t
donor management in, 707-708, 709t
donor recovery in, 708-710, 710t
education prior to, 714
genetic factors related to, 684-685
grafts in, types of, 666t
for hepatitis B virus, 358-359
for hepatitis C virus, 361
for hepatitis D virus, 362
histocompatibility testing in, 687-688
historical perspectives on, 661-666, 664t
surgery, immunobiology, and law in, 663-664, 664t, 665t
HLA inheritance, 687, 687f
immunologic aspects of, 667-683
immunosuppressive agents in, 688-689, 689t, 690t-691t. *See also* specific agent, e.g., Methylprednisolone
indications for, 756-757, 756t
infection following, 697-707
bacterial infections, 697t, 698-699
causes of, 697
fungal infections, 697t, 704-705
host protection from, 698
nursing considerations regarding, 707
opportunistic infections, 697-698
parasitic infections, 697t, 705-706
prevalence of, 697
sites of, 698
time of, 698
time table approach to, 706-707
types of, 697t, 698
viral infections, 697t, 699-704, 699t
introduction to, 663
living-related, 761-762, 761t
MHC in, 685-687, 685t, 686f, 687t
National Organ Sharing System in, 666, 666t
organ donation for, 707
pancreas. *See* Pancreas transplantation
for patients with HBV, 704
postoperative management and nursing care in, 762-765
preservation time in, 709, 710t
recipient evaluation prior to, 758-760, 758t, 759t
recipient selection for, 754, 756-757, 756t, 757t
regulatory activity related to, 808
rehabilitation and, 414
rejection following, 695-697
accelerated rejection, 725
acute rejection, 695-697, 695t, 696f, 725-726
causes of, 697, 698
chronic rejection, 695t, 697, 726-727, 730
hyperacute rejection, 695, 695t, 725
initiation of, 695
types of, 695, 695t, 725
split, described, 761
stressors associated with, 271, 271t
surgical procedure for, 760-762, 760f, 761t
survival rates following, 754
Living-related donors (LRD), in renal transplantation, 715
Living-related liver transplant donor evaluation, 761t, 762
Living-related liver transplantation (LRLTx), described, 761-762, 761t
Lobbying, process of, 788
Logic of nursing, 47
Loop diuretics, in renal failure patients, 315
Loop of Henle, 170-171, 170f
calcium transport in, 152
composition of filtrate as passes through, 142-143
described, 131f, 132
Lymphocele(s), posttransplant, 730
Lymphocyte(s). *See also* B lymphocytes; T lymphocytes
cell classes of, 671-672
characteristics of, 672t
function of, 672t
uremic syndrome and, 255
values of, 672t
Lymphokine activated killer (LAK) cells, function of, 683
Lymphoproliferative disease, EBV-mediated, posttransplant, 701-702
Lysosomal enzymes, characteristics of, 677t
Lysozyme(s), described, 669

M

Macro level, of professional responsibility, 89-90, 89t
Macroangiopathy, diabetes mellitus and, 472
Macrophage(s)
of mononuclear phagocyte system, 673-674, 674t
values, characteristics, and function of, 672t
Mag-3 radiology study, in renal transplantation, goal and interpretation of, 721t
Magnesium
functions of, 156-157
renal control of, 156-157, 156f
renal handling of, 156f, 157
transport of, in thick ascending limb, 156f, 157
Magnesium balance, alterations in, in acute and chronic renal failure, 245-246, 246t
Magnesium excretion, regulation of, 157
Magnesium homeostasis, 157
Magnesium reabsorption, regulation of, 157
Maintenance factors, 44-45
Major histocompatibility complex (MHC)
described, 669
in renal transplantation, 685-687, 685t, 686f, 687t
Malignancy(ies), posttransplant, 746
Malin, N., 76
Malnutrition
and dialysis, 294, 296t, 296-298, 297t
in ESRD, 296, 296t
in peritoneal dialysis patients, 652-653
Management, nursing opportunities in, 40
Mannitol, for ARF, 227t
Marshall, N.L., 48-49
Maslow's Hierarchy of Needs, 44, 44t
in patient education, 841-842
Mast cells, values, characteristics, and function of, 672t
Maturational state, renal failure effects on, 316t
Mayfield, P., 495
McBride, A.B., 116
McCloskey, J.C., 46, 48, 49
McDonald, M., 91-92, 92t
Medicaid, for children with renal failure, 461
Medical assessment, in diabetic nephropathy management, 472-473
Medicare, for children with renal failure, 461
Medicare amendments for 1993 and 1994, 808
Medicare ESRD program, in CRF treatment, 33
Medulla, described, 130f, 131, 131f
Medullary sponge kidney, 185
Membrane excitability, potassium and calcium effects on, 240f
Membrane permeability, defined, 609
Membrane plasma exchange circuit, 593f
Membrane plasma separators, in therapeutic plasma exchange, 592-593, 593f
Membranous glomerulopathy, in nephrotic syndrome, 180
Mendelssohn, D.C., 278
Menke, E.M., 274
Menopause, renal failure effects on, 318t
Meperidine, in renal failure patients, 319
6-Mercaptopurine (6-MP), in kidney transplantation, history of, 333
Mesangial cells, of glomerulus, 136
Meso level, of professional responsibility, 89-90, 89t
Metabolic acidosis, 246-247, 247t
nursing management of, 9
Metabolic alkalosis, 247, 247t
nursing management of, 9
Metabolic bone disease, following liver transplantation, 768
Metabolic complications, following liver transplantation, 767
Metabolic defects, posttransplant, 747
Metabolic system, diabetic effects on, 749t
Metabolism
diabetes mellitus effects on, 472
disturbances in, nursing management of, 10
peritoneal dialysis effects on, 650-651
of pharmacologic agents, 312-313, 312t
enzymes in, 312, 312t
hepatic blood flow effects on, 312t, 313
hepatocytes in, 312
rate of, 312t, 313
renal failure in children effects on, 441
Metals, renal insufficiency due to, 191
Methicillin-resistant *Staphylococcus aureus*, 389-392, 393-394
Methodological issues, in gerontological research, 507
Methylprednisolone
purpose, dose, administration, and side effects of, 333t

in renal transplantation, 690t
MHC. *See* Major histocompatibility complex
Miconazole, in renal failure patients, 323
Micro level, of professional responsibility, 89, 89t
Microangiopathy, diabetes mellitus and, 472
β_2 Microglobulin, deposition of, renal failure in children and, 441
Miller, M.P., 69
Minimal change disease, nephrotic syndrome and, 179-180
Mission statements, of nonprofit organizations, 51t, 52
Mixed leukocyte culture, 688
Mixed lymphocyte crossmatch, 688
Mixed lymphocyte culture, in renal transplantation, 714, 714t
Mofetil, in renal transplantation, 691t
Molzahn, A.E., 113, 114, 116, 118-119, 119, 276-277
Moncreif, J., in peritoneal dialysis, 605
Monitor(s), in hemodialysis, 535
Monoclonal antibody(ies)
in kidney transplantation, 338
purpose, dose, administration, and side effects of, 333t
Monocyte(s)
of mononuclear phagocyte system, 673-674, 674t
values, characteristics, and function of, 672t
Mononuclear phagocyte(s), values, characteristics, and function of, 672t
Mononuclear phagocyte system, 673-674, 674t
Moody, L.E., 116
Moonshine alcohol, renal insufficiency due to, 191
Morbidity, defined, 654
Morbidity rate, defined, 353
Morphine sulfate, in renal failure patients, 319
Mortality, defined, 654
Mortality rate, defined, 353
Motherhood, nurses and, 48-49
Motivation
process of, 44
in rehabilitation process, 410
Motivational factors, 45
Motivational theories, 44
Moving, in NANDA taxonomy classification system for nursing diagnoses, 825t, 827t-828t
Muromonab-CD3 (OKT3)
in kidney transplantation, 338-339
in renal transplantation, 691t
Muscle aches, OTC medications for, 340t
Muscle cramps, hemodialysis and, 558t, 564
Musculoskeletal disease, posttransplant, 746
Musculoskeletal system
aging effects on, 487t
uremic syndrome effects on, 258f, 259-260
nursing management of, 17-18
Mycobacterium tuberculosis, peritonitis due to, 641
Mycophenolate mofetil
in kidney transplantation, 335t, 338
purpose, dose, administration, and side effects of, 332t
in renal transplantation, 691t
Myogenic theory, of autoregulatory phenomena, 138-139

N

Nail changes, in chronic dialysis patients, 257
Narcotics, in renal failure patients, 319
National Association of Nephrology Technologists and Technicians (NANT), address for, 858t
National Core Indicators Project, 857
National Kidney Dialysis and Kidney Transplantation Study (NKDKTS), 405
National Kidney Foundation Inc., address for, 858t
National Kidney Foundation-Dialysis Outcomes Quality Initiative (NFK-DOQI), 811, 811t
National Organ Transplant Act of 1984, 804
National Renal Diet, 299t, 300t, 300-301
Natural killer (NK) cells, function of, 683
Needs, Maslow's Hierarchy of, 44, 44t
in patient education, 841-842
Nelson, M., 495
Neonate(s), hemodialysis in, 449
Neoplasms. *See* Tumor(s)
Neoral. *See* Cyclosporine
Nephralgia, conditions associated with, 203t
Nephritic syndrome, 180-181
symptoms of, 180
Nephritis, interstitial
acute, 182-183
chronic, 183
Nephrology, development of, overview of, 27
Nephrology community, 853-859. *See also* Nephrology nursing
components of, 857
industry and, 859
international, 859
national, 857-859
network system in, 857
regional, 857
renal coalition in, 858-859, 858t
Nephrology nurse. *See under* Nurse
Nephrology nursing, 853-859
beginning of, 6-7
certification in, 38
continuous quality improvement in, 857-858
described, 27
history of, 5, 25-42. *See also* History, of nephrology nursing
nursing practice for, scope of, 856f
practitioners in, 855
as a specialty, 3-23
conceptual framework for, 9-13, 10t-12t
definition of, 7-8
development of, 6-7
evolution of, 5-6, 13-21, 16f, 17t-19t
factors influential in, 7
foundation for, 7-13
in United States, 855
Nephrology nursing assessment tool, development of, 71, 72t-75t
Nephrology Nursing Certification Board (NNCB)
described, 5, 17-19
eligibility criteria of, 17, 17t
history of, 17-19
objectives of, 19-20, 19t
Nephrology Nursing Clinical Ladder Programs, 15
Nephrology nursing interventions, typology of, development of, 71, 76
Nephrology nursing practice, ethical foundations for, 84-85
Nephrology nursing practice base, model for, 8f, 9
Nephrology Nursing Standards of Clinical Practice, 14
Nephrology organizations, address for, 858t
Nephron(s)
described, 131, 131f
distal, potassium handling by, cellular model for, 146-147, 146f
Nephropathy
analgesic, described, 315
diabetic, 188. *See* Diabetic nephropathy
HIV-associated, 188-189, 189t
IgA, 180-181
obstructive, 185-188, 186f, 187t
toxic, 189-191, 190t
Nephrosclerosis
control of, 519-520
defined, 519
hypertensive, 184
Nephrotic syndrome, 179-180
defined, 179
membranous glomerulopathy in, 180
minimal change disease and, 179-180
Nephrotoxic agents, 224t
renal failure due to, 189-190, 190t
Nervous system, aging effects on, 486t
Net ultrafiltration, defined, 611
Neuman's Systems Model, 68-69
overview of, 64t
Neurologic system
diabetic effects on, 749t
uremic syndrome effects on, 250-252
nursing management of, 12
Neuromuscular system, renal failure in children effects on, 441
Neuropathy, peripheral, defined, 472
Neutropenia, hemodialysis and, 561t, 569-570
Neutrophil(s)
described, 679
values, characteristics, and function of, 672t
Neutrophil chemotactic factor of anaphylaxis (NCFA), characteristics of, 677t
Nicardipine, for hypertension in renal failure, 520
Nifedipine, for hypertension in renal failure, 520
Nightingale, F., 5-6, 62, 90, 91
on environmental effects on therapeutic outcome, 457
Nightly intermittent peritoneal dialysis (NIPD), described, 614-615, 614t
NIPD. *See* Nightly intermittent peritoneal dialysis
NNCB Bylaws, 21
NNCB Policy & Procedure Manual, 21
NNCB's Guide to Recertification by Continuing Education Credit, 21
Nocturia, conditions associated with, 203t
Noddings, N., 88
Non-anastomotic strictures, following liver transplantation, 767
Noncompliance, in CRF patients, 272-273
Non-insulin-dependent (NIDDM), described, 467
Nonmaleficence, defined, 86-87

Nonprofit organizations
  Board of Directors of, role of, 52-53, 52t
  described, 52
  mission statements of, 51t, 52
  paid staff members of, roles of, 53
  volunteers of, roles of, 53
Nonstreptococcal postinfectious acute glomerulonephritis, 182
Norris, M.K.G., 69
North American Nursing Diagnosis Association (NANDA), taxonomy, classification system for nursing diagnosis, 825-829, 825t, 826t-828t
Northwest Kidney Center in Seattle, 85
Nurse(s). *See also under* History, of nephrology nursing
  career opportunities for, 39-41
    in advanced practice nursing, 40
    in case management, 40
    in conservative management, 39
    in corporate/government arena, 40-41
    in education, 40
    in hemodialysis, 39
    in management, 40
    in peritoneal dialysis, 39
    in renal transplantation, 39
    in research, 40
  current status of, 38-40
  in early treatment of nephrology, roles of, 33-36, 33f-35f
  epidemiology and, 352-353
  gender predilection of, 47
  job satisfaction of, 48
  opportunities for, in pediatric nephrology, 39-40
  professional roles of, 43-57, 855
    accountability in, 46
    acquiring of, 45
    administrative roles, 51
    behavior patterns, 45, 46-48
    clinical roles, 49-51, 50t
    contradictory job expectations and, 48
    descriptions of, 52t, 53-54
    educators, 51-52
    evaluation of, 54
    functional roles, 49-51, 50t
    inference in, 46
    interpersonal domain, 45
    motherhood and, 48-49
    nonprofit organization, 51t, 52-53
    overload due to, 49
    personal domain, 45
    relationships between, 48-49, 49t
    strain in, 49
    stress in, 49, 49t
    system domain, 45-46
    theoretical foundations of, 44-45, 44t
    types of, 45-46, 49-52, 50t, 51t
    volunteer role, 51t, 52
  as successful teachers, 847-850, 849t-851t
  working with health care team, 855-856, 856f
Nurse administrators, described, 51
Nurse educators, 51-52
Nurse practitioners, described, 51
Nursing
  challenges facing, 5
  complications associated with, 5
  described, 5
  history of, 27
    Nightingale in, 5-6
  nephrology, history of, 25-42. *See also* History, of nephrology nursing
  organized, history of, 6
  professional, origin of, 5-6
  specialization in
    evolution of, 5-6
    recognition of, 6
Nursing - A Social Policy Statement, 13
Nursing behaviors, patterns of, 47-48
Nursing diagnosis(es)
NANDA taxonomy classification system for, 825-829, 825t, 826t-828t
  in standards of care, 825-829, 825t, 826t-828t
  taxonomy of, 825-829, 825t, 826t-828t
Nursing homes, for elderly patients with renal disease, 484
Nursing practice, logic and content of, 47
Nursing process
  documentation and, 824-833
  standards of care and, 821, 822t
Nursing profession, image of, 47
Nursing record formats, 831t
Nutrition
  in the elderly, 497-498
    environmental considerations in, 498
    issues related to, addressing of, 498
    pathological considerations in, 498
    physiological considerations in, 497-498
    psychosocial considerations in, 498
  following renal failure in children, 456
  intradialytic parenteral, for malnutrition in dialysis patients, 296-298, 297t
  intraperitoneal, for malnutrition in dialysis patients, 298
  physiology of, 287
  for renal patients, 285-303
    assessment of patient in, 292-294, 293f, 294f
      anthropometric measurements, 294, 294f, 295f
      biochemical data, 294
      medical history, 292
    cultural diversity among, 300
    effects of, 287
    National Renal Diet in, 299t, 300t, 300-301
    patient education in, 299-301, 299t, 300t
    registered dietitian in, 287
  renal transplantation and, 292
Nutritional state, renal failure effects on, 316t
Nutritional status
  in peritoneal dialysis adequacy, 637
  in peritoneal dialysis patients, 652-653

O

OBRA. *See under* Omnibus Budget Reconciliation Act
O'Brien, M.E., 69, 275
Obstructive nephropathy, 185-188, 186f, 187t
Obstructive uropathy, 185-188, 186f, 187t
OKT3
  in kidney transplantation, 336-337
  purpose, dose, administration, and side effects of, 331t
Oliguria, conditions associated with, 203t
Olsson, H.M., 45
Omnibus Budget Reconciliation Act (OBRA) of 1981, 803-804
Omnibus Budget Reconciliation Act (OBRA) of 1986, 804-805, 805f
Omnibus Budget Reconciliation Act (OBRA) of 1987, 805-806
Omnibus Budget Reconciliation Act (OBRA) of 1989, 806
Omnibus Budget Reconciliation Act (OBRA) of 1990, 806-807
Omnibus Budget Reconciliation Act (OBRA) of 1993, 807-808
Omnibus Budget Reconciliation Act (1986), 405
Oncotic pressure, colloid, described, 610
Opportunistic infections
  in AIDS patients, 383-384, 384t
  described, 364
  posttransplant, 697-698
Oral cavity, aging effects on, 486t
Oral iron preparations, for anemia of renal failure, 323-324
Oregon Experiment, 101-102
Orem's Self-Care Framework, 69
  overview of, 65t
Organ donation, 707
Organ Procurement and Transplant Act, 664
Organ Procurement Transplant Network (OPTN), 666
Organic factors, described, 408
Orthoclone. *See* Muromonab-CD3
Orthotropic graft, described, 666t
OSHA's Bloodborne Pathogens Regulations, 379-381
  cleaning of potentially contaminated work areas and handling of infectious waste in, 381
  described, 379
  engineering controls in, 381
  exposure determination in, 379
  hepatitis B vaccination for staff at risk for occupational exposure to hepatitis B virus in, 381
  laundry practices in, 381
  management of percutaneous exposure to blood and other infectious body fluids in, 381
  personal protective equipment in, 381
  record-keeping requirements in, 381
  staff training in, 379
  universal precautions in, 380-381
Osmolality, renal regulation of, 164-173
Osmosis
  defined, 610
  factors affecting, 612t
  reverse, in water purification, 537, 537f
  in solute removal and transport, 610-612, 611f, 612t
Osmotic pressure, colloid, described, 610
Osteodystrophy, renal
  control of, in renal failure management, 521-522
  uremic syndrome and, 259-260
OTC medications. *See* Over-the-counter (OTC) medications
Outcome identification, in patient education, 840-841
Over-the-counter (OTC) medications, for transplant recipients, 340t, 342

P

P450 enzyme system, drugs affecting, 312, 312t
Pain
abdominal, peritoneal dialysis and, 648-649
back, peritoneal dialysis and, 649
chest, hemodialysis and, 558t, 564-565
OTC medications for, 340t
shoulder, peritoneal dialysis and, 649
Painter, P., 410
Pancreas, normal function of, 749
Pancreas transplantation, 748-754
approaches to, 748
clinical future of, 751
goal of, 748
historical perspectives on, 664t
indications for, 748
postoperative management and nursing care for, 751-754, 753t
prevalence of, 748
recipient evaluation for, 750t, 751
recipient selection for, 751
surgical procedure for, 751
types of, 750-751
Pancreas-kidney transplantation, long-term management following, 754
Pancreatic cells, function of, 749, 749t
Pancreatic graft survival, defined, 748
"Panel Holds Life or Death Vote in Allotting of Artificial Kidney," 29
Paradigm. *See* Conceptual models of nursing
Paradoxical pulse, in uremic syndrome, checking for, 252t
Parallel plate hemodialyzer, 531, 531f
Parasitic infections, posttransplant, 697t, 705-706
Parathyroid hormone (PTH), calcium transport in, 152f, 153
Parenchyma, regions of, 130-131, 130f
Passive diluting segment, described, 143
Patient assessment, in diabetic nephropathy management, 472
Patient Bill of Rights, 839
Patient education, 837-852
assessment and diagnosis in, 840
assumptions for, 841-842
considerations in, 842-844
defined, 839
in diabetic nephropathy management, 471
evaluation in, 841
goals of, 840
levels of learning in, 841, 841t
nephrology health care team's role in, 839-840
nurses' role in, 839-840
in nutritional care in renal patients, 299-301, 299t, 300t
patient learning in, 844-850. *See also* Patient learning
planning and outcomes identification in, 840-841
planning steps for written material in, 849-850, 851t
as process, 839
process of, 840-841, 841t
teaching barriers, 849
teaching methods and media in, 841, 841t
teaching strategy in, 847-849, 849t-850t
for vascular access, 846t
Patient history, in renal failure assessment, 202-203, 203t
Patient learning, 844-850. *See also* Learning
assumptions for, 846-847
goals of, 844-846
literacy skills and, 847, 848t
theories of, 843t, 844
Patient profile, in renal failure assessment, 202-203
Patient Self-Determination Act, 277-278
Patrick, D.L., 412, 420, 422
Pediatric nephrology, nursing opportunities in, 39-40
Pediatric nephrology care, brief history of, 437-439
Pediatric renal nursing, philosophy of, 437
Pellegrino, E., 85, 87, 88
Penicillin(s), in renal failure patients, 323
Perceiving, in NANDA taxonomy classification system for nursing diagnoses, 825t, 828t
Perfusion rates, renal failure effects on, 318t
Pericarditis, uremic, 252-253
Peripheral neuropathy, defined, 472
Peripheral system, uremic syndrome effects on, nursing management of, 12-13
Peripheral vascular disease, in diabetic patients, 475
Peritoneal cavity
access to, in peritoneal dialysis, 620-625
host defenses for, 608
lymphatic drainage of, in peritoneal dialysis, 607-608
Peritoneal dialysis, 603-657
access issues in, 452, 452f
access to peritoneal cavity in, 620-625
acute catheters in, 620
chronic catheters in, 620-625
adequacy of, 634, 636-637, 636t
APD, 614t, 615
automated
described, 614t, 615
for renal failure in children, 450, 452
Baxter worldwide survey on, 606f
CAPD, 614, 614t
CCPD, 614, 614t
complications of
abdominal pain, 648-649
back pain, 649
blood pressure elevation, 649
catheter insertion-related, 646-647
catheter malfunction/malposition-related, 647-648
endocrine-related, 651-652
exit site infections, 643-645, 645t
fluid volume changes, 649-650, 650t
hydrothorax, 649
increased intra-abdominal pressure, 648
infectious, 639-646
malnutrition, 652-653
metabolic, 650-651
noninfectious, 646-653
nutritional status, 652-653
peritonitis, 639-643
reproductive system-related, 651-652
shoulder pain, 649
tunnel infections, 645-646
continuous ambulatory, for renal failure in children, 450
continuous cycling, for renal failure in children, 450, 452
contraindications to, 618-619
COPD and, 619
creatinine clearance effects on, 637
delivery systems for, 615-618, 615f, 616f, 617t
assist devices, 617
cyclers, 618
disconnect systems, 615-616, 615f, 617t
straight systems, 616-617, 616f, 617t
development of, 606t
in diabetic(s), insulin requirements for, 651-652
in diabetic nephropathy management, 475-476
diverticular disease and, 619
in the elderly, 496-497
versus hemodialysis, comparison of, 606-607, 607t
historical perspectives of, 605
history of
1900-1959, 28-29
1960-1972, 29-30
1973-present, 30-31
home management of patients on, 632-634, 633t, 635t
individualization of, 637-639
changes in clearance over time and, 638-639
modifications to initial prescription, 638
tools in, 639
intermittent, for renal failure in children, 450
intra-abdominal vascular graft and, 619
IPD, 614-615, 614t
Kt/V in, 636-637, 636t
lymphatic drainage of peritoneal cavity in, 607-608
metabolic control following, 653
modality selection for, factors affecting, 619, 619t
modality survival in, 653
morbidity associated with, 654
mortality associated with, 654
NIPD, 614-615, 614t
nurses' role in, 36
nursing interventions and procedures in, 631-632, 632t
nursing opportunities in, 39
nutritional status effects on, 637
optimal, defined, 634
patient outcome following, 653-654
patient selection for, 618-619
preferred option, 618
prescription for, 625-631. *See also* Peritoneal dialysis prescription
prevalence of, 605
principles of, 606-618
process of
cycle in, 614
delivery systems, 615-618, 615f, 616f, 617t
described, 613-618
exchange in, 614
for renal failure in children, 450-453
complications of, 452-453
incenter *versus* home, 453
techniques, 450, 451f, 452

in solute removal and transport, 608-613
clearance in, 612-613, 613f, 613t
convective transport in, 612
diffusion in, 608-610, 609t, 610t
ultrafiltration in, 610-612, 612t
TPD, 614t, 615
transfer set change in, 631
types of, 614-615, 614t
utilization of, 605-606, 606f
Peritoneal dialysis exchange, 614
Peritoneal dialysis prescription, 625-631
dialysis solution in, 629-631, 629t, 630t
nursing considerations with, 630-631, 630t
preparation of, 630, 630t
elements of, 625t, 628-629, 628t
membrane classification applied to, 626-628
modifications of, 638
peritoneal equilibration test in, 625-626, 625t, 626t, 627f
peritoneal function test in, 626
Peritoneal equilibration test (PET), in peritoneal dialysis prescription, 625-626, 625t, 626t, 627f
Peritoneal function test (PFT), in peritoneal dialysis prescription, 626
Peritoneal lavage, for renal failure in children, 438
Peritoneal membrane
anatomy and physiology of, 607-608, 608f
characteristics of, evaluation of, in peritoneal dialysis prescription, 625-626, 625t, 626t, 627f
Peritoneum, purpose of, 607
Peritonitis
"chemical," described, 640
defined, 639
diagnostic criteria for, 639-640, 641t
episode of, described, 640
home instruction sheet for, 851t
peritoneal dialysis and, 639-643
causative organisms, 640-641
clinical course of, 641-642
incidence of, 639
nursing management in, 642-643
portals of entry of, 640
rates of, 643, 643t
signs and symptoms of, 640
recurrent, described, 640
relapsing, described, 640
Perras, S., 69
Perry, L.D., 278
Personal domain, roles in, 45
Pettengill, M.M., 118
pH
defined, 158
normal, 158
urinary, renal failure effects on, 318t
Phagocyte(s)
described, 671, 673t
mononuclear, values, characteristics, and function of, 672t
Phagocytosis, described, 671, 673t
Pharmacodynamics, described, 315-316
Pharmacokinetics, described, 314
Pharmacologic agents, 307-327. *See also* under Drug
absorption of, 310t, 311
activity of, normal, process of, 309, 309f
acute interstitial nephritis due to, 316
acute tubular necrosis due to, 316-324
ARF due to, 316-317
clearance of, 315, 315t
dialyzability of, 327
distribution of, 311-312, 311t
effect on liver P450 enzyme function, 312, 312t
effect on sexuality in the elderly, 490
for elderly renal disease patients, 498-501, 500t
elimination of, 309-314, 313-314, 313f
through artificial clearance, 315, 315t
metabolism of, 309-314, 312-313, 312t
nonnarcotic, in renal failure patients, 319
pharmacodynamics of, 315-316
pharmacokinetics of, 314-316, 315t
protein binding of, 311-312, 311t
renal disease due to, 316-317, 318t
in renal failure patients, 317-324
$alpha_1$-receptor blockers, 320
analgesics, 319
antacids, 322
antianemics, 325-326
antidiabetic agents, 324
antihypertensives, 319-321
antimicrobial agents, 322-323
antituberculosis antibiotics, 324
antiviral agents, 323-324
beta-adrenergic blockers, 320
calcium channel blockers, 320
cardiotonics, 321
cathartics, 322
centrally acting $alpha_2$-agonists, 320-321
diuretics, 317, 319
electrolyte supplements, 321
histamine H_2 receptor antagonists, 322
hypnotics, 322
hypoglycemics, 324
phosphate binders, 321-322
renal failure effects on, 320
sedatives, 322
stool softeners, 322
vasodilators, 321
vitamin replacements, 321-322
vitamins, 322
in transplant patients, 329-344. *See also* Kidney transplantation, drugs in
volume of distribution of, 314-315
Pharmacology, in renal disease, 307-327. *See also* under Drug; Pharmacologic agents
Phenacetin, in renal failure patients, 319
Phosphate binders, in renal failure patients, 321-322
Phosphate excretion, regulation of, 156
Phosphate reabsorption, regulation of, 154f, 155-156
Phosphate restriction, in renal failure management, 522
Phosphorous
described, 241
Phosphorous balance, alterations in, in acute and chronic renal failure, 241-246
Phosphorus
in dialysis patients, 290
functions of, 154-155
renal control of, 154-156, 154f
renal handling of, 154f, 155-156
Phosphorus homeostasis, 155
Phosphorus restriction, in renal failure management, 521
Physical examination
in diabetic nephropathy diagnosis, 469
in rehabilitation process, 409
in renal failure assessment, 203, 205t, 206-207
Physical issues, in rehabilitation process, 409-412
Physical therapy, in rehabilitation process, 410
Physiological changes, in elderly patients with renal disease, 484-488, 486t-487t
Physiological mode, of Roy Adaptation Model, 70
Physiology, renal, 127-175
Pinholt, E.M., 418
Planning
in patient education, 1676-1677
in standards of care, 829
Plasma clearance, defined, 612
Platelet(s), in mononuclear phagocyte system, 674
Platelet activating factor (PAF), characteristics of, 677t
Platelet dysfunction, uremic syndrome and, 254-255, 255t
Play, as factor in children with renal failure, 459-460
Pleuritis, uremic syndrome and, 254
PLISSIT model, in sexual counseling of geriatric nephrology patient, 490-491, 490t
Pneumocystis carinii infection, posttransplant, 697t, 705
Pneumonia, posttransplant infections due to, 707
Pneumonitis, uremic, factors contributing to, 253f
Podocyte(s), described, 136
Political action, nurses and, 788-791
Polyclonal antibody(ies)
in kidney transplantation, 338
purpose, dose, administration, and side effects of, 333t
Polycystic kidney disease, 184-185
Polymerase chain reaction (PCR), in tuberculosis detection, 374
Polymorphonuclear granulocytes, values, characteristics, and function of, 672t
Polyuria
conditions associated with, 203t
with renal insufficiency, 521
Popovich, R., in peritoneal dialysis, 605
Portal vein thrombosis, following liver transplantation, 766
Positions of life, described, 45-46
Postinfectious acute glomerulonephritis (PSGN), 181-182
Postrenal failure, 218-221
causes of, 218-219, 218t
clinical features of, 219-220
laboratory findings in, 217t, 219-220
pathophysiology of, 218-219, 219f
prevention of, 220-221
treatment of, 220
Poststreptococcal glomerulonephritis, 181-182
Potassium
changes in, ECG abnormalities associated with, 240f
in dialysate, 550
in dialysis patients, 288, 289t
effects on membrane excitability, 240f

functions of, 145
internal, extrarenal regulation of, 146
renal handling of, 145-150, 145f-148f
secretion of, regulation of, 148-149, 148f
segmental handling of, 146-147, 146f
transport of, cellular model for, 147-148, 147f
Potassium balance, alterations of, in acute and chronic renal failure, 238-241, 239t, 240f, 241t
Potassium imbalance, posttransplant, infection following, 722-723, 722t
Potassium-sparing diuretics, in renal failure patients, 319
Powerlessness, CRF-related, 271-272
Prednisolone, in renal transplantation, 690t
Prednisone
purpose, dose, administration, and side effects of, 332t-333t
in renal transplantation, 690t
Pre-ESRD, treatment of, 298t
Pregnancy
ARF in, 192
diabetes mellitus effects on, 472
posttransplant, 747-748
preexisting renal disease and, 191-192
renal disease in, 191-192, 191t
renal failure effects on, 318t
renal function changes during, 191, 191t
Prepathogenesis, stages of, 350, 350t
Prerenal azotemia, 214-218. *See also* Prerenal failure
Prerenal failure, 214-218
causes of, 214-216, 215t
clinical features of, 216-217
laboratory findings in, 216-217, 217t
pathophysiology of, 214-216, 216f
prevention of, 218
treatment of, 217-218
Presensitization, in renal transplantation, 715
Preservation time, in transplantation, 709, 710t
President, in federal government, action of, 786
Pressly, K.B., 69
Pressure monitors, in hemodialysis, 533
Primary arteriovenous fistula, in hemodialysis, 542-545, 542f, 544t
Primary nonfunction, following liver transplantation, 766
Principlism, period of, of ethical theory development, 85t, 86
Professional behaviors, patterns of, 46-47, 46t
Professional characteristics, 46-47, 46t
Professional responsibility, levels of, 89-91, 89t
Prograf. *See* Tacrolimus
Propranolol, for hypertension in renal failure, 520
Proportioning system, dialysate, 535
Propositions, defined, 62
Prostaglandins
for ARF, 227t
characteristics of, 677t
Protein
in dialysis patients, 291
restriction of, in diabetic nephropathy management, 471
Protein metabolism
abnormal, nursing management of, 10
alterations of, in acute and chronic renal failure, 248
Protein restriction, in renal failure management, 521
Proteinase(s), characteristics of, 677t
Proximal tubule
calcium transport in, 152
described, 132
reabsorption in, 169-170, 169f
Pruritis, in renal failure patients, 522
Pruritus, chronic, treatment of, 256t
Pseudohyponatremia, 236
Pseudomonas sp., peritonitis due to, 641
Psychologic response, renal failure effects on, 318t
Psychomotor learning, 845-846, 846t
Psychosocial assessment, in renal transplant recipient evaluation, 714
Psychosocial care, of children in renal failure, 458-459
Psychosocial changes, in elderly patients with renal disease, 488-491, 490t
Psychosocial development, renal failure in children effects on, 444
Psychosocial issues
described, 408
in dietary restrictions in the elderly, 498
in rehabilitation process, 412
in renal disease, 269-283. *See also under* Chronic renal failure
nursing care in relation to, 279-280
Psychosocial problems, posttransplant, 748
Psyllium, for transplant recipients, 340
PTH. *See* Parathyroid hormone
Public Law 92-603, 404
Public Law 92-603 (H.R. 1), 30
Pulmonary complications, following liver transplantation, 766
Pulmonary edema, uremic syndrome and, 254
Pulmonary evaluation, in renal transplant recipient evaluation, 713
Pulmonary function, monitoring of, post transplant, of renal transplant recipient, 724
Pyelonephritis, acute uncomplicated, 188
Pyrazinamide, for tuberculosis, 375-377, 376t

Q

Quality assurance, in standards of care, 832-833
Quality index, 117
Quality of life
in care of elderly patients, 503
with ESRD, 277
low, dealing with patients with, 277-279, 278t, 283t
Quality of life (QoL) domains, in rehabilitation process, 408
Quantitative overload, 48
Quinton Instrument Company, 31

R

R561443. *See* Mofetil
Race
as factor in hypertension, 184
renal failure effects on, 318t
Radioimmunoassay (RIA), in cyclosporine monitoring, 334, 336t
Radiologic studies, in renal failure assessment, 212, 213t
Raimondo, J.M., 69
Ranitidine, in renal failure patients, 322
Rapamycin, in kidney transplantation, 339
Rapidly progressive glomerulonephritis (RPGN), 182
Raven's Progressive Matrices, 442
Rawls' Theory of Justice, 86t, 87
Reabsorption, described, 134
Recurrent peritonitis, described, 640
REDY system, for hemodialysis, flow path for, 571f
Regulatory cells, function of, 682
Rehabilitation, 403-429. *See also* Rehabilitation process
assessment in, 424
behavioral adaptation in, 423-424
for children, 415-417, 416t
defined, 407
for diabetics, 415
effectiveness of, 424
in elderly patients, 417-420, 418t, 419t, 504-506
components of, 505-506
education in, 505
employment in, 505-506
evaluation in, 506
exercise in, 505
implementation of, 506
epidemiology in, 424
ESRD treatment modality and, 414-415
historical perspective of, 404-407
outcomes assessment for, 420-421
research related to, 423
domains of science relevant to, 406t
for special populations, 413-420
specification and measurement of health outcomes, 421-422, 422t
systems approach to, 405f
for transplant patients, 414
whole body system response to, 423
Rehabilitation process
conceptual model of, 405f, 407-413, 411t
contact with community programs for referral of patients in, 410
disability classification and, 407
domains of science and, 406t, 408-409
exercise in, 409-410
in-center program for, 410
life span issues in, 405f, 408
motivation in, 410
personal background factors in, 408
physical examination in, 409
physical issues in, 409-412
physical therapy for, 410
psychosocial issues in, 412
quality of life domains in, 408
systems approach to, 405f
vocational issues in, 412-413
Reilly, 67
Reischman, F., 270
Rejection. *See also* Allograft rejection
posttransplant, 695-697, 725-727
accelerated rejection, 725
acute rejection, 695-697, 695t, 696f, 725-726
causes of, 697, 698
chronic rejection, 695t, 697, 726-727, 730
hyperacute rejection, 695, 695t, 725
accelerated, 725
types of, 695, 695t, 725

Relapsing peritonitis, defined, 640
Relating, in NANDA taxonomy classification system for nursing diagnoses, 825t, 827t
Renal. *See also under* Kidney
Renal absorption, mechanisms of, 168-172, 169f-172f
Renal acidification, 157-164, 158f-161f
Renal artery disorders, 183-184
Renal artery stenosis (RAS), 183
  posttransplant, 728, 728t, 731
Renal artery thrombosis, posttransplant, 728, 728t
Renal biopsy, in renal failure assessment, 213-214
Renal blood flow
  ADH in, 140
  angiotensin II in, 139f, 140
  autoregulation in, 138-139
  dopamine in, 140
  drug metabolism effects of, 311
  EDRF in, 140-141
  eicosanoid synthesis in, 139-140
  endothelin in, 140
  extrinsic factors affecting, 140-141
  histamine in, 140
  intrinsic factors affecting, 138-140
  kallikrein-kinin synthesis in, 140
  mechanisms controlling, 138-142
  renin-angiotensin mechanism in, 139, 139f
  sympathetic nervous system in, 139f, 140
Renal cell carcinoma, 192-193
Renal circulation, described, 134f, 135-136
Renal clearance, described, 136-137
Renal colic, conditions associated with, 203t
Renal disease. *See* Kidney disease
Renal failure, 199-264
  acidemia in, 521
  acute. *See* Acute renal failure
  anemia of, drugs for, 325-326
  in children, 435-465. See also Children, renal failure in
  chronic
    anemia of, iron metabolism and, 290
    defined, 201
    peritoneal dialysis for, 603-657. *See also* Peritoneal dialysis
  clinical assessment of, 201-214
  clinical presentation of, 201-202
  diagnostic tests in, 206t, 207-214, 207t-211t, 213t
    blood analyses, 206t, 207t, 208
    creatinine clearance, 212
    radiologic studies, 212, 213t
    renal biopsy, 213-214
    urinalysis, 208-211, 208t-211t
    urinary electrolytes, 211-212, 211t
    urine volume, 212
  effects on physiologic characteristics, 318t
  family history in, 202
  glucose intolerance in, 520
  high-risk patients for, identification of, 519
  hyperparathyroidism in, development of, 258f
  management of
    blood pressure control in, 519-520
    conservative, 517-524
      described, 519
      nursing plan for, 519
      control of anemia in, 521
      control of renal osteodystrophy in, 521-522
    diabetes mellitus control in, 520
    dietary control in, 520-521
    drugs, 317-324
      ACE inhibitors, 320
      alpha$_1$-receptor blockers, 320
      analgesics, 319
      antacids, 322
      antianemics, 325-326
      antidiabetic agents, 324
      antihypertensives, 319-321
      antimicrobial agents, 322-323
      antituberculosis antibiotics, 324
      antiviral agents, 323-324
      beta-adrenergic blockers, 320
      calcium channel blockers, 320
      cardiotonics, 321
      cathartics, 322
      centrally acting alpha$_2$-agonists, 320-321
      diuretics, 317, 319
      electrolyte supplements, 321
      histamine H_2 receptor antagonists, 322
      hypnotics, 322
      hypoglycemics, 324
      narcotics, 319
      NSAIDs, 319
      phosphate binders, 321-322
      sedatives, 322
      stool softeners, 322
      vasodilators, 321
      vitamin(s), 322
      vitamin replacements, 321-322
    infection prevention in, 522
    integumentary care in, 522
  nephrotoxic agents and, 189-190, 190t
  nursing management of, 3-18
  outcome goals for, 407
  patient history in, 202-203, 203t
  patient profile in, 202-203
  physical examination in, 203, 205t, 206-207
  progression of
    causes of, 519
    diet and, 287-288
Renal failure index (RFI), 211-212
Renal function
  clinical manifestations of, 233-234, 234t
  continuum of, 201, 201t
  normal, defined, 201
  posttransplant, of renal transplant recipient, 719-720, 720t, 721t
  during pregnancy, 191, 191t
Renal insufficiency
  following liver transplantation, 766
  in infants and children, growth retardation due to, 651
  polyuria in, 521
Renal ischemia, acute tubular necrosis due to, 221
Renal osteodystrophy
  control of, in renal failure management, 521-522
  uremic syndrome and, 259-260
Renal palpation, in renal failure assessment, 207
Renal Physicians Association (RPA), address for, 858t
Renal processes, 134-135
  excretion, 134-135
  glomerular filtration, 134
  reabsorption, 134
  secretion, 134
Renal replacement therapy
  for ARF, 229t
  in diabetic nephropathy management, 472-477
    contraindications for, 474
    indications for, 474
    medical assessment in, 472-473
    patient assessment in, 472
    social-family issues in, 473-474
  in the elderly, 495-497
    hemodialysis, 495-496
    peritoneal dialysis, 496-497
    selection process, 497
  rehabilitation due to, 403-429. *See also* Rehabilitation
Renal reserve, diminished, defined, 201
Renal sarcoma, 193
Renal system
  aging effects on, 487t, 488
  components of, 130, 130f
  hemodynamics of, 138-142
    control factors in, 141-142, 141f
    hemorrhage in, 141-142, 141f
  physiology of, 127-175
    overview of, 129-130
Renal tenderness, in renal failure assessment, 207
Renal transplantation, 710-748
  ABO blood group testing in, 714
  allograft dysfunction following, differential diagnosis of, 720t
  in children, 710
  complications following
    early, 725-730
      infection, 727-728
      lymphatic, 730
      rejection, 725-727
      urologic, 729-730, 729t
      vascular, 728-729, 728t
    late, 730-732, 731t, 746-748
      anxiety, 748
      avascular necrosis, 746-747
      depression, 748
      hepatitis, 732, 746
      malignancies, 746
      metabolic defects, 747
      musculoskeletal disease, 746
      psychosocial problems, 748
      recurrent diseases, 731t
      steroid-induced diabetes, 747
      weight gain, 747
  in diabetic nephropathy management, 476-477
    complications of, 476
    described, 476
    prognosis of, 476
  in diabetic patients
    advantages of, 473t
    disadvantages of, 473t
  diagnostic studies in, analysis of, 721t
  donor evaluation and selection in, 715-717, 716t
  drugs in, 329-348, 331. *See also specific drug*, e.g, Cyclosporine
    antifungal agents, oral, 341
    antihypertensives, 341
    antiulcer medication, 340
    bowel medications, 341
    calcium channel blockers, 341
    electrolyte supplements, 340

immunosuppressants, 331-346. *See also* Immunosuppressant(s)
over-the-counter medications, 340t, 342
TMP-SMZ, 341
in the elderly, 497
history of
1900-1959, 29
1960-1972, 30
1973-present, 31
HLA testing in, 714
immunologic considerations in, 714-715, 714t
indications for, 710-711, 711t
mixed lymphocyte culture in, 714, 714t
monoclonal, in kidney transplantation, 336
nurses' role in, 35-36
nursing opportunities in, 39
nutrition and, 292
postoperative management and nursing care of recipient, 719-725
cardiovascular problems, 724-725
fluid and electrolyte monitoring, 720-723, 722t
gastrointestinal problems, 724-725
pulmonary function, 724
renal function, 719-720, 720t, 721t
urinary tract problems, 723
pregnancy following, 747-748
presensitization in, 715
prevalence of, 710
recipient care in, 733t-745t
recipient considerations pretransplant, 717
recipient evaluation prior to, 711-714, 712t
recipient selection for, 710-711, 711t
recurrent diseases following, 731t
for renal failure in children, 438-439, 455
sexuality following, 747
surgical procedure for, 717-719, 718f
white cell crossmatching in, 714-715
Renal ultrasound, in renal transplantation, goal and interpretation of, 721t
Renal vein thrombosis (RVT), posttransplant, 728, 728t
Renin-angiotensin mechanism, in renal blood flow, 139, 139f
Renovascular hypertension, 183
Reports of Medical Cases, 28
Reproductive system, peritoneal dialysis effects on, 651-652
Research, 111-123
form of, 113-114
analytical observational studies, 122
descriptive studies, 122
designs for, 122
development of, factors influencing, 112-113
establishment of research grant program, 119
in ethical decision making, 101
experimental studies, 122
funding for, 113, 114t
future directions for, 120
gerontological, 506-507, 508t, 509t
historical overview of, 112
historical studies, 122
methodologic studies, 122
nursing opportunities in, 40
phenomena studied, 114-116
quality of literature in, 116-118, 117f
recent, 113-118, 114t, 115t, 117f
rehabilitation-related, domains of science relevant to, 406t
researchers in, 113
study designs, 116
theoretical base for, 116
utilization of, 118-119
volume of, 113-114
Research utilization, 283
Researchers, in nephrology nursing, 113
Resource allocation, public and health care provider dialogue about, in ethical decision making, 101-102
Respiratory system
aging effects on, 487t, 488
renal failure in children effects on, 441
uremic syndrome effects on, 253f, 254
nursing management of, 14
Retinopathy, defined, 472
Reuben, D., 417
Reverse osmosis, in water purification, 537, 537f
Rifampin, for tuberculosis, 375-377, 376t
Right to vote, importance of, 782
Risk management, in standards of care, 832
Robinson, R.R., 404
Rogers' Science of Unitary Human Beings, 69
overview of, 65t
Role(s)
defined, 45
of nephrology nurse, 43-57. *See also* Nurse, professional roles of
Role conflict, 48
Role description, defined, 53-54, 53t
Role function mode, of Roy Adaptation Model, 70
Role overload, 49
Role strain, 49, 49t
Role stress, 49
Rose, B.D., 178
Ross, W., 86
Rotating drum kidney, history of, 31
Roy Adaptation Model
described, 70-71
functions of, 67, 69-70
overview of, 66t
Roy Adaptation Model assessment tool for adult hemodialysis patient, 72t-75t
Roy Adaptation Model-based typology of nursing interventions, for hemodialysis patients, 77t-79t

S

Sandimmune. *See* Cyclosporine
purpose, dose, administration, and side effects of, 332t
Sarcoma(s), renal, 193
Satisfiers, 45
Sausage casing membrane, history of, 31
School, as factor in children with renal failure, 460
Science, and rehabilitation process, 406t, 408-409
Scope of Practice for Nephrology Nursing, 13
Scribner, B., 31, 85
SCUF. *See* Slow continuous ultrafiltration
Seattle, Washington, Northwest Kidney Center in, 85
Seattle Artificial Kidney Center, 29
Secretion, described, 134
Sedative(s), in renal failure patients, 322
Seizure(s), hemodialysis and, 560t, 568-569
Self-concept mode, of Roy Adaptation Model, 70
Self-esteem, enhancement of, in psychological stability of the elderly, 494f
Semipermeable membrane, for hemodialysis, described, 527, 527f
Senate, in federal government, action of, 786
Sensory changes, in elderly patients with renal disease, 485, 486t
Seropositivity, described, 699
Serotonin, characteristics of, 677t
Sexual counseling, of geriatric nephrology patient, PLISSIT model, 490-491, 490t
Sexual dysfunction
in endocrine disorders, 249
in renal failure patients, 522
Sexual function, aging effects on, 487t
Sexual maturation, renal failure in children effects on, 442-443
Sexuality
and CRF, 273-274, 274t, 275t
in the elderly, 489-491, 490t
aging physiology effects on, 489
chronic illness effects on, 489-490
educational background and, 490
lack of partner or spouse impact on, 490
medications/drugs and alcohol effects on, 490
sexual counseling related to, 490-491, 490t
societal attitudes and myths related to, 489
as stressor, 489
posttransplant, 747
Shebelski, D., 35
Shoulder pain, peritoneal dialysis and, 649
Shunt(s), arteriovenous, external, in hemodialysis, 541-542, 541f
Simultaneous pancreas/kidney (SPK) transplants, survival rates for, 748
Singer, P.A., 278
Single needle devices, in hemodialysis, 536
Sinus congestion, OTC medications for, 339t
Siu, A., 417
Skeletal system, renal failure in children effects on, 441
Skin
aging effects on, 486t
diabetic effects on, 749t
renal failure in children effects on, 440
uremic syndrome effects on, nursing management of, 16
Skinfold thickness, measurement of, calibrated skinfold caliper in, 294, 295f
Slit pores, described, 135f, 136
Slow continuous ultrafiltration (SCUF). *See* Continuous renal replacement therapy
for ARF, 581
Smell, aging effects on, 486t
Smyth, A.M., 34
Social issues, in diabetic nephropathy management, 473-474
Social Security, desktop guide to, 411t
Social Security Amendments of 1972, 798-803, 799t-802t

Social support, for CRF, 274-276
Social support networks, in psychological stability of the elderly, 494
Socialization of employees, process of, 45
Societal attitudes, sexuality among the elderly and, 489
Sodium
  body requirements for, 164-165, 164t
  in dialysate, 550
  in dialysis patients, 288
  in hemodialysis, 535-536
  homeostatic control of, 165-168, 165t, 166f
Sodium balance, alterations in, in acute and chronic renal failure, 236-238, 237t, 238t
Sodium excretion, control of, 166f
Sodium filtration, control of, 166-167
Sodium reabsorption
  control of, 167-168
  in early distal tubule, 171-172, 171f
  in early proximal tubule, 169-170, 169f
  hollow fiber, 530-531, 530f
  in late distal tubule and collecting ducts, 172, 172f
  parallel plate, 531, 531f
  in thick ascending limb of Henle, 170f, 171
  types of, 531-532, 532t
Sodium-potassium ATPase pump, 145-146, 145f
Solu-Medrol. *See* Methylprednisolone
Solute(s)
  defined, 608
  molecular weight of, 609t
  removal and transport of
    factors affecting, 608-610, 610t
    in peritoneal dialysis, 608-613. *See also* Peritoneal dialysis, in solute removal and transport
Solvent, defined, 608
Sorbent hemodialysis, 571, 571f
Sowell, R., 91
Sphygmomanometer, for paradoxical pulse, 252t
Spirituality, among the elderly, 491
Spironolactone, in renal failure patients, 317
Split liver transplantation, described, 761
Standard(s)
  defined, 819
  versus guidelines, 822
  of nursing profession. *See* Standards of care of professional performance, 820-821
Standards of care, 817-837
  assessment in, 825
  benefits derived from, 821-822
  clinical practice guidelines for, 822-824. See also Clinical practice guidelines
  continuous quality improvement and, 832-833
  described, 819-820, 820t
  documentation and, 824-833
  evaluation of, 830-832
  historical background of, 820
  implementation of, 829-830, 830t, 831t
  legal aspects of, 832
  nursing diagnosis in, 825-829, 825t, 826t-828t
  nursing process and, 821, 822t
  planning in, 829
  quality assurance and, 832-833
  recording of, purposes of, 830, 830t
  risk management and, 832
Standards of Clinical Practice for Nephrology Nursing, 14
Standards of Clinical Practice for the Nephrology Patient, 13-14
Staphylococcus aureus
  methicillin-resistant, 389-392, 393-394
  peritonitis due to, 640-641
Starr, P., 90
Stavudine, for HIV infection, 366
Stead, W.W., 404
Steal syndrome, described, 544
Steroid(s), in kidney transplantation, 337-338
  history of, 330, 333
  side effects of, 335t, 337-338
Stewart, R., 32
Stineman, M., 505
Stool softeners, in renal failure patients, 322
Straight systems, in peritoneal dialysis, 616-617, 616f, 617t
Strain, role, 49, 49t
Strauss, A.L., 270
Streptomycin, for tuberculosis, 375-377, 376t
Stress, of nurses, 49, 49t
Stressors
  of aging, 489
  CAPD-related, 271, 271t
  CRF-related, 271, 271t
  hemodialysis-related, 271, 271t
  transplantation-related, 271, 271t
Strong, M., 69
Strongyloides stercoralis infection, post-transplant, 706
Studies. *See* under Research
Styles, M., 9
Subclavian vein catheters, in hemodialysis, 538-540, 538f
Subcommittees, in federal government, 785-786
Supplemental Security Income (SSI), for children with renal failure, 461
Supplemental Security Income (SSI) work incentives, 411t
Support groups, in psychological stability of the elderly, 494
Suppressor T cells, function of, 683
Surgery, in renal transplantation history, 663, 664t
Surveillance, defined, 378
Survival issues, described, 408
Swan Neck Missouri catheter with flange and bead at preperitoneal cuff, 621f
Sympathetic nervous system, in renal blood flow, 139f, 140
Syngraft, described, 666t
System domain, roles in, 45-46
Systemic amyloidosis, 180
Systemic atherosclerosis, renal disease and, 183-184

T

T cell subsets, 682-683
T cells. *See* T lymphocytes
T lymphocytes (T cells)
  in cellular immunity, 682-683
  cytotoxic
    function of, 683
    in immune response, 684
  described, 671-673
  helper
    function of, 683
    in immune response, 684
  suppressor, function of, 683
  values, characteristics, and function of, 672t
Tacrolimus
  administration of, 332t
  dose of, 332t
  drug interactions with, 337
  in kidney transplantation, 336-337
    history of, 336
    indications for, 336-337
  purpose of, 332t
  in renal transplantation, 690t
  side effects of, 332t, 335t, 337
Tarule, J.M., 116
Teaching, defined, 1675
Teasdale, K., 76
Teflon shunt, arteriovenous, history of, 31
Temperature, body
  during hemodialysis, monitoring of, 557
  renal failure effects on, 318t
Tenckhoff, H., in peritoneal dialysis, 605
Tenove, S., 118
Tetracycline(s), in renal failure patients, 321
Thalhimer, W., 31
The Core Curriculum for Nephrology Nursing, 14, 19
The Nurse Manager and The Law, 824
Therapeutic apheresis, historical review of, 590-591, 591f
Therapeutic plasma exchange (TPE), 589-600
  cascade plasma filtration, 594, 594f
  complications requiring, 596
  continuous flow centrifugation, 592, 592f
  equipment and supplies for, 595
  hemodialysis and, comparison of, 594-597, 595t
  hemodialysis during, 596-597
  historical review of, 590-591, 591f
  indications for, 594
  intermittent flow centrifugation, 591
  intraprocedural monitoring for, 595-597
  membrane plasma separators in, 592-593, 593f
  nursing literature related to, 597-598
  postprocedural nursing care, 597
  pretreatment nursing assessment in, 594
  research related to, 597-598
  specific therapies, development of, 591-594, 592f-594f
  vascular accesses in, 594-595
Thrombocyte(s). *See* Platelet(s)
Thrombosis
  hepatic artery, following liver transplantation, 765
  portal vein, following liver transplantation, 766
  renal artery, posttransplant, 728, 728t
Thrush, *Candida albicans* and, 704-705
Thurstone, I., 118
Tidal peritoneal dialysis (TPD), described, 614t, 615
Tissue typing, 688
TMP-SMZ. *See* Trimethoprim-sulfamethoxazole
TPD. *See* Tidal peritoneal dialysis
TPE. *See* Therapeutic plasma exchange
Transforming growth factor (TGF), functions of, 679t
Transplant Amendments Act of 1990, 807

Transplant rejection, 695-697. *See also* Transplantation, rejection following
Transplantation
  islet cell, described, 750
  kidney. *See* Renal transplantation
  kidney-pancreas
    described, 750-751
    in diabetic nephropathy management, 477
  laboratory tests prior to, 759, 759t
  liver. *See* Liver transplantation
  pancreas-kidney, survival rates for, 748
Travel, as factor in children with renal failure, 460
Treatment, described, 46
Trimethoprim-sulfamethoxazole (TMP-SMZ), for transplant recipients, 341
Trousseau's sign, position of hand in, 243f
Tuberculosis, 367-368
  BCG vaccine for, 369-370
  causes of, 367-368
  diagnosis of, 373-374
  drug-resistant, treatment of, 377
  extrapulmonary, treatment of, 377
  HIV infection and, treatment of, 377
  infectivity with, 377-378
  medical conditions precipitating, 370-371, 370t
  multi-drug resistant, 367, 369
  nursing management of, 384-389
  pathophysiology of, 368-369
  posttransplant, 697t, 698
  prevalence of, 367
  pulmonary, treatment of, 375-377
  risk factors for, 370-371, 370t, 371t
  screening methods for, 370-373, 370t-372t
    candidates for, 371-371t
  signs and symptoms of, 369
  treatment of, 374-378, 376t
    drugs in, 374-378, 376t
    preventive, 374-375
Tuberculosis skin testing, 371-373, 372t
Tubular processes, in urinary concentration and dilution, 142-143
Tubular system
  collecting tubule in, 133
  components of, 132-133
  described, 132-133
  distal tubule in, 132-133
  loop of Henle in, 131f, 132
  proximal tubule in, 132
Tubuloglomerular feedback theory, of autoregulatory phenomena, 138-139
Tumor(s)
  of kidney, 192-193
  Wilm's, 193
Tumor necrosis factor (TNF), functions of, 679t
Tunnel infections, peritoneal dialysis and, 645-646
Turner, 69

U

Ullman, E., 663
Ultrafiltration
  defined, 610
  factors affecting, 612t
  in hemodialysis, 528-530, 529f
  isolated, hemodialysis with, 571-572
  net, defined, 611
  in solute removal and transport, 610-612, 612t
Ultrafiltration (UF) controller, in hemodialysis, 535
Ultrafiltration rate (UFR), calculation of, 580, 580t
Ultrasound, renal, in renal transplantation, goal and interpretation of, 721t
Underutilization skills, 48
Uniform Anatomical Gift Act, 664
Uniform Determination of Death Act, 664
United Network for Organ Sharing (UNOS), 666
  address for, 858t
  in liver transplantation, 760
United States, nephrology nursing in, 855
United States Renal Data System (USRDS), 405
Urea, molecular weight of, 609t
Urea clearance, defined, 612
Uremia. *See also* Uremic syndrome
  acute
    clinical findings in, 225t
    pathophysiology of, 225t
  defined, 250
Uremic frost, 256-257
Uremic pericarditis, 252-253
Uremic pneumonitis, factors contributing to, 253f
Uremic syndrome
  in ARF and CRF, 250-260
    autonomic manifestations of, nursing management of, 13
    cardiovascular manifestations of, 251f, 252-254, 252t
      nursing management of, 13-14
    dermatologic manifestations of, 256-257, 256t
      nursing management of, 16
    gastrointestinal manifestations of, 257-259, 257f
      nursing management of, 16-17
    hematologic manifestations of, 254-256, 255t
      nursing management of, 15
    leukocyte function effects of,
      nursing management of, 15-16
    musculoskeletal manifestations of, 258f, 259-260
      nursing management of, 17-18
    neurologic manifestations of, 250-252
      nursing management of, 12
    paradoxical pulse in, 252t
    peripheral manifestations of, nursing management of, 12-13
    respiratory manifestations of, nursing management of, 14
    respiratory manifestations of, 253f, 254
  bleeding time in, pharmacologic reduction of, 255t
  nursing management of, 12-18
Ureter(s), described, 130, 130f
Ureteral obstruction, posttransplant, 729-730, 729t
Urgency, conditions associated with, 203t
Urinalysis
  in diabetic nephropathy diagnosis, 469
  in renal failure assessment, 208-211, 208t-211t
  variables measured by dipstick in, 209t, 210
Urinary bladder, described, 130, 130f
Urinary electrolytes, in renal failure assessment, 211-212, 211t
Urinary flow rates, renal failure effects on, 316t
Urinary pH, renal failure effects on, 318t
Urinary system, organizational plan of, 130f
Urinary tract infections (UTIs), 188
  posttransplant, 727
  recurrent, posttransplant, 731
Urinary tract obstruction, 185-188, 186f, 187t
  bilateral, renal responses to, 219f
  causes of, 185-186, 186f, 187t
  classification of, 187t
  development of, 186f
  diagnosis of, 186-187
  symptoms of, 186
  treatment of, 186-187
Urinary tract problems, posttransplant, of renal transplant recipient, 723
Urine
  bloody, conditions associated with, 203t
  casts in, 211
  cloudy, conditions associated with, 203t
  color variations of, 208t, 210
  concentrated, formation of, 145
  concentration of, 142-145
  crystals in, 211
  dilute, formation of, 145
  frothy, conditions associated with, 203t
  sediment in, clinical significance of, 210t, 211
  specific gravity of, 210
Urine tests, in diabetic nephropathy diagnosis, 469-470
Urine volume, in renal failure assessment, 212
Urokinase, for anemia of renal failure, 326
Uropathy, obstructive, 185-188, 186f, 187t
Utilitarian(s), described, 86
Utilitarian theories, 86t, 87
UTIs. *See* Urinary tract infections

V

VA hospital dialysis program, in CRF treatment, 32
Vaccine(s)
  Bacille Calmette-Guérin, for tuberculosis, 369-370
  for HIV infection, 365
Valuing, in NANDA taxonomy classification system for nursing diagnoses, 825t, 827t
Vancomycin
  in renal failure patients, 323
  as risk factor for vancomycin-resistant enterococci, 392-393
Vancomycin-resistant enterococci (VRE), 392, 394-395
Varicella-zoster virus (VZV), posttransplant, 697t, 703
Vascular access, patient teaching for, 1682t
Vascular complications, following liver transplantation, 765
Vascular diseases, renal, 183-184
Vascular system, diabetic effects on, 749t
Vasodilator(s), in renal failure patients, 319
Vesicoureteral reflux (VUR), 187-188
Vineland Adaptive Behavior Scales, 442

Viral infections, posttransplant, 697t, 699-704, 699t
  causes of, 699

characteristics among, 699
CMV, 697t, 699-701, 699t
Epstein-Barr virus, 697t, 701-702
hepatitis, 697t, 703-704
HSV infection, 697t, 702-703
presentation of, 699
VZV, 697t, 703
Virtue ethics, 88
Vision, aging effects on, 486t
Visking membrane, history of, 31
Vitamin(s), in renal failure patients, 322
Vitamin C, in dialysis patients, 290
Vitamin D
in dialysis patients, 290
in renal failure patients, 321-322
Vitamin D3, calcium transport in, 153-154
Vitamin replacements, in renal failure patients, 321-322
Vividiffusion device, history of, 31
Vocational issues, in rehabilitation process, 412-413
Volume of distribution, of pharmacologic agents, 314-315
Volume status, monitoring of, posttransplant, of renal transplant recipient, 721-722
Volunteer(s), roles of, 51t, 52, 53
Volunteer organizations
elements of, 51t, 52
members of, roles of, 53
VUR. *See* Vesicoureteral reflux
VZV. *See* Varicella-zoster virus

W

Ware, J.E., Jr., 422
Water
body requirements for, 164-165, 164t
in hemodialysis, 536-537, 537f
homeostatic control of, 165-168, 165t, 166f
impurities in, 536
Water excretion, control of, 166f, 168
Water softening, in water purification, 537
Weight
gain in, posttransplant, 747
monitoring of, posttransplant, of renal transplant recipient, 720
Weschler Intelligence Scale for Children (WISC), 442
Westinghouse Corporation, 31
White blood cells (WBCs), values, characteristics, and function of, 672t
White cell crossmatching, 688, 714-715
Winslow, G., 90
World Council of Renal Care (WCRC), 859
Wound infections, posttransplant, 706-707, 727-728
Wrubel, J., 47

X - Z

Xenograft, described, 666
X-ray(s), chest, in tuberculosis detection, 373

Zadai, C.C., 419
Zalcitabine, for HIV infection, 366
Zappacosta, A., 69
Zinc, in dialysis patients, 290
Zinn, 69
Zwolski, K., 48

